Synopsis of Neurology, Psychiatry, and Related Systemic Disorders

Synopsis of Neurology, Psychiatry, and Related Systemic Disorders

EDITED BY

Alan B. Ettinger
Former Professor of Clinical Neurology, Albert Einstein College of Medicine, Bronx, NY
President, Professional Advisory Board, EPIC – Epilepsy Foundation of Long Island, East Meadow, NY

Deborah M. Weisbrot
Department of Psychiatry, Stony Brook School of Medicine, Stony Brook, NY

Casey E. Gallimore
Associate Professor, University of Wisconsin School of Pharmacy, Madison, WI

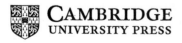
CAMBRIDGE
UNIVERSITY PRESS

CAMBRIDGE
UNIVERSITY PRESS

University Printing House, Cambridge CB2 8BS, United Kingdom

One Liberty Plaza, 20th Floor, New York, NY 10006, USA

477 Williamstown Road, Port Melbourne, VIC 3207, Australia

314–321, 3rd Floor, Plot 3, Splendor Forum, Jasola District Centre, New Delhi – 110025, India

79 Anson Road, #06-04/06, Singapore 079906

It furthers the University's mission by disseminating knowledge in the pursuit of
education, learning, and research at the highest international levels of excellence.

www.cambridge.org
Information on this title: www.cambridge.org/9781107069565
DOI: 10.1017/9781107706866

First published 2019

Printed and bound in Great Britain by Clays Ltd, Elcograf S.p.A.

A catalogue record for this publication is available from the British Library.

Library of Congress Cataloging-in-Publication Data

Names: Ettinger, Alan B., editor. | Weisbrot, Deborah M., 1954- editor. |
    Gallimore, Casey, editor.
Title: Synopsis of neurology, psychiatry and related systemic disorders /
    edited by Alan B. Ettinger, Deborah Weisbrot, Casey Gallimore.
Description: Cambridge, United Kingdom ; New York, NY : Cambridge University
    Press, 2019. | Includes bibliographical references and index.
Identifiers: LCCN 2019007592 | ISBN 9781107069565 (hardback)
Subjects:| MESH: Nervous System Diseases—diagnosis | Nervous System
    Diseases—epidemiology | Mental Disorders—diagnosis | Mental
    Disorders—epidemiology | Comorbidity | Diagnosis, Differential
Classification: LCC RC346 | NLM WL 141 | DDC 616.8—dc23 LC record available at https://lccn.loc.gov/2019007592

ISBN 978-1-107-06956-5 Hardback

To Dave Jones,
A truly wise and loving man. We have been so blessed to have had him in our lives and will be grateful to him forever.
Deborah and Alan

To Cynthia,
Who stood by my side and helped me fight for what was right.
Deborah

To Mom, Dad, and Terry,
Thank you for all the inspiration, laughter, and support. I love you always.
Casey

Contents

List of Contributors   *xi*

Preface   *xxi*

SECTION 1   Diagnostics   **1**

Entries A–Z   1

SECTION 2   Medication Adverse Effects   **707**

Cardiovascular and Renal Medications   **709**

Angiotensin-Converting Enzyme (ACE) Inhibitors   709

Angiotensin Receptor Blockers (ARBs)   709

Antiarrhythmics   709

  Amiodarone   709

  Digoxin   710

  Procainamide   710

  Other Antiarrhythmics   710

Anticoagulants   711

Antiplatelets   711

Beta-Blockers   712

Calcium Channel Blockers   712

  Dihydropyridines   712

  Nondihydropyridines   713

Diuretics   713

  Loop Diuretics   713

  Potassium-Sparing Diuretics   713

  Thiazide and Thiazide-Like Diuretics   714

Lipid Lowering   714

  Bile Acid Sequestrants   714

  Ezetimibe   714

  Fibric Acid Derivatives   715

  HMG CoA Reductase Inhibitors (Statins)   715

  Niacin   716

Methyldopa   716

Orlistat   716

Reserpine   717

Vasodilators   717

  Endothelin Receptor Antagonists and Prostanoids   717

  Nitrates and Peripheral Vasodilators   717

Medications to Treat Diabetes   **719**

Alpha-Glucosidase Inhibitors (AGIs)   719

Amylinomimetics   719

Biguanides   719

Dipeptidyl Peptidase-4 Inhibitors (DPP-4 inhibitors)   720

Glucagon-Like Peptide-1 Receptor Agonists (GLP-1RA)   720

Sodium Glucose Cotransporter-2 Inhibitors (SGLT2 Inhibitors)   721

Sulfonylureas and Other Secretagogues (Meglitinides)   721

Thiazolidinediones (TZDs)   721

Hormones and Medications to Treat Endocrine and Bone Disorders   **722**

Alpha Receptor Blockers   722

Androgenic Anabolic Steroids   722

Bisphosphonates   723

Calcitonin   723

Cinacalcet   724

Hormonal Contraceptives   724

Hormone Replacement Therapy (HRT)   724

Parathyroid Hormone   725

Phosphodiesterase-5 (PDE-5) Inhibitors   725

Thyroid Supplement   726

Gastrointestinal Medications   **727**

Antacids   727

H_2 Antagonists   727

Metoclopramide   728

Proton Pump Inhibitors (PPIs)   728

Scopolamine   729

Vitamins and Minerals   **730**

Iron Preparations   730

Isotretinoin   730

Vitamin A   731

Vitamin B Complex   731

Vitamin D   732

Vitamin E   732
Zinc   733

Medications to Treat Asthma and Allergies   **734**
Anticholinergic Bronchodilators   734
Antihistamines   734
Decongestants   735
Leukotriene Antagonists   735
Long-Acting Beta Agonists (LABA)   736
Methylxanthines   736
Short-Acting Beta Agonists (SABA)   736

Antimicrobial Medications   **738**
Aminoglycosides   738
Amphotericin B   738
Antivirals   738
Azole Antifungals   739
Aztreonam   739
Beta-Lactam/Beta-Lactamase Inhibitors   740
Carbapenems   740
Cephalosporins   741
Clindamycin   741
Daptomycin   741
Echinocandins   742
Ethambutol   742
Fidaxomicin   742
Fluoroquinolones   742
Fosfomycin   743
Glycopeptides   743
Isoniazid   743
Macrolides   744
Metronidazole   744
Neuraminidase Inhibitors   745
Nitrofurantoin   745
Oxazolidinones   745
Penicillins   746
Pyrazinamide   746
Rifampin   746
Sulfamethoxazole-Trimethoprim   747
Tetracyclines   747

Antiretroviral Medications   **748**
Entry Inhibitors (Chemokine Receptor Inhibitors and Fusion Inhibitors)   748
Integrase Strand Transfer Inhibitors   748
Non-Nucleotide Reverse Transcriptase Inhibitors (NNRTIs)   749
Nucleoside Reverse Transcriptase Inhibitors (NRTIs)   749
Protease Inhibitors   750

Immunosuppressive Medications   **751**
Alemtuzumab   751
Antithymocyte Globulin   751
Azathioprine   751
Basiliximab   751
Calcineurin Inhibitors   752
Corticosteroids   752
Mycophenolic Acid Derivatives   753
Proliferation Signal Inhibitors (Mammalian Target of Rapamycin Inhibitors)   753

Oncology and Hematology Medications   **754**
Blinatumomab   754
Cytarabine (Ara-C) (Intravenous)   754
Erythropoiesis-Stimulating Agents   755
Fluoropyrimidine Antimetabolites   755
Granulocyte Colony-Stimulating Factors (G-CSF) and Granulocyte-Macrophage Colony-Stimulating Factors (GM-CSF)   756
Interferon   756
Intrathecal Chemotherapy   757
Ipilimumab   757
Ixabepilone   757
Nelarabine   758
Nitrosoureas   758
Oxazaphosphorines   759
Platinum Analogs   759
Proteasome Inhibitors   760
Selective Serotonin Receptor Modulators   760
Taxanes   761
Thalidomide Analogs   761
Vascular Endothelial Growth Factor (VEGF) Signaling Inhibitors   762
Vinca Alkaloids   762

Disease-Modifying Antirheumatic Medications (DMARDs)   **764**
Abatacept   764
Hydroxychloroquine   764
IL-1 Inhibitors   764
Leflunomide   765
Methotrexate   765
Sulfasalazine   766
Tumor Necrosis Factor-Alpha (TNF-α) Inhibitors   766

Medications to Treat Neurodegenerative Diseases   **767**
Amantadine   767
Anticholinergics   768

Catechol-O-Methyl Transferase (COMT) Inhibitors 768
Cholinesterase Inhibitors 769
Dopamine Agonists 769
Dopamine Precursors 770
Memantine 771
Natalizumab 771
Riluzole 772
Tetrabenazine 773

Medications to Treat Epilepsy 774
Brivaracetam 774
Carbamazepine (and Related Agents) 774
Ethosuximide 775
Felbamate 775
Gabapentin 775
Lacosamide 776
Lamotrigine 776
Levetiracetam 776
Perampanel 777
Phenytoin 777
Pregabalin 778
Rufinamide 778
Tiagabine 778
Topiramate 778
Valproate Products 779
Vigabatrin 779
Zonisamide 780

Medications to Treat Headache and Migraine 781
Antiemetics 781
Cannabinoids 781
Dopamine Receptor Antagonists 781
Neurokinin Receptor Antagonists 782
Serotonin Receptor Antagonists 782
Botulinum Toxin A injections 783
Butalbital 783
Caffeine 783
Ergotamines 784
Dihydroergotamine 784
Ergotamine 784
Isometheptene Mucate 785
Muscle Relaxants 785
Nonsteroidal Anti-inflammatory Drugs (NSAIDs) 786

Opiates/Opioids 786
Salicylates 787
Serotonin 1D/1B Selective Agonists (Triptans) 788

Medications to Treat Mental Health and Substance Abuse Disorders 790
Acamprosate 790
Alpha-2 Adrenergic Agonists 790
Antidepressants 791
Amoxapine 791
Bupropion 791
Mirtazapine 792
Monoamine Oxidase Inhibitors (MAOIs) 792
Serotonin–Norepinephrine Reuptake Inhibitors (SNRIs) 793
Selective Serotonin Reuptake Inhibitors (SSRIs) 793
Trazodone 794
Tricyclic Antidepressants (TCAs) 794
Vilazodone 795
Vortioxetine 795
Antipsychotics 796
First-Generation (Typical) Antipsychotics (FGAs) 796
Second-Generation (Atypical) Antipsychotics (SGAs) 796
Atomoxetine 797
Benzodiazepines 797
Buprenorphine 798
Buspirone 799
Disulfiram 799
Lithium Carbonate 800
Lorcaserin 800
Melatonin Receptor Agonists 801
Nicotine Replacement Therapy 801
Opioid Antagonists 801
Sedative Hypnotics Non-Benzodiazepine Type 802
Sodium Oxybate 802
Stimulants 803
Suvorexant 804
Varenicline Tartrate 804

Index 807

Contributors

Section 1 Edited by

Alan B. Ettinger, MD, MBA, FAAN, FAES
Former Professor of Clinical Neurology at Albert
Einstein College of Medicine
Bronx NY, USA and
President, Professional Advisory Board, EPIC-
Epilepsy Foundation of Long Island
East Meadow NY, USA

Deborah M. Weisbrot, MD, DFAACAP
Clinical Professor of Psychiatry, Stony Brook
University, Stony Brook NY, USA

Section 2 Edited by

Casey E. Gallimore, PharmD, MS
Associate Professor, University of Wisconsin School
of Pharmacy
Madison WI, USA

Section 1 (Diagnostics) Authors by Topic

Cardiac Disorders

Brandon Needelman, MD
Research Intern in Electrophysiology/Cardiology,
NYU-Winthrop University Hospital
Mineola NY, USA

Todd J. Cohen, MD
Director of Electrophysiology, NYU-Winthrop
University Hospital
Mineola NY, USA

Dementing and Degenerative Disorders

Chen Zhao, MD
Fellow in Aging and Dementia, Columbia University
New York NY, USA

Howard Crystal, MD
Professor of Psychiatry and Pathology, State
University of New York Downstate
Brooklyn NY, USA

Demyelinating Disorders

Intazam U. Khan, MD
Clinical Assistant Professor of Neurology and
Neuroscience, Cornell University
New York NY, USA and
Attending Neurologist, Donald and Barbara Zucker
School of Medicine at Hofstra/Northwell
Hempstead NY, USA

Tanya Kapoor, DO
North Shore University Hospital
Manhasset, NY and Donald and Barbara Zucker
School of Medicine at Hofstra/Northwell
Hempstead NY, USA

Endocrine Disorders

Zianka Huzailyn Fallil, MD
Attending Neurologist, Rochester Regional Health
Rochester NY, USA

Gastrointestinal Disorders

Mohammad A. Khoshnoodi, MD
Assistant Professor of Neurology, Johns Hopkins
School of Medicine
Baltimore MD, USA

Vinay Chaudhry, MD, MBA, CPE, FAAN, FRCP
Professor of Neurology, Johns Hopkins University
School of Medicine
Baltimore MD, USA

Headache

James Y. Soh, MD, PhD
Resident in Neurology, State University of New York
Downstate Brooklyn NY, USA

Susan W. Law, DO, MPH
Director of Stroke Services, Kings County Hospital
and Clinical Associate Professor of Neurology, State
University of New York (SUNY) Downstate Medical
Center, Brooklyn NY, USA

Ira Turner, MD,
Neurologist, Island Neurological Associates
Plainview NY, USA

Hematologic Disorders

Shamik Bhattacharyya, MD, MS
Attending Neurologist, Brigham and Women's
Hospital, Harvard Medical School
Boston MA, USA

Martin Samuels, MD
Chair, Department of Neurology, Brigham and
Women's Hospital and
Professor of Neurology, Harvard Medical School
Boston MA, USA

Heredofamilial Disorders

Lead authors

Amy Goldstein, MD
Clinical Director, Mitochondrial Medicine Frontier
Program at Children's Hospital of Philadelphia and
Associate Professor of Clinical Pediatrics, Perelman
School of Medicine at the University of Pennsylvania
Philadelphia PA, USA

Neil Datta, MD,
Fellow in Neurophysiology, Beth Israel Deaconess Medical
Center/Harvard Medical School, Boston MA, USA

Co-authors

Maria Luisa Escolar, MD, MS
Associate Professor of Pediatrics, University of
Pittsburgh School of Medicine, Pittsburgh PA, USA

Alan B. Ettinger, MD, MBA, FAAN, FAES
Former Professor of Clinical Neurology at Albert
Einstein College of Medicine
Bronx NY, USA and
EPIC-Epilepsy Foundation of Long Island
East Meadow NY, USA

Infectious Disorders

Lead authors

Shazia Alam, DO
Attending Neurologist, NYU-Winthrop Hospital
Mineola NY, USA

Antenor P. Vilceus, MD, MBA
Attending NeuroHospitalist, NYU-Winthrop
Hospital
Mineola NY, USA

Daniel Torres, MD
Clinical Assistant Professor of Neurology,
NYU School of Medicine
New York NY, USA

Aparna M. Prabhu, MD, MRCP
Clinical Assistant Professor of Neurology, Sidney
Kimmel Medical School,
Thomas Jefferson University and
Associate Program director for Neurology Residency,
Albert Einstein Medical Center, Philadelphia PA, USA

Neil Datta, MD
Fellow in Neurophysiology, Beth Israel Deaconess
Medical Center/Harvard Medical School, Boston MA,
USA

Co-authors

Nissah Vilceus, BS, MA
[No affiliation]

Alan B. Ettinger, MD, MBA, FAAN, FAES
Former Professor of Clinical Neurology at Albert
Einstein College of Medicine,
Bronx NY, USA and
EPIC-Epilepsy Foundation of Long Island, East
Meadow NY, USA

Saman Zafar, MD, MRCP
Neurology Resident, Albert Einstein Medical Center
Philadelphia PA, USA

Annie Hsieh, MD, PhD
Neurology Resident, Albert Einstein Medical Center
Philadelphia PA, USA

Sridhara S. Yaddanapudi, MBBS, MD
Specialist in Vascular Neurology, Hypertension and
Internal Medicine, Christiana Care Health Services
Newark DE, USA

Inflammatory Non-Infectious Disorders

Lead authors

Patricia Coyle, MD
Director, MS Comprehensive Care Center, and
Professor and Vice Chair of Clinical Affairs,
Stony Brook Neurosciences Institute, State
University of New York at Stony Brook
Stony Brook NY, USA

Amit M. Shelat, DO, MPA, MS, FACP
Assistant Professor of Clinical Neurology, Stony
Brook University School of Medicine
Stony Brook NY, USA and
Attending Neurologist, Medsurant Holdings, LLC
Teaneck NJ, USA

Co-authors

Imad R. Khan, MD
Fellow, Neurocritical Care, University of Maryland
Medical Center
Baltimore MD, USA

Metabolic Disorders

Lead authors

Derek Cheng, DO
Neurology Resident, Donald and Barbara Zucker
School of Medicine at Hofstra/Northwell
Hempstead NY, USA

Chilvana Patel, MD
Assistant Professor of Neurology, University of Texas
Medical Branch
Galveston TX, USA

Co-authors

Elizabeth Ng, MD
Attending Child Neurologist, Pediatric Epileptologist
and Clinical Neurophysiologist, Connecticut
Children's Medical Center,
Hartford CT, USA

Scott J. Stevens, MD
Assistant Professor of Neurology, Donald and Barbara
Zucker School of Medicine at Hofstra/Northwell
Hempstead NY, USA

Purvesh Patel, MD
Assistant Professor of Medicine, Baylor College of
Medicine Houston TX, USA

Alan B. Ettinger, MD, MBA, FAAN, FAES
Former Professor of Clinical Neurology at Albert
Einstein College of Medicine
Bronx NY, USA and
EPIC-Epilepsy Foundation of Long Island
East Meadow NY, USA

Pediatric Metabolic Disorders

Gidon N. Winter, MBBS
Pediatric Neurologist, Shaare-Zedek Medical Centre
and Maccabi Health Services Jerusalem, Israel

Movement Disorders

Lead authors

Nora L. Chan, MD
Director of the Movement Disorders Division,
NYU Winthrop University Hospital
Mineola NY, USA and
Clinical Assistant Professor, School of Medicine at
State University of New York,
Stony Brook NY, USA

Matthew S. Goldfinger
Medical student, New York Institute of
Technology–College of Osteopathic Medicine
Old Westbury NY, USA

Co-authors

Sachin Kapur, MD
Medical Director of Movement Disorders, Advocate
Christ Medical Center
Oak Lawn IL, USA

Raminder Parihar, MD
Assistant Professor, Donald and Barbara Zucker
School of Medicine at Hofstra/Northwell
Hempstead NY, USA

Vinny Sharma, DO
Neurology resident, University of Illinois–Chicago
College of Medicine
Chicago IL, USA

Mohammad S. Hussain, MS
Medical student, New York Institute of
Technology–College of Osteopathic Medicine
Old Westbury NY, USA

Jayme Mancini, DO, PhD
Medical student, New York Institute of
Technology–College of Osteopathic Medicine
Old Westbury NY, USA

George Koutsouras, MPH
Medical student, New York Institute of
Technology–College of Osteopathic Medicine
Old Westbury NY, USA

Matthew A. Goldstein
Medical student, New York Institute of
Technology–College of Osteopathic Medicine
Old Westbury NY, USA

Adena N. Leder, DO
Medical Director, Parkinson's Center, and Assistant
Professor of Neurology, New York Institute of
Technology–College of Osteopathic Medicine
Old Westbury NY, USA

Myopathic Disorders

Neil Datta, MD
Fellow in Neurophysiology, Beth Israel Deaconess
Medical Center/Harvard Medical School
Boston MA, USA

Lucas Meira Benchaya, MD
Neurologist, University of Connecticut and Hartford
Hospital
Hartford CT, USA

Erica Schuyler, MD
Assistant Professor and Neurology Residency
Program Director, University of Connecticut and
Hartford Hospital
Hartford CT, USA

Neoplastic Disorders

Lead authors

Sridhara S. Yaddanapudi, MBBS, MD
Specialist in Vascular Neurology, Hypertension and
Internal Medicine, Christiana Care Health Services
Newark DE, USA

Patrick Drummond, MD
Resident, Department of Neurology, New York
University Medical Center
New York NY, USA

Maninder Kaur, MD
Fellow in Vascular Neurology, University of Tennessee
Memphis TN, USA

Co-authors

Dilip Jayaraman, MD
Fellow in Vascular Neurology, University of
Massachusetts Medical School
Worcester MA, USA

Ylec Mariana Cardenas, MD
Neurology Resident, Albert Einstein Medical Center
Philadelphia PA, USA

Aparna M. Prabhu, MD, MRCP
Clinical Assistant Professor of Neurology, Sidney
Kimmel Medical School,
Thomas Jefferson University and Albert Einstein
Medical Center
Philadelphia PA, USA

Doria Gold, MD
Fellow in Neuro-ophthalmology, New York University
Medical Center
New York NY, USA

Nina Kim, MD
Resident, Department of Neurology, New York
University Medical Center
New York NY, USA

Andrea Lee, MD
Resident, Department of Neurology, New York
University Medical Center
New York NY, USA

Nicole S. Morgan, MD
Resident, Department of Neurology, New York
University Medical Center
New York NY, USA

Lynda Nwabuobi, MD
Movement Disorders Fellow, Columbia University
Medical Center
New York NY, USA

Danielle Stember, MD
Movement Disorders Fellow, New York University
Medical Center
New York NY, USA

Vanessa Tiongson, MD
Assistant Professor of Neurology, Mount Sinai
Medical Center
New York NY, USA

Jonathan Tiu, MD
Neurology Resident, New York University Medical Center
New York NY, USA

Arielle M. Kurzweil, MD
Clinical Assistant Professor of Neurology, New York
University Medical Center
New York NY, USA

Tajinder Kaur, MD
Director of Clinical Coordination and Quality, All
Medical Care IPA
Brooklyn NY, USA

Joseph C. Landolfi, DO
Chief of Neurology; Director of Neuro-oncology and
Gamma Knife, JFK Health System
Edison NJ, USA

Ophthalmologic Disorders

Peter W. MacIntosh, MD
Assistant Professor, Department of Ophthalmology
and Visual Sciences, University of Illinois at Chicago
Chicago IL, USA

Mei P. Zhou, MD
Ophthalmologist, Department of Ophthalmology &
Visual Sciences, University of Illinois at Chicago
Chicago IL, USA

Heather E. Moss, MD, PhD
Assistant Professor of Ophthalmology and of
Neurology, Stanford University Medical Center and
Byers Eye Institute at Stanford
Palo Alto CA, USA

Orthopedic/Spine Conditions

Padmaja Aradhya, MD
Neurologist
Massapequa NY, USA

Peripheral Nerve Disorders

Lead authors

Steven Ender DO
Neurologist
Bethpage NY, USA

Nuttawan Vongveeranonchai, MD
Neuromuscular Fellow, University Hospitals
Cleveland Medical Center and
Case Western Reserve University, School of Medicine
Cleveland OH, USA

Li-Fen Chen, MD
Assistant Professor of Neurology, Donald and Barbara
Zucker School of Medicine at Hofstra/Northwell
Hempstead NY, USA

Co-authors

Saima Ali, MD
Neurologist, North Shore University Hospital
Manhasset NY, USA

Michael Nissenbaum, MD
Neurologist, New York Neurologic Associates
New Hyde Park NY, USA

Amy Hua, DO
Neurologist, White Plains Hospital Physician
Associates
Armonk NY, USA

Songkit Supakornnumporn, MD
Neuromuscular Research Fellow, University
Hospitals Cleveland Medical Center and
Case Western Reserve University, School of Medicine
Cleveland OH, USA

Saba Saeed, MD
Neuromuscular Fellow, University Hospitals
Cleveland Medical Center and
Case Western Reserve University, School of Medicine
Cleveland OH, USA

Trixy Suy, DO
Neuromuscular Fellow, University Hospitals
Cleveland Medical Center and
Case Western Reserve University, School of Medicine
Cleveland OH, USA

Bashar Katirji, MD, FACP
Director, Neuromuscular Center & EMG Laboratory,
University Hospitals Cleveland Medical Center and
Professor of Neurology,
Case Western Reserve University, School of
Medicine
Cleveland OH, USA

Pregnancy-Related Disorders

Christine Lu, MD
Resident in Neurology, Mount Sinai Medical Center
New York NY, USA

Cynthia Harden, MD
Therapeutic Area Head in Epilepsy, Xenon
Pharmaceuticals, Inc. and
Neurologist, East 14th Street Medical Arts Center
New York NY, USA

Psychiatric Disorders

Lead authors

Juliana Lockman, MD
Clinical Assistant Professor,
Stanford University School of Medicine
Stanford CA, USA

Aaron M. Pinkhasov, MD
Chairman, Department of Behavioral Health, NYU-
Winthrop Hospital, Mineola NY, USA

Co-authors

Anna Frenklach Rief, MD
Psychiatrist, Palo Alto Medical Foundation
Palo Alto CA, USA

Deepan Singh, MD
Attending in Child, Adolescent and Adult Psychiatry,
NYU-Winthrop University Hospital
Mineola NY, USA

Glenn T. Werneburg
Fellow in Molecular Genetics and Microbiology, Stony
Brook University
Stony Brook NY, USA

Gregory Gunyan, MD
Attending Psychiatrist, NYU-Winthrop University
Hospital
Mineola NY, USA

Substance Abuse

Mehrdad Golzad, MD
Neurologist
Queens NY, USA

Fabian Rentas, PA
Surgical Critical Care Physician Assistant, Saint
Barnabas Hospital
Bronx NY, USA

Alan B. Ettinger, MD, MBA, FAAN, FAES
Former Professor of Clinical Neurology at Albert
Einstein College of Medicine,
Bronx NY, USA and
EPIC-Epilepsy Foundation of Long Island
East Meadow NY, USA

Sleep Disorders

Annamaria Iakovou, MD
Fellow, Sleep Medicine, Donald and Barbara Zucker
School of Medicine at Hofstra/Northwell
Hempstead NY, USA

Stella Hahn, MD
Fellow, Pulmonary and Critical Care Medicine,
Donald and Barbara Zucker School of Medicine at
Hofstra/Northwell
Hempstead NY, USA

Yonatan Greenstein, MD
Fellow, Pulmonary and Critical Care Medicine,
Donald and Barbara Zucker School of Medicine at
Hofstra/Northwell
Hempstead NY, USA

Preethi Rajan, MD
Assistant Professor of Medicine, Donald and
Barbara Zucker School of Medicine at Hofstra/
Northwell
Hempstead NY, USA

Harly Greenberg, MD, FCCP, FAASM
Medical Director of the Northwell Sleep Disorders
Center, Donald and Barbara Zucker School of
Medicine at Hofstra/Northwell
Hempstead NY, USA

Seizure-Related Disorders

Nadia Sotudeh, MD
Resident, Department of Neurology, Northwell
Health System
Great Neck NY, USA

Sean T. Hwang, MD
Epileptologist, Northwell Health System
Great Neck NY, USA

David J. Anschel, MD
Director, Comprehensive Epilepsy Center of Long
Island at St. Charles Hospital
Port Jefferson NY, USA

Toxin-Related Disorders

Jaimin Shah, MD
Assistant Professor of Neurology, University of Florida College of Medicine
Jacksonville FL, USA

Michael T. Pulley, MD, PhD
Clinical Associate Professor of Neurology, University of Florida College of Medicine
Jacksonville FL, USA

Alan R. Berger, MD
Professor and Chairman, Department of Neurology, University of Florida College of Medicine
Jacksonville FL, USA

Transplant-Related Disorders

Rishi Garg, MD, MBA
Attending Neurologist, Edward Hines, Jr. VA Hospital
Hines IL, USA

Jasvinder Chawla, MD, MBA, FAAN
Chief, Neurology Service, Edward Hines, Jr. VA Hospital
Hines IL, USA

Alan B. Ettinger, MD, MBA, FAAN, FAES
Former Professor of Clinical Neurology at Albert Einstein College of Medicine,
Bronx NY, USA and
EPIC-Epilepsy Foundation of Long Island
East Meadow NY, USA

Vaccine-Related Complications

Hind Kettani, MD
Neurologist (Epileptologist), Premier Neurology and Wellness Center Stuart FL, USA

Janine Harewood, MD
Resident, NY Presbyterian Queens
Queens NY, USA

Hadi Zein, MD
Physician, NY Presbyterian Queens, Queens NY, USA

Danial Arshed, MD
Fellow, Pulmonary Disease/Critical Care Medicine, NY Presbyterian Queens
Queens NY, USA

Vascular Disorders

Lead authors

Jacob R. Hascalovici, MD, PhD
Assistant Professor, Saul R. Korey Department of Neurology, Albert Einstein College of Medicine, Montefiore Medical Center
Bronx NY, USA

Aparna M. Prabhu, MD, MRCP
Clinical Assistant Professor of Neurology, Sidney Kimmel Medical School,
Thomas Jefferson University and
Associate Program Director for Neurology Residency, Albert Einstein Medical Center, Philadelphia PA, USA

Michael Guido III, MD
Co-Director, Stony Brook Comprehensive Cerebrovascular & Stroke Center,
Associate Professor of Neurology, State University of New York at Stony Brook
Stony Brook NY, USA

Co-authors

Elizabeth Chernyak, MD
Resident, Columbia University Medical Center
New York NY, USA

Stephen Briggs, MD, PhD
Neurology Resident, Vanderbilt University Medical Center
Nashville TN, USA

Samuel Ahn, MD
Resident, UCLA
Los Angeles CA, USA

Michael Tau, MD
Resident in Psychiatry, Albert Einstein College of Medicine
Bronx NY, USA

Mark Stevens Jacobs, MD
Resident in Internal Medicine, Jackson Memorial Hospital
Miami FL, USA

Nina M. Massad, MD
Resident, Columbia University Medical Center
New York NY, USA

Arjun Seth, MD
Resident, Johns Hopkins School of Medicine
Baltimore MD, USA

Steven A. Sparr, MD, FAAN
Professor of Clinical Neurology and Assistant
Professor of Rehabilitation Medicine, Albert Einstein
College of Medicine
Bronx NY, USA

Sridhara S. Yaddanapudi, MBBS, MD
Specialist in Vascular Neurology, Hypertension and
Internal Medicine, Christiana Care Health Services
Newark DE, USA

Yongwoo Kim, MD
Assistant Professor of Neurology, Lewis Katz School
of Medicine, Temple University
Philadelphia PA, USA

George C. Newman, MD, PhD
Professor and Chairman, Neurosensory Sciences,
Albert Einstein Medical Center
Philadelphia PA, USA

Vestibular Disorders

Eric Smouha, MD
Clinical Professor of Otolaryngology, Icahn School of
Medicine at Mount Sinai
New York NY, USA

Enrique Perez, MD
Resident, Department of Otolaryngology,
Mount Sinai Hospital
New York NY, USA

Daniel Carlton, MD,
Resident, Mount Sinai Hospital
New York NY, USA

Neurodegenerative and Miscellaneous Disorders

Hamada Hamid Altalib, MD
Co-Director, Epilepsy Center of Excellence,
Connecticut VA Healthcare System and
Assistant Professor, Departments of Neurology &
Psychiatry, Yale School of Medicine
New Haven CT, USA

Paola Ayora, MD
Fellow in Child and Adolescent Psychiatry,
Montefiore Medical Center
Bronx NY, USA

Arman Fesharaki-Zadeh, MD
Instructor of Psychiatry and Neurology, Yale
University Memory Clinic
New Haven CT, USA

Alan Ettinger, MD, MBA, FAAN, FAES
Former Professor of Clinical Neurology at Albert
Einstein College of Medicine,
Bronx NY, USA and
EPIC-Epilepsy Foundation of Long Island
East Meadow NY, USA

Section 2 (Medication Adverse Effects) Authors by Topic

Cardiovascular and Renal Medications

Jeff Freund, PharmD, BCACP
Clinical Pharmacist, Froedtert Health
Milwaukee WI, USA

Heather LaRue, PharmD
Clinical Pharmacist, UW Health University Hospital
Madison WI, USA

Greta Nemergut, PharmD, BCCCP
Clinical Pharmacist, UW Health University Hospital
Madison WI, USA

Medications to Treat Diabetes

Curtis L. Triplitt, PharmD, CDE
Associate Professor of Medicine, University of Texas
Health Science Center
San Antonio TX, USA

Hormones and Medications to Treat Endocrine and Bone Disorders

Emily Zimmerman, PharmD, BCPS
Clinical Pharmacist, UW Health University Hospital
Madison WI, USA

Casey E. Gallimore, PharmD, MS
Associate Professor, University of Wisconsin School
of Pharmacy
Madison WI, USA

Gastrointestinal Medications

Christi Ann Albert, PharmD, BCPS
Clinical Pharmacist, UW Health University Hospital
Madison WI, USA

Casey E. Gallimore, PharmD, MS,
Associate Professor, University of Wisconsin School
of Pharmacy
Madison WI, USA

Vitamins and Minerals

Chris Hulstein, PharmD
Clinical Pharmacy Specialist, Providence Health and
Services
Portland OR, USA

Casey E. Gallimore, PharmD, MS,
Associate Professor, University of Wisconsin School
of Pharmacy
Madison WI, USA

Medications to Treat Asthma and Allergies

Christi Ann Albert, PharmD, BCPS
Clinical Pharmacist, UW Health University Hospital
Madison WI, USA

Megan Bauer, PharmD, BCPS,
2500 Overlook Terrace,
Madison WI, USA

Antimicrobial Medications

Susanne G. Barnett, PharmD, BCPS
Associate Professor, University of Wisconsin School
of Pharmacy
Madison WI, USA

Jennifer C. Dela-Pena, PharmD, BCPS
Infectious Diseases/Antimicrobial Stewardship
Pharmacist, Advocate Health Care
Chicago IL, USA

Tyler Liebenstein, PharmD, BCPS-AQ ID
Clinical Pharmacist, UW Health University Hospital
Madison WI, USA

Eileen Shannon, PharmD
Clinical Pharmacist, UW Health University Hospital
Madison WI, USA

Antiretroviral Medications

Anthony T. Podany, PharmD
Assistant Professor, University of Nebraska Medical
Center
Omaha NE, USA

Uriel Sandkovsky, MD MS, FIDSA
Physician, North Infectious Disease Consultants
Dallas TX, USA

Caroline Jamison, PharmD
Clinical Pharmacist, University of Nebraska Medical
Center
Omaha NE, USA

Immunosuppressive Medications

Heather J. Johnson, PharmD, BCPS
Assistant Professor, University of Pittsburgh School of
Pharmacy
Pittsburg PA, USA

Oncology and Hematology Medications

Latha Radhakrishnan, PharmD, BCPS, BCOP
Clinical Assistant Professor, University of Illinois at
Chicago College of Pharmacy
Chicago IL, USA

Scott M. Wirth, PharmD, BCOP
Clinical Assistant Professor, University of Illinois at
Chicago College of Pharmacy
Chicago IL, USA

Disease-Modifying Antirheumatic Medications (DMARDs)

Rebecca Fiore, PharmD
Clinical Pharmacy Specialist, Rockford VA
Community Based Outpatient Clinic (CBOC)
Rockford IL, USA

Daniel J. Langenburg, PharmD
Clinical Pharmacy Specialist, Portland VA
Medical Center
Portland OR, USA

Medications to Treat Neurodegenerative Diseases

Angela M. Hill, PharmD, BCPP, CPh
Professor and Chair, Department of
Pharmacotherapeutics and Clinical Research,
University of South Florida College of Pharmacy
Tampa FL, USA

Jasmine B. R. Cutler, PharmD, CPh
Assistant Professor, University of South Florida
College of Pharmacy
Tampa FL, USA

Kristin Robinson, PharmD
Assistant Professor, Florida Agricultural and
Mechanical University, Tallahassee FL, USA

Medications to Treat Epilepsy

Jeannine Conway, PharmD, BCPS
Assistant Dean for Professional Education, University
of Minnesota College of Pharmacy
Minneapolis MN, USA

Medications to Treat Headache and Migraine

F. Michael Cutrer, MD
Neurologist, Mayo Clinic College of Medicine
Rochester MN, USA

Aaron A. Bubolz, DO
Neurologist, Aurora Health Care Medical Group
Green Bay WI, USA

Medications to Treat Mental Health and Substance Abuse Disorders

Kelly N. Gable, PharmD, BCPP
Associate Professor, Department of
Pharmacy Practice, SIUE School of
Pharmacy
Edwardsville IL, USA

Mei T. Liu, PharmD, BCPP
Clinical Assistant Professor, Ernest Mario School of
Pharmacy
Piscataway Township NJ, USA

Megan Maroney, PharmD, BCPP
Clinical Associate Professor, Ernest Mario School of
Pharmacy
Piscataway Township NJ, USA

Preface

Neurologic Differential Diagnosis: A Case-Based Approach (A. B. Ettinger and D. Weisbrot, eds., Cambridge University Press), published in 2014, emphasizes a pragmatic and quick-reference approach to achieving a comprehensive differential diagnosis. Using this text, the clinician can efficiently look up specific symptoms and signs such as "dizziness," "mental status change," "diplopia," "foot drop," or "psychosis" to immediately generate diagnostic possibilities. Each chapter outlines key features of clinical presentations and quickly reminds the clinician what diagnoses to consider.

While our prior textbook helps the clinician to rapidly generate a differential diagnosis, an additional approach would also be invaluable. Symptoms and signs in neurology and psychiatry do not typically occur in isolation; rather, they present in the clinical context of other underlying conditions. For example, a physician evaluating a 40-year-old male with change in mental status could utilize *Neurologic Differential Diagnosis: A Case-Based Approach* to review a diverse list of potential underlying diagnoses. However, if it is known, for example, that this patient carries a diagnosis of HIV, the clinician would also consider what complications of HIV are associated with mental status changes. These include AIDS dementia complex, central nervous system (CNS) lymphomas, cryptococcal meningitis, CMV superinfections, neurosyphilis, toxoplasmosis, and other conditions that occur in immunocompromised states. Having a checklist of these conditions enables the clinician to quickly access information on the neurologic and psychiatric complications of co-existing conditions such as HIV, and this further enhances the busy clinician's attempt to provide a comprehensive evaluation.

What about a 30-year-old woman with epilepsy who now complains of headaches? While the broad differential diagnosis as described in our earlier textbook includes seizures and postictal states or nonepileptic conditions such as migraine or subarachnoid hemorrhage, this patient happens to have been recently started on lamotrigine to treat seizures. Could lamotrigine be responsible for the headaches? A review of a succinct summary of lamotrigine's neurologic or psychiatric adverse effects would describe headaches, including uncommonly encountered aseptic meningitis. This in turn would lead the clinician to perform additional investigations.

Consider a 39-year-old male with Down syndrome who presents with gait instability. Examination reveals diffuse hyperreflexia and our prior text has chapters on gait alteration and on myelopathy that inform differential diagnosis. However, if the clinician wonders whether there may be a relationship between Down syndrome and gait disturbances, wouldn't it be helpful if the clinician had an additional reference to quickly review the neurologic and psychiatric complications of Down syndrome? Such a reference would cite the predisposition of patients with Down syndrome to experience atlanto-axial instability and knowing this could lead to ordering emergent neuroimaging.

How about the case of a 40-year-old man referred to rule out seizures because of episodic feelings of derealization? Seizures are listed in our earlier textbook but other entities, including panic attacks, are also cited with a brief description. Seeking a more detailed description of the characteristics of panic attacks, the clinician would then have an easily accessible succinct summary of panic attack features. This in turn would lead the clinician to inquire about symptoms such as palpitations, diaphoresis, sensations of smothering or choking, shortness of breath, and fear of dying. Positive endorsements of many of these symptoms could lead to additional testing and referral to a psychiatrist.

Yet another example concerns a 50-year-old male with carpal tunnel syndrome and Addison's disease. While the neurologist has a vague recollection of the latter diagnosis, she can benefit from the availability of a summary of the neurologic and psychiatric complications of Addison's disease. This helps ensure that its features do not have any relationship to the patient's current neurologic complaints.

In this spirit, *Synopsis of Neurology, Psychiatry, and Related Systemic Disorders* was designed to provide concise summaries of neurologic, psychiatric, and medical diagnoses with a focus on neurologic and psychiatric implications. A separate pharmacology section provides a consolidated review of potential neurologic and psychiatric adverse effects of medications. All entries are listed alphabetically for quick access, and diagnostic conditions follow a stereotyped order of presentation including epidemiology and demographics, highlights of each disorder, neurologic and psychiatric symptoms and signs, secondary complications, and potential neurologic or psychiatric complications of treatments.

We hope that *Synopsis of Neurology, Psychiatry, and Related Systemic Disorders*, like its predecessor, *Neurologic Differential Diagnosis: A Case-Based Approach*, will be an invaluable resource for a broad medical audience. For the experienced neurologist or psychiatrist, the book can provide quick reminders of the main highlights of underlying neurologic and psychiatric conditions as well as medical conditions that may be associated with neurologic or psychiatric complications. For other healthcare providers, *Synopsis of Neurology, Psychiatry, and Related Systemic Disorders* may introduce the clinician to the interface between neurology and psychiatry with co-existing medical conditions. For the medical student, resident, junior neurologist, or psychiatrist preparing for board examinations, this text can be a very useful guide to approaching the neurologic and psychiatric aspects of medical disorders and medication therapies. Pharmacists may also find great value in the succinct summaries in the medication section of the text.

The process of developing this book required many hours of hard work on the part of the editors and by the many authors who labored to complete their submissions on top of undoubtedly very busy clinical obligations. While we strove to be as comprehensive as possible in the selection of conditions to include in this book, many disorders, especially in the realm of pediatrics or rare genetic syndromes, could not unfortunately be included and would be best left for references that specialize in these specific topics.

Finally, we would like to express our appreciation to the staff of Cambridge University Press (including Mr. Nicholas Dunton, Ms. Anna Whiting, and Mr. Nigel Graves) for their kind and vigorous support and patience throughout the book development process. We would also like to thank Ms. Penny Lyons for her careful attention to detail during her painstaking copy-editing work.

Alan B. Ettinger, MD, MBA, FAES
Deborah M. Weisbrot, MD,
Distinguished Fellow, American Academy
of Child & Adolescent Psychiatry
Casey Gallimore, PharmD

SECTION 1   # Diagnostics

Entries A–Z

A

Absence Seizures (Petit Mal or Generalized Nonconvulsive Seizures)

Epidemiology and Demographics: Typical absence seizures account for 10% of epileptic seizures in children. Annual incidence is estimated at 0.7–4.6/100,000 in the general population, and up to 6–8/100,000 in children aged 0–15 years. Associated with a variety of generalized epilepsy syndromes. Age of onset varies depending on the coinciding syndrome, generally in the first two decades. Early onset more consistent with childhood absence epilepsy or myoclonic astatic epilepsy, whereas presentation near puberty supports juvenile absence epilepsy or juvenile myoclonic epilepsy. May occur among other seizure types in more severe epilepsy syndromes, such as Lennox–Gastaut syndrome.

Disorder Description: Nonconvulsive generalized seizure type characterized by brief episodes of abrupt loss of consciousness, lasting 10–20 seconds, which may occur on a frequent, recurrent basis. Associated with subtle freezing or oral or manual automatisms. Of shorter duration than complex partial seizures, and a postictal period is not present. Events can be mistaken for daydreaming, which may contribute to delay in diagnosis. Typical absence seizures have a 3-Hz generalized spike and wave pattern on the EEG, often provoked by hyperventilation. Ethosuximide is used when absence seizures occur in isolation, valproate when there is co-occurrence with generalized tonic–clonic seizures (GTCS).

Atypical absence seizures have less abrupt onset and offset and may be prolonged. Often presenting with a loss of muscle tone (a gradual slump) and subtle myoclonic jerks. Loss of awareness may be incomplete, with physical activity continuing more slowly or with frequent errors. Atypical absence seizures are associated with a generalized slow spike and wave pattern of <2.5 Hz, and typically occur in the setting of more severe epilepsy syndromes with intellectual impairment.

Symptoms

Localization site	Comment
Cerebral hemispheres	Sudden interruption of consciousness. Automatisms, in the form of lip-smacking, chewing, and fumbling movements of the fingers. Mild tonic stiffening
Mental status and psychiatric aspects/complications	Deficits in global cognitive function, attention and focus, visual-spatial functions, and visual memory most pronounced during active disease. Cognitive status depends on underlying syndrome

Secondary Complications: Attentional issues may result in decreased school performance. Increased risk of accidental injury associated with driving or operating heavy machinery.

Treatment Complications: Some antiepileptic drugs (AEDs), such as vigabatrin, gabapentin, phenytoin, phenobarbital, or carbamazepine and their derivatives, can worsen seizures and should be avoided for certain epilepsy types. Valproate side effects include hyperactivity, weight gain, transaminitis, thrombocytopenia, pancreatitis, and known teratogenic effects. Ethosuximide most commonly causes dizziness and gastrointestinal complaints. Rare side effects include psychosis.

Bibliography

Fong GC, Shah PU, Gee MN, et al. Childhood absence epilepsy with tonic-clonic seizures and electroencephalogram 3–4-Hz spike and multispike-slow wave complexes: linkage to chromosome 8q24. *Am J Hum Genet.* 1998;63(4):1117–29.

Guerrini R, Belmonte A, Genton P. Antiepileptic drug-induced worsening of seizures in children. *Epilepsia.* 1998;39 Suppl 3:S2–10.

Pavon P, Bianchini R, Trifiletti RR, et al. Neuropsychological assessment in children with absence epilepsy. *Neurology.* 2001;56(8):1047–51.

Schwartzkroin PA. *Brain development and epilepsy.* New York: Oxford University Press; 1995. xii, 337 p.

Acquired Hepatocerebral Degeneration

Epidemiology and Demographics: Acquired hepatocerebral degeneration (AHD) is a rare condition that occurs in about 1% of patients with cirrhosis. This condition can occur in patients with severe and decompensated chronic liver failure and can happen at any age.

Disorder Description: AHD is associated with portosystemic shunting, either iatrogenic or spontaneous. Clinical presentation of AHD closely resembles Wilson's disease and therefore it is sometimes called non-Wilsonian hepatocerebral degeneration. Patients often have hepatic encephalopathy, followed by extrapyramidal symptoms such as rigidity, bradykinesia, tremor, and choreoathetosis. MRI of the brain often shows hyperintense signal changes on T1-weighted images and hypointense or normal signal on T2-weighted images in the basal ganglia and cerebellum.

Symptoms

Localization site	Comment
Cerebral hemispheres	Hepatic encephalopathy Parkinsonism
Cerebellum	Ataxia

Bibliography

Burkhard PR, Delavelle J, Du Pasquier R, Spahr L. Chronic parkinsonism associated with cirrhosis: a distinct subset of acquired hepatocerebral degeneration. *Arch Neurol.* 2003;60(4):521–8.

Fernández-Rodriguez R, Contreras A, De Villoria JG, Grandas F. Acquired hepatocerebral degeneration: clinical characteristics and MRI findings. *Eur J Neurol.* 2010;17(12):1463–70.

Saporta MA, Andre C, Bahia PR, et al. Acquired hepatocerebral degeneration without overt liver disease. *Neurology.* 2004;63:1981–2.

Victor M, Adams RD, Cole M. The acquired (non-Wilsonian) type of chronic hepatocerebral degeneration. *Medicine (Baltimore).* 1965;44:345–96.

Actinomycosis

Epidemiology and Demographics: Actinomycosis affects males more so than females, between 20 and 60 years old.

Disorder Description: Actinomycosis is a slowly progressive bacterial infection, most commonly caused by the gram-positive, anaerobic, or microaerophilic rod *Actinomyces israelii*. It normally resides in the nasopharyngeal, gastrointestinal, and female genital tracts. Infection may spread by cervicofacial infections (most common) or hematogenous spread. Risk factors for infection include poor oral hygiene or dental procedures, trauma, use of contraceptive intrauterine devices (IUDs), or immunocompromised state.[1]

Symptoms

Localization site	Comment
Cerebral hemispheres	Brain abscesses (most common) Meningitis Encephalitis Subdural empyema Dural sinus thrombosis[2]
Base of skull	Basilar meningitis
Spinal cord	Epidural abscess causing cord compression Myelopathy[3]
Syndromes with combined spinal cord and peripheral nerve lesions	Myeloradiculopathy[3]

Secondary Complications: Chronic meningitis may develop from brain abscesses, which may lead to hydrocephalus.

Treatment Complications: Response to medication may be slow and take months to take effect.

References

1. Ham H, Jung S, Jung T, Heo S. Cerebral actinomycosis: unusual clinical and radiological findings of an abscess. *J Korean Neurosurg Soc.* 2011;50(2):147.
2. Bradley W. Actinomycosis. *Neurology in clinical practice.* Philadelphia: Butterworth-Heinemann; 2004. p. 1505.
3. Dua R, Bhat D, Indira D. Spinal actinomycosis: a rare disease. *Neurol India.* 2010;58(2):298.

Acute Brachial Neuritis (Parsonage–Turner Syndrome)

Epidemiology and Demographics: More common among middle-aged men (70%); average age 41.4 years. Mostly unilateral onset, involving the dominant limb.

Disorder Description: Acute brachial neuritis, also known as Parsonage–Turner syndrome, brachial plexus neuritis, or neuralgic amyotrophy, is an immune-mediated, multifocal peripheral nervous system disorder. Most lesions are axonal but some may be demyelinating. Targets predominantly proximal motor axons. Most commonly affected nerves include the long thoracic, suprascapular, axillary, and musculocutaneous. The diagnosis is difficult, with single nerve involvement; local compression may be suspected first. The symptoms include sudden onset of severe pain in the shoulder or scapular area that radiates down the arm or up the neck. The pain often awakens patient from sleep. The pain usually resolves within a few weeks. Weakness becomes evident as the pain resolves and the limb is being used more frequently. Can lead to muscle atrophy. Paresthesia is less intense than the pain. The treatment includes analgesics, including narcotics and neuropathic pain medications. Oral corticosteroid course may also be beneficial in reducing the pain. After pain has been controlled, physical and occupational therapies are recommended. Recovery rates of 36% at 1 year, 75% at 2 years, and 89% at 3 years have been reported.

Symptoms

Localization site	Comment
Plexus	Brachial plexus, trunk, cord, nerve branches
Mononeuropathy or mononeuropathy multiplex	Can present as single or multiple nerve involvement
Muscle	Atrophy and weakness

Treatment Complications: Narcotic analgesics used for painful crises can lead to sedation or depressed mentation.

Bibliography

Ferrante M. Brachial plexopathies. *CONTINUUM* 2014;20(5):1323–42.

Acute Disseminated Encephalomyelitis (ADEM)

Epidemiology and Demographics: Acute disseminated encephalomyelitis (ADEM) has an incidence of 0.2–0.4/100,000 per year in North America. There are no clear data suggesting higher prevalence in one race. However, it is found to be slightly more common in males than females, given a gender ratio of 1.3:1. The median age of onset is 5–8 years, and in North America its peak incidence is in the winter and spring months.

Disorder Description: An autoimmune demyelinating disease involving the central nervous system. It is usually preceded by viral infection or immunizations. It usually presents immediately after an infectious illness, or several days later. The onset is usually acute to subacute. Symptoms present over hours or 1 to 2 days. There are encephalitic and myelitic types. Encephalitic symptoms include confusion, seizures, fever, somnolence, headache, and neck stiffness. Rarely, choreoathetosis occurs. Patients can experience decerebrate rigidity and coma. Patients with myelitic type experience loss of sensation, bowel/bladder paralysis, and varying degrees of extremity weakness, paraplegia, or quadriplegia.

Symptoms

Localization site	Comment
Cerebral hemispheres	Seizures, confusion, coma, meningeal irritation
Mental status and psychiatric aspects/complications	Confusion, lethargy
Brainstem	Decerebrate rigidity, coma
Cranial nerves	Optic neuritis
Spinal cord	Quadriplegia, paraplegia, sensory disturbance, bowel/bladder dysfunction

Treatment Complications: Steroid therapy can lead to psychosis, confusion, weight gain, hyperglycemia, myopathy, glaucoma, cataracts, osteoporosis, or vertebral fractures.

Plasma exchange complications include anaphylaxis, hypocalcemia, and depletion of immunoglobulins and coagulation factors.

Bibliography

Banwell B, Kennedy J, Sadovnick D, et al. Incidence of acquired demyelination of the CNS in Canadian children. *Neurology*. 2009; 72(3):232–9.

Leake JA, Albani S, Kao AS, et al. Acute disseminated encephalomyelitis in childhood: epidemiologic, clinical and laboratory features. *Pediatr Infect Dis J*. 2004;23(8):756–64.

Murthy SN, Faden HS, Cohen ME, Bakshi R. Acute disseminated encephalomyelitis in children. *Pediatrics*. 2002;110(2 Pt 1):e21.

Pohl D, Hennemuth I, von Kries R, Hanefeld F. Paediatric multiple sclerosis and acute disseminated encephalomyelitis in Germany: results of a nationwide survey. *Eur J Pediatr*. 2007;166(5):405–12.

Ropper AH, Samuels MA, Klein JP. Multiple sclerosis and other inflammatory demyelinating diseases. In *Adams & Victor's principles of neurology*. 10th ed. New York: McGraw-Hill; 2014.

Torisu H, Kira R, Ishizaki Y, et al. Clinical study of childhood acute disseminated encephalomyelitis, multiple sclerosis, and acute transverse myelitis in Fukuoka Prefecture, Japan. *Brain Dev*. 2010;32(6):454–62.

Acute Inflammatory Demyelinating Polyneuropathy (AIDP) and Miller Fisher Variant of Guillain–Barré Syndrome

Epidemiology and Demographics: Acute inflammatory demyelinating polyneuropathy (AIDP) has a worldwide incidence of 0.6–4.0/100,000 with a mean age of onset of 40 years. Overall incidence is lower in children, 0.34–1.34/100,000, and higher in people over age 50, 1.7–3.3/100,000. It is more common in males, with a male-to-female ratio of 1.7:1. It is found in all races. It has no predilection for a specific time of year; however, summer epidemics of the axonal variant have been reported in northern China. Two-thirds of cases are preceded by upper respiratory infection or diarrhea due to *Campylobacter jejuni*. Has been associated with swine flu H1N1 vaccine.

Disorder Description: AIDP is an autoimmune attack of peripheral nerve myelin with secondary axonal loss. It typically presents as a symmetric ascending weakness, mild sensory loss, and hypo- or areflexia following a viral illness and, in some cases, more specifically with infection with *C. jejuni*. Its onset occurs over several days to 2 weeks. Proximal muscles can be affected before distal. The most common initial symptom is numbness of the toes. Weakness usually starts in the legs, ascends to the arms, and at times can lead to facial diplopia and respiratory failure. It can also lead to autonomic dysfunction including tachycardia, bradycardia, facial flushing, and fluctuating blood pressure. Urinary retention occurs in 15% of patients. Recovery occurs over weeks to months. Most patients recover with mild residual motor and sensory deficits. However, 10% of patients are left with disability.

Severe respiratory muscle weakness requiring ventilator support develops in 10–30% of patients, paresthesia (and sometimes pain) in the hands and feet occurs in up to 80% of patients. Dysautonomia occurs in 70% of patients, presenting as tachycardia (most common), urinary retention, and alternating hypertension/hypotension, and can be associated with sudden death.

Miller Fisher syndrome is a variant of Guillain–Barré syndrome (GBS)/AIDP. It presents as a descending paralysis. The most common manifestations are ophthalmoplegia, ataxia, and areflexia. Eighty-five percent to 90% of patients with Miller Fisher syndrome have antibodies against GQ1b, a ganglioside nerve component.

Diagnosis is clinical, confirmed with cerebrospinal fluid (CSF) studies and electromyography/nerve conduction velocity (EMG/NCV) tests. Time course is about 4 weeks and self-limiting. Other conditions to consider in the differential diagnosis include vitamin B1 deficiency, acute arsenic poisoning, n-hexane exposure, vasculitis, Lyme disease, tick paralysis, porphyria, sarcoidosis, leptomeningeal disease, paraneoplastic disease, critical illness myopathy, and chronic inflammatory demyelinating polyneuropathy (CIDP).

Symptoms

Localization site	Comment
Cerebral hemispheres	Confusion, coma in variants of GBS, i.e., Bickerstaff encephalitis
Mental status and psychiatric aspects/complications	Confusion, coma in variants of GBS, i.e., Bickerstaff encephalitis
Brainstem	Confusion, coma, ophthalmoplegia, ataxia in variants of GBS, i.e., Bickerstaff encephalitis

Localization site	Comment
Cranial nerves	Cranial nerves III–VII and IX–XII may be involved, diplopia, ophthalmoplegia, dysphagia, dysarthria, facial droop
Peripheral nerve/muscle	Sensory disturbance, symmetric limb weakness, areflexia, respiratory failure, bulbar muscle weakness, myalgias
Unclear localization	Dysautonomia due to involvement of parasympathetic and sympathetic systems

Secondary Complications: Respiratory failure leading to mechanical ventilation and aspiration pneumonia. Immobilization leading to ileus, pulmonary embolus, or deep vein thrombosis. There can be residual weakness, sensory loss, or neuropathic pain. Death occurs in 3–5% of cases.

Treatment Complications: Initial treatment is supportive care – monitoring in the ICU setting, close respiratory monitoring (negative inspiratory force [NIF]/vital capacity [VC]), and ventilator support if necessary. For patients with dysautonomia, cardiac and blood pressure monitoring may be necessary. Main therapies include intravenous immunoglobulin (IVIG) or plasma exchange, which shortens the time to walking independently by 40–50%. Plasma exchange is recommended over IVIG for patients who are nonambulatory. There is a reported residual neuropathic pain in 40–50% of patients during the course of GBS.

Plasma exchange complications include anaphylaxis, hypocalcemia, and depletion of immunoglobulins and coagulation factors.

Adverse effects from IVIG include local injection site reaction. More serious side effects include anaphylaxis, from IgA deficiency, chest pain, myocardial infarction, tachycardia, hyponatremia, hemolysis, hemolytic anemia, thrombosis, hepatitis, anaphylaxis, backache, severe headache, aseptic meningitis, proteinuria, acute renal failure, hypokalemic nephropathy, pulmonary embolism, and transfusion-related lung injury. Plasmapheresis potential problems include mild allergic reaction, anaphylaxis, infection, or hypotension.

Bibliography

Chiba A, Kusunoki S, Obata H, et al. Serum anti-GQ1b IgG antibody is associated with ophthalmoplegia in Miller Fisher syndrome and Guillain-Barré syndrome: clinical and immunohistochemical studies. *Neurology.* 1993;43:1911.

Dimachkie MM, Barohn RJ. Guillain-Barré syndrome and variants. *Neurol Clin.* 2013;31(2):491–510.

Ropper AH, Samuels MA, Klein JP. Diseases of the peripheral nerves. In *Adams & Victor's principles of neurology.* 10th ed. New York: McGraw-Hill; 2014.

Willison HJ, Veitch J, Paterson G, Kennedy PG. Miller Fisher syndrome is associated with serum antibodies to GQ1b ganglioside. *J Neurol Neurosurg Psychiatry.* 1993; 56:204.

Acute Stress Disorder

Epidemiology and Demographics: Prevalence rate is dependent on the nature and severity of the preceding traumatic event as well as the criteria used to define the disorder. Estimates range from 20 to 50% with interpersonal trauma (e.g., assault, rape, witnessing a mass shooting) and less than 20% with other forms of trauma (e.g., accidents, mild traumatic brain injury, burns). More common in women.

Disorder Description: Acute stress disorder is characterized by development of significant distress or functional impairment post exposure to a traumatic event. Per DSM-5, a traumatic event is defined as "exposure to actual or threatened death, serious injury or sexual violence."[1] To meet criteria, symptoms must be present within 3 days to 1 month after the traumatic exposure. Symptoms include intrusive memories and/or dreams, dissociative reactions (e.g., flashbacks), negative mood, dissociative symptoms (e.g., amnesia for aspects of the event), avoidance symptoms, and hyperarousal, including sleep disturbance, irritability, unprovoked anger or aggression, and/or exaggerated startle response. Symptoms are not better accounted for by effects of a substance, medical condition, or brief psychotic disorder. Risk factors include pre-existing psychiatric disorder, high severity of exposure, presence of prior traumatic exposure, and female gender.

Symptoms

Localization site	Comment
Mental status and psychiatric aspects/complications	Intrusive thoughts, flashbacks, dissociative symptoms (e.g., amnesia), nightmares, deficits in attention, concentration and declarative memory, hyperarousal symptoms (e.g., sleep disturbances, irritability, unprovoked anger/aggression, exaggerated startle response), anhedonia

Secondary Complications: Posttraumatic stress disorder, alcohol/substance abuse, depressive disorders, anxiety disorders, sleep disorders.

Treatment Complications: Treatment with benzodiazepines may improve hyperarousal symptoms. However, there is risk for sedation and development of dependence and tolerance if used chronically.

Reference

1. American Psychiatric Association. *Diagnostic and statistical manual of mental disorders: DSM-5.* 5th ed. Washington, DC: American Psychiatric Association; 2013.

Suggested Reading

Kessler RC, Sonnega A, Bromet E, et al. Posttraumatic stress disorder in the national comorbidity survey. *Arch Gen Psychiatry.* 1995;52(12):1048–60.

Adenovirus

Epidemiology and Demographics: Worldwide distribution and infections occur in every season. Causes 5–10% of all febrile illnesses in infants and young children.[1]

Central nervous system (CNS) dysfunction was identified in 3.3% of children with adenovirus infection, mostly occurring in those younger than 5 years.[2]

Disorder Description: Adenoviruses are nonenveloped viruses with double-stranded DNA that most commonly cause upper respiratory tract illness, but may cause other systemic illness. Risk factors for infection include immunosuppression, people who live in close quarters (those in military barracks or college dormitories). Adenoviruses tend to be more prevalent in day-care centers and in households with young children. Transmission may be via aerosol droplets, fecal–oral route, transplants, vertical transmission during vaginal birth, and by contact with contaminated fomites.[3]

Symptoms

Localization site	Comment
Cerebral hemispheres	Meningitis[2]
	Encephalitis
	Seizures
	Hydrocephalus
Mental status and psychiatric aspects/complications	Altered mental status
	Visual hallucinations
Spinal cord	Transverse myelitis
Anterior horn cells	Flaccid paralysis

Secondary Complications: Seizure disorder may be a complication.

Treatment Complications: Ribavirin may cause hyperammonemia, which may suppress mental status.

References

1. Flomenberg P, Kojaoghlanian T. Epidemiology and clinical manifestations of adenovirus infection. In Hirsch M, ed. *UpToDate.* Waltham, MA: Wolters Kluwer.
2. Huang Y, Huang S, Chen S, et al. Adenovirus infection associated with central nervous system dysfunction in children. *J Clin Virol.* 2013;57(4):300–4.
3. Centers for Disease Control and Prevention. *Adenovirus.* Atlanta, GA: CDC; 2015. Accessed Jan 20, 2016. Available from www.cdc.gov/adenovirus/hcp/clinical-overview.html

Adenylosuccinate Lyase Deficiency

Epidemiology and Demographics: 1/70,000 live births; rare, autosomal recessive. Second-most common urea cycle disorder. Druze community in Israel has carrier frequency 1/41, with 20 cases also being diagnosed in Finland. Associated with high morbidity and mortality rates. A low-protein diet initiated early may prevent neurologic sequelae. ASL gene maps to 7q11.21

Disorder Description: Argininosuccinate (ASA) lyase deficiency results in defective cleavage of ASA and argininosuccinic aciduria. It leads to deficiency of both ureagenesis and nitric oxide (NO) production. Like all urea cycle disorders, it has a propensity to cause hyperammonemia in affected individuals.

Adenylosuccinate lyase (ASL) deficiency presents in two main forms – a severe neonatal form and late-onset form.

The severe neonatal form is indistinguishable from other urea cycle disorders, characterized by the triad of hyperammonemia, encephalopathy, and respiratory alkalosis. Vomiting, lethargy, and hypothermia present a few days after birth, and if left untreated or unrecognized, can result in death.

Late-onset forms are characterized by episodic hyperammonemia, triggered by acute infection, stress, or dietary noncompliance. Patients may also display chronic symptoms such as episodic vomiting, mental status changes, lethargy, and behavioral abnormalities associated with hyperammonemia. Some patients may present with cognitive impairment, behavioral abnormalities, or learning disabilities in the absence of any documented episodes of hyperammonemia. A pathognomonic phenotype includes a combination of neurocognitive deficiency, hepatitis with cirrhosis, trichorrhexis nodosa (friable hair), and systemic hypertension (due to NO deficiency).

ASA is an intermediate in the pathway of urea synthesis from ammonia and is split into arginine and fumarate in a reaction catalyzed by argininosuccinate lyase. As a result of this enzyme defect, patients have increased ammonia, both ASA and citrulline accumulate in the blood, and ASA is excreted in the urine. There is considerable phenotypic variability. Symptoms related to the central nervous system (CNS) are due to the toxic effects of hyperammonemia, although some have suggested a possible direct toxic effect of argininosuccinic acid on the brain.

Symptoms

Localization site	Comment
Cerebral hemispheres	In acute setting of hyperammonemia – delirium, somnolence, obtundation, coma, cerebral edema, seizures
	Long term – delayed development, intellectual disabilities, behavioral difficulties, learning difficulties, attention deficit hyperactivity disorder
Basal ganglia/cerebellum	Hypotonia, ataxia, tremor, choreoathetotic movement disorder

Secondary Complications: Hepatic failure may lead to a hepatic encephalopathy. Secondary coagulopathy may lead to intracranial hemorrhage.

Treatment Complications: Treatment of metabolic crises consists of withdrawal of protein from diet; promotion of anabolism (supplementing oral intake with intravenous lipids, glucose, and intravenous insulin); and sodium benzoate (intravenous nitrogen scavenging therapy).

Long-term interventions include lifelong dietary management (protein restriction), arginine base supplementation, and oral nitrogen scavenging therapy.

Complications of treatments include electrolyte disturbances or dehydration.

Bibliography

Ficicioglu C, Mandell R, Shih VE. Argininosuccinate lyase deficiency: longterm outcome of 13 patients detected by newborn screening. *Mol Genet Metab.* 2009;98:273–7. DOI: 10.1016/j.ymgme.2009.06.011

Nagamani SCS, Erez A, Lee B. Argininosuccinate lyase deficiency. Feb 3, 2011 [Updated Feb 2, 2012]. In Pagon RA, Adam MP, Ardinger HH, et al., eds. *GeneReviews®* [Internet]. Seattle, WA: University of Washington, Seattle; 1993–2017. Available from www.ncbi.nlm.nih.gov/books/NBK51784/

Summar ML, Koelker S, Freedenberg D, et al. The incidence of urea cycle disorders. *Mol Genet Metab.* 2013;110:179–80.

Adjustment Disorder

Epidemiology and Demographics: Adjustment disorder (AD) is diagnosed in an estimated 5–20% of individuals in outpatient mental health settings and up to 50% of inpatient psychiatric consultations.

Disorder Description: AD is defined in DSM-5 as the manifestation of marked, disproportionate distress and/or impaired function referable to an identifiable stressor. Symptoms must be clinically significant, with onset within 3 months of the stressor and continue no more than 6 months post-resolution of the stressor or associated consequences. Symptoms must not be better accounted for by bereavement, another mental disorder, or exacerbation of a preexisting condition.

Can be associated with anxiety, depressed mood, conduct disturbance, or a combination of these. Classified as acute (duration less than 6 months) versus chronic (duration greater than 6 months). Commonly occurs in setting of coexisting psychiatric and/or medical illness.

Symptoms

Localization site	Comment
Mental status and psychiatric aspects/complications	Depressed mood, anxiety, rage, antisocial behavior

Secondary Complications: AD with depressed mood carries an increased risk for attempted and completed suicide. When disturbance of conduct is associated, there can be reckless and/or aggressive behavior toward property or others.

Treatment Complications: Both brief supportive psychotherapy and short-term use of benzodiazepines and antidepressant medication may be considered. Side effects of benzodiazepines include risk for sedation and development of dependence and tolerance if used chronically. Selective serotonin reuptake inhibitor (SSRI) medications have rare potential to increase risk of suicide; therefore, they should be monitored with caution.

Bibliography

American Psychiatric Association. *Diagnostic and statistical manual of mental disorders: DSM-5.* 5th ed. Washington, DC: American Psychiatric Association; 2013.

Fabrega H Jr, Mezzich JE, Mezzich AC. Adjustment disorder as a marginal or transitional illness category in DSM-III. *Arch Gen Psychiatry.* 1987;44(6):567–72.

Foster P, Oxman T. A descriptive study of AD diagnoses in general hospital patients. *Isr J Psychol Med.* 1994;11:153–7.

Popkin MK, Callies AL, Colón EA, Stiebel V. Adjustment disorders in medically ill patients referred for consultation in a university hospital. *Psychosomatics.* 1990;31(4):410–4.

Portzky G, Audenaert K, van Heeringen K. Adjustment disorder and the course of the suicidal process in adolescents. *J Affect Disord.* 2005;87(2–3):265–70.

Adrenal Insufficiency

Epidemiology and Demographics: Secondary adrenal insufficiency is more common than primary adrenal insufficiency (Addison's disease), with an estimated prevalence of 150–280 per million, affecting more women than men, usually in the sixth decade of life.[1]

Disorder Description: Life-threatening disorder caused by primary or secondary adrenal insufficiency due to a dysfunction of the hypothalamic–pituitary axis. Most cases of primary adrenal insufficiency (failure of the adrenal glands to produce sufficient cortisol and sometimes aldosterone) are caused by autoimmune adrenalitis. Secondary adrenal insufficiency is usually caused by any process that interferes with corticotropin secretion that involves the pituitary gland.[2]

Symptoms

Localization site	Comment
Cerebral hemispheres	Seizures precipitated by hyponatremia/hypoglycemia
Mental status and psychiatric aspects/complications	Memory impairment, depression, psychosis[3] more common in primary adrenal insufficiency Confusion or disorientation seen in the acute setting of bilateral adrenal injury
Cranial nerves	External ophthalmoplegia as seen in Kearns–Sayre syndrome
Pituitary gland	Severe headache and visual symptoms with organic injury to the pituitary gland
Muscle	Myalgias and joint pain[4]; weakness; flexion contractures

Secondary Complications: General decompensation during an adrenal crisis may include depressed mental status and is often accompanied by generalized weakness, nausea, and vomiting.

Treatment Complications: Potential side effects of corticosteroid supplementation described ubiquitously throughout this book.

References

1. Charmandari E, Nicolaides NC, Chrousos GP. Adrenal insufficiency. *Lancet*. 2014;383(9935):2152–67. DOI: 10.1016/S0140-6736(13)61684-0
2. Arlt W, Allolio B. Adrenal insufficiency. *Lancet*. 2003;361:1881–93.
3. Leigh H, Kramer SI. The psychiatric manifestations of endocrine disease. *Adv Intern Med*. 1984;29:413.
4. Ebinger G, Six R, Bruyland M, Somers G. Flexion contractures: a forgotten symptom in Addison's disease and hypopituitarism. *Lancet*. 1986;2(8511):858.

Adrenoleukodystrophy (ALD)

Epidemiology and Demographics: Incidence of adrenoleukodystrophy (ALD) is 1/21,000 in the United States. The peak age for the childhood form is 7 years in boys. Adrenomyeloneuropathy (AMN) occurs in men aged 20 to 40. Adrenal insufficiency only subtype usually presents in males before 7.5 years of age but can occur between age 2 and adulthood. ALD is more common in males, but female carriers can present with symptoms in adulthood, with frequency of symptoms increasing with age.

Disorder Description: ALD is an X-linked peroxisomal disorder that occurs as a result of the accumulation of very long chain fatty acids in tissues; most commonly affecting the central nervous system, testes, and adrenal glands. It has three main types: childhood cerebral form, AMN, and Addison's disease or adrenal insufficiency only.

Childhood cerebral form presents as learning and behavior problems, commonly misdiagnosed as attention deficit hyperactivity disorder. It can present as seizure, cognitive decline, blindness, and, in some cases, quadriparesis. It is rapidly progressive, usually leading to death within 5 to 10 years. AMN predominantly presents as spinal cord dysfunction, but rarely can have cerebral involvement. Adrenal insufficiency only can present as weakness, unexplained vomiting, coma, or hyperpigmented skin.

Symptoms

Localization site	Comment
Cerebral hemispheres	Epilepsy, aphasia, visual loss, hemiparesis
Mental status and psychiatric aspects/complications	Dementia, behavioral disturbances, cognitive decline, psychosis
Brainstem	Ataxia, hemiparesis, visual disturbance
Cerebellum	Ataxia
Pituitary gland	Adrenal failure, hyperpigmented skin
Spinal cord	Paralysis, sensory disturbance, spastic paraparesis, impotence, sphincter disturbances
Dorsal root ganglia	Inhibits adrenocorticotropic hormone-producing cells in DRG contributing to adrenal failure, sensory disturbances

Treatment Complications: Corticosteroid therapy used for adrenal insufficiency can lead to psychosis, confusion, weight gain, hyperglycemia, myopathy, glaucoma, cataracts, osteoporosis, or vertebral fractures.

Bibliography

Bezman L, Moser AB, Raymond GV, et al. Adrenoleukodystrophy: incidence, new mutation rate, and results of extended family screening. *Ann Neurol*. 2001;49:512–7.

Engelen M, Barbier M, Dijkstra IM, et al. X-linked adrenoleukodystrophy in women: a cross-sectional cohort study. *Brain*. 2014;137:693–706.

Moser HW, Moser AB, Steinberg SJ. X-linked adrenoleukodystrophy. In Pagon RA, Adam MP, Ardinger HH, et al., eds. *GeneReviews®* [Internet]. Seattle, WA: University of Washington; 1993–2018. Accessed Feb 6, 2015. Available from www.genetests.org

Moser HW, Raymond GV, Dubey P. Adrenoleukodystrophy: new approaches to a neurodegenerative disease. *JAMA*. 2005;294:3131–4.

Percy AK, Rutledge SL. Adrenoleukodystrophy and related disorders. *Ment Retard Dev Disabil Res Rev.* 2001;7:179–89.

van Geel BM, Bezman L, Loes DJ, et al. Evolution of phenotypes in adult male patients with X-linked adrenoleukodystrophy. *Ann Neurol.* 2001;49:186–94.

Advanced Sleep–Wake Phase Disorder

Epidemiology and Demographics: Exact prevalence is unknown. Advanced sleep–wake phase disorder (ASWPD) is estimated to be much less prevalent than delayed sleep-wake phase disorder (DSWPD). No known sex predominance.

Familial ASWPD is a lifelong condition, while advancement of circadian rhythm may be a physiologic consequence of aging.

Disorder Description: The endogenous circadian period length (tau) is approximately 24.2 hours long and is entrained to the external 24-hour light–dark cycle. Patients with ASWPD have sleep onset and offset that begin several hours earlier than the light–dark cycle would dictate. Patients often report excessive evening sleepiness, early sleep onset, and early morning awakening. The earlier timing of sleep onset and offset has a self-perpetuating effect whereby the early sleep–wake timing leads to reduced exposure to phase-delaying evening light and increased phase-advancing morning light, which can perpetuate the ASWPD.[1]

Diagnosis of ASWPD is made if the patient meets the following criteria: (1) there is an advance in the phase of the major sleep episode in relation to the desired or required sleep time and wake-up time as evidenced by difficulty staying awake until the desired or required bedtime and an inability to remain asleep until the desired or required awakening time; (2) the symptoms are present for ≥3 months; (3) when patients are allowed to choose their own schedule, they will exhibit improved sleep quality and duration via advanced timing of the major sleep episode; (4) sleep log for ≥7 days demonstrates an advance in the timing of the habitual sleep period; and (5) the sleep disturbance is not better explained by another disorder or medication.[2]

Sleep logs and actigraphy are key instruments and 7–14 days of data are needed to ensure that working and non-working days are included. Although not necessary, biologic markers of endogenous circadian timing such as salivary or plasma dim light melatonin onset can provide important information.

Symptoms

Localization site	Comment
The exact mechanism responsible is unknown	The main site of the endogenous circadian rhythm is in the suprachiasmatic nuclei; however, circadian clocks also exist in peripheral cells

Secondary Complications: Social dysfunction is common from early evening sleepiness.

Treatment Complications: Treatment is necessary only if the patient desires a change in schedule. Potential modalities include evening bright light exposure and low-dose melatonin given in the morning.

References

1. Paine SJ, Fink J, Gander PH. Identifying advanced and delayed sleep phase disorders in the general population: a national survey of New Zealand adults. *Chronobiol Int.* 2014;31:627–36.
2. Sateia M, Berry RB, Bornemann MC, et al. *International classification of sleep disorders.* 3rd ed. Darien, IL: American Academy of Sleep Medicine; 2014.

Suggested Reading

Auger RR, Burgess HJ, Emens JS, et al. Clinical practice guideline for the treatment of intrinsic circadian rhythm sleep-wake disorders: advanced sleep-wake phase disorder (ASWPD), delayed sleep-wake phase disorder (DSWPD), non-24-hour sleep-wake rhythm disorder (N24SWD), and irregular sleep-wake rhythm disorder (ISWRD) an update for 2015. *J Clin Sleep Med.* 2015;11:1199–236.

Bjorvatn B, Pallesen S. A practical approach to circadian rhythm sleep disorders. *Sleep Med Rev.* 2009;13:47–60.

Sack RL, Auckley D, Auger RR, et al. Circadian rhythm sleep disorders: part II, advanced sleep phase disorder, delayed sleep phase disorder, free-running disorder, and irregular sleep-wake rhythm. *Sleep.* 2007;30:1484–501.

Schrader H, Bovim G, Sand T. The prevalence of delayed and advanced sleep phase disorders. *J. Sleep Res.* 1993;2:51–5.

Aerosol Inhalation Abuse (also see Specific Agents Such As Nitrous Oxide or Solvents)

Epidemiology and Demographics: More commonly abused by male children and adolescents. Higher rate of episodes among Native American children.

Disorder Description: These inhalants produce an effect within seconds that typically lasts 15 to 45 minutes. There have been rare cases of prolonged symptoms when large quantities have been inhaled. Household products that are abused, which contain hydrocarbons, include solvents, aerosol sprays (e.g., butane, propane), gases, nitrates, methylene chloride or toluene in paint thinners, nitrous oxide ("laughing gas"), trichloroethylene (in spot removers), and benzene in gasoline.

Symptoms

Localization site	Comment
Cerebral hemispheres	Seizures (acute)
	Toxic leukoencephalopathy (chronic)
Mental status and psychiatric aspects/complications	Hallucinations (acute)
	Violent behavior (acute)
Cerebellum	Ataxia (acute)
Cranial nerves	Cranial neuropathies (acute)
Muscle	Myopathy (chronic)

Secondary Complications: Indirect effects on nervous system via respiratory complications. Respiratory arrest results in cerebral ischemia.

Bibliography

Perry H. Inhalant abuse in children and adolescents. In Burns MM, ed. *UpToDate*. Waltham, MA: Wolters Kluwer; 2018. Available from www .uptodate.com/contents/inhalant-abuse-in-children-and-adolescents?source=search_result&search=aerosol%20inhalation%20abuse&selectedTitle=2~133

Afferent Pupillary Defect (Marcus Gunn Pupil, Poorly Reactive Pupil)

Epidemiology and Demographics: Afferent pupillary defects can affect all races/ethnicities of either sex at any age.

Disorder Description: This entry addresses abnormal pupil reactivity to light due to afferent (i.e., visual pathway) dysfunction. In most cases, it is associated with measurable visual loss. This is distinct from pupils that are poorly reactive to light due to dysfunction of the efferent pathway (see entry *Tonic Pupil*). Unilateral or asymmetric afferent pupillary defects are apparent on exam as a pupil that constricts less during direct light stimulation (i.e., shining light in the affected eye) than to indirect light stimulation (i.e., shining light in the unaffected eye). This can best be perceived using the swinging flashlight test, during which the eyes are alternately illuminated. When moving the light from the unaffected to the affected eye, the affected pupil is observed to dilate. When moving the light from the affected eye to the unaffected eye, the unaffected pupil is observed to constrict. There is no anisocoria unless there is concurrent efferent pupillary dysfunction (see entries *Tonic Pupil* and *Miosis*).

Symptoms

Localization site	Comment
Cranial nerves	Dysfunction of the retinal ganglion cells that make up the optic nerve is the most common cause of afferent pupillary defects. There is typically associated decrease in central or peripheral vision and altered color perception. Demyelinating optic neuropathies can cause afferent pupillary defects out of proportion to vision loss
	Etiologies include glaucoma, optic neuropathies, optic chiasm injury, and optic tract injury. The latter is distinguished from the former by homonymous visual field defects
Pituitary gland	Macroadenomas of the pituitary gland are the most common cause of compressive chiasmal lesions. If asymmetrically compressing one side more than the other, these lesions can cause a relative afferent lesion on that side compared with the other
Unclear localization	Severe vision loss due to ophthalmic disease can cause afferent pupillary defects even if it does not affect the optic nerve, such as in dense cataract, severe and diffuse retinal pathology, or dense vitreous hemorrhage. In these cases, there should be profoundly reduced visual acuity

Bibliography

Leavatin P. Pupillary escape in diseases of the retina or optic nerve. *Arch Ophthalmol.* 1959;62:768–79.

Air Embolism

Epidemiology and Demographics: Venous air emboli occur in approximately 0.13% of patients receiving a central venous catheter, 10% of patients undergoing neurosurgical procedures, and 4–14% of patients with severe lung trauma. There is no predilection for age, sex, or race.

Disorder Description: Air embolism occurs with the introduction of atmospheric gas into the circulation, most commonly the venous circulation (venous air embolism). There must be direct communication between the vessel and the air source, with a pressure gradient favoring entry of air from the source into the circulation. Most cases are iatrogenic, but barotrauma can also be seen in divers, astronauts, or aviators. Common iatrogenic causes include surgical introduction (most commonly neurosurgery), central venous catheterization, trauma, excessive positive pressure ventilation, thoracentesis, dialysis, and diagnostic studies that require radiocontrast injection. Air emboli generally result in severe morbidity and mortality, with severity depending upon volume of air entry, rate of accumulation, and position at time of embolus formation (i.e., sitting position usually leads to retrograde air flow). Arterial air emboli occur with right to left intracardiac shunting (i.e., patent foramen ovale [PFO]). Usually more than 5 mL/kg of air entry is needed to create symptoms, but as little as 2–3 mL of air reaching the cerebral circulation can be fatal. Air emboli occlude blood vessels, causing cerebral ischemic/infarction and symptoms similar to those seen in stroke.

Symptoms

Localization site	Comment
Cerebral hemispheres	Seizures, stroke, coma (secondary to cerebral edema), dysarthria
Mental status and psychiatric aspects/complications	Acute altered mental status, diminished arousal, anxiety, agitation, disorientation, sense of "impending doom"
Cranial nerves	Blurry vision
Cerebellum	Ataxia
Vestibular system (and nonspecific dizziness)	Dizziness, lightheadedness, vertigo, nausea
Meninges	Headache

Secondary Complications: Ischemia to all other end organs, e.g., acute renal injury, pulmonary infarction.

Bibliography

Hartveit F, Lystad H, Minken A. The pathology of venous air embolism. *Br J Exp Pathol.* 1968;49: 81–6.

Heckmann JG, Lang CJ, Kindler K, et al. Neurologic manifestations of cerebral air embolism as a complication of central venous catheterization. *Crit Care Med.* 2000;28:1621–5.

Mirski MA, Lele AV, Fitzsimmons L, Toung TJ. Diagnosis and treatment of vascular air embolism. *Anesthesiology.* 2007;106(1):164–77.

Alcohol Intoxication and Chronic Abuse

Epidemiology and Demographics: Ethyl alcohol (ETOH) abuse affects about 14 million Americans, with the highest level in the 18–29 age-group; it is more common in men, with no race or ethnicity predilection.

Disorder Description: Prolonged drinking episodes of excessive amounts of alcoholic beverages (consumption of five or more drinks on an occasion for men or four or more drinks on an occasion for women) within a 12-month period, during which an individual has:

- prioritized drinking over other major relationships and obligations;
- engaged in physically endangering situations;
- experienced withdrawal symptoms.

Ethanol is obtained from a fermentation process of by-products of foods such as barley or grapes. The ethanol contributes to the depressive effects that a person experiences with intoxication or chronic use. The toxic effect of ethanol on the nervous system can be either direct or indirect.

Alcohol, Poison of Neuronal Mass Destruction: Ethanol directly affects every single component of the central nervous system (CNS) as well as the peripheral neuromuscular structures (PNS). Alcohol exerts detrimental effects on skeletal muscles, neuromuscular junctions, motor and sensory nerves, the spinal cord, and the supra- as well as infratentorial components of the brain. Alcoholic hemispheric dysfunction results in behavioral abnormalities including disinhibition, violent conduct, and social, family, and occupational disorders.

Symptoms

Localization site	Comment
Cerebral hemispheres	Chronic-diffuse cerebral degeneration and atrophy
	Korsakoff syndrome (acute rare), psychosis with associated memory dysfunction
	Marchiafava–Bignami syndrome: demyelination, subsequent atrophy of the corpus callosum (rare, chronic)
	Ischemic and hemorrhagic stroke (acute and chronic)
	Seizures, ischemic and hemorrhagic stroke, neuronal degeneration damage due to N-methyl-D-aspartate (NMDA) excitotoxicity; nerve spasticity alteration due to oxidative stress of neurons
	Increased occurrences of motor vehicle accidents and traumatic brain injuries
Mental status and psychiatric aspects/ complications	Mental and physical impairments (acute and chronic)
	Wernicke encephalopathy: thiamine deficiency resulting in abnormal eye movements, unsteady gait with associated mental confusion
	Executive dysfunction (acute and chronic)
	Depressed mood (acute and chronic)
	Dementia (chronic)
	Violent behavior (acute and chronic)
Family, social, and occupational consequences	Family discord, increased rate of divorce, detachment from children, occupational instability, unemployment, violent behavior and criminality, motor vehicle accidents, social alienation
Brainstem	Altered consciousness, dysregulation of respiratory rate and heart rate (acute)
	Central pontine myelinolysis (acute or chronic, rare)

Localization site	Comment
Cerebellum	Cerebellar degeneration with glial cell loss
	Acquired cerebellar syndrome
	Cerebellar gait ataxia (chronic)
	Wernicke and Korsakoff syndromes (chronic)
Vestibular system (and nonspecific dizziness)	Positional nystagmus (acute)
	Postural instability (acute and chronic)
Cranial nerves	Polyneuropathy (chronic)
	Wernicke encephalopathy (rare, acute)
Pituitary gland	Hyperactivity of the HPA axis (hypothalamus–pituitary–adrenal axis and its production of corticotropin-releasing factor [CRF], chronic)
Spinal cord	Increased excitability to stimuli, myelopathy (acute/chronic)
Anterior horn cells	Alcoholic polyneuropathy (chronic)
Dorsal root ganglia	Ataxia (acute and chronic effect)
Conus medullaris	Alcoholic polyneuropathy (chronic)
Cauda equina	Alcoholic polyneuropathy (chronic)
Specific spinal roots	Alcoholic neuropathy (chronic effect)
Plexus	Alcoholic neuropathy (chronic effect)
Mononeuropathy or mononeuropathy multiplex	Sensory neuropathy (chronic)
	Motor neuropathy (chronic)
Peripheral neuropathy	Polyneuropathy (motor, sensory, and autonomic due to thiamine deficiency; chronic effect)
Muscle	Alcoholic myopathy (chronic), acute necrotizing myopathy (acute)
Neuromuscular junction	Inhibition of neuromuscular junction (acute and chronic)
Syndromes with combined upper and lower motor neuron deficits	Alcoholic polyneuropathy (chronic)
Syndromes with combined spinal cord and peripheral nerve lesions	Alcoholic polyneuropathy (chronic)

Secondary Complications: Indirectly, via its harmful effect on other organ systems alcohol can inflict significant damage on CNS/PNS.

- **Cardiovascular** effects: Dilated cardiomyopathy and dysrhythmia result in embolic complications and stroke.
- **Coagulation** dysfunction, combined with hypertensive effect result in hemorrhagic strokes.
- **Hepatic** complications:
  - acute liver failure may result in brain edema, amplified by hypoglycemia, hypoxia, and seizures;
  - hepatic myelopathy with rapidly progressing spastic paraparesis;
  - severe fatigue, cognitive dysfunction, and mood disorder.
- **Gastritis and pancreatitis** may lead to chronic malnutrition and widespread CNS/PNS dysfunction.
- **Nutritional consequences:**
  - The relatively high caloric content in alcohol (which ranks second only to the caloric content of various forms of fat) can easily lead to weight gain.
  - The increased nutritional demands of alcohol processing can lead to significant deficiencies in:
    - all members of the B vitamin family, particularly B9 and B12, but also B1 (thiamine), B2 (riboflavin), B3 (niacin), B5 (pantothenic acid), and B6 (pyridoxine). All these vitamins are indispensable to normal functioning of the peripheral and central nervous systems;
    - vitamin A and the mineral calcium.

Treatment Complications: Disulfiram (Antabuse) has been associated with reports of neuropathy, psychotic symptoms, and optic neuritis. Naltrexone may be associated with withdrawal symptoms in opiate-dependent patients. Topiramate may cause cognitive impairments and rarely acute glaucoma.

Bibliography

Driessen M, Lange W, Junghanns K, Wetterling T. Proposal of a comprehensive clinical typology of alcohol withdrawal – a cluster analysis approach. *Alcohol Alcohol.* 2005;40(4):308–13.

Jesse S, Brathen G, Ferra M, et al. Alcohol withdrawal syndrome: mechanisms, manifestations, and management. *Acta Neurol Scand.* 2016;135:4–16.

Alcohol Withdrawal

Epidemiology and Demographics: In the United States, 8.5% of the population are users of alcohol (ETOH). Higher prevalence among individuals greater than 18 years of age. No gender or ethnicity predilection.

Disorder Description: The basis of ETOH withdrawal can be explained through a phenomenon called *kindling*. This process can be described as a chemical stimulus triggering behavior responses that were previously absent. Withdrawal symptoms in alcoholics are derived from neurochemical imbalance when consumption is reduced abruptly. Symptoms should be treated when they first appear to prevent any further cognitive deterioration of the individual.

Symptoms

Localization site	Comment
Cerebral hemispheres	Seizures (acute), Wernicke encephalopathy
Mental status and psychiatric aspects/complications	Hallucinations (acute), confusion (acute), anxiety (acute)
	Delirium tremens – altered mental status (global confusion) and sympathetic overdrive (autonomic hyperactivity), which can progress to cardiovascular collapse
	Dysphoria (acute)
Brainstem	Insomnia (chronic)
Vestibular system (and nonspecific dizziness)	Ataxia (acute)
Pituitary gland	Neuroendocrine dysregulation, increases in hypothalamus–pituitary–adrenal (HPA) activation (chronic)
Muscle	Tremors, decreased muscle tone (chronic)
Neuromuscular junction	Increase of excitatory neurotransmitters
	Decrease in inhibitory neurotransmitters

Treatment Complications: Benzodiazepines, which are the treatment of choice for withdrawal, are high risk for addiction. They may cause sedation, altered mentation, or unsteadiness.

Bibliography

Becker HC. Kindling in alcohol withdrawal. *Alcohol Health Res World*. 1998;22(1):25–33. Available from http://pubs.niaaa.nih.gov/publications/arh22-1/25-34.pdf

National Institute on Alcohol Abuse and Alcoholism. Alcohol Alert: Alcohol withdrawal syndrome. *Alcohol Alert*. Washington, DC: National Institute on Alcohol Abuse and Alcoholism No. 5 PH 270. August 1989. Available from http://pubs.niaaa.nih.gov/publications/aa05.htm

Alpers Disease (Alpers–Huttenlocher Syndrome [AHS])

Epidemiology and Demographics: Alpers disease (Alpers–Huttenlocher syndrome [AHS]) occurs in 1/50,000–100,000 live births, and is a rare and severe form of mitochondrial DNA (mtDNA) depletion syndrome, caused by mutations of the mitochondrial DNA gamma polymerase enzyme (POLG). It is characterized by a triad of progressive developmental regression, intractable seizures, and hepatic dysfunction.

Disorder Description: The POLG gene (15q24) encodes a mitochondrial DNA polymerase subunit, which is involved in the replication and repair of mtDNA. Alterations in enzyme activity result in mitochondrial DNA deletions, with phenotypic heterogeneity. While POLG mutations can be inherited in a dominant or recessive fashion, AHS is inherited in an autosomal recessive manner only. Mutations in polymerase gamma may manifest in multiple organ systems. Incidental infections and drugs such as valproic acid can accelerate the onset of symptoms and exaggerate the phenotype. mtDNA depletion leads to energy failure and cell death, affecting predominantly the nervous system and liver.

Clinical: Hallmark is a triad of **intractable seizures, developmental regression,** and **liver dysfunction.** Onset usually between ages of 2 and 4 years and up to age 25–35 (usually with pre-existing developmental delays in adults). Seizures can be the first sign of AHS in about 50% of affected children, and can be simple focal, generalized, or myoclonic. In some instances, it can present as epilepsia partialis continua. There is associated developmental delay, hypotonia, ataxia, cortical blindness, and hepatic failure. Disease progression is variable, with life expectancy ranging from months to 12 years from first onset of symptoms.

Diagnosis: The triad of clinical hepatocerebral symptoms and seizures, when combined with 2 of the following 11 features, constitute the clinical diagnosis of Alpers–Huttenlocher syndrome: (1) brain MRS showing reduced N-acetylaspartate (NAA) and elevated lactate; (2) elevated cerebrospinal fluid (CSF) protein; (3) cerebral volume loss; (4) EEG showing multifocal paroxysmal activity with high-amplitude delta slowing; (5) cortical blindness or optic atrophy; (6) abnormal visual evoked potential (VEP) and normal electroretinogram; (7) quantitative mitochondrial DNA depletion in skeletal muscle or liver; (8) deficiency in POLG enzyme activity (<10% of normal) in skeletal muscle or liver; (9) elevated blood or CSF lactate (3 mM); (10) complex IV or combination of multiple (I, III, IV) electron transport complex defects (<20% N) in liver respiratory chain testing; (11) a known sibling diagnosed with the condition.

Useful diagnostic tests include liver function tests, lactic acid levels in blood and cerebrospinal fluid, EEG, and MRI. POLG gene sequencing is used to confirm the diagnosis, demonstrating homozygous or compound heterozygous mutations.

Symptoms

Localization site	Comment
Cerebral hemispheres	Seizures – including generalized tonic–clonic seizure (GTCS), myoclonic and epilepsia partialis continua. Worsening with sodium valproate
	Headaches with visual auras reflecting occipital lobe dysfunction
	Cognitive dysfunction – episodic regression (especially during infection)
	Cortical visual loss
	Imaging – cerebral volume loss (central > cortical, with gliosis especially in occipital lobe region)
Cranial nerves	Retinitis pigmentosa, optic atrophy, hearing loss
Basal ganglia/ cerebellar	Movement disorder – myoclonus and choreoathetosis
	Palatal myoclonus
	Ataxia, nystagmus
Neuropathy	Areflexia (early)
	Spastic paraparesis (late) – loss of cortical neuronal function

Secondary Complications: Hepatic failure may lead to a hepatic encephalopathy. Secondary coagulopathy may lead to intracranial hemorrhage.

Treatment Complications: Treating the seizures with valproic acid can cause the rapid onset of liver failure and should be avoided.

Bibliography

Cohen BH, Chinnery PF, Copeland WC. POLG-related disorders. In Pagon RA, Adam MP, Ardinger HH, et al., eds. *GeneReviews®* [Internet]. Seattle, WA: University of Washington; 1993–2017. Available from www.ncbi.nlm.nih.gov/books/NBK26471/

Gordon N. Alpers syndrome: progressive neuronal degeneration of children with liver disease. *DMCN.* 2006;48:1001–3.

Saneto RP, Cohen BH, Copeland WC, Naviaux RK. Alpers-Huttenlocher syndrome: a review. *Pediatr Neurol.* 2013;48(3):167–78.

Alzheimer's Disease

Epidemiology and Demographics: Alzheimer's disease (AD) is the most common neurodegenerative disorder in the United States,[1] with an estimated lifetime prevalence of 9.7%.[2] Symptom onset is typically after age 65, and age is the greatest risk factor for AD. Even after adjusting for women's longer life expectancy, AD may be more prevalent in women.[1] Other risk factors for AD include low levels of educational and occupational attainment[3] and comorbid hypertension and/or diabetes.[4]

Disorder Description: Alzheimer's dementia is a clinical diagnosis, based on a supportive clinical history featuring prominent early impairment in memory, a supportive non-focal neurologic exam, and a negative reversible dementia workup, which includes neuroimaging. The typical Alzheimer's dementia patient presents with memory impairment, such as complaints of forgetting recent events or misplacing objects. Long-term memory, semantic memory, and working memory are typically preserved until later in the disease course. Neurologic exam in these patients is typically non-focal. If gait failure, poor balance, and/or extrapyramidal signs are present early in presentation, either the patient has AD and another disorder that will account for these signs, or AD is not the likely cause of the cognitive impairment. Late in the disease course, patients develop gait impairment and in final stages may decompensate into a mute, bedbound state.

The American Academy of Neurology (AAN) recommends checking vitamin B12 and thyroid-stimulating hormone (TSH) levels, in addition to obtaining basic labs (CBC, comprehensive metabolic panel [CMP]), as part of the basic reversible dementia workup. Screening for depression is also important, as it can present as a pseudodementia. The AAN recommends against routine screening for syphilis as part of a dementia workup, unless the patient has specific risk factors for syphilis. Similarly, there is no evidence to support obtaining lumbar puncture or EEG in a routine workup for dementia.[5] Neuroimaging – either a CT head or MRI brain – is essential to rule out structural lesions such as subdural hematoma, normal pressure hydrocephalus, or frontal lobe tumor.

Less than 1% of all cases of AD are autosomal dominant.[6] Patients with these mutations usually present in their 30s to 50s. Mutations are found in the amyloid precursor protein gene (APP on chromosome 21), the presenilin 1 gene (PSEN1 on chromosome 14), or the presenilin 2 gene (PSEN2 on chromosome 1). These mutations increase the level of beta-amyloid in the brain and provide support for the amyloid hypothesis, which posits that beta-amyloid deposition in the brain causes AD. Of note, the presence of amyloid pathology found on autopsy does not necessarily imply a clinical diagnosis of dementia, and some cognitively intact individuals are found postmortem to have a high amyloid burden. Conversely, neurofibrillary tangle burden shows a stronger association with cognitive impairment, and a specific, consistent pattern of spread has been described (Braak staging I to VI).[7] Nevertheless, the amyloid hypothesis has spawned a variety of anti-amyloid therapeutic efforts, which have been largely unsuccessful to date. Amyloid deposition occurs decades prior to onset of symptoms, prompting some to question whether anti-amyloid therapies during this prodromal phase may be of more benefit.

Atypical variants of AD include frontal variant of AD, posterior cortical atrophy, and logopenic variant of primary progressive aphasia (lvPPA). Frontal variant of AD presents with predominant behavioral changes such as disinhibited and impulsive behavior that is out of proportion to memory impairment. Posterior cortical atrophy presents with visuospatial dysfunction, such as dressing apraxia, or with elements of Balint syndrome or Gerstmann syndrome. lvPPA due to AD presents with early language dysfunction, with nonfluent, effortful speech, but preserved grammar and preserved single-word comprehension.[1]

In early-onset Alzheimer's, or atypical variants of Alzheimer's, further testing by a dementia specialist can provide additional support for a diagnosis of Alzheimer's. Lumbar puncture can be useful in atypical presentations, to rule out infectious causes of cognitive decline and to confirm Alzheimer's. In Alzheimer's, CSF beta-amyloid is decreased, and CSF hyperphosphorylated tau is increased. Genetic testing in early-onset cases is often helpful. Both deoxyglucose and "amyloid" PET scans provide useful data, but both types of studies lack specificity.[8,9] If effective, but toxic, therapies for AD are developed, a battery of diagnostic tests possibly including lumbar puncture would improve specificity. Until such therapies are available, lumbar puncture and/or PET scans are rarely indicated in typical, late-onset cases.

The presence of the APOE4 allele is another major risk factor for Alzheimer's: one copy increases the risk about 3-fold, and two copies may increase risk 9- to 10-fold.[1]

Symptoms

Localization site	Comment
Entorhinal cortex and hippocampus, then cerebral hemispheres (especially association cortices)	Neurofibrillary tangles accumulate in the transentorhinal cortex initially, then spread to involve limbic structures including the hippocampus, before spreading to involve more extensive neocortical regions (Braak stages I–VI)[6]

Secondary Complications: Late in the disease course, the individual becomes bedbound and susceptible to decubitus ulcers and assorted infections, as well as severe malnourishment. Decisions concerning the best ways to provide nutrition are challenging and require repeated discussion with family members over several visits. Referral to specialists such as social workers, family clergy, and support groups can be invaluable.

Treatment Complications: No treatments are available to slow the course of disease. Symptomatic treatment options include cholinesterase inhibitors (donepezil, rivastigmine, and galantamine are approved

in the United States), and the partial N-methyl-D-aspartic acid (NMDA) receptor blocker memantine. Management of neuropsychiatric issues/behavioral symptoms is important for improving quality of life.[1]

Donepezil may cause bradycardia and may precipitate cardiogenic syncope in an elderly patient on beta-blockers or other medications that prolong the PR interval. In the United States, all antipsychotics carry "black box warnings" for use with demented patients because they may increase the risk of stroke. These risks vary among antipsychotics, and judicious use may be helpful in selected cases.

References

1. Apostolova LG. Alzheimer disease. *Continuum (Minneap Minn)*. 2016;22:419–34.
2. Plassman BL, Langa KM, Fisher GG, et al. Prevalence of dementia in the United States: the aging, demographics, and memory study. *Neuroepidemiology.* 2007;29:125–32.
3. Stern Y, Gurland B, Tatemichi TK, et al. Influence of education and occupation on the incidence of Alzheimer's disease. *JAMA.* 1994;271:1004–10.
4. Beeri MS, Ravona-Springer R, Silverman JM, Haroutunian V. The effects of cardiovascular risk factors on cognitive compromise. *Dialogues Clin Neurosci.* 2009;11:201–12.
5. American Academy of Neurology. Detection, diagnosis and management of dementia. AAN Guideline Summary for Clinicians. Available from http://tools.aan.com/professionals/practice/pdfs/dementia_guideline.pdf
6. Bateman RJ, Aisen PS, De Strooper B, et al. Autosomal-dominant Alzheimer's disease: a review and proposal for the prevention of Alzheimer's disease. *Alzheimers Res Ther.* 2011;3.
7. Braak H, Braak E. Neuropathological stageing of Alzheimer-related changes. *Acta Neuropathol (Berl).* 1991;82:239–59.
8. Beach TG, Schneider JA, Sue LI, et al. Theoretical impact of florbetapir (18F) amyloid imaging on diagnosis of Alzheimer dementia and detection of preclinical cortical amyloid. *J. Neuropathol Exp Neurol.* 2014;73:948–53.
9. Zhang S, Han D, Tan X, et al. Diagnostic accuracy of 18 F-FDG and 11 C-PIB-PET for prediction of short-term conversion to Alzheimer's disease in subjects with mild cognitive impairment. *Int J Clin Pract.* 2012;66:185–98.

Amaurosis Fugax

Epidemiology and Demographics: The incidence of amaurosis fugax (AF) is estimated to be 14/100,000 per year and, it is more prevalent among males and adults >50 years.

Disorder Description: Brief period of monocular visual loss due to transient ophthalmic artery (OA) occlusion. AF is most commonly due to embolism from the internal carotid artery (ICA) to the OA. AF can be a complication of carotid endarterectomy caused by dislodging a plaque. Risk factors include diabetes mellitus, hypertension, and hyperlipidemia.

Symptoms

Localization site	Comment
Cerebral hemispheres	Similar to transient cerebral ischemic attack, AF is often a harbinger of stroke
Cranial nerves	Optic nerve infarction, optic neuropathy

Secondary Complications: Blindness, retinal artery occlusion, transient ischemic attacks, strokes.

Treatment Complications: Treatment with antiplatelet medications can lead to bleeding complications. Endarterectomy can be complicated by stroke, local hematoma formation, myocardial infarction.

Bibliography

Andersen CU, Marquardsen J, Mikkelsen B, et al. Amaurosis fugax in a Danish community: a prospective study. *Stroke.* 1988;19:196–9.

Bacigalupi M. Amaurosis fugax: a clinical review. *IJAHSP.* 2006;4:1–6.

Amoebiasis

Epidemiology and Demographics: There were 133 primary amebic meningoencephalitis (PAM) infections from 1962 through 2014 in the United States. Of these infections, 112 (84%) were in children, with median age of 11 years and range of 8 months to 66 years, with >75% infections in males.[1] Only a few hundred cases have been reported of *Balamuthia mandrillaris* granulomatous amebic encephalitis (GAE), mostly in Peru, and in Hispanic males.[2]

Disorder Description: Free living amoeba have been known to cause two types of encephalitis: PAM or GAE.[3]

PAM (also known as the "brain eating amoeba") is commonly caused by *Naegleria fowleri*; however, recently *Paravahlkampfia francinae* has also been implicated. It has been detected in Australia, Europe, Asia, Africa, and southern-tier North America. Risk factors include swimming, diving, or washing in warm, fresh water, and nasal or sinus irrigation – all of which may cause contaminated water to migrate into the nose and subsequently into the brain.[3]

GAE is commonly associated with *Acanthamoeba* spp., *B. mandrillaris*, and *Sappinia* spp. and is usually associated with autoimmune conditions, immunocompromised states, alcoholism, and pregnancy. *B. mandrillaris* has also been seen to be transmitted via organ transplants.[3]

Symptoms

Localization site	Comment
Cerebral hemispheres	Meningitis Encephalitis Seizures Hemiparesis Hydrocephalus Vasculitis, causing ischemic or hemorrhagic strokes
Mental status and psychiatric aspects/complications	Behavioral changes Personality changes Coma
Cerebellum	Ataxia
Cranial nerves	Cranial nerve palsies. Distortion of taste and smell often seen in PAM

Secondary Complications: Of the 133 PAM infections from 1962 through 2014 in the United States, only 3 patients survived.[1] Survivors may develop vision impairment or hearing loss.[2]

Treatment Complications: Amphotericin B may cause seizures, vision changes, or paresthesias.

References

1. Centers for Disease Control and Prevention. *Primary amebic meningoencephalitis (PAM): sources of infection and risk factors.* Atlanta, GA: CDC; 2013. Accessed Jan 20, 2016. Available from www.cdc.gov/parasites/naegleria/infection-sources.html

2. DynaMed Plus [Internet]. *Amebic brain diseases*. Ipswich, MA: EBSCO Information Services; 1995. Record No. 900886. Available from www.dynamed.com/login .aspx?direct=true&site=DynaMed&id=900886 [Registration and login required.]
3. Chow F, Glaser C. Emerging and reemerging neurologic infections. *Neurohospitalist*. 2014;4(4):173–84.

Amyloidosis

Epidemiology and Demographics: Worldwide incidence for all causes of amyloidosis is reported as "five to nine cases per million patient-years"[1] predominantly affecting people between the ages of 60 and 80.[2] Overall, more common in men.

Disorder Description: Acquired or genetic disorder that leads to protein misfolding resulting in deposition of abnormally folded protein known as fibrils in tissue. Earlier classifications were focused on localized versus systemic forms but more recent classification emphasizes the amyloid protein types. Amyloidosis is associated with a wide array of potential neurologic clinical manifestations[2] and often involves assorted organ enlargements due to amyloid deposition.

Symptoms

Localization site	Comment
Mental status and psychiatric aspects/ complications	(Amyloidosis should be distinguished from the concept of central nervous system amyloid plaques that occur in some dementing illnesses)
Peripheral neuropathy	Focal, multifocal, or diffuse neuropathy, usually a sensory motor polyneuropathy with symptoms of numbness and pain occasionally leading to weakness if advanced. Symptoms are first noted in the feet with progression to the upper extremities. Carpal tunnel syndrome is the most common focal neuropathy. May also cause an autonomic neuropathy with predominant gastrointestinal symptoms
Muscle	Enlargement of the muscles from amyloid deposition may occur, resulting in subsequent atrophy and weakness

Treatment Complications: Treatment is contingent on the specific type of amyloidosis. Some types may be responsive to chemotherapeutic agents and subsequent autologous blood stem cell transplant, while others may warrant consideration for liver transplant. Amyloidosis associated with inflammatory disorders can be treated in part with anti-inflammatory agents. Please see Section 2: Medication Adverse Effects, for discussion of potential adverse events.

References

1. Real de Asúa D, Costa R, Galván JM, et al. Systemic AA amyloidosis: epidemiology, diagnosis, and management. *Clin Epidemiol*. 2014;6:369–77. DOI: 10.2147/CLEP.S39981
2. Kyle RA, Linos A, Beard CM, et al. Incidence and natural history of primary systemic amyloidosis in Olmsted County, Minnesota, 1950 through 1989. *Blood*. 1992;79(7):1817–22.

Suggested Reading

Arvanitakis Z, Leurgans SE, Wang Z, et al. Cerebral amyloid angiopathy pathology and cognitive domains in older persons. *Ann Neurol*. 2011; 69:320–7.

Bellotti V, Nuvolone M, Giorgetti S, et al. The workings of the amyloid diseases. *Ann Med*. 2007;39:200–7.

Greenberg SM, Vonsattel JP, Stakes JW, et al. The clinical spectrum of cerebral amyloid angiopathy: presentations without lobar hemorrhage. *Neurology*. 1993;43:2073–9.

Shin SC, Robinson-Papp J. Amyloid neuropathies. *Mt Sinai J Med*. 2012;79:733–48.

Tsourdi E, Därr R, Wieczorek K, et al. Macroglossia as the only presenting feature of amyloidosis due to MGUS. *Eur J Haematol*. 2014;92:88–9.

Amyotrophic Lateral Sclerosis (ALS)– Parkinsonism-Dementia Complex

Epidemiology and Demographics: Amyotrophic lateral sclerosis (ALS)–parkinsonism-dementia complex (ALS-PDC) is primarily seen in the Chamorro population on the island of Guam. There have been non-Chamorros that inhabited the Mariana and Caroline Islands who have also been found to have the ALS and parkinsonism-dementia complex.[1] A review in 1990 found males affected twice as frequently as females. In the 1950s, the incidence of ALS-PDC was higher on Guam than anywhere else in the world. From the late 1960s to the early 1980s, the incidence decreased.[2] The rapid decrease in incidence is likely due to changes brought about by rapid westernization of Guam.[3] Age of onset is 32–64 years, with a mean age of 52 years.[4,5]

Disorder Description: This is an extrapyramidal disorder coupled with a progressive dementia and upper motor neuron signs. Prior to 2010, this condition had only been reported in islands of the Guam archipelago, the Kii peninsula of Japan, and Western New Guinea. This condition has now been reported in four unrelated Czech patients.

Tau-immunoreactive neurofibrillary tangles are present and have a distinctive neuroanatomic distribution that is different from Alzheimer's disease. Significant olfactory dysfunction has been found in this population compared with Chamorro controls.[1]

There are several possible risk factors that may contribute to the development of this condition. High concentrations of aluminum in the island's soil is one possible consideration for the cause. Ingesting the toxin beta-N-methylamino-L-alanine (BMAA) from the seeds of the cycad plant is another possible risk factor. A more recent study re-examined cycads as a possible cause of the ALS-PDC. High levels of zinc (which is a potential neurotoxin) have been found in the flour made from *Cycas circinalis*,[5] which is used in traditional Chamorros cooking. Another potential cause of the disorder is related to the Chamorros' diet of eating flying foxes (*Pteropus*). These animals feed on the cycads.

Patients present with akinesia with a mask-like face and stooped posture with a slow and shuffling gait that resembles that of Parkinson's disease. There is poor coordination and significant slowing of movements. Tremor was not a major characteristic of the cases that were originally studied. If tremor was present, it occurred when the patient was excited or during action, rather than a rest tremor, which is usual for Parkinson's. Rigidity was also not a prominent feature. All patients had mental deterioration, described as a mental slowness and poor memory, which was appreciated by the family rather than the patient. They became indifferent, and depression was also common among patients. There were some who experienced hallucinations that involved old friends and past events.[4,6]

Symptoms

Localization site	Comment
Cerebral hemispheres	Cerebral atrophy, most prominent in frontal and temporal lobes with characteristic memory loss
Mental status and psychiatric aspects/complications	Hallucinations, mental slowing, depression, memory loss
Brainstem	Parkinsonian features from basal ganglion degeneration
Cranial nerves	CN I: olfactory bulbs affected, causing anosmia
Spinal cord	Neurofibrillary tangles found within the spinal cord
Anterior horn cells	Degeneration occurs, causing features of ALS
Syndromes with combined upper and lower motor neuron deficits	Classic upper and lower motor neuron (brisk reflexes with weakness) as seen in ALS

Secondary Complications: Decubiti and pneumonia as end-stage complications of the disorder due to inability to move.

Treatment Complications: No treatment aside from supportive.

References

1. Elizan TS, Chen KM, Mathai KV, Dunn D, Kurland LT. Amyotrophic lateral sclerosis and parkinsonism-dementia complex. A study in non-Chamorros of the Mariana and Caroline Islands. *Arch Neurol.* 1966;14:347–54.
2. Rodgers-Johnson P, Garruto RM, Yanagihara R, et al. Amyotrophic lateral sclerosis and parkinsonism-dementia on Guam: a 30-year evaluation of clinical and neuropathologic trends. *Neurology.* 1986;36:7–13.

3. Plato CC, Garruto RM, Galasko D, et al. Amyotrophic lateral sclerosis and parkinsonism-dementia complex of Guam: changing incidence rates during the past 60 years. *Am J Epidemiol.* 2003;157(2):149–57.
4. Hirano A, Kurland LT, Krooth RS, Lessell S. Parkinsonism-dementia complex, an endemic disease on the island of Guam. I. Clinical features. *Brain.* 1961;84:642–61.
5. Khabazian I, Bains JS, Williams DE, et al. Isolation of various forms of sterol B-D-glucoside from the seed of *Cycas circinalis*: neurotoxicity and implications for ALS-parkinsonism dementia complex. *J Neurochem.* 2002;82: 516–28.
6. Hirano A, Kurland LT, Krooth RS, Lessell S. Parkinsonism-dementia complex, an endemic disease on the island of Guam. II. Pathological features. *Brain.* 1961;84:662–70.

Anderson–Tawil Syndrome (ATS; Periodic Paralysis, Potassium-Sensitive Cardiodysrhythmic Type, Andersen Cardiodysrhythmic Periodic Paralysis)

Epidemiology and Demographics: Andersen–Tawil syndrome (ATS) typically presents in the first or second decade with periodic paralysis or cardiac manifestations (palpitations/syncope). Prevalence of ATS is unknown, but it accounts for less than 10% of all cases of primary periodic paralysis.

Disorder Description: ATS has three main features: periodic paralysis (flaccid muscle weakness), cardiac issues (ventricular arrhythmias, prolonged QT interval), and congenital anomalies (low-set ears, widely spaced eyes, small mandible, fifth-digit clinodactyly, 2,3-syndactyly, small hands and feet). In addition, skeletal features include short stature and scoliosis. Learning disability and other cognitive features may be present.

ATS is an autosomal dominant disorder, caused by mutations in *KCNJ2* on chromosome 17q24.3, which encodes the inward rectifier potassium channel 2 protein (Kir2.1). Fifty percent are inherited from an affected parent and 50% are *de novo*.

Symptoms

Localization site	Comment
Mental status and psychiatric aspects/complications	Mild learning difficulties with deficits in executive function and abstract reasoning without intellectual disability[1,2]

Secondary Complications: Periodic paralysis episodes may lead to mild permanent weakness.

Potassium abnormalities have been reported, both hypokalemia and hyperkalemia, and may require treatment.

Syncope may need to be treated with an implantable cardioverter-defibrillator.

Ventricular arrhythmias may need to be treated with flecainide, especially when accompanied by left ventricular dysfunction.

References

1. Davies NP, Imbrici P, Fialho D, et al. Andersen-Tawil syndrome: new potassium channel mutations and possible phenotypic variation. *Neurology.* 2005;65:1083–9.
2. Yoon G, Quitania L, Kramer JH, et al. Andersen-Tawil syndrome: definition of a neurocognitive phenotype. *Neurology.* 2006;66:1703–10.

Suggested Reading

Statland JM, Tawil R, Venance SL. Andersen-Tawil syndrome. Nov 22, 2004 [Updated Sep 3, 2015]. In Pagon RA, Adam MP, Ardinger HH, et al., eds. *GeneReviews*® [Internet]. Seattle, WA: University of Washington; 1993–2016. Available from www.ncbi.nlm.nih.gov/books/NBK1264/

Aneurysm – Cerebral

Epidemiology and Demographics: Overall prevalence is estimated as 3.2% (95% CI 1.9–5.2), mean age of 50 years. For populations <50 years of age, there is an even gender distribution, but for ages >50 the ratio of male-to-female is 2:1.

Disorder Description: Acquired condition that can be due to an underlying connective tissue disorder. Aneurysms usually form as thin wall protrusions from intracranial arteries due to thin or absent media and elastic lamina layers (saccular), but may also be caused by full-circumference (fusiform) dilation of the vessel or infectious emboli from infectious endocarditis. Cigarette smoking, hypertension, and connective tissue disorders such as Ehlers–Danlos syndrome and familial polycystic kidney disease can be contributory factors. Turbulent and high-flow states may cause degeneration of the vessel and aneurysm formation. Cerebral aneurysm is most likely to form at branch points in the circle of Willis because of inherent weakness in the vessel walls at those sites. Subarachnoid hemorrhage can occur if ruptured.

Symptoms

Localization site	Comment
Mental status and psychiatric aspects/complications	Altered consciousness (ruptured cerebral aneurysm)
Brainstem	Pyramidal tract dysfunction
Cranial nerves	Mass effect may cause visual acuity loss, loss of ipsilateral adduction, elevation and depression of the eye, and facial pain due to II, III, and V cranial nerve compression. Other cranial neuropathies may occur
Pituitary gland	Pituitary apoplexy or stimulation due to compression (rare)
Unclear localization	Headache due to meningeal irritation from sentinel bleed or subarachnoid hemorrhage

Secondary Complications: Subarachnoid hemorrhage can occur if the aneurysm ruptures. Additionally, mass effect from an expanding cerebral aneurysm often causes compression of cranial nerves. Vasospasm can cause focal or diffuse brain infarctions.

Treatment Complications: Treatment of the aneurysm by clipping or endovascular coiling can lead to aneurysm rupture, arterial occlusion, or intraoperative bleeding.

Bibliography

Dority JS, Oldham JS. Subarachnoid hemorrhage: an update. *Anesthesiol Clin.* 2016;34:577–600.

Vlak MH, Algra A, Brandenburg R, et al. Prevalence of unruptured intracranial aneurysms, with emphasis on sex, age, comorbidity, country, and time period: a systematic review and meta-analysis. *Lancet Neurology.* 2011;10:626–36.

Angelman Syndrome

Epidemiology and Demographics: Prevalence of between 1/10,000 and 1/20,000 individuals. Most cases of Angelman syndrome (AS) are not inherited, particularly those caused by a deletion in the maternal chromosome 15 or by paternal uniparental disomy. These genetic changes occur as random events during the formation of reproductive cells (eggs and sperm) or in early embryonic development. Affected people typically have no family history of the disorder.

Disorder Description: A neurodevelopmental disorder whose main features are intellectual disability, lack of speech, seizures, and a characteristic behavioral profile. The behavioral features of AS include a happy demeanor, easily provoked laughter, short attention span, hypermotoric behavior, mouthing of objects, sleep disturbance, and an affinity for water. Microcephaly and subtle dysmorphic features, as well as ataxia and other movement disturbances, are also seen in most affected individuals.

Findings Typically Present in Affected Individuals

- Normal prenatal and birth history, head circumference at birth, laboratory profiles, and no major birth defects.
- Normal brain imaging, although mild cortical atrophy or dysmyelination may be observed.
- Delayed attainment of developmental milestones without loss of skills but evidence of developmental delay by age 6 to 12 months, eventually classified as severe.
- Speech impairment, with minimal to no use of words; receptive language skills and nonverbal communication skills higher than expressive language skills.

- Movement or balance disorder, usually ataxia of gait and/or tremulous movement of the limbs.
- Behavioral uniqueness, including any combination of frequent laughter/smiling; apparent happy demeanor; excitability, often with hand-flapping movements; hypermotoric behavior; short attention span.

Findings in More Than 80% of Affected Individuals

- Delayed growth in head circumference.
- Seizures, usually starting before age 3 years with an abnormal EEG, with a characteristic pattern of large-amplitude slow-spike waves.

Findings in Less Than 80% of Affected Individuals

- Flat occiput.
- Occipital groove.
- Protruding tongue.
- Tongue thrusting; suck/swallowing disorders.
- Feeding problems and/or muscle hypotonia during infancy.
- Prognathia.
- Wide mouth, wide-spaced teeth.
- Frequent drooling.
- Excessive chewing/mouthing behaviors.
- Strabismus.
- Hypopigmented skin, light hair and eye color (compared with family); seen only in those with a deletion.
- Hyperactive lower-extremity deep-tendon reflexes.
- Uplifted, flexed arm position especially during ambulation.
- Wide-based gait with out-going ankles.
- Increased sensitivity to heat.
- Abnormal sleep–wake cycles and diminished need for sleep.
- Attraction to/fascination with water; fascination with crinkly items such as certain papers and plastics.
- Abnormal food-related behaviors.
- Obesity (in the older child; more common in those who do not have a deletion).
- Scoliosis.
- Constipation.

Symptoms

Localization site	Comment
Cerebral hemispheres	Mild atrophy and dysmyelination might be observed on brain MRI. Seizures usually before age 3 years. Abnormal EEG with characteristic pattern of large-amplitude slow-spike waves
Mental status and psychiatric aspects/ complications	Severely delayed milestones by age 6 to 12 months without loss of skills. Speech impairments: receptive language and nonverbal communication better than expressive. Frequent laughter/smiling, happy demeanor, excitability, hand-flapping and tremulous movements, hypermotor behavior, short attention span
Cerebellum	Gait ataxia
Cranial nerves	Strabismus
Spinal cord	Hyperreflexia

Secondary Complications: Obesity.

Treatment Complications: Children with AS are at risk for medication overtreatment because their movement abnormalities can be mistaken for seizures and because EEG abnormalities can persist even when seizures are controlled.

Bibliography

Bird LM. Angelman syndrome: review of clinical and molecular aspects. *Appl Clin Genet*. 2014;7:93–104.

Dagli AI, Mueller J, Williams CA. Angelman syndrome. In Pagon RA, Adam MP, Ardinger HH, et al., eds. *GeneReviews®* [Internet]. Seattle, WA: University of Washington; 1993–2018.

Williams CA, Driscoll DJ, Dagli AI. Clinical and genetic aspects of Angelman syndrome. *Genet Med*. 2010;12(7):385–95.

Angiostrongyliasis

Epidemiology and Demographics: There is no predominant age or gender frequency.

Disorder Description: *Angiostrongylus cantonensis*, also known as the "rat lungworm," is a parasitic nematode that is considered to be the most common infectious cause of eosinophilic meningitis in humans. Ingested larvae may invade farther into the brain parenchyma and cause focal neurologic deficits. Abnormal skin sensations (such as tingling or painful feelings) are more common than in other types of meningitis.[1] Infection spontaneously resolves within in a few weeks and is rarely fatal.[2]

Infection occurs by consuming infected snails, slugs, or freshwater shrimp, crabs, fish, and frogs; however, contaminated produce or raw juices have also been implicated. Infected larvae migrate to the central nervous system hematogenously. Most described cases have occurred in Southeast Asia and tropical Pacific islands; however, cases have been reported in Hawaii, the Caribbean, and Latin America.[1-3]

Symptoms

Localization site	Comment
Cerebral hemispheres	Meningitis
	Encephalitis
	Cerebritis
	Focal neurologic deficits
	Weakness, tremors, sensory abnormalities
	Seizures
	Vision changes
	Headache
Mental status and psychiatric aspects/complications	Encephalopathy
	Lethargy, confusion
	Coma (rare)
Cerebellum	Ataxia
Cranial nerves	Cranial nerve palsies
Spinal cord	Myelitis (rare)
	Bowel/bladder dysfunction
	Autonomic dysfunction
Specific spinal roots	Radiculitis, weakness, paresthesias, hyperesthesias
	Hypo/areflexia
Syndromes with combined spinal cord and peripheral nerve lesions	Radiculomyelitis

Secondary Complications: Paresthesias, blindness, weakness, cognitive deficits, headaches, and seizures may persist.[1,2]

Treatment Complications: Use of anti-helminthics is controversial, as it has been postulated that they may cause more harm by rapidly killing the worms and subsequently leading to an increased immune response.[3]

References

1. Hochberg N, Blackburn B, Park S, et al. Eosinophilic meningitis attributable to *Angiostrongylus cantonensis* infection in Hawaii: clinical characteristics and potential exposures. *Am J Trop Med Hyg.* 2011;85(4):685–90.
2. Graeff-Teixeira C, da Silva A, Yoshimura K. Update on eosinophilic meningoencephalitis and its clinical relevance. *Clin Microbiol Rev.* 2009;22(2):322–48.
3. Murphy GS, Johnson S. Clinical aspects of eosinophilic meningitis and meningoencephalitis caused by *Angiostrongylus cantonensis*, the rat lungworm. *Hawaii J Med Public Health.* 2013;72(6)Suppl 2:35–40.

Anorexia Nervosa

Epidemiology and Demographics: The prevalence of anorexia nervosa in young females is approximately 0.4%; less is known about the prevalence in males. Much more common in females, with a 10:1 female:male ratio in clinical populations. Risk factors include pre-existing anxiety disorders or obsessional traits in childhood, occupations that value thinness (e.g., modeling, elite athletics), and first-degree relatives with eating disorders and/or mood disorders.

Disorder Description: Characterized by three core features: (1) persistent energy intake restriction leading to a significantly low body weight; (2) intense fear of gaining weight or becoming fat, or persistent behavior that interferes with weight gain; and (3) a disturbance in self-perceived weight or shape. Per the DSM-5, a significantly low body weight is defined as a weight that is less than minimally normal, or for children and adolescents, less than minimally expected. Anorexia nervosa can be further characterized by the subtype (restricting versus binge-eating/purging type) and remission status, as well as severity as defined by BMI (or BMI percentile for children and adolescents).

Symptoms

Localization site	Comment
Mental status and psychiatric aspects/ complications	Depressive symptoms including depressed mood, social withdrawal, irritability, insomnia, decreased sex drive. Obsessive-compulsive features. Higher rates of impulsivity and alcohol/substance abuse in binge-eating/purging type. Elevated suicide risk (12/100,000 per year)

Secondary Complications: Physiologic disturbances due to malnutrition and dehydration, mood disorders, anxiety disorders, alcohol/substance abuse, death due to medical complications or suicide.

Treatment Complications: While weight gain is the cornerstone of treatment for patients with anorexia nervosa, refeeding syndrome can occur as a result of fluid and electrolyte shifts during aggressive nutritional rehabilitation of malnourished patients. Complications of refeeding syndrome are potentially fatal.

Bibliography

American Psychiatric Association. *Diagnostic and statistical manual of mental disorders: DSM-5.* 5th ed. Washington, DC: American Psychiatric Association; 2013.

Attia E, Walsh BT. Anorexia nervosa. *Am J Psychiatry.* 2007;164(12):1805–10.

Mehanna HM, Moledina J, Travis J. Refeeding syndrome: what it is, and how to prevent and treat it. *BMJ.* 2008;336(7659):1495–8.

Preti A, Rocchi MB, Sisti D, et al. A comprehensive meta-analysis of the risk of suicide in eating disorders. *Acta Psychiatr Scand.* 2011;124(1): 6–17.

Anoxic Encephalopathy

Epidemiology and Demographics: Survivors of cardiac arrest are susceptible to developing anoxic encephalopathy. Various factors influence the development of brain injury: duration of arrest and underlying rhythm during the arrest, as well as comorbidities. Arrest due to asystole and pulseless electrical activity is associated with a worse prognosis and higher occurrence of anoxic injury.

Disorder Description: Anoxic encephalopathy can evolve to a persistent vegetative state and subsequent brain death, or partial recovery. Some clinical signs have been correlated with poor prognosis such as absent pupillary or corneal reflexes and absent somatosensory evoked responses after 3 days. It is imperative to distinguish anoxic encephalopathy from other causes such as metabolic or drug-induced encephalopathies, because the latter have better outcomes. Therapeutic hypothermia is the standard of care to improve neurologic outcomes and prevent anoxic encephalopathy in resuscitated patients who remain unresponsive after cardiac arrest.

Symptoms

Localization site	Comment
Cerebral hemispheres	Myoclonic status epilepticus Brain death
Mental status and psychiatric aspects/ complications	Mental status ranges from brain death to persistent vegetative state to recovery If recovered: Diffuse cognitive deficits, amnesic and executive impairments, apathy and anosognosia; complete functional dependence
Brainstem	Brain death: absence of brainstem reflexes – absent pupillary reflexes, no oculocephalic reflexes or corneal reflexes, no jaw reflex, no pharyngeal or tracheal reflexes
Cerebellum	Ataxia
Cranial nerves	All cranial nerves could be affected, depending on the region affected by the hypoxia/anoxia, causing respective absent reflexes
Spinal cord	Movements originating from the spinal cord such as upper limb pronation extension reflex, widespread fasciculations of trunk and extremities
Muscle	Intention myoclonus

Secondary Complications: Impaired cognition and dementia, persistent vegetative state, seizures, and brain death.

Treatment Complications: Therapeutic hypothermia can induce coagulopathies (increased risk of bleeding), arrhythmias (mostly bradycardia), hyperglycemia and cold diuresis leading to hypokalemia, hypomagnesemia, and hypophosphatemia.

Bibliography

Adams RD, Victor M, Ropper AH, eds. The acquired metabolic disorders of the nervous system. In *Principles of neurology*. 6th ed. New York: McGraw-Hill; 1997, pp. 1108–37.

Adams, RD, Victor M, Ropper AH, Daroff, RB. Principles of neurology. *Cogn Behav Neurol.* 1997;10(3):220.

Hypothermia after Cardiac Arrest Study Group. Mild therapeutic hypothermia to improve the neurologic outcome after cardiac arrest. *N Engl J Med.* 2002;346:549–56.

Levy DE, Caronna JJ, Singer BH, et al. Predicting outcome from hypoxic-ischemic coma. *JAMA.* 1985;253(10):1420–6.

Mateen FJ, Josephs KA, Trenerry MR, et al. Long-term cognitive outcomes following out-of-hospital cardiac arrest: a population-based study. *Neurology.* 2011;77(15):1438–45.

Anterior Cerebral Artery (ACA), Right Infarction

Epidemiology and Demographics: Anterior cerebral artery (ACA) infarction is the least common large vessel stroke syndrome, accounting for ~1.3–3% of all strokes. African Americans and Hispanics are at higher risk for an ACA infarct.

Disorder Description: ACA infarction may occur as a result of cardiogenic emboli, emboli originating from the internal carotid artery and in situ atherosclerosis. The ACA commonly supplies the parasagittal motor, sensory and prefrontal cortices, and the supplemental motor areas. Infarction to these areas may present as acute confusional state, behavioral abnormalities, left-sided weakness and sensory loss (leg > arm), aprosodia, alien limb, and left hemispatial/sensory neglect. Hypertension, hyperlipidemia, diabetes, atrial fibrillation, history of myocardial infarction, and smoking are risk factors for ACA stroke.

Symptoms

Localization site	Comment
Cerebral hemispheres	Left hemiparesis and left-sided sensory loss (leg > arm), frontal release signs (grasp), aprosodia, left hemisensory/spatial neglect
Mental status and psychiatric aspects/complications	Acute confusional state, frontal lobe behavioral disorder

Secondary Complications: Increased intracranial pressure, left-sided weakness, left-sided sensory loss.

Treatment Complications: Complications of thrombolysis, i.e., intracerebral hemorrhage, systemic bleeding, and angioedema.

Bibliography

Bogousslavsky J, Regli F. Anterior cerebral artery territory infarction in the Lausanne Stroke Registry. Clinical and etiologic patterns. *Arch Neurol.* 1990;47(2):144–50.

Gacs G, Fox AJ, Barnett HJ, Vinuela F. Occurrence and mechanisms of occlusion of the anterior cerebral artery. *Stroke.* 1983;14(6):952–9.

Kumral E, Bayulkem G, Evyapan D, Yunten N. Spectrum of anterior cerebral artery territory infarction: clinical and MRI findings. *Eur J Neurol.* 2002;9(6):615–24.

Anterior Choroidal Artery (AChA) Infarction

Epidemiology and Demographics: Anterior choroidal artery (AChA) infarction has been found in 8.3% of patients with cerebral infarction.

Disorder Description: The AChA supplies the ipsilateral optic tract, posterior limb of the internal capsule, lateral thalamus, and lateral aspects of the midbrain. Infarction of the AChA territory can cause hemiparesis, hemianopia, and hemisensory symptoms. Infrequently, pseudobulbar mutism and abulia have been described in bilateral AChA infarction. Arteriosclerosis and atherosclerosis are the most common causes of AChA disease, followed by cardioembolism.

Symptoms

Localization site	Comment
Cerebral hemispheres	Weakness, spasticity, hemisensory loss, thalamic pain syndrome, visual loss
Brainstem	Ischemia to midbrain can cause tremor (red nucleus), hemiparesis

Secondary Complications: Visual loss.

Treatment Complications: Intracerebral hemorrhage, systemic bleeding, and angioedema if tissue plasminogen activator is administered.

Bibliography

Helgason C, Caplan LR, Goodwin J, Hedges T III. Anterior choroidal artery-territory infarction: report of cases and review. *Arch Neurol.* 1986;43(7):681–6.

Ois A, Cuadrado-Godia E, Solano A, Perich-Alsina X, Roquer J. Acute ischemic stroke in anterior choroidal artery territory. *J Neurol Sci.* 2009;281(1–2):80–4.

van Son B, Vandevenne J, Viaene P. Bilateral anterior choroidal artery infarction presenting with progressive somnolence. *J Stroke Cerebrovasc Dis.* 2014;23(8):e409–10.

Anterior Spinal Artery Disease (Beck's Syndrome)

Epidemiology and Demographics: Spinal cord ischemia is rare, accounting for 5–8% of all acute myelopathies and 1–2% of all neurovascular disease.

Disorder Description: Acquired condition caused by anterior spinal artery (ASA) occlusion. Ischemia and infarction of the ASA territory, which includes the anterior two-thirds of the spinal cord, can cause loss of motor function and sensory modalities (pain and temperature) that travel in the anterior columns below the level of the lesion. Proprioception is unaffected. Most often seen with aortic artery aneurysms and dissections, but may also be caused by thrombosis or hypotension.

Symptoms

Localization site	Comment
Spinal cord	Ischemic myelopathy with paraplegia below the level of infarct; loss of spinothalamic tract sensory modalities (pain and temperature) at and below level of infarct, bladder dysfunction

Secondary Complications: Autonomic dysfunction including orthostatic or frank hypotension, bladder and bowel dysfunction, and sexual dysfunction.

Treatment Complications: Mostly due to surgical repair of aortic aneurysm/dissection when these are the etiology.

Bibliography

de Seze J, Stojkovid T, Breteau G, et al. Acute myelopathies: clinical, laboratory and outcome profiles in 79 cases. *Brain.* 2001;124:1509–21.

Nedeltchev K, Loher TJ, Stepper F, et al. Long-term outcomes of acute spinal cord ischemia syndrome. *Stroke.* 2014;35(2):560–5.

Anticholinergic Poisoning

Epidemiology and Demographics: Anticholinergic poisoning is rare; more common in elderly patients and "naturopaths."

Disorder Description: Medications and natural herbs (*Datura stramonium* – jimsonweed; *Lamprocapnos spectabilis* – bleeding heart) that are antagonists at muscarinic cholinergic receptors may result in parasympathetic block in the peripheral nervous system (PNS) and cause tremors, confusion, euphoria, or seizures when the central nervous system (CNS) receptors are affected. Mild manifestations related to peripheral anticholinergic effects of medications are common, but development of the full-blown syndrome is rare.

Symptoms

Localization site	Comment
Cerebral hemispheres	Bilateral – delirium and cognitive impairment, coma, seizures
Mental status and psychiatric aspects/complications	Delirium and cognitive impairment, coma. Visual, auditory, and sensory hallucinations
Brainstem	Diplopia
Cranial nerves	Pupillary dilation (autonomic), blurred vision
Autonomic nervous system	Parasympathetic blockade with dry mouth, urinary retention, pupillary dilation, increased body temperature, tachycardia

Bibliography

Chan TY. Herbal medicines induced anticholinergic poisoning in Hong Kong. *Toxins (Basel).* 2016;8(3). PMID: 26999208

Ludolph AC. *Datura stramonium.* In Spencer PS, Schaumburg HH, eds. *Experimental and clinical neurotoxicology.* 2nd ed. New York: Oxford University Press; 2000. pp. 466–7.

Anti-Hu Syndrome

Epidemiology and Demographics: Anti-Hu is a paraneoplastic syndrome found predominantly in patients with small cell lung carcinoma. Like many autoimmune conditions, it is more frequent in women (55%). The median age at onset is 60 years. However, it has been reported in childhood as well, the youngest patient being a 4-year-old girl with neuroblastoma and bulbar dysfunction.

Disorder Description: Anti-Hu is an immune-mediated paraneoplastic disorder mainly presenting as a painful sensory neuropathy. The neurologic symptoms usually precede the diagnosis of cancer. The presentation is usually asymmetric dysesthesias and sensory loss in the limbs. The sensory symptoms later progress to involve the torso and the face. Other symptoms include sensory ataxia, with inability to walk, stand, or even sit without support due to prominent proprioception loss. Hu is a family of RNA-binding proteins (HuD, HuC, and Hel-N1), which are only expressed in neurons. These same proteins are also usually expressed by cancer cells, triggering the patient's antibodies to cross-react with the Hu proteins in the dorsal root ganglion. Sensory neuronopathy is the most common manifestation; however, limbic encephalitis, seizures, brainstem encephalitis (vestibular, ophthalmoparesis, bulbar palsy, or hearing loss), asymmetric weakness, cerebellar ataxia, autonomic failure, myelitis, and rarely opsoclonus–myoclonus syndrome can also be present. There are two types of treatments: first is to treat the cancer and the second is immune suppression with use of corticosteroids, cyclophosphamide, azathioprine, plasma exchange, and intravenous immunoglobulin. However, most cases are unresponsive to treatment.

Symptoms

Localization site	Comment
Autonomic failure	Orthostatic hypotension, abnormal pupillary responses, urinary retention, cardiac arrhythmias
Mental status and psychiatric aspects/complications	Limbic encephalitis: confusion, disordered affect, cognitive decline, hallucinations, and short-term memory loss
Brainstem	Brainstem encephalitis: diplopia, oscillopsia, dysarthria, dysphagia, supra- and internuclear gaze abnormalities, sensorineural deafness, facial numbness, or palsy
Cerebellum	Cerebellar degeneration: cerebellar ataxia and tremors
Motor neuron involvement	Muscle atrophy and fasciculation associated with asymmetric loss of strength
Dorsal root ganglia	Dysesthesias and sensory loss of the distal extremities, proprioceptive and nociceptive sensory loss, sensory ataxia

Secondary Complications: Autonomic signs: intestinal pseudo-obstruction, orthostatic hypotension, and cardiac arrhythmias.

Treatment Complications: Complications of the treatment include the associated side effects of the medications used.

Bibliography

Hauser A. Guillain-Barre syndrome and other immune-mediated neuropathies. In Hauser SL, ed. *Harisson's neurology in clinical medicine.* 3rd ed. New York: McGraw-Hill Education/Medical; 2013.

Senties-Madrid H, Vega-Boada F. Paraneoplastic syndromes associated with Anti-Hu antibodies. *IMAJ.* 2001;3:94–103.

Anti-MAG Paraproteinemic Demyelinating Polyneuropathy

Epidemiology and Demographics: Limited data on incidence. Mean age of onset is 61.

Disorder Description: Paraproteinemic neuropathy is caused by the presence of homogeneous immunoglobulin in the serum. Abnormal clonal proliferation of B lymphocytes or plasma cells produces increased production of immunoglobulins. Anti-MAG paraproteinemic demyelinating polyneuropathy is an immune-mediated polyneuropathy with antibodies against myelin-associated glycoprotein, ultimately causing damage to Schwann cells. It is a slowly progressive distal acquired demyelinating symmetric sensory and motor neuropathy. It presents with minimal weakness, distal sensory ataxia, and frequent tremor.

Symptoms

Localization Site	Comment
Peripheral neuropathy	Distal sensory ataxia, minimal weakness

Secondary Complications: Twenty-four percent of patients are disabled after 10 years from onset.

Treatment Complications: Rituximab can lead to hepatitis B reactivation, JC virus (John Cunningham virus) infection, and subsequent progressive multifocal leukoencephalopathy (PML), or death.

Intravenous immunoglobulin complications include anaphylaxis secondary to IgA deficiency, renal failure, proteinuria, severe headache, and aseptic meningitis.

Steroid therapy can lead to psychosis, confusion, weight gain, hyperglycemia, myopathy, glaucoma, cataracts, osteoporosis, or vertebral fractures.

Bibliography

Launay M, Delmont E, Benaim C, et al. Anti-MAG paraproteinemic demyelinating polyneuropathy: a clinical, biological, electrophysiological and anatomopathological descriptive study of a 13-patients' cohort. *Rev Neurol (Paris)*. 2009;165(12):1071–9.

Niermeijer JM, Fischer K, Eurelings M, et al. Prognosis of polyneuropathy due to IgM monoclonal gammopathy: a prospective cohort study. *Neurology*. 2010;74(5):406–12.

Rison RA. Paraproteinemic neuropathy: a practical review. *BMC Neurology*. 2016;16:13.

Antithrombin Deficiency

Epidemiology and Demographics: Prevalence rates of inherited antithrombin deficiency range from 1/500 to 1/5000 depending on assay and confirmation. Equal occurrence in males and females.

Disorder Description: Antithrombin inhibits clotting factors thrombin and factor Xa and is activated physiologically a thousand times in the presence of heparin. In inherited forms, heterozygous mutations lead to decreased quantity or reduced activity of antithrombin. Acquired forms result from reduced production of antithrombin, such as in liver cirrhosis, or increased losses, such as in nephrotic syndrome or protein-losing enteropathy.

Symptoms

Localization site	Comment
Cerebral hemispheres	Cerebral venous sinus thrombosis – increases relative risk by three-fold, with associated venous infarction or hemorrhage. Whether there is increased risk of arterial ischemic stroke is unclear

Secondary Complications: There is high risk of venous thromboembolism systemically (50-fold increased risk) that can complicate recovery from initial neurologic injury.

Treatment Complications: Because heparin potentiates antithrombin for anticoagulation, higher doses of heparin may be required to achieve similar partial thromboplastin time (PTT) values.

Bibliography

Martinelli I, Passamonti SM, Bucciarelli P. Thrombophilic states. *Handb Clin Neurol*. 2014;120:1061–71.

Patnaik MM, Moll S. Inherited antithrombin deficiency: a review. *Haemophilia*. 2008;14:1229–39.

Anxiety Disorder Due to Another Medical Condition

Epidemiology and Demographics: Prevalence of anxiety disorder due to another medical condition is unclear; however, there appears to be an elevated prevalence in patients with medical conditions including asthma, hypertension, ulcers, and arthritis. Late age of onset, atypical symptoms, and absence of a personal or family history of anxiety disorders suggest the need for a thorough evaluation for potential medical conditions that may be causing anxiety.

Disorder Description: The defining feature of anxiety disorder due to another medical condition is clinically significant anxiety that is best explained as a physiologic effect of another medical condition that is known to include anxiety as a symptomatic manifestation and preceded the onset of anxiety. Symptoms may include prominent anxiety or panic attacks. Symptoms do not occur exclusively within the course of delirium and are not better explained by the effects of a substance/medication or primary psychiatric disorder, such as adjustment disorder with anxiety in which the stressor is a medical condition.

Symptoms

Localization Site	Comment
Mental status and psychiatric aspects/complications	Prominent anxiety, panic attacks

Secondary Complications: Depressive disorders, alcohol/substance abuse, sleep disorders.

Treatment Complications: Treatment of anxiety disorder due to another medical condition relies on appropriate treatment of the underlying medical condition. Symptomatic treatment with benzodiazepines may be helpful for panic symptoms; however, caution must be used given the risks of sedation, potential worsening of the underlying medical condition, and cognitive side effects, as well as tolerance and dependence if used chronically.

Bibliography

American Psychiatric Association. *Diagnostic and statistical manual of mental disorders: DSM-5.* 5th ed. Washington, DC: American Psychiatric Association; 2013.

Kessler RC, Ormel J, Demler O, Stang PE. Comorbid mental disorders account for the role impairment of commonly occurring chronic physical disorders: results from the National Comorbidity Survey. *J Occup Environ Med.* 2003;45(12): 1257–66.

Aortic Arteritis/Aortitis

Epidemiology and Demographics: May vary based on etiology of the arteritis/aortitis.

Disorder Description: Aortic arteritis/aortitis is inflammation of the aorta that occurs as a result of infectious or noninfectious causes. Infectious causes include bacteria (from seeding due to trauma, bacterial endocarditis, impaired immunity, and infection of the vasa vasorum) and syphilis. Most common causative bacteria are *Staphylococcus aureus* and *Salmonella*. Rarer causes include *Pseudomonas, Klebsiella, Bacteroides fragilis,* and *Neisseria gonorrhoeae*. Noninfectious causes include Takayasu disease and giant cell arteritis. Other, less common causes include Bechet's disease, rheumatoid arthritis, systemic lupus erythematosus, Crohn's disease, and sarcoidosis.

Symptoms

Localization site	Comment
Mental status and psychiatric aspects/complications	Aortic arteritis secondary to infection can be associated with a variety of symptoms. If etiology is septic emboli, patients can get confusion, stroke, renal dysfunction, pulmonary emboli, and other symptoms
	In temporal arteritis, patients can present with depression, dementia, ataxia, auditory and visual hallucinations, cognitive decline, and ischemic mononeuropathy because of multiple artery involvement
	Syphilis causing aortitis is considered tertiary syphilis. Neurosyphilis can also occur and patients may present with confusion, dementia, hallucinations, or psychosis
Syndromes with combined spinal cord and peripheral nerve lesions	Syphilis at tertiary stage can cause not only aortitis but also tabes dorsalis and general paresis
Unclear localization	Aortic arteritis secondary to infection can be associated with a variety of symptoms. If etiology is septic emboli, can get confusion, stroke, renal dysfunction, and other symptoms
	In giant cell arteritis, nonspecific headaches, visual loss, jaw claudication, transient ischemic attacks, cerebral infarction, and acute confusional states can occur

Secondary Complications: In giant cell arteritis, visual loss and strokes may occur. In syphilis, permanent paresis and sensory ataxia can result if not treated appropriately. With aortitis due to bacterial infections, sepsis can develop and result in death.

Bibliography

Caselli RJ, Hunder GG. Neurologic aspects of giant cell (temporal) arteritis. *Rheum Dis Clin North Am.* 1993;19(4):941–53.

Johnson H, Bouman W, Pinner G. Psychiatric aspects of temporal arteritis: a case report and review of the literature. *J Geriatr Psychiatry Neurol.* 1997;10(4):142–5.

Nyatsanza F, Tipple C. Syphilis: presentations in general medicine. *Clin Med (Lond).* 2016;16(2):184–8.

Aortic Coarctation

Epidemiology and Demographics: Coarctation of the aorta has a prevalence of approximately 4/10,000 live births and represents about 5% of congenital heart defects. Incidence is greater in males (~60%) vs. females (~40%). Thirty percent of patients with Turner syndrome have coarctation of the aorta as well.

Disorder Description: Narrowing of the descending aorta occurs, typically distal to the left subclavian artery, at or around the insertion of the ductus arteriosus. Most cases are congenital (likely secondary to diminished intrauterine blood flow leading to underdevelopment of the fetal aortic arch), but genetic (Turner) and acquired cases (i.e., Takayasu's arteritis) occur as well. Intrauterine compensation for decreased blood flow through the descending aorta is achieved via the foramen ovale and ductus arteriosus, but at birth, shunt closure leads to hemodynamic changes that may range from mild systolic hypertension to severe heart failure, depending on the severity of aortic narrowing and other cardiac anomalies. Left ventricular hypertrophy will often develop from increased pressure, along with increased collateral flow through intercostal, internal mammary, and scapular vessels. Absent or delayed femoral pulse with an elevated brachial pulse (brachial–femoral delay) is a diagnostic finding, and cyanosis of lower extremities from right-to-left shunting can be seen with a patent ductus arteriosus (PDA) and severe coarctation. Less severe cases may present with hypertension in younger age groups.

Symptoms

Localization site	Comment
Cerebral hemispheres	Intracranial aneurysms, especially more common in older patients or in those with more severe coarctation and/or hypertension; mycotic aneurysms in those with previous endocarditis (patients with coarctation are at increased risk for infective endocarditis); intracerebral and intraventricular hemorrhages with resultant complications of stroke; cerebral abscess
Vestibular system (and nonspecific dizziness)	Vertigo, usually secondary to intracranial aneurysms
Spinal cord	Spinal cord compression secondary to dilated collateral arteries within spinal canal

Secondary Complications: Ruptured intracranial aneurysms can lead to hemorrhagic stroke.

Treatment Complications: Septic emboli can spread through cerebral vasculature during coarctation repair. Aneurysms may develop, enlarge, or rupture during stenting procedures. Intraoperative sacrifice of intercostal arteries can worsen spinal cord ischemia and cause subsequent paralysis in a patient who already has poor collateral circulation.

Bibliography

Hartveit F, Lystad H, Minken A. The pathology of venous air embolism. *Br J Exp Pathol.* 1968;49:81–6.

Leblanc FE, Charrette EP, Dobell AR, Branch CL. Neurological complications of aortic coarctation. *Can Med Assoc J.* 1968;99(7):299–303.

Aortic Dissection

Epidemiology and Demographics: Estimated 2.6–3.5/100,000 person-years, with higher incidence and lower mean age of onset in men (60 years vs. 67 years in women).

Disorder Description: Primary event involves tear in aortic intima; blood passes through tear into aortic media, causing separation of intima from surrounding media/adventitia and creation of a false lumen, which can spread proximally or distally. Compression and loss of perfusion can lead to symptoms from affected structures (coronary, cerebral, spinal, visceral). Hypertension is the most important predisposing factor but other risk factors include collagen vascular disorders (e.g., Marfan, Ehlers–Danlos), prior aortic aneurysm, bicuspid aortic valve, aortic instrumentation, aortic coarctation, Turner syndrome, vasculitis, trauma, and pregnancy and delivery.

Symptoms

Localization site	Comment
Cerebral hemispheres	Cerebral ischemia/infarction from direct extension of dissection into carotid arteries or diminished carotid blood flow
Cranial nerves	Hoarseness from vocal cord paralysis due to compression of left recurrent laryngeal nerve
Spinal cord	Acute paraplegia from spinal cord ischemia, from interruption of intercostal vessels
Syndromes with combined spinal cord and peripheral nerve lesions	Horner syndrome from compression of superior cervical ganglion

Secondary Complications: Alterations in consciousness or syncope can result from hypotension, aortic insufficiency, cardiac tamponade due to rupture into pericardium.

Treatment Complications: Risk of periprocedural stroke and paraplegia with endovascular surgical repair.

Bibliography

Hagan PG, Nienaber CA, Isselbacher EM, et al. The International Registry of Acute Aortic Dissection (IRAD): new insights into an old disease. *JAMA*. 2000;283:897–903.

Nallamothu BK, Mehta RH, Saint S, et al. Syncope in acute aortic dissection: diagnostic, prognostic, and clinical implications. *Am J Med*. 2002;113:468–71.

Nienaber CA, Fattori R, Mehta RH, et al. Gender-related differences in acute aortic dissection. *Circulation*. 2004;109:3014–21.

Aortic Regurgitation

Epidemiology and Demographics: The rate of development of symptoms in aortic regurgitation (AR) is greater in patients over the age of 60 years. Including mild or trace cases, overall prevalence rates between 9 and 13% have been estimated.

Disorder Description: The primary causes of AR include aortic stenosis that resulted from calcification of the aortic valve, aortic root disease, infective endocarditis, rheumatic fever, and a complication of valvuloplasty. Patients experience enlargement of the left ventricle because AR results in an increase in left ventricular output. Symptoms may be indolent and may take many years to develop.

Symptoms

Localization site	Comment
Cerebral hemispheres	Severe AR may result in cerebral hemispheric hypoperfusion
Mental status and psychiatric aspects/complications	Severe AR with associated heart failure may lead to confusion/disorientation as a result of cerebral hypoperfusion
Brainstem	Same as above
Cerebellum	Same as above
Vestibular system (and nonspecific dizziness)	Same as above

Secondary Complications: AR may lead to heart failure caused by the hypertrophied heart muscles, which leads to an inability to properly supply the body with blood. The aorta may also enlarge, creating areas with increased proclivity to aortic aneurysm.

Treatment Complications: Complications of aortic valve replacement include death, stroke, blood loss, myocardial infarction, atrial fibrillation, and atrial flutter, and complications of the prosthetic valve include thrombosis and infective endocarditis.

Bibliography

American Heart Association. Problem: aortic valve regurgitation. 2014. Available from www .heart.org/HEARTORG/Conditions/More /HeartValveProblemsandDisease/Problem-Aortic-Valve-Regurgitation_UCM_450611_Article.jsp. Accessed Oct 5, 2018.

Otto CM, Bonow RO. Valvular heart disease. In Mann DL, Zipes DP, Libby P, Bonow RO, Braunwald E, eds. *Braunwald's heart diseases: A textbook of cardiovascular medicine.* 10th ed. Philadelphia: Elsevier/Saunders; 2015. pp. 1409–10.

Aortic Stenosis (AS)

Epidemiology and Demographics: Prevalence increases with age (0.2% ages 50–59, 1.3% ages 60–69, 3.9% ages 70–79, 9.8% ages 80–89). A common cause of aortic stenosis (AS) is congenital bicuspid aortic valve, which is seen in about 1% of the population and is the most common cause in children.

Disorder Description: Left ventricular outflow obstruction across abnormal aortic valve. Stenosis can be due to valvular (most common), supravalvular (high frequency in Williams syndrome), or subvalvular disease (e.g., dynamic obstruction of hypertrophic cardiomyopathy).

The primary causes of AS include calcification of a congenital bicuspid valve or normal aortic valve and/or rheumatic fever that results in rheumatic disease. A decrease in size of the opening of the aortic valve, which results in an outflow tract obstruction of the left ventricle, is the consequence of AS.

Symptomatic disease presents with dyspnea on exertion, presyncope/syncope, and exertional angina, though these are nonspecific. Heart failure, syncope, and angina reflect end-stage disease. Primary causes of valvular aortic stenosis include a congenitally abnormal valve with superimposed calcification, calcific disease of a trileaflet valve, and rheumatic valve disease (most common worldwide, most patients also have mitral disease). Risk factors for progression of disease are increased aortic jet velocity and decreased valve area, degree of valve calcification, older age, male gender, hyperlipidemia, renal insufficiency, hypercalcemia, smoking, metabolic syndrome, and diabetes mellitus.

Symptoms

Localization site	Comment
Cerebral hemispheres	Exertional dizziness (presyncope) and syncope; result of decreased cerebral perfusion. Proposed mechanisms include hypotension from exercise-induced vasodilation in presence of obstruction with fixed cardiac output; postexertional transient bradyarrhythmia; inability to appropriately increase blood pressure due to abnormal baroreceptor response; arrhythmia is uncommon cause

Secondary Complications: Sudden cardiac death, arrhythmia (atrial fibrillation), infective endocarditis, embolic events, coronary artery disease.

Treatment Complications: In patients undergoing valve replacement: bleeding, shock, low cardiac output during and following deployment, annular rupture, valve leaflet thrombosis, myocardial injury, heart block, aortic regurgitation, stroke, death.

Bibliography

American Heart Association. Aortic valve stenosis (AVS). 2015. Available from www.heart.org/en/health-topics/congenital-heart-defects/about-congenital-heart-defects/aortic-valve-stenosis-avs. Accessed Oct 10, 2018.

Eveborn GW, Schirmer H, Heggelund G, et al. The evolving epidemiology of valvular aortic stenosis. The Tromsø study. *Heart.* 2013;99:396.

Faggiano P, Aurigemma GP, Rusconi C, Gaasch WH. Progression of valvular aortic stenosis in adults: literature review and clinical implications. *Am Heart J.* 1996;132:408.

Nishimura RA, Otto CM, Bonow RO, et al. 2014 AHA/ACC guideline for the management of patients with valvular heart disease: a report of the American College of Cardiology/American Heart Association Task Force on Practice Guidelines. *Circulation.* 2014;129(23):2440–92.

Otto CM, Bonow RO. Valvular heart disease. In Mann DL, Zipes DP, Libby P, Bonow RO, Braunwald E, eds. *Braunwald's heart diseases: a textbook of cardiovascular medicine.* 10th ed. Philadelphia: Elsevier/Saunders; 2015. pp. 1448–58.

Aortic Surgeries and Other Procedures, Including Abdominal Aortic Aneurysm Repair, Sympathectomy, Aortography, and Intra-aortic Balloon Assistance

Procedure Descriptions: *Abdominal aortic aneurysm repair* with endovascular grafts or open surgery can lead to a variety of complications, including paralysis, paresis, and stroke.

Sympathectomy involves cauterizing, severing, or clipping the sympathetic chain or nerves and is used as treatment for patients with debilitating primary focal hyperhidrosis, ischemic rest pain secondary to peripheral artery disease, or Raynaud's phenomenon.

Aortography involves catheter placement in the aorta and injection of contrast material while x-ray images are captured; previously the gold standard to diagnose aortic dissections.

Intra-aortic balloon assistance is used to support cardiac output and oxygenation or blood in a variety of conditions, including cardiogenic shock or complications from myocardial infarctions.

Symptoms

Localization site	Comment
Cerebral hemispheres	Ischemic strokes can occur with abdominal aneurysm repair. Embolic strokes can occur from intra-aortic balloon assistance
Spinal cord	Paraplegia and paraparesis do occur with abdominal aneurysm repair, and occur largely because of ischemia to the spinal cord. Schemia to spinal cord after intra-aortic balloon pump or aortography may occur as well, but is rare
Unclear localization	Cholesterol embolization causing livedo reticularis, acute kidney injury, intestinal ischemia can occur secondary to plaque embolization. Infections can occur with procedures. With thoracic sympathectomies, complications such as pneumothorax or hemothorax can occur. With intra-aortic balloon pumps, arterial dissection can occur

Secondary Complications: Hematoma, anemia, thrombocytopenia, endograft migration after abdominal aneurysm repair, surgical complications post sympathectomy, infection, death.

Bibliography

Achneck HE, Rizzo JA, Tranquilli M, Elefteriades JA. Safety of thoracic aortic surgery in the present era. *Ann Thorac Surg.* 2007;84:1180–5.

Dharmaraj B, Kosai NR, Gendeh H, Ramzisham AR, Das S. A prospective cohort study on quality of life after endoscopic thoracic sympathectomy for primary hyperhidrosis. *Clin Ter.* 2016;167:67–71.

Messé SR, Bavaria JE, Mullen, et al. Neurologic outcomes from high risk descending thoracic and thoracoabdominal aortic operations in the era of endovascular repair. *Neurocrit Care.* 2008;9(3):344–51.

Aortic Trauma

Epidemiology and Demographics: The majority of aortic trauma occur secondary to motor vehicle accidents, causing blunt thoracic trauma. It is a major cause of death from blunt trauma. It occurs more frequently in men than women, but women have a greater risk of death or major complications from the aortic trauma. Risk factors include age greater than 60 years, front seat occupancy, and not wearing a seat belt.

Disorder Description: Aortic trauma in the setting of blunt thoracic injury usually occurs due to rapid deceleration and high-energy impact. The most common cause includes motor vehicle accidents, but other causes include falls, crush injuries, motorcycle and aircraft crashes, and collision with a motor vehicle. There are often several associated injuries, including head and neck injuries, cardiac and lung contusions, bone and pelvic fractures, intra-abdominal hemorrhages, and diaphragmatic rupture.

Symptoms

Localization site	Comment
Mental status and psychiatric aspects/complications	Abnormal Glasgow Coma Scale
Spinal cord	Paraplegia can occur and has been reported to occur postoperatively during aortic repair
Unclear localization	Head injury/trauma, difficulty breathing/swallowing, abdominal trauma, splenic rupture, bone fractures can all occur in the setting of blunt trauma. Other findings that can assist with diagnosis of aortic injury/trauma include midscapular back pain, upper extremity hypertension, bilateral femoral pulse deficit, or unexplained hypotension

Secondary Complications: Death, paraplegia, head trauma, coma.

Bibliography

Benjamin ER, Tillou A, Hiatt JR, Cryer HG. Blunt thoracic aortic injury. *Am Surg.* 2008;74(10):1033–7.

Cowley RA, Turney SZ, Hankins JR, et al. Rupture of thoracic aorta caused by blunt trauma. A fifteen-year experience. *J Thorac Cardiovasc Surg.* 1990;100:652–60.

Fabian TC, Richardson JD, Croce MA, et al. Prospective study of blunt aortic injury: multicenter trial of the American Association for the Surgery of Trauma. *J Trauma.* 1997;42:374–80.

Kram HB, Appel PL, Wohlmuth DA, Shoemaker WC. Diagnosis of traumatic thoracic aortic rupture: a 10-year retrospective analysis. *Ann Thorac Surg.* 1989;47:282–6.

Aqueductal Stenosis

Epidemiology and Demographics: In children, 15–60% of cases of hydrocephalus are attributed to aqueductal stenosis. In adults, 10–40% of cases of hydrocephalus are attributed to aqueductal stenosis. There are two peaks of distribution for age: one in the first year of life and the other in adolescence. There is a slight male prevalence for this condition.

Disorder Description: Aqueductal stenosis is due to narrowing of the aqueduct of Sylvius, causing blockage of flow of cerebrospinal fluid and resulting in hydrocephalus, which may be congenital and/or obstructive. CT scan and MRI are typically used to diagnose this condition.

Causes

Adapted in part from CheckOrphan.[1]

- Tumor compression mainly in the pineal region: tectal glioma is one example.
- Narrow aqueduct: a defect from birth, can be due to abnormal folding of the neural plate.
- Forking: aqueduct split into multiple separate channels as a result of incomplete fusion of the median fissure.
- Septum formation through gliosis of membrane or glial cells develops across the aqueduct. This abnormal membrane forms at the lower and distal portion of the aqueduct, causing obstruction predominantly.
- Gliosis: aqueduct begins as partially blocked. To compensate for the blockage, pressure is increased in the third ventricle, which in turn increases cerebrospinal flow to normal rates. There is an increase in the third ventricle. Therefore, the increase in velocity is noted. This in turn increases the shear stress in the aqueduct, causing more damage to epithelial cell linings and ventricles, and resulting in gliosis and proliferation of glial cells.
- Bickers–Adams–Edwards syndrome or X-linked hydrocephalus: caused by point mutation in the gene for neural cell adhesion. Males with this disorder have severe hydrocephalus, adducted thumbs, spastic motion, and intellectual delays.
- Bacterial meningitis.
- Giant fusiform aneurysm of basilar artery can cause pressure on the aqueduct and cause obstruction.
- Neurofibromatosis, nontumoral aqueductal stenosis in 5% of children with neurofibromatosis I.

Symptoms

Localization site	Comment
Cerebral hemispheres	Headaches, deterioration of the patient level of consciousness, upward gaze palsy, and developmental delay. The developmental delay can range from mild to severe to the extent that the child may be unable to use spoken language or control movements or interact with others. Tremors have been reported rarely
Cranial nerves	Upward gaze palsy in which a person has difficulty looking up

Treatment Complications: An extracranial shunt, either ventriculoperitoneal or ventriculoatrial, can be placed. An endoscopic surgery with low mortality rate can also be used. There is a 50% failure rate in 2 years. Shunt malfunctions and associated complications can lead to a death rate of 1.2% per year. Secondary surgery sometimes needed to repair mechanical failure, incorrect catheter size, valve drainage pressure problems, and mechanical difficulties that could predispose to infection. Change in mental status can be seen when shunt malfunction occurs.

Reference

1. CheckOrphan. Aqueductal stenosis. 2006–2018. Available from www.checkorphan.org/diseases/ hydrocephalus-due-congenital-stenosis-aqueduct-sylvius. Accessed Aug 1, 2018.

Bibliography

Cinalli G, Spennato P, Nastro A, et al. Hydrocephalus in aqueductal stenosis. *Childs Nerv Sys.* 2011;27(10):1621–42.

Arachnoid Cysts

Epidemiology and Demographics: Arachnoid cysts are seen in about 1% of the population. Male-to-female gender distribution is 2:1.

Disorder Description: Arachnoid cysts are cerebrospinal fluid sacs lined with arachnoid cells and collagen that develop between the surface of the brain and the cranial base. They are congenital. Most arachnoid cyst cases manifest themselves as early as infancy. They can occur on the brain or on the spine. Spinal arachnoid cysts may be extradural or intradural as well as perineural. The exact cause is not known, although developmental malformation is suspected. Diagnosis is with neuroimaging.

Symptoms

Localization site	Comment
Cranium	Cranium deformation or macrocephaly in children
Suprasellar region in children	Bobbing and nodding of head, called bobble-head doll syndrome
Left middle cranial fossa	Attention deficit hyperactivity disorder, alexithymia, psychosis
Temporal lobe	Headaches
Cerebral hemisphere	Seizures, increased intracranial pressure, hydrocephalus, developmental delay, hemiparesis, musical hallucinations, pre-senile dementia
Supratentorial	Ménière's disease
Frontal lobe	Depression
Specific spinal roots	Radiculopathies are reported

Secondary Complications: Minor head injury can cause damage to cyst, causing the fluid within the cyst to leak. Arachnoid cyst secondary to Marfan syndrome, arachnoiditis, or agenesis of corpus callosum has been described.

Treatment: Most of the arachnoid cysts do not require any treatment. If symptomatic, an internal or external shunt may be placed. Fenestration involves drainage by needle aspiration or burr hole. Surgery can resolve psychiatric manifestation in some patients.

Bibliography

Gelabert-Gonzalez M. Intracranial arachnoid cyst. *Rev Neurol.* 2004;39(12):1161–6.

Millichap JG. Temporal lobe arachnoid cyst-attention deficit disorder syndrome. Role of the electroencephalogram and diagnosis. *Neurology.* 1997;48(5):1435–9.

Arachnoiditis

Epidemiology and Demographics: Most common age of onset is between 40 and 60 years. No clear gender or race predisposition is apparent, though may be higher in females, as a result of spinal and epidural anesthesia prior to giving birth. Precise incidence is unknown, but is reported to be as high as 1.6–3% following spinal procedures.

Disorder Description: Nonspecific inflammation of the arachnoid layer with consequent membrane thickening and nerve root adhesions. Arachnoid layer is susceptible to poor healing due to lack of vascularization. Most common etiologies include myelography with oil-based agents and surgical trauma/procedures of the lumbar spine. Additional causes include subarachnoid hemorrhage, infections, and tumors. The condition and symptoms progress over 6–18 months because of tethering of the spinal cord.

Symptoms

Localization site	Comment
Specific spinal roots	Radiculopathy – low back pain, mono- and multiradicular pain
Syndromes with combined spinal cord and peripheral nerve lesions	Partial or complete paralysis of the lower extremities. Urinary urgency, frequency, incontinence. Spasms of the back and lower extremities. Paresthesias, hypoesthesia, dysesthesia. Unexplained skin rashes and itching. Burning of ankles and feet

Secondary Complications: Late complications include cauda equina syndrome, ossification of the spinal meninges, and failed back syndrome resulting in worsening of pain and neurologic symptoms.

Treatment Complications: Treatment options are limited to symptomatic pain relief and rare surgical intervention. Chronic pain and opioid use may lead to chronic fatigue, major depression, addiction, opioid-induced constipation.

Bibliography

Postacchini F. *Lumbar disc herniation*. New York: Springer; 1999.

Wright MH, Denney LC. A comprehensive review of spinal arachnoiditis. *Orthop Nurs*. 2003;22:215–9.

Arteriovenous Fistula

Epidemiology and Demographics: Brain arteriovenous (AV) malformations occur in about 0.1% of the population. Ninety percent of brain AV fistulas are supratentorial. Patients usually present between ages 10 and 40 years. Higher prevalence in patients with hereditary hemorrhagic telangiectasia (Osler–Weber–Rendu syndrome). Overall annual hemorrhage rate of 3%. Spinal dural AV fistula makes up about 70% of all spinal AV malformations and is the most frequent of all spinal vascular diseases. Brain AV fistulas account for 1–2% of all strokes, 3% of strokes in young adults, and 9% of subarachnoid hemorrhages.

Disorder Description: Characterized by abnormal shunting of blood between arterial and venous systems, without the presence of the normal capillary bed in between. AV malformations cause neurologic symptoms through reduction of oxygen delivery to neurologic tissue, hemorrhage, or compression or displacement of parts of the brain or spinal cord. Abnormally rapid rate of blood flow from arterial to venous circulation leads to chronically elevated venous pressure, reduced oxygenation, and structural changes such as aneurysm formation. Vascular steal is also one of the mechanisms that is known to cause clinical symptoms. Increased risk of hemorrhage in patients with associated aneurysms, exclusive deep venous drainage, and deep brain location.

Symptoms

Localization site	Comment
Cerebral hemispheres	Intracranial hemorrhage, symptoms depending on anatomic location
Mental status and psychiatric aspects/ complications	Headaches related to stretching of dural structures, venous thrombosis/hemorrhage, seizures (focal or generalized). Repetitive microbleeds over time can lead to increased risk of dementia
Brainstem	Impaired consciousness
Cerebellum	Dizziness, tremors, impaired coordination
Cranial nerves	Cranial nerve involvement related to anatomic location (e.g., headaches from pressure on CN V, diplopia from CN III, IV, or VI)
Spinal cord	Myeloradiculopathy related to venous hypertension is most common clinical presentation of dural AV fistulas. Usually present in the fifth decade of life, more common in men
Unclear localization	Compression causing impaired cerebrospinal fluid flow leading to hydrocephalus

Secondary Complications: Risk of cerebral sinus thrombosis from dural AV fistulas, leading to intracranial hemorrhage, venous infarction, seizure, altered mental status, intracranial hypertension.

Treatment Complications: With stereotactic radiosurgery, there is a risk of hemorrhage during lesion obliteration, and later radiation necrosis causing new neurologic deficits.

Bibliography

AlShahi R, Warlow C. A systematic review of the frequency and prognosis of arteriovenous malformations of the brain in adults. *Brain*. 2001;124:1900–26.

American Society of Neuroradiology. Arteriovenous fistulae of the CNS. *AJNR AM J Neuroradiol*. 2001;22: S22–5.

da Costa L, Wallace MC, Ter Brugge KG, et al. The natural history and predictive features of hemorrhage from brain arteriovenous malformations. *Stroke*. 2009;40:100–5.

Gross BA, Du R. Natural history of cerebral arteriovenous malformations: a meta-analysis. *J Neurosurg*. 2013;118:437–43.

Lev N, Maimon S, Rappaport ZH, Melamed E. Spinal dural arteriovenous fistulae: a diagnostic challenge. *Isr Med Assoc J.* 2001;3:492–6.

Mohr JP, KejdaScharler J, PileSpellman J. Diagnosis and treatment of arteriovenous malformations. *Curr Neurol Neurosci Rep.* 2013;13:324.

Stapf C, Mast H, Sciacca RR, et al. Predictors of hemorrhage in patients with untreated brain arteriovenous malformation. *Neurology.* 2006;66:1350–5.

Tsai LL. Intracranial dural arteriovenous fistulas with or without cerebral sinus thrombosis: analysis of 69 patients. *J Neurol Neurosurg Psychiatry.* 2004;75:1639–41.

Arteriovenous Malformations (AVMs)

Epidemiology and Demographics: Incidence for arteriovenous malformations (AVMs) is approximately 2/100,000 person-years, with most cases revealed in adulthood despite the congenital nature of the lesion. Death rates in those with ruptured arteriovenous malformations are 10–15%. Rupture is more likely to occur in men, and this risk increases in both sexes by about 1–3% per year. About 66% of patients with AVMs have comorbid learning disabilities.

Disorder Description: AVMs are complex networks of aberrant blood vessels in the brain. Blood travels directly from artery to vein, without intermediary capillary connections. The nidus is characterized by arteries lacking a muscularis layer, absent capillary bed, and dilated veins with increased intravascular pressure. No specific cause for AVMs has been elucidated, but there is an increased prevalence of AVMs in patients with certain genetic disorders, including neurofibromatosis and Osler–Weber–Rendu, Sturge–Weber, and von Hippel–Lindau syndromes. Neurologic dysfunction caused by AVMs usually results from hemorrhages or progressive decline in blood flow secondary to steal phenomenon. AVMs can by themselves cause localization-related seizures as well. AVMs can occur anywhere along the neuroaxis, and symptoms depend predominantly on the involved location. Patients with a history of prior AVM rupture are at increased risk for re-rupture. AVMs are classified as true AVMs, occult/cryptic AVMs or vascular malformations, venous malformations, hemangiomas, or dural fistulas. For all types, the Spetzler–Martin grading scheme is used to assess surgical treatment risks, assigning points based on AVM size, location, and absence or presence of venous drainage; higher scores correlate to greater surgical risks. Surgical options include resection, super selective embolization, radiosurgery, or any combination thereof.

Symptoms

Localization site	Comment
Cerebral hemispheres	Seizure (usually simple, partial, or secondarily generalized) seen in about 50% of patients with AVM; hemorrhagic stroke secondary to bleeding or rupture of the AVM, producing deficits characteristic of the area of subsequent ischemia (i.e., language, corticospinal tract). Bleeding can be parenchymal, subarachnoid, or intraventricular. Blood flow may be reduced to other areas of the brain via a "steal phenomenon" in which flow is reduced to brain tissue adjacent to unruptured AVM
Mental status and psychiatric aspects/complications	Minor learning disability seen in approximately 66% of patients
Brainstem	Dysarthria, dysphagia, vertigo
Cerebellum	Ataxia, gait instability
Meninges	Headache
Cranial nerves	Optic nerve/optic radiations compression, producing deficits in vision

Secondary Complications: Kinking of draining veins from an AVM can promote thrombus formation, which can spread to brain parenchyma and cause an ischemic stroke.

Treatment Complications: Antiepileptic drugs (AEDs) are used to treat seizures in patients with unruptured AVMs. Neurologic side effects of AEDs are agent-dependent but broadly include sedation, fatigue, dizziness, dyscoordination, tremor, cognitive deficits, and behavioral disturbances.

Surgical management includes resection, embolization, or radio-ablation. All carry risk of hemorrhage and brain ischemia. Embolization procedures can inadvertently induce embolization and subsequent ischemia to nearby healthy parenchyma.

Radiosurgery can produce white matter edema and radiation-induced necrosis. Radiotherapy can also induce thrombosis of the arterial feeders of an AVM, which can in turn promote re-hemorrhage of the already weak arteries of the AVM. Seizure frequency has also been found to be increased in patients after radiotherapy. Finally, radiotherapy is a risk factor for atherosclerosis.

Bibliography

Al-Shahi R, Warlow C. A systematic review of the frequency and prognosis of arteriovenous malformations of the brain in adults. *Brain*. 2001;124:1900.

American Heart Association. What is an arteriovenous malformation (AVM)? Reviewed Oct 23, 2012. Available from www.strokeassociation.org/STROKEORG/ AboutStroke/TypesofStroke/HemorrhagicBleeds/ What-Is-an-Arteriovenous-Malformation-AVM_UCM_310099_Article.jsp#.VpLPKvkrLIU. Accessed Oct 5, 2018.

Gross BA, Du R. Natural history of cerebral arteriovenous malformations: a meta-analysis. *J Neurosurg*. 2013;118:437.

Ross J, Al-Shahi Salman R. Interventions for treating brain arteriovenous malformations in adults. *Cochrane Database Syst Rev*. 2010;(7):CD003436.

Arteritic Anterior Ischemic Optic Neuropathy (AAION)

Epidemiology and Demographics: The incidence of arteritic anterior ischemic optic neuropathy (AAION) increases with age and is approximately 0.36/100,000 in the United States. The disease is most prevalent in the 50-year and older age group. It is more common in women (2:1) and in Caucasian ethnicities, i.e., Scandinavian, German, and other European ancestry.

Disorder Description: For a description of anterior ischemic optic neuropathy, see entry for *Non-arteritic Anterior Ischemic Optic Neuropathy (NAION)*.

AAION is most often a form of giant cell arteritis (GCA), affecting the ophthalmic artery, central retinal artery, and/or the distal posterior ciliary arteries. Pathologically, affected blood vessels demonstrate focal granulomatous inflammation with giant cells.

Elevated serum erythrocyte sedimentation rate and C-reactive protein are commonly found. AAION can be seen in other vasculitides, including polyarteritis nodosa, systemic lupus erythematosus, and others.

Symptoms

Localization site	Comment
Cerebral hemispheres	Stroke involving the large intracranial vessels when GCA is diffuse
Cranial nerves	Unilateral and bilateral visual loss (50% of cases), with chalky white, pale, and swollen disc seen on funduscopic exam; diplopia secondary to extraocular muscle ischemia; facial pain secondary to jaw claudication
Other	Prominent temporal arteries to palpation, polymyalgia rheumatica

Treatment Complications: Temporal artery biopsy is helpful for suspected AAION. Risks of biopsy include damage to facial nerve.

Pulse IV steroids are the mainstay of treatment when visual loss is present. Neurologic complications of steroids include mood disturbance, decreased concentration, and insomnia.

Bibliography

Miller NR, ed. Anterior ischemic optic neuropathy. In *Walsh and Hoyt's clinical neuro-ophthalmology*. 4th ed. Vol 1. Baltimore: Williams & Wilkins;1982. pp. 212–26.

Russo E, Ciriaco M, Ventrice P, et al. Corticosteroid-related central nervous system side effects. *J Pharmacol Pharmacother*. 2013;4(Suppl 1):S94–8.

Aspergillosus

Epidemiology and Demographics: Mean age 42.6 years (range 2 days to 78 years), with male predominance.[1] Central nervous system (CNS) aspergillosis accounts for less than 5% of all CNS infections.[2]

Disorder Description: *Aspergillus* species are ubiquitous septated fungi in soil, water, or decaying vegetation and are generally opportunistic and angio-invasive. *A. fumigatus* is the most commonly identified human pathogen.[1] Infection is commonly by airborne spores via lungs or paranasal sinuses. Intracranial spread may be involved through hematogenous spread or as a result of direct invasion from adjacent structures and may occur in 10–20% of cases, with focal abscesses being the most common sequelae.[1,3]

Risk factors for development include immunosuppression, especially in HIV or AIDS, solid organ transplantation, hematologic malignancies, prior brain pathology, or autoimmune diseases.[1-3]

It affects immunocompromised hosts worldwide, but affected immunocompetent hosts have also been reported in India, Sudan, Pakistan, Saudi Arabia, UAE, and some African countries.[1]

Symptoms

Localization site	Comment
Cerebral hemispheres	Abscesses
	Cerebritis
	Headaches
	Mycotic aneurysms, may cause subarachnoid hemorrhage
	Meningitis
	Seizures
	Vision changes
	Vasculitis
	Ischemic stroke (anterior cerebral artery or middle cerebral artery mostly involved)
	Hemorrhagic stroke
Mental status and psychiatric aspects/complications	Encephalopathy
Brainstem	Abscesses
	Strokes
	Hemorrhages
Cerebellum	Abscesses
	Strokes
	Hemorrhages
Base of skull	Meningitis
	Cavernous sinus thrombosis
Cranial nerves	Cranial neuropathies
Spinal cord	Epidural abscesses (rare)

Secondary Complications: Long-term complications include seizures or hydrocephalus.

Treatment Complications: Amphotericin B has nephrotoxic side effects, which may further depress mental status. Voriconazole may lead to visual disturbances or hallucinations.

References

1. Kourkoumpetis T, Desalermos A, Muhammed M, Mylonakis E. Central nervous system aspergillosis. *Medicine*. 2012;91(6):328–36.
2. Shamim M, Enam S, Ali R, Anwar S. Craniocerebral aspergillosis: a review of advances in diagnosis and management. *J Pak Med Assoc*. 2010;60(7):573–9.
3. Panackal A, Williamson P. Fungal infections of the central nervous system. *CONTINUUM (Minneap Minn)*. 2015;21:1662–78.

Astrocytomas

Disorder Description: Astrocytomas arise from specific glial cells called astrocytes that form the supportive tissue of the brain. Astrocytomas can appear in various parts of the brain and nervous system, including the cerebellum, the cerebrum, the central areas of the brain, the brainstem, and the spinal cord. There are varying types of astrocytomas: pilocytic, diffuse, anaplastic, grade IV, and subependymal giant cell.

WHO Classification of Diffuse Astrocytic/ Oligodendroglial Tumors

Grade I: Pilocytic astrocytomas, subependymal giant cell astrocytomas

Grade II: Pleomorphic xanthoastrocytoma, diffuse astrocytoma (isocitrate dehydrogenase [IDH] mutant), oligodendroglioma (IDH mutant and 1p/19q co-deleted)

Grade III: Anaplastic astrocytoma (IDH-mutant), anaplastic oligodendroglioma (IDH mutant and 1p/19q co-deleted), anaplastic pleomorphic xanthoastrocytoma

Grade IV: Glioblastoma (IDH mutant and IDH wild type)

Descriptions of Various Astrocytic Tumors

Pilocytic astrocytoma *(also called juvenile pilocytic astrocytoma)* – Grade I astrocytomas that rarely spread out from origin site and are considered the "most benign" of all the astrocytomas. Other grade I astrocytomas are cerebellar astrocytoma and desmoplastic infantile astrocytoma. Histologically, most pilocytic astrocytomas form cysts or are enclosed within one; slow growing, but can become very large.

Diffuse astrocytoma *(also called low-grade or astrocytoma grade II)* – Although growth rate is slow, they tend to invade adjoining structures. The labels *fibrillary, gemistocytic, protoplasmic* describe their operational and histologic preferences. They are more likely to contain microcysts and mucus-like fluid.

Anaplastic astrocytoma – A grade III tumor. They form projectile appendages, invade into surrounding tissues; rare.

Astrocytoma grade IV *(also called glioblastoma, previously labeled glioblastoma multiforme, grade IV glioblastoma, and GBM)* – There are two types of astrocytoma grade IV: primary, or *de novo*, and secondary. Primary tumors are very aggressive and the most common form of astrocytoma grade IV. The secondary tumors are those that originate as a lower-grade tumor and evolve into a grade IV tumor. May contain cystic material, calcium deposits, blood vessels, and/or a mixed grade of cells.

Subependymal giant cell astrocytoma – These astrocytomas are ventricular tumors associated with tuberous sclerosis.

Astrocytoma, Cerebellum: Pilocytic

Epidemiology and Demographics: The overall adult incidence rate of primary malignant brain tumors (including gliomas: oligodendrocytes, glioblastomas, etc.) is 7.23/100,000. Females in the United States have higher rates of overall malignant and non-malignant brain and central nervous system (CNS) tumors; this varies from worldwide incidence, in which males have higher incidence rate as compared with females.[1]

Pediatric and adolescent incidence rate (0–19 years) is 5.57/100,000 for primary malignant and nonmalignant brain and CNS tumors, with higher rates in males than females.

Disorder Description: Rates of primary malignant brain tumors are higher in developed countries. Only a few specific factors have been convincingly linked with the risk of incurring a glioma. For example, therapeutic or high-dose radiation, particularly in the presence of a genetic predisposition such as germline polymorphisms leading to reduced thiopurine methyltransferase activity, can increase the risk of developing a brain neoplasm.[2] Several studies have shown lower incidence rates in patients with higher IgE levels, e.g., with asthma or allergies.

Glioblastoma

Epidemiology and Demographics: This tumor represents about 15.4% of all primary brain tumors and about 60–75% of all astrocytomas. Glioblastomas increase in frequency with age, and affect more men than women; they generally affect adults aged 45–65. Only 3% of childhood brain tumors are glioblastomas. Most common of all the brain cancers and most aggressive (Grade IV).

Disorder Description: Uncommon risk factors include genetic disorders such as neurofibromatosis and Li–Fraumeni syndrome and previous radiation therapy. Associated with viruses SV40 and HHV6 and cytomegalovirus. Some studies have linked glioblastoma with malaria, either the disease or the immunosuppressive therapy used in malaria.

Astrocytoma Glioma, Cerebellum

Epidemiology and Demographics: They are the second most common childhood tumor (15–20% of all pediatric tumors). More common in children, presenting from childhood to adolescence.

Disorder Description: The majority of brain tumors are not hereditary. Brain tumors caused by a genetically inherited syndrome, such as neurofibromatosis, Li–Fraumeni, von Hippel–Lindau and Turcot syndromes, and tuberous sclerosis, affect only 5% of patients.

Symptoms

Localization site	Comment
Mental status and psychiatric aspects/ complications	Vary from mild to severe; memory deficit, slurry speech, nausea, vomiting, vertigo, unsteadiness, uncoordinated limb movements, headache possible in occipital, frontal, or upper cervical areas
Cerebellum	Difficulties with walking, clumsiness, nausea, headache, and vomiting
Unclear	Depending on the location in the cerebral hemispheres

Localization site	Comment
Focal	Focal signs: hemiparesis, sensory loss, visual loss, aphasia
Cerebellum	Headaches, nausea and vomiting, poor coordination and difficulty walking (ataxia)
Spinal cord	Symptoms depend on the location of the tumor

Treatment Complications: Wide range of potential complications such as incurring new focal neurologic deficits as result of therapies including surgery and radiation. Chemotherapy may cause depressed blood cell counts which in turn can predispose to coagulopathies and immunosuppression, which themselves can ultimately result in systemic and neurologic complications.

References

1. Central Brain Tumor Registry of the United States. www.CBTRUS.org. Accessed Oct 10, 2018.
2. Schwartzbaum JA, Fisher JL, Aldape KD, Wrensch M. Epidemiology and molecular pathology of glioma. *Nat Clin Pract Neurol.* 2006;2:494–503.

Suggested Reading

Davis FG, Bruner JM, Surawicz TS. The rationale for standardized registration and reporting of brain and central nervous system tumors in population-based cancer registries. *Neuroepidemiology.* 1997;16:308–16.

Pan E, Prados MD. Glioblastoma multiforme and anaplastic astrocytoma. In Kufe DW, Pollock RE, Weichselbaum RR, et al., eds. *Holland-Frei cancer medicine.* 6th ed. Hamilton, ON: BC Decker; 2003. Available from www.ncbi.nlm.nih.gov/books/NBK12526/

Smith MA Freidlin B Gloeckler Ries LA Simon R. Trends in reported incidence of primary malignant brain tumors in children in the United States. *J Natl Cancer Inst.* 1998;90:1269–77.

Watanabe T, Katayama Y, Yoshino A, et al. Treatment of low-grade diffuse astrocytomas by surgery and human fibroblast interferon without radiation therapy. *J Neurooncol.* 2003;61(2):171–6.

Atlantoaxial Subluxation (Atlanto-Occipital Instability)

Epidemiology and Demographics: Atlantoaxial instability/subluxation is rare without predisposing factors. In patients with Down syndrome, frequency of asymptomatic atlantoaxial insufficiency is about 13.1%. Symptomatic atlantoaxial insufficiency in Down syndrome is about 1.5%. Odontoid fractures are associated with severe atlantoaxial insufficiency with a 2-fold increase in mortality. In patients with rheumatoid arthritis, the frequency is 20–49%. Rheumatoid arthritis affects women more than men.

Disorder Description: Sometimes atlantoaxial subluxation is a congenital condition, but in adults it is mainly caused by acute trauma or degenerative disease due to inflammatory pannus of rheumatoid arthritis. Superimposed infection can contribute to instability. Congenital conditions include Down syndrome, osteogenesis imperfecta, and neurofibromatosis. Congenital abnormalities do not become symptomatic before the third decade of life.

Grisel syndrome is defined as atlantoaxial subluxation following inflammation of adjacent soft tissues after a pharyngeal infection or surgical intervention. It is seen in children aged 5 to 12 years, though some cases are reported in adults. In patients with Down syndrome, the primary etiology of atlantoaxial instability is a laxity of the transverse ligament.

Diagnosis is facilitated through use of neuroimaging including x-ray, CT scan, or MRI.

Symptoms

Localization site	Comment
Cranial nerves	Lower cranial neuropathies
Cerebellum	Vertigo
Spinal cord	Myelopathy
Pyramidal signs	Hyperreflexia, positive Babinski, proprioceptive loss
Specific spinal roots	Radiculopathy

Treatment Complications: Unless symptoms of spinal cord compression present, no treatment is necessary. If symptomatic, cervical spine stabilization C1–C2 fusion can be considered. Postsurgical complications are possible.

Bibliography

Boden SD, Dodge LD, Bohlman HH, Rechtine GR. Rheumatoid arthritis of the cervical spine. A long-term analysis with predictors of paralysis and recovery. *J Bone Joint Surg Am.* 1993;75(9):1282–97.

Pueschel SM, Scola FH. Atlantoaxial instability in individuals with Down syndrome. Epidemiological, radiographic and clinical studies. *Pediatrics.* 1987;80(4):555–60.

Atonic Seizures (Akinetic Seizures or Drop Attacks)

Epidemiology and Demographics: Atonic seizures often begin in childhood, often in the context of multiple seizure types as part of certain types of epilepsy syndromes.

Disorder Description: Brief abrupt loss of muscle tone secondary to an epileptic seizure, with or without loss of consciousness; typically duration of <15 seconds. May result in falls or dropping of the head. Associated with generalized epilepsy syndromes, most commonly Lennox–Gastaut syndrome. Rarely the sole seizure type. EEG may show electrodecrement or slow, repetitive polyspike wave complexes. Valproate, lamotrigine, topiramate, rufinamide, and clobazam appear to be helpful, as well as corpus callosotomy or vagal nerve stimulation.

Symptoms

Localization site	Comment
Cerebral hemispheres	Drop attacks (abrupt loss of tone during seizures)

Secondary Complications: Injuries including head trauma, fractures, and dental damage secondary to unprotected falls.

Treatment Complications: Valproate side effects include weight gain, hyperactivity, transaminitis, thrombocytopenia, pancreatitis. The combination of valproate acid and lamotrigine may increase the risk of Stevens–Johnson syndrome. Topiramate is commonly associated with weight loss. Felbamate is associated with aplastic anemia and hepatic failure. Vagal nerve stimulation is most commonly associated with hoarseness. Corpus callosotomy may be associated with a disconnection syndrome.

Bibliography

Machado VH, Palmini A, Bastos FA, Rotert R. Long-term control of epileptic drop attacks with the combination of valproate, lamotrigine, and a benzodiazepine: a "proof of concept," open label study. *Epilepsia.* 2011;52(7): 1303–10.

Atrial Fibrillation

Epidemiology and Demographics: Atrial fibrillation (AF) is the most common arrhythmia seen, as approximately 33% of hospitalizations for arrhythmias are for AF. The incidence of AF in patients under the age of 40 years is 0.1%, while in patients over the age of 80 years, the incidence is over 1.5% for women and over 2.0% for men.

Disorder Description: Atrial fibrillation is a very rapid and irregular tachycardia of the atria leading to ineffective movement of blood into the ventricles. AF can run in families and is linked to several polymorphisms that affect proper conduction in the heart. Etiologies of AF include hyperthyroidism, mitral valve disease, myocardial ischemia/infarction, hypertension, hypertrophic obstructive cardiomyopathy, status post-open heart surgery, alcohol abuse, and other direct and indirect insults/abnormalities of the myocardium.

Symptoms

Localization site	Comment
Cerebral hemispheres	Embolic events that result from atrial fibrillation may cause focal injury and infarction to the following areas (*). In addition unabated rapid atrial fibrillation may cause presyncope/syncope
Mental status and psychiatric aspects/complications	*
Brainstem	*
Cerebellum	*
Vestibular system (and nonspecific dizziness)	*
Base of skull	*

Secondary Complications: When untreated, there is a 4- to 5-fold increase in thromboembolic events and a 2-fold increase in mortality associated with problems of the heart.

Treatment Complications: Complications of treatment include bleeding as a result of anticoagulation and thromboembolic events/cerebrovascular accidents/transient ischemic attacks as a result of a left atrial thrombus dislodging and traveling to the central nervous system. Anticoagulation either with warfarin or novel oral anticoagulants may help lower the incidence of cerebrovascular events in patients with AF. In addition, devices such as the Watchmen® (Boston Scientific) could be placed percutaneously via the transseptal approach and plug the left atrial appendage. In addition, the LARIAT® device (Sentreheart) may be used percutaneously to tie off the left atrial appendage using a pericardial and transseptal approach.

Bibliography

American Heart Association. What is atrial fibrillation (AFib or AF)? 2014. Available from www.heart.org/HEARTORG/Conditions/Arrhythmia/AboutArrhythmia/What-is-Atrial-Fibrillation-AFib-or-AF_UCM_423748_Article.jsp. Accessed Oct 5, 2018.

Morady F, Zipes DP. Atrial fibrillation: clinical features, mechanisms, and management. In Mann DL, Zipes DP, Libby P, Bonow RO, Braunwald E, eds. *Braunwald's heart disease: a textbook of cardiovascular medicine.* 10th ed. Philadelphia: Elsevier/Saunders; 2015. pp. 798–811.

Atrial Septal Defect

Epidemiology and Demographics: Disorders of the atrial septum occur in approximately 2/1000 live births, accounting for about 13% of congenital heart disorders. Most occur sporadically and are isolated defects; however, some are genetic (e.g., Holt–Oram syndrome). Foramen ovale does not completely seal in about 25% of adults.

Disorder Description: Congenital heart defect in which blood flows between the atria of the heart. Primum atrial septal defect (ASD) and secundum ASD are the two most common types of atrial septal defects. Pathophysiology depends on size of the defect, relationship between pulmonary and systemic resistances, and compliance of right and left ventricles. Differing pressure gradients between right and left atria may occur transiently, with oxygenated blood from left atrium recirculating into right atrium, or deoxygenated blood from right atrium entering into systemic circulation. Increases in right atrial pressure occur during early ventricular systole, during Valsalva maneuver, and with repetitive cough. In adults with an atrial septal defect, emboli from systemic circulation can pass through ASD (paradoxical embolus) and result in embolic stroke through right to left shunting. Additionally, patients with hemodynamically significant atrial septal defects may develop arrhythmias (e.g., atrial fibrillation), which is another source of emboli. While 25–40% of strokes are cryptogenic, identification of atrial septal defect in a patient does not prove a cause–effect relationship, as many patients have multiple potential sources for embolization. Therefore, stroke due to ASD is typically a diagnosis of exclusion. Should be considered as a cause of cryptogenic embolic stroke or transient ischemic attack in patients ≤60 years of age with no other identifiable cause. Risk factors include history of Valsalva maneuver (e.g., straining) prior to embolic event, history of multiple strokes, and hypercoagulable state.

Symptoms

Localization site	Comment
Cerebral hemispheres	Embolic stroke phenomenon, neuroimaging reveals infarcts in multiple vascular territories, or a single wedge-shaped infarct involving cortex and underlying subcortical white matter. Neurologic deficit is typically maximal from onset with a tendency to improve quickly

Secondary Complications: Arrhythmias, Eisenmenger syndrome, migraine with aura (possible link with right to left shunt, although evidence is conflicting).

Treatment Complications: Risk of intracerebral hemorrhage due to anticoagulation or antithrombotic therapy after stroke; acute deep vein thrombosis, pulmonary embolism. Closure of atrial septal defect for secondary prevention of recurrent stroke has not been established.

Bibliography

Anzola GP, Magoni M, Guindani M, et al. Potential source of cerebral embolism in migraine with aura: a transcranial Doppler study. *Neurology.* 1999;52:1622.

Del Sette M, Angeli S, Leandri M, et al. Migraine with aura and right-to-left shunt on transcranial Doppler: a case-control study. *Cerebrovasc Dis.* 1998;8:327.

Harvey JR, Teague SM, Anderson JL, et al. Clinically silent atrial septal defects with evidence for cerebral embolization. *Ann Intern Med.* 1986;105:695.

Kumar, V, Abbas AK, Fausto N, Mitchell RN, eds. *Robbins basic pathology.* 8th ed. Philadelphia: Saunders/Elsevier; 2007. p. 384.

Lamy C, Giannesini C, Zuber M, et al. Clinical and imaging findings in cryptogenic stroke patients with and without patent foramen ovale: the PFOASA Study. Atrial Septal Aneurysm. *Stroke.* 2002;33:706.

Meissner I, Whisnant JP, Khandheria BK, et al. Prevalence of potential risk factors for stroke assessed by transesophageal echocardiography and carotid ultrasonography: the SPARC study. Stroke Prevention: Assessment of Risk in a Community. *Mayo Clin Proc.* 1999;74:862.

Vaughan CJ, Basson CT. Molecular determinants of atrial and ventricular septal defects and patent ductus arteriosus. *Am J Med Genet.* 2000;97:304.

Attention Deficit Hyperactivity Disorder (ADHD)

Epidemiology and Demographics: Attention deficit hyperactivity disorder (ADHD) occurs in most cultures in approximately 5% of children and 2.5% of adults. More frequent in males than females, with a male to female ratio of 2:1 in children and 1.6:1 in adults. Females are more likely to present with inattentive features. Rarely, a genetic etiology can be identified (e.g., fragile X syndrome, 22q11 deletion syndrome).

Disorder Description: Defined by a persistent pattern of inattention and/or hyperactivity–impulsivity that has been present for at least 6 months and significantly interferes with functioning or development. Symptoms must be present prior to age 12 and occur in two or more settings (e.g., home, school, work). Furthermore, symptoms must be inconsistent with developmental level and are not better explained by another psychiatric disorder or the effects of a substance. Comorbid disorders are frequent and may include depression, anxiety, obsessive-compulsive disorder, tic disorders, autism spectrum disorders, substance use disorders, oppositional defiant disorder, conduct disorder (adolescents), or antisocial personality disorder (adults).

Symptoms

Localization site	Comment
Mental status and psychiatric aspects/complications	Inattention, hyperactivity, impulsivity, low frustration tolerance, irritability, mood lability, suicidality. Mild delays in speech, motor, or social development may occur

Secondary Complications: Depression, anxiety, substance use disorders, social rejection, interpersonal conflict, frequent injuries, impaired academic or work performance, unemployment, increased risk of suicide attempts by adulthood particularly when comorbid with mood, conduct, or substance use disorders.

Treatment Complications: Stimulants frequently used for the treatment of ADHD may result in insomnia, weight loss, worsening or new onset of tics, cardiovascular side effects, mood changes (e.g., irritability, dysphoria), psychosis (rare), as well as misuse and/or addiction.

Bibliography

American Psychiatric Association. *Diagnostic and statistical manual of mental disorders: DSM-5.* 5th ed. Washington, DC: American Psychiatric Association; 2013.

Polanczyk G, de Lima MS, Horta BL, et al. The worldwide prevalence of ADHD: a systematic review and metaregression analysis. *Am J Psychiatry.* 2007;164(6):942–48.

Atypical Facial Pain

Epidemiology and Demographics: Limited data available on frequency of atypical facial pain. Trigeminal neuralgia, a related form of this condition, is a more common form of this facial neuralgia. Trigeminal neuralgia has an incidence of 5/100,000 people. Another variant of this neuralgia is burning mouth syndrome, and the incidence is more common in middle-aged and older women with a prevalence rate of 0.6–12.22%.

Disorder Description: Atypical facial pain is also called persistent idiopathic facial pain (PIFP) and involves the territory of the trigeminal nerve. The etiology of this condition is unknown and the diagnosis is given when there is persistent facial pain with no known pain mechanism or underlying cause discovered. The pain is often described as deep in nature, poorly localized, and typically unilateral – often in the nasolabial fold or side of the chin. The pain does not follow classic dermatomal patterns and may spread to upper or lower jaw or a wider area of the face and neck. The pain is continuous, unlike other forms of neuralgia, with no periods of remission. There are no autonomic symptoms associated with this condition. The Headache Classification Subcommittee also defines this condition as having no association with sensory loss or other physical sign and no laboratory or imaging abnormalities.

Symptoms

Localization site	Comment
Cerebral hemispheres	Some studies suggest the role of dopaminergic pathways and their involvement in pain symptoms, especially in the basal ganglia. Often associated with depression and anxiety
Cranial nerves	Some studies suggest involvement of trigeminal nerve, but often the symptoms do not fit the classic dermatome and distribution of pain is diffuse

Secondary Complications: There are no established treatment modalities for this condition. Often, if the patient is not well informed on the pathophysiology of this disease, they are prone to seek multiple medical professionals for advice and diagnostic workup.

Treatment Complications: The mainstay of treatment is tricyclic antidepressants. Side effects associated with any tricyclic antidepressant can be a complication of treatment.

Bibliography

Macfarlane TV, Blinkhorn AS, Davies RM, et al. Oro-facial pain in the community: prevalence and associated impact. *Community Dent Oral Epidemiol.* 2002;30(1):52–60.

Obermann M, Holle D, Katsarava Z. Trigeminal neuralgia and persistent idiopathic facial pain. *Expert Rev Neurother.* 2011;11(11):1619–29.

Weiss AL, Ehrhardt KP, Tolba R. Atypical facial pain: a comprehensive, evidence-based review. *Curr Pain Headache Rep.* 2017;21(8):8.

Zakrzewska JM. Differential diagnosis of facial pain and guidelines for management. *Br J Anaesth.* 2013;111(1):95–104.

Atypical Parkinsonism (Parkinson's-Plus)

Epidemiology and Demographics: Of new patients seeking evaluation by movement disorder clinics in the United States, 71.5% are diagnosed with Parkinson's disease (PD), while the majority of the other 28.5% are diagnosed with Parkinson's-plus syndromes.[1] Parkinson's plus specifically means that patients have parkinsonism with coexisting signs and symptoms that are not typical for idiopathic Parkinson's disease. Parkinson's-plus syndromes include progressive supranuclear palsy (PSP), multiple system atrophy (MSA)/(formerly, Shy–Drager syndrome), corticobasal ganglionic degeneration (CBD), dementia with Lewy bodies (DLB), and parkinsonism–dementia–amyotrophic lateral sclerosis complex of Guam (PDACG) (see entries for *Parkinson's Disease* and *Amyotrophic Lateral Sclerosis (ALS)–Parkinsonism-Dementia Complex* for more information). The age-adjusted prevalence of PSP is estimated to be 1.39/100,000 in the United States, 1 to 6.5/100,000 in the United Kingdom, and 5.82/100,000 in Yonago, Japan.[2] The age-adjusted prevalence of MSA is estimated as being up to 4.4/100,000.[2] MSA is more common in men than women with symptoms typically beginning in the sixth decade. Smoking tobacco is significantly less frequent in MSA. Farming has been considered an independent risk factor for MSA. The prevalence of DLB among the general population is not clear, but DLB prevalence is estimated to be 3.8–4.5% of all diagnosed dementias.[2] CBD is a rare disease of unknown distribution.[1]

Disorder Description: Parkinson's-plus syndromes are hypokinetic neurodegenerative diseases pathologically associated with either a tauopathy or a synucleinopathy affecting multiple systems. Parkinson's-plus syndromes include PSP, MSA with subtypes MSA-P (formerly striatal nigral degeneration) or MSA-C (formerly, olivopontocerebellar atrophy), CBD, DLB, and PDACG. The main motor feature of Parkinson's-plus syndromes is bradykinesia with decrement and degradation of repetitive movements.[1]

PSP accounts for approximately 5% of parkinsonian patients in a typical movement disorder center. PSP is considered a tauopathy. It appears to be sporadic rather than genetic. It is often misdiagnosed as PD in the early stages because of marked rigidity and bradykinesia. However, unlike idiopathic PD, PSP presents with pronounced axial rigidity (especially in the neck) that is more pronounced than appendicular rigidity. A tremor may be present in 5–10%, but it is more common with action rather than at rest. Generally, the eye movement abnormalities, which are the hallmark of this condition, do not become evident until approximately 4 years after the onset of the disease.[3] Although the eye movements will eventually be affected in all directions of gaze, it begins as an impairment of down gaze. Another component to this diagnostic challenge is that in the early stages of PSP, approximately 40–50% of patients will have a mild transient response to levodopa.[3]

Gait and balance impairment with postural instability may occur early in the course of the disease, especially with frequent falls. Cognitive disturbance is also a prominent but early feature. There may be mental slowing, irritability, social withdrawal, and pseudobulbar affect or depression. Bradykinesia can manifest as start hesitation, freezing, motor blocks, and festinating gait. The cranial manifestations include stuttering, hypophonia, blepharospasm, eyelid apraxia, and severe dysarthria and dysphagia later in the course of the disease.[1,4] The typical appearance of a patient with PSP is that of a hyperextended neck and contracted facial muscles with a distinctive look of surprise.[1] In terms of diagnostic imaging, atrophy of the pons is better quantified on MRI by measuring the area on sagittal projection (less than 105 mm^2).[2] Pathologically, this condition has neurofibrillary tangles rather than Lewy bodies.

MSA is a sporadic synucleinopathy characterized by adult onset, progressive parkinsonism, dysautonomia, and cerebellar ataxia. These aspects of the disorder occur in combinations of varying severity, and MSA may be subcategorized by the predominant area affected. The dysautonomia-dominant condition was temporarily classified as MSA-A in 1996 and named Shy–Drager syndrome (SDS) prior to that (see entry for *Multiple System Atrophy [MSA; Shy-Drager Syndrome]* for more information).

As all patients diagnosed with MSA have progressive dysautonomia, this subtype has been dissolved into the other two subtypes. The parkinsonism-dominant type is MSA-P, which was previously named striatonigral degeneration (SND). Finally, the cerebellar ataxia-dominant subtype is MSA-C, which was previously identified as olivopontocerebellar atrophy (OPCA). Features of MSA-P include parkinsonism, with bradykinesia and rigidity, which is asymmetric at onset, and postural instability. As in other Parkinson's-plus syndromes, there is absence of classic tremor at rest. The onset is typically after age 40 years in the absence of a family history, and disease duration is typically less than 10 years. Approximately one-third to one-half of patients may have a good levodopa response at some point in their condition. Other features that distinguish MSA-P from PD include early onset of falling, severe dysarthria and dysphonia, obstructive sleep apnea, respiratory stridor, hyperreflexia, and extensor plantar responses. Survival ranges from 3 to 8 years. In MSA-C, there is progressive parkinsonism and cerebellar ataxia (wide gait) as well as atrophy of the ventral pons, inferior olives, and cerebellar cortex. Dystonia, specifically anterocollis, is not uncommonly seen in MSA.[1,2,5] Neuroimaging can be helpful in distinguishing MSA from other Parkinson's-plus disorders. The classic MRI in MSA reveals cruciform hyperintensity of the pontocerebellar fibers while sparing the corticospinal tracts on T2-weighted (T2W) MR. In MSA-P, there may also be infratentorial hyperintensity and cerebellar atrophy. In MSA-C neuroimaging, there typically is middle cerebellar peduncle atrophy and 4th ventricle dilation in addition to signs of cerebellar atrophy.[2] On positron emission tomography (PET), the pattern of neurodegeneration is often diagnostic.

Anal sphincter EMG indicates denervation secondary to loss of anterior horn cells in Onuf's nucleus. It is therefore a sensitive and specific diagnostic test for MSA.[3] With regard to pathology, glial cytoplasmic inclusions (GCIs), which are found in oligodendrocytes, are considered to be pathognomonic for MSA.[3]

Corticobasal ganglionic degeneration (CBD) is a tauopathy. It often presents as asymmetric hand clumsiness, which is the most common presenting symptom. It is characterized by asymmetric focal rigidity and dystonic posturing of the arm and hand with or without tremor. When tremor is present, it occurs with action, improves with rest, and may be associated with myoclonic jerking (which is stimulus sensitive). Ideomotor apraxia occurs commonly with this condition. Alien limb phenomenon occurs in about half of patients later on in the course of the disease.[3] This condition may be as simple as levitation, or more complex, where the limb is performing actions without the patient's voluntary control. The cognitive decline or cortical dementia may not always precede the motor symptoms. Other symptoms include cortical sensory deficit, language and speech changes, frontal lobe impairment, depression, apathy, irritability, and agitation. Survival ranges from 2.5 to 12.5 years.[1,2] Neuroimaging may reveal neurodegeneration predominantly in the frontoparietal cortex, basal ganglia, and substantia nigra and asymmetric enlargement of the lateral ventricles contralateral to the more affected side.[2]

DLB is the second most common cause of dementia in the elderly. DLB patients manifest parkinsonism and dementia with or without psychosis. The three essential features of DLB are fluctuations in cognitive performance, visual hallucinations, and parkinsonism. Fluctuations are a marked variation in a patient's cognition or decreased responsiveness fluctuating with lucidity.[3] Although visual hallucinations may be seen frequently with antiparkinsonian medication use, the visual hallucinations in DLB may also be attributable to the hypoperfusion of the occipital areas. Patients with DLB may be less responsive to levodopa or more susceptible to side effects. The cognitive problems of DLB have been classified as a subcortical dementia. Deficits in memory, attention, language, executive functions, and visuospatial and visuoconstructional abilities are prevalent. Supportive features include repeated falls, syncope, transient loss of consciousness, neuroleptic sensitivity, and systematized delusions and other aspects of psychosis. REM sleep behavior disorder is often associated with this condition.[3]

As in typical PD, there is neuronal loss in the substantia nigra in DLB as well as other subcortical structures.[2,6] On neuroimaging, the mesial temporal lobe, including the hippocampus, is relatively spared compared with imaging of patients with Alzheimer's dementia. Studies have found changes in the subcortical regions with striatal and putaminal atrophy as well as hypoperfusion of the occipital lobes on functional imaging.[2]

Symptoms

Localization site	Comment
Cerebral hemispheres	CBD – ideomotor apraxia in supplemental motor area
	CBD – degeneration of cortical sensory and motor areas. Focal cortical myoclonus, mirror movements, hyperreflexia, Babinski sign
Mental status and psychiatric aspects/ complications	MSA-P associated with mild memory and executive function impairment
	MSA-C associated with emotionality, anxiety, and a tendency toward depression with or without a cognitive decline
Brainstem	CBD – oculomotility disturbance in the form of impaired convergence, vertical and horizontal gaze palsy – increased horizontal saccade latency
	PSP – pons atrophy and dilated 3rd ventricle on sagittal neuroimaging, referred to as the "hummingbird" or "penguin silhouette" sign
	MSA – cruciform hyperintensity referred to as "hot cross bun" sign on transverse T2W neuroimaging due to degeneration of pontocerebellar fibers while sparing the corticospinal tracts
Cerebellum	Cerebellar ataxia in MSA-C and middle cerebellar peduncle atrophy with 4th ventricle dilation
Vestibular system (and nonspecific dizziness)	Dizziness seen with MSA may be secondary to orthostasis

Depression and anxiety are often comorbid with these disorders and can often precede the motor symptoms, making the diagnosis challenging. Visual hallucinations are also prominent in diffuse Lewy body dementia and can therefore be mistaken for psychosis.

Secondary Complications: Aspiration pneumonia can result from dysphagia, and complications sustained from a fall are the usual causative factors that lead to mortality.

Treatment Complications: Please refer to complications in the entry *Parkinson's Disease* with regard to medication use.

References

1. Jankovic J, Rajput AH, McDermott MP, Perl DP. The evolution of diagnosis in early Parkinson disease. Parkinson Study Group. *Arch Neurol.* 2000;57(3):369–72.
2. Dąbrowska M, Schinwelski M, Sitek EJ, et al. The role of neuroimaging in the diagnosis of the atypical parkinsonian syndromes in clinical practice. *Neurol Neurochir Pol.* 2015;49(6):421–31.
3. Mark M. Lumping and splitting the Parkinson plus syndromes. *Neurol Clin.* 2001;19(3):607–27.
4. Arena J, Weigand SD, Whitwell JL, et al. Progressive supranuclear palsy: progression and survival. *J Neurol.* 2016;263(2):380–9.
5. Köllensperger M, Geser F, Ndayisaba JP, et al. Presentation, diagnosis, and management of multiple system atrophy in Europe: final analysis of the European multiple system atrophy registry. *Mov Disord.* 2010;25(15):2604–12.
6. McKeith IG, Dickson DW, Lowe J, et al. Diagnosis and management of dementia with Lewy bodies. Third report of the DLB consortium. *Neurology.* 2005;65;1863–72.

Autism Spectrum Disorder

Epidemiology and Demographics: Prevalence numbers for autism spectrum disorder (ASD) have progressively increased over recent decades. It is unclear how much of this is due to a truly increased prevalence rate versus increased awareness and identification of cases and inclusion of more subtle cases. Currently, ASD is felt to affect approximately 1% of the population[1] and is more common in males. Symptoms develop in the early developmental period but may not be appreciated until later in life. The term "spectrum" connotes the wide range of severity and presentations that fit within this disorder.

Disorder Description: Autism spectrum disorder is a clinical diagnosis based on the identification of specific symptoms and signs that meet criteria for the condition. As described in DSM-5,[2] ASD is characterized by "persistent deficits in social communication and social interaction." This involves problems in "social reciprocity, nonverbal communicative behaviors used for social interactions, and skills in developing, maintaining, and understanding relationships." These may be subtle as in "failure of normal back-and-forth conversation" or "failure to initiate or respond to social interactions." Impairments in

communication may be verbal and non-verbal such as abnormal eye contact and failure to comprehend or use communicative gestures. Varying severity of impairment in "developing, maintaining and understanding relationships" is noted.

DSM-5 also describes "restricted, repetitive patterns of behavior, interests, or activities." Repetitive motor activity and stereotypies may occur. Other features include ritualized behaviors, excessive fixations and highly restricted interests, and exaggerated or severely diminished reactions to sensory input.

Symptoms impair daily functioning. DSM-5 envelops disorders previously cited in DSM-IV such as Asperger's disorder (high functioning autism), pervasive developmental disorder not otherwise specified (PDD-NOS), and childhood disintegrative disorder.[1]

There is no unifying etiology or theory of pathogenesis, although a complex interaction between genetics and environmental factors is posited.[3] There is no evidence to support the notion that vaccines are etiologically responsible.

Symptoms

Impairment	Comment (examples)
Social communication	Failure to exhibit normal facial expressions, bodily movements, or verbal responses expected in social communication. Appearing not to appreciate needs or social experiences of others
Communication	Verbal skills acquired late or never acquired. Language production sounds abnormal and lacks spontaneous fluidity. Diverse abnormalities such as abnormal sound quality or repetitive nonsensical-sounding word or phrase repetition. Words or sounds that are incomprehensible. Abnormal social use of language
Restricted behaviors and interests	Stereotypies such as repetitive hand clapping or flapping are classic. Rigid adherence to eating the same kind of food or peculiar preoccupations. Attachments to odd types of objects
Cognition	Often impaired to varying degrees and often with more severe deficits in some domains compared with others

Adapted from discussion in reference 1.

Secondary Complications: Numerous potential comorbidities with assorted degrees of severity in areas including intellectual impairments, language deficits, behavioral problems, and the symptoms and signs that may accompany associated potential "medical/genetic or environmental/acquired" conditions.[2] These may include deficits in many neurologic functions including motoric, sensory, cognitive, language-based, and coordination systems. Hyperactivity, attentional difficulties, and impulsive behaviors are common. There is a heightened risk of seizures with widely varying estimates depending in part on other coexisting conditions. One series suggests that 44% of children with ASD will ultimately receive a diagnosis of epilepsy.[4]

Treatment Complications: Psychosocial interventions are often instituted and intensive language and behavioral interventions early on in life may be helpful.[5] Psychopharmacologic interventions can be helpful to treat the comorbidities associated with autism (e.g., attention deficit hyperactivity disorder). However, there are numerous potential adverse effects of pharmacotherapy used for aberrant behaviors and emotional symptoms. The reader is directed to the pharmacology section of this text for reviews of adverse events associated with drug classes including neuroleptics, anxiolytics (e.g., benzodiazepines), selective serotonin reuptake inhibitors (SSRIs), and selective serotonin-norepinephrine reuptake inhibitors (SNRIs). Antiepileptic drugs such as valproate are also sometimes tried.[6]

References

1. Bostic JQ, Prince JB, Buxton DC. Child and adolescent psychiatric disorders. In Stern T, Fava M, Wilens T, Rosenbaum J, eds. *Massachusetts General Hospital comprehensive clinical psychiatry*. London: Elsevier; 2015. pp. 741–45.
2. American Psychiatric Association. Autism spectrum disorder. In *Diagnostic and statistical manual of mental disorders: DSM-5*. 5th ed. Washington, DC: American Psychiatric Association; 2013. pp. 50–9.
3. Rutter M. Changing concepts and findings on autism. *J Autism Dev Disorder*. 2013;43:1749–57.
4. Kasari C. Update on behavioral interventions for autism and developmental disabilities. *Curr Opin Neurol*. 2015;28:124–9.
5. Jokiranta E, Sourander A, Suominen A, et al. Epilepsy among children and adolescents with autism spectrum disorders: a population-based study. *J Autism Dev Disord*. 2013;44(10):2547–57.
6. Baribeau DA, Anagnostou E. An update on medication management of behavioral disorders in autism. *Curr Psych Rep*. 2014;16:437–50.

Avoidant/Restrictive Food Intake Disorder

Epidemiology and Demographics: Prevalence of avoidant/restrictive food intake disorder varies from 5% to 23% in tertiary treatment settings. More common in children than adults. Equal in males and females in the general population; more common in males when comorbid with autism spectrum disorder. Increased risk with anxiety disorders, obsessive-compulsive disorder, neurodevelopmental disorders (e.g., autism spectrum disorders, attention deficit hyperactivity disorder, intellectual disability), gastrointestinal disease, and child abuse/neglect.

Disorder Description: Avoidance or restriction of food intake manifested by persistent failure to meet appropriate nutritional and/or energy needs associated with one or more of the following: significant weight loss (or failure to achieve expected weight gain), significant nutritional deficiency, dependence on enteral feeding or oral nutritional supplements, or marked interference with psychosocial functioning. The symptoms are not better explained by developmentally normal behaviors, lack of available food, cultural practices, underlying medical condition, or another psychiatric or eating disorder.

Symptoms

Localization site	Comment
Mental status and psychiatric aspects/complications	Lack of interest in eating or food, heightened sensitivity to textures of food, fear of consequences of eating (e.g., choking), anxiety, obsessive-compulsive traits, emotional rigidity

Secondary Complications: Physiologic disturbances due to malnutrition and dehydration, impaired development and learning, anorexia nervosa (rare), death due to medical complications.

Treatment Complications: During aggressive nutritional rehabilitation of malnourished patients, fluid and electrolyte shifts can cause refeeding syndrome, which is potentially fatal.

Bibliography

American Psychiatric Association. *Diagnostic and statistical manual of mental disorders: DSM-5.* 5th ed. Washington, DC: American Psychiatric Association; 2013.

Mairs R, Nicholls D. Assessment and treatment of eating disorders in children and adolescents. *Arch Dis Child.* 2016;101(12):1168–75.

Babesiosis

Epidemiology and Demographics: Median age 62, range of age <1 to 103. Approximately two-thirds are male.[1] Babesiosis may occur in all seasons, but mostly in spring and summer when ticks thrive.[1,2]

Disorder Description: Babesiosis is caused by intraerythrocytic protozoa that are transmitted by ixodid ticks. Most common is *Babesia microti*, which is found in the northeastern and midwestern United States and in Europe. Infection is either through cytokine inflammation or adherence to vascular endothelium.[1,2]

Risk factors include being bitten by an infected tick in outdoor activities, congenitally through vaginal delivery, blood transfusions, or immunocompromised states.[2]

Symptoms

Localization site	Comment
Cerebral hemispheres	Headache
Mental status and psychiatric aspects/ complications	Coma (rare) Lethargy
Muscle	Myalgias

Secondary Complications: Complications may include disseminated intravascular coagulation (DIC), which may cause intracranial hemorrhage or other systemic bleeding.[1,2]

Treatment Complications: Clindamycin and quinine may cause vertigo and hearing loss.[3]

References

1. Centers for Disease Control and Prevention. *Babesiosis*. Atlanta, GA: CDC; 2014. Available from www.cdc.gov/parasites/babesiosis/data-statistics/index.html.
2. Usmani-Brown S, Halperin J, Krause P. Neurological manifestations of human babesiosis. *Handb Clin Neurol*. 2013;114:199–203.
3. Krause P, Lepore T, Sikand V, et al. Atovaquone and azithromycin for the treatment of babesiosis. *N Engl J Med*. 2000;343(20):1454–58.

Back Strain/Sprain

Epidemiology and Demographics: In the United States 7–13% of all sports injuries in college athletes are of the low back, the most common being muscle strain 60% and disc injury 7%. American football and gymnastics participants are at high risk of low back injury.

Disorder Description: Sprains are caused by a sudden violent contraction, which results in ligamentous injuries. All major components can sustain sprain, but longitudinal ligaments are more prone. Trauma, disease, and surgery are further causes.

Symptoms

Localization site	Comment
Lower back	Pain and spasms localized over the posterior lumbar spine muscles. Range of motion may be restricted and flexion in particular is usually painful and decreased

Workup usually not indicated in routine cases. However, x-rays can be done to rule out degenerative or neoplastic causes. If no response to treatment, CT scan/MRIs can be performed.

Secondary Complications: Chronic low back pain has been associated with depression.

Treatment Complications: Physical therapy, nonsteroidal anti-inflammatories, and lightweight lumbosacral corset. Robaxin, which is used as a muscle relaxant, can cause drowsiness, light-headedness, seizures, and sedation.

Bibliography

Gourmelen J, Chastang JF, Ozguler A, et al. Frequency of low back pain among men and women age 30 to 64 years in France. Results of two national surveys. *Med Phys*. 2007;50(8):640–4.

Noonan DJ, Garrett WE Jr. Muscle sprain injury diagnosis and treatment. *J Am Acad Orthop Surg*. 1999;7(4):262–9.

Bacteroides

Epidemiology and Demographics: Meningitis occurs mostly in the very young or elderly people.[1]

Disorder Description: *Bacteroides* species are anaerobic, bile-resistant, non-spore-forming, gram-negative rods that are components of the normal flora of the mucous membranes.[2] Infection usually occurs when mucosal barriers break down or immune defense is compromised. *Bacteroides* infections can develop in all body sites, including the central nervous system. Its capsule is thought to initiate an immune response, resulting in abscess formation.[1,2] Brain abscesses may be formed by *Bacteroides* species from spread of infection from the paranasal sinuses. Risk factors include ventriculoperitoneal shunts and poor oral hygiene.

Symptoms[1,3]

Localization site	Comment
Cerebral hemispheres	Abscesses
Spinal cord	Epidural abscess

Secondary Complications: Seizures.

References

1. Ngan C, Tan A. *Bacteroides fragilis* meningitis. *Singapore Med J.* 1994;35:283–5.
2. Wexler H. *Bacteroides*: the good, the bad, and the nitty-gritty. *Clin Microbiol Rev.* 2007;20(4):593–621.
3. Miller N, Burton F, Walsh F, Hoyt W. *Walsh and Hoyt's clinical neuro-ophthalmology*. Philadelphia: Wolters Kluwer Health/Lippincott Williams & Wilkins; 2004. p. 2714.

Balint Syndrome

Epidemiology and Demographics: The epidemiology of Balint syndrome is unclear.

Disorder Description: Balint syndrome refers to a triad of simultagnosia, ocular apraxia, and optic ataxia, described classically in patients with bilateral lesions of the parieto-occipital cortex. Causes include watershed infarctions, tumor, trauma, neurodegenerative causes such as Alzheimer's disease, and infectious causes such as Creutzfeldt–Jakob disease.

Simultagnosia refers to an inability to attend to multiple visual stimuli simultaneously, and in particular impaired switching of attention between local details and global structure. Specifically, Mevorach et al. posit that a failure of top-down directed attention causes simultagnosia, through impaired ability to shift attention from one level of processing to another.[1] For example, a patient with simultagnosia when presented with the American flag, may identify stars and stripes without being able to identify the entire object as a flag. To assess for simultagnosia, the patient can be asked to describe a complex visual scene such as the Boston Cookie Theft picture, or a hierarchical figure such as Navon's figure (a large number or letter made up of smaller numbers or letters). Significantly, simultagnosia may cause impairment with reading (alexia), and the patient may be able to read single letters, but not words.[2] Computational models predict that a disconnection between the dorsal "where/how" visual pathway and the ventral "what" visual pathway could cause this syndrome.[3]

Ocular apraxia, initially termed by Balint a "psychic paralysis of gaze,"[4] refers to an inability to voluntarily direct eye movements to a new visual target. When asked to look at an object, the patient is unable to follow the command. The deficit in eye movement is not due to neglect and not confined to a particular side. Indeed, the patient's eyes can move spontaneously in all quadrants.[2]

Optic ataxia refers to an inability to reach the hand toward an object under visual guidance, despite intact motor function and intact visual acuity. To assess for optic ataxia, the patient can be asked to touch the examiner's ear, while looking at the examiner's nose.[5]

The three features of Balint syndrome may occur in isolation or in combination with each other, suggesting distinct underlying physiologic substrates. As we gain more understanding of these underlying mechanisms, the existence of Balint syndrome as a fixed triad archetype is increasingly called into question.[4]

Symptoms: Simultagnosia, ocular apraxia, and optic ataxia.

Secondary Complications: The higher-order perceptual deficits of Balint syndrome can cause significant difficulties with activities of daily living (ADLs), as well as profound difficulties with ambulation, leading to falls and injuries. Occupational therapy and adaptive strategies are important for preventing these complications.

Treatment Complications: Balint syndrome deficits are managed symptomatically, and adaptive measures are critical for recovery of function and maintenance of independence. Examples of adaptive strategies include putting bright yellow tape on edges of objects such as cabinets to distinguish them from the background, putting toothpaste directly in the mouth rather than on the toothbrush, and using audiobooks to compensate for alexia.[6]

References

1. Mevorach C, Shalev L, Green RJ, et al. Hierarchical processing in Balint's syndrome: a failure of flexible top-down attention. *Front Hum Neurosci.* 2014;8:113.
2. Finney GR. Perceptual-motor dysfunction. *Continuum (Minneap Minn).* 2015;21: 678–89.
3. O'Reilly RC, Munakata Y, Frank MJ, et al. *Computational cognitive neuroscience.* Wiki Book. Available from http:/ccnbook .colorado.edu
4. Moreaud O. Balint syndrome. *Arch Neurol.* 2003;60:1329.
5. Cavina-Pratesi C, Connolly JD, Milner AD. Optic ataxia as a model to investigate the role of the posterior parietal cortex in visually guided action: evidence from studies of patient M.H. *Front Hum Neurosci.* 2013;7:336.
6. Cuomo J, Flaster M, Biller J. Right brain: a descriptive account of two patients' experience with and adaptations to Balint syndrome. *Neurology.* 2012;79:e95–96.

Bariatric Surgery

Epidemiology and Demographics: Obesity is a problem in the United States, with an estimated 30% prevalence. Bariatric surgery is considered one of the most effective long-term treatments for obesity and thus has been gaining popularity. The number of procedures done in the United States has been increasing over recent years, estimated at more than 180,000 procedures done per year.

Disorder Description: The incidence of neurologic complications after bariatric surgery has been estimated at between 2 and 5%. Mechanisms by which neurologic complications happen are nutritional deficiencies (most common by far) and mechanical and entrapment neuropathies during the procedure or as a result of rapid weight loss.

Symptoms and Psychiatric Aspects/Complications

Localization site	Comment
Cerebral hemispheres	Wernicke's encephalopathy (vitamin B1) Korsakoff syndrome (vitamin B1)
Cranial nerves	Optic neuropathy
Spinal cord	Myelopathy
Specific spinal roots	Polyradiculoneuropathy
Plexus	Plexopathy
Mononeuropathy or mononeuropathy multiplex	Entrapment neuropathies
Peripheral neuropathy	Distal symmetric polyneuropathy Small fiber neuropathy
Muscle	Myopathy

Bibliography

Becker DA, Balcer LJ, Galetta SL. The neurological complications of nutritional deficiency following bariatric surgery. *J Obes.* 2012;2012:608534.

Juhasz-Pocsine K, Rudnicki SA, Archer RL, Harik SI. Neurologic complications of gastric bypass surgery for morbid obesity. *Neurology.* 2007;68(21):1843–50.

Koffman BM, Greenfield LJ, Ali II, Pirzada NA. Neurologic complications after surgery for obesity. *Muscle Nerve.* 2006;33(2):166–76.

Landais A. Neurological complications of bariatric surgery. *Obes Surg.* 2014;24(10):1800–7.

Basilar Invagination

Epidemiology and Demographics: Basilar invagination is a very rare condition. Specific epidemiologic information is not available.

Disorder Description: Basilar invagination is defined as infolding of the base of the skull that occurs when the top of the C2 vertebra migrates upward. It can cause narrowing of the foramen magnum. It can be present at birth. If after birth, it is usually the result of injury or disease. Motor vehicle and bicycle accidents can result in basilar invagination. Basilar invagination can be seen in rheumatoid arthritis, osteomalacia, Paget's disease, Ehlers–Danlos syndrome, Marfan syndrome, osteogenesis imperfecta. Workup includes x-rays, CT/MRI.

Platybasia is a developmental anomaly of the cranium or an acquired softening of the cranial bones such that the floor of the posterior cranial fossa bulges upward in the region around the foramen magnum.

Symptoms

Localization site	Comment
Cerebral hemispheres	Confusion
Mental status and psychiatric aspects	Confusion
Brainstem	Dysarthria, deficits of lower cranial nerves
Cerebellum	Vertigo
Cervical spine	Lhermitte sign, pain, pseudo-ulnar hand with tingling and numbness in the fourth and fifth digits

Treatment Complications: If no neurologic symptoms, consider treatment with nonsteroidal anti-inflammatories (see *Medication Adverse Effects* section for potential complications). Cervical collar and/or traction is recommended. If symptomatic, surgery is recommended

Bibliography

Chaudrhry NS, Ozpinar A, Bi WL, et al. Basilar invagination: case report and literature review. *World Neurosurg.* 2015;83:e7–111.

Smith JS, Shaffrey CI, Abel MF, Menezes AH. Basilar invagination. *Neurosurgery.* 2010;66:A39–A47.

Becker Muscular Dystrophy

Epidemiology and Demographics: Becker muscular dystrophy (BMD) is an X-linked disease that has an incidence reported as approximately one-tenth to one-fifth that of Duchenne muscular dystrophy (DMD). Boys are more affected than girls. Weakness may begin as early as 5 to 6 years of age or may start in the fifth or sixth decade. There is no major geographic distribution for BMD.

Disorder Description: BMD and DMD occur as a result of mutations (mainly deletions) in the dystrophin gene DMD. Variable phenotypic expression relates mainly to the type of mutation and its effects on the production of dystrophin.

BMD is an X-linked recessive mutation in the DMD gene located at Xp21.2. Mutations lead to a defect in the protein dystrophin, which results in progressive muscle degeneration. Diagnosis is based on genetic analysis.

Symptoms

Localization site	Comment
Cerebral hemispheres	In BMD, intellectual function is generally normal, although learning disabilities are slightly more common
Muscles	Delayed motor milestones and falls, along with difficulty running and jumping starting at age 5–6 years. By convention, at age of 12 years should be ambulatory. Less severe than DMD. On average, older onset of disease correlates with slower progression of weakness. Patient also can present with isolated hyperCKemia, limb-girdle phenotype

Secondary Complications: Less common than in DMD; however, they can present with joint contractures, cardiac involvement that is not correlated with the degree of muscle weakness, and respiratory dysfunction that tends to be milder in BMD than in DMD.

Treatment Complications: There is no cure for BMD, and management is largely supportive. There is some discussion of whether steroids can slow the progression, but usually they are not used.

Management of BMD requires a multidisciplinary health care team as in DMD. Mean life span is shortened for men with major cardiac and diaphragmatic involvement. Corticosteroids are not typically indicated.

Bibliography

Bushby K. Diagnosis and management of Duchenne muscular dystrophy, part 1: diagnosis, and pharmacological and psychosocial management. *Lancet Neurol.* 2010;9:77–93.

Hendriksen JG, Vles JS. Neuropsychiatric disorders in males with Duchenne muscular dystrophy: frequency rate of attention-deficit hyperactivity disorder (ADHD), autism spectrum disorder, and obsessive compulsive disorder. *J Child Neurol.* 2008;23(5):477–81.

Benign Epilepsy of Childhood with Centrotemporal Spikes (BECTS; Rolandic Epilepsy)

Epidemiology and Demographics: Incidence of benign epilepsy of childhood with centrotemporal spikes (BECTS) is 1–2/10,000, occurring between 1 and 14 years of age, peak incidence 7–10 years. Male-to-female ratio is 3:2.

Disorder Description: Hemifacial sensorimotor partial seizures often with oropharyngolaryngeal or brachial involvement, anarthria, and hypersalivation. May progress to loss of consciousness and more hemi- or full-body convulsive activity. Most frequently occurring during non-REM sleep. Syndrome linked to chromosomes 11p13 and 15q14. Remission before age 16 years. Neurologic examination and neuroimaging typically normal, though Todd's paralysis may occur. Antiepileptic drugs (AEDs) may be deferred in relatively milder cases, though rescue medications such as benzodiazepines may be considered.

Symptoms

Localization site	Comment
Cerebral hemispheres	Focal sensorimotor, complex partial, and secondarily generalized seizures originating from the Rolandic cortex Postictal paresis may occur EEG with bilaterally independent centrotemporal epileptiform discharges. MRI normal
Mental status and psychiatric aspects/complications	Mild linguistic, cognitive, and behavioral disturbances may be observed around the time that seizures manifest. Prognosis for later development and social and occupational functioning is excellent

Treatment Complications: AEDs, if utilized, are associated with a number of idiosyncratic reactions. Opercular focal status epilepticus has been precipitated with the use of lamotrigine or carbamazepine in this condition. Benzodiazepines may be associated with excessive sedation, hypotension, or respiratory depression.

Bibliography

Berkovic SF. Genetics of epilepsy in clinical practice. *Epilepsy Curr.* 2015;15(4):192–6.

Benign Familial Infantile Convulsions and Choreoathetosis (ICCA)

Epidemiology and Demographics: Rare. Onset between birth and 17 months. Autosomal dominant inheritance, though sporadic mutations may occur.

Disorder Description: Infantile onset convulsions that resolve by age 2, then paroxysmal kinesigenic dyskinesias occurring later in childhood or adolescence. Movements may include choreoathetosis, ballism, or dystonia induced by abrupt voluntary action lasting 5 seconds to 5 minutes. Due to mutations in the proline-rich transmembrane protein 2 (PRRT2) gene on chromosome 16, affecting synaptic neurotransmitter release. Mutations in PRRT2 may also be responsible for the syndromes of benign familial infantile seizures (BFIS), paroxysmal kinesigenic dyskinesia (in the absence of seizures), and hemiplegic migraine. Both seizures and dyskinesias may respond to phenytoin, carbamazepine, and topiramate.

Symptoms

Localization site	Comment
Cerebral hemispheres	Focal and secondarily generalized convulsions in infancy. Interictal EEG usually normal, though focal epileptiform discharges may be observed
Mental status and psychiatric aspects/complications	Intellectual disability is uncommon, but may occur with biallelic mutations
Basal ganglia	Kinesigenic choreoathetosis, ballism, or dystonia
Unclear localization	Migraines with aura may occur

Treatment Complications: Antiepileptic drugs may be associated with a number of idiosyncratic reactions. Phenytoin and carbamazepine may cause rash or abnormalities in blood counts, hepatic function, and bone density. Topiramate may cause metabolic acidosis, anorexia, closed angle glaucoma, and nephrolithiasis.

Bibliography

Becker F, Schubert J, Striano P, et al. PRRT2-related disorders: further PKD and ICCA cases and review of the literature. *J Neurol*. 2013;260(5):1234–44.

Ebrahimi-Fakhari D, Saffari A, Westenberger A, et al. The evolving spectrum of PRRT2-associated paroxysmal diseases. *Brain*. 2015;138(Pt 12):3476–95.

Benign Familial Neonatal Infantile Seizures (BFNIS)

Epidemiology and Demographics: Onset between 2 days and 7 months old. Autosomal dominant inheritance.

Disorder Description: Generalized afebrile convulsions in early infancy, which usually resolve by age 12 months. Associated with mutations in the sodium channel neuronal type 2 alpha subunit (SCN2A) gene on chromosome 2. Antiepileptic drugs (AEDs) often successful at reducing seizures, repetitive convulsions, and risk for status epilepticus. Long-term treatment is not usually necessary.

Genetically distinguished from the phenotypically similar autosomal dominant syndromes of benign familial infantile seizures (BFIS) with focal onset seizures in later infancy due to mutations on chromosomes 1, 16, or 19; and benign familial neonatal seizures (BFNS) with convulsions in the first week of life due to mutations in the voltage-gated potassium channel.

Symptoms

Localization site	Comment
Cerebral hemispheres	Focal and generalized convulsions in infancy. Interictal EEG normal, sometimes with posterior temporal parietal epileptiform discharges
Mental status and psychiatric aspects/complications	Intellectual development normal

Treatment Complications: AEDs may be associated with a number of idiosyncratic reactions, including multiorgan issues, and possible long-term cognitive effects.

Bibliography

Alam S, Lux AL. Epilepsies in infancy. *Arch Dis Child*. 2012;97(11):985–92.

Nabbout R, Dulac O. Epileptic syndromes in infancy and childhood. *Curr Opin Neurol*. 2008;21(2):161–6.

Benign Familial Neonatal Seizures (BFNS)

Epidemiology and Demographics: Occurring in the first week of life and remitting by 4 months. Autosomal dominant inheritance.

Disorder Description: Familial neonatal focal or generalized convulsions, which may be associated with ocular findings or apnea. Linked to abnormalities in the voltage-gated potassium channel genes KCNQ2 on chromosome 20q13.3 and KCNQ3 on chromosome 8q24, resulting in neuronal hyperexcitability. Antiepileptic drugs (AEDs) such as phenytoin, phenobarbital, or valproate are often successful at reducing seizures, repetitive convulsions, and risk for status epilepticus. Long-term treatment is not usually necessary. Childhood seizures may develop in 10–15% of cases.

Symptoms

Localization site	Comment
Cerebral hemispheres	Focal or generalized seizures. EEG may be normal or show transient multifocal abnormalities
Mental status and psychiatric aspects/complications	Neurocognitive development is usually normal
Unclear localization	Apnea

Treatment Complications: AEDs may be associated with a number of idiosyncratic reactions, including multiorgan issues, and possible long-term cognitive effects.

Bibliography

Cilio MR. Neonatal seizures. *Paediatr Child Health*. 2009;19:S28–S31.

Benign Fasciculation Syndrome

Epidemiology and Demographics: Fasciculations are common, and spontaneous fasciculations can occur in up to 70% of people. Some of these patients will have relatively frequent fasciculations that may be widespread or relatively focal and may be accompanied by cramps (see entry for *Muscle Cramps*). There is no sex, age, or geographic predominance.

Disorder Description: Fasciculations are defined as a brief, spontaneous contraction affecting a small number of muscle fibers, often causing a flicker of movement under the skin. While it can be associated with motor neuron disease, it can occur spontaneously and is benign in most people.

Benign fasciculation syndrome is likely metabolic in origin, although exact etiology is not clear. Magnesium deficiency has been thought to contribute. Medication side effect is possible.

Nerve conduction studies will be normal, as will electromyography for the most part. There should be no clinical weakness.

Symptoms

Localization site	Comment
Mental status and psychiatric aspects/complications	It can cause distress/anxiety to some patients
Muscle	Benign fasciculations, **not** associated with weakness

Treatment: Magnesium supplementation has been used to treat benign fasciculation syndrome, though there are no supporting studies. Most of treatment is based on anxiety control.

Bibliography

Amato AA, Russell JA. *Neuromuscular disorders*. New York: McGraw-Hill; 2008. pp. 143–56.

Blexrud MD, Windebank AJ, Daube JR. Long-term follow-up of 121 patients with benign fasciculations. *Ann Neurol.* 1993;34:622.

Longo DL, Kasper DL, Fauci A, et al., eds. *Harrison's principles of internal medicine*. 17th ed. New York: McGraw-Hill; 2016. pp. 1292, 1412, 1462–1464

Benign Paroxysmal Positional Vertigo (BPPV; Benign Positional Vertigo)

Epidemiology and Demographics: Sporadic disorder of the inner ear. Usually idiopathic but may follow head concussion or chronic otitis media. Equal gender distribution. The prevalence of benign paroxysmal positional vertigo (BPPV) in the United States is approximately 64/100,000.

Disorder Description: Brief episodes of spinning vertigo, lasting less than 1 minute, elicited by the head-hanging position with the affected ear down. Vertigo typically occurs when turning in bed, reaching for the top shelf, or stooping. Some cases are preceded by a typical episode of acute vestibular neuritis (see entry for *Vestibular Neuritis*).

The pathophysiology is canalithiasis, or microparticles of calcium entrapped within the limb of the posterior semicircular canal. These calcium particles are dislodged otoliths from the utricle or saccule. Variants include cupulolithiasis, in which particles adhere to the vestibular end-organ, and lateral and anterior semicircular canal BPPV, in which the inciting position varies.

Symptoms

Localization site	Comment
Inner ear	Canalithiasis, or microparticles of calcium carbonate, trapped within lumen of the posterior semicircular canal
Cranial nerves	The cochleovestibular nerve is not affected
Central nervous system	The central nervous system is not affected

Secondary Complications: Sudden onset of positional vertigo may pose risk of injury from falling, and may create a hazard for driving.

Treatment Complications: BPPV is effectively treated with a particle repositioning procedure ("Epley maneuver," named for its originator) in which the head is placed in the inciting position and then rotated 180 degrees, so as to redistribute the particles out of the posterior semicircular canal. Untreated cases will usually resolve spontaneously after about 3 months. Surgical occlusion of the posterior semicircular canal can be performed in refractory cases. Physical therapy can cause neck injury. Surgical therapy can cause sensorineural hearing loss or prolonged continuous vertigo.

Bibliography

Epley JM. The canalith repositioning procedure: for treatment of benign paroxysmal positional vertigo. *Otolaryngol Head Neck Surg.* 1992;107:399–404.

Furman JM, Cass SP. Benign paroxysmal positional vertigo. *N Engl J Med.* 1999;341(21):1590–6.

Fife TD, Iverson DJ, Lempert T, et al. Practice parameter: therapies for benign paroxysmal positional vertigo (an evidence-based review): report of the Quality Standards Subcommittee of the American Academy of Neurology. *Neurology.* 2008;70(22):2067–74.

Smouha EE. Time course of recovery after Epley maneuvers for benign paroxysmal positional vertigo. *Laryngoscope.* 1997;107:187–91.

Binge Eating Disorder

Epidemiology and Demographics: Female predominance, with lifetime prevalence of 3.5% in women versus 2% in men. Binge eating behaviors have been observed in children and are commonly seen in adolescents and young adults.

Disorder Description: Characterized per the DSM-5 as recurrent episodes of binge eating as defined by eating a significantly larger portion of food within a discrete time period (e.g., 2 hours) along with lack of sense of control of eating behavior. Episodes are associated with three or more of the following: (1) eating much faster than normal, (2) eating until uncomfortably full, (3) eating large amounts when not feeling hungry, (4) eating alone because of embarrassment about quantity of food intake, (5) feeling disgusted with self, depressed, or excessively guilty after episode. Frequency of episodes is at least 1 per week for 3 months, with marked distress regarding behaviors. No compensatory measures such as in bulimia nervosa and it does not occur exclusively in the context of anorexia or bulimia nervosa.

Causes are unknown, but there is a probable heritable component. Seen in similar frequency across industrialized countries. Risk factors are poorly defined but may include those that predispose to psychiatric illness as well as obesity.

Symptoms

Localization site	Comment
Mental status and psychiatric aspects/ complications	Hyperphagia during discrete time period, depressed mood, anxiety, guilt. Can demonstrate cognitive rigidity, perfectionistic tendencies, ritualistic behaviors around food. Symptoms related to comorbid disorders such as bipolar, depressive, and anxiety disorders, as well as substance use

Secondary Complications: Isolating behavior, especially around meals, which can be part of wider range of psychosocial functional impairment. Increased use of health care services as well as increased risk for obesity.

Treatment Complications: Treatments include medications such as selective serotonin reuptake inhibitors (SSRIs), norepinephrine/dopamine reuptake inhibitors, cognitive behavioral therapy. Side effects of pharmacotherapy depend on the agent and can include headache, insomnia, anxiety, and gastrointestinal disturbance and/or hemodynamic changes that require monitoring.

Bibliography

American Psychiatric Association. *Diagnostic and statistical manual of mental disorders: DSM-5.* 5th ed. Washington, DC: American Psychiatric Association; 2013.

Hudson JI, Hiripi E, Pope HG, et al. The prevalence and correlates of eating disorders in the National Comorbidity Survey Replication. *Biol Psychiatry.* 2007;61:348–58.

Hudson JI, Lalonde JK, Coit CE, et al. Longitudinal study of the diagnosis of components of the metabolic syndrome in individuals with binge-eating disorder. *Am J Clin Nutr.* 2010;91(6): 1568–73.

Binswanger's Disease

Epidemiology and Demographic: Binswanger's disease is most frequently seen in the sixth and seventh decades of life but can still be seen in those aged 50 or above 80. Men and women are affected equally. Most commonly seen in patients with chronic hypertension, diabetes, history of stroke, obesity, states of malnourishment (alcoholics), and smokers, but can be seen in any disease in which small artery flow is disturbed, e.g., antiphospholipid syndrome and cerebral amyloidosis.

Disorder Description: Binswanger's disease, also known as subcortical leukoencephalopathy, subcortical ischemic encephalopathy, or subcortical arteriosclerotic encephalopathy, is a type of vascular dementia associated with white matter disease and atrophy. The clinical phenotype is variable but includes intellectual/executive dysfunction, short-term memory loss, and behavioral changes. Ischemia to the subcortical white matter secondary to atherosclerosis to arterioles is seen in this condition. Histologically, myelin loss, diffuse gliosis, and axon loss are observed. CT or MRI demonstrates leukoaraiosis – attenuation of white matter (CT) or white matter hyperintensities (MRI T2 images). The disease was first defined by Binswanger in 1894 with gross findings of atherosclerotic cerebral arteries, lesioned white matter, large ventricles, and preserved cortex. The disease progresses gradually, often in a stepwise manner with sudden changes, but may show some gradual changes as well. For diagnosis of Binswanger's disease, a proposed scheme involves:

Confirmation of dementia via clinical exam/ Montreal Cognitive Assessment (MOCA).
At least two of the following:
history of hypertension, coronary artery disease, or peripheral vascular disease;
evidence of cerebrovascular disease (i.e., stroke);
subcortical brain dysfunction.
Bilateral subcortical leuokoaraiosis on CT or MRI.

Symptoms

Localization site	Comment
Cerebral hemispheres	Any region of subcortex can be affected, including basal ganglia, pons, and white matter, producing deficits in short-term memory, attention, and motivation (executive functions); urinary incontinence; clumsiness; gait disorder; seizures
Mental status and psychiatric aspects/complications	Potential positive psychotropic effects: forgetfulness (though not as severe as in Alzheimer's disease), mood changes (most commonly apathy, abulia, irritability, depression, but can see psychosis, hallucinations, delusions, paranoia, euphoria)
Brainstem	Reflex asymmetries, hemiparesis, rigidity, pseudobulbar palsy including pathologic laughing/crying
Cerebellum	Limb and gait ataxia

Treatment Complications: Treatment is largely symptomatic, i.e., antidepressants or antipsychotics for mood changes. Complications reflect the adverse effects of individual antidepressants or psychotropics.

Bibliography

Caplan LR. Binswanger's disease – revisited. *Neurology*. 1995;45:626–33.
Olsen C, Clasen M. Senile dementia of the Binswanger's type. *Am Fam Physician*. 1998;58(9):2068–74.
Roman GC. Senile dementia of the Binswanger type: a vascular form of dementia in the elderly. *JAMA*. 1987;258:1782–8.

Biotinidase Deficiency (BTD) (Late-Onset Biotin-Responsive Multiple Carboxylase Deficiency, Late-Onset Multiple Carboxylase Deficiency)

Epidemiology and Demographics: The incidence of biotinidase deficiency (BTD) is 1/137,401 for profound BTD; 1/109,921 for partial BTD; and 1/61,067 for the combined incidence of profound and partial BTD. In the United States, incidence is estimated at 1/80,000 births and that of partial BTD between 1/31,000 and 1/40,000. Incidence is higher in populations with a high rate of consanguinity. Carrier frequency in the general population is approximately 1/120.

Disorder Description: Autosomal recessively inherited disorder of biotin recycling that is associated with neurologic and cutaneous consequences. The initial clinical presentation and expression of profound BTD are variable, even within the same family. Affected individuals may have features ranging from multiple mild episodes of seizures and ataxia to severe metabolic compromise, which can result in coma or death. Patients with profound BTD have 10% mean normal serum activity, whereas patients with the partial BTD variant have 10–30% of mean normal serum activity and are largely asymptomatic.

Symptoms in untreated patients usually appear between 2 and 5 months of age, but may not be evident until several years of age. Seizures and hypotonia are frequently the first features. Children may also exhibit rash or alopecia before diagnosis and treatment. Other common symptoms include: ataxia, developmental delay, conjunctivitis, visual problems, and hearing loss. The hearing loss, visual abnormalities, and developmental delay do not seem to be reversible with biotin therapy once they occur. When symptoms develop later in childhood or during adolescence, they exhibit motor limb weakness, spastic paresis, and visual problems, such as loss of acuity and scotoma. Biochemically, untreated individuals may exhibit metabolic ketoacidosis, lactic acidosis, and/or hyperammonemia.

Older age of onset presentations include progressive spastic paraparesis and myelopathy. Neuroimaging findings may reveal cortical and/or cerebellar atrophy and basal ganglia abnormalities.

Symptoms

Localization site	Comment
Cerebral hemispheres	Seizures usually myoclonic, but epilepsy may be generalized or focal. Some children with infantile spasms. Diffuse cerebral atrophy. Frontoparietal leukoencephalopathy. Basal ganglia involvement
Mental status and psychiatric aspects/complications	Cognitive impairment and neurodevelopmental delays
Cerebellum	Ataxia. Diffuse atrophy or atrophy of the superior vermis
Cranial nerves	Visual loss, scotoma, optic atrophy (cranial nerve II), sensorineural hearing loss (cranial nerve VIII)
Spinal cord	Progressive spastic paraparesis, myelopathy
Conus medullaris	Signal abnormalities
Peripheral neuropathy	Axonal motor polyneuropathy
Muscle	Muscle atrophy, weakness
Other	Respiratory difficulties. Untreated disease may progress to coma and death

Secondary Complications: Biotin supplementation seems to prevent the development of symptoms in presymptomatic children with profound BTD, and all symptomatic children that are treated show improvements. Seizures and ataxia resolve within hours to days, and the cutaneous manifestations resolve within weeks. Patients with partial BTD may develop symptoms when under stress (infection or starvation), but these resolve with biotin therapy.

The lack of the biotinidase enzyme prevents recycling and therefore deficiency of biotin, which is needed for biotin-dependent carboxylases that participate in gluconeogenesis, amino acid catabolism,

and fatty acid synthesis. Metabolic consequences include acidosis, elevated lactate (in blood and cerebrospinal fluid), elevated urine organic acids (3-hydroxyisovaleric acid), and hyperammonemia. These metabolic derangements may cause altered mental status.

Treatment Complications: Treatment is necessary with lifelong biotin supplementation. Biotin will not reverse all manifestations; vision loss may require additional visual aids and hearing loss may require aids or cochlear implants. Developmental delay should be treated with appropriate therapies and rehabilitative equipment.

Biotin has not shown any adverse effects and is well tolerated.

Bibliography

Chedrawi AK, Ali A, Al Hassnan ZN, Faiyaz-Ul-Haque M, Wolf B. Profound biotinidase deficiency in a child with predominantly spinal cord disease. *J Child Neurol*. 2008;23(9):1043–8. DOI: 10.1177/0883073808318062

Cowan TM, Blitzer MG, Wolf B; Working Group of the American College of Medical Genetics Laboratory Quality Assurance Committee. Technical standards and guidelines for the diagnosis of biotinidase deficiency. *Genet Med*. 2010;12(7):464–70.

Grunewald S, Champion MP, Leonard JV, et al. Biotinidase deficiency: a treatable leukoencephalopathy. *Neuropediatrics*. 2004;35(4):211–6.

Raha S, Udani V. Biotinidase deficiency presenting as recurrent myelopathy in a 7-year-old boy and a review of the literature. *Pediatr Neurol*. 2011;45(4):261–4. DOI: 10.1016/j.pediatrneurol.2011.06.010

Wolf B. Biotinidase deficiency should be considered in individuals exhibiting myelopathy with or without and vision loss. *Mol Genet Metab*. 2015;116(3):113–8. DOI: 10.1016/j.ymgme.2015.08.012

Wolf B. The neurology of biotinidase deficiency. *Mol Genet Metab*. 2011;104(1–2):27–34. DOI: 10.1016/j.ymgme.2011.06.001. Epub 2011 Jun 12.

Wolf B. Biotinidase deficiency. In Pagon RA, Adam MP, Ardinger HH, et al., eds. *GeneReviews*® [Internet]. Seattle, WA: University of Washington; 1993–2015.

Wolf B. Biotinidase deficiency: "if you have to have an inherited metabolic disease, this is the one to have." *Genet Med.* 2012;14(6):565–75.

Bipolar I Disorder

Epidemiology and Demographics: The 12-month prevalence in the United States is 0.6% with a 1.1:1 male-to-female ratio. Strong genetic component with a 10-fold increased risk among adult relatives of individuals with bipolar I and II disorders.

Disorder Description: Bipolar I disorder requires at least one lifetime manic episode, which is defined as a distinct period of abnormally and persistently elevated, expansive, or irritable mood and persistently increased activity or energy lasting at least 1 week (or any duration if hospitalization is necessary). The mood disturbance must be sufficiently severe as evidenced by marked impairment in social or occupational functioning, hospitalization to prevent harm to self or others, or associated psychotic features. The manic episode may have been preceded or followed by hypomanic or major depressive episodes; however, these are not required for a diagnosis of bipolar I disorder. The manic episode is not better attributable to the effects of a substance, medication, or another medical condition. However, a full manic episode that emerges during antidepressant treatment but persists beyond the physiologic effect of that treatment is sufficient evidence for the diagnosis of a manic episode.

Symptoms

Localization site	Comment
Mental status and psychiatric aspects/ complications	Symptoms of mania may include elevated, expansive, or irritable mood; mood lability; increased energy; increased goal-directed activity; inflated self-esteem or grandiosity; decreased need for sleep; rapid and/or pressured speech; racing thoughts (flight of ideas); distractibility; psychomotor agitation; impulsivity; poor judgment and insight; increased involvement in activities that have a high potential for painful consequences (e.g., shopping sprees, sexual indiscretions); antisocial behavior; psychosis; suicidality
	Symptoms of depression may also occur during the course of bipolar I disorder

Secondary Complications: Substance use disorders, cognitive impairment, occupational difficulties, high rates of serious and/or untreated co-occurring medical conditions, increased lifetime suicide risk with estimates of at least 15 times that of the general population.

Treatment Complications: Mood stabilization with lithium can result in lithium toxicity due to its narrow therapeutic index. Long-term use of lithium can adversely affect cognitive, cardiac, kidney, and thyroid functions. Anticonvulsants used for mood stabilization including valproic acid and carbamazepine have been associated with an increased risk of suicide and should be monitored closely in this population. Antipsychotics are also commonly used for mood stabilization and can result in varying degrees of extrapyramidal symptoms and metabolic syndrome. Benzodiazepines can be useful as adjunctive treatment for insomnia, agitation, and anxiety; however, they pose the risk of dependence and tolerance if used chronically. Because of the risk of inducing a hypomanic/manic episode, significant caution should be exercised when using antidepressants for the treatment of depression in bipolar disorder and they should only be considered in combination with adequate doses of a mood stabilizer. Finally, special consideration should be given to the pharmacologic treatment of bipolar I disorder during pregnancy due to the teratogenic risks associated with many of these agents, particularly lithium and anticonvulsants.

Bibliography

American Psychiatric Association. *Diagnostic and statistical manual of mental disorders: DSM-5.* 5th ed. Washington, DC: American Psychiatric Association; 2013.

Lichtenstein P, Yip BH, Björk C, et al. Common genetic determinants of schizophrenia and bipolar disorder in Swedish families: a population-based study. *Lancet.* 2009;373(9659):234–9.

Marangell LB, Bauer MS, Dennehy EB, et al. Prospective predictors of suicide and suicide attempts in 1,556 patients with bipolar disorders followed for up to 2 years. *Bipolar Disord.* 2006;8(5 Pt 2):566–75.

Merikangas KR, Akiskal HS, Angst J, et al. Lifetime and 12-month prevalence of bipolar spectrum disorder in the National Comorbidity Survey replication. *Arch Gen Psychiatry.* 2007;64(5):543–52.

Bipolar II Disorder

Epidemiology and Demographics: The 12-month prevalence of bipolar II disorder in the United States is approximately 0.8%. Findings on gender differences are mixed and range from no evidence of gender difference to a female predominance. Approximately 5–15% of individuals with bipolar II disorder will eventually develop a manic episode, which converts the diagnosis to bipolar I disorder.

Disorder Description: Bipolar II disorder requires at least one lifetime hypomanic episode **and** one or more major depressive episode. To meet diagnostic criteria, the hypomanic episode must last at least 4 days and the major depressive episode must last at least 2 weeks. In contrast to a manic episode, the hypomanic episode is not associated with psychotic symptoms and is not severe enough to impair social or occupational functioning or necessitate hospitalization. The hypomanic episode is not better attributable to the effects of a substance, medication, or another medical condition. However, a full hypomanic episode that emerges during antidepressant treatment but persists beyond the physiologic effect of that treatment is sufficient evidence for the diagnosis of a hypomanic episode. Compared with individuals with bipolar I disorder, individuals with bipolar II disorder have greater chronicity of illness and spend more time on average in the depressive phase of their illness.

Symptoms

Localization site	Comment
Mental status and psychiatric aspects/ complications	Symptoms of hypomania may include elevated, expansive, or irritable mood; mood lability; increased energy; increased goal-directed activity; inflated self-esteem or grandiosity; decreased need for sleep; rapid and/or pressured speech; racing thoughts (flight of ideas); distractibility; psychomotor agitation; impulsivity; poor judgment and insight; increased involvement in activities that have a high potential for painful consequences (e.g., shopping sprees, sexual indiscretions); antisocial behavior; suicidality
	Symptoms of depression may include depressed mood, anhedonia, changes in appetite and/or weight, insomnia or hypersomnia, psychomotor agitation or retardation, fatigue, poor concentration, indecisiveness, guilt, worthlessness, hopelessness, suicidality

Secondary Complications: Substance use disorders, cognitive impairment, occupational difficulties, increased risk of suicide attempts, increased lethality of suicide attempts in individuals with bipolar II disorder compared with bipolar I disorder.

Treatment Complications: Mood stabilization with lithium can result in lithium toxicity due to its narrow therapeutic index. Long-term use of lithium can adversely affect cognitive, cardiac, kidney, and thyroid functions. Anticonvulsants used for mood stabilization including valproic acid and carbamazepine have been associated with an increased risk of suicide and should be monitored closely in this population. Antipsychotics are also commonly used for mood stabilization and can result in varying degrees of extrapyramidal symptoms and metabolic syndrome. Benzodiazepines can be useful as adjunctive treatment for insomnia, agitation, and anxiety, however pose the risk of dependence and tolerance if used chronically. Due to the risk of inducing a hypomanic/manic episode, significant caution should be exercised when using antidepressants for the treatment of depression in bipolar disorder and should be considered only in combination with adequate doses of a mood stabilizer. Finally, special consideration should be given to the pharmacologic treatment of bipolar II disorder during pregnancy because of the teratogenic risks associated with many of these agents, particularly lithium and anticonvulsants.

Bibliography

American Psychiatric Association. *Diagnostic and statistical manual of mental disorders: DSM-5.* 5th ed. Washington, DC: American Psychiatric Association; 2013.

Judd LL, Akiskal HS, Schettler PJ, et al. The comparative clinical phenotype and long term longitudinal episode course of bipolar I and II: a clinical spectrum or distinct disorders? *J Affect Disord.* 2003;73(1–2):19–32.

Merikangas KR, Jin R, He JP, et al. Prevalence and correlates of bipolar spectrum disorder in the world mental health survey initiative. *Arch Gen Psychiatry.* 2011;68(3):241–51.

Tondo L, Lepri B, Baldessarini RJ. Suicidal risks among 2826 Sardinian major affective disorder patients. *Acta Psychiatr Scand.* 2007;116(6): 419–28.

Bipolar and Related Disorder Due to Another Medical Condition

Epidemiology and Demographics: Prevalence of bipolar and related disorder due to another medical condition is unclear and depends on the underlying medical condition. Gender differences also pertain to those associated with the underlying medical condition. Medical conditions best known to cause hypomania/mania are Cushing's disease, hyperthyroidism, multiple sclerosis, stroke, brain tumors, traumatic brain injuries, tertiary neurosyphilis, and neurodegenerative disorders.

Disorder Description: Characterized by a prominent and persistent period of abnormally elevated, expansive, or irritable mood and abnormally increased activity or energy that is attributable to another medical condition. The mood disturbance must be sufficiently severe as evidenced by marked impairment in social or occupational functioning, hospitalization to prevent harm to self or others, or associated psychotic features. Furthermore, the mood disturbance is not better explained by another psychiatric disorder and does not occur exclusively within the course of delirium.

Symptoms

Localization site	Comment
Mental status and psychiatric aspects/complications	Symptoms of hypomania or mania may include elevated, expansive, or irritable mood; mood lability; increased energy; increased goal-directed activity; inflated self-esteem or grandiosity; decreased need for sleep; rapid and/or pressured speech; racing thoughts (flight of ideas); distractibility; psychomotor agitation; impulsivity; poor judgment and insight; increased involvement in activities that have a high potential for painful consequences (e.g., shopping sprees, sexual indiscretions); antisocial behavior; suicidality
	Depressive symptoms may also occur; however, they do not predominate in the clinical picture

Secondary Complications: Bipolar symptoms may exacerbate impairments associated with the underlying medical condition as well as interfere with the necessary medical treatment.

Treatment Complications: Treatment of bipolar and related disorder due to another medical condition relies on appropriate treatment of the underlying medical condition. Acute symptomatic treatment with antipsychotics and/or benzodiazepines may be helpful; however, caution should be used given the risks of extrapyramidal symptoms as well as sedation and tolerance/dependence, respectively.

Bibliography

American Psychiatric Association. *Diagnostic and statistical manual of mental disorders: DSM-5.* 5th ed. Washington, DC: American Psychiatric Association; 2013.

Haskett RF. Diagnostic categorization of psychiatric disturbance in Cushing's syndrome. *Am J Psychiatry.* 1985;142(8):911–6.

Joffe RT, Lippert GP, Gray TA, et al. Mood disorder and multiple sclerosis. *Arch Neurol.* 1987;44: 376–8.

Mustafa B, Evrim O, Sari A. Secondary mania following traumatic brain injury. *J Neuropsychiatry Clin Neurosci.* 2005;17(1):122–4.

Robinson RG. Neuropsychiatric consequences of stroke. *Annu Rev Med.* 1997;48:217–29.

Black Widow Spider Envenomation (Latrotoxin)

Epidemiology and Demographics: Within the United States, black widow spider envenomation (latrotoxin) is most frequent in the southeastern states but is present in every state except Alaska. More frequent in September in the United States, least likely in January and February. Small children and the elderly are more likely to develop symptoms.

Disorder Description: Adult female spiders only are toxic; males and juveniles are harmless. The spiders are shiny black with a red hourglass or anvil-shaped mark on the underside of the abdomen. The toxin causes release of acetylcholine from the motor nerve terminal with depolarization of the peripheral nerves and neuromuscular junction. Can cause severe abdominal pain mimicking acute abdomen. Motor activity manifests as tremor, rigidity, spasms, and paralysis, while sensory and autonomic overactivity also can occur.

Majority of cases are mild (two-thirds). If muscle cramps happen, the person should probably be taken to the emergency room. The bite is rarely fatal (far less than 1%), with no deaths reported in the United States during the past 10 years.

Symptoms

Localization site	Comment
Peripheral nerve	Depolarization of peripheral nerves with generalized pain and hyperesthesia
Autonomic nervous system	Salivation, lacrimation, priapism, sweating, tachycardia
Neuromuscular junction	Alpha-latrotoxin causes spontaneous release of acetylcholine from the presynaptic terminal with resultant overactivity of muscles with rigidity and pain. Once transmitter is exhausted, paralysis ensues

Treatment Complications: Anti-venom has a risk of systemic hypersensitivity in 3–4% of cases, and very few cases really need to be treated with anti-venom.

Bibliography

Gorio A, Di Giulio AM. Black widow spider venom. In Spencer PS, Schaumburg HH, eds. *Experimental and clinical neurotoxicology.* 2nd ed. New York: Oxford University Press; 2000. pp. 239–43.

Isbister GK, Page CB, Buckley NA, et al. Randomized controlled trial of intravenous antivenom versus placebo for latrodectism: the second Redback Antivenom Evaluation (RAVE-II) Study. *Ann Emerg Med.* 2014;64:620–8.

Monte AA, Bucher-Bartelson B, Heard KJ. A US perspective of symptomatic *Latrodectus* spp. envenomation and treatment: a National Poison Data System review. *Ann Pharmacother.* 2011;45(12):1491–8.

Bladder Cancer

Epidemiology and Demographics: Bladder cancer accounts for approximately 5% of all newly diagnosed cancers and is the fourth most common cancer in men; less common in women in the United States. The incidence is 3 times higher in men than women and 2 times higher in whites than blacks. The median age of diagnosis is 73.

Disorder Description: Bladder cancers start in the innermost lining of the bladder, which is called the *urothelium* or *transitional epithelium*. As the cancer grows into or through the other layers in the bladder wall, it becomes more advanced. Urothelial carcinoma, also known as *transitional cell carcinoma* (TCC), is by far the most common type of bladder cancer.

Urothelial cells also line other parts of the urinary tract, such as the part of the kidney that connects to the ureter, the ureters, and the urethra. Over time, the cancer might grow outside the bladder and into nearby structures, lymph nodes, or other organs. (If bladder cancer spreads, it often goes first to distant lymph nodes, the bones, the lungs, or the liver.) Squamous cell carcinoma is an infrequent but second most common form of bladder cancer. Even rarer types include adenocarcinoma, small cell carcinoma, and sarcoma. Hematuria is the most common symptom for all bladder cancers.

Cigarette smoking has a strong link and smokers are three times more likely to develop bladder cancer. The following drugs or chemicals are linked to bladder cancer: benzidine; beta-napthylamine; organic chemical exposure in industries of rubber, leather, textiles, paint products, machinists, printers, hairdressers, truck drivers. Aristolochic acid has also been linked with higher risk of bladder cancer along with pioglitazone for more than 1 year of use, although the latter is still an area of active research. Arsenic in drinking water can also increase risk of bladder cancer along with positive family history, past cyclophosphamide use for treatment, and personal history of bladder cancer.

Symptoms

Localization site	Comment
Unclear localization	Small cell carcinoma can rarely lead to paraneoplastic syndromes such as ectopic adrenocorticotropic hormone secretion and hypercalcemia

Treatment Complications: Rarely, intravesical Bacillus Calmette–Guérin treatment may produce a systemic illness that may require antituberculin therapy. Gemcitabine and cisplatin treatment sometimes can lead to anemia and thrombocytopenia.

Bibliography

American Cancer Society. Bladder cancer. Available from www.cancer.org/cancer/bladdercancer/#. Accessed Oct 8, 2018.

Mayo Clinic Staff. Bladder cancer. Dec 22, 2017. Available from www.mayoclinic.org/diseases-conditions/bladder-cancer/basics/definition/con-20027606. Accessed Oct 8, 2018.2018.

Blastomycosis

Epidemiology and Demographics: Blastomycosis has an incidence of 1–2 cases/100,000 people.[1] Forty percent of patients with AIDS who have blastomycosis have concomitant neurologic disease.[2]

Disorder Description: Blastomycosis is caused by the dimorphic fungus *Blastomyces dermatitidis*, which lives in soil, is associated with decaying vegetation, and is endemic to the midwestern and southwestern United States and Canada, but also ocurs worldwide. Most commonly, the lungs are the primary site of infection because of inhalation of spores; however, accidental skin penetration or dog bites may also cause cutaneous infections. Infection may disseminate to other parts of the body such as bones, urinary tract, and central nervous system (CNS).[1]

CNS blastomycosis has mostly been associated with concomitant infection of other sites; however, isolated infections have been reported. CNS involvement represents 5–10% of cases of disseminated blastomycosis and 33% on autopsy.[3]

Risk factors include diabetes, immunosuppression, solid organ or stem cell transplantation. Farmers, forestry workers, hunters, and campers are also at higher risk because of their exposure to wooded areas.[1,3]

Symptoms

Localization site	Comment
Cerebral hemispheres	Abscess
	Headache
	Hydrocephalus
	Meningitis
	Seizures
	Vision changes
	Focal neurologic deficit

Localization site	Comment
Mental status and psychiatric aspects/complications	Altered mental status
Cerebellum	Dysfunction due to basilar meningitis
Base of skull	Basilar meningitis
Cranial nerves	Optic neuropathy causing vision loss
	Diplopia due to increased intracranial pressure
Spinal cord	Intramedullary lesion causing myelopathy (rare)
	Abscess
	Epidural abscess causing compression
Specific spinal roots	Radiculopathy

Secondary Complications: Seizures, hydrocephalus.

Treatment Complications: Nephrotoxicity is a common adverse effect of amphotericin B use, which may further depress mental status.[2]

References

1. Centers for Disease Control and Prevention. *Blastomycosis*. Atlanta, GA: CDC; 2016. Available from www.cdc.gov/fungal/diseases/blastomycosis/index.html. Accessed Oct 8, 2018.
2. Chapman S, Dismukes W, Proia L, et al. Clinical practice guidelines for the management of blastomycosis: 2008 update by the Infectious Diseases Society of America. *Clin Infect Dis*. 2008;46(12):1801–12.
3. Bariola J, Perry P, Pappas P, et al. Blastomycosis of the central nervous system: a multicenter review of diagnosis and treatment in the modern era. *Clin Infect Dis*. 2010;50(6): 797–804.

Blepharospasm

Epidemiology and Demographics: Blepharospasm has a prevalence of 3–13/100,000 with a 3:1 female preponderance and presents usually in the 5th to 7th decades of life.

Disorder Description: Blepharospasm is characterized by involuntary, bilateral, and symmetric spasms of the orbicularis oculi muscles that lead to partial or total eyelid closure. The spasms may be triggered by bright lights, chewing, or speaking, and they may be lessened by attention, such as during a doctor's exam.

Symptoms

Localization site	Comment
Basal ganglia	Parkinson's disease is associated with apraxia of eyelid opening and blepharospasm
Cranial nerves	Hemifacial spasm (HS) is distinguished from blepharospasm by being unilateral and involving other muscles of facial expression. HS can result from neurovascular compression of the facial nerve at the root exit zone as it leaves the brainstem
Muscle	Meige syndrome is a segmental craniocervical dystonia affecting the head and neck that can include features of blepharospasm

Secondary Complications: Severe blepharospasm may lead to functional blindness as a result of occlusion of the visual axis.

Treatment Complications: The mainstay of treatment of blepharospasm is botulinum toxin injections, the main complication being eyelid ptosis from toxin diffusing across the septum and affecting the levator muscle. This ptosis is reversible, as the toxin wears off in 3–4 months.

Bibliography

Defazio G, Hallett M, Jinnah HA, et al. Development and validation of a clinical scale for rating the severity of blepharospasm. *Mov Disord.* 2015;30(4):525–530.

Hellman A, Torres-Russotto D. Botulinum toxin in the management of blepharospasm: current evidence and recent developments. *Ther Adv Neurol Disord.* 2014;8(2):82–91.

Rana AQ, Kabir A, Dogu O, Patel A, Khondker S. Prevalence of blepharospasm and apraxia of eyelid opening in patients with parkinsonism, cervical dystonia and essential tremor. *Eur Neurol.* 2012;68(5):318–21.

Body Dysmorphic Disorder

Epidemiology and Demographics: In the United States, point prevalence is 2.4% with slight predominance in females. Most commonly, onset is between 12 and 13 years of age, with two-thirds demonstrating criteria for disorder by age 18.

Disorder Description: Characterized by preoccupation with one's physical appearance, with perception of defects not noticed by others or found to be minor. Per the DSM-5, repetitive behaviors occur and may include checking oneself in mirrors, frequent grooming, picking at skin, and eliciting reassurance from others. May excessively compare appearance with that of others. Must cause significant distress or functional impairment and not better represent the type of body perceptual disturbance seen in an eating disorder. There are additional specifiers for muscle dysmorphia (present mostly in males) and degree of insight.

Similar rates of cross-cultural representation. Risk factors include childhood abuse, family history of the disorder, obsessive-compulsive disorder (OCD) and tendency toward perfectionism.

Symptoms

Localization site	Comment
Mental status and psychiatric aspects/complications	Anxiety, depressed mood, delusional beliefs about body appearance, suicidal ideation, cognitive rigidity (perfectionism), avoidance
	Executive and visual processing dysfunction
	When comorbid with depression, OCD, substance abuse, symptoms of those disorders may be present

Secondary Complications: Increased risk of suicidal ideation and attempts, additive risk when comorbid with depressive disorders. Many pursue cosmetic surgery, which may not improve condition and may worsen it. May have significant impairment in social and occupational realms. Many have hospitalization history.

Treatment Complications: Supportive psychotherapy and cognitive behavioral therapy found to be helpful, as well as treatment of psychiatric comorbidity when present.

Bibliography

American Psychiatric Association. *Diagnostic and statistical manual of mental disorders: DSM-5.* 5th ed. Washington, DC: American Psychiatric Association; 2013.

Dunai J, Labuschagne I, Castle DJ, et al. Executive function in body dysmorphic disorder. *Psychol Med.* 2010;40(9):1541–8.

Feusner JD, Moody T, Hembacher E, et al. Abnormalities of visual processing and frontostriatal systems in body dysmorphic disorder. *Arch Gen Psychiatry.* 2010;67(2): 197–205.

Koran LM, Abujaoude E, Large MD, Serpe RT. The prevalence of body dysmorphic disorder in the United States adult population. *CNS Spectr.* 2008;13(4):316–22.

Phillips KA, Wilhelm S, Koran LM, et al. Body dysmorphic disorder: some key issues for DSM-V. *Depress Anxiety.* 2010;27(6):573–91.

Botulism

Epidemiology and Demographics: According to CDC, an average of 110 cases of botulism are reported each year in the United States. About 72% of these cases are infant botulism.

Disorder Description: Botulism is a rare syndrome caused by toxin released by *Clostridium botulinum*, an anaerobic gram-positive, spore-forming rod. The toxin enzymatically cleaves proteins essential for the release of the excitatory neurotransmitter acetylcholine (ACh) from the presynaptic cholinergic nerve terminals at the neuromuscular junction (NMJ) and the autonomic nerve terminals (sympathetic and parasympathetic). The most common cause of botulism is ingestion of improperly prepared food containing the toxin. Botulism spores may also germinate in wounds. In infants, the pores usually germinate in the gastrointestinal (GI) tract and release the toxin. The typical presentation is bulbar weakness (diplopia, dysphagia, and dysarthria). The weakness may spread to limbs and, in severe cases, the diaphragm, causing respiratory failure. The deep tendon reflexes may be normal early in the disease but then diminish as disease progresses. Mentation and sensation are usually intact. Autonomic findings include constipation, urinary retention, hypotension, bradycardia, and poorly reactive pupils; dry mouth and skin may be present. Treatment is usually supportive with ventilator support and nutrition. Antitoxin should be given as early as possible to be effective.

Symptoms

Localization site	Comment
Muscle	Diffuse muscle weakness from lack of ACh at NMJ
Brainstem	Ptosis, ophthalmoparesis, dysphagia, dysarthria
Neuromuscular junction	Inhibition of ACh release

Secondary Complications: Respiratory failure, nutritional deficiencies, deep venous thrombosis.

Treatment Complications: Possible pneumonia caused by ventilator support, discomfort due to deep vein thrombosis prophylaxis injection.

Bibliography

Hauser S, Amato A. Guillain-Barre syndrome and other immune-mediated neuropathies. In Hauser SL, Josephson SA, eds. *Harrison's neurology in clinical medicine.* 3rd ed. New York: McGraw-Hill Education/Medical; 2013. pp. 612–3.

Pegram P, Stone S. Botulism. In Post TW, ed. *UpToDate.* Waltham, MA. Accessed Jan 21, 2016. www.uptodate.com/contents/botulism. Accessed Oct 12, 2018.

Bovine Spongiform Encephalopathy (BSE)

Epidemiology and Demographics: Bovine spongiform encephalopathy (BSE) occurred chiefly in the United Kingdom. Epidemic peaked around 1992–1993 and had been controlled by early 2000s.[1] By the end of 2010, more than 184,500 cows with BSE were confirmed in the United Kingdom alone.[2]

Disorder Description: BSE, also known as "mad cow disease," is a fatal neurodegenerative disease seen in cattle. It is thought to have occurred because of the practice of feeding cattle infected sheep products, which were contaminated with the prion disease scrapie. It is thought that the outbreak was amplified and spread throughout the United Kingdom cattle industry by feeding prion-infected bovine meat-and-bone meal to young calves.[1,2]

There is a strong causal association with the human disease variant Creutzfeldt–Jakob disease (vCJD); 231 cases reported. The disease can be transmitted to humans via ingestion of meat from infected cattle.[1]

Symptoms

Localization site	Comment
Mental status and psychiatric aspects/complications	Progressive dementia (aggression in cows)

Secondary Complications: May cause vCJD-like disease in humans.[1]

References

1. Geschwind M. Prion diseases. *Continuum (Minneap Minn)*. 2015;21:1612–38.
2. Centers for Disease Control and Prevention. Bovine spongiform encephalopathy (BSE), or mad cow disease. 2015. Available from www.cdc.gov/prions/bse/index.html. Accessed Oct 10, 2018.

Brachial Plexopathy

The plexus is formed from the C5–T1 nerve roots that then run distally to form the trunks, divisions, cords, branches, and nerves. The C5 and C6 have the largest percentages of motor fibers and the least are from C7 and T1 roots. The greatest number of sensory fibers is from the C7 root and the remainder are from C5–C6 and C8–T1 nerve roots. Postganglionic sympathetic nerve fibers from the vertebral ganglia travel through the brachial plexus.

Epidemiology and Demographics: Rare. About 0.4% of plexopathies are associated with cancer, and 2–5% of those treated with radiation. Idiopathic brachial plexopathy has estimated annual incidence of 2–3/100,000. Reported male-to-female ratio is 2:1. Nerve compression is uncommon because the plexus is protected by surrounding bony structures.

Disorder Description: The causes of brachial plexopathy include: compression, inflammation, metabolic abnormalities, neoplasia, and ischemia. Trauma is the most common cause in children and adults, with contact sports the most common etiology. Diabetes mellitus is the most common metabolic abnormality leading to plexus dysfunction. The most common symptoms include pain, numbness, and weakness. On exam, muscle weakness, atrophy, sensory loss, and reduced reflexes may be detected. Diagnostic tools include electromyography and radiologic images. The management and outcome vary depending on the etiology of the dysfunction.

Location

Localization site	Comment
Plexus	Brachial plexus

Secondary Complications: Deep vein thrombosis.
Treatment Complications: Narcotic used for pain management may result in altered mental status.

Bibliography

Bromberg MB. Brachial plexus syndrome. In Post TW, ed. *UpToDate*. Waltham, MA; 2016.

Brachial Plexopathy (Burner Syndrome)

Epidemiology and Demographics: Common. Reported in up to 52% of college football players in a single season. About 70% of college football players have experienced Burner syndrome.

Disorder Description: Burner syndrome, or "stingers," is a result of upper plexus traction injury, which can be caused by force applied to the head or shoulder, creating deviation away from each other. The symptoms include sudden pain and numbness along the neck and shoulder, radiating down to forearm and hand. The majority of injuries occur in males playing contact sports, i.e., football or rugby. All athletes complaining of burning should be examined thoroughly for injury to the spine and shoulder. If symptoms persist beyond a few minutes, then radiologic tests including MRI should be considered to exclude disc herniation or other compression injury. If symptoms continue for 2–3 weeks, then EMG should be considered. Treatment includes rehab exercises to strengthen the muscles. Prognosis is usually favorable.

Potential Sites of Involvement: Plexus, brachial plexus.

Bibliography

Bowen BC, Seidenwurm DJ; for the Expert Panel on Neurologic Imaging. Plexopathy. *Am J Neuroradiol*. 2008;29(2):400–2.

Wittenberg KH, Adkins MC. MR imaging of nontraumatic brachial plexopathies: frequency and spectrum of findings. *RadioGraphics*. 2000;20(4).

Brachial Plexopathy (Neoplasm Related)

Epidemiology and Demographics: Rare. Incidence is about 0.5% of breast cancer patients. After radiation-induced fibrosis, metastatic lung and breast cancers are the most common nontraumatic causes of brachial plexopathy.

Disorder Description: Pain in the shoulder and axilla and radiating down the arm is the most common presenting symptom, with the lower plexus more commonly involved then the upper portion. Pancoast syndrome is a result of non-small-cell lung cancer in the apex of the lung invading the lower trunk of the brachial plexus. Often this is associated with Horner syndrome (miosis, ptosis, and anhidrosis) with weakness and sensory loss in the distribution of the lower plexus. Radiation therapy leading to fibrosis can also affect the plexus and is difficult to distinguish from malignant spread from lymph nodes or bone. This can occur from months to years after treatment. Primary plexus tumors, i.e., schwannomas or neurofibromas, are less common. The diagnostic modalities include chest x-ray, CT, or MRI. Management is predominantly geared toward pain management and primary tumor treatment.

Location

Localization Site	Comment
Plexus	Brachial plexus – lower more common than the upper plexus

Secondary Complications: Neoplasms are associated with hypercoagulable state and deep vein thrombosis.

Treatment Complications: Narcotic analgesic use may lead to altered mental status. Chemotherapies have neurotoxic effects.

Bibliography

Bromberg MB. Brachial plexus syndrome. In Post TW, ed. *UpToDate*. Waltham, MA; 2016.

Kannan T, Sivaram Naik G, Sreedhar Babu KV, Vijayalakshim Devi B. Metastatic brachial plexopathy in breast cancer. *J Clin Sci Res*. 2012;1:196–8.

Brain Metastasis

Epidemiology and Demographics: Brain metastases are the most common direct neurologic complication of systemic cancer. They are more common than the primary brain tumors. The exact incidence is not known, but the risk of brain metastasis varies with the primary tumor type. For example, the brain metastasis rate for lung cancer is between 18 and 63% and for breast cancer between 20 and 30%.

Disorder Description: Brain metastases are tumors that have spread to the brain from primary tumors elsewhere in the body. The most common primary site is lung. Other common primary sources of brain metastases are melanoma, renal, breast, and colorectal cancers. Eight-five percent of brain metastases are found in the cerebral hemisphere, 10–15% in the cerebellum, and 1–3% are in the brainstem. Hemorrhagic metastases account for 3–14% of all brain metastases. They are most commonly from melanoma, choriocarcinoma, thyroid, renal cell, hepatocellular carcinoma, lung, and breast (as lung and breast are extremely common although they hemorrhage less).

Symptoms

Localization site	Comment
Cerebral hemispheres	Seizures, hemiparesis, aphasia (dominant), neglect (nondominant), homonymous hemianopia
Mental status and psychiatric aspects/complications	Progressive worsening of memory and functioning
Brainstem	Cranial nerve palsies (meningeal carcinomatosis usually), depending on the extent involved Reduced level of consciousness, interruption of reticular activating system fibers
Cerebellum	Unsteadiness and gait disturbances

Localization site	Comment
Cerebellum	Obstructive hydrocephalus if effacement and obstruction of fourth ventricle with drowsiness, nausea, vomiting
Unclear localization	Headache, nuchal rigidity, and photophobia indicate meninges involvement (meningeal carcinomatosis)

Treatment Complications

Surgical resection (in isolated metastasis or cerebellar metastasis causing obstructive hydrocephalus) can lead to permanent focal deficits.

Chemotherapy-related side effects depend on regimen chosen for primary tumor.

Radiation therapy may lead to dementia (leukoencephalopathy), secondary brain tumors, stroke (accelerated atherosclerosis).

Bibliography

Bernardi D, Tomassi O, Stefani M, Di Giacobbe A. Comment on "Clinical features and course of brain metastases in colorectal cancer: an experience from a single institution." *Curr Oncol.* 2013;20(3):e278.

Freilich RJ, Krol G, Deangelis LM. Neuroimaging and cerebrospinal fluid cytology in the diagnosis of leptomeningeal metastasis. *Ann Neurol.* 1995;38(1):51–7.

Brainstem Concussion

Epidemiology and Demographics: Central vestibular dysfunction secondary to brainstem injury arising in patients with varying degrees of head trauma. The incidence of traumatic brainstem injury varies between 8 and 52% of head injuries.

Disorder Description: Mild to severe head trauma leads to shearing forces on the cranial nerve root entry zone resulting in petechial hemorrhages. These hemorrhages occur in the brainstem and specifically in the vestibular nuclei. MRI can display the hemorrhages.

Patients have symptoms of vertigo, unsteadiness, and imbalance with a limited ability for central compensation. The damage to the vestibular nucleus prevents central compensation from occurring, resulting in perpetual vestibular dysfunction.

Symptoms

Localization site	Comment
Inner ear	Not affected
Cranial nerves	CN VIII is subject to shearing and stretching
Central nervous system	Damage to the vestibular nuclei

Secondary Complications: These patients are at risk for falls due to the perpetual nature of the disorder.

Treatment Complications: There is no treatment for the condition other than vestibular therapy. The results of therapy depend on the ability for central compensation to occur, and thus recovery may be incomplete in severe cases. There are no complications associated with vestibular rehabilitation.

Bibliography

Fife TD, Giza C. Posttraumatic vertigo and dizziness. *Semin Neurol.* 2013;33(3):238–43.

Fitzgerald D. Head trauma: hearing loss and dizziness. *J Trauma Inj Infect Crit Care.* 1996;40(3):488–96.

Katz DI, Cohen SI, Alexander MP. Mild traumatic brain injury. *Handb Clin Neurol.* 2015;127: 131–56.

Breast Cancer

Epidemiology and Demographics: Metastases occur in 10–16% of breast cancer patients. Female predominance. Most common cancer in women worldwide. White women are more likely to develop breast cancer than are African American women.

Disorder Description: Risk factors include family history, some genetic mutations (BRCA1/BRCA2/p53), prolonged exposure to endogenous estrogens (early menarche, late menopause, late age at first childbirth), Western diet, radiation to chest. Danaei et al. calculated that 21% of worldwide breast cancer deaths are related to alcohol use, overweight/obesity, physical inactivity.[1]

Incidence rates vary: WHO reported 19.3/100,000 women in eastern Africa compared with 89.7/100,000 women in western Europe. In developing regions, 40/100,000. WHO also reported that lowest incidence rates occur in most African countries, but these rates are increasing.[2]

Symptoms

Localization	Comment
Mental status and psychiatric aspects/ complications	Less common symptoms include changes in behavior, confusion, memory problems Difficulty with speech
Cerebellar	Paraneoplastic cerebellar degeneration
Cerebral hemisphere	Limbic encephalitis
Paraneoplastic and associated syndromes	Syndrome of inappropriate secretion of antidiuretic hormone Hypercalcemia Paraneoplastic neurologic syndrome Dermatomyositis Sweet syndrome Paraneoplastic granulocytosis Subacute (peripheral) sensory neuropathy Polymyalgia rheumatica Eosinophilia, granulocytosis, thrombocytosis
Unclear localization	Headache, nausea and/or vomiting, fatigue, weakness or feeling numb down one side of the body, unsteadiness, seizures (fits), double or wavy vision. Symptoms vary depending on the site of metastasis

Treatment Complications: Chemotherapy/radiation side effects, hormone treatment side effects, surgical complications.

References

1. Danaei G, VanderHoorn S, Lopez AD, et al. Causes of cancer in the world: comparative risk assessment of nine behavioural and environmental risk factors. *Lancet*. 2005;366:1784–93.
2. World Health Organization. Breast cancer: prevention and control. www.who.int/cancer/detection/breastcancer/en/. Accessed Oct 15, 2018.

Further Reading

American Cancer Society. Leading new cancer cases and deaths – 2016 estimates. Available from www.cancer.org/research/cancerfactsstatistics/cancerfactsfigures2016/index. Accessed May 4, 2016.

AskMayoExpert. *Breast cancer*. Rochester, MN: Mayo Foundation for Medical Education and Research; 2015.

National Cancer Institute. SEER stat fact sheet: Female breast cancer. Available from http://seer.cancer.gov/statfacts/html/breast.html. Accessed May 4, 2016.

National Comprehensive Cancer Network. *Breast cancer*. Fort Washington, PA: National Comprehensive Cancer Network. Available from www.nccn.org/professionals/physician_gls/f_guidelines.asp. Accessed Oct 10, 2018.

Pelosof LC, Gerber DE. Paraneoplastic syndromes: an approach to diagnosis and treatment. *Mayo Clin Proc*. 2010;85(9),838–54. Available from http://doi.org/10.4065/mcp.2010.0099

Brief Psychotic Disorder

Epidemiology and Demographics: Brief psychotic disorder is rare, with limited epidemiologic data. Higher incidences have been reported in developing countries compared with developed countries. Twice as common in females than males.

Disorder Description: Brief psychotic disorder involves the sudden onset of at least one positive psychotic symptom such as delusions, hallucinations, disorganized speech, or grossly disorganized or catatonic behavior. Symptoms must be present for at least 1 day with full remission of all symptoms within 1 month, and are not better explained by another psychiatric disorder, the effects of a substance or medication, or another medical condition. The disturbance may be preceded by marked stressors such as stressful life events, immigration, or the peripartum period.

Symptoms

Localization site	Comment
Mental status and psychiatric aspects/ complications	Delusions including persecutory, grandiose, referential, somatic, jealous, erotomanic, nihilistic, control, mixed, or unspecified types; hallucinations most commonly occur as auditory hallucinations, however may occur in any sensory modality; disorganized speech as evidenced by derailment, loose associations, tangentiality, or "word salad"; disorganized behavior, agitation, or catatonia; poor judgment and cognitive impairment

Secondary Complications: Increased risk of suicide, particularly during the acute episode. Many individuals who initially meet criteria for a brief psychotic disorder go on to develop other primary psychotic disorders or affective disorders with psychosis.

Treatment Complications: Antipsychotics are recommended for the treatment of psychotic symptoms; however, they can result in varying degrees of extrapyramidal symptoms and metabolic syndrome. Benzodiazepines may be useful for treating acute agitation; however, they pose the risk of dependence and tolerance if used chronically.

Bibliography

American Psychiatric Association. *Diagnostic and statistical manual of mental disorders: DSM-5.* 5th ed. Washington, DC: American Psychiatric Association; 2013.

Pillmann F, Balzuweit S, Haring A, et al. Suicidal behavior in acute and transient psychotic disorders. *Psychiatry Res.* 2003;117(3): 199–209.

Susser E, Wanderling J. Epidemiology of non-affective acute remitting psychosis vs schizophrenia: sex and sociocultural setting. *Arch Gen Psychiatry.* 1994;51(4): 294–301.

Brucellosis

Epidemiology and Demographics: More than 500,000 new cases occur annually. In 2010, there were 115 cases of brucellosis reported in the United States. Persons of any age can be affected and peak incidence is during spring and summer in developing countries.[1] The frequency of neurobrucellosis has been reported as 0.5–25%.[2]

Disorder Description: Brucellosis is the most common zoonotic disease in the world, caused by *Brucella* bacteria, a family of gram-negative, facultative intracellular coccobacilli. Transmission occurs to humans by direct contact with infected animals, through cuts and abrasions, or inhalation of contaminated aerosols, or by ingestion of unpasteurized milk or milk products.[1,2]

Brucellosis is endemic in the Middle East, Mediterranean basin, India, eastern Europe, Mexico, and Central/South America.

Symptoms

Localization site	Comment
Cerebral hemispheres	Abscess
	Granuloma
	Encephalitis
	Meningitis
	Subarachnoid hemorrhage
	Headache
	Seizures
	Vasculitis (rare), may cause ischemic or hemorrhagic strokes[2,3]
Mental status and psychiatric aspects/complications	Encephalopathy
	Behavioral changes
	Agitation
	Depression[3]
Cranial nerves	Cranial neuropathies
Spinal cord	Epidural abscess causing compression
	Intramedullary abscess
Conus medullaris	Abscess
Specific spinal roots	Radiculopathy/polyradiculopathy
Syndromes with combined spinal cord and peripheral nerve lesions	Myeloradiculoneuritis

Secondary Complications: Seizures and hydrocephalus may be complications.

Treatment Complications: Rifampin may be added to antibacterials; however, it may lead to hepatotoxicity or blood dyscrasias.[1]

References

1. Abdullayev R, Kracalik I, Ismayilova R, et al. Analyzing the spatial and temporal distribution of human brucellosis in Azerbaijan (1995–2009) using spatial and spatio-temporal statistics. *BMC Infect Dis.* 2012;12:185. DOI:10.1186/1471-2334-12-185.

2. Guven T, Ugurlu K, Ergonul O, et al. Neurobrucellosis: clinical and diagnostic features. *Clin Infect Dis.* 2013;56(10):1407–12.

3. Gul H, Erdem H, Bek S. Overview of neurobrucellosis: a pooled analysis of 187 cases. *Int J Infect Dis*. 2009;13(6):e339–43.

Suggested Reading

Centers for Disease Control and Prevention. Brucellosis. Updated Sep 13, 2017. Available from www.cdc.gov/brucellosis/index.html. Accessed Oct 16, 2018.

NIH. Brucellosis. Updated Dec 12, 2014. Available from https://rarediseases.info.nih.gov/diseases/5966/brucellosis. Accessed Oct 16, 2018.

World Health Organization. Brucellosis. Available from www.who.int/zoonoses/diseases/brucellosis/en/. Accessed Oct 16, 2018.

Buckthorn Fruit (*Karwinskia humboldtiana*)

Epidemiology and Demographics: Children and livestock are more susceptible to poisoning by the buckthorn fruit plant.

Disorder Description: Most common in the southwestern United States and Mexico. Symptoms may be delayed 5–20 days after ingestion. Fleshy part of the fruit does not seem to be toxic; seeds and the stone are responsible. Weakness is the primary manifestation and can involve bulbar muscles.

Symptoms

Localization site	Comment
Cranial nerves	Bulbar muscle weakness due to involvement of motor cranial nerves
Peripheral nerve	Segmental demyelination and axonal degeneration preferentially in motor nerves results in weakness and areflexia

Bibliography

Calderon-Gonzalez R, Rizzi-Hernandez H. Buckthorn polyneuropathy *N Engl J Med*. 1967;277:69–71.

Weller RO. *Karwinskia humboldtiana*. In Spencer PS, Schaumburg HH, eds. *Experimental and clinical neurotoxicology*. 2nd ed. New York: Oxford University Press; 2000. pp. 705–7.

Bulimia Nervosa

Epidemiology and Demographics: The 12-month prevalence among young females is 1–1.5%. Prevalence peaks in older adolescence and young adulthood. More common in females, with an approximately 10:1 female-to-male ratio. Risk factors include depression, social anxiety disorder, overanxious disorders of childhood, low self-esteem, internalization of a thin body ideal, childhood obesity, early pubertal maturation, childhood sexual or physical abuse, and family history of bulimia nervosa.

Disorder Description: As defined by the DSM-5, a diagnosis of bulimia nervosa requires three essential features: (1) recurrent episodes of binge eating; (2) recurrent inappropriate compensatory behaviors to prevent weight gain; and (3) self-evaluation that is unduly influenced by body shape and weight. An episode of binge eating is characterized by eating an amount of food that is larger than what most individuals would eat in a similar period of time as well as an associated sense of lack of control. Compensatory behaviors may include self-induced vomiting, fasting, excessive exercise, or misuse of laxatives, diuretics, or other medications. Episodes of binge eating and inappropriate compensatory behaviors must occur at least once per week for 3 months, on average. Finally, the disturbance does not occur exclusively during episodes of anorexia nervosa.

Symptoms

Localization site	Comment
Mental status and psychiatric aspects/ complications	Symptoms of depression, anxiety, low self-esteem, impulsivity, perfectionism, compulsivity. Higher rates of comorbid psychiatric disorders including mood and anxiety disorders, posttraumatic stress disorder, body dysmorphic disorder, personality disorders, and substance abuse. Elevated suicide risk (6–8 times greater in patients with bulimia nervosa)

Secondary Complications: Complications from repeated vomiting may occur including electrolyte disturbances, esophageal tears, gastric rupture, and cardiac arrhythmias. Increased risk for substance abuse, all-cause mortality, and suicide.

Treatment Complications: Bupropion is contraindicated in patients with active symptoms of bulimia nervosa given the increased risk of seizures in this patient population.

Bibliography

American Psychiatric Association. *Diagnostic and statistical manual of mental disorders: DSM-5.* 5th ed. Washington, DC: American Psychiatric Association; 2013.

Smink FR, van Hoeken D, Hoek HW. Epidemiology of eating disorders: incidence, prevalence, and mortality rates. *Curr Psychiatry Rep.* 2012;14(4):406–14.

Steinhausen HC, Weber S. The outcome of bulimia nervosa: findings from one-quarter century of research. *Am J Psychiatry.* 2009;166(12):1331–41.

Suokas JT, Suvisaari JM, Gissler M, et al. Mortality in eating disorders: a follow-up study of adult eating disorder patients treated in tertiary care, 1995–2010. *Psychiatry Res.* 2013;210(3):1101–6.

Burkitt Lymphoma

Epidemiology and Demographics: Burkitt lymphoma occurs endemically in Africa, sporadically in the United States and Western Europe (primarily in children; peak incidence at age 11), and in association with immunosuppression such as with HIV infection or following bone marrow transplantation. The incidence of sporadic disease is 3 cases/million per year. Central nervous system (CNS) involvement is present in 15% of sporadic cases at presentation.

Disorder Description: Burkitt lymphoma is associated with translocation and unregulated expression of *c-myc* oncogene. The tumor is rapidly growing, with doubling time of approximately 1 day. Endemic forms primarily present with jaw or facial bone tumor with secondary spread. Sporadic forms usually arise in the abdomen. Reports of primary CNS Burkitt lymphoma also exist but are rarer.

Symptoms

Localization site	Comment
Cerebral hemispheres	Can present as solitary or multifocal masses in the cerebral hemispheres. Symptoms related to site of involvement. Hydrocephalus from meningeal or ventricular involvement can also cause secondary hemispheric dysfunction
Cerebellum	Can present as cerebellar mass
Base of skull	Dural masses can compress associated structures such as the sella or destroy the overlying bone
Cranial nerves	Cranial neuropathy can occur either from leptomeningeal involvement or compression from masses
Pituitary gland	Sellar compression can cause pituitary dysfunction
Spinal cord	Spinal epidural masses causing cord compression
Specific spinal roots	Radiculopathy either from compression or leptomeningeal disease

Secondary Complications: Because sporadic disease commonly arises in the abdomen, there can be associated ascites, gastrointestinal obstruction, or bleeding. Endemic disease affecting the jaw can cause difficulty eating and is disfiguring.

Treatment Complications: Intrathecal chemotherapy is often given with methotrexate and cytarabine for prophylaxis or treatment of CNS disease. Both intrathecal methotrexate and cytarabine can cause arachnoiditis or neurologic dysfunction including somnolence and confusion.

Bibliography

Blum KA, Lozanski G, Byrd JC. Adult Burkitt leukemia and lymphoma. *Blood.* 2004;104:3009–20.

Gu Y, Hou Y, Zhang X, Hu F. Primary central nervous system Burkitt lymphoma as concomitant lesions in the third and the left ventricles: a case study and literature review. *J Neurooncol.* 2010;99:277–81.

Campylobacter Enteritis

Epidemiology and Demographics: Annual cases of campylobacter enteritis diagnosed at 14/100,000, but many are undiagnosed or unreported. Estimated to affect more than 1.3 million persons every year. Tends to occur much more frequently in the summer months. Males more frequently affected, with infants and young adults affected the most; however, bimodal distribution has also been suggested with increased number of cases in the elderly.[1,2]

Disorder Description: Campylobacter enteritis is an infection of the intestine caused by the gram-negative Campylobacteraceae family and is the leading cause of bacterial enteritis in the world. Most infections are caused by *C. jejuni* or *C. coli*. Infection is usually food-borne via raw poultry, fresh produce, or contaminated water or milk (mostly unpasteurized). Infection can also be fecal–oral. While infection is found worldwide, risk of infection is highest in Africa and South America.[1]

Campylobacter infection is the most identifiable preceding infection associated with the development of Guillain–Barré syndrome (GBS), an immune-mediated demyelinating polyneuropathy. Twenty-five to 40% of GBS patients worldwide suffer from a preceding *C. jejuni* infection; however, only 1/1000 patients who have campylobacter infection actually develops GBS. Mechanism leading to GBS is thought to be through molecular mimicry and a cross-reactive immune response with antibodies to gangliosides, resulting in damage to the peripheral nerves.[2]

Symptoms

Localization site	Comment
Cranial nerves	May precede cranial neuropathy (Miller–Fisher syndrome)
Specific spinal roots	May precede GBS, which may cause polyradiculopathy
Peripheral neuropathy	May precede GBS, leading to either demyelinating or axonal neuropathy

Secondary Complications: Dehydration, bacteremia, or septicemia may occur. As mentioned above, may lead to GBS.

Treatment Complications: Resistance to fluoroquinolones is common.

References

1. Centers for Disease Control and Prevention. *Campylobacter*. Atlanta, GA: CDC; 2017. Available at www.cdc.gov/campylobacter/index.html. Accessed Oct 10, 2018.
2. Nyati K, Nyati R. Role of *Campylobacter jejuni* infection in the pathogenesis of Guillain-Barré syndrome: an update. *Biomed Res Int*. 2013;2013: 1–13.

Candida

Epidemiology and Demographics: Incidence rate is 72.8 cases/million/year for all *Candida* infections; invasive candidemia (IC) is 22–24 infections/100,000 population/year. IC-associated mortality has remained stable, at approximately 0.4 deaths/100,000 population, since 1997. The highest rates of candidemia are found in infants younger than 1 year and in adults older than 65 years, with blacks noted to have higher rates.[1] Half of patients with candidemia have central nervous system (CNS) involvement.[2]

Disorder Description: Most disseminated infections to the CNS are due to *Candida albicans*, but *C. parapsilosis*, *C. tropicalis*, and *C. glabrata* have also been isolated. A primary risk factor for disseminated candidiasis is neutropenia, but other risk factors include immunosuppression, diabetes, solid organ transplantations, certain genetic disorders, malignancy, prolonged hospitalizations, indwelling catheters, injectable drug use, total parenteral nutrition, and infected hardware or prosthetics. There is a higher risk in premature neonates and those that undergo neurosurgery or procedures. CNS infection is due to hematogenous dissemination, or direct access through craniotomy procedures and device implantation.[2]

Symptoms

Localization site	Comment
Cerebral hemispheres	Headache
	Meningitis (acute in neonates, chronic in adults)
	Ventriculitis
	Encephalitis
	Abscesses (usually small)
	Vasculitis, causing ischemic or hemorrhagic strokes
	Subarachnoid hemorrhage due to mycotic aneurysm formation
Mental status and psychiatric aspects/complications	Encephalopathy
Cranial nerves	Cranial neuropathy
Spinal cord	Myelopathy (rare)

Secondary Complications: Seizures or hydrocephalus may result.

Treatment Complications: Amphotericin B may cause hepatotoxicity, further depressing mental status. Flucytosine may cause thrombocytopenia or neutropenia.[1] In complicated cases, intrathecal amphotericin B may be used, but adverse effects include headache, radicular pain, cranial nerve palsies, myelopathy, foot drop, vision changes, and sphincter dysfunction.[2]

References

1. Pfaller M, Diekema D. Epidemiology of invasive candidiasis: a persistent public health problem. *Clin Microbiol Rev*. 2007;20(1):133–63.
2. Henao N, Vagner B. Infections of the central nervous system by candida. *J Infect Dis Immun*. 2011;3(5):79–84.

Cannabis Intoxication and Chronic Abuse

Epidemiology and Demographics: After alcohol, cannabis is the most frequently used psychoactive compound in the United States. Cannabis use affects a growing number of Americans, with the highest level in the 20–29 age-group; more common in men, with no race or ethnicity predilection. Parallel to increased usage, there has been a significant increase in marijuana-related medical emergencies since 2009–2011.

Disorder Description: Cannabis users smoke marijuana and sometimes mix it with food or brew it as a tea. Tetrahydrocannabinol (THC) and other related compounds in the hemp plant *Cannabis sativa* act on specific brain cell receptors that ordinarily react to natural THC-like chemicals. The short-term effects include altered mental status, increased tolerance to pain, impaired memory and concentration, altered sense of time, changes in mood, impaired body movement, and difficulty with thinking and problem solving. Long-term use affects brain development; especially when used in early teenage years, it leads to deterioration of higher cognitive functions and loss of an average of eight IQ points. Some individuals using this substance will ultimately go on to use other illicit drugs. An estimated 182 million individuals worldwide use cannabis.

Symptoms

Localization site	Comment
Cerebral hemispheres	Gray matter degeneration – diffuse, especially areas with cannabinoid receptor (chronic)
	Cerebral ischemia (acute)
Mental status and psychiatric aspects/complications	Confusion (acute), amnesia (chronic), delusions (acute), hallucinations (acute), anxiety (acute), and agitation (acute), paranoia panic disorder, dysphoria
	Cognitive dysfunction (chronic/acute)
	Decrease in executive function (chronic/acute)
	Schizophrenia (chronic)
	Mood disorder (chronic)
Brainstem	Dysregulation of pain sensation (acute)

Localization site	Comment
Cerebellum	Gray matter degeneration (chronic) Ataxia (acute)
Vestibular system (and nonspecific dizziness)	Ataxia (acute)
Cranial nerves	Paresis of fourth cranial nerve (chronic)
Pituitary gland	Neuroendocrine dysregulation increase in hypothalamic–pituitary–adrenal axis activation
Spinal cord	Analgesic effect (acute)
Anterior horn cells	Decreased motor coordination (acute)
Dorsal root ganglia	Analgesic – dysregulation of sensory stimuli (acute)
Specific spinal roots	Analgesic effects (acute)
Plexus	Analgesic effects (acute)
Mononeuropathy or mononeuropathy multiplex	
Peripheral neuropathy	Analgesic – dysregulation of sensory stimuli (anesthetic)
Muscle	Muscle weakness
Neuromuscular junction	Dysregulation of cannabinoid receptors in brain, leading to decreased functional capacity of naturally occurring cannabinoids Dysregulation of dopamine and norepinephrine

Secondary Complications

Indirect effects on nervous system.

Cardiovascular complications: Dysrhythmias resulting in subsequent stroke risk.

Respiratory complications: Respiratory compromise results in cerebral ischemia.

Treatment Complications: Benzodiazepines sometimes used in marijuana withdrawal or anxiety have potential adverse events of sedation, ataxia or confusion, or risk of addiction.

Bibliography

Coleman JH, Tacker HL, Evans WE, Lemmi H, Britton EL. Neurological manifestations of chronic marihuana intoxication. Part I: paresis of the fourth cranial nerve. *Dis Nerv Syst.* 1976;37(1):29.

Macleod J, Oakes R, Copello A, et al. Psychological and social sequelae of cannabis and other illicit drug use by young people: a systematic review of longitudinal, general population studies. *Lancet.* 2004;363(9421):1579–88.

Solowij N, Battisti R. The chronic effects of cannabis on memory in humans: a review. *Curr Drug Abuse Rev.* 2008;1(1):81–98.

Steinherz K, Vissing T. The medical effects of marijuana on the brain. *21st Century.* 1997–1998(Winter):59–69.

Cannabis Withdrawal

Epidemiology and Demographics: Predominant users are 16–30 years of age; no gender or ethnicity predilection.

Disorder Description: An individual will experience a variety of symptoms and physiologic, behavioral, and psychologic effects, such as anxiety, decreased appetite, depressed mood, disturbed sleep, gastrointestinal symptoms, and irritability.

Symptoms

Localization site	Comment
Cerebral hemispheres	Cerebral perfusion (chronic), abnormalities in cerebral cortical activity
Mental status and psychiatric aspects/complications	Anxiety (acute and chronic) Depressed mood (chronic) Irritability (chronic) Mood swings (chronic)
Brainstem	Insomnia (chronic)
Cerebellum	Ataxia (acute)
Vestibular system (and nonspecific dizziness)	Nonspecific dizziness (acute)
Muscle	Tremors (chronic)
Neuromuscular junction	Dysregulation of dopamine receptors (chronic)

Bibliography

Herning RI, Better W, Cadet JL. EEG of chronic marijuana users during abstinence: relationship to years of marijuana use, cerebral blood flow and thyroid function. *Clin Neurophysiol.* 2008;119(2):321–31. Available from www .ncbi.nlm.nih.gov/pmc/articles/PMC2234454/

Tracey N. Marijuana withdrawal and managing marijuana withdrawal symptoms. Healthy Place. 2016. Available from www.healthyplace.com/ addictions/marijuana-addiction/marijuana-withdrawal-and-managing-marijuana-withdrawal-symptoms/. Accessed Oct 10, 2018.

CANOMAD Syndrome

Epidemiology and Demographics: Chronic ataxic neuropathy, ophthalmoplegia, IgM paraprotein, cold agglutinins, and anti-disialosyl antibodies (CANOMAD) syndrome is a rare disorder with fewer than 30 cases reported in the literature. Prevalence is unknown.

Disorder Description: An immune-mediated demyelinating polyneuropathy. It presents as chronic neuropathy with sensory ataxia and areflexia. Motor function is preserved in the extremities; however, motor weakness may occur in the oculomotor and bulbar muscles in either a relapsing–remitting or fixed course. It is associated with anti-GQ1b and anti-disialosyl antibodies; it is similar to Miller–Fisher syndrome but symptoms follow a chronic time course.

Symptoms

Localization site	Comment
Cranial nerves	Oculomotor and bulbar weakness
Peripheral neuropathy	Sensory ataxia, areflexia

Treatment Complications: Plasma exchange complications include anaphylaxis, hypocalcemia, and depletion of immunoglobulins and coagulation factors.

Intravenous immunoglobulin complications include anaphylaxis secondary to IgA deficiency, renal failure, proteinuria, severe headache, and aseptic meningitis. Steroid therapy can lead to psychosis, confusion, weight gain, hyperglycemia, myopathy, glaucoma, cataracts, osteoporosis, or vertebral fractures.

Bibliography

Fontaine B. CANOMAD syndrome. *Orphanet.* March 2007.

Capillary Telangiectasia

Epidemiology and Demographics: Capillary telangiectasia accounts for 4–12% of vascular malformations. Estimated prevalence by autopsy studies is 0.68%. May be associated with other vascular disorders such as Osler–Weber–Rendu disease.

Disorder Description: Capillary telangiectasias of the brain are congenital vascular malformations that are usually asymptomatic. They are best seen by contrast-enhanced MRI, and usually found incidentally. One series found 28.6% of large (>1 cm) capillary telangiectasias become symptomatic, likely because of hemorrhage or compression of neighboring tissue. Most commonly found in the pons, but have also been seen in the temporal cortex, basal ganglia, medulla, and spinal cord.

Symptoms: Capillary telangiectasias are usually asymptomatic, and found incidentally on imaging. Symptomatic cases listed below:

Localization site	Comment
Cerebral hemispheres	Headache, seizures, confusion. Rarely hemorrhage
Brainstem	Headache, disequilibrium, dizziness or vertigo, tinnitus, facial or limb weakness, gait abnormality, hearing loss, slurred speech, transient aphasia

Secondary Complications: Rare hemorrhage.

Treatment Complications: Usually no treatment is indicated.

Bibliography

Barr RM, Dillon WP, Wilson CB. Slow-flow vascular malformations of the pons: capillary telangiectasias? *AJNR Am J Neuroradiol.* 1996;17(1):71–8.

Lee RR, Becher MW, Benson ML, Rigamonti D. Brain capillary telangiectasia: MR imaging appearance and clinicohistopathologic findings. *Radiology.* 1997;205(3):797–805.

Sarwar M, McCormick WF. Intracerebral venous angioma. Case report and review. *Arch Neurol.* 1978;35(5):323–5.

Sayama CM, Osborn AG, Chin SS, Couldwell WT. Capillary telangiectasias: clinical, radiographic, and histopathological features. Clinical article. *J Neurosurg*. 2010;113(4):709–14.

Carbon Disulfide Toxicity

Epidemiology and Demographics: Most exposures are occupational, classically in the viscose rayon industry, and the toxin is absorbed by inhalation or dermal contact.

Disorder Description: Acute, high-level exposure causes central nervous system dysfunction while chronic lower-level exposure causes neuropathy. The neuropathy is length dependent and axonal.

Symptoms

Localization site	Comment
Mental status and psychiatric aspects/complications	Confusion, hallucinations, memory impairment and emotional lability with acute, high-level exposure
Corticospinal tracts	Spasticity
Basal ganglia	Tremor, rigidity, and bradykinesia have been reported
Peripheral neuropathy	Chronic low-level exposure causes distal sensorimotor neuropathy. Axonal swellings are seen on nerve biopsy

Bibliography

Graham D, Valentine WM. Carbon disulfide. In Spencer PS, Schaumburg HH, eds. *Experimental and clinical neurotoxicology*. 2nd ed. New York: Oxford University Press; 2000. pp. 315–7.

Pulley M, Berger AR. Disorders of the peripheral nervous system (carbon disulfide). In Rosenstock L, Cullen MR, Brodkin CA, Redlich CA, eds. *Textbook of clinical occupational and environmental medicine*. 2nd ed. Philadelphia: Elsevier Saunders; 2005. pp. 674–5.

Carbon Monoxide Poisoning

Epidemiology and Demographics: Leading cause of poisoning mortality in the United States and possibly half of all poisoning deaths worldwide. Exposure happens with suicide attempts using automobile exhaust or accidentally with faulty heating systems, fires, or heaters.

Disorder Description: Carbon monoxide occupies oxygen-binding sites on hemoglobin, creating carboxyhemoglobin. Symptoms are usually nonspecific with headache, nausea, and fatigue but can progress to confusion, lethargy, and coma. Respiratory failure, cardiac arrhythmia, and cardiac arrest may occur. There is controversy about the role of hyperbaric oxygen therapy in the treatment of carbon monoxide poisoning in terms of whether there is any benefit. Also, whether carboxyhemoglobin levels are useful in clinical evaluation is unclear.

Symptoms

Localization site	Comment
Cerebral hemispheres	Headache
Mental status and psychiatric aspects/complications	Fatigue, lethargy, and coma

Bibliography

Crystal HA, Ginsberg MD. Carbon monoxide. In Spencer PS, Schaumburg HH, eds. *Experimental and clinical neurotoxicology*. 2nd ed. New York: Oxford University Press; 2000. pp. 318–29.

Kao LW, Nañagas KA. Carbon monoxide poisoning. *Emerg Med Clin North Am*. 2004;22(4):985–1018.

Carcinoid Tumor

Epidemiology and Demographics: Each year, about 8000 adults in the United States are diagnosed with a carcinoid tumor in the gastrointestinal tract (GI) tract, the most common site being the small intestine. African American men are more affected compared with white men, as well as compared with African American women. White males and white females are equally affected. Average age at diagnosis is 55–65. Average age for diagnosis in the appendix is 40 and in the lung is between 45 and 55; children are rarely affected.

Disorder Description: The cause of carcinoid tumors is unknown, and no avoidable risk factors have been found. However, the following factors may raise a person's risk of developing a carcinoid tumor: multiple endocrine neoplasia type 1; age and sex as described above; any condition that leads to decreased stomach acid content.

Symptoms

Localization site	Comment
Mental status and psychiatric aspects/complications	Neurosis and psychosis associated with carcinoid syndrome
Unclear localization	GI carcinoid: diarrhea, abdominal pain, asthma, rash, heart disease, intestinal bleeding, pellagra, melena, facial flushing
	Lung carcinoid: cough with or without sputum production, wheezing, post-obstructive pneumonia
	Carcinoid syndrome: GI carcinoid symptoms plus shortness of breath, heart murmur, palpitations, weakness, secondary diabetes, increased body and facial hair. Carcinoid crisis: above-mentioned symptoms occur together

Treatment Complications

Surgical complications
Liver metastases such as hepatic artery occlusion/
    embolization can have severe side effects
Lymph node dissection: risk of spreading the cancer
Radiation and chemotherapy side effects
Immunotherapy side effects

Bibliography

Buda A, Giuliani D, Montano N, Perego P, Milani R. Primary insular carcinoid of the ovary with carcinoid heart disease: unfavourable outcome of a case. *Int J Surg Case Rep*. 2012;3(2):59–61. Available from http://doi.org/10.1016/j.ijscr.2011.10.014

Miller JK. Carcinoid syndrome and the APUD concept. *Semin Anesth*. 1987;3:228–37.

Palaniswamy C, Frishman WE, Aronow WS. Carcinoid heart disease. *Cardiol Rev*. 2012;20:1167–76. Available from www.ncbi.nlm.nih.gov/pubmed/22314145

Stewart MJ, Willis RA, Saram GSW. Argentaffin carcinoma arising in ovarian teratomas – a report of two cases. *J Pathol Bacteriol*. 1939;49:207–12.

Telerman A. Germ cell tumor of the ovary. In Kurman RJ, ed. *Blaunstein's pathology of the female genital tract*. New York: Springer-Verlag; 2002. pp. 1006–8.

Carcinomatous Meningitis

Epidemiology and Demographics: Overall, about 5/100 people who have cancer (5%) develop carcinomatous meningitis. It happens most often with some types of leukemia and lymphomas. It can also happen with melanomas and lung and breast cancers.

The incidence of clinically diagnosed leptomeningeal metastases (LM) in patients with solid tumors is approximately 5%, but the incidence of undiagnosed or asymptomatic LM may be 20% or more with many solid tumors. Three affected domains of neurologic function: cerebral hemisphere (15%), cranial nerves (35%), spinal cord and roots (60%).

Disorder Description: The most common causes of solid tumor-related LM include: breast cancer (12–35%), lung cancer (10–26%), melanoma (5–25%), gastrointestinal cancer (4–14%), and cancers of unknown primary (1–7%).

In breast cancer, risk factors for LM include an infiltrating lobular carcinoma and cancers negative for estrogen receptor (ER) and progesterone receptor (PR). Triple-negative status of breast cancer (human epidermal growth factor receptor 2 [HER2]/neu negative; ER negative; PR negative) has been reported to be a risk factor for LM.

Symptoms

Localization site	Comment
Mental status and psychiatric aspects/complications	Vary from mild to severe; memory deficit, dysarthria, nausea, vomiting, vertigo, unsteadiness, uncoordinated limb movements, headache possible in occipital, frontal or upper cervical areas, depression, somnolence

Localization site	Comment
Cerebellum	Ataxia
	Increased intracranial pressure symptoms
	Encephalopathy
	Seizures
	Stroke
	Hemiparesis
	Aphasias
Vestibular system (and nonspecific dizziness)	Vertigo
Brainstem	Gait ataxia
	Diabetes insipidus
Cranial nerves	Cranial nerve palsies
	Diplopia
Spinal cord	Radiculopathy
	Atonic bladder
	Circular necrosis of white matter in the periphery or spinal cord
	Dorsal radiculopathy
	Other symptoms
Mononeuropathy or mononeuropathy multiplex	Multiple mononeuropathy-like symptoms associated with lymphomas
Peripheral nerve	Produces symptoms when lymphomas infiltrate

Secondary Complications:

Hydrocephalus, increased intracranial pressure, and associated symptoms

Aseptic meningitis: mimics bacterial meningitis

Acute/subacute encephalopathy: seizures, confusion, etc.

Myelopathy

Acute cerebellar syndrome

Delayed leukoencephalopathy

Bibliography

Chamberlain MC. Combined-modality treatment of leptomeningeal gliomatosis. *Neurosurgery.* 2003;52:324.

Chamberlain MC, Tsao-Wei D, Groshen S. Neoplastic meningitis-related encephalopathy: prognostic significance. *Neurology.* 2004;63:2159.

Lee SH, Kong DS, Seol HJ, et al. Ventriculoperitoneal shunt for hydrocephalus caused by central nervous system metastasis. *J Neurooncol.* 2011;104:545.

Le Rhun E, Taillibert S, Chamberlain MC. Carcinomatous meningitis: Leptomeningeal metastases in solid tumors. *Surg Neurol Int.* 2013;4(Suppl 4):S265–88. Available from http://doi.org/10.4103/2152-7806.111304

Omuro AM, Lallana EC, Bilsky MH, DeAngelis LM. Ventriculoperitoneal shunt in patients with leptomeningeal metastasis. *Neurology.* 2005;64:1625.

Cardiac Arrhythmia

Epidemiology and Demographics: Can be congenital or acquired. Arrhythmia in infancy occurs in about 24.4/100,000 live births. Atrial fibrillation is present in 1–2% of population; lifetime risk 25%, mean age at presentation 75 years.

Disorder Description: Causes can be pathogenic (congenital, acquired) or iatrogenic (e.g., atrioventricular [AV] nodal blocking agents). They include myocardial infarction, structural heart disease, coronary artery disease, thyroid abnormalities, substance-induced (e.g., medication, caffeine, alcohol, illicit substances), sleep apnea, infection, metabolic derangements (e.g., hyperkalemia, hypomagnesemia). Tachyarrhythmias can be regular or irregular, narrow or wide QRS complex. AV block bradyarrhythmias include first-degree, second-degree Mobitz I (Wenckebach), second-degree Mobitz II, third-degree (complete). Ischemic heart disease accounts for about 40% of cases of AV block. Common causes in children include atrioventricular reentry tachycardia, complete AV block, and atrial flutter.

Symptoms

Localization site	Comment
Cerebral hemispheres	Cardioembolic or ischemic strokes leading to varying degrees of neurologic deficit. Hypoxic–ischemic brain injury in sudden cardiac arrest

Localization site	Comment
Mental status and psychiatric aspects/complications	Light-headedness, dizziness, presyncope, syncope in both brady- and tachyarrhythmias. Arrhythmias account for about 15% of all causes of syncope. Anxiety is a common symptom in tachyarrhythmias
Vestibular system (and nonspecific dizziness)	Dizziness from cerebral hypoperfusion

Secondary Complications: Risk of intracerebral hemorrhage following ischemic stroke.

Treatment Complications: Conversion of tachyarrhythmia to sinus rhythm carries risk of left atrial thrombus causing embolic phenomena. Patients receiving anticoagulation for stroke prevention are at increased risk of intracerebral hemorrhage. Rate/rhythm control medications (e.g., verapamil, diltiazem, digoxin, beta blockers, amiodarone) and radiofrequency catheter ablation used to treat various tachyarrhythmias may secondarily cause bradyarrhythmias with related neurologic complications.

Bibliography

Chow GV, Marine JE, Fleg JL. Epidemiology of arrhythmias and conduction disorders in older adults. *Clin Geriatr Med.* 2012;28(4):539–53.

Morady F. Radio-frequency ablation as treatment for cardiac arrhythmias. *N Engl J Med.* 1999;340:534.

Sekar RP. Epidemiology of arrhythmias in children. *Indian Pacing Electrophysiol J.* 2008;8(Suppl 1): S8–13.

Turner CJ, Wren C. The epidemiology of arrhythmia in infants: A population-based study. *J Paediatr Child Health.* 2013;49:278–81.

Zoom M, Smith KS. The aetiology of complete heart-block. *Br Med J.* 1963;2:1149.

Cardiac Embolus/Cardioembolic Stroke

Epidemiology and Demographics: Approximately 20% of all ischemic strokes are of cardioembolic origin. Can occur at any age, but risk increases with age. Incidence of cardioembolic stroke is 30/100,000. It has a prevalence of 5/1000 above the age of 65.

Disorder Description: Cardiac embolism may occur in the setting of atrial fibrillation and mechanical and bioprosthetic heart valves without appropriate anticoagulation, as well as in endocarditis and myocardial infarction (MI) with mural thrombus. Emboli form in the heart as a result of turbulent blood flow or stasis and exit to the brain and other structures, causing blood vessel occlusion. Age, hypertension, and diabetes are important risk factors for the development of cardioembolic stroke.

Symptoms

Localization site	Comment
Cerebral hemispheres	Large vessel cortical stroke
Mental status and psychiatric aspects/complications	Altered consciousness, loss of speech or memory, and hemineglect due to ischemic stroke
Brainstem	Altered consciousness, diplopia, locked-in syndrome
Cerebellum	Cerebellar stroke, dysmetria and vertigo
Vestibular system (and nonspecific dizziness)	Vertigo
Cranial nerves	Optic neuropathy due to retinal artery embolism
Spinal cord	Anterior/posterior spinal artery syndrome (rare)

Secondary Complications: Rapid atrial fibrillation, limb ischemia, mesenteric ischemia.

Treatment Complications: Treatment of cardiac embolus is usually preventative. Warfarin, heparin, and novel oral anticoagulant (NOAC) use can lead to intracranial and severe systemic bleeding, such as gastrointestinal bleeding.

Bibliography

Arboix A, Alio J. Cardioembolic stroke: clinical features, specific cardiac disorders and prognosis. *Curr Cardiol Rev.* 2010;6(3):150–61.

Hornung M, Franke J, Gafoor S, Sievert H. Cardioembolic stroke and postmyocardial infarction stroke. *Cardiol Clin.* 2016;34(2):207–14.

Cardiac Surgery

Epidemiology and Demographics: Incidence of neurologic complications of cardiac surgery is estimated to be about 6%. Advanced age is a dominant risk factor.

Disorder Description: Most neurologic problems related to cardiac surgery occur as stroke, neuropsychiatric abnormalities/encephalopathies, or peripheral neuropathies. Causes include cerebral hypoperfusion, atheroembolization, gaseous embolization, renal failure, hepatic failure, thyroid abnormalities, metabolic disturbances (e.g., hyponatremia, hypoglycemia), drug toxicity, postoperative hyperthermia, and surgery (e.g., sternal retraction, artery harvesting, hemodynamic changes during cardiac bypass). Risk factors include hypertension, carotid disease, advanced age, previous stroke, and underlying pulmonary disease.

Symptoms

Localization site	Comment
Cerebral hemispheres	Ischemic, hemorrhagic stroke. Associated with poorer outcome compared with those cardiac surgery patients without a stroke
Mental status and psychiatric aspects/complications	Disturbances in memory, executive function, motor speed, attention, seizures, delirium, and coma
Brainstem	Supranuclear gaze palsy (ischemic injury)
Cranial nerves	Retinal infarctions, ischemic optic neuropathy (rare)
Plexus	Brachial plexus injury; numbness, weakness, pain, diminished reflexes, discoordination in upper extremity. Symptoms improve or resolve within 3 weeks (suggesting a neuropraxic injury caused by disruption of myelin sheath)
Peripheral neuropathy	Phrenic neuropathy; prolonged ventilator dependence Intercostal neuropathy (pain and dysesthesia in a localized distribution in the lateral chest wall) caused by harvesting of the internal thoracic artery

Secondary Complications: Intracerebral hemorrhage secondary to ischemic stroke. Greater in-hospital mortality rates.

Treatment Complications: Risk of hemopericardium when antithrombotic therapy initiated for ischemic stroke.

Bibliography

Boyd WC, Hartman GS. Neurologic dysfunction in cardiac surgery. *New Horiz.* 1999;7:504.

Cheung AT, Stecker MM. Neurologic complications of cardiac surgery. *Prog Anaesthesiol.* 1998;12:3.

Gardner TJ, Horneffer PJ, Manolio TA, et al. Stroke following coronary artery bypass grafting: a ten-year study. *Ann Thorac Surg.* 1985;40:574.

Cardiogenic Syncope

Epidemiology and Demographics: Neurocardiogenic syncope occurs in about 25–40% of patients with syncope, representing the most common cause of all types of syncope. It has an overall prevalence of 22% in the general population. Classic neurocardiogenic syncope is often linked to an identifiable trigger, such as an emotional stimulus. Genetics are thought to play a role in the "non-classical" neurocardiogenic syncope, which appears to be familial and without an identifiable trigger. The classical type most often occurs in the elderly and is associated with micturition, cough, defecation, and deglutition. Neurocardiogenic syncope in general is not restricted by age or sex.

Disorder Description: Neurocardiogenic syncope, also known as vasovagal syncope, is one type of syncope that results from complex interactions between the autonomic nervous system, the body's peripheral vascular resistance, the heart, and the brain. Mechanistically, the reflex begins with a low blood pressure in the setting of blood pooling in the lower extremities, i.e., after standing for a prolonged period. This leads to inadequate blood supply to the brain. A sympathetic response ensues, with the heart appropriately responding by increasing the heart rate and stroke volume. In those with neurocardiogenic syncope, the increased activity in the left ventricle stimulates the Bezold–Jarisch reflex in which mechanoreceptors of the left ventricle stimulate paradoxical vasodilation and increased vagal tone, leading to decreased end-diastolic volume, bradycardia, and subsequent syncope. Passing out allows one to be supine, which is thought to bring adequate blood supply to the brain in this position. Clinically, it is observed to occur in predisposed individuals following prolonged periods of upright posture, warm environments (hot weather, crowded rooms, hot shower/baths), pain, vomiting, intense emotion/tense psychologic states (i.e., fearful situations like blood draws), dehydration, heavy alcohol intake, or in some patients, after heavy meals.

Symptoms

Localization site	Comment
Cerebral hemispheres	Seizure-like activity may be seen, though this is nonepileptic
Mental status and psychiatric aspects/ complications	Alterations in alertness, cognition, orientation, speech, memory, mood, anxiety; psychotic symptoms such as delusions or hallucinations, suicidal ideation. During the prodromal phase of the syncopal event, there may be an associated diaphoresis, pallor, disorientation, and nausea. Following the syncopal event, patients often express feeling depressed, delayed, fatigued, cloudy, light-headed, with difficulty concentrating. Fatigue is the most common complaint after an episode and may last for a number of days
Vestibular system (and nonspecific dizziness)	Recurrent dizziness (prodromal or post-syncope)
Muscles	Diffuse muscle aches, pain
Meninges	Headache

Treatment Complications: There is no well-established pharmacotherapy for this disease. Reassurance, reduction of anxiety, and physical counter-pressure are helpful. Other considerations for treatment include cardiac pacing or closed loop stimulation, volume maintenance therapies, i.e., support stockings, high salt intake, fludrocortisone, midodrine, and beta-blockade. Other medications include selective serotonin reuptake inhibitors (SSRIs), disopyramide, clonidine, and desmopressin, all of which have their associated adverse effects, i.e., fatigue and decreased libido in SSRIs, anticholinergic effects of disopyramide and clonidine, and orthostatic hypotension, taste alterations, and hyperkalemia with desmopressin.

Bibliography

Chen-Scarabelli C. Neurocardiogenic syncope. *BMJ*. 2004;329(7461):336–41.

Grubb BP. Neurocardiogenic syncope and related disorders of orthostatic intolerance. *Circulation*. 2005;111(22):2997–3006.

Carotid Artery Aneurysm

Epidemiology and Demographics: An estimated 3.2% of the population without comorbidity have an unruptured intracranial saccular aneurysm. The mean age is 50 years and split evenly between genders. Risk of intracranial aneurysm increases with a positive family history or in patients with autosomal dominant polycystic kidney disease and connective tissue disease.

Disorder Description: Aneurysms are abnormal dilations of a blood vessel wall that arise due to defects, disease, or injury to the vessel. The majority of carotid aneurysms occur intracranially at the bifurcation of the internal carotid and posterior communicating artery but can occur in the cervical carotid, especially as a result of trauma. Aneurysms may be saccular (sac-like protrusion from the vessel) or fusiform (involving entire circumference of involved vessel).

Symptoms

Localization site	Comment
Cerebral hemispheres	Severe acute headache (sign of acute aneurysm rupture; pain is severe and comparable to subarachnoid hemorrhage), often lateralized to side of aneurysm; focal neurologic symptoms if brain tissue is damaged
Mental status and psychiatric aspects/complications	Associated with acute headache, loss of consciousness, and altered mental status/confusion; alterations in speech possible depending on location and severity of rupture
Brainstem	Respiratory dysfunction (sign of brainstem compression from acute rupture)
Cranial nerves	Oculomotor (CN III) nerve palsy: diplopia, ptosis, enlarged pupil; facial pain (if aneurysm involves cavernous sinus); visual symptoms, specifically blurry vision

Secondary Complications: After an aneurysm rupture, vasospasm can also occur, limiting perfusion and even causing delayed cerebral ischemia.

Treatment Complications: Treatment of unruptured aneurysms by procedural intervention is possible; however, there is an associated risk of morbidity and mortality. Endovascular repair has been found to have lower mortality than surgical repair. Overall, small unruptured carotid artery aneurysms typically do not warrant intervention; for larger aneurysms, intervention should be considered based on aneurysm size, symptoms, age, and functional status of the patient.

Bibliography

Sonobe M, Yamazaki T, Yonekura M, Kikuchi H. Small unruptured intracranial aneurysm verification study: SUAVE Study, Japan. *Stroke.* 2010;41:1969.

Vlak MH, Algra A, Brandenburg R, Rinkel GJ. Prevalence of unruptured intracranial aneurysms, with emphasis on sex, age, comorbidity, country, and time period: a systematic review and meta-analysis. *Lancet Neurol.* 2011;10:626.

Carotid Artery Dissection

Epidemiology and Demographics: Incidence of spontaneous carotid artery dissection is 1.72/100,000. Average age of those with dissection is 44–46 years based on North American and European studies, with no predisposition related to gender or ethnicity. Patients with connective tissue disorders are at increased risk of spontaneous dissection.

Disorder Description: Dissection is caused by the tearing or separation of arterial wall layers. It occurs after the formation of a tear in the tunica intima layer of the artery, allowing arterial blood to enter into the vessel wall. These subintimal dissections cause stenosis or possibly occlusion of the vessel and increase the risk of thrombus formation, which may embolize distally. Dissections can be secondary to trauma or spontaneous.

Symptoms

Localization site	Comment
Cerebral hemispheres	Headache pain, typically more gradual in onset, however can be acute, throbbing; focal weakness
Visual system	Painless loss of vision (amaurosis fugax)

Localization site	Comment
Vestibular system (and nonspecific dizziness)	Pulsatile tinnitus
Base of skull	Painful Horner syndrome (ptosis, miosis, anhidrosis) from sympathetic fiber involvement
Cranial nerves	Facial pain (CN V), facial palsy (CN VII), oculomotor (CN III) symptoms

Secondary Complications: After conservative treatment, most carotid artery dissections have complete symptom resolution. Transient ischemic attack and acute ischemic stroke are possible, which can have permanent consequences depending on severity, duration, and location of ischemia.

Treatment Complications: Treatment depends on location and severity of dissection. In cases of thrombus, anticoagulation is often used, complications of which include bleeding. Angioplasty or stenting can be done in case of failed medical management and have lower risk of complication compared with surgical treatment but may cause stroke.

Bibliography

Lee VH, Brown RD Jr, Mandrekar JN, Mokri B. Incidence and outcome of cervical artery dissection: a population-based study. *Neurology.* 2006;67:1809.

Mitsias P, Ramadan NM. Headache in ischemic cerebrovascular disease. Part I: Clinical features. *Cephalalgia.* 1992;12:269.

Müller BT, Luther B, Hort W, et al. Surgical treatment of 50 carotid dissections: indications and results. *J Vasc Surg.* 2000;31:980.

Carotid Artery Endarterectomy or Stent

Epidemiology and Demographics: Carotid artery endarterectomy and stenting are both utilized in patients with carotid artery stenosis for prevention of stroke, which is currently the fourth leading cause of death in the United States and where 20% of strokes are secondary to carotid artery stenosis. In patients with asymptomatic carotid artery stenosis, the risk of ipsilateral stroke is 0.5–1% per year.

Disorder Description: Carotid artery stenosis is a result of atherosclerosis. Surgical intervention for carotid stenosis, either by endarterectomy or stenting, can be considered in symptomatic patients with over 70% stenosis. In symptomatic patients with less than 70% stenosis, intervention has questionable benefit compared with medical treatment and carries risks. In patients with asymptomatic carotid atherosclerosis, intervention can be considered if stenosis is greater than 60%. Carotid atherosclerosis can cause symptoms either by decreased flow due to stenosis or artery-to-artery embolism.

Symptoms

Localization site	Comment
Cerebral hemispheres	Transient ischemic attacks, stroke: can present as focal deficits such as sudden weakness, numbness, difficulty speaking, etc. Hemiparesis, aphasia, neglect; headache
Mental status and psychiatric aspects/complications	Confusion, altered mental status, or loss of consciousness
Visual system	Amaurosis fugax. Ocular ischemia: unilateral blindness with absent pupillary response, often ischemic retinal damage
Vestibular system (and nonspecific dizziness)	Tinnitus, dizziness
Cranial nerves	Diplopia, dysarthria

Treatment Complications: When indicated, both carotid endarterectomy and stenting have been proved beneficial overall, although complications can occur. In terms of primary outcomes of stroke, myocardial infarction and death, endarterectomy and stenting appear to have similar risks of adverse outcomes. Perioperatively, stenting is associated with higher risk of stroke, while endarterectomy is associated with higher risk of myocardial infarction. Hyperperfusion syndrome can occur after carotid artery stenting or endarterectomy and is characterized by severe headache and hypertension. Patients who develop hyperperfusion syndrome often had diagnoses of very severe or bilateral stenosis.

Bibliography

Abou-Chebl A, Yadav JS, Reginelli JP, et al. Intracranial hemorrhage and hyperperfusion syndrome following carotid artery stenting: risk factors, prevention, and treatment. *J Am Coll Cardiol.* 2004;43:1596.

Perkins WJ, Lanzino G, Brott TG. Carotid Stenting vs Endarterectomy: New Results in Perspective. *Mayo Clin Proc.* 2010;85:1101–8.

Rosenfield K, Matsumura JS, Chaturvedi S, et al. Randomized trial of stent versus surgery for asymptomatic carotid stenosis. *N Engl J Med.* 2016;374:10113.

Silver FL, Mackey A, Clark WM, et al. Safety of stenting and endarterectomy by symptomatic status in the Carotid Revascularization Endarterectomy versus Stenting Trial (CREST). *Stroke.* 2011;42:6754.

Carotid–Cavernous Fistula

Epidemiology and Demographics: Traumatically induced carotid–cavernous fistula is primarily seen in young males, as this is the population with the highest rates of head trauma. These occur in 0.2% of all patients with head trauma and in 3.8% of patients with a basilar skull fracture.

Disorder Description: The internal carotid artery forms a fistula with the cavernous sinus, shunting blood away from the brain and into the venous circulation. The higher arterial blood pressure subjects the wall of the cavernous sinus to substantial mechanical forces. The most common etiology for fistula formation is head trauma, while the remainder are "spontaneous" carotid–cavernous fistulae, thought to arise from ruptured carotid aneurysms within the cavernous sinus.

Symptoms

Localization site	Comment
Cranial nerves	CN III, IV, V1, V2, and VI pass through the cavernous sinus and can be impaired when cavernous sinus disease is present, causing unilateral visual loss, proptosis, chemosis, eye pain, diplopia, ophthalmoplegia, orbital bruit, headache

Secondary Complications: Risk of hemorrhage is present in traumatic carotid–cavernous fistula, especially among those with vascular risk factors.

Treatment Complications: In most settings, the current preferred treatment is endovascular embolization. Embolization carries the risk of cerebral infarction, diabetes insipidus, decreased visual acuity, orbital ecchymosis, retroperitoneal hematoma, and deep vein thrombosis.

Bibliography

Ellis JA, Goldstein H, Connolly ES Jr., Meyers PM. Carotid-cavernous fistulas. *Neurosurg Focus.* 2012;32:E9.

Liang W, Xiaofeng Y, Weiguo L, et al. Traumatic carotid cavernous fistula accompanying basilar skull fracture: a study on the incidence of traumatic carotid cavernous fistula in the patients with basilar skull fracture and the prognostic analysis about traumatic carotid cavernous fistula. *J Trauma.* 2007;63:1014–20

Meyers PM, Halbach VV, Dowd CF, et al. Dural carotid cavernous fistula: definitive endovascular management and long-term follow-up. *Am J Ophthalmol.* 2002;134:85–92.

Carotid Sinus Hypersensitivity

Epidemiology and Demographics: Incidence is related to age; prevalence is 2.4% among those aged 50–59 years and up to 40.4% in those >80 years. Rarely seen in those <50 years. More common in females at 4:1.

Disorder Description: Carotid sinus hypersensitivity is defined as a decrease in heart rate (at least 3-second asystole, "cardioinhibitory type") or blood pressure (>50 mmHg systolic pressure drop, "vasodepressor type") or both ("mixed type") in response to carotid sinus massage. Syncope and near syncope, provoked by head turning, a tight collar, or shaving, are the most common presentations. Risk factors include age and atherosclerotic disease. Pathogenesis may be related to carotid sinus atherosclerosis, sternocleidomastoid proprioceptive denervation, or autonomic dysfunction.

Symptoms

Localization site	Comment
Mental status and psychiatric aspects/complications	Recurrent syncope, near syncope, light-headedness

Secondary Complications: This condition can cause falls in the elderly.

Treatment Complications: Treatment involves placement of a permanent cardiac pacemaker. Risks for this procedure include palpitations, infection, bleeding, pacemaker lead dislodgement, and pacemaker malfunction.

Bibliography

Amin V, Pavri BB. Carotid sinus syndrome. *Cardiol Rev.* 2015;23:130–4.

Connolly SJ, Sheldon R, Roberts RS, Gent M. The North American Vasovagal Pacemaker Study (VPS). A randomized trial of permanent cardiac pacing for the prevention of vasovagal syncope. *J Am Coll Cardiol.* 1999;33:16–20.

Sutton R. Carotid sinus syndrome: Progress in understanding and management. *Glob Cardiol Sci Pract.* 2014;2014:1–8.

Carpal Tunnel Syndrome

Epidemiology and Demographics: Carpal tunnel syndrome (CTS) is a very common disorder. The estimated annual incidence for women is 324–542/100,000 population and 125–303/100,000 for men. The estimated prevalence is about 1–5%. The prevalence is higher among obese women. The female-to-male ratio for CTS is estimated to be 3:1.

Disorder Description: CTS is a result of median nerve compression at the carpal tunnel. The patients present with pain, paresthesia, numbness, and possible weakness in the median nerve distribution. The median nerve emerges from the fifth cervical to the first thoracic roots, but is mainly formed from the sixth cervical root. The median nerve supplies four muscles in the forearm (pronator teres, flexor carpi radialis, palmaris longus, and flexor digitorum superficialis). The median nerve enters the hand through the carpal tunnel. Within the tunnel is the tendon of the flexor pollicus longus and four tendons of the flexor digitorum superficialis and profundus muscles. Distal to the tunnel the median nerve branches into the motor and sensory fibers. The motor branch usually supplies the abductor pollicis brevis, opponens pollicis, and the first and second lumbrical muscles (sometimes the flexor pollicus brevis muscle). The sensory palmar digital branches supply sensation to the palmar aspect of D1–D3 and half of D4. The palmar cutaneous nerve arises proximal to the carpal tunnel and supplies the skin over the thenar eminence.

Anatomical compression and/or inflammation are the most common causes of carpal tunnel syndrome. Risk factors include repetitive use of the hand, obesity, female gender, pregnancy, diabetes mellitus, rheumatoid arthritis, hypothyroidism, and workplace factors.

Symptoms are usually worse at night. Phalen maneuver and Tinel's signs at the wrist are useful in the diagnosis, with sensitivity of up to 50% but higher specificity.

Treatment includes symptomatic relief with a wrist splint, nonsteroidal anti-inflammatory drugs (NSAIDs), glucocorticoid injections, and oral glucocorticoids. Treatment of underlying condition if present, such as rheumatoid arthritis and hypothyroidism, is usually helpful. Treatment for severe cases is decompression of the median nerve at the carpal tunnel.

Symptoms

Localization site	Comment
Peripheral neuropathy/ mononeuropathy	Median nerve distribution sensory and motor symptoms
Muscle	Atrophy of abductor pollicis brevis

Treatment Complications: Oral glucocorticoid treatment should not extend beyond 4 weeks due to deleterious side effects of chronic therapy. Glucocorticoid injection risks include: exacerbation of the compression, accidental injection into the median or ulnar nerves, and digital flexor tendon rupture. Surgical complications include permanent nerve damage and infection.

Bibliography

Kothari M. Carpal tunnel syndrome: etiology and epidemiology. In Post TW, ed. *UpToDate*. Waltham, MA. Accessed Jan 21, 2016.

Ropper A, Samuels M. Disease of the peripheral nervous system. In *Adams and Victor's principles of neurology*. 9th ed. New York: McGraw-Hill Education/Medical; 2009. pp. 1314–5.

Cassava Root Toxicity (Konzo)

Epidemiology and Demographics: Cyanide poisoning occurring within hours of ingesting raw or inadequately processed cassava. It is almost exclusively seen in poor populations in famine conditions.

Disorder Description: Cyanogens from consumption of insufficiently processed bitter roots release cyanide, which causes acute poisoning with onset within a half to several hours with nausea, vomiting, diarrhea, and weakness. This may progress to collapse

and even death. Interestingly, although other forms of cyanide poisoning have been shown to cause basal ganglia damage and parkinsonism with severe toxicity, this has not been reported with cassava root poisoning, probably because those stricken do not survive. Tropical ataxic neuropathy develops slowly as a result of chronic consumption of cassava root and is associated with sensory loss in the lower extremities and optic atrophy. It is most commonly seen in Nigeria. Konzo is an upper motor neuron disorder originally described in Zaire. *Konzo* means "tired legs" and refers to the resultant spastic gait. Interestingly the cyanide exposure is higher in konzo than in tropical ataxic neuropathy, and the onset is abrupt.

Symptoms

Localization site	Comment
Cerebral hemispheres	Konzo causes upper motor neuron damage with spastic paraparesis. Rarely, there may also be spastic dysarthria, but it usually resolves
Cranial nerves	Optic atrophy with tropical ataxic neuropathy
Peripheral neuropathy	Tropical ataxic neuropathy causes distal sensory loss

Bibliography

Howlet WP, Brubaker GR, Mlingi N, Rosling H. Konzo, an epidemic upper motor neuron disease studied in Tanzania. *Brain*. 1990;113:223–35.

Rosling H, Tyklesklar T. Cassava. In Spencer PS, Schaumburg HH, eds. *Experimental and clinical neurotoxicology*. 2nd ed. New York: Oxford University Press; 2000. pp. 338–43.

Cataract

Epidemiology and Demographics: In 2010, the World Health Organization estimated cataract was the most common cause of blindness worldwide, affecting approximately 22 million people across the globe. Cataract surgery is the most common surgical procedure performed in the developed world. Cataracts can affect patients of any age, but most often are age related or congenital. Certain metabolic conditions such as diabetes can contribute to cataract formation. In developing countries, cataracts occur earlier in life and the incidence is higher. Additionally, the amount of visual disability attributable to cataract is greater in developing countries where there are fewer surgeons to perform cataract extraction surgery than in developed countries.

Disorder Description: A cataract is defined as an opacification of the natural crystalline ocular lens. Cataracts are categorized by which part of the lens structure is affected. Age-related or so-called senile cataracts are the most common and cause the lens nucleus to become larger and more brunescent (yellow or brown). Diabetes, hypertension, UV light, smoking, and alcohol have all been identified as risk factors but knowledge of cataract is incomplete. Age is the greatest risk factor as there is cumulative exposure to toxins and increased risk of disease. Despite the common co-existence of senile cataracts with some degree of cognitive impairment, there is no clear-cut causative relationship between senile cataracts and dementia. Less commonly, cataracts can be seen in a number of systemic disorders with neurologic complications.

Symptoms: The degree of cataract and cataract morphology affects patient symptomatology. Patients typically complain of decreased vision, decreased contrast sensitivity, and glare, particularly with nighttime driving. Other symptoms include refractive changes, monocular diplopia, glare, and changes in color vision.

Localization site	Comment
Mental status and psychiatric aspects/ complications	**Wilson's disease** is an inherited disorder of copper metabolism in which excess copper accumulates throughout the body. It is associated with psychiatric symptoms. In the lens, the copper deposits in the anterior capsule and cortex in a petaloid, "sunflower"-like configuration. The basal ganglia are the most commonly affected sites in the brain
Basal ganglia	As per above
Vestibular system (and non-specific dizziness)	**Neurofibromatosis type 2** is associated with posterior subcapsular cataracts and acoustic neuromas
Peripheral neuropathy	**Diabetes mellitus** is associated with many types of cataracts and the earlier development of age-related cataracts. Peripheral neuropathy is among the most common complications of diabetes and is thought to occur as a result of damage to peripheral nerves secondary to prolonged exposure to elevated blood glucose levels

Localization site	Comment
Muscle	**Myotonic dystrophy**, characterized by progressive muscle wasting and weakness, is associated with characteristic polychromic cortical cataracts (also known as "Christmas tree cataracts")

Secondary Complications: Cataracts are a major cause of geriatric vision loss. Patients with vision loss from cataracts are at increased risk for nursing home placement, falls, and hip replacement surgery.

Release visual hallucinations (sometimes termed Charles Bonnet syndrome) may occur in patients with dense bilateral cataracts and severe vision loss. These patients will report seeing geometric shapes, small characters, or faces, but they have insight into the hallucinations and recognize that they are not real. These patients do not have psychiatric disease, but may be disturbed by the images and afraid to admit that they see them for fear of being labeled with psychiatric disease. The term "release hallucinations" stems from the concept that interruption of normal visual input is associated with release of brain activity. These hallucinations are usually seen in elderly patients with central vision loss from macular degeneration, diabetic retinopathy, or cataracts but have also been described in those with visual field deficits and children. Charles Bonnet syndrome is a diagnosis of exclusion and requires careful evaluation for psychiatric disease, drug use, and seizure activity.

Treatment Complications: Complications of modern cataract surgery are rare but include vision loss, visual distortion, pain, and diplopia. In a meta-analysis of 90 studies on cataract extraction with intraocular lens implantation, the incidence of sight-threatening complications was less than 2% regardless of lens extraction technique.

Bibliography

Brian G, Taylor H. Cataract blindness – challenges for the 21st century. *Bull World Health Org.* 2001;79(3):249–56.

Frick KD, Foster A. The magnitude and cost of global blindness: an increasing problem that can be alleviated. *Am J Ophthalmol.* 2013;135(4):471–6.

Pascolini D, Mariotti SP. Global estimates of visual impairment: 2010. *Br J Ophthalmol.* 2012;96(5):614–8.

Shiels A, Bennett TM, Fielding Hejtmancik J. Cat-map: putting cataract on the map. *Mol Vis.* 2010;16:2007–15.

Catatonia

Epidemiology and Demographics: May be underrecognized in clinical practice; however, catatonia has been reported to occur in approximately 10% of acutely ill psychiatric inpatients. More common in patients with unipolar major depression, bipolar disorder, psychotic disorders, autism spectrum disorder, and delirium, as well as many general medical conditions including infectious, metabolic, neurologic, and rheumatologic disorders.

Disorder Description: Behavioral syndrome characterized by significant psychomotor disturbance, which can occur in the context of a variety of underlying psychiatric and general medical disorders. The syndrome can present with heterogeneous signs and symptoms; however, the most common include immobility, rigidity, mutism, posturing, excessive motor activity, stupor, negativism, staring, and echolalia. Based on the clinical presentation, three primary subtypes exist: retarded, malignant, and excited catatonia.

Symptoms

Localization site	Comment
Mental status and psychiatric aspects/ complications	Immobility including hypokinetic or akinetic behavior, stupor, staring, mutism, negativism, posturing (catalepsy), excitement (impulsive, frantic, and stereotypic behavior that may result in harm to self or others), echophenomena (echolalia, echopraxia), speech mannerisms (robotic speech, feigned foreign accent, verbigeration), behavioral mannerisms (odd, purposeful movements), stereotypy (grimacing, teeth/tongue clicking, rocking, sniffing, biting, automatically touching or tapping), ambitendency, automatic obedience, waxy flexibility, stimulus-bound behavior

Secondary Complications: Complications may include dehydration, malnutrition, deep vein thrombosis and pulmonary embolism, contractures, pressure ulcers, or injury to self or others. In some cases, life-threatening malignant catatonia can develop with fever, autonomic instability, delirium, and rigidity.

Treatment Complications: Antipsychotics and other dopamine-blocking agents should generally be avoided in patients with catatonia because of the risk of precipitating neuroleptic malignant syndrome in this patient population. Antipsychotics are contraindicated in malignant catatonia.

Bibliography

American Psychiatric Association. *Diagnostic and statistical manual of mental disorders: DSM-5.* 5th ed. Washington, DC: American Psychiatric Association; 2013.

Bush G, Fink M, Petrides G, et al. Catatonia. I. Rating scale and standardized examination. *Acta Psychiatr Scand.* 1996;93:129.

Fink M, Taylor MA. *Catatonia: a clinician's guide to diagnosis and treatment.* Cambridge: Cambridge University Press; 2003.

Fink M, Taylor MA. The catatonia syndrome: forgotten but not gone. *Arch Gen Psychiatry.* 2009;66(11):1173.

Cat Scratch Disease (CSD)

Epidemiology and Demographics: Disease occurs worldwide. Eighty percent of cat scratch disease (CSD) patients are younger than 21 years of age. Estimated 22,000 cases/year in the United States.[1] Neurologic complications account for 1–2% of cases of CSD.[2]

Disorder Description: Commonly known as "cat scratch fever," CSD is a bacterial infection caused by the gram-negative rod *Bartonella henselae*. Patients typically present with painful regional lymphadenopathy with fever following an animal bite or scratch, generally occurring 2 weeks later. Severe cases may spread to the central nervous system.[1]

Greater than 90% of risk for infection is contact with cats, mainly kittens; however, tick or flea bites, rodents, sheep, monkeys, cows, foxes, coyotes, porcupines, and dogs have been reported. Needle-stick transmission has also been reported. Veterinary professionals, groomers, animal rescue workers, and pet owners are at risk for infection.[1,3]

Symptoms

Localization site	Comment
Cerebral hemispheres	Meningitis
	Encephalitis
	Seizures (status epilepticus has been reported)
	Vasculitis
Mental status and psychiatric aspects/complications	Encephalopathy[3]
	Behavioral abnormalities
	Hallucinations
Cranial nerves	Neuroretinitis, presenting as visual field loss due to optic nerve edema
	Optic neuropathy
	Bell's palsy (rare)
Spinal cord	Transverse myelitis
Specific spinal roots	Radiculitis
Peripheral neuropathy	Polyneuropathy, Guillain–Barré syndrome[3]

Secondary Complications: Seizures or vision loss due to neuroretinitis or optic neuropathy may result.

Treatment Complications: Rifampin may cause blood dyscrasias or hepatotoxicity.

References

1. Nervi SJ. Cat scratch disease (cat scratch fever) clinical presentation. Updated Jul 24, 2017. Available from https://emedicine.medscape.com/article/214100-clinical. Accessed Oct 16, 2018.
2. Lamas C, Curi A, Bóia M, Lemos E. Human bartonellosis: seroepidemiological and clinical features with an emphasis on data from Brazil – a review. *Mem Inst Oswaldo Cruz*. 2008;103(3).
3. Breitschwerdt E, Sontakke S, Hopkins S. Neurological manifestations of bartonellosis in immunocompetent patients: a composite of reports from 2005–2012. *J Neuroparasitol*. 2012;3:1–15.

Cauda Equina Syndrome

Epidemiology and Demographics: Cauda equina syndrome affects about 2% of herniated lumbar disc cases.

Disorder Description: The cauda equina is composed of nerve roots distal to the conus medullaris. Cauda equina syndrome is a combination of symptoms and signs that include low back pain, radicular pain, motor weakness, saddle anesthesia, and bowel or bladder dysfunction resulting from cauda equina compression. It is a surgical emergency. Etiologies of cauda equina syndrome include trauma, acute disc herniation, degenerative spine disease with or without congenital stenosis, primary central nervous system tumors, metastatic disease, abscesses, archnoiditis, or epidural anesthesia. An MRI is the study of choice to evaluate for a compressive lesion and to determine if there is a surgical emergency since timely surgical intervention is the key to prognostic outcome.

Symptoms

Localization site	Comment
Cauda equina	Nerves arising from cauda equina
Mononeuropathy or mononeuropathy multiplex	Single nerve may be affected

Secondary Complications: Urinary tract infection from urinary retention.

Treatment Complications: Postsurgical complications including altered mental status from anesthesia.

Bibliography

Gitelman A, Hishme S, Morelli BN, et al. Cauda equina syndrome: a comprehensive review. *Am J Orthop*. 2008;37(11):556–62.

Cavernous Angioma

Epidemiology and Demographics: Cerebral cavernous angioma has a prevalence of about 0.6% in the general population. About half are inherited (autosomal dominant with variable penetrance). The average age of presentation is 30.6 years.

Disorder Description: Angiomas (also known as cavernous hemangiomas, cavernomas, and cerebral cavernous malformations) are collections of aberrant dilated blood vessels. They are most commonly located in the white matter tissue. Angioma expansion can occur spontaneously and can cause symptomatic or asymptomatic microhemorrhages.

Symptoms

Localization site	Comment
Cerebral hemispheres	Seizure, focal neurologic deficit, headache, hemorrhage
Brainstem	Seizure, focal neurologic deficit, headache, hemorrhage, cranial neuropathy
Cerebellum	Ataxia, headache, hemorrhage
Spinal cord	Stepwise or gradual motor or sensory deficits below the level of the lesion

Secondary Complications: Intracerebral hemorrhage may be a presenting symptom, or may occur later.

Treatment Complications: Surgical and interventional radiologic treatment of symptomatic and asymptomatic cavernous angiomas share similar risks, such as causing neurologic deficits (motor, sensory, ataxia) depending on the location. These occur with a similar incidence between surgical and non-surgical intervention, at about 6 serious events per 100 person-years.

Bibliography

Al-Holou WN, O'Lynnger TM, Pandey AS, et al. Natural history and imaging prevalence of cavernous malformations in children and young adults. *J Neurosurg Pediatr*. 2012;9:198–205.

Maraire JN, Awad IA. Intracranial cavernous malformations: lesion behavior and management strategies. *Neurosurgery*. 1995;37:591–605.

Poorthuis MH, Klijn CJ, Algra A, Rinkel GJ, Al-Shahi Salman R. Treatment of cerebral cavernous malformations: a systematic review and meta-regression analysis. *J Neurol Neurosurg Psychiatry*. 2014;85:1319–23.

Cavernous Sinus Thrombophlebitis

Epidemiology and Demographics: Approximately 3–4 cases of cerebral venous thrombosis occur per million people per year. Females account for 75% of cases. Can occur across all age ranges, with a mean age of presentation of 22 years.

Disorder Description: Acquired condition in which a blood clot forms in the cavernous sinus at the base of the brain, usually due to infection with *Staphylococcus aureus*. This may cause interference with structures in the cavernous sinus, including cranial nerves III, IV, V1, V2, and VI. Use of anticoagulation is controversial and may exacerbate the spread of infection. The infection and thrombosis is considered life threatening and requires immediate treatment.

Symptoms

Localization site	Comment
Cranial nerves	CN III, IV, V, VI nerve palsies with diplopia or facial pain/numbness. Unilateral visual loss (optic nerve ischemia)
Pituitary gland	Pituitary insufficiency
Unclear localization	Headache

Secondary Complications: Inflammation and edema can cause damage to surrounding structures including carotid artery and pituitary. Additionally, emboli (septic and otherwise) can occur and cause tissue infarction.

Treatment Complications: Allergic reaction to antibiotics (i.e., nafcillin, cefotaxime, and metronidazole) used for empiric treatment. Anticoagulants used may cause bleeding.

Bibliography

Agostoni E, Aliprandi A, Longoni M. Review. Cerebral venous thrombosis. *Expert Rev Neurother*. 2009;9:553–64.

Cavernous Sinus Thrombosis (CST)

Epidemiology and Demographics: Cavernous sinus thrombosis (CST) is a rare condition, with no epidemiologic data available.

Disorder Description: Most commonly occurs in the setting of venous stasis, endovascular injury, and hypercoagulability. Direct spread of *Streptococcus*, *Staphylococcus*, or *Pneumococcus* species from a paranasal sinus infection, abscess, or orbital cellulitis can cause CST. Aseptic cavernous sinus thrombosis is usually from a tumor or aneurysm causing venous stasis within the cavernous sinus.

Symptoms

Localization site	Comment
Base of skull	Unilateral progressing to bilateral: eye pain, chemosis, and proptosis. Lateral gaze palsy progressing to ophthalmoplegia. Diplopia, vision loss. Headache, nausea, vomiting, chills, diaphoresis, seizures

Secondary Complications: Dissemination of infection can cause blindness, focal seizures, hemiparesis, intracranial or systemic infection/abscess, cerebral edema, vascular steal, and hypopituitarism.

Treatment Complications: As CST is a rare disease, there is no rigorously tested treatment regime for these patients. For septic causes, antibiotics or antimicrobials are the primary therapy, with anticoagulation in selected patients. Antithrombotics and corticosteroids may be used in aseptic cases, with surgical resection possible if there is a tumor. These carry the risk of hemorrhage.

Bibliography

Bousser M-G, Barnett HJM. Cerebral venous thrombosis. In Mohr J, Grotta J, Wolf P, Choi D, Weir B, eds. *Stroke.* 4th ed. Philadelphia: Churchill Livingstone; 2004. pp. 301–25.

Cockerham KP. Orbital and ocular manifestations of neurological disease. In Aminoff MJ, ed. *Neurology and general medicine.* 4th ed. Philadelphia: Churchill Livingstone; 2008. pp. 483–501.

Ebright JR, Pace MT, Niazi AF. Septic thrombosis of the cavernous sinuses. *Arch Intern Med.* 2001;161:2671–6.

Cavernous Sinus Tumor

Epidemiology and Demographics: Cavernous sinus tumor is considered a rare disease; little is known about incidence or prevalence.

Disorder Description: Many tumors can invade the cavernous sinus, including primary meningioma or neurofibroma as well as metastatic disease. The mechanical blockage of venous outflow through the cavernous sinus causes fluid to build up and put pressure on the cranial nerves that pass through the cavernous sinus. The result is called cavernous sinus syndrome, a constellation of neurologic and ophthalmologic signs and symptoms.

Symptoms

Localization site	Comment
Base of skull	Ophthalmoplegia, chemosis, proptosis. Cranial nerve palsies of CN II, III, IV, V, VI

Secondary Complications: Benign tumors may expand locally and compromise cranial nerves in the cavernous sinus. Malignant tumors can metastasize to the brain or elsewhere.

Treatment Complications: Radiosurgery or surgery can be used to shrink or remove the tumor. Complications of each include damage to the adjacent cranial nerves.

Bibliography

Keane JR. Cavernous sinus syndrome. Analysis of 151 cases. *Arch Neurol.* 1996;53:967–71.

Kuo JS, Chen JC, Yu C, et al. Gamma knife radiosurgery for benign cavernous sinus tumors: quantitative analysis of treatment outcomes. *Neurosurgery.* 2004;54:1385–93

Newman S. A prospective study of cavernous sinus surgery for meningiomas and resultant common ophthalmic complications (an American Ophthalmological Society thesis). *Trans Am Ophthalmol Soc.* 2007;105:392–447.

Celiac Disease

Epidemiology and Demographics: Celiac disease is found in about 1% of the population. The incidence of celiac disease has a bimodal distribution, with one peak during the first decade of life and a second one between 40 and 50 years of age. Women are affected more often than men (2:1).

Disorder Description: Celiac disease is caused by an immune reaction to the cereal grain protein gluten, which causes small bowel injury resulting in malabsorption. Postprandial bloating, steatorrhea, and weight loss are cardinal features of this disease. Pathologic studies of the small intestine often show villus atrophy and intraepithelial lymphocytic infiltrate. Anti-endomysial antibodies, anti-tissue transglutaminase antibodies, and anti-gliadin antibodies are main serologic markers of this disease.

Symptoms

Localization site	Comment
Cerebral hemispheres	Seizure
Mental status and psychiatric aspects/complications	Schizophrenia
	Depression
	Anxiety
	Autism spectrum disorder
	Attention deficit hyperactivity disorder

Localization site	Comment
Brainstem	Brainstem encephalitis
Cerebellum	Cerebellar ataxia Cerebellar degeneration
Spinal cord	Myelopathy
Mononeuropathy or mononeuropathy multiplex	Mononeuritis multiplex
Peripheral neuropathy	Distal symmetric axonal sensorimotor polyneuropathy
Neuromuscular junction	Myasthenia gravis
Muscle	Polymyositis Dermatomyositis Inclusion body myositis
Unclear localization	Migraine

Secondary Complications: Malabsorption can lead to deficiency of vitamins and essential micronutrients. Copper deficiency for example can cause myelopathy, neuropathy, and optic neuropathy. Vitamin B12 deficiency can cause optic neuropathy or syndrome of subacute combined degeneration.

Bibliography

Briani C, Zara G, Alaedini A, et al. Neurological complications of celiac disease and autoimmune mechanisms: a prospective study. *J Neuroimmunol.* 2008;195(1–2):171–5.

Fasano A, Catassi C. Current approaches to diagnosis and treatment of celiac disease: an evolving spectrum. *Gastroenterology.* 2001;120(3): 636–51.

Hadjivassiliou M, Grünewald RA, Chattopadhyay AK, et al. Clinical, radiological, neurophysiological, and neuropathological characteristics of gluten ataxia. *Lancet.* 1998;352:1582–5.

Hadjivassiliou M, Grünewald RA, Davies-Jones GA. Gluten sensitivity as a neurological illness. *J Neurol Neurosurg Psychiatry.* 2002;72(5): 560–3.

Jackson JR, Eaton WW, Cascella NG, Fasano A, Kelly DL. Neurologic and psychiatric manifestations of celiac disease and gluten sensitivity. *Psychiatr Q.* 2012;83(1):91–102.

Central Pontine Myelinolysis

Epidemiology and Demographics: Exact incidence is unknown; however, incidence is highest among alcoholics and liver transplant recipients. It occurs most often between age 30 and 50 years.

Disorder Description: Central pontine myelinolysis is an uncommon neurologic disorder that occurs as a result of damage to the myelin sheath of neurons. It affects the pontine white matter tracts, but can also cause extrapontine lesions (extrapontine myelinolysis). Extrapontine lesions include involvement of the basal ganglia, lentiform nucleus, internal and external capsule, and thalamus. The exact pathophysiology is unknown, but it is associated with rapid correction of hyponatremia. It has been found to occur in alcoholics and liver transplant recipients. It has also been associated with severe hypophosphatemia, severe burns, Wilson's disease, hyponatremia, hypokalemia, renal failure, diabetes, hyperemesis gravidarum, anorexia nervosa, and systemic lupus erythematosus. It presents as seizures or encephalopathy that progresses to dysarthria, dysphagia, oculomotor dysfunction, or quadriparesis, and sometimes patients may experience locked-in syndrome.

Symptoms

Localization site	Comment
Cerebral hemispheres	Encephalopathy, seizures
Mental status and psychiatric aspects/ complications	Acute confusion; behavioral changes; mania; deficits in short-term memory, attention/concentration, and learning ability
Cerebellum	Rare extension to cerebellum can lead to ataxia
Brainstem	Dysarthria, dysphagia, oculomotor dysfunction, quadriparesis, locked-in syndrome

Secondary Complications: Can lead to long-term dystonia, slow choreoathetotic movements, tremor, and neuropsychologic deficits including problems with short-term memory, attention/concentration, and learning ability.

Bibliography

Musana A, Yale SH. Central pontine myelinolysis: case series and review. *WMJ.* 2005;104(6):56–60.

Singh TD, Fugate JE, Rabinstein AA. Central pontine and extrapontine myelinolysis: a systematic review. *Eur J Neurol*. 2014;21:1443–50.

Vermetten E. Neuropsychiatric and neuropsychological manifestations of central pontine myelinolysis. *Gen Hosp Psychiatry*. 2005;21(4):296–302.

Central Retinal Artery Occlusion (CRAO; or Branch Retinal Artery Occlusion)

Epidemiology and Demographics: Central retinal artery occlusion (CRAO) is a relatively rare disease, with an incidence of ~1/10,000. The vast majority of patients have unilateral occlusion, but 1–2% have bilateral involvement. The mean age of patients with central retinal artery occlusion is 60–65 years. Men are affected more frequently than women. Patients with CRAO have higher prevalence of comorbidities such as hypertension, diabetes, and smoking, and often have undiagnosed vascular risk factors. Patients with inflammatory disease such as giant cell arteritis are also more likely to have CRAO.

Disorder Description: Central retinal artery occlusion is characterized by acute painless monocular loss of vision, along with retinal ischemia on funduscopic exam. This occlusion is typically secondary to embolism or atherosclerosis. Visual loss occurs because of occlusion of the central retinal artery, which is the first intraorbital branch of the ophthalmic artery. This leads to ischemia of the inner layer of the retina, pyknosis, and eventual necrosis of the retina. Recovery of vision is very unlikely without emergent intervention; definitive intervention typically involves revascularization.

Symptoms

Localization site	Comment
Cerebral hemispheres	Headache (presence suggests giant cell arteritis as etiology); motor or sensory symptoms might suggest carotid artery disease as associated etiology
Visual system	Acute, severe loss of vision (typically monocular), typically painless

Secondary Complications: If plaque is present in the internal carotid artery, further embolization to the brain can occur.

Treatment Complications: The goal of intervention with CRAO involves restoring blood flow to the retina, and neovascularization can occur if enough retina survives. Treatment complications can occur. Vitreous hemorrhage is possible; however, this occurs in less than 1/50 patients. Neovascular glaucoma is also possible and is more common; this can be extremely painful and may even require eventual removal of the affected eye.

Bibliography

Leavitt JA, Larson TA, Hodge DO, Gullerud RE. The incidence of central retinal artery occlusion in Olmsted County, Minnesota. *Am J Ophthalmol*. 2011;152:820.

Rudkin AK, Lee AW, Aldrich E, et al. Clinical characteristics and outcome of current standard management of central retinal artery occlusion. *Clin Exp Ophthalmol*. 2010;38:496.

Central Retinal Vein Occlusion (CRVO)

Epidemiology and Demographics: Central retinal vein occlusion (CRVO) is uncommon with studies citing 0.1% prevalence in the general population. Most patients with CRVO are >50 years old and men are at a slightly increased risk.

Disorder Description: CRVO causes venous outflow obstruction from the central retinal vein. Acutely, this condition presents as painless, unilateral vision loss. Risk factors include age, a history of hypercoagulable diseases, and cardiovascular risk factors, such as diabetes, obesity, and hypertension.

Symptoms

Localization site	Comment
Cranial nerves	Monocular visual loss. Can see an afferent pupillary defect if the optic nerve is affected

Secondary Complications: Neovascularization of the iris, anterior chamber angle, and the retina causing glaucoma and blindness.

Treatment Complications: Complications of retinal photocoagulation, such as macular edema, transient visual loss, and color vision changes.

Bibliography

Klein R, Klein BE, Moss SE, Meuer SM. The epidemiology of retinal vein occlusion: the Beaver Dam Eye Study. *Trans Am Ophthalmol Soc.* 2000;98:133–43.

The Eye Disease Case-Control Study Group. Risk factors for central retinal vein occlusion. *Arch Ophthalmol.* 1996;114:545–54.

Central Serous Choroidopathy

Epidemiology and Demographics: Incidence of central serous choroidopathy is 1/10,000 for men and 1.7/100,000 for women in the United States. Men are affected up to 10 times more often than women. The mean age of presentation is 49.8 years. Patients may present with choroidopathy after age 50, although these patients are often found to have bilateral disease.

Disorder Description: Central serous choroidopathy, or chorioretinopathy, is an ophthalmologic disease that is caused by serous detachment of the retina due to fluid accumulation in the subretinal space. This leakage occurs because of breaks in the retinal pigment epithelium. Patients present with acute visual loss and distorted or blurred vision. Patients also can present with decreased central vision or scotoma. Prognosis is generally very good once fluid accumulation has resolved.

Symptoms

Localization site	Comment
Visual system	Acute visual loss and metamorphopsia, scotoma, and decreased central vision; more subtle visual symptoms include impaired color saturation and sensitivity to contrast

Secondary Complications: Complications of central serous chorioretinopathy include pigment epithelial detachment and subretinal neovascularization. The neovascularization is understood to be a result of the leakage itself and of laser treatment. Retinal detachment can occur in patients with central serous choroidopathy who are otherwise healthy; however, corticosteroid use has been found to increase likelihood of this complication.

Treatment Complications: Laser photocoagulation has been found to increase the risk of subretinal neovascularization.

Bibliography

Burumcek E, Mudun A, Karacorlu S, Arslan MO. Laser photocoagulation for persistent central serous retinopathy: results of long-term follow-up. *Ophthalmology.* 1997;104:616–22.

Kitzmann AS, Pulido JS, Diehl NN, Hodge DO, Burke JP. The incidence of central serous chorioretinopathy in Olmsted County, Minnesota, 1980–2002. *Ophthalmology.* 2008;115:169–73.

Liew G, Quin G, Gillies M, Fraser-Bell S. Central serous chorioretinopathy: a review of epidemiology and pathophysiology. *Clin Exp Ophthalmol.* 2012;41:201–14.

Central Sleep Apnea Due to High-Altitude Periodic Breathing

Epidemiology and Demographics: Virtually anyone who ascends to an altitude >4000 m and approximately 25% of individuals who ascend to 2500 m will have periodic breathing during sleep.

Predisposing Factors: Increased hypoxic ventilatory response to high-altitude hypoxia predisposes to hyperventilation, which drives the arterial partial pressure of carbon dioxide ($Paco_2$) below the apneic threshold, resulting in central apnea during sleep. The more rapid the ascent, the more likely periodic breathing is to occur.

Disorder Description: Periodic breathing at high altitude is characterized by repetitive oscillations consisting of hyperpnea followed by hypopnea or central apnea, which occurs during rapid eye movement (REM) and non-rapid eye movement (NREM) sleep. These hyperpneas induce arousals that disturb sleep.

Periodic breathing due to high altitudes occurs as an individual reaches an altitude that exposes them to hypoxia, and compensatory hyperventilation ensues in an attempt to correct the hypoxemia. When sleeping at altitude in a hypoxic environment, tidal volume oscillates and $Paco_2$ falls to a level at or below the apneic threshold. The periodic breaths occur in short cycles of 15–25 seconds followed by apneas of 5 to 15 seconds.

Diagnosis of CSA due to high-altitude periodic breathing is made if the patient meets the following criteria:

1. Recent ascent to high altitude (typically at least 2500 m).
2. The presence of one or more of the following:
   a. sleepiness;
   b. difficulty initiating or maintaining sleep, frequent awakenings, or nonrestorative sleep;
   c. awakening with shortness of breath or morning headache;
   d. witnessed apnea.
3. The symptoms are clinically attributable to high-altitude periodic breathing or polysomnogram demonstrates recurrent central apneas or hypopneas.

Symptoms are worse during the initial ascent to altitude (first few nights) and tend to improve over time with acclimatization.

Symptoms

Localization site	Comment
Brainstem	Ventral medullary respiratory control centers
Mental status and psychiatric aspects/complications	Sleepiness, insomnia, fragmented sleep

Secondary Complications: Daytime somnolence, effects of sleep deprivation in the setting of sleep fragmentation, and insomnia.

Treatment Complications: The most effective treatment of CSA due to high altitude periodic breathing is to descend to a lower altitude. Acetazolamide widens the difference between eupneic and apneic threshold $PaCO_2$, resulting in improvement in periodic breathing while at altitude. Inhalation of supplemental oxygen decreases periodic breathing as well. Despite acclimatization at altitude, evidence exists to suggest that periodic breathing persists. Acetazolamide may worsen dehydration and cause paresthesias.

Bibliography

Eckert DJ, Jordan AS, Merchia P, et al. Central sleep apnea: pathophysiology and treatment. *Chest*. 2005;131:595–607.

Jahaveri S. Central sleep apnea. *Clin Chest Med*. 2010;31:235–48.

Jahaveri S, Dempsey JA. Central sleep apnea. *Compr Physiol*. 2013;3:141–63.

Küpper T, Schöffl V, Netzer N. Cheyne Stokes breathing at high altitude: a helpful response or a troublemaker? *Sleep Breath*. 2008;12(2):123–7.

Sateia M, Berry RB, Bornemann MC, et al. *International classification of sleep disorders*. 3rd ed. Darien, IL: American Academy of Sleep Medicine; 2014.

Tellez HF, MacDonald-Nethercott E, Neyte X, et al. Sleep-related periodic breathing does not acclimatize to chronic hypobaric hypoxia: a 1-year study at high altitude in Antarctica. *Am J Respir Crit Care Med*. 2014;190:114–6.

Central Sleep Apnea Secondary to Medications or Substance Abuse

Epidemiology and Demographics: Estimating the true prevalence of central sleep apnea (CSA) secondary to medications or other substances is difficult. Opioids are the most studied substances that induce CSA. A meta-analysis of seven studies found the mean prevalence of opioid-induced CSA to be 24% (range 4–60%). There is no known sex predominance and no specific age at onset.

Opioids of any dose may induce CSA; however, potent and long-acting opioids are the most likely to exert this effect. A direct relationship between the dose of opioids and the development and severity of CSA has been reported. Both benzodiazepines and antidepressants have been shown to worsen the severity of opioid-induced CSA. Body mass index is inversely related to the severity of CSA.

Disorder Description: This disorder is typically seen after opioids have been used for >2 months; methadone is the most common causative agent. These drugs can cause hypoventilation and obstructive apneas in addition to CSA. The drug-induced central apneas can vary in respiratory pattern and include periodic breathing with multiple central apneas followed by several normal breaths of short cycle time. The patient's underlying respiratory pattern may be ataxic, which is characterized by a variable tidal volume and irregular rhythm.

Diagnosis of CSA due to a medication or substance is made if the patient meets the following criteria:

1. Must be taking an opioid or other respiratory depressant.

2. Must have one or more of the following:
   a. sleepiness;
   b. difficulty initiating or maintaining sleep, frequent awakenings, or nonrestorative sleep;
   c. awakening short of breath;
   d. snoring;
   e. witnessed apneas.
3. Has a polysomnogram consistent with CSA.
4. The disorder occurs as a consequence of an opioid or other respiratory depressant.
5. The disorder is not better explained by another sleep disorder.

Symptoms

Localization site	Comment
Medulla	Mu receptors of the ventral medulla in the pre-Botzinger complex (putative respiratory pattern generator) as well other medullary ventilatory control areas
Mental status and psychiatric aspects/complications	Sleepiness, depression, social dysfunction. Effects may also be due to the effects of the underlying condition requiring opioids

Secondary Complications: Daytime somnolence, depression, social and workplace dysfunction may occur in the setting of sleep fragmentation.

Treatment Complications: Withdrawal of the medication causing the apneas may resolve the CSA. Polysomnography should be performed to establish the diagnosis and to ensure no other sleep disorder such as obstructive sleep apnea is present. If dose reduction or withdrawal of opioids causing CSA is not possible, positive airway pressure (PAP) therapy including bilevel in the spontaneous timed mode or adaptive servo-ventilation may be tried.

Bibliography

Alattar MA, Scharf SM. Opioid-associated central sleep apnea: a case series. *Sleep Breath.* 2009;13:201–6.
Correa D, Farney RJ, Chung F, et al. Chronic opioid use and central sleep apnea: a review of the prevalence, mechanisms, and perioperative considerations. *Anesth Analg.* 2015;120: 1273–85.
Davis MJ, Livingston M, Scharf SM. Reversal of central sleep apnea following discontinuation of opioids. *J Clin Sleep Med.* 2012;8(5):579–80.
Jahaveri S, Dempsey JA. Central sleep apnea. *Compr Physiol.* 2013;3:141–63.
Sateia M, Berry RB, Bornemann MC, et al. *International classification of sleep disorders.* 3rd ed. Darien, IL: American Academy of Sleep Medicine; 2014.
Walker JM, Farney RJ, Rhondeau SM, et al. Chronic opioid use is a risk factor for the development of central sleep apnea and ataxic breathing. *J Clin Sleep Med.* 2007;3(5):455–61.

Central Sleep Apnea with Cheyne–Stokes Respiration

Epidemiology and Demographics: Up to 40% of patients with chronic congestive heart failure have been reported to have central sleep apnea with Cheyne–Stokes respiration (CSA-CSR). There is a male predominance in patients with heart failure. CSA-CSR is generally seen in patients >60 years.

Most patients with CSA-CSR have systolic heart failure (left ventricular ejection fraction of <40%), diastolic heart failure, or atrial fibrillation/flutter. CSA-CSR may also be observed after cerebral vascular accident or other neurologic disorders.

Disorder Description: CSA-CSR is characterized by a crescendo-decrescendo ventilatory pattern alternating with central apneas or hypopneas. Each CSA-CSR cycle is typically more than 45 seconds in duration with cycle time correlating with circulation time. It most often occurs during relaxed wakefulness, stages N1 and N2, and usually resolves during rapid eye movement (REM) sleep.

Diagnosis of CSA with Cheyne–Stokes respiration is made if the patient meets the following clinical criteria:
1. The presence of one or more of the following:
   a. sleepiness;
   b. difficulty initiating or maintaining sleep, frequent awakenings, or nonrestorative sleep;
   c. awakening short of breath;
   d. snoring;
   e. witnessed apneas.

2. Polysomnogram with episodes of three or fewer consecutive central apeas and/or hypopneas separated by a crescendo and decrescendo change in breathing amplitude with a cycle length of 40 seconds or less. There must also be five or more central apneas and/or central hypopneas per hour of sleep associated with the crescendo/decrescendo breathing pattern recorded over 2 or more hours of monitoring. Cycle length is the time from the beginning of a central apnea to the end of the next crescendo/decrescendo respiratory phase.
3. The number of central apneas and/or central hypopneas is more than 50% of the total number of apneas and hypopneas.
4. There is no evidence of daytime or nocturnal hypoventilation.
5. The disorder is not better explained by another sleep disorder, medical or neurologic disorder, medication use, or substance use disorder.

Symptoms

Localization site	Comment
Mental status and psychiatric aspects/complications	Sleepiness, depression, social dysfunction

Secondary Complications: Daytime somnolence, insomnia, and nocturnal dyspnea.

Treatment Complications: First-line treatment relates to optimization of the underlying cardiac disorder. Positive airway pressure has been most extensively studied in patients with CSA and chronic heart failure. In this population, continuous positive airway pressure (CPAP) has been shown to attenuate CSR-CSA in some patients, improve nocturnal oxygenation and left ventricular ejection fraction, and lower plasma norepinephrine levels without benefit to transplantation-free survival, number of hospitalizations, or quality of life. Adaptive servo-ventilation (ASV) more effectively treats CSR-CSA, but does not improve mortality, need for lifesaving cardiovascular intervention, or hospitalizations for worsening heart failure. In one study, ASV increased all-cause mortality and cardiovascular mortality in patients with a left ventricular ejection factor (LVEF) <45% and a predominance of CSA. Other treatments include nocturnal oxygen supplementation or acetazolamide. The optimal treatment of this condition has not been established.

Treatment complications include intolerance of positive airway pressure modalities. Tachyphylaxis and paresthesias with acetazolamide may occur.

Bibliography

Bradley TD, Logan AG, Kimoff RJ, et al. Continuous positive airway pressure for central sleep apnea and heart failure. *N Engl J Med*. 2005;353: 2025–33.

Cowie MR, Woehrle H, Wegscheider K, et al. Adaptive servo-ventilation for central sleep apnea in systolic heart failure. *N Engl J Med*. 2015;373:1095–105.

Dempsey JA, Smith CA, Przybylowski T, et al. The ventilator responsiveness to CO_2 below eupnoea as a determinant of ventilator stability in sleep. *J Physiol*. 2004;560: 1–11.

Eckert DJ, Jordan AS, Merchia P, et al. Central sleep apnea: pathophysiology and treatment. *Chest*. 2007;131:595–607.

Jahaveri S, Dempsey JA. Central sleep apnea. *Compr Physiol*. 2013;3:141–63

Sateia M, Berry RB, Bornemann MC, et al. *International classification of sleep disorders*. 3rd ed. Darien, IL: American Academy of Sleep Medicine; 2014.

Central Visual Impairment

Central Visual Impairment/Cortical Visual Impairment/Cortical Blindness/Higher-Order Visual Processing Disturbance

Epidemiology and Demographics: Cortical visual impairment can affect any race/ethnicity of either sex at any age. In adults, the most common cause is ischemic or hemorrhagic stroke. In children, the most common cause is tumors.

Disorder Description: Central visual impairment refers to vision loss related to dysfunction of the visual pathways distal to the lateral geniculate nucleus. The visual pathways anterior to the injury (i.e., eye, optic nerves, chiasm, optic tract) are normal. Vision loss can range from homonymous visual field loss (i.e., same in each eye) to complete blindness. Bilateral hemispheric damage is necessary to cause complete blindness.

Symptoms

Localization site	Comment
Cerebral hemispheres	Unilateral ischemic or hemorrhagic stroke affecting the parietal lobe is associated with contralateral inferior visual field loss in both eyes. Typical associated symptoms include contralateral hemiparesis, aphasia (dominant hemisphere), or neglect (nondominant hemisphere)
	Unilateral stroke affecting the temporal lobe is associated with contralateral superior visual field loss in both eyes. Typical associated symptoms include aphasia and memory deficits. Mass lesions in these areas can cause similar visual field changes, usually in association with other neurologic symptoms
	Unilateral lesions (most commonly stroke or tumor) affecting the occipital lobes can cause isolated contralateral hemianopia or quadrantanopia. Loss of ability to read but not write is associated with left occipital lobe lesions (right homonymous hemianopias). Loss of color vision in the contralateral hemifield is associated with inferior occipital lobe injury (upper quadrant visual field loss)
	Focal injury to the occipital pole – for example, related to trauma or tumor – can exclusively impair central vision. Ischemic strokes typically spare the occipital pole and are associated with normal central vision
	Complete cerebral blindness is rare from ischemic stroke due to sparing of central vision. Diffuse hypoxic injury or carbon monoxide poisoning can cause cerebral blindness, typically with associated alteration in consciousness. Posterior reversible leukoencephalopathy syndrome can cause acquired cortical blindness with a less striking encephalopathy in patients who are hypertensive, postpartum, or on certain medications such as cyclosporine or tacrolimus
	Infantile causes of cerebral vision loss often present with nystagmus and are associated with other neurologic deficits and/or developmental delay. These include periventricular leukomalacia, hypoxic injury, cortical dysplasia, and stroke. Delayed visual maturation can present in an isolated fashion
	Childhood presentations of cerebral vision loss not associated with mass lesions include mitochondrial disorders and adrenoleukodystrophy
	Cerebral hemispheric processes can affect visual processing without damaging the optic radiations or primary visual cortex. Inability to recognize objects or faces (agnosia) or recognize motion localizes to the occipital temporal lobes. Inability to interpret visual scenes or navigate space visually localizes to the occipital parietal region
	Important causes of cortical blindness or visual processing disturbances without prominent findings on MRI include neurodegenerative diseases such as Creutzfeldt–Jakob disease, posterior cortical atrophy variant of Alzheimer's disease, and Lewy body disease

Localization site	Comment
Mental status and psychiatric aspects/complications	Temporal lobe lesions are associated with mood and behavioral changes in addition to contralateral superior visual field loss
	Visual hallucinations can occur in the setting of bilateral vision loss from any cause, including cerebral vision loss due to "release" of the deafferented visual system. Patients typically have insight into these
	Riddoch phenomenon is the perception of motion in a blind field and is thought to reflect persistence of visual pathway connections that bypass the primary pathways
	Complete cerebral blindness is associated with Anton syndrome, with lack of insight into vision loss and confabulation of the visual environment
	Progressive cognitive change following presentation with cerebral visual disturbances without a lesion raises suspicion for Alzheimer's disease, Lewy body disease, and Creutzfeldt–Jakob disease

Secondary Complications: Patients with unilateral visual field loss can have difficulty with both distance and near tasks. At distance, navigation can be challenging and driving with visual field loss is prohibited in many states. At near, reading can be challenging due to difficulty tracking lines of text and identifying text margins. Associated other neurologic symptoms can make both of these activities more challenging. Higher-order visual processing disturbances can be very disabling even in the absence of central or peripheral vision loss.

Treatment Complications: Surgical treatment of any lesion near cerebral visual pathways can cause injury to these with resultant vision loss. Both acute and delayed radiation injury can occur to cause further vision loss in cases treated with radiation therapy.

Bibliography

Fazzi E, Signorini SG, Bova SM, et al. Spectrum of visual disorders in children with cerebral visual impairment. *J Child Neurol.* 2007;22(3):294–301.

Centronuclear Myopathy (Formerly, Myotubular Myopathy)

Epidemiology and Demographics: Centronuclear myopathies (CNMs) are a heterogeneous group of disorders. They are rare disorders, with exact prevalence/incidence unknown. There are at least three major forms that present at different ages: (1) an X-linked, severe form that presents in the neonate and is usually fatal; (2) a slowly progressive form, which is the most common and presents in infancy to early childhood; and (3) a third form that occurs in late childhood or at adult onset. Other than male predominance in the X-linked form, there is no overt sex predominance in the other forms. There is no overt geographic distribution.

Disorder Description: The fatal neonatal form is X-linked recessive, with defects in MTM1 encoding myotubularin 1. The slowly progressive infantile form can be autosomal dominant or recessive. Most of the mutations are membrane movement and remodeling genes; the most common gene is DNM2. The autosomal-dominant mutations are found in the genes DNM2 (dynamin 2), BIN1 (amphiphysin 2), and CCDC78 (coiled-coil domain containing protein 78). The autosomal-recessive mutations are found in BIN1, MTMR14 (hJumpy), RYR1 (skeletal muscle ryanodine receptor), TTN (titin), and SPEG (striated muscle preferentially expressed protein kinase). The late-childhood to early-adult onset form is primarily due to DNM2 mutations. However, there is a late-onset MTM1 form that presents with milder symptoms at about 20 years of age.

Serum creatine kinase is usually normal or slightly elevated. Nerve conduction studies are normal for both sensory and motor modalities. Electromyography is significantly abnormal, demonstrating increased insertional and spontaneous activity, with positive sharp waves, fibrillation potentials, complex repetitive discharges, and even myotonic discharges. This is particularly evident in the X-linked neonatal/infantile onset form. Affected muscles in the other forms may also have early recruitment of short-duration, small-amplitude motor unit action potentials (MUAPs). Muscle biopsy is the critical diagnostic modality and can show a variable degree of endomysial fibrosis and adipose tissue replacement, but most important, the hallmark finding is muscle fibers with one or more centrally placed nuclei with a surrounding clear area due to the absence of myofibrils.

Symptoms

Localization site	Comment
Cerebral hemispheres	In the slowly progressing infantile form, seizures may occur
Mental status and psychiatric aspects/ complications	In the slowly progressive infantile form, cognitive disability may be present
Muscle	The frequently fatal X-linked form presents at birth with severe hypotonia and generalized weakness. Respiratory muscle weakness, facial/bulbar weakness, ptosis, and extraocular muscle weakness are common
	Later onset forms can include motor dysfunction, exercise intolerance, and fatigable weakness
	There can be myasthenic features as well

Secondary Complications: In the X-linked form, respiratory and nutritional difficulties are evident early. Rarely, there can be ambiguous genitalia or severe hypospadias. Prior to birth, polyhydramnios is noted in 50–60% of cases. In the more common infantile form, intellectual disabilities and seizures are possible. In general, some can present with myasthenic features.

Treatment Complications: In the X-linked form, neonates frequently need respiratory support and feeding tube nutritional support for life support. In the more common infantile form, antiepileptics may need to be added. For those with myasthenic features, use of pyridostigmine has demonstrated significant improvement.

As treatment is limited and supportive, there are no major complications. However, should pyridostigmine be utilized, adverse effects include sweating, diarrhea, nausea, vomiting, tearing, salivation, pupillary constriction, and facial flushing.

Bibliography

Amato AA, Russell JA. *Neuromuscular disorders*. New York: McGraw-Hill; 2008. pp. 578, 582–3.

Mah JK, Joseph JT. An overview of congenital myopathies. *Continuum (Minneap Minn)*. 2016;22(6):1932–53.

Cerebral Amyloid Angiopathy (CAA)

Epidemiology and Demographics: The prevalence of cerebral amyloid angiopathy (CAA) increases with age and approaches 50% in patients older than 80 years. Eighty percent to 90% of patients with Alzheimer's disease (AD) have concomitant CAA.

Disorder Description: CAA is caused by amyloid deposition in small and medium-sized leptomeningeal and cerebral arteries. Protein deposition is thought to modify the blood vessel compliance, resulting in micro-tears and intracranial hemorrhage. CAA is most often sporadic but several genetic mutations including apolipoprotein E2 and E4 alleles are associated with increased prevalence of this disease.

Symptoms

Localization site	Comment
Cerebral hemispheres	Transient and permanent motor, sensory, and/or behavioral symptoms due to cortical microhemorrhages and larger hematomas. Bleeding may be multicentric
Brainstem	Small perforating vessels are unaffected by CAA and therefore brainstem is typically spared
Cerebellum	Decreased arousal can occur if a hematoma is large enough to exert mass effect

Secondary Complications: Cortical hemorrhages and associated acute complications including elevated intracranial pressure, herniation, and seizures. Cognitive decline is seen in patients with CAA and concurrent AD.

Treatment Complications: Complications associated with surgical decompression of life-threatening hematomas.

Bibliography

Izumihara A, Ishihara T, Iwamoto N, Yamashita K, Ito H. Postoperative outcome of 37 patients with lobar intracerebral hemorrhage related to cerebral amyloid angiopathy. *Stroke*. 1999;30(1):29.

Maxwell SS, Jackson CA, Paternoster L, et al. Genetic associations with brain microbleeds: systematic review and meta-analyses. *Neurology*. 2011;77(2):158.

Yamada M. Cerebral amyloid angiopathy: emerging concepts. *J Stroke*. 2015;17(1):17–30.

Cerebral Autosomal Dominant Arteriopathy with Subcortical Infarcts and Leukoencephalopathy (CADASIL)

Epidemiology and Demographics: The prevalence of cerebral autosomal dominant arteriopathy with subcortical infarcts and leukoencephalopathy (CADASIL) is 2/100,000. The age of onset is typically adulthood, and men and women are equally affected.

Disorder Description: CADASIL is a genetic disease caused by a mutation in the NOTCH3 gene that leads to diseased blood vessels within the subcortical white matter. Migraines with aura, recurrent small vessel strokes, and progressive cognitive impairment are common in patients with CADASIL.

Symptoms

Localization site	Comment
Cerebral hemispheres	Manifestations of lacunar syndromes such as hemiparesis, sensory symptoms
Mental status and psychiatric aspects/complications	Subcortical dementia, i.e., progressive deficits in executive function and processing speed. Depression, bipolar, adjustment and panic disorders, and/or apathy
Brainstem	Brainstem lacunar syndromes

Secondary Complications: Progressive stepwise cognitive decline, gait disturbance, and urinary incontinence.

Treatment Complications: Medication related, i.e., excessive bruising and bleeding caused by antiplatelets and anticoagulants.

Bibliography

Adib-Samii P, Brice G, Martin RJ, Markus HS. Clinical spectrum of CADASIL and the effect of cardiovascular risk factors on phenotype: study in 200 consecutively recruited individuals. *Stroke*. 2010;41(4):630–4.

Razvi SS, Davidson R, Bone I, Muir KW. The prevalence of cerebral autosomal dominant arteriopathy with subcortical infarcts and leucoencephalopathy (CADASIL) in the west of Scotland. *J Neurol Neurosurg Psychiatry*. 2005;76(5):739–41.

Cerebral Palsy

Epidemiology and Demographics: In developed countries, estimated prevalence of cerebral palsy is 2–2.5/1000 live births. Prevalence of cerebral palsy among preterm babies is very much higher. In the developing countries, information is not well established, but approximate estimates are anywhere from 1.5 to 5.6/1000 live births. All races are affected. It is a leading cause of childhood disability. Lower socioeconomic status and male sex may be risk factors for cerebral palsy.

Disorder Description: Cerebral palsy is described as nonprogressive brain lesions involving motor or postural abnormalities noted during early development. Cerebral palsy is often accompanied by disturbances of sensation, cognition, communication, perception, and/or behavior and/or a seizure disorder.

With respect to evaluation, the 2003 American Academy of Neurology Practice Parameters recommends lab studies only if atypical features noted or any abnormalities on MRI. If hereditary or neurodegenerative disorders are suspected, screening for an underlying metabolic or genetic disorder should be done.

Symptoms

Localization site	Comment
Cerebral hemispheres	Seizures, speech and language disturbance, oromotor dysfunction, spastic hemiplegia 20–30%, spastic diplegia 30–40%, spastic quadriplegia 10–15%, abnormal muscle tone, psychiatric manifestation, intellectual disabilities, which is increasingly associated with spastic quadriplegia, attention deficit hyperactivity disorder, learning disability, depression, increased prevalence of progressive development disorder or autism
Extrapyramidal sites	Choreoathetoid and dystonic movements
Cranial nerves	Hearing loss, visual field abnormalities

Treatment Complications: Treatment is usually supportive for spasticity. Botox with or without casting is recommended. Antiparkinsonian, anticonvulsant, antidopaminergic, and antidepressant agents can be used. Intrathecal baclofen, selective dorsal rhizotomies, and stereotactic basal ganglia and orthopedic surgical intervention can also be offered. Multidisciplinary approach is required for management of this condition. Muscle relaxants can cause drowsiness, seizures (baclofen). Benzodiazepines can cause sedation and may worsen swelling problems.

Bibliography

Capute AJ, Accardo PJ. *Developmental disabilities in infancy and childhood.* Vol 2. 2nd ed. EDS. Baltimore, MD; Brooks Publishing; 2001.

Monster D, Wilcox AJ, Vollset SE, Markestad T, Lie RT. Cerebral palsy long-term and post-term births. *JAMA.* 2010;304(9):976–82.

Shevell MI, Bodensteiner JB. Cerebral palsy: defining the problem. *Semin Pediatric Neurol.* 2004;11(1):2–4.

Volpe JJ. *Neurology of the newborn.* 4th ed. Philadelphia, PA: WB Saunders; 2001. p. 41.

Cerebral Venous Thrombosis (CVT)

Epidemiology and Demographics: Cerebral venous thrombosis (CVT) accounts for 0.5% of all strokes with an approximate incidence of 3–4/million population. CVT can occur at any age, but in young adults it predominates among women in relation to oral contraceptives, pregnancy, and puerperium.

Disorder Description: Blood return from the brain is through cerebral veins, which drain into venous sinuses, which in turn empty mostly into the internal jugular veins. Occlusion of the venous sinuses by thrombus leads to the constellation that is cerebral venous sinus thrombosis.

Symptoms

Localization site	Comment
Cerebral hemispheres	Headache, thunderclap headache, aphasia, hemiparesis, hemisensory loss, seizures (generalized or focal), stroke, intracranial hemorrhage
Mental status and psychiatric aspects/complications	Altered mental status/coma (deep cerebral vein thrombosis)
Base of skull	Cranial neuropathy (jugular vein thrombosis can affect CN IX, XI, XII)
Cranial nerves	Cranial neuropathies (sixth nerve common), papilledema, proptosis, chemosis (cavernous sinus thrombosis)

Treatment Complications: Anticoagulation can lead to systemic bleeding, causing altered mental status (anticoagulation may be given even with intracranial hemorrhage).

Bibliography

Caplan LR, van Gijn J, eds. *Stroke syndromes*. 3rd ed. Cambridge: Cambridge University Press; 2012.

Cerebrotendinous Xanthomatosis

Epidemiology and Demographics: Data are limited. Prevalence of cerebrotendinous xanthomatosis (CTX) is 1.9/100,000 in Caucasians of European ancestry. However, it has been found in many countries around the world. Spinal variant is less common but usually presents between ages 20 and 35.

Disorder Description: A rare autosomal recessive demyelinating disease due to mutation in CYP27A1 gene. This leads to inactive sterol 27-hydroxylase and buildup of sterol intermediates in lipophilic tissues. CTX presents as cataracts and diarrhea in childhood followed by tendon xanthomas and progressive neurologic dysfunction. Neurologic manifestations include cerebellar dysfunction, neuropathy, myelopathy, seizures, neuropsychiatric disease, and intellectual disabilities. Spinal variant is less common, but presents as a slowly progressive myelopathy with corticospinal tract and dorsum column demyelination. It has a less aggressive course and usually patients have bilateral cataracts, but are spared from the other manifestations of CTX.

Symptoms

Localization site	Comment
Cerebral hemispheres	Seizures, parkinsonism, dystonia
Mental status and psychiatric aspects/complications	Cognitive decline, intellectual disabilities, dementia, hallucinations, depression, agitation
Cerebellum	Ataxia
Spinal cord	Myelopathy, spastic paraparesis
Peripheral neuropathy	Sensory neuropathy

Secondary Complications: Can lead to fractures, skeletal abnormalities due to decreased calcium reabsorption. Buildup of cholestanol (sterol intermediate) and cholesterol leads to cardiovascular disease and atherosclerosis.

Treatment Complications: Chenodeoxycholic acid is the main treatment for CTX. Little is known about the side effects of this medication; however, it is found to be associated with increased diarrhea, hypercholesterolemia, and increased liver enzyme levels.

Bibliography

Dunbar K. Cerebrotendinous xanthomatosis: a treatable genetic disease not to be missed. *J Clin Rheumatol*. 2016;22(2):92–3.

Lorincz MT, Rainier S, Thomas D, Fink JK. Cerebrotendinous xanthomatosis: possible higher prevalence than previously recognized. *Arch Neurol*. 2005;62:1459.

Cerebrovascular Disorders and Pregnancy

Epidemiology and Demographics: The incidence of pregnancy-related strokes is approximately 25–34/100,000, about three times more common than in the same nonpregnant age-group. Of these, 6–64% are the result of sinus venous thrombosis. Hemorrhagic strokes have an incidence of 5–35/100,000, with a relative risk of 2.5 during pregnancy. Highest risk of cerebrovascular disease occurs in the puerperium.

Other vascular entities, including pre-eclampsia, eclampsia, reversible cerebral vasoconstriction syndrome (RCVS), and posterior reversible leukoencephalopathy (PRES), are discussed elsewhere in this text.

Predisposing Factors: Pre-eclampsia and eclampsia are the greatest risk factors and are present in 10–47% of all pregnancy-related strokes. Pregnant women with ischemic strokes tend to be younger and less likely to have hypertension compared with their nonpregnant counterparts.

Arteriovenous malformations and aneurysms increase the risk of hemorrhagic strokes. Aneurysms are more prone to rupture during pregnancy in the late third trimester, likely due to remodeling of vascular tissue and loss of elasticity in blood vessel walls.

Disorder Description: There are several cardiovascular and hematologic changes that occur during pregnancy in order to accommodate the growing fetus and to prepare for delivery. First, there is an increase in renin activity, which increases volume retention. Heart rate and stroke volume (cardiac output) also increase by about 30%. Blood pressure first drops and then rises in the third trimester until term to slightly above normal. Finally, blood vessels become less elastic and possibly more vulnerable to pressure.

Coagulation factor levels (factors I, VII, IX, X, XII, and XIII) increase and coagulation inhibitor levels (protein S) decrease, contributing to a hypercoagulable state. These changes make the mother more prone to clot formation, resulting in ischemic strokes. In most cases, the stroke is of either cardioembolic origin or venous sinus thrombosis. Amniotic fluid embolism is very rare but should be considered if the patient also has pulmonary embolism.

Stroke is a clinical diagnosis, with the help of CT scans to differentiate between ischemic and hemorrhagic stroke. A filling defect in the venous sinus may be seen on a regular CT to suggest a venous sinus thrombosis, or a CT venogram can be used to confirm the diagnosis.

Symptoms

Localization site	Comment
Cerebral hemispheres	Ischemic or hemorrhagic stroke: • Sudden onset of focal neurologic deficit, usually without a change in the level of consciousness at time of onset • Headache may be present, especially in hemorrhagic strokes with surrounding edema and mass effect • Hypoglycemia and hyperglycemia (glucose less than 50 mg/dL or greater than 400 mg/dL, respectively) can cause focal neurologic deficits and finger-stick glucose should first be checked Venous thrombosis: • Characterized by a nonspecific unrelenting headache, seizures, focal symptoms such as weakness or numbness, and signs of increased intracranial pressure • It should be considered in the differential of pregnant women presenting with a new headache Subarachnoid hemorrhage: • Sentinel headache with leaking cerebral aneurysm precede the hemorrhage in 50% cases • Exam findings of a posterior circulation aneurysm include cranial nerve III palsy, retro-orbital pain, and a dilated pupil

Secondary Complications: Strokes with significant neurologic deficits are very disabling. Untreated stroke increases the mother's morbidity and mortality. Large territory strokes can cause compression of surrounding structures by mass effect and midline shift. Amniotic fluid embolism, although a rare phenomenon, can be fatal, with a mortality rate of about 20%.

Treatment Complications: Standard management of ischemic arterial stroke should be carried out without delay, as would occur with nonpregnant patients, including urgent CT head, CT angiography, and intravenous tissue plasminogen activator (tPA) with or without thrombectomy or clot retrieval. Pregnant women were excluded in the ischemic stroke trials, but case reports have found the same therapy to be generally safe in pregnant women, without fetal complications. Specifically, tPA does not cross the placenta in animal models.

However, in the setting of pre-eclampsia/eclampsia, hypertensive encephalopathy increases the risk of cerebral hemorrhage significantly and therefore tPA is not recommended.

Hemorrhagic strokes are managed with neurosurgical consultation, blood pressure control, and reversal of anticoagulant therapy if applicable.

Venous thrombosis is treated with anticoagulation. Most trials were conducted using heparin and demonstrated clear benefits even in patients with hemorrhagic conversions.

As described in case series of pregnant patients who received tPA for ischemic stroke, hemorrhagic conversion of the infarct can occur. One case of intrauterine hematoma has been reported. The data regarding stroke treatment in pregnant women are very limited, as these women were excluded from most major trials, but the general practice is to treat, given the high morbidity and mortality in untreated cases.

Bibliography

Leffert LR, Clancy CR, Bateman BT, et al. Treatment patterns and short-term outcomes in ischemic stroke in pregnancy or postpartum period. *Am J Obstet Gynecol.* 2016;214(6):723.e1–723.e11.

Mas JL, Lamy C. Stroke in pregnancy and the puerperium. *Neurology.* 1998;245(6–7):305–13.

Tang SC, Jeng JS. Management of stroke in pregnancy and the puerperium. *Expert Rev Neurother.* 2010;10(2):205–15.

Cervical Arthritis

Epidemiology and Demographics: In the United States, the incidence in men is 7% and in women 9.4%. It is common in people who have mentally and physically stressful jobs. It is also more common in people who are current smokers.

Disorder Description: Cervical arthritis predominantly presents with neck pain. This pain radiates into the shoulder or between the shoulder blades. Pain and stiffness are worse in the morning, improving as the patient starts to move but returning at the end of the day. Rest helps. It may be associated with occipital localized headache.

Symptoms

Localization site	Comment
Cervical spine	Neck pain radiating into the shoulders or into the shoulder blades
Neck stiffness	Decreased range of motion
Cervical cord	Cervical spinal cord myelopathy can be noted if there is compression. Symptoms of myelopathy include weakness in the extremities and may or may not involve bowel or bladder dysfunctions

Treatment Complications: Rest, nonsteroidal anti-inflammatory drugs (NSAIDs), and muscle relaxants. Physical therapy including traction and neck exercises, cortisone injection, heat and cold therapy, and activity modification. Cervical arthritis is rarely progressive and rarely requires surgery. If progressive, cervical laminectomy or cervical spinal fusion is indicated. Osteophytes are predominantly noted, which can cause nerve impingement. Muscle relaxants can cause drowsiness and dizziness; NSAIDs may cause gastrointestinal symptoms such as nausea and vomiting, as well as cerebrovascular events rarely.

Bibliography

Praemer A, Furner S, Rice D. *Musculoskeletal conditions in the United States*. Rosemont, IL: AAOS; 1992. p 23.

Cervical Disc Disorders

Epidemiology and Demographics: Asymptomatic disc herniations are seen in 10% of patients younger than 40 years and in 5% of those older than 40 years. Approximately 51–67% of adults experience neck and back pain at some point in their lifetime. Male-to-female ratio is 1:1 for disc herniation. In patients under age 40, herniated nucleus pulposus is noted. In patients older than 40 years, degenerative disc disease is more likely.

Disorder Description: Cervical disc disorders include herniated nucleus pulposus, degenerative disc disease, and internal disc disruption. The cervical radiculopathy can result from nerve root injury due to disc disease resulting in motor, sensory, or reflex abnormality in affected nerve root distribution.

Workup includes checking for rheumatologic conditions with lab studies, x-rays, CT scan and MRI, and electrodiagnostic testing.

Symptoms

Localization site	Comment
C2–C3 discs	Rare trauma induced. Nonspecific shoulder pain is noted
C5 disc	Radiculopathy, weakness of shoulder abduction, external rotation, elbow flexion, and supination of the wrist. Sensory symptoms are noted in the shoulder area
C6 disc	Similar to C5; in addition, weakness may involve extension of the elbow (triceps) pronation and extension of the wrist (extensor carpi radialis). Numbness localized to the thumb
C7 disc	Pain or sensory symptoms radiating down the arm into the middle digit, weakness of the elbow extension and wrist flexion or finger extension, decreased triceps reflex noted
C8–T1	Sensory disturbance affecting the medial aspect of the hand and forearm along with hand weakness
Multiple cervical discs	Combination of the above

Treatment Complications: Conservative treatment includes cervical stabilization, postural training, and strengthening. Surgery is warranted when there is neurogenic bowel and bladder dysfunction, deteriorating neurologic function, or intractable radicular or discogenic neck pain. Nonsteroidal anti-inflammatories, short-term corticosteroids, and muscle relaxants can be used.

Steroids can cause weight gain, psychosis, increased blood sugar; muscle relaxants can cause sedation.

Bibliography

Amato AA, Russell JA. *Neuromuscular disorders.* 2nd ed. New York: McGraw-Hill Education/Medical; 2015.

Carette F, Fehlings MG. Clinical practice: Cervical radiculopathy. *N Engl J Med.* 2005;353(4):392–9.

Cervical Dystonia (CD)

Epidemiology and Demographics: Cervical dystonia (CD) is the most common form of adult-onset isolated focal dystonia. The overall prevalence is 5–20/100,000 individuals, with an increased incidence in the Caucasian population. There is a female predominance (74%) with a mean age of 49 years at symptom onset. The most commonly reported subtype is torticollis, followed by laterocollis.

Disorder Description: CD is a focal dystonia of the head, neck, and shoulder that causes abnormal postures or repetitive twisting movements due to sustained cocontractions of opposing agonist and antagonist muscles. It may be associated with overlying muscle spasm resembling tremor. The abnormal postures include turning of the head (torticollis), lateral flexion (laterocollis), forward flexion (anterocollis), neck extension (retrocollis), anterior/posterior sagittal shifts, and lateral displacement. There may also be shoulder elevation and displacement. The postures may be complex, involving a combination of muscles. There may also be a dynamic component, with different combinations of muscle activation more prominent during specific activities. There are often sensory tricks that improve symptoms. CD may be idiopathic or secondary with an identifiable genetic or acquired etiology. Toxic exposures, medications, structural lesions, and degenerative diseases may be associated with secondary CD. The pathophysiology of primary CD is unknown but may involve dysfunction in the basal ganglia-thalamo-cortical circuits

Symptoms

Localization site	Comment
Mental status and psychiatric aspects/ complications	Depression, anxiety, panic disorders, obsessive-compulsive symptoms, social phobia, loss of self-confidence, substance abuse
Specific spinal roots	Secondary radiculopathy
Muscle	Painful muscle spasms
Unclear localization	Sleep disturbances: insomnia and fragmented sleep Sensory abnormalities with temporal and spatial discrimination abnormalities

Secondary Complications: Patients may develop structural changes along the cervical spine including arthritis, radiculopathies, and cervical stenosis.

Treatment Complications: First line treatment is focused botulinum toxin injections. The most common side effect is dysphagia. Patients may also experience unintended weakness in the muscles and spread of toxin to surrounding areas, resulting in neck weakness. Refractory cases may respond to deep brain stimulation, but gait disorders and parkinsonism have been reported from chronic stimulation.

Bibliography

Bledsoe IO, Comella CL. Botulinum toxin treatment of cervical dystonia. In *Seminars in neurology.* Stuttgart: Thieme Medical; 2016.

Contarino MF, Smit M, van den Dool J, Volkmann J, Tijssen MAJ. Unmet needs in the management of cervical dystonia. *Front Neurol.* 2016;7:165.

Klingelhoefer L, Martino D, Martinez-Martin P, et al. Nonmotor symptoms and focal cervical dystonia: observations from 102 patients. *Basal Ganglia.* 2014;4:117–20.

LeDoux MS, Vemula SR, Xiao J, et al. Clinical and genetic features of cervical dystonia in a large multicenter cohort. *Neurol Genet.* 2016;2:e69.

Patel S, Martino D. Cervical dystonia: from pathophysiology to pharmacotherapy. *Behav Neurol.* 2013;26:275–82.

Cervical Facet Syndrome

Epidemiology and Demographics: The prevalence of cervical facet joint pain has been described as low as

26% or as high as 65%. After a whiplash injury, the prevalence is about 54%.

Disorder Description: Cervical facet pain is characterized by tenderness to palpation over the facet joints or paraspinal muscles, pain with cervical extension or rotation, and absent neurologic abnormalities. X-rays may be performed.

Symptoms

Localization site	Comment
Cervical spine	Neck pain, headaches, limited range of motion, dull aching, discomfort in the posterior neck that sometimes radiates to the shoulder or mid back regions

Secondary Complications: Persistent pain.
Treatment Complications: Physical therapy, which includes manual therapy, joint mobilization, soft tissue massage and manual stretching, intra-articular facet joint injections, percutaneous radiofrequency, and neurotomy. Medication treatments include nonsteroidal anti-inflammatories, tricyclic antidepressants, antiseizure medications, and muscle relaxants. Tricyclic antidepressants can cause sedation, drowsiness, urinary obstruction in older men with prostate problems. Antiseizure medications can cause sedation and dizziness among many other potential adverse effects. Muscle relaxants can cause sedation and dizziness.

Bibliography

Bovim G, Schrader H, Sand T. Neck pain in the general population. *Spine.* 1994;19(12):1307–9.
Friedenberg ZB, Miller WT. Degenerative disc disease of the cervical spine. *J Bone Joint Surg Am.* 1963;45:1171–8.

Cervical Myofascial Pain Syndrome

Epidemiology and Demographics: Twenty-one percent of patients seen in orthopedic clinics have myofascial pain. At specialty pain management centers, 85–93% can have myofascial pain. This condition is more common in women. Recurrence is common.
Disorder Description: Cervical myofascial pain syndrome associated pain is attributed to muscle and its surrounding tissue. Cervical myofascial pain is probably due to overuse or trauma of the muscles supporting the shoulder and back. Trigger points are located in the skeletal muscles on palpation.

Treatment includes proper exercises, home exercise program, improved posture awareness, improved body mechanics with focus on improving activities of daily living.

Symptoms

Localization site	Comment
Cervical spine, trapezius, levator scapulae, rhomboids, supraspinatus and infraspinatus	Pain

Bibliography

Travell JG, Simons DG. *Myofascial pain and dysfunction.* Vol. 2. Baltimore, MD: Lippincott Williams & Wilkins; 1992.

Cervical Odontoid Fracture

Epidemiology and Demographics: Incidence of odontoid fracture is 15% of all cervical spine fractures.
Disorder Description: Important to rule out associated C1 anterior ring fracture. There are three types of odontoid fractures:

Type I fracture occurs in less than 5% of cases. It is an oblique fracture through the upper part of the odontoid; occasionally associated with gross instability.
Type II fracture occurs in 60% of cases. It is a fracture occurring at the base of the odontoid as it attaches to the body of C2.
Type III fracture occurs in 30% of cases. The fracture line extends through the body of the axis.

Symptoms

Localization site	Comment
Cervical spine	Upper myelopathic symptoms and signs including perception of instability, quadriparesis or quadriplegia with respiratory deficits, cervical radiculopathy, four limb motor and sensory deficits of varying degrees

Secondary Complications: Nonunion of cervical spine, malunion, pseudoarthrosis formation, infection, neurovascular injury, acute airway complications, and hardware failure.

Bibliography

Trafton PG. Spinal cord injuries. *Surg Clin North Am.* 1982;62(1):61–72.

Cervical Spondylosis

Epidemiology and Demographics: Average annual incidence of cervical spondylosis is 107.3/100,000 in men and 63.5/100,000 in women. Average age at diagnosis is 47.9 years.

Disorder Description: Cervical spondylosis is the medical term for "wear and tear" chronic degeneration of cervical spine vertebral bodies and intervertebral discs. It is often caused by long-standing abnormal pressure in the cervical region due to joint subluxation or poor posture. Abnormal stress promotes the formation of new bone to compensate for the new weight distribution.

Cervical spondylosis is associated with disc herniation leading to calcification, degenerative arthritis, and osteophytic outgrowths. This can cause impingement on nerve roots or compression and vascular insufficiency to the spinal cord leading to myelopathy. It presents as neck or occipital pain with radicular pain down the arms at times. It can present as weakness in the arms or legs with dermatomal sensory loss. The most common areas affected are the C5 and C6 nerve roots leading to decreased biceps and brachioradialis reflexes; however, reflexes may be increased if there is an associated myelopathy. Cervical spondylosis is the most common cause of nontraumatic spastic paraparesis and quadriplegia.

Diagnosis is suspecting through findings on physical examination including abnormalities on the cervical compression test, and documentation of reduced range of motion. MRI and CAT scan of the spine may be helpful in demonstrating the associated anatomical abnormalities.

Symptoms

Localization site	Comment
Spinal cord	Weakness of lower and upper extremities, hyperreflexia, increased tone, clonus, gait dysfunction, loss of balance, loss of bowel function, bladder dysfunction. Lhermitte's sign may be present
Spinal roots	Radiculopathy, dermatomal sensory loss, decreased reflexes of affected root, weakness in upper extremity muscles supplied by root

Secondary Complications: Secondary vertebrobasilar insufficiency may occur. Movement or further injury to neck can lead to worsening weakness or paralysis.

Treatment Complications: Treatment consists of physical therapy or pain control with nonsteroidal anti-inflammatory drugs (NSAIDs), tricyclic antidepressants, or steroids. These medications can have potential central nervous system adverse effects. Depending on the degree of impingement and if there is bladder involvement, assorted surgical interventions may be indicated which can sometimes result in worsened or new neurologic deficits.

Bibliography

Aminoff MJ, Greenberg DA, Simon RP. Motor disorders. In Aminoff MJ, Greenberg DA, Simon RP, eds. *Clinical neurology.* 9th ed. New York: McGraw-Hill; 2015.

Radhakrishnan K, Litchy WJ, O'Fallon WM, Kurland LT. Epidemiology of cervical radiculopathy. A population-based study from Rochester, Minnesota, 1976 through 1990. *Brain.* 1994;117(Pt 2):325.

McCormack BM, Weinstein PR. Cervical spondylosis. An update. *West J Med.* 1996;165(1–2):43–5.

Cervical Trauma

Epidemiology and Demographics: About 2.4% of blunt trauma victims can experience cervical spine trauma. Usually, it is due to accident, fall or motor vehicle collisions. It is more common in patients who are older than 65 years, male, and Caucasian.

Disorder Description: Cervical spine trauma is common with a wide range of severity from minor ligamentous injury to frank osteoligamentous instability with spinal cord injury.

Symptoms

Localization site	Comment
Cranial nerves	Cranial nerves VI, VII, IX, X, and XI as well as XII nerve abnormality can occur in association with upper cervical cord injuries. Horner's syndrome, ataxia, dysmetria, contralateral pain, and temperature loss due to Wallenberg syndrome can also be seen

Localization site	Comment
Occipitocervical dissociation	• Anterior subluxation • Vertical distraction greater than 2 mm of the atlanto-occipital joint • Posterior dislocation Above can cause spinal cord compression
Extension injury causing spinal cord compression	Central cord syndrome, which involves greater motor impairment of the upper extremities with concomitant bladder dysfunction and variable sensory disturbance
Vertebral artery	Quadriplegia, brainstem/cerebellar infarction, dysphagia, diplopia, blurred vision, or nystagmus

Bibliography

Hu R, Mustard CA, Burns C. Epidemiology of incidental CT spinal fracture in a complete population. *Spine*. 1996;21:492–9.

Torretti JA, Sengupta DK. Cervical spine trauma. *Indian J Orthop*. 2007;41(4):255–67.

Chagas Disease (American Trypanosomiasis)

Epidemiology and Demographics: Chagas disease can affect either sex and any age group. It is endemic to South America but has occurred in the southern United States and Spain. According to the World Health Organization, Chagas disease infections afflict 8 million people worldwide, with 10,000 Chagas disease-related deaths occurring each year.

Disorder Description: Chagas disease is also known as "American Trypanosomiasis" and is a protozoan parasitic disease. It is spread by the Triatominae subfamily of hematophagous (blood-consuming) insects. It can also be transmitted hematogenously (through transfusions, transplants, or intrauterine) or orally (through consumption of contaminated food/drink).

Chagas disease is caused by the protozoan *Trypanosoma cruzi*. Risk factors for contracting the parasite are largely exposure driven; i.e., exposure to endemic areas. In the absence of adequate treatment, it can be life-long in duration. Immunocompromise, especially HIV co-infection, results in high risk of cerebral involvement.

Diagnosis is confirmed through identification of the parasite in a blood smear observed under the microscope. MRI imaging can help evaluate for Chagas meningoencephalitis, potentially demonstrating multiple, T2-hyperintense lesions with ring enhancement (possibly nodular as well) in the corpus callosum, periventricular white matter, cerebellum, or spinal cord.

Symptoms

Localization site	Comment
Cerebral hemispheres	Signs of infarctions, sensory or motor deficits
Mental status and psychiatric aspects/complications	Acute meningitis/encephalitis, confusion/encephalopathy, dementia (less likely)
Cerebellum	Involvement in meningoencephalitis
Spinal cord	Involvement in meningoencephalitis
Outside CNS	Myocarditis

Secondary Complications: Secondary complications from cardiac involvement can result in cardioembolic infarctions.

Treatment Complications: Chagas disease, especially with CNS involvement, is treated with benzidazole or nifurtimox; the former is usually better tolerated. Patients with cardiac involvement may be considered for surgical treatment or anticoagulation. Complications of treatment are largely limited to adverse/side effects of the aforementioned antihelminthics; these include gastrointestinal symptoms, headache, dizziness, fever, or chills

Bibliography

Finsterer J, Auer H. Parasitoses of the human central nervous system. *J Helminthol*. 2013;87(3):257–70.

Salvana EMT, Salata RA, King CH. Parasitic infections of the central nervous system. In Aminoff MJ, Josephson SA, eds. *Aminoff's neurology and general medicine*. 5th ed. London: Academic Press; 2014: pp. 947–68.

World Health Organization. Chagas disease (American trypanosomiasis). www.who.int/chagas/epidemiology/en/. Accessed Oct 11, 2018.

Cheyne–Stokes Respiration

Epidemiology and Demographics: The total prevalence is unknown but increases with advancing age over 60 years. Cheyne–Stokes respiration has been reported in 25–40% of patients with heart failure and in 10% of patients who have had a stroke. There is a male predominance.

Disorder Description: Cheyne–Stokes respiration is a type of central sleep apnea. It is observed clinically as a crescendo–decrescendo cyclic breathing pattern with three phases: the apnea phase, which is then followed by gradually increasing respiratory rate and tidal volume, and then a gradually decreasing respiratory rate and tidal volume until the next apneic period.

Symptoms

Localization site	Comment
Cerebral hemispheres	Unilateral/bilateral hemispheric infarcts
Mental status and psychiatric aspects/complications	Insomnia, disrupted sleep, excessive daytime sleepiness, poor subjective sleep quality, fatigue, inattention, moodiness, decreased libido, and impotence
Brainstem	Brainstem infarcts
Cerebellum	Ataxia
Vestibular system	Dizziness
Cranial nerves	Cranial nerve deficits
Unclear localization	Paroxysmal nocturnal dyspnea, morning headaches, and nocturnal angina
Muscle	Weakness

Secondary Complications: Pulmonary hypertension, cor pulmonale, cardiac arrhythmias, and death.

Treatment: Treatment involves treatment of primary underlying condition, respiratory stimulants, respiratory depressants, oxygen, and continuous positive airway pressure.

Bibliography

Cherniack NS, Longobardo G, Evangelista CJ. Causes of Cheyne-Stokes respiration. *Neurocrit Care.* 2005;3(3):271–9.

Giannoni A, Emdin M, Passino C. Cheyne-Stokes respiration, chemoreflex, and ticagrelor-related dyspnea. *N Engl J Med.* 2016;375(10):1004–6. DOI: 10.1056/NEJMc1601662.

Naughton MT. Pathophysiology and treatment of Cheyne-Stokes respiration. *Thorax.* 1998;53:514–8. DOI: 10.1136/thx.53.6.514.

Orr JE, Malhotra A, Sands SA. Pathogenesis of central and complex sleep apnoea. *Respirology.* 2017;22(1):43–52. DOI: 10.1111/resp.12927. Epub 2016 Oct 31.

Wang Y, Cao J, Feng J, Chen BY. Cheyne-Stokes respiration during sleep: mechanisms and potential interventions. *Br J Hosp Med (Lond).* 2015;76(7):390–6. DOI: 10.12968/hmed.2015.76.7.390.

Child Abuse (Both Vascular-Trauma and Psych Complications)

Epidemiology and Demographics: Child abuse affects 1/8 children in the United States annually. Increased risk with the following factors: parent/caregiver with a personal history of physical illness, mental illness, alcohol/substance abuse, or childhood abuse; family stress (e.g., marital conflict, domestic violence, single parenting); child in the family with developmental or physical disability; financial stress; family isolation.

Disorder Description: Broadly defined as the maltreatment of a child under the age of 18 by a parent or caretaker. Child abuse may take many forms including physical abuse, sexual abuse, psychologic abuse, fabricated or induced illness, or neglect, which may be co-occurring. Often, the abuse is committed by someone whom the child knows and trusts.

Symptoms

Localization site	Comment
Mental status and psychiatric aspects/complications	Depression, anxiety, low self-esteem, shame, guilt, fear, withdrawal from friends or previously enjoyed activities, aggression, anger, hostility, hyperactivity, changes in school performance, frequent absences from school, avoidance of home, attempts to run away, rebellious or defiant behavior, suicidality

Localization site	Comment
Neurologic manifestations	Specific neurologic signs and symptoms are diverse and can occur anywhere along the neuro-axis depending on the type of abuse. Physical injuries are often unexplained and/or do not match the provided explanation

Secondary Complications: Depression, anxiety, attachment disorders, posttraumatic stress disorder, substance abuse, eating disorders, personality disorders, sleep disturbances, learning disabilities, attention deficit hyperactivity disorder, oppositional or antisocial behaviors, poor growth or weight gain, poor hygiene, difficulty forming or sustaining close relationships, difficulty sustaining employment, abuse of others, unintended and/or teen pregnancy, sexually transmitted infections, physical disability, death due to physical injuries, suicidal behavior.

Treatment Complications: Selective serotonin reuptake inhibitors may be used to treat co-occurring depression and/or anxiety; however, caution is recommended given the associated black box warning for increased suicidality in children, adolescents, and young adults.

Bibliography

American Psychiatric Association. *Diagnostic and statistical manual of mental disorders: DSM-5.* 5th ed. Washington, DC: American Psychiatric Association; 2013.

Ferrara P, Guadagno C, Sbordone A, et al. Child abuse and neglect: A review of the literature. *Curr Pediatr Rev.* 2016;12(4):301–10.

National Institute for Health and Care Excellence (NICE). Clinical Guideline. Child maltreatment: when to suspect maltreatment in under 18s. July 2009. www.nice.org.uk/guidance/cg89. Accessed Aug 15, 2018.

Cholesterol Embolism

Epidemiology and Demographics: Cholesterol embolism is a disorder of middle-aged patients, typically older than 50 years, with atherosclerotic disease in the large vessels. It does not have to be temporally related to a procedure.

Disorder Description: Caused by either spontaneous plaque rupture or rupture related to procedures (angiography, cardiac surgery, aortic surgery or manipulation, thrombolysis). Multiple cholesterol emboli may be released into the circulation, which cause end organ damage as a result of vessel occlusion and an inflammatory cascade.

Symptoms

Localization site	Comment
Cerebral hemispheres	Cerebral embolism may lead to hemiparesis, aphasia, hemisensory loss, hemianopia
Mental status and psychiatric aspects/complications	Delirium may result from cerebral embolism, acute kidney injury or hypoxia due to acute respiratory distress syndrome
Brainstem	Cranial nerve palsy with contralateral hemiplegia (cerebral embolism)
Cerebellum	Ataxia (cerebral embolism)
Cranial nerves	Monocular vision loss (Hollenhorst plaque in the retina)
Muscle	Myalgia
Unclear localization	Foot pain (embolism-livedo reticularis & blue toes)

Treatment Complications: Thrombolysis, antiplatelets, or anticoagulants used to treat cerebral embolism can worsen the embolism due to further plaque rupture. They can cause intracerebral hemorrhage leading to worsening mental status and neurologic deficits.

Bibliography

Kirkland L. Cholesterol embolism clinical presentation. Medscape. Oct 5, 2017.

Kronzon I. Cholesterol embolization syndrome. *Circulation.* 2010;122:631–41. DOI: 10.1161/CIRCULATIONAHA.109.886465

Chorea Gravidarium (CG)

Epidemiology and Demographics: Chorea gravidarum (CG) is a rare movement disorder of pregnancy with a varied etiology. Its true prevalence is unknown as it has been reported only in a few case series and individual case reports. Historically, the most common cause of CG has been rheumatic heart disease (86%). However, since the availability of antibiotics, its incidence has decreased and it is reported rarely in developing countries. In developed countries, CG is more associated with systemic conditions including systemic lupus erythematosus and antiphospholipid antibody syndrome.

Disorder Description: Chorea in CG manifests as quick, involuntary, irregular, non-rhythmic movements that typically begin in the first trimester. Thirty percent of cases may spontaneously remit before delivery. Most patients have complete remission after delivery. Chorea with subsequent pregnancies has been described. The exact pathophysiology is unknown but likely involves hormonal fluctuations acting on dysfunctional basal ganglia circuitry.

Symptoms

Localization site	Comment
Cerebral hemispheres	Ischemic and hemorrhagic stroke
Mental status and psychiatric aspects/complications	Psychosis, personality changes, depression, hypnic hallucinations, delirium, cognitive changes
Muscle	Rhabdomyolysis

Secondary Complications: CG was once associated with a high mortality due to maternal rhabdomyolysis. Miscarriages have also been documented. When CG is associated with rheumatic fever from group A beta hemolytic streptococcal infection, cardiac complications such as cardiac failure and valvular disease may arise if patients are not treated with appropriate antibiotics.

Treatment Complications: Fortunately, most cases are mild and may not require treatment. Treatment with dopamine receptor blockade is to be avoided in the first trimester and reserpine is a known teratogen. There have been reports of infants born with extrapyramidal signs or dyskinesias after maternal treatment with dopamine receptor blockade. However, if treatment is required, haloperidol is generally preferred and seems to be safe at low doses. Additionally, patients who have experienced CG and/or Sydenham's chorea are likely to develop chorea again when treated with oral contraception.

Bibliography

Cardoso F. Chorea gravidarum. *Arch Neurol.* 2002;59(5):868–70.

Kranick SM, Mowry EM, Colcher A, Horn S, Golbe LI. Movement disorders and pregnancy: a review of the literature. *Mov Disord.* 2010;25(6):665–71.

Maia DP, Fonseca PG, Camargos ST, et al. Pregnancy in patients with Sydenham's chorea. *Parkinsonism Relat Disord.* 2012;18(5):458–61.

Robottom BJ, Weiner WJ. Chorea gravidarum. *Handb Clin Neurol.* 2011;100:231–5.

Chronic Inflammatory Demyelinating Polyneuropathy (CIDP)

Epidemiology and Demographics: Prevalence of chronic inflammatory demyelinating polyneuropathy (CIDP) is 1.9–7.7/100,000. It is more common in patients with diabetes.

Disorder Description: CIDP is an acquired, immune-mediated inflammatory demyelinating polyneuropathy, not usually preceded by infection as in acute inflammatory demyelinating polyneuropathy (AIDP). It can be symmetric or asymmetric and is present in upper extremities predominantly. It is slowly progressive, reaching its peak after several months, and may present in a relapsing fashion. A small percentage of patients with AIDP or Guillain–Barré syndrome (GBS) may have slowly worsening symptoms, which may progress to CIDP. Symptoms can improve with corticosteroids. It presents as limb weakness, proximal more so than distal, paresthesia, and areflexia.

Diabetic chronic inflammatory demyelinating polyneuropathy may be difficult to distinguish from diabetic neuropathy; however, there are a few differentiating features that may help aid in the diagnosis of diabetic CIDP. Diabetic polyneuropathy is due to damage of small unmyelinated fibers, leading to distal numbness and tingling. Proprioception loss and damage to large myelinated fibers point more toward CIDP. Diabetic polyneuropathy is usually a result of chronic hyperglycemia. Recent well-controlled diabetes mellitus (DM) presenting with polyneuropathy would be more indicative of diabetic CIDP. Diabetic polyneuropathy affects lower extremities more than upper extremities; the opposite is true in CIDP. It is important to distinguish between the two as diabetic CIDP would require treatment with corticosteroids, intravenous immunoglobulin (IVIG), plasmapheresis, or other immunomodulatory agents.

Symptoms

Localization site	Comment
Cerebral hemispheres	Confusion, coma in variants of GBS, i.e., Bickerstaff encephalitis
Mental status and psychiatric aspects/complications	Confusion, coma in variants of GBS, i.e., Bickerstaff encephalitis
Brainstem	Confusion, coma, ophthalmoplegia, ataxia in variants of GBS, i.e., Bickerstaff encephalitis
Cranial nerves	Cranial nerves III–VII and IX–XII may be involved, diplopia, ophthalmoplegia, dysphagia, dysarthria, facial droop
Peripheral nerve/muscle	Sensory disturbance, limb weakness, areflexia, myalgias
Unclear localization	Dysautonomia due to involvement of parasympathetic and sympathetic systems, less common than in AIDP

Treatment Complications: Plasma exchange complications include anaphylaxis, hypocalcemia, and depletion of immunoglobulins and coagulation factors.

IVIG complications include anaphylaxis in IgA deficiency, renal failure, proteinuria, severe headache, and aseptic meningitis.

Steroid therapy can lead to psychosis, confusion, weight gain, hyperglycemia, myopathy, glaucoma, cataracts, osteoporosis, or vertebral fractures.

Bibliography

Laughlin RS, Dyck PJ, Melton LJ III, et al. Incidence and prevalence of CIDP and the association of diabetes mellitus. *Neurology.* 2009;73:39.

Lotan I, Hellman MA, Steiner I. Diagnostic criteria of chronic inflammatory demyelinating polyneuropathy in diabetes mellitus. *Acta Neurol Scand.* 2015;132:278–83.

Ropper AH, Samuels MA, Klein JP. Diseases of the peripheral nerves. In *Adams & Victor's principles of neurology.* 10th ed. New York: McGraw-Hill; 2014.

Chronic Otitis Media (COM)

Epidemiology and Demographics: Acute otitis media is nearly universal, affecting 85% of children at least once, and 50% multiple times. Chronic OM occurs sporadically, and most frequently in indigenous populations. There is a male predominance, and it often affects preschool children. COM is likely secondary to eustachian tube dysfunction.

Disorder Description: Chronic otitis media (COM) is a term used to describe irreversible damage of the middle ear secondary to infection or inflammation. COM is most often associated with a permanent tympanic membrane (TM) perforation and recurring otorrhea but may also be seen with TM retraction pockets and/or atelectasis, ossicular chain erosion, middle ear granulation, and cholesteatoma. Otorrhea and conductive hearing loss are the most common presenting symptoms. The presence of otorrhea implies active infection. The presence of a polyp in the external canal of an ear with COM usually indicates an underlying cholesteatoma. *Pseudomonas aeruginosa* and *Staphylococcus aureus* are the two most common pathogens.

Symptoms

Localization site	Comment
Inner ear	Unaffected, in the classical case
Cranial nerves	Cochleovestibular nerve is not affected
Central nervous system	CNS is not affected

Secondary Complications: The "aural" complications of COM include mastoiditis with bony coalescence, labyrinthitis causing vertigo and/or sensorineural hearing loss, facial nerve paresis, and petrositis (inflammation of the petrous apex) causing sixth nerve palsy and retrobulbar headache. Intracranial complications of COM include meningitis, epidural or brain abscess, sigmoid sinus thrombophlebitis, and otitic hydrocephalus. Complications of COM generally require systemic antibiotics and urgent surgery.

Treatment Complications: The primary goal of COM treatment is to achieve a "safe ear" with low risk for further complications. Symptomatic relief and hearing restoration are secondary goals. Initial medical management consists of topical drops containing a quinolone antibiotic with or without steroid, as well as dry ear precautions. If a dry TM perforation is encountered and there are no concerns for cholesteatoma, tympanoplasty surgery with or without ossicular chain reconstruction (OCR) can be performed. TM retraction pockets can initially be managed with pressure-equalizing tubes (PETs). A cartilage-graft tympanoplasty with or without PETs may be performed in cases with significant TM atelectasis or adhesive COM. COM with cholesteatoma will require tympanomastoidectomy surgery. The mastoidectomy can be canal-wall-up or canal-wall-down, depending on the anatomic size of the mastoid and extent of the disease.

The prolonged use of topical steroid–antibiotic drops can result in fungal superinfection. Aminoglycoside-containing drops can result in ototoxicity and permanent hearing loss. PETs carry the risk of otorrhea or permanent TM. Tympanomastoidectomy surgery carries the risks of recurrent perforation, conductive or sensorineural hearing loss, vertigo, recurrent otorrhea, meatal stenosis, facial nerve injury, and the need for cleaning if a cavity is created. The most common risk associated with cholesteatoma is recurrence of the disease despite adequate surgery.

Bibliography

Bojrab DI, Smouha E. Tympanic membrane perforation and tympanoplasty. In Lalwani A, ed. *Sataloff's comprehensive textbook of otolaryngology.* Philadelphia, PA: JP Medical; 2015.

Smouha EE, Bojrab DI. *Cholesteatoma.* New York: Thieme; 2011. Chapter 1.

Smouha E, Bojrab DI. Cholesteatoma. In Lalwani A, ed. *Sataloff's comprehensive textbook of otolaryngology.* Philadelphia, PA: JP Medical; 2015.

Chronic Respiratory Failure

Epidemiology and Demographics: The incidence and prevalence of chronic respiratory failure vary among different countries; however, it is predominant among males. The overall prevalence worldwide is estimated to be approximately 8.4% with values varying depending on stratification method used. The incidence worldwide is estimated to be 2.8/1,000 patients/year.

Disorder Description: Chronic respiratory failure in this context represents emphysema, chronic bronchitis, and asthma; all of these diseases follow an obstructive pattern. The resulting increased pCO_2 levels are responsible for a wide array of downstream effects and in this context, hypercapneic encephalopathy. The complete pathophysiology of increased pCO_2 and resulting hypercapnic encephalopathy is not completely understood, but some of its effects have been demonstrated. The decreased pH results in vasodilation of cerebral arteries, decreased acetylcholine, impaired Kreb's cycle metabolism of glucose, and cerebral hypoxia from systemic hypoxemia. Increased amino acid metabolism is also seen resulting in increased levels of ammonium and glutamine. The resulting decrease in systemic pH also results in electrolyte abnormalities seen on serum chemistries.

Symptoms

Localization site	Comment
Cerebral hemispheres	Hypercapnic encephalopathy, CO_2 narcosis CSF acidosis, hypoxia, increased intracranial pressure
Mental status and psychiatric aspects/complications	Headache, drowsiness, confusion, stupor and coma, cognitive dysfunction, memory impairment, depression
Muscle	Asterixis, skeletal muscle weakness, myoclonus
Cerebrospinal fluid (CSF)	Decreased pH, papilledema

Secondary Complications: Worsening respiratory function will lead to respiratory arrest, CO_2 narcosis, coma, and possible endotracheal intubation.

Treatment Complications: Treatment of chronic respiratory failure or acute-on-chronic respiratory failure begins with noninvasive positive-pressure ventilation (NIPPV) if possible; however, mouth intermittent positive pressure ventilation (MPPV) may be necessary if NIPPV cannot be utilized or fails. In addition, while therapeutic, MPPV carries multiple risks including ventilator-associated pneumonia, barotrauma, and complications from endotracheal tube placement. Sedation required during mechanical ventilation may be complicated by delirium. Other treatment complications include side effects from both inhaled and systemic glucocorticoids.

Bibliography

Butterworth RF. Hypercapnic encephalopathy. In Siegel GJ, Agranoff BW, Albers RW, et al., eds. *Basic neurochemistry: molecular, cellular and medical aspects.* 6th ed. Philadelphia: Lippincott-Raven; 1999. Available from: www.ncbi.nlm.nih.gov/books/NBK28164/

Incalzi RA, Gemma A, Marra C, et al. Verbal memory impairment in COPD. *Chest.* 1997;112(6):1506–13. DOI:10.1378/chest.112.6.1506

Ropper AH, Samuels MA, Klein JP. The acquired metabolic disorders of the nervous system. In *Adams & Victor's principles of neurology,* 10th ed. New York, NY: McGraw-Hill; 2014. pp. 1132–60.

Rycroft CE, Heyes A, Lanza L, Becker K. Epidemiology of chronic obstructive pulmonary disease: a literature review. *Int J Chron Obstruct Pulmon Dis.* 2012;7:457–94. DOI:10.2147/COPD.S32330.

Scala R. Hypercapnic encephalopathy syndrome: A new frontier for non-invasive ventilation? *Respir Med.* 2011;105(8):1109–17. DOI:10.1016/j.rmed.2011.02.004

Thakur N, Blanc PD, Julian LJ, et al. COPD and cognitive impairment: the role of hypoxemia and oxygen therapy. *Int J Chron Obstruct Pulmon Dis.* 2010;5:263–9.

Ciguatera Poisoning

Epidemiology and Demographics: The most common food-borne illness caused by a chemical toxin in the United States, and the most common related to fish consumption in the world. It has been estimated that there are 10,000–50,000 cases/year but only about 10% are reported. Most frequent in the South Pacific, Hawaii, Florida, and the Caribbean.

Disorder Description: The toxin is produced by dinoflagellates, consumed by herbivorous fish, and eventually concentrated in higher-level carnivorous fish such as grouper, red snapper, and barracuda. The toxin causes increased membrane permeability to sodium and membrane depolarization. Neurologic symptoms begin with or after a 1- to 2-day bout of gastroenteritis with paresthesias in the perioral area or distal extremities. Paradoxical burning from cold exposure is a classic manifestation but myalgias, arthralgias, and itching are also common. Although weakness is described, it appears to be more of a generalized asthenia than paralysis. Dental pain is considered a classic feature but is seen in a minority of cases. Cardiac manifestations also occur with hypotension, arrhythmia, or bradycardia.

Symptoms

Localization site	Comment
Cerebral hemispheres	Headache
Mental status and psychiatric aspects/complications	Memory and concentration problems Depression and hallucinations
Peripheral neuropathy	Paresthesias in the distal extremities and perioral area; pruritis
Muscle	Myalgias

Secondary Complications: There may be residual symptoms for weeks or months. There appears to be sensitization with more prominent symptoms on re-exposure to the toxin.

Treatment Complications: Treatment with mannitol has been reported to improve symptoms and shorten duration but has the risk of further dehydration.

Bibliography

1. Friedman MA, Fleming LE, Fernandez M, et al. Ciguatera fish poisoning: treatment, prevention and management. *Mar Drugs.* 2008;6(3):456–79. PMCID: PMC2579736.

2. Kaplan JG. Ciguatoxin. In Spencer PS, Schaumburg HH, eds. *Experimental and clinical neurotoxicology.* 2nd ed. New York: Oxford University Press; 2000. pp. 386–90.

Citrobacter

Epidemiology and Demographics: *Citrobacter* species account for about 4–6% of all Gram-negative meningitis cases in infants, predominantly *C. koseri,* which causes brain abscesses in 75% of patients with meningitis.[1] Mortality may be high in these patients (up to 30%).[1] Central nervous system (CNS) disease is found mostly in neonates and infants, but also in adults >65 years.[2]

Disorder Description: *Citrobacter* species are facultatively anaerobic, lactose-fermenting, gram-negative bacilli and are part of the Enterobacteriaceae family.[2] They are commonly found in soil and water, and in the intestinal tracts of animals and humans and may cause a wide spectrum of infections in humans, including CNS infection.[2] *C. koseri* is the most common (>90%) species.[2]

Risk factors for infection include history of head trauma or neurosurgical procedure, bacteremia, diabetes, urinary tract infection, immunosuppression, or in debilitated adults >65 years. Bacteria can also be transmitted vertically from mother to neonate.[2]

Symptoms

Localization site	Comment
Cerebral hemispheres	Neonatal meningitis
	Abscesses (usually neonates and infants, but cases in adults have been reported)
	Ventriculitis
	Headache
	Seizures
	Cerebral infarction[3]
Mental status and psychiatric aspects/complications	Encephalopathy

Secondary Complications: A third of patients with CNS infections die, and >50% have residual neurologic deficits.[2]

Other complications include hydrocephalus and seizures.

Treatment Complications: Quinolone use may cause arthropathy in weight-bearing joints and should be restricted in neonates and young children.[1] Aminoglycosides cause hearing loss and nephrotoxicity.[3]

References

1. Plakkal N, Soraisham A, Amin H. Citrobacter freundii brain abscess in a preterm infant: a case report and literature review. *Pediatr Neonatol.* 2013;54(2):137–40.
2. Liu H, Chang C, Hsieh C. Brain abscess caused by Citrobacter koseri infection in an adult. *Neurosciences.* 2015;20(2):170–2.
3. Marecos C, Ferreira M, Ferreira M, Barroso M. Sepsis, meningitis and cerebral abscesses caused by Citrobacter koseri. *BMJ Case Rep.* 2012;2012.

Clostridium

Epidemiology and Demographics: *Clostridium botulinum* is found worldwide with 2943 cases reported. In the United States, 110 cases of botulism are reported annually, 75% of which are in infants.[1]

C. tetani causes 800,000 to 1 million deaths worldwide each year from tetanus, with half of the deaths in neonates. The highest number of fatal cases occur in Africa and Southeast Asia.[1]

C. perfringens affects children and adults worldwide.[2]

Disorder Description: *Clostridium* species are anaerobic, gram-positive rod-shaped bacilli that are capable of producing toxins. They are generally found in soil, freshwater and marine sediments, and intestines of humans and animals. Most common neurologic infections are caused by *C. botulinum*, *C. tetani*, and *C. perfringens*.[1]

C. botulinum may cause botulism. Transmission may occur by toxin in foodstuffs (usually canned goods or honey), infected wounds, intravenous drug abuse with black tar heroin, or inhalation of aerosolized spores. Infants <1 year are at risk of infection, due to the lack of fully established normal bowel flora at this age.[1]

C. tetani may cause tetanus. Risk factors for infection include deep penetrating wounds, burns, ulcers, intramuscular injections, snakebites, tattooing, or poor umbilical hygiene in neonates.[1]

C. perfringens is frequently present in the intestines of humans and animals, and its spores persist in soil, food, and decaying vegetation. It may cause single organ infection or spread and involve both the central and peripheral nervous systems. Risk factors for central nervous sytem infection include recent spinal surgery or neurosurgery, or local trauma. Risk factors for peripheral nervous system infection include trauma, or recent surgery.[2]

Symptoms

Localization site	
Cerebral hemispheres	*C. perfringens* – meningitis, encephalitis (with or without pneumocephalus), plexitis, cerebral abscess, subdural empyema[2]
Cranial nerves	*C. botulinum* can cause symmetric cranial nerve palsies, usually ophthalmoplegia, ptosis, dysphagia, facial palsy
	C. tetani may cause facial palsy or ophthalmoplegia
Peripheral neuropathy	*C. perfringens* may cause sensorimotor polyneuropathy (rare)
Muscle	*C. perfringens* – myonecrosis, myositis, rhabdomyolysis
Neuromuscular junction	*C. botulinum* – botulism *C. tetani* – tetanus
Unclear localization	*C. tetani* may cause autonomic dysfunction

Secondary Complications: Botulism may result in respiratory paralysis.[1] Tetanus may also cause loss of airway protection due to excessive bronchial secretions, hypersalivation, laryngeal spasms, and dysphagia. Limb contractures, bed sores, seizures, myoclonus, and sleep disturbances may be complications.[1]

Treatment Complications: In patients with tetanus, high doses of penicillins may act synergistically with the toxin to block GABA neuronal activity, causing hyperexcitability and convulsions. Anti-tetanus immunoglobulin (passive vaccination), which may shorten the course and severity of disease, may cause anaphylactic reactions.[1]

References

1. Goonetilleke A. Clostridial neurotoxins. *J Neurol Neurosurg Psychiatry*. 2004;75(Suppl 3):iii35–iii39.
2. Finsterer J, Hess B. Neuromuscular and central nervous system manifestations of Clostridium perfringens infections. *Infection*. 2007;35(6):396–405.

Cluster Headache

Epidemiology and Demographics: Studies suggest a prevalence of 0.1% in the general population. A preference for male over female is seen in this condition with a ratio of 2.5:1. However, this bias tends to equalize with increasing age.

Disorder Description: This condition is characterized by acute, severe stabbing pain. Most studies show that cluster headache localizes to the retro-orbital territory in a unilateral fashion. However, some reports suggest that the side of onset can switch during the attack. Less frequently, temporal territory is also affected. Pain has been reported over the forehead, jaw, cheek, upper and lower teeth. Areas around ears, nose, neck, shoulder, and other regions of the hemicranium are less frequently associated with cluster headache. Some reports suggest that the pain originates from the V1 trigeminal dermatome.

Symptoms

Localization site	Comment
Cerebral hemispheres	Can involve unilateral or bilateral hemispheres
Cranial nerves	Involvement of V1 trigeminal nerve dermatome
Hypothalamus	Some studies suggest a role for this area of the brain as the origin of cluster headache symptoms
Eye	Most cases report involvement of retro-orbital territory as localized pain

Secondary Complications: There are no reported secondary complications associated with cluster headaches.

Treatment Complications: Established guidelines for treatment of acute cluster headache involve sumatriptan (oral, subcutaneous, or intravenous) and high-flow oxygen. In patients who have history of vascular disease in neck and head, the use of sumatriptan is cautioned as these patients are at high risk of developing strokes.

Bibliography

Bahra A, May A, Gaodsby PJ. Cluster headache: a prospective clinical study with diagnostic implications. *Neurology*. 2002;58:354–61.

Kudrow L. *Cluster headache: mechanisms and management*. Oxford: Oxford University Press; 1980.

Manzoni GC. Gender ratio of cluster headache over the years: a possible role of changes in lifestyle. *Cephalalgia*. 1998;18:138–42.

Coagulopathy

Epidemiology and Demographics: Coagulopathy can be divided into hyper- or hypocoagulable disorders, which can be further divided into inherited (genetic) or acquired (medications, liver cirrhosis, kidney failure, cancer, autoimmune, etc.)

Disorder Description: Hypercoagulable disorders are characterized by thrombosis that is arterial or venous with symptoms determined by where the thrombosis is located. In contrast, hypocoagulable disorders are characterized by excessive bleeding with symptoms related to blood loss or location of the hematoma. The modes of inheritance and demographics vary widely.

Symptoms

Localization site	Comment
Cerebral hemispheres	Headache, thunderclap headache, aphasia, hemiparesis, hemisensory loss, seizures (generalized or focal), stroke, cerebral vein thrombosis. In hypocoagulable disorders, subarachnoid hemorrhage, subdural or epidural hematoma, or parenchymal hemorrhage
Mental status and psychiatric aspects/ complications	Delirium or coma (intracranial hemorrhage, seizures, strokes, liver failure from hepatic vein thrombosis, hypoxia from pulmonary embolism)
Brainstem	Hemorrhage may produce cranial nerve palsy with contralateral hemiplegia
Cerebellum	Ataxia (stroke or hemorrhage)
Vestibular system (and non-specific dizziness)	Vertigo or dizziness (stroke, anemia due to blood loss)
Base of skull	Cranial neuropathy (jugular vein thrombosis 9, 11, 12)
Cranial nerves	Cranial neuropathy (6th nerve common), papilledema, proptosis, chemosis (cavernous sinus thrombosis)
Spinal cord	Cord compression (epidural hematoma)
Plexus	Lumbosacral plexopathy (retroperitoneal hematoma)
Muscle	Weakness and pain (compartment syndrome due to arterial embolism)

Treatment Complications: Blood product transfusion related infections, antibodies to factor transfusion in hypocoagulable states, antiepileptic drug side effects for seizure treatment, excessive bleeding from antiplatelet and anticoagulants, and excessive clotting from clotting factor infusions.

Bibliography

Lancé MD. A general review of major global coagulation assays: thrombelastography, thrombin generation test and clot waveform analysis. *Thromb J.* 2015;13:1.

Cocaine Abuse

Epidemiology and Demographics: No race or ethnicity predilection. More common users range from 18 to 25 years old and are more often male.

Disorder Description: Cocaine, a natural alkaloid, is extracted from leaves of an Andean shrub, *Erythroxylon coca*. This substance is abused particularly via insufflation (snorting/sniffing), inhalation (smoking), and injection. Its prevalence in the United States has increased drastically, and its use has also grown in Central American countries, Europe, and parts of Asia. Globally, 100 million people are believed to be cocaine users.

Symptoms

Localization site	Comment
Cerebral hemispheres	Cerebral ischemia (acute)
	Cerebral atrophy (chronic)
	Cerebral hemorrhage (acute)
	Aneurysm rupture (acute)
	Seizures (acute)
	Coma (acute)
Mental status and psychiatric aspects/complications	Depression, suicidal ideation, paranoia (acute and chronic)
	Cognitive dysfunction (chronic)
	Violent antisocial behavior (chronic)
Cerebellum	Decreased synapses (chronic)
Cranial nerves	Cocaine-induced third nerve palsy
Pituitary gland	Dysfunction of the release of anterior pituitary hormones (acute)

Localization site	Comment
Spinal cord	Spinal cord infarction (acute)
Anterior horn cells	Destruction of the anterior horn cells (chronic)
Dorsal root ganglia	Destruction of the dorsal root ganglia (chronic)
Specific spinal roots	Spinal cord infarction (acute)
Plexus	Spinal cord infarction (acute)
Mononeuropathy or mononeuropathy multiplex	Cocaine-induced neuropathy (chronic)
Peripheral neuropathy	Cocaine-induced neuropathy (chronic)
Muscle	Rhabdomyolysis (acute) Dystonia (acute) Tic disorder (acute)
Neuromuscular junction	Increased dopaminergic aggregation and hyperactivity (acute and chronic) Increased norepinephrine, in smooth muscle junction (acute and chronic)
Syndromes with combined spinal cord and peripheral nerve lesions	Anterior spinal artery syndrome (acute)

Secondary Complications: Indirect effects on neurologic system via the following:

- **Cardiovascular** complications – Cocaine causes systolic and diastolic dysfunction, arrhythmias, and atherosclerosis, which ultimately contribute to strokes.
- **Coagulation effect** – Cocaine causes elevation of von Willebrand factor and erythrocytes, which leads to increase in viscosity that results in thrombosis leading to cerebral infarction.
- **Hepatic complications** – Hepatic failure resulting in rhabdomyolysis.
- **Gastritis and pancreatitis** result in chronic malnutrition and widespread central nervous system/peripheral nervous system dysfunction.

Bibliography

Agarwal P. Neurologic effects of cocaine. Medscape. http://emedicine.medscape.com/article/1174408-overview#a6. Accessed Aug 15, 2018.

Enevoldson TP. Recreational drugs and their neurological consequences. http://jnnp.bmj.com/content/75/suppl_3/iii9.full. Accessed Aug 15, 2018.

Kuriyama H, Suyama A. Multiple actions of cocaine on neuromuscular transmission and smooth muscle cells of the guinea-pig mesenteric artery. *J Physiol*. 1983;337:631–54. http://onlinelibrary.wiley.com/doi/10.1113/jphysiol.1983.sp014646/pdf.

Schwartz BG, Rezkalla S, Kloner RA. Cardiovascular effects of cocaine. *Circulation*. 2010;122:2558–69.

Siegel AJ, Sholar MB, Mendelson JH, et al. Cocaine-induced erythrocytosis and increase in von Willebrand factor: evidence for drug-related blood doping and prothrombotic effects. *Arch Intern Med*. 1999;159(16):1925–9. DOI:10.1001/archinte.159.16.1925.

Venton BJ, Seipel AT, Phillips PEM, et al. Cocaine increases dopamine release by mobilization of a synapsin-dependent reserve pool. *J Neurosci*. 2006;26(12):3206–9.

Coccidioides immitis

Epidemiology and Demographics: The number of *Coccidioides immitis* infections has risen to ~150,000 per year. Extrapulmonary complications estimated at 0.5% of infections in Caucasians, and 30–50% of infections in heavily immunosuppressed patients.[1]

Tends to occur more in those of Asian or African descent.

Disorder Description: *C. immitis* is a dimorphic yeast species of the genus *Coccidioides*, a member of the Onygenaceae family. It usually exists in soil, and it is endemic to the southwestern United States and parts of Central and South America.[1,2]

Infection is through inhalation of spores and most often causes pneumonia. Disseminated disease may lead to rash, skeletal lesions, or meningitis. A lesser cause of infection is through solid organ transplantation or percutaneous inoculation.[2]

Risk factors include living in endemic areas, being exposed to dust or dirt with spores, or occupations involving aerosolization of soil. Risk factors for severe disease include immunosuppression, pregnancy, autoimmune conditions, malignancy, solid organ transplantation, older age, male sex, or underlying genetic disease. After reaching its human host, it will change to yeast form.[2]

Symptoms

Localization site	Comment
Cerebral hemispheres	Abscess
	Headache
	Meningitis, which may become complicated by vasculitis causing intracerebral hemorrhage or ischemic stroke
Base of skull	Basilar meningitis
Specific spinal roots	Radiculopathy (rare)

Secondary Complications: Complications may include hydrocephalus or central nervous system vasculitis.[1,3]

Treatment Complications: Despite adequate therapy, hydrocephalus may result, requiring shunt placement. Also, patients may require lifelong treatment with fluconazole.[3]

References

1. Galgiani J, Ampel N, Blair J, et al. Coccidioidomycosis. *Clin Infect Dis.* 2005;41(9):1217–23.
2. DynaMed Plus [Internet]. Record No. 116164, Coccidioidomycosis. Updated Oct 26, 2015. Ipswich,MA: EBSCO InformationServices. 1995. Available from www.dynamed.com/login .aspxdirect=true&site=DynaMed&id=116164. Accessed Jan 29, 2016. Registration and login required.
3. Zunt J, Baldwin K. Chronic and subacute meningitis. *Continuum (Minneap Minn).* 2012;18:1290–318.

Complex Regional Pain Syndrome (formerly, Reflex Sympathetic Dystrophy)

Epidemiology and Demographics: Complex regional pain syndrome (CRPS) usually affects women in their 40s or 50s. The incidence is 5.5/100,000 and the prevalence is 21/100,000 for CRPS type 1.

Disorder Description: How the disease comes about is not known. However, theories include inflammation of the nerves and their surroundings, and hypersensitivity in perception of pain in the brain.

Patients may experience excruciating pain, numbness, hypersensitivity, weakness, excessive sweating, and changes in hair distribution. There may or may not be a prior history of trauma. The anxiety caused by the condition and comorbid psychiatric disorder may delay or even hamper adequate treatment.

Symptoms

Localization site	Comment
Cerebral hemispheres	Somatosensory cortex affected
Mental status and psychiatric aspects/complications	Anxiety and depression, posttraumatic stress disorder
Spinal cord	Remodeling
Dorsal root ganglia	Peripheral sensitization
Autonomic nervous system	Vasomotor and sudomotor dysfunction including alterations in sweating, skin color, temperature, trophic changes in the skin, hair, or nails

Secondary Complications: Anxiety from chronic pain, weakness in the extremities from pain limitation. Decreased range of motion in the limb due to disuse.

Treatment Complications: Neuropathic medications such as gabapentin can cause sedation. Transdermal lidocaine patches may cause skin irritation.

Bibliography

Bussa M, Gutilla D, Lucia M, et al. Complex regional pain syndrome type 1: a comprehensive review *Acta Anaesthesiol Scand.* 2015;59(6):685–97.

Guthmiller K, Dulebohn S. Pain, complex regional pain syndrome (reflex sympathetic dystrophy, RSD, CRPS). In *StatPearls* [Internet]. Treasure Island, FL: StatPearls Publishing; 2017. www .ncbi.nlm.nih.gov/books/NBK430719/

Sandroni P, Benrud-Larson LM, McClelland RL, Low PA. Complex regional pain syndrome type I: incidence and prevalence in Olmsted county, a population-based study. *Pain.* 2003;103 (1–2):199–207.

Compression Fracture, Vertebral

Epidemiology and Demographics: Vertebral compression fractures are seen in approximately 25% of all postmenopausal women in the United States. Motor vehicle accidents account for these fractures in younger patients, and they are seen more often in men than woman in younger age groups.

Disorder Description: A compression fracture is the collapse of a vertebra. It can be due to trauma or weakening of the vertebra. Weakening can be seen in patients with osteoporosis or osteogenesis imperfecta, lytic lesions from metastatic or primary tumors, or infection.

Symptoms

Localization site	Comment
Acute fracture	Severe pain

Treatment Complications: Treatment includes back braces, opioids, calcitonin, kyphoplasty, and vertebroplasty. Opioids can cause sedation, falls in elderly patients, confusion, and addiction.

Bibliography

Brant WE, Helmes Clyde A. *Benign compression fracture. Fundamentals of diagnostic radiology.* 3rd ed. Philadelphia: Lippincott Williams & Wilkins; 2007. p. 302.

Confusional Arousals

Epidemiology and Demographics: The prevalence of confusional arousal varies by age group: 3–13 years 17.3%, >15 years 2.9–4.2%, and lifetime risk of 18.5%. There is equal sex predominance. The age at onset is most often in early childhood at around 2 years.

Predisposing factors include priming factors of sleep deprivation and situational stress. Hyperthyroidism, migraines, head injury, encephalitis, and stroke are rarer potential priming factors.

Precipitating factors include conditions that cause sleep fragmentation or deprivation resulting in increased homeostatic sleep pressure, thus increasing the opportunity for slow-wave sleep parasomnias to arise. Obstructive sleep apnea (OSA) and other sleep-related respiratory events may be precipitants of disorders of arousal. Other triggers include environmental stimuli (e.g., telephone calls, pagers, electronic devices, noise, light), internal stimuli (distended bladder), travel, sleeping in unfamiliar surroundings, febrile illness in children, physical emotional stress, premenstrual period in women, and psychotropic medications (e.g., lithium carbonate, phenothiazines, anticholinergics, sedative/hypnotic agents). Literature on the relationship between alcohol and disorders of arousal is mixed.

Disorder Description: Confusional arousals are characterized by confusion or disoriented behavior during an arousal without terror or ambulation outside of the bed. Confusional arousals typically last less than 5 minutes, but episodes can occasionally last longer. Patients typically have poor recollection of the events the following day.

Polysomnography is not routinely indicated for evaluation of confusional arousals but may show high-amplitude hypersynchronous delta waves and frequent arousals from slow-wave sleep. It may also be helpful in ruling out other disorders such as REM behavior disorder, nocturnal epilepsy, or associated sleep disordered breathing. Pharmacologic treatment is generally not indicated and management should focus on reassurance, avoidance of precipitating factors, and maintenance of a safe sleep environment to minimize risk of injury. Benzodiazepines and serotonin reuptake inhibitors may be effective in extreme cases.

Symptoms

Localization site	Comment
Unclear localization	Majority of individuals with disorders of arousal do not have neurologic or psychologic pathology. Rare reported cases of confusional arousals associated with brain lesions in areas involving arousal (posterior hypothalamus, midbrain reticular area, and periventricular gray matter). Functional abnormality in the brain may be possible that leaves some regions (hippocampus and frontal cortices) asleep, while other parts of the brain (motor, cingulate, insular, amygdala, and temporopolar cortices) are awake. Disorders of arousal represent a dissociation of different regions of the brain in addition to activation of locomotor centers/central pattern generators, accompanied by sleep inertia and sleep state instability

Treatment Complications: Benzodiazepines may result in morning somnolence and may exacerbate underlying sleep disordered breathing.

Bibliography

American Academy of Sleep Medicine. *International classification of sleep disorders*. 3rd ed. Darien, IL: American Academy of Sleep Medicine; 2014.

Howell MJ. Parasomnias: an updated review. *Neurotherapeutics*. 2012;9:753–75.

Mahowald M. Non-REM arousal parasomnias. In Kryger MH, Roth T, Dement WC, eds. *Principles and practice of sleep medicine*. 5th ed. Philadelphia: Saunders; 2010. pp. 1075–82.

Congenital Central Alveolar Hypoventilation Syndrome

Epidemiology and Demographics: Congenital central alveolar hypoventilation syndrome is rare with unknown prevalence. Occurs equally among the sexes and all ethnic/racial groups. It is a genetic condition that is present from birth, although some patients present later in life.

Disorder Description: Congenital central alveolar hypoventilation syndrome is a congenital genetic disorder characterized by autonomic dysfunction and failure of the automatic central control of breathing. The PHOX2B gene has been implicated in its pathogenesis; this gene plays a role in the development of the autonomic nervous system and central respiratory control pathways. The disease usually results from a de novo mutation.

Patients typically present with hypoventilation, usually present at birth, and require ventilatory support at varying levels, depending on the severity of the disease. Some patients with a milder mutation may present later in life.

It is diagnosed when sleep-related hypoventilation is present and when mutation of the PHOX2B gene is present. The gene is dominant, and patients are at risk of having children with congenital central alveolar hypoventilation syndrome.

Symptoms

Localization site	Comment
Mental status and psychiatric aspects/ complications	Headaches, hypersomnolence related to chronic hypoventilation, mood disturbances

Secondary Complications: Occurs in association with autonomic abnormalities in a subset of patients, such as Hirschsprung disease, autonomic dysfunction with decreased heart rate variability or hypotension, neural tumors, such as ganglioneuromas or ganglioneuroblastomas, and ocular abnormalities.

Treatment Complications: Treatment includes the use of invasive or noninvasive ventilation in the form of bilevel or average volume-assured pressure support. Diaphragm pacing has also been used.

Discomfort and noncompliance with noninvasive ventilation as well as complications of invasive ventilator support.

Bibliography

American Academy of Sleep Medicine. *International classification of sleep disorders*. 3rd ed. Darien, IL: American Academy of Sleep Medicine; 2014.

Paton JY, Swaminathan S, Sargent CW, Hawksworth A, Keens TG. Hypoxic and hypercapnic ventilatory responses in awake children with congenital central hypoventilation syndrome. *Am Rev Respir Dis*. 1989;140:368–72.

Congestive Heart Failure

Epidemiology and Demographics: In people over the age of 65, the incidence of congestive heart failure (CHF) is approximately 1%. CHF is seen equally in men and women but the incidence in African Americans is approximately 1.5 times greater. Mortality is seen in more than 50% of patients within 5 years of developing CHF.

Disorder Description: CHF results from damage to the myocardium due to coronary artery disease, hypertension, diabetes, and other disorders that lead to ischemia. CHF may result in an inability to sufficiently pump blood through both the systemic and pulmonary circulations, as well as an increase in filling pressures. The increase in pressure may give rise to pulmonary vascular congestion as fluid fills the interstitial space of the bronchioles and other lung structures.

Symptoms

Localization site	Comment
Cerebral hemispheres	Hypoperfusion from lack of cardiac output may result in light-headedness, dizziness, tiredness, and fatigue

Localization site	Comment
Mental status and psychiatric aspects/ complications	Patients may get depressed and experience limitations in their functionality due to the cerebral hypoperfusion. They may also become confused, disoriented, and anxious. Severe cases may result in hallucinations and delirium
Cerebellum	May have balance issues due to hypoperfusion of the cerebellum
Vestibular system (and nonspecific dizziness)	Same as above

Secondary Complications: CHF may result in pulmonary edema and problems with the heart, liver, and kidneys.

Treatment Complications: Treatment of CHF may result in hypotension including presyncope and syncope, for example as a result of afterload reduction with ACE inhibitors and/or aldosterone receptor blockers.

Bibliography

Cohen TJ. Congestive heart failure. In *Practical electrophysiology*. Malvern, PA: HMP Communications; 2009. pp. 207–11.

Emory Healthcare. Heart failure statistics. 2015. Available from www.emoryhealthcare.org/heart-failure/learn-about-heart-failure/statistics.html. Accessed July 6, 2015.

Mayo Clinic Staff. Heart failure. 2015. Available from www.mayoclinic.org/diseases-conditions/heart-failure/basics/complications/con-20029801. Accessed July 7, 2015.

PubMed Health. Heart failure. June 11, 2014. Available from www.ncbi.nlm.nih.gov/pubmedhealth/PMH0063056/. Accessed July 6, 2015.

Copper Deficiency Myeloneuropathy

Epidemiology and Demographics: The age range for copper deficiency myeloneuropathy is 30 to 82 years. Affects women more than men.

Disorder Description: Copper is important for normal structure and function of the nervous system. It allows electron transfer in enzymatic pathways. Animal studies of copper deficiency reveal neuronal loss in the cerebellum and spinal tracts with extensive demyelination. Risk factors for copper deficiency include excessive zinc ingestion, gastric surgery, and malabsorption due to inflammatory bowel disease, celiac disease, and other gastrointestinal disorders. Rarely, overtreatment of Wilson's disease can also result in copper deficiency. Neurologic manifestations include subacute gait disorder with sensory ataxia, spasticity, myelopathy, impaired vibration and position sense, positive Rhomberg's sign, and peripheral neuropathy in a stocking and glove distribution. Rarely, patients also experience bladder dysfunction. Some patients may have bilateral vision loss due to optic nerve involvement.

Symptoms

Localization site	Comment
Cranial nerves	Subacute bilateral vision loss, optic nerve involvement
Spinal cord	Spasticity, positive Babinksi's, hyperreflexia, myelopathy, (dorsal columns) – impaired vibration and position sense
Dorsal root ganglia	Sensory ataxia, pseudoathetosis, allodynia, sensory ganglionopathy, asymmetric sensory loss in face, trunk, and limbs
Peripheral neuropathy	Hyporeflexia, decreased sensation in stocking and glove distribution, wrist drop, foot drop
Syndromes with combined spinal cord and peripheral nerve lesions	Impaired vibration and position sense, positive Rhomberg's sign, peripheral neuropathy with hyporeflexia (typically ankle jerks), and hyperreflexia

Secondary Complications: Physical injury due to difficulty walking and loss of vision.

Bibliography

Danks DM. Copper deficiency in humans. *Annu Rev Nutr*. 1988;8:235.

Jaiser SR, Winston GP. Copper deficiency myelopathy. *J Neurol*. 2010;257:869.

Kumar N, Gross JB Jr, Ahlskog JE. Copper deficiency myelopathy produces a clinical picture like subacute combined degeneration. *Neurology.* 2004;63:33.

Naismith RT, Shepherd JB, Weihl CC, et al. Acute and bilateral blindness due to optic neuropathy associated with copper deficiency. *Arch Neurol.* 2009;66:1025.

Cortical Dysplasia

Epidemiology and Demographics: Cortical dysplasia is one of the most common causes of intractable epilepsy in children, accounting for 25–40% of cases. Epilepsy can occur at any age, but usually presents in early childhood. Reported incidence and prevalence are variable and increasing with advances in neuroimaging techniques.

Disorder Description: Focal cortical dysplasia (FCD) is a developmental malformation of the cerebral cortex that occurs secondary to disruption of normal neuronal cytoarchitecture. Sporadic disorder with few defined family pedigrees; the pathogenesis remains unknown. Studies have suggested that mutations affecting *DEPDC5*, mTOR signaling may be responsible.

The Internal League Against Epilepsy has proposed a 3-tier classification system based on clinico-pathologic features:

Type I – characterized by abnormal cortical layering with radial microcolumns. Has three subtypes.

Type II – common among epilepsy surgical series and in the extratemporal areas, particularly the frontal lobe. Characterized by dysmorphic and cytomegalic neurons. Has two subtypes.

Type III – pathologic changes adjacent to or associated with substantive brain lesions (such as vascular malformations and tumors). Has four subtypes.

Neuroimaging, mainly MRI, is important to identify FCD. Common findings include: increased cortical thickness, subtle changes in the smoothness of gyri or sulci, and changes in subcortical white matter signal. Focal rhythmic epileptiform discharges may be seen on EEG, sometimes activated by non-rapid eye movement sleep. Intermittent or continuous focal slowing may also be noted.

Treatment may require physical, occupational, and speech therapy. Epilepsy surgery is often required because of medication-resistant seizures.

Symptoms

Localization site	Comment
Cerebral hemispheres	Focal seizures. Other deficits such as motor or language impairments depend on localization and extent of lesion
Mental status and psychiatric aspects/complications	Cognitive impairments may occur. Psychiatric comorbidity more common in patients with early-onset epilepsy and posterior cerebral lesions

Secondary Complications: Refractory epilepsy occurring as a result of FCD is commonly associated with cognitive, psychiatric, and social comorbidities.

Treatment Complications: Antiepileptic drugs may be associated with a number of idiosyncratic reactions including multi-organ dysfunction, cognitive or psychiatric effects, and drug interactions. Postoperative complications of surgical resection may include nondisabling visual field defects, often transient sensorimotor deficits, and meningitis.

Bibliography

Crino PB. Focal cortical dysplasia. *Semin Neurol.* 2015;35(3):201–8.

Gaitanis JN, Donahue J. Focal cortical dysplasia. *Pediatr Neurol.* 2013;49(2):79–87.

Lee SK, Kim DW. Focal cortical dysplasia and epilepsy surgery. *J Epilepsy Res.* 2013;3(2):43–7.

Corticobasal Degeneration

Epidemiology and Demographics: In a recent review by Armstrong and colleagues,[1] mean age of onset of corticobasal degeneration (CBD) was 63.7 years (range 45 to 77.2), with mean disease duration of 6.6 years (range 2 to 12.5).

Disorder Description: The classic clinical presentation of CBD (sometimes called corticobasal syndrome or CBS) is a slowly progressive syndrome with asymmetric rigidity, limb apraxia and alien limb, cortical sensory loss, and cognitive impairment.[1–3] The classic neuropathologic criteria are tau-positive neuronal and glial lesions with astrocytic plaques in the cerebral cortex and basal ganglia with asymmetric cell loss.[4] Unfortunately, the mapping between these clinical and pathologic diagnoses is poor.[3,5,6] Many patients with CBD pathology present with a progressive supranuclear palsy-like clinical syndrome or frontotemporal dementia clinical syndrome. Some patients with the classic clinical syndrome have Parkinson's disease, dementia lacking distinctive histology, Alzheimer's disease, or Creutzfeld–Jacob disease on brain examination, but not classic CBD pathology. An effort to broaden the spectrum of clinical presentations was associated with poor specificity against pathologic diagnoses.[6]

In our judgment, the clinical utility of the CBD concept is to give a clinical diagnosis to patients who present with some combination of gradually progressive asymmetric limb rigidity or akinesia, limb dystonia, limb myoclonus, orobuccal or limb apraxia, cortical sensory deficit, and/or alien limb phenomenon. The clinician should be aware that classic CBD pathology is the most likely substrate, but other neurodegenerative pathologies are possible. Asymmetric parietal atrophy on MRI scan supports the diagnosis. Progressive cognitive impairment is part of the syndrome, but may be subtle at presentation and overshadowed by apraxia or an alien limb. Similar to other atypical Parkinson syndromes, CBD responds poorly to levodopa, though a small benefit may be observed at higher doses (1200 mg daily for 2 to 3 months).[2] No effective disease-modifying therapy for CBD exists, and treatment is largely supportive.

Symptoms

Localization site	Comment
Cerebral hemispheres – asymmetric frontoparietal degeneration	Limb rigidity (85%)
	Bradykinesia or clumsy limb (76%)
	Cognitive impairment (70%)
	Limb apraxia (57%)
	Behavioral changes (55%)
	Aphasia (52%)
	Alien limb (30%)
	Myoclonus (27%)
	Cortical sensory loss (27%)

Secondary Complications: Gait instability may lead to falls and further disability. Physical and occupational therapy are essential for maximizing functionality and delaying disability.

Treatment Complications: Side effects of levodopa include dyskinesias and gastrointestinal distress.

Clonazepam used for myoclonus and baclofen used for dystonia can both cause lethargy.

References

1. Armstrong MJ, et al. Criteria for the diagnosis of corticobasal degeneration. *Neurology.* 2013;80:496–503.
2. McFarland NR. Diagnostic approach to atypical parkinsonian syndromes. *Continuum (Minneap Minn).* 2016;22:1117–42.
3. Ling H, et al. Does corticobasal degeneration exist? A clinicopathological re-evaluation. *Brain.* 2010;133:2045–57.
4. Dickson DW, et al. Office of Rare Diseases neuropathologic criteria for corticobasal degeneration. *J Neuropathol Exp Neurol.* 2002;61(11):935–46.
5. Boeve BF, et al. Pathologic heterogeneity in clinically diagnosed corticobasal degeneration. *Neurology.* 1999;53:795–800.
6. Alexander SK, et al. Validation of the new consensus criteria for the diagnosis of corticobasal degeneration. *J Neurol Neurosurg Psychiatry.* 2014;85(8):925–9. DOI: 10.1136/jnnp-2013-307035.

Coxsackievirus

Epidemiology and Demographics: Infants, children, and adolescents account for 90% of Coxsackie B virus infections, with 75% of cases occuring in infants <1 year old and toddlers aged 1–4 years. Most infections tend to occur in the summer and fall.[1]

Disorder Description: Coxsackieviruses are non-enveloped viruses with linear single-stranded RNA that belong to the family Picornaviridae and the genus *Enterovirus*. They are further divided into group A and group B.[1]

Group A viruses tend to infect skin and mucous membranes, typically causing hand, foot, and mouth disease. Group B viruses tend to infect the heart, pleura, liver, and pancreas. Both groups can cause aseptic meningitis. The leading serotypes associated with central nervous system diseases are B1 to B6, A7, and A9.[1]

Risk factors include close skin contact with an infected person, and the virus can be transmitted by the fecal–oral route, vertically during pregnancy, and via respiratory secretions.[1]

Symptoms[1,2]

Localization site	Comment
Cerebral hemispheres	Meningitis
	Encephalitis
	Headache
	Seizures
	Myoclonus
Anterior horn cells	Flaccid paralysis
Syndromes with combined upper and lower motor neuron deficits	Motor neuron disease (rare)

Secondary Complications: Seizures, post-encephalitic parkinsonism, and acute disseminated encephalomyelitis may be complications.[2]

References

1. DynaMed Plus [Internet]. Record No. 901254, Coxsackie virus B (CVB) infection. Ipswich, MA: EBSCO Information Services. 1995. Updated Nov 20, 2015 [about 5 screens]. Available from direct=true&site=DynaMed&id=901254. Accessed Jan 21, 2016. Registration and login required.
2. Berger J, Chumley W, Pittman T, Given C, Nuovo G. Persistent Coxsackie B encephalitis: Report of a case and review of the literature. *J Neurovirol.* 2006;12(6):511–16.

Craniofacial Tremor

Epidemiology and Demographics: Facial tremor is rarely seen in isolation and its prevalence is unknown.

Disorder Description: Facial tremor is rarely an isolated phenomenon. It usually occurs as part of another neurologic disorder such as essential tremor (ET) or Parkinson's disease (PD). Tremor of the chin is more common in PD, while tremor of the jaw is more common in ET. The "rabbit syndrome," seen in elderly patients maintained on neuroleptics, involves fine rhythmic tremor of the oral, paranasal, and masticatory muscles.

Treatment Complications: Medications used to treat PD are varied and may be associated with side effects including dyskinesia, gastrointestinal distress, impulse control disorders, and sedation among others. Medications used to treat ET are also varied and

may cause light-headedness, bradycardia, changes in cognition, etc.

Bibliography

Balasubramaniam R, Ram S. Orofacial movement disorders. *Oral Maxillofac Surg Clin North Am.* 2008;20(2): 273–85.

Evidente VGH, Adler CH. Hemifacial spasm and other craniofacial movement disorders. *Mayo Clin Proc.* 1998;73(1):67–71.

Kraft SP, Lang AE. Cranial dystonia, blepharospasm and hemifacial spasm: clinical features and treatment, including the use of botulinum toxin. *CMAJ.* 1988;139(9):837–44.

Creutzfeldt–Jakob Disease (CJD)

Epidemiology and Demographics: Incidence of Creutzfeldt–Jakob disease (CJD) is 1–1.5 cases per million per year in developed countries. Approximately 400 cases of prion disease are diagnosed per year in the United States,[1] of which 80–95% are sporadic form, 10–15% are genetic (familial), and <1% are acquired.[1]

The mean age at onset of symptoms of sporadic CJD is 64 years and median survival time is about 6 months from disease onset, with 85–90% of patients dying within 1 year.[2] Familial CJD has an onset usually between 30 and 55 years and is most prevalent in Jews of Libyan and Tunisian descent, and Slovakians.[2]

Two hundred and twenty-nine cases of variant CJD have been reported worldwide, most of them occurring in the UK or France, but the United States and Canada have also had cases.[1]

Disorder Description: CJD is a rapidly progressive dementia, caused by the conversion of normal prion protein (PrP^C) into an abnormal misfolded form (PrP^{Sc}).[1]

Three mechanisms exist: sporadic, genetic (familial), and acquired. In sporadic CJD, which is the most common form, the conversion of PrP^C to PrP^{Sc} is considered to be spontaneous or through a somatic mutation of *PRNP*. In the familial form, mutations in the prion protein gene, *PRNP*, make the PrP^C more susceptible to misfolding into PrP^{Sc}. In the acquired form, PrP^{Sc} is accidentally transmitted to a person, causing their endogenous PrP^C to misfold.[1]

Acquired CJD is either iatrogenic or variant. Iatrogenic infections are transmitted from human to human via contamination with tissue from an infected person, usually as a result of a medical procedure. These include corneal and meningeal transplants and human-derived hormonal therapies. Variant CJD occurs from dietary exposure, most notably from cattle infected with bovine spongiform encephalopathy.[1,2]

Symptoms[3]

Localization site	
Cerebral hemispheres	Extrapyramidal symptoms
	Pyramidal symptoms
	Tremors
	Myoclonus
	Sleep disturbances
	Headache
	Seizures
	Sensory disturbance
	Visual disturbances (blurring, visual field defects, perception abnormalities)
Mental status and psychiatric aspects/ complications	Subacute progressive dementia[3]
	Visuospatial difficulties
	Memory loss
	Inattention
	Apraxia
	Hemineglect
	Akinetic mutism
	Psychiatric
	Agitation/irritability
	Personality changes
	Hallucinations
	Depression
Cerebellum	Gait abnormalities, ataxia
Cranial nerves	Oculomotor dysfunction
Unclear localization	Myoclonus

Secondary Complications: Patients with dysphagia may develop aspiration pneumonia, which is the most common cause of death.[2]

Treatment Complications: No current available treatment.

References

1. Geschwind M. Prion diseases. *Continuum (Minneap Minn)*. 2015;21:1612–38.

2. DynaMed Plus [Internet]. Record No. 114980, Creutzfeldt-Jakob disease. Ipswich, MA: EBSCO Information Services. 1995. Updated May 01, 2015 [about 17 screens]. Available from www.dynamed .com/login.aspx?direct=true&site=DynaMed& id=114980. Accessed Jan 18, 2016. Registration and login required.

3. Rabinovici G, Wang P, Levin J, et al. First symptom in sporadic Creutzfeldt-Jakob disease. *Neurology*. 2006;66(2):286–7.

Critical Illness Myopathy

Epidemiology and Demographics: Critical illness myopathy (CIM) is a common condition in critically ill patients, affecting more than 25% of patients in the intensive care unit (ICU) who have been mechanically ventilated for at least 7 days. No clear sex predominance is known. No clear age link is known. There is no geographic or ethnic predilection.

Disorder Description: CIM is thought to be a toxic effect myopathy that affects ICU patients. It results in diffuse weakening from muscle degeneration, but is reversible. The etiology of CIM is unclear; it typically occurs in patients with steroid and neuromuscular junction (NMJ) blockade, and at this time, is thought to result from toxicity due to those agents. High-dose intravenous corticosteroid administration is a well-known risk factor, especially with NMJ blocking agent administration, which is common in status asthmaticus patients (who are typically intubated and ventilated in the ICU). Longer NMJ blockade (over 24–48 hours), as well as higher dose/longer course steroids, increase the likelihood of CIM. Major systemic inflammatory responses accompanying critical injuries/illnesses may also play a part.

With respect to diagnostic testing, elevated serum creatine kinase level is typically present early in the course, but normalizing later. Electrodiagnostic studies are critical to diagnosis. In short, sensory and NMJ studies will be normal, but motor unit studies will be abnormal. Nerve conduction studies will show low compound muscle action potential (CMAP) amplitudes, but without any signs of demyelination (conduction velocities and distal latencies will be normal, though some patients can have CMAPs of long duration). Similarly, sensory studies should be normal (excluding comorbid issues, or a critical illness polyneuropathy). Needle electromyography will show spontaneous short-duration, low-amplitude muscle unit action potentials, with some evidence of denervation, but normal recruitment despite the clinical weakness. Repetitive stimulation will be normal. Muscle biopsy can be done, but is rarely used; histopathology shows largely myopathy and myosin loss.

Sensation/sensory distribution is spared

Symptoms

Localization site	Comment
Cranial nerves	Bifacial weakness (uncommon), extraocular weakness (unusual/rare)
Spinal cord	Areflexia (diffuse, typically distal)
Muscle	Generalized weakness, often flaccid, typically distal

Secondary Complications: Secondary complications of CIM are largely related to the difficulties and complications in treating comorbid or underlying issues. For instance, it will delay extubation due to respiratory weakness. It can be associated with critical illness polyneuropathy.

Treatment Complications: Treatment largely involves reducing or discontinuing steroids, and avoiding NMJ blockade. CIM is usually reversible over weeks to months. Glycemic control as treatment has been controversial and is not standard of care.

Complications are largely due to delayed treatment of underlying issue (i.e., status asthmaticus, sepsis, etc.) or ventilator-associated complications from delayed extubation. In effect, CIM leads to prolonged ICU stays and increased length of hospital stay in general.

Bibliography

Bolton CF. Neuromuscular manifestations of critical illness. *Muscle Nerve.* 2005;32:140.

Latronico N, Shehu I, Seghelini E. Neuromuscular sequelae of critical illness. *Curr Opin Crit Care.* 2005;11:381.

Preston DC, Shapiro BE. *Electromyography and neuromuscular disorders: clinical-electrophysiologic correlations.* 3rd ed. New York: Saunders; 2013. pp. 556–61.

Critical Illness Neuropathy/Polyneuropathy (CIP)

Epidemiology and Demographics: Critical illness neuropathy/polyneuropathy (CIP) affects up to 45% of critically ill patients admitted to intensive care units (ICUs). About 70% of patients with sepsis or systemic inflammatory response syndrome (SIRS) develop CIP. Seen in up to 58% of those receiving mechanical ventilation for at least 4–7 days and 77% of those with ICU stays more than 7 days. More common in females, though precise gender predisposition is unknown.

Disorder Description: Complication of severe illness involving sensorimotor axons, frequently affecting skeletal muscle (critical illness myopathy). The causes of axonal degeneration, atrophy, and necrosis of myofibers are not fully understood, but are believed to involve microcirculatory abnormalities, metabolic derangements, reversible channelopathy, and bioenergetic dysfunction. Major risk factors include severity of illness, duration of organ dysfunction, duration of ICU stay, acute respiratory distress syndrome, sepsis, SIRS, and hyperglycemia. Corticosteroid and neuromuscular blocking agents may contribute as well. As both respiratory and limb muscles can be affected, the condition results in prolonged weaning from mechanical ventilation and physical rehabilitation.

Symptoms

Localization site	Comment
Cerebral hemispheres	Early response to critical illness: diffuse encephalopathy
Cranial nerves	Rarely: ophthalmoplegia, facial weakness
Peripheral neuropathy	Mostly symmetric involvement of lower extremities sensorimotor axons, phrenic nerve involvement, distal loss of sensitivity to pain, temperature, vibration
Muscle	Frequently associated with critical illness myopathy. Mostly symmetric lower extremity weakness/paralysis Diaphragmatic, intercostal, and other accessory respiratory weakness/paralysis

Secondary Complications: Extended ICU stay, prolonged mechanical ventilation, immobility leading to increased rates of delirium, infection, thromboembolism, and increased mortality.

Treatment Complications: Treatment is primarily preventive and includes early and aggressive treatment of sepsis, minimizing duration and dosages of corticosteroids and neuromuscular blocking agents, glycemic control, and rehabilitation programs and careful positioning. Complications include potential ventilation dependency and antibiotic-resistant infections.

Bibliography

Hermans G, De Jonghe B, Bruyninckx F, Van den Berghe G. Clinical review: Critical illness polyneuropathy and myopathy. *Crit Care.* 2008;12(6):238.

Zhou C, Wu L, Ni F, et al. Critical illness polyneuropathy and myopathy. a systematic review. *Neural Regen Res.* 2014;9:101–10.

Crohn's Disease

Epidemiology and Demographics: The annual incidence of Crohn's disease is about 20/100,000 in North America. The highest incidence occurs in the second to fourth decade of life, and the risk is equal in men and women.

Disorder Description: Crohn's disease is a chronic relapsing-remitting condition that can affect any part of the gastrointestinal tract, but most commonly colon and distal ileum. The cardinal features of Crohn's disease include chronic diarrhea, abdominal pain, presence of blood or mucus in stool, and weight loss. Extraintestinal involvement is common. The exact etiology is unknown and a complex interaction between genetic (e.g., NOD2/CARD15 gene) and environmental factors (diet, antibiotics, gut microbiome) influence the clinical presentation and severity.

Symptoms

Localization site	Comment
Cerebral hemispheres	Thromboembolic events causing transient ischemic attacks or strokes. Venous sinus thrombosis. There is increased incidence of demyelinating disorders such as MS
Mental status and psychiatric aspects/complications	Depression, anxiety, fatigue, and restless leg syndrome
Cranial nerves	Sensorineural hearing loss
	Melkersson–Rosenthal syndrome (recurrent facial nerve palsy)
	Optic neuritis
	Isolated microvascular 6th nerve palsy
Cauda equina	Spinal epidural abscess presenting as cauda equina syndrome
Peripheral neuropathy	Small fiber sensory neuropathy
	Axonal sensorimotor polyneuropathy
	Demyelinating neuropathies
Neuromuscular junction	Myasthenia gravis
Muscle	Inflammatory myopathy

Secondary Complications: Nutritional deficiencies such as vitamins B12 and B1 or copper deficiencies can lead to neuropathy, myelopathy, or encephalopathy. Hypercoagulable state can lead to thromboembolic or venous strokes even when the disease is not clinically active. Rapid weight loss can put patients at risk of entrapment mononeuropathies.

Treatment Complications: Biologic treatment used in treating Crohn's disease such as natalizumab can increase the risk of progressive multifocal leukoencephalopathy caused by John Cunningham virus. Posterior reversible encephalopathy syndrome has been reported with infliximab infusion. A case of central nervous system (CNS) vasculitis has been reported with adalimumab. There are reports of cases with multiple sclerosis associated with biologic treatment for Crohn's disease. Metronidazole can cause peripheral neuropathy. Tumor necrosis factor alpha antagonists have been reported to be associated with demyelinating neuropathies. Immunosuppressive therapy is associated with increased risk of CNS infections and malignancies. Cyclosporine can cause optic neuropathy, ophthalmoplegia, and nystagmus.

Bibliography

Gondim FA, Brannagan TH III, Sander HW, Chin RL, Latov N. Peripheral neuropathy in patients with inflammatory bowel disease. *Brain.* 2005;128:867–79.

Gupta G, Gelfand JM, Lewis JD. Increased risk for demyelinating diseases in patients with inflammatory bowel disease. *Gastroenterology* 2005;129:819–26.

Leibowitz G, Eliakim R, Amir G, Rachmilewitz D. Dermatomyositis associated with Crohn's disease. *J Clin Gastroenterol*. 1994;18:48–52.

Lossos A, River Y, Eliakim A, Steiner I. Neurologic aspects of inflammatory bowel disease. *Neurology*. 1995;45:416–21.

Molodecky NA, Soon IS, Rabi DM, et al. Increasing incidence and prevalence of the inflammatory bowel diseases with time, based on systematic review. *Gastroenterology*. 2012;142:46–54.

Singh S, Kumar N, Loftus EV, Kane SV. Neurologic complications in patients with inflammatory bowel disease: increasing relevance in the era of biologics. *Inflamm Bowel Dis*. 2013; 19:864–72.

Crutch Use Neuropathy

Epidemiology and Demographics: May affect any individual using axillary crutches though more common when poorly fitted and in children and patients who are either not properly trained or are mentally or physically incapable of using crutches properly. Precise incidence is unknown.

Disorder Description: Crutch use neuropathy is a well known, albeit an extremely rare, complication of axillary crutch use. Pathology is believed to result from compression that produces differential pressure along the nerve trunk of the brachial plexus, resulting in invagination of the nodes of Ranvier, as opposed to nerve ischemia. Incorrect use of axillary crutches leads to a seven-fold increase in force on the axilla. In addition to neurologic symptoms, the patient may exhibit signs of chronic irritation near the axilla, such as hyperpigmentation and skin hypertrophy. Most patients exhibit full recovery within 2–3 months, with length of recovery time postulated to relate to duration of nerve compression.

Physical therapy is primarily preventive by ensuring correct length and use of crutches. Treatment is limited to cessation of axillary crutch use and physical therapy.

Localization site	Comment
Plexus	Posterior cord of brachial plexus
Peripheral neuropathy	Most common: • Radial nerve – weakness of triceps and forearm/wrist/finger extensors. Paresthesias in radial distribution may be observed • Axillary nerve – weakness of shoulder abduction. Paresthesias near shoulder Less common: • Median nerve • Ulnar nerve • Suprascapular nerve • Long thoracic nerve

Secondary Complications: Rarely, improper crutch use can result in aneurysm of the axillary artery and embolism due to repetitive trauma.

Treatment Complications: Good prognosis and therefore no treatment complications.

Bibliography

Chang IT, Depold Holder A. Bilateral radial nerve compression (crutch palsy): a case report. *J Neurol Neurophysiol*. 2012;3:3.

Raikin S, Froimson MI. Bilateral brachial plexus compressive neuropathy (crutch palsy). *J Orthop Trauma*. 1997;11:136–8.

Cryoglobulinemia

Epidemiology and Demographics: Cryoglobulinemia typically occurs in the context of three disease groups: monoclonal gammopathy, chronic viral infections such as hepatitis C virus (HCV) or HIV, and chronic inflammatory disorders such as Sjögren syndrome. Within these populations, laboratory evidence of cryoglobulins is present in 10–20% or more. Clinically symptomatic cryoglobulin disease is present in far fewer, particularly in those with low cryocrits.

Disorder Description: Cryoglobulins are proteins that precipitate from serum and plasma at temperatures less than 37°C. There are three types of cryoglobulins: (a) Type I associated with paraproteinemia consists of monoclonal immunoglobulin such as from multiple myeloma; (b) Type II associated with HCV consists of polyclonal immunoglobulin plus a monoclonal antibody with rheumatoid factor activity (typically IgM reacting to IgG); and (c) Type III associated with chronic inflammatory autoimmune disorders consists of polyclonal immunoglobulin without a monoclonal component. Type I cryoglobulins cause disease by hyperviscosity and thrombosis while Types II and III cause inflammatory disease such as vasculitis.

Symptoms

Localization site	Comment
Cerebral hemispheres	Diffuse effects with hyperviscosity from Type I cryoglobulinemia. Brain usually not affected by Type II or III cryoglobulinemia
Mental status and psychiatric aspects/complications	Headache and confusion are common symptoms of hyperviscosity syndrome
Cranial nerves	Blurry vision and visual loss from hyperviscosity with Type I cryoglobulinemia
Mononeuropathy or mononeuropathy multiplex	Type II or III cyroglobulinemia can cause vasculitic neuropathy with multiple mononeuropathies
Peripheral neuropathy	Type II or III can also present as painful or burning paresthesia with gradual motor involvement

Secondary Complications: Type I cryoglobulins and associated hyperviscosity can cause intratubular cryoprecipitation and rapidly progressive renal failure. Type II or III cryoglobulinemia often has accompanying fever, arthralgia, and palpable purpura (54–82% of cases).

Treatment Complications: Clinically significant cryoglobulinemia is treated with immunosuppression, which has infectious complications especially in patients who have altered baseline immunity. Plasma exchange carries risk of thrombosis.

Bibliography

Ramos-Casals M, Stone JH, Cid MC, Bosch X. The cryoglobulinaemias. *Lancet*. 2012;379:348–60.

Tedeschi A, Baratè C, Minola E, Morra E. Cryoglobulinemia. *Blood Rev* 2007; 21: 183–200.

Cryptococcal Meningitis (*Cryptococcus neoformans*)

Epidemiology and Demographics: Worldwide distribution. Prevalence of 10% in the United States and 30% in sub-Saharan Africa.[1]

Disorder Description: Cryptococcal meningitis is caused by the encapsulated yeast organism *Cryptococcus neoformans* and is considered to be the most common systemic fungal infection in immunocompromised patients. It is usually found in contaminated soil, avian excrement, or certain tree bark. Infection usually occurs by inhalation, which may cause a respiratory infection or dissemination. Patients are typically immunocompromised or have had an environmental exposure.[1,2]

It has become increasingly prevalent in immunocompromised patients. Risk factors include HIV, immunosuppression from solid organ transplants, sarcoidosis, corticosteroid use, and hepatorenal failure.[2]

Symptoms

Localization site	Comment
Cerebral hemispheres	Gait disturbances due to dopaminergic involvement Cryptococcomas/granulomas Non-obstructive hydrocephalus Meningitis Vision changes due to increased intracranial pressure (ICP)
Mental status and psychiatric aspects/complications	Cognitive decline/dementia Depression
Vestibular system (and non-specific dizziness)	Pseudo-Ménière disease
Base of skull	Basilar meningitis
Cranial nerves	Cranial neuropathies

Secondary Complications: Complications include hydrocephalus, increased ICP, seizures, or blindness.

Treatment Complications: Immune reconstitution inflammatory syndrome may occur more commonly in HIV patients. Also, during initial therapy, increased intracranial pressures are commonly seen and may require serial lumbar punctures.[2]

References

1. Zunt J, Baldwin K. Chronic and subacute meningitis. *Continuum (Minneap Minn)*. 2012;18:1290–318.
2. Panackal A, Williamson P. Fungal infections of the central nervous system. *Continuum (Minneap Minn)*. 2015;21:1662–78.

Cuban Epidemic Neuropathy

Epidemiology and Demographics: Affected more than 50,000 of the Cuban population predominantly in the early 1990s. Most were adults aged 45–64 years, 75% of whom drank alcohol and smoked cigarettes regularly. The incidence from 1992 to 1994 was 566.7/100,000 in women and 368.5/100,000 in men.

Disorder Description: The epidemic is believed to be mainly the result of nutritional deficiencies. Risk factors included low body mass index, low percentage of body fat, less than 50% of recommended daily intake of protein, pyridoxine, thiamine, vitamin E and vitamin A, and consumption of alcohol and tobacco. Other suspected etiologic factors included chronic exposure to methanol and cyanide.

Symptoms

Localization site	Comment
Mental status and psychiatric aspects/complications	Irritability Encephalopathy and decreased alertness
Cranial nerves	Optic neuropathy – decrease in visual acuity and color vision Sensorineural deafness, dysphagia, dysphonia
Spinal cord	Dorsolateral myeloneuropathy – loss of proprioception, vibration, and light touch sensation
Peripheral neuropathy	Peripheral neuropathy – predominantly pain (sharp and burning), hypoesthesia, and weakness of the extremities
Syndromes with combined spinal cord and peripheral nerve lesions	Urinary urgency, nocturia, frequency, incontinence, constipation, sexual impotence

Secondary Complications: May lead to falls and injury secondary to decreased visual acuity, sensory ataxia, and neuropathy.

Treatment Complications: The Cuban government distributed vitamins A, B, and E in May 1993 at the peak of the epidemic. By July 1993, the incidence had sharply declined. There are no known complications of treatment.

Bibliography

Dobbs M. *Clinical neurotoxicology*. Philadelphia: Elsevier; 2009.

Ordúñez-García PO, Nieto FJ, Espinosa-Brito AD, Caballero B. Cuban epidemic neuropathy, 1991 to 1994: history repeats itself a century after the "amblyopia of the blockade." *Am J Public Health*. 1996;86:738–43.

Cushing Disease (Cushing's Syndrome)

Epidemiology and Demographics: Estimated 10–15 cases per million people per year. Usually affects younger adults aged 20–50 years, and is more common in women.

Disorder Description: Excess glucocorticoid, usually from exogenous administration rather than endogenous causes due to pituitary or ectopic corticotropin secretion. Systemic manifestations are broad, affecting adipose distribution (central obesity), bone resorption and osteoporosis, weakened immune system, skin and connective tissue catabolism, and neuropsychologic function. Primary neurologic dysfunctions are limited.

Symptoms

Localization site	Comment
Cerebral hemispheres	Processing speed, attention, working memory impairment
Mental status and psychiatric aspects/complications	Mood instability, agitation, anxiety, depression, mania, paranoia, insomnia
Cranial nerves	Glaucoma
Pituitary gland	Adrenocorticotropic hormone (ACTH)-related Cushings (more common than ectopic ACTH)
Muscle	Myopathy, weakness

Secondary Complications: Obesity, hypertension, and glucose intolerance can increase the risk of stroke.

Treatment Complications: Adrenal crisis or Addisonian condition may cause seizures or impaired consciousness.

Bibliography

Haskett R. Diagnostic categorization of psychiatric disturbance in Cushing's syndrome. *Am J Psychiatry*. 1985;142(8):911.

Loosen P, Chambliss B, DeBold C, Shelton R, Orth D. Psychiatric phenomenology in Cushing's disease. *Pharmacopsychiatry*. 1992;25(4):192.

Newell-Price J, Bertagna X, Grossman A, Nieman L. Cushing's syndrome. *Lancet*. 2006;367(9522):1605–17.

Nieman L, Biller B, Findling J, et al. The diagnosis of Cushing's syndrome: an Endocrine Society Clinical Practice Guidline. *J Clin Endocrinol Metab*. 2008;93(5):1526–40.

Cyclic Vomiting Syndrome (CVS, Abdominal Migraine)

Epidemiology and Demographics: The true prevalence of cyclic vomiting syndrome (CVS) is unknown; estimates range from 4 to 2000/100,000 children, with an incidence of approximately 3/100,000 children per year. Median age at onset is 5 years. In children of elementary school age it more often affects girls than boys. A family history of migraine is present in 67–82% of cases.

Disorder Description: Idiopathic disorder characterized by stereotypical recurrent, explosive bouts of severe nausea and bilious emesis punctuated by symptom-free periods. It is defined by symptom-based criteria and the absence of positive laboratory, radiographic, and endoscopic testing. Episodes most often during the night or in the early morning, a high peak frequency of vomiting every 10 to 15 minutes, associated with nausea, retching, abdominal pain, lethargy, anorexia and pallor, and then rapid complete resolution. Attacks can last from an hour to 10 days. Common triggering factors include stress, emotional excitement, fasting, certain foods or alcohol, and infections. The natural history of CVS is variable: some patients will ultimately cease to have emetic episodes, some switch from having vomiting episodes to having migraine headaches, whereas some continue to have vomiting episodes. The median age at resolution of symptoms is 10 years.

Early reports also linked CVS to epilepsy, as in rare cases, vomiting may be the sole manifestation of recurrent epileptic seizures. Progressive or focal neurologic findings as well as new-onset ataxia, abnormal eye movements, papilledema, motor asymmetry, gait abnormality, developmental regression or stagnation, or recent personality changes are not typical of CVS and should alert the clinician to evaluate for increased intracranial pressure or a metabolic disorder.

Potential neuroendocrine mediators such as corticotropin-releasing factor and related downstream effector pathways – cortisol production and prostaglandin E2 – as well as autonomic alterations may initiate or sustain vomiting.

The ROME III Criteria for CVS diagnosis (must include all of the following):

IV. Stereotypical episodes of vomiting regarding onset (acute) and duration (less than 1 week).
V. Three or more discrete episodes in the prior year.
VI. Absence of nausea and vomiting between episodes.

- Supportive criterion: History or family history of migraine headaches.

North American Society for Pediatric Gastroenterology, Hepatology, and Nutrition diagnostic criteria (must include all of the following):

- At least five attacks in any interval, or a minimum of three attacks during a 6-month period.
- Episodic attacks of intense nausea and vomiting lasting from 1 hour to 10 days and occurring at least 1 week apart.
- Stereotypical pattern and symptoms in the individual patient.
- Vomiting during attacks occurs at least four times/hour for at least 1 hour.
- Return to baseline health between episodes.
- Not attributed to another disorder.

Symptoms

Localization site	Comment
Cerebral hemispheres	Migraines, seizures. Functional 15 O-PET brain imaging in adults with CVS suggest alterations in brain areas that deal with heightened awareness and anxiety (the cingulate cortices) as well as those that deal with pain and pleasure (the inferior frontal cortex)
Mental status and psychiatric aspects/complications	Anxiety and depression are frequent

Secondary Complications: Migraine headaches, gastro-oesophageal reflux disease, irritable bowel syndrome, gallbladder disease, and insulin-dependent diabetes mellitus.

Treatment Complications: Antihistamines associated with increased appetite, weight gain, and sedation. Beta blockers associated with lethargy, reduced exercise intolerance. Amitriptyline associated with constipation, sedation, arrhythmia, behavioral changes.

Bibliography

Abell TL, et al. Cyclic vomiting syndrome in adults. *Neurogastroenterol Motil.* 2008;20(4):269–84.

Abu-Arafeh I, Russell G. Cyclical vomiting syndrome in children: a population-based study. *J Pediatr Gastroenterol Nutr.* 1995;21(4):454–8.

Li BU, et al. North American Society for Pediatric Gastroenterology, Hepatology, and Nutrition consensus statement on the diagnosis and management of cyclic vomiting syndrome. *J Pediatr Gastroenterol Nutr.* 2008;47(3): 379–93.

Cyclothymic Disorder

Epidemiology and Demographics: Lifetime prevalence is approximately 0.4–1%; prevalence in mood disorder clinics may range from 3 to 5%. Equally common in males and females in the general population; however, females may be more likely to present for treatment in clinical settings. May be more common in first-degree relatives of individuals with bipolar I disorder.

Disorder Description: As per the DSM-5, cyclothymic disorder is defined as a chronic, fluctuating mood disorder of at least 2 years' duration involving numerous hypomanic and depressive periods that are distinct from each other. The hypomanic and depressive symptoms must not meet full criteria for a hypomanic/manic or major depressive episode, respectively. Furthermore, symptoms must be present for at least half of the 2-year duration of illness, cause clinically significant distress or impaired functioning, and are not better attributable to another psychiatric disorder, substance, medication, or another medical condition.

Symptoms

Localization site	Comment
Mental status and psychiatric aspects/ complications	Symptoms of hypomania may include elevated, expansive, or irritable mood, mood lability, increased energy, increased goal-directed activity, inflated self-esteem or grandiosity, decreased need for sleep, rapid and/or pressured speech, racing thoughts (flight of ideas), distractibility, psychomotor agitation, impulsivity, poor judgment and insight, increased involvement in activities that have a high potential for painful consequences (shopping sprees, sexual indiscretions), antisocial behavior, suicidality
	Symptoms of depression may include depressed mood, anhedonia, changes in appetite and/or weight, insomnia or hypersomnia, psychomotor agitation or retardation, fatigue, poor concentration, indecisiveness, guilt, worthlessness, hopelessness, suicidality

Secondary Complications: Alcohol/substance abuse, sleep disorders. Approximately 15–50% risk that an individual with cyclothymic disorder will go on to develop bipolar I or II disorder.

Treatment Complications: Similar complications may occur with the treatment of cyclothymic disorder as with the treatment of other bipolar spectrum disorders. Most notably, special consideration should be given to the following potential treatment complications: side effects of lithium including lithium toxicity as well as cognitive, cardiac, kidney, and thyroid abnormalities; increased risk of suicide with anticonvulsants; extrapyramidal symptoms and metabolic syndrome with antipsychotics; sedation and dependence/tolerance with benzodiazepines; and the potential teratogenic risks associated with many of these agents. Please see treatment complications for Bipolar I Disorder and Bipolar II Disorder for further discussion.

Bibliography

American Psychiatric Association. *Diagnostic and statistical manual of mental disorders: DSM-5.* 5th ed. Washington, DC: American Psychiatric Association; 2013.

Regeer EJ, ten Have M, Rosso ML, et al. Prevalence of bipolar disorder in the general population: a reappraisal study of the Netherlands Mental Health Survey and Incidence Study. *Acta Psychiatr Scand.* 2004;110(5):374–82.

Cysticercosis

Epidemiology and Demographics: Cysticercosis infection occurs worldwide and affects both males and females, with peak incidence among middle-aged adults. Neurocysticercosis tends to be more severe in women.[1]

Disorder Description: Cysticercosis is a tissue infection caused by the pork tapeworm *Taenia solium* and is the most common helminthic infection of the central nervous system (CNS). Transmission occurs by ingesting undercooked pork, infected water, food (mainly uncooked vegetables), soil, or water. Spread of tapeworm eggs may also be fecal–oral, which may be a large source of human–human transmission.[1–3]

After ingestion, eggs develop into larvae and penetrate the intestinal wall and disseminate via blood. Areas affected may include skin, eye, central nervous system, and muscle.[2] Once in the CNS (called neurocysticercosis), it may degenerate and cause an inflammatory response and lead to seizures or other focal deficits.[1] Seventy-five percent of these patients may also develop muscle involvement.[2]

Neurocysticercosis is endemic in Latin America, sub-Saharan Africa, the Indian subcontinent, Indonesia, Vietnam, Korea, and China. Cases reported in other countries are mainly due to immigration from endemic countries rather than local transmission.[1,3]

Symptoms

Localization site	Comment
Cerebral hemispheres	Encephalitis (occurs commonly in children and young women)
	Seizures
	Hydrocephalus
	Intracranial cysts; these may calcify
	Strokes
	Focal neurologic deficits

Localization site	Comment
Mental status and psychiatric aspects/complications	Cognitive decline[3]
Cranial nerves	Cranial nerve palsies, mainly ophthalmoplegia
Spinal cord	Myelopathy
Specific spinal roots	Radiculopathy
Muscle[2]	Myopathy/myositis
	Myalgias
	Intramuscular lesions
	Pseudomuscular pseudo hypertrophy (massive parasite burden may lead to symmetric enlargement and weakness of skeletal muscle)

Secondary Complications: Focal deficits, blindness, or epilepsy may result.

Treatment Complications: Cysticidal drugs should be avoided in cysticercotic encephalitis, as these drugs may worsen the inflammatory response within the brain parenchyma.[1] Steroids may also cause psychosis.

References

1. Del Brutto OH. Neurocysticercosis. *Continuum (Minneap Minn).* 2012;18:1392–416.
2. El-Beshbishi S, Ahmed N, Mostafa S, El-Ganainy G. Parasitic infections and myositis. *Parasitol Res.* 2011;110(1):1–18.
3. Garcia H, Nash T, Del Brutto O. Clinical symptoms, diagnosis, and treatment of neurocysticercosis. *Lancet Neurol.* 2014;13(12):1202–15.

Cytomegalovirus (CMV)

Epidemiology and Demographics: Cytomegalovirus (CMV) affects about 45–100% of the world's population. Increased seropositivity seen in the elderly, nonwhite race/ethnicity, females, and in low socioeconomic groups. Higher prevalence also seen in male homosexuals and residents of developing countries.[1]

Disorder Description: CMV is a double-stranded DNA virus, which is a member of the Herpesviridae family. Acute infection in immunocompetent people is usually asymptomatic, but may also be associated with a mild febrile illness. It then remains latent unless significant immunocompromise occurs, when chances of reactivation are higher.[1]

CMV is spread by close contact with a person who has the virus in his or her saliva, urine, or other body fluids. Thus, blood transfusions, organ or stem cell transplants, working in a childcare center, or sexual intercourse may all be sources of CMV acquisition and transfer. In addition, it may be transmitted from a pregnant woman to her fetus during pregnancy or delivery.[1]

It is a big concern in patients with HIV and other opportunistic diseases.[2,3]

Congenital CMV is the leading infectious cause of hearing loss and intellectual disabilities in developing countries.

Symptoms[2,3]

Localization site	Comment
Cerebral hemispheres	Encephalitis
	Meningitis
	Ventriculitis
	Cerebral venous thrombosis
Mental status and psychiatric aspects/complications	Alzheimer's dementia (increased risk)
	Subacute dementia in HIV patients
Spinal cord	Transverse myelitis
Cauda equina	Cauda equina syndrome
Specific spinal roots	Polyradiculitis
Mononeuropathy or mononeuropathy multiplex	Mononeuropathy multiplex
Peripheral neuropathy	Peripheral neuropathy
Syndromes with combined spinal cord and peripheral nerve lesions	Polyradiculomyelitis

Secondary Complications: CMV infection may precede Guillain–Barré syndrome.[1]

Treatment Complications: Ganciclovir may cause neuropathy.[1] Valganciclovir may cause renal failure, which may suppress mental status. Both these medications may cause blood dyscrasias, which can cause intracranial hemorrhage.

References

1. DynaMed Plus [Internet]. Record No. 906245, Cytomegalovirus (CMV) infection in immunocompetent patients. Ipswich, MA: EBSCO Information Services. 1995. Updated Mar 9, 2015 [about 9 screens]. Available from www.dynamed.com/login .aspx?direct=true&site=DynaMed&id=906245. Accessed Jan 20, 2016. Registration and login required.
2. Mamidi A, DeSimone J, Pomerantz R. Central nervous system infections in individuals with HIV-1 infection. *J Neurovirol.* 2002;8(3):158–67.
3. Anders H, Goebel F. Neurological manifestations of cytomegalovirus infection in the acquired immunodeficiency syndrome. *Int J STD AIDS.* 1999;10(3):151–61.

Dandy–Walker Syndrome

Epidemiology and Demographics: Seen in 1 in 30,000 live births; it is a rare condition.

Disorder Description: Congenital brain malformation involving the cerebellum and the fourth ventricle. It is characterized by agenesis or hypoplasia of the cerebellar vermis, cystic dilatation of the fourth ventricle, and enlargement of the posterior fossa. Workup includes MRI, CAT scans, and ultrasound.

Symptoms

Localization site	Comment
Non-CNS-related symptoms	Orofacial deformities including hypertelorism and cleft palate. Polydactyly and syndactyly on the left side, cardiac anomalies, polycystic kidneys, cataracts, retinal degeneration Vascular facial hemangioma
Neurologic symptoms, cerebral hemispheres	Slow motor development, hydrocephalus, increased cerebral spinal fluid pressure with irritability, vomiting
Cerebellum	Unsteadiness and lack of muscle coordination, nystagmus, increased skull circumference, bulging at the base of the skull

Treatment Complications: Hydrocephalus should be treated with ventriculoperitoneal shunt, physical therapy, occupational therapy, speech therapy, and specialized education. Surgical complications, including incurring new neurologic deficits, could occur.

Bibliography

Osenbach RK, Menezes AH. Diagnoses and management of the Dandy Walker Malformation: 30 years of experience. *Pediatr Neurosurg.* 1992;18(4):179–89.

Decompression Sickness (DCS)

Epidemiology and Demographics: Due to variability in reporting and collection of information, mainstream medical journal publication of diving-related injury statistics is inconsistent. However, it appears that men are at greater risk than women, and there is no age or geographic predominance.

Disorder Description: Decompression sickness (DCS) encompasses all clinical manifestations induced by a rapid decrease of environmental pressure, sufficient to cause the formation of inert gas bubbles previously loaded within tissues or blood as a soluble phase. Based on clinical symptoms, DCS can be classified as type I or type II. Type I DCS generally presents with joint pain, skin rash, skin marbling, or localized edema. Scuba divers with type I DCS have more serious symptoms, usually characterized by myelopathy. The symptoms most often appear 10 to 30 minutes after surfacing, at times beginning with a feeling of malaise and gradually progressing to paresthesias or paralysis. Spinal cord injury occurs in 20 to 50% of type II DCS. Brain and spinal cord injury result from nitrogen bubbles causing either arterial occlusion, venous infarction, or in situ nitrogen toxicity. The treatment is supportive with hyperbaric oxygen therapy.

Rapid surfacing during deep diving is a major risk factor; this is particularly a risk for inexperienced divers. Travelling by airplane soon after scuba diving increases the risk of decompression sickness.

Diagnosis is largely clinical and based on history.

Symptoms

Localization site	Comment
Cerebral hemispheres	Encephalopathy, stroke-like symptoms, seizures
Spinal cord	Thoracic cord segments are predominately affected. Symptoms mimic spinal cord trauma. Low back pain may start within a few minutes to hours after the dive and may progress to paresis, paralysis, paresthesia, loss of sphincter control, and girdle pain of the lower trunk. Neurologic deficits after a spinal cord injury can be multifocal. Sensory and motor disturbances can present independently, often resulting in a situation of dissociation

Secondary Complications: Residual weakness, neuropathic pain, and neurogenic bladder are possible.

Treatment Complications: In general, treatment for DCS hinges on reduction of gas embolism and the effects of gas embolism. Primarily, this includes hydration, administration of 100% oxygen (preferably hyperbaric chamber oxygen therapy), and positioning the patient in the left lateral decubitus (Durant's maneuver) and mild Trendelenburg position in an effort to restore forward blood flow.

Some patients can develop complications related to hyperbaric oxygen therapy. Patients can report ear pain or discomfort and, rarely, seizures.

Bibliography

Elliott DH, Moon RE. *Manifestations of the decompression disorders: the physiology and medicine of diving.* 4th ed. London: Saunders; 1993. p. 481.

Kamtchum Tatuene J, Pignel R, Pollak P, et al. Neuroimaging of diving-related decompression illness: current knowledge and perspectives. *AJNR Am J Neuroradiol.* 2014;35:2039–44.

Kei PL, Choong CT, Young T, et al. Decompression sickness: MRI of the spinal cord. *J Neuroimag.* 2007;17:378–80.

Newton HB. Neurologic complications of scuba diving. *Am Fam Physician.* 2001;63:2211–8.

Degenerative Disc Disease

Epidemiology and Demographics: As many as 80% of adults in the United States have experienced at least one episode of low back pain during their lifetime, and 5% experience chronic problems. It is more common with increasing age.

Disorder Description: Degeneration of one or more intravertebral disc of the spine resulting in chronic neck or low back pain. Radiologic findings include disc space narrowing, vacuum disc, endplate sclerosis, and osteophyte formation. Workup includes neuroimaging (x-ray, CT, MRI).

Symptoms

Localization site	Comment
Cervical spine	Neck pain, which may radiate to the head, shoulders, arms, and hands. Tingling of hands and fingers is sometimes noted
Lumbar spine	Low back pain, which may radiate to hips, or there is pain in the buttocks or thighs while walking. Occasional tingling and numbness is noted in the knees and weakness through the knees

Treatment Complications: Treatment includes physical therapy, range of motion exercises, postural training, pain management, and spinal fusion. Loss of weight, particularly in degenerative disc disease involving lumbosacral spine, is strongly recommended.

Bibliography

Modic MT, Ross JS. Lumbar degenerative disc disease. *Radiology.* 2007;245(1):43–61.

Delayed Sleep–Wake Phase Disorder

Epidemiology and Demographics: Exact prevalence is unknown. In the general population, 0.17% of individuals are estimated to have delayed sleep–wake phase disorder (DSWPD); in the adolescent and young adult population, disparate reports of prevalence range from 1 to 16%. Approximately 10% of patients who present to sleep medicine clinics with complaints of insomnia have DSWPD. No known sex predominance. Most commonly occurs in adolescents who have reached puberty.

Disorder Description: Polymorphisms in several circadian clock genes including hPer3 are associated with DSWPD. The timing of exposure to light, changes in work and social schedules, travel across time zones, and stimulants such as caffeine may exacerbate DSWPD. The endogenous circadian period length (tau) is approximately 24.2 hours long and is entrained to the external 24-hour light–dark cycle. Patients with DSWPD have sleep onset that begins much later than the light–dark cycle would dictate. Patients present with complaints of difficulty initiating sleep, trouble awakening in the morning, and excessive daytime sleepiness. This disorder typically first manifests during adolescence. Clock times vary; however, for many individuals sleep is delayed by 2–6 hours compared with individuals who sleep at conventional times, and wake time occurs in the late morning or afternoon. Individuals may wake up earlier than desired during work or school days resulting in truncated sleep time due to delayed bedtime with resulting daytime sleepiness. When sleep is unrestricted, delayed bedtime and wake-up time allows adequate sleep hours with no resulting daytime sleepiness. Bright light exposure (commercially available light boxes or natural sunlight) in the morning, and behavioral and pharmacologic treatments can advance the timing of sleep hours, but there is usually a continued preference for delayed sleep hours.

Diagnosis of DSWPD is made if the patient meets the following criteria: (1) there is a significant delay in the phase of the major sleep episode in relation to the desired or required sleep time and wake-up time as evidenced by the inability to fall asleep and difficulty awakening at a desired or required time; (2) the symptoms are present for ≥3 months; (3) when patients are allowed to choose their own schedule, they will exhibit improved sleep quality and duration, but will maintain a delayed phase of the sleep–wake pattern; (4) sleep log for ≥7 days demonstrates a delay in the timing of the habitual sleep period; and (5) the sleep disturbance is not better explained by another disorder or medication.

Sleep logs and actigraphy are key instruments and 7–14 days of data are needed to ensure that working and non-working days are included. Although not necessary, biologic markers of endogenous circadian timing such as salivary or plasma dim light melatonin onset can provide important information.

Symptoms

Localization site	Comment
The exact mechanism responsible is unknown	The main site of the endogenous circadian rhythm is in the suprachiasmatic nuclei and circadian clocks in peripheral cells. Polymorphisms in the circadian clock genes such as hPer3 are associated with DSWPD
Mental status and psychiatric aspects/ complications	In adolescents may present with school absences, chronic tardiness, and academic failure

Secondary Complications: Social dysfunction and isolation, with increased risk of daytime sleepiness when forced to awaken early.

Treatment Complications: A multimodality approach to treatment of DSWPD is required. This includes evening sunlight avoidance, morning bright light exposure, and low-dose melatonin treatment approximately 5 hours prior to bedtime. Chronotherapy involves progressive delay in the sleep schedule until the desired evening bedtime is reached. The effect of light on circadian rhythms follows a phase-response curve (PRC) whereby light exposure before the nadir core body temperature causes a phase delay, and light after nadir produces a phase advance. In the case of DSWPD, avoidance of evening light exposure helps to avoid an unwanted phase delay, and bright light exposure in the morning after the nadir core body temperature produces a desired phase advance. Exogenous melatonin has phase shifting properties that are about 12 hours out of phase with the PRC of light. Since the shift in the PRC to light (nadir of core body temperature) is delayed in DSWPD and may occur during the later morning hours, early awakenings for work or school with sunlight exposure at that time may contribute to further phase delay.

Bibliography

Bjorvatn B, Pallesen S. A practical approach to circadian rhythm sleep disorders. *Sleep Med Rev.* 2009;13:47–60.

Nesbitt AD, Dijk DJ. Out of synch with society: an update on delayed sleep phase disorder. *Curr Opin Pulm Med.* 2014;20:581–7.

Sack RL, Auckley D, Auger RR, et al. Circadian rhythm sleep disorders: Part II, Advanced sleep phase disorder, delayed sleep phase disorder, free-running disorder, and irregular sleep-wake rhythm. *Sleep.* 2007;30:1484–501.

Sateia M, Berry RB, Bornemann MC, et al. *International classification of sleep disorders.* 3rd ed. Darien, IL: American Academy of Sleep Medicine; 2014.

Schrader H, Bovim G, Sand T. The prevalence of delayed and advanced sleep phase disorders. *J Sleep Res.* 1993;2:51–5.

Delirium

Epidemiology and Demographics: Prevalence is highest among hospitalized older individuals and has been estimated to be 10–30% in older individuals presenting to emergency departments, 15–53% in older individuals post-operatively, 70–87% in intensive care settings, and up to 60% in nursing homes or post-acute care settings. Increased risk associated with older age, underlying neurocognitive disorder, underlying medical illness, functional impairment, immobility, history of falls, low levels of activity, and use of drugs and medications with psychoactive properties (particularly alcohol and anticholinergics).

Disorder Description: The DSM-5 defines delirium as a disturbance in attention and awareness that develops over a short period of time, represents a change from baseline, tends to fluctuate in severity during the day, and is associated with at least one additional disturbance in a cognitive domain such as memory, orientation, language, visuospatial, or perception. The disturbance is not better explained by another neurocognitive disorder. Evidence from the history, physical examination, or laboratory findings demonstrates that the disturbance is a direct physiologic result of another medical condition, substance intoxication or withdrawal, toxin exposure, or multiple etiologies. Based on the level of psychomotor activity, mood lability, and/or agitation, delirium can be classified as hyperactive, hypoactive, or mixed. Delirium may not be diagnosed in the context of coma.

Symptoms

Localization site	Comment
Mental status and psychiatric aspects/ complications	Inattention, disorientation, distractibility, memory deficits, language alterations, and perceptual distortions including misinterpretations, illusions, or hallucinations (most frequently visual). Sleep–wake disturbances including daytime sleepiness, nighttime agitation, and complete reversal. Emotional disturbances including depression, anxiety, fear, apathy, euphoria, irritability, anger, agitation, and lability

Secondary Complications: Prolonged hospitalizations, functional and cognitive decline, increased risk for institutionalization, higher overall mortality.

Treatment Complications: Antipsychotics are frequently used for the treatment of delirium; however, caution must be used given the risk of extrapyramidal symptoms as well as increased risk of mortality associated with antipsychotics when used in patients with dementia. Additionally, providers should be aware of the risk for QTc prolongation associated with haloperidol, which is frequently used for the treatment of delirium. Physical restraints should be used only as a last resort, if at all, as they frequently increase agitation and may cause loss of mobility, pressure ulcers, aspiration, and prolonged delirium. Benzodiazepines should be avoided due to concern for worsening confusion and sedation.

Bibliography

American Psychiatric Association. *Diagnostic and statistical manual of mental disorders: DSM-5.* 5th ed. Washington, DC: American Psychiatric Association; 2013.

Inouye SK. Delirium in older persons. *N Engl J Med.* 2006;354(11):1157–65.

Robinson TN, Raeburn CD, Tran ZV, et al. Postoperative delirium in the elderly: risk factors and outcomes. *Ann Surg.* 2009;249(1):173.

Witlox J, Eurelings LS, de Jonghe JF, et al. Delirium in elderly patients and the risk of postdischarge mortality, institutionalization, and dementia: a meta-analysis. *JAMA.* 2010;304(4):443.

Delusional Disorder

Epidemiology and Demographics: Overall rates are similar between genders, with lifetime prevalence of 0.2%. More common in older age groups. Prevalence estimates are limited by low rates of presentation to health care providers.

Disorder Description: As per the DSM-5, one or more delusions must be present for at least 1 month. Hallucinations can occur, but are uncommon. If present, they are congruent with the content of delusions and do not fulfill criteria for schizophrenia. Odd behaviors are absent. Psychosocial function is often mostly intact; however, areas of work or home life can be impacted. Duration of delusions typically spans longer than any comorbid mood episodes (depressive or manic). Symptoms must not be better accounted for by the effects of a substance or another mental or medical condition. There are several subtypes, including persecutory (most common), erotomanic, grandiose, jealous, somatic, mixed, and unspecified. There are also specifiers for bizarre content and course.

There may be a higher rate of schizophrenia and/ or schizotypal personality disorder in families of individuals with delusional disorder. In determining whether thoughts are delusional, the role of cultural norms must be considered.

Symptoms

Localization site	Comment
Mental status and psychiatric aspects/complications	Delusional content of thought, congruent hallucinations (uncommon)

Secondary Complications: Delusions can be significant enough to affect function, impacting work and relationships. There is small but increased risk of development of schizophrenia.

Treatment Complications: Due to diminished insight, individuals may resist accepting treatment. Treatment is typically a combination of antipsychotic medication and psychotherapy. Antipsychotics carry risk of weight gain, metabolic syndrome, and extrapyramidal side effects.

Bibliography

American Psychiatric Association. *Diagnostic and statistical manual of mental disorders: DSM-5*. 5th ed. Washington, DC: American Psychiatric Association; 2013.

de Portugal E, González N, Haro JM, et al. A descriptive case-register study of delusional disorder. *Eur Psychiatry*. 2008;23(2):125–33.

Kendler KS, McGuire M, Gruenberg AM, et al. The Roscommon Family Study, II: the risk of nonschizophrenic nonaffective psychoses in relatives. *Arch Gen Psychiatry*. 1993;50(8):645–52.

Perälä J, Suvisaari J, Saarni SI, et al. Lifetime prevalence of psychotic and bipolar I disorders in a general population. *Arch Gen Psychiatry*. 2007;64(1):19–28.

Salvatore P, Baldessarini RJ, Tohen M, et al. McLean-Harvard International First-Episode Project: two-year stability of ICD-10 diagnoses in 500 first-episode psychotic disorder patients. *J Clin Psychiatry*. 2011;72(2):183–93.

Dematiaceous Fungi

Epidemiology and Demographics: Usually in the second and third decades of life with male predominance. *Rhinocladiella mackenziei* affects adults, with median age of 62 years.[1]

Disorder Description: Dematiaceous fungi are darkly pigmented fungi that contain melanin in their wall and produce spores that can cause phaeohyphomycosis. Found in soil and decaying vegetation worldwide, but mostly found in tropical and subtropical regions. Emerging as infections in individuals with or without immunocompromised states, particularly in brain abscesses. The most frequently isolated species, *Cladophialophora bantiana*, has historically caused central nervous system (CNS) disease in most of the cases, but other species have also been reported. The presence of melanin may be the reason for their pathogenic potential.[2,3]

CNS infection is thought to occur by hematogenous infections from other primary sites or via direct extension from the sinuses after inhalation of spores. Other infections may occur due to penetrating head trauma or contaminated wounds. Recently, an outbreak occurring in patients receiving steroid epidural injections has been reported as another potential cause of infection.[2,3]

Risk factors for disease include immunosuppression, malignancy, intravenous drug abuse, and agricultural workers; however, many of those affected do not have any underlying immunodeficiency or risk factor.[2]

Symptoms

Localization site	Comment
Cerebral hemispheres	Abscess (most common)
	Meningitis/encephalitis
	Focal neurologic deficit
	Headache
	Seizures
Mental status and psychiatric aspects/complications	Altered mental status
Spinal cord	Epidural abscess, causing cord compression

Secondary Complications: Mortality rate is 100% without treatment and 65–73% despite aggressive treatment.[1]

Treatment Complications: Amphotericin B may cause hepatotoxicity, which may further depress mental status. Surgical resection may cause permanent neurologic deficit if lesion is in eloquent area.

References

1. Jung N, Kim E. Cerebral phaeohyphomycosis: a rare cause of brain abscess. *J Korean Neurosurg Soc*. 2014;56(5):444.
2. Revankar S, Sutton D, Rinaldi M. Primary central nervous system phaeohyphomycosis: a review of 101 cases. *Clin Infect Dis*. 2004;38(2):206–16.

3. Cox M. Central nervous system infections due to dematiaceous fungi (cerebral phaeohyphomycosis). In Kaufman C, ed. *UpToDate*. Waltham, MA. Accessed Jan 29, 2016.

Dengue Virus

Epidemiology and Demographics: The global incidence of dengue virus is estimated to range between 50 million and 200 million population; however; using cartographic approaches, recent estimate is close to almost 400 million population.[1] Transmission is present in every World Health Organization region of the world and more than 125 countries are known to be dengue endemic. Dengue infection has expanded geographically and is expected to increase due to factors such as more dynamic climate change, globalization, travel, trade, socioeconomic factors, settlement, and viral evolution. It is the most prominent acute mosquito-borne viral infection and places a significant socioeconomic and disease burden on many tropical and subtropical regions of the world.

Disorder Description: Dengue virus, a member of the genus *Flavivirus*, is a single-stranded, positive-sense RNA virus with four antigenically distinct serotypes, each of which has been found to cause dengue epidemics and severe disease.[1-3] Infection with one serotype does not provide immunity to the other serotypes, and secondary dengue infections or particularly virulent viral strains are due to factors thought to be associated with increased risk of severity. The main arthropod vector for transmission of the dengue virus serotypes is *Aedes aegypti*, which is well renowned for its efficient vectorial capacity including features such as a high affinity for human blood, high susceptibility to the four dengue virus serotypes, and high adaptivity to urban living.[2] The second but less effective vector is *Aedes albopictus*. Humans are the main cause of spread of dengue between communities.

Clinicians typically describe symptomatic dengue infections as either undifferentiated fever type, dengue fever (DF), or dengue haemorrhagic fever (DHF).[2,3] This classification has enabled clinicians to capture severe cases of dengue that require treatment in intensive-care units. The initial features of dengue infection are characterized by fever accompanied by headache, vomiting, myalgia, joint pain, and occasionally a transient macular rash. Certain warning signs indicative of significant vascular leakage and impending clinical deterioration often precede severe dengue. These warning signs include persistent vomiting, increasingly severe abdominal pain, tender hepatomegaly, a high or increasing hematocrit level coupled with a rapid decrease in the platelet count, serosal effusions, mucosal bleeding, and lethargy or restlessness. The criteria for severe dengue are either severe plasma leakage leading to shock and fluid accumulation with respiratory distress, or severe bleeding, or severe organ involvement including liver, central nervous system involvement, impaired consciousness, and heart or other organ involvement. Laboratory diagnosis of dengue is established directly by detection of viral components in serum or indirectly by serologic means.

The majority of people experience a self-limiting clinical course, which does not progress to the severe forms of dengue, dengue hemorrhagic fever (DHF) or dengue shock syndrome (DSS). There are no effective antiviral agents to treat dengue infection. Current treatment is supportive and careful fluid management. Blood transfusion can be lifesaving for patients with severe bleeding. Vasopressor and inotropic therapies, renal replacement therapy, and further treatment of organ impairment may be necessary for severe dengue. Effective vector control is the mainstay of dengue prevention and control.

Symptoms[3-5]

Localization site	Comment
Cerebral hemisphere	***Acute encephalopathy:*** Diminished consciousness precipitated by prolonged shock, anoxia, cerebral edema, metabolic disturbances, systemic or cerebral hemorrhages, acute liver failure, or renal failure. CSF analyses are normal
	Encephalitis: Diminished consciousness, headache, disorientation, seizures and behavioral symptoms due to central nervous system (CNS) invasion characterized by pleocytosis and high viral load in CSF without blood contamination
	Hemorrhagic stroke is more common than ischemic stroke
	Acute disseminated encephalomyelitis: has been reported in the convalescence stage of dengue virus infection with areas of high signal on T2-weighted and gadolinium enhancement on T1-weighted images

Localization site	Comment
Mental status and psychiatric aspects/ complications	One case of organic mania characterized by increased psychomotor activity, pressure of speech, irritable mood, a delusion of grandiosity has been reported on the 6th day of dengue illness
	Another episode of mania characterized by overactivity, overtalkativeness, argumentativeness, abusiveness, religiosity, sexual preoccupation has been reported after an acute attack of dengue infection[4,5]
Brainstem	Miller–Fisher variant
Spinal cord	*Neuromyelitis optica* with many high-intensity lesions on T2-weighted images of the spine following dengue infection
	Transverse myelitis following dengue infection[3]
Mononeuropathy or mononeuropathy multiplex	Phrenic neuropathy, long thoracic neuropathy, isolated Bell's palsy, abducens nerve palsy, and oculomotor palsy[3]
Peripheral neuropathy	Guillain–Barré syndrome has been described in case reports and case series with acute onset of limb weakness and areflexia following dengue virus infection. CSF shows increased protein concentrations without pleocytosis[3]
Muscle	Transient myalgia, benign acute viral myositis, and rhabdomyolysis[3]

Secondary Complications: Dengue encephalopathy is believed to be a consequence of systemic infection while dengue encephalitis is secondary to neuroinvasion of the viruses into the CNS.

References

1. Murray NEA, Quam MB, Wilder-Smith A. Epidemiology of dengue: past, present and future prospects. *Clin Epidemiol*. 2013;5:299–309.
2. Simmons CP, Farrar JJ, Vinh Chau NV, Wills B. Dengue. *New Engl J Med*. 2012;366:1423–32.
3. Carod-Artal FJ, Wichmann O, Farrar J, Gascon J. Neurological complications of dengue virus infection. *Lancet Neurol*. 2013;12:906–19.
4. Tripathi SM, Mishra N. Late onset mania in dengue fever. *Immunol Infect Dis*. 2014;2:1–3.
5. Srivastawa S, Jhanjee A. Organic mania in dengue. *J Clin Diagn Res*. 2013;7:566–7.

Dental Disease

Epidemiology and Demographics: Oral conditions collectively are highly prevalent worldwide, affecting 3.9 billion people. The global prevalence of untreated caries in permanent teeth is 35% for all ages combined, while severe periodontitis and untreated caries in deciduous teeth affect 11% and 9% of the global population, respectively.[1]

Disorder Description: The two most common dental disorders are dental caries and periodontal disease.

Dental caries,[2] also known as dental decay, is one of the most common chronic diseases and is of medical, social, and economic importance. Bacteria and sugar play an important role in the pathogenesis of dental caries, where microorganisms ferment sugar into acids capable of destroying tooth enamel. There are periods of acid attack and mineral loss interspersed with periods of remineralization. Major tooth destruction only occurs if mineral loss is greater than healing. Removing dental plaque, altering dental plaque to prevent metabolism of dietary sugars to acid, neutralizing the acids within plaque, and removing and reducing dietary sugars are ways to prevent dental caries. The widespread use of fluoride prevents dental caries by:

1. causing the enamel to become more acid resistant;
2. altering the shape of the fissures in tooth crowns during tooth formation;
3. reducing demineralization and enhancing remineralization;
4. preventing metabolism of sugars into acids.

Periodontal disease[3] is a group of inflammatory diseases affecting the periodontium or the tissues that surround and support the teeth. It runs the gamut from localized gingivitis, severe gingival inflammation, periodontitis (separation of gingival tissue from the tooth), to severe periodontitis eventually resulting in tooth loss. The primary etiology of gingivitis is adherence and growth of microbacterial species on the surface of the teeth, forming dental plaque. The dental plaque, if left untreated, accumulates and calcifies to form **calculus**, which then leads to chronic inflammation of the periodontal tissues. The main periodontal pathogens are gram-negative bacteria, which orchestrate inflammatory periodontitis through interactions with oral commensal microbiota and the complement system. The risk factors for periodontal disease include lack of oral hygiene, smoking, genetic susceptibility, poor nutrition, age, and immunodeficiency. Prevention and treatment of periodontitis are aimed at controlling the bacterial biofilm and other risk factors, arresting progressive disease, and restoring lost tooth support. Periodontal surgery may be needed to stop progressive bone loss. There is substantial evidence linking periodontitis to increased inflammation in the body, as indicated by increased C-reactive protein and interleukin-6, and a 1.2- to 6-fold increased risk of cardiovascular disease.

Symptoms

Localization site	Comment
Cerebral hemispheres	Studies suggest a strong association between periodontal disease and ischemic stroke[4]

References

1. Marcenes W, Kassebaum NJ, Bernabe E, et al. Global burden of oral conditions in 1990–2010: a systematic analysis. *J Dent Res*. 2013;92:592–7.
2. Rugg-Gunn A. Dental caries: strategies to control this preventable disease. *Acta Med Acad*. 2013;42:117–30. DOI: 10.5644/ama2006-124.80
3. Khan SA, Kong EF, Meiller TF, Jabra-Rizk MA. Periodontal diseases: bug induced, host promoted. *PLoS Path*. 2015;11(7):e1004952. DOI:10.1371/journal.ppat.1004952.
4. Slowik J, Wnuk MA, Grzech K, et al. Periodontitis affects neurologic deficit in acute stroke. *J Neurol Sci*. 2010;297: 82–4.

Dentatorubral-Pallidoluysian Atrophy (DRPLA)

Epidemiology and Demographics: Dentatorubral-pallidoluysian atrophy (DRPLA) is quite a rare disease in the general population, but it is relatively more common in the Japanese population with the reported prevalence of 2–7 in 1,000,000.

Disorder Description: It is a rare autosomal dominant neurodegenerative disease, characterized by various degrees of cerebellar ataxia, choreoathetosis, myoclonus, epilepsy, dementia, and psychiatric symptoms. DRPLA is caused by an unstable CAG trinucleotide repeat expansion on the short arm of chromosome 12 encoding a polyglutamine tract in the atrophin-1

protein. The clinical features of DRPLA can be quite heterogeneous, and vary depending on the age of onset and degree of genetic anticipation. Before the age of 20, DRPLA resembles progressive myoclonus epilepsy (PME), which is characterized by progressive ataxia, seizures, myclonus, and intellectual deterioration. If the onset is after age 20 years, the patients can present with cerebellar ataxia, choreoathetosis, and dementia, which could be clinically quite similar to Huntington's disease (HD).

Symptoms

Localization site	Comment
Cerebellum	Cerebellar vermis is often affected, and the degree of cerebellar as well as brainstem involvement often correlates with age of onset as well as the size of CAG repeats
Brainstem	Size of CAG repeat and the degree of brainstem involvement are also correlated
Cerebral white matter	Cerebral white matter lesions are often seen in patients with adult onset (>20 years old). Autopsy of white matter lesions has demonstrated diffuse myelin pallor, axonal preservation, and reactive astrogliosis
Basal ganglia	Rigidity

Secondary Complications: The late-onset group of DRPLA could be diagnostically challenging, since it closely resembles HD, and can often lead to misdiagnosis of DRPLA patients. The caudate involvement would favor the diagnosis of HD.

Treatment Complications: There are no specific treatments that are currently approved for DRPLA. Hence, the main therapy is focused on individual symptoms. Antiepileptic drugs are recommended in patients with seizures, and haloperidol can be given to patients with choreoathetosis.

Bibliography

Koide R, Ikeuchi T, Onodera O, et al. Unstable expansion of CAG repeat in hereditary dentarubral-pallidoluysian atrophy (DRPLA). *Nat Genet*. 1994;6:9–13.

Licht DJ, Lynch DR. Juvenile dentatorubral-pallidoluysian atrophy: new clinical features. *Pediatr Neurol*. 2002;26:51–4.

Tsui S. Dentatorubral-pallidoluysian atrophy. *Handb Clin Neurol*. 2012;103:587–94.

Depersonalization/Derealization Disorder

Epidemiology and Demographics: Cross-cultural studies estimate a prevalence of 0.8 to 2.8%. Affects males and females equally. Average age of onset is in the teens, with lower prevalence with increasing age.

Disorder Description: Defined by DSM-5 as recurrent episodes of depersonalization or derealization and as feelings of detachment or unreality with regard to self or environment, respectively. In depersonalization, one feels separate from or like an outside observer of the self or aspects of the self, such as thoughts, emotions, body, or sensations. There may be loss of control of self or aspects of the self. In derealization, there is sense of disconnection or unfamiliarity with the world or the people or objects in it. During these episodes, an individual's ability to distinguish reality is intact. There may be perceptual disturbances and distortions, and often difficulty describing symptoms in words. Onset can be acute or gradual and course can be episodic, relapsing and remitting, or persistent. The condition must cause distress or impairment in several realms of functioning and is not better accounted for by effects of a substance, or another mental or medical condition.

Environmental causes include exposure to trauma, such as that in childhood abuse or growing up with a mentally ill caregiver. Can also be related to stress linked to death of loved one, or conflict in family or at work. Depression and anxiety, among other mental conditions, are common comorbidities. It is also associated with use of various substances. In some, however, there are no overt risk factors. In evaluating for the disorder, the role of cultural norms must be considered.

Symptoms

Localization site	Comment
Cerebral hemispheres	Distinguish symptoms from temporal lobe seizures, vestibular pathology, sleep apnea
Mental status and psychiatric aspects/complications	May have flat affect that may be incongruent with mood
	May report perceptual alterations in setting of intact reality testing

Secondary Complications: Many have impairments in multiple realms of functioning. There may be increased risk of suicide; however, it can be challenging to distinguish the degree to which comorbid psychiatric conditions contribute.

Bibliography

American Psychiatric Association. *Diagnostic and statistical manual of mental disorders: DSM-5.* 5th ed. Washington, DC: American Psychiatric Association; 2013.

Hunter EC, Sierra M, David AS. The epidemiology of depersonalisation and derealisation: a systematic review. *Soc Psychiatry Psychiatr Epidemiol.* 2004;39:9.

Ross CA, Joshi S, Currie R. Dissociative experiences in the general population: a factor analysis. *Hosp Community Psychiatry.* 1991;42:297.

Spiegel D, Loewenstein RJ, Lewis-Fernández R, et al. Dissociative disorders in DSM-5. *Depress Anxiety.* 2011;28(9):824–52. DOI: 10.1002/da.20874

De Quervain's Tenosynovitis

Epidemiology and Demographics: De Quervain's tenosynovitis is the second most common entrapment tendonitis of the hand and wrist, the first being the trigger digit. This can be due to direct trauma to the area of the first dorsal compartment. Common in new mothers and daycare workers who repetitively lift infants.

Disorder Description: Entrapment tendonitis of the tendons contained within the first dorsal compartment at the wrist causing pain during the thumb motion. Tendons of the abductor pollicis longus and the extensor pollicis brevis are tightly secured against the radial styloid by the overlying extensor retinaculum. Any thickening of the tendons from acute or repetitive trauma limits the movement of the tendons through the sheath. Workup includes x-rays to differentiate from osteoarthritis.

Symptoms

Localization site	Comment
Thumb and wrist	Pain resulting from thumb and wrist motion along with tenderness and thickening at the radial styloid

Treatment complications: Splinting of the thumb and wrist is recommended. Injection of corticosteroids into the sheath of the first dorsal compartment reduces tendon thickening and inflammation. Surgical release of the first dorsal compartment can be done if conservative treatment fails.

Complications due to corticosteroid injections such as fat and dermal atrophy can be seen. Superficial radial nerve injury can also be noted. Subluxation of release of tendons may occur.

Bibliography

Weiss AP, Akelman E, Tabatabai M. Treatment of De Quervain's disease. *J Hand Surg Am.* 1994;19(4):595–8.

Dermatomyositis

Epidemiology and Demographics: The annual incidence of dermatomyositis has been estimated to be about 1–2/100,000. There is an increased incidence of dermatomyositis in women compared with men. There is no clear geographic predominance.

Disorder Description: Dermatomyositis presents with muscle weakness that is greater in the proximal muscles than distal muscles and in the legs more than the arms. Dysphagia occurs in a third of patients. It is associated with skin manifestations such as heliotrope rash, Gottron papules, and sun-sensitive rash. Interstitial lung disease occurs in approximately 10–20% of patients. Cancer is present in 6–45% of adult cases.

This disorder is an acquired inflammatory myopathy.

In diagnostic tests, serum CK is elevated in approximately 70% of patients, but serum CK levels do not correlate with the severity of weakness and can be normal. AntiYJo-1 antibodies are present in at least 50% of interstitial lung disease cases. EMG shows signs of myopathy (short duration, low-amplitude, polyphasic motor unit action potentials) associated with spontaneous activity (fibrillation potentials, positive sharp waves). MRI may demonstrate signal abnormalities in affected muscles secondary to inflammation, replacement by fibrotic tissue, or atrophy. Muscle biopsy will show perifascicular atrophy and perivascular inflammatory cells.

Symptoms

Localization site	Comment
Muscles	Proximal muscle weakness more than distal, and more involvement of the leg compared with the arm. Dysphagia occurs in one-third of patients. Presentation could be acute or gradual

Secondary Complications: Cancer is present in 6–45% of the patients. Poor prognosis increases with age, and there is an association with interstitial lung disease and cardiac disease (conduction defects and arrhythmias, pericarditis, myocarditis, and eventual congestive heart failure). Five-year survival rates range from 70 to 93%.

Treatment Complications: Treatment largely hinges on corticosteroid therapy for immune suppression, and it is first-line treatment of choice for dermatomyositis.

Patients can develop complications related to steroid therapy (hyperglycemia, osteoporosis, cataracts, infections, weight gain, steroid-induced myopathy).

Bibliography

Amato AA, Greenberg SA. Inflammatory myopathies. *Continuum (Minneap Minn).* 2013;19(6):1615–33.

Diabetic Autonomic Neuropathy

Epidemiology and Demographics: Reported prevalence varies widely based on cohort studied. In randomly selected cohorts of asymptomatic individuals with diabetes, approximately 20% had cardiovascular autonomic dysfunction.

Disorder Description: Diabetic autonomic neuropathy is a subtype of the peripheral neuropathies of diabetes and can involve the entire autonomic nervous system. It is manifested by dysfunction of one or more organ systems (cardiovascular, gastrointestinal, genitourinary, sudomotor, ocular). Clinical symptoms generally occur in the later stages of diabetes, though subclinical autonomic dysfunction may occur within 1 year of diagnosis in type 2 diabetes and 2 years in type 1 diabetes. Etiologies hypothesized include metabolic insult to nerve fibers, neurovascular insufficiency, autoimmune damage, and neuro-hormonal growth factor deficiency. Early observation suggests that prevention with glycemic control is the most effective intervention. Non-pharmaceutical treatment includes increased hydration, avoiding alcohol, support stockings, an exercise program focused on improving conditioning, and teaching physical maneuvers to avoid orthostatic hypotension. Pharmaceutical therapy includes sodium supplement, fludrocortisone, midodrine, or pyridostigmine.

Symptoms and Secondary Complications

Cardiovascular

- Resting tachycardia
- Exercise intolerance
- Orthostatic hypotension
- Silent myocardial ischemia

Gastrointestinal

- Esophageal dysmotility
- Gastroparesis diabeticorum
- Constipation
- Diarrhea
- Fecal incontinence

Genitourinary

- Neurogenic bladder (diabetic cystopathy)
- Erectile dysfunction
- Retrograde ejaculation
- Female sexual dysfunction (e.g., loss of vaginal lubrication)

Metabolic

- Hypoglycemia unawareness
- Hypoglycemia-associated autonomic failure

Sudomotor

- Anhidrosis
- Heat intolerance
- Gustatory sweating
- Dry skin

Pupillary

- Pupillomotor function impairment (e.g., decreased diameter of dark adapted pupil)
- Argyll–Robertson pupil

Complications of Treatment: Associated symptoms due to complications of treatment of the disorder: supine hypertension, hypokalemia, congestive heart failure, edema, and headache.

Bibliography

Low PA, Singer W. Management of neurogenic orthostatic hypotension: an update. *Lancet Neurol.* 2008;7(5):451–8.

Vinik AI, Maser RE, Mitchell BD, Freeman R. Diabetic autonomic neuropathy. *Diabetes Care.* 2003;26:1553–79.

Diabetic Cranial Mononeuropathy

Epidemiology and Demographics: Seen in an estimated 1% of all diabetic patients. In one large study, 13.7% of oculomotor nerve palsies were associated with diabetes. Oculomotor and abducens palsies are estimated to be equal in prevalence.

Disorder Description: The most common diabetic cranial neuropathies are oculomotor, abducens, and facial nerve palsies. Oculomotor palsy occurs due to centrofascicular ischemia of the nerve in the intracavernous portion with relative sparing of the periphery of the nerve trunk. Transient frontal pain precedes the clinical manifestations in about 50% of cases. Onset of cranial neuropathy is usually abrupt with progression occurring over 1–2 days. Patients recover spontaneously within 2–3 months, though relapses on the contralateral side may occur. Treatment includes glycemic control. A short course of steroids for facial nerve palsy if acute, and use of optical prisms until spontaneous recovery.

Symptoms

Localization site	Comment
Cranial nerves	Oculomotor palsy:
	• Paresis of the superior, inferior, medial recti, and inferior oblique
	• Ptosis from involvement of levator palpebrae
	• Pupil sparing
	Abducens palsy:
	• Paresis of lateral rectus
	Facial palsy:
	• Paresis of ipsilateral forehead and face

Secondary Complications: Complications of oculomotor and abducens palsy include diplopia, difficulty walking, and poor depth perception. Facial nerve palsy may result in corneal dryness, abrasions, or infection.

Treatment Complications: Treatment with steroids usually leads to poorly controlled blood sugar.

Bibliography

Said G. Diabetic neuropathy: a review. *Nat Clin Pract Neurol.* 2007;3:331–40.

Tracy JA, Dyck JB. The spectrum of diabetic neuropathy. *Phys Med Rehabil Clin N Am.* 2008;19:1–26.

Diabetic Ketoacidosis

Epidemiology and Demographics: More commonly found in patients less than 65 years of age, mostly affecting children and young adults. The incidence is slightly higher in females and whites.

Disorder Description: Potentially fatal medical emergency characterized by hyperglycemia, ketoacidosis, and ketonuria. It primarily results from an acute complication of type 1 diabetes mellitus, although sometimes seen in type 2 diabetes when insufficient insulin causes impaired uptake of glucose. Acidic ketones are used as an alternative source of energy with the side effect of acidosis. Precipitating factors include acute insulin deficiency (missed doses or noncompliance), infections, trauma, and emotional stress.

Symptoms

Localization site	Comment
Cerebral hemispheres	Cerebral arterial infarctions, venous sinus thrombosis may cause severe headaches, encephalopathy, stroke-like symptoms. Cerebral edema may cause decreased level of consciousness, as well as headache. Seizures are rare
Brainstem	Deep rapid Kussmaul's respirations
Cranial nerves	Blurred vision may result from rapid osmotic shifts in and out of orbits

Secondary Complications: Cerebral edema; less commonly: cerebral arterial infarctions, venous sinus thrombosis, CNS infections.

Treatment Complications: Infusion of insulin may drive intracellular uptake of potassium causing hypokalemia.

Bibliography

Kitabchi AE, Umpierrez GE, Miles JM, Fisher JN. Hyperglycemic crises in adult patients with diabetes. *Diabetes Care.* 2009;32:1335.

Steenkamp DW, Alexanian SM, McDonnell ME. Adult hyperglycemic crisis: a review and perspective. *Curr Diab Rep.* 2013;13:130–7.

Diabetic Mononeuropathy

Epidemiology and Demographics: In the Rochester Diabetic Neuropathy cohort, electrophysiologic evidence of median neuropathy at the wrist was found in 22% of type 1 diabetes mellitus and in 29% of type 2 diabetes mellitus patients without any symptoms. Clinical evidence for median neuropathy at the wrist was found in 9% of type 1 and 4% of type 2 diabetic patients.

Disorder Description: Several mononeuropathies appear in greater frequency in diabetic patients than in the general population. These include median neuropathy at the wrist, ulnar neuropathy at the elbow, and peroneal neuropathy at the fibular head. The mechanism for the increased risk for carpal tunnel syndrome in diabetic patients is unclear and may relate to compression or to increased stiffness of connective tissue. Multiple mononeuropathies is referred to as mononeuropathy multiplex.

Symptoms

Localization site	Comment
Mononeuropathy or mononeuropathy multiplex	Most common mononeuropathies: • Median neuropathy – carpal tunnel syndrome • Ulnar neuropathy • Peroneal neuropathy

Secondary Complications: Peroneal neuropathy may result in foot drop, leading to falls and injury.

Treatment Complications: Complications of treatment are limited, as treatment is supportive with glycemic control, wrist splints, and orthotics.

Bibliography

Tracy, JA, Dyck, JB. The spectrum of diabetic neuropathy. *Phys Med Rehabil Clin N Am.* 2008;19:1–26.

Diabetic Neuropathy

Epidemiology and Demographics: Diabetic neuropathy is the most common cause of neuropathy in the Western world and affects 20–30 million people worldwide. It is estimated that about 50% of patients with diabetes will develop neuropathy.

Disorder Description: Diabetic neuropathy is divided into distinct clinical syndromes:

- Distal symmetric polyneuropathy
- Autonomic neuropathy
- Thoracic and lumbar nerve root disease
- Individual cranial and peripheral nerve involvement
- Mononeuropathy multiplex

Distal symmetric polyneuropathy is often considered synonymous with diabetic neuropathy. More than 80% of patients with diabetic neuropathy have the distal symmetric form. Signs and symptoms of sensory dysfunction first begin most distally at the feet and progress to affect more proximal parts of the lower limbs before involving the hands and forearms, indicating that the longest fibers are affected first. If severe, may progress to involve the anterior trunk and in most severe cases, the scalp. Affects all modalities of sensation (e.g., light, touch, vibration, pain, temperature, proprioception) and in later stages results in distal weakness and atrophy. Treatment is limited to strict glycemic control to lower the risk of deterioration. Medication for neuropathic pain is beneficial for symptoms that interfere with daytime activities or sleep.

Symptoms

Cranial nerves	Most common – cranial nerves III, VI, VII
Mononeuropathy or mononeuropathy multiplex	Most common – median, ulnar, peroneal nerves
Peripheral neuropathy	Distal symmetric polyneuropathy – numbness, burning feet, pins and needles sensations, lightning pains, weakness

Secondary Complications: Diabetic symmetric polyneuropathy may lead to painless burns, foot ulcers, neuropathic osteoarthropathy (Charcot foot), lower extremity infections, and amputations.

Treatment Complications: Complications and side effects from the various medications for neuropathic pain.

Bibliography

Said G. Diabetic neuropathy: a review. *Nat Clin Pract Neurol.* 2007;3:331.

Diabetic Polyradiculopathy

Epidemiology and Demographics: Usually found in patients older than 50 years with diabetes mellitus type 2 and often associated with weight loss.

Disorder Description: Presents with pain (reported as burning, stabbing, belt-like, or aching) in the abdominal or chest wall of the thoracic or upper lumbar roots. Usually unilateral, may be bilateral or patchy. Allodynia from light touch and clothing. May present with weakness in the abdominal wall muscles (bulging of the wall with coughing) or lower extremity weakness.

Symptoms: Pain and allodynia usually respect thoracic dermatomes, most commonly associated with distal distribution of the intercostal nerves. Diagnosed with EMG/nerve conduction velocity (NCV), which reveals fibrillations of the paraspinal or abdominal wall muscles that are commonly associated with a distal symmetric polyneuropathy. Commonly misdiagnosed as shingles without a rash, as distribution is dermatomal. Treatment is with symptomatic pain management. Sensory symptoms persist for weeks to months, with gradual resolution.

Secondary Complications: Interrupted sleep and depression from neuropathic pain.

Treatment Complications: Complications from analgesic medication or steroids due to misdiagnosis as shingles.

Bibliography

1. Pasnoor M, Dimachkie MM, Barohn RJ. Diabetic neuropathy Part 2: proximal and asymmetric phenotypes. *Neurol Clin.* 2013;31(2):447–62. DOI:10.1016/j.ncl.2013.02.003.

Dialysis Dementia

Epidemiology and Demographics: Demographics reflect the chronic dialysis patient population. The risk of dementia from vascular disease is also highly correlated in this group. Up to 37% of hemodialysis patients have been reported to have severe cognitive impairment.

Disorder Description: Cognitive impairment associated with chronic hemodialysis. It may be caused by dialysate metal impurities, particularly aluminum, or may be related to uremic and metabolic disturbances in chronic kidney disease. Cerebrovascular disease causing vascular dementia may also occur at a higher frequency immediately post-dialysis.

Symptoms

Localization site	Comment
Cerebral hemispheres	Seizures (EEG with diffuse slowing and spike-and-wave patterns)
Mental status and psychiatric aspects/ complications	Dysarthria, mutism, stuttered speech, progressive cognitive impairment

Secondary Complications: Dialysis may cause transient cerebral ischemia, acute delirium, rapid fluid shifts and metabolic derangements, and cardiopulmonary compromise.

Treatment Complications: Chelation therapy for aluminum toxicity from dialysis may cause temporary exacerbation of neurologic problems. Benzodiazepines for acute delirium may cause respiratory depression.

Bibliography

Murray A. Cognitive impairment in the aging dialysis and chronic kidney disease populations: an occult burden. *Adv Chronic Kidney Dis.* 2008;15(2):123–32.

Naganuma T, Takemoto Y, Shoji T, et al. Factors associated with cerebral white matter hyperintensities in haemodialysis patients. *Nephrology (Carlton).* 2012;17:561–8.

Seliger S, Gillen D, Longstreth W, Kestenbaum B, Stehman-Breen C. Elevated risk of stroke among patients with end-stage renal disease. *Kidney Int.* 2003;64(2):603.

Dialysis Disequilibrium Syndrome

Epidemiology and Demographics: Epidemiologic data are limited though incidence has been declining with preventative measures. Demographics reflect chronic dialysis patient population.

Disorder Description: Constellation of neurologic signs and symptoms that occur within 24 hours after dialysis – usually self limited. Etiology is related to cerebral edema from electrolyte and fluid shifts. Patients new to dialysis and those with marked blood urea nitrogen levels are most susceptible.

Symptoms

Localization site	Comment
Cerebral hemispheres	Cerebral edema may cause headaches, dizziness, nausea, blurry vision, papilledema, seizures
Mental status and psychiatric aspects/ complications	Disorientation, acute delirium, decreased level of consciousness, coma (rare)

Secondary Complications: Small increased risk of intracranial bleeding in subset of patients with history of bleeding disorders.

Treatment Complications: Self-limited and spontaneously resolves in 48 hours post-dialysis.

Bibliography

Arieff A. Dialysis disequilibrium syndrome: current concepts on pathogenesis and prevention. *Kidney Int.* 1994;45(3):629.

Bagshaw SM, Peets AD, Hameed M, et al. Dialysis dysequilibrium syndrome: brain death and acute renal failure – A case report. *BMC Nephrol.* 2004;5:9.

Diffuse Idiopathic Skeletal Hyperostosis (DISH)

Epidemiology and Demographics: Diffuse idiopathic skeletal hyperostosis (DISH) occurs in 19% of men and 4% of women older than 50 years.

Disorder Description: There is a tendency toward ossification of ligaments predominantly affecting the spine. It may be completely asymptomatic, and the cause is unknown. Thoracic vertebrae are involved in 100%, lumbar vertebrae in 68–90%, and cervical vertebrae in 65–78% of affected individuals. It may not be limited to the spine, as it may occur in tendons, ligaments, or joint capsule insertions.

Symptoms

Localization site	Comment
Esophagus	Dysphagia
Spine	Reduction in range of spinal motion

Secondary Complications: Overgrowth of ligamentous calcification could impinge on other structures like the esophagus and cause dysphagia. Posterior longitudinal ligament ossification may impinge on the spinal cord rarely. It reduces vertebral column flexibility, predisposing to vertebral fracture.

Bibliography

Miyazawa A. Ossification of the ligamentum flavum of the cervical spine. *J Neurosurg Sci.* 2007;51(3):139–44.

Ono M, Russell WJ, Kudo S, et al. Ossification of the thoracic posterior longitudinal ligament in a fixed population. Radiological and neurosurgical manifestations. *Radiology.* 1982;143(2):469–74.

Diphtheria

Epidemiology and Demographics: Diphtheria occurs worldwide, particularly in tropical areas. In the 1990s, a major epidemic of diphtheria occurred in the countries of the former Soviet Union with more than 157,000 cases and at least 5000 deaths. From 1990 through 1995, the countries of the former Soviet Union accounted for more than 90% of all diphtheria cases reported to the World Health Organization. From 1980 through 2011, only 55 cases were reported in the United States, while globally, reported cases of diphtheria have declined from 11,625 in 2000 to 4880 in 2011.[1–3]

Disorder Description: The toxin produced by *Corynebacterium diphtheriae,*[1–3] an aerobic gram-positive bacillus, causes diphtheria. It is produced only when *C. diphtheriae* is itself infected by a specific virus carrying the tox gene. Only *C. diphtheriae* containing the tox gene can cause severe disease. Once produced by the organism, the toxin inhibits cellular protein, causes local tissue destruction, induces pseudomembrane formation, absorbs into the circulation, and damages remote organs resulting in severe disease and potentially death.

Diphtheria can affect any mucous membrane. The anatomic area of mucous membrane involved is most characteristic of the severity and evolution of clinical diphtheria. Anterior nasal diphtheria, which is indistinguishable from the common cold, is usually of mild severity because of poor systemic absorption of the toxin, while pharyngeal and tonsillar diphtheria, manifesting itself by early symptoms of malaise, sore throat, anorexia and low-grade fever,

can cause extensive pseudomembrane formation resulting in respiratory obstruction. Pharyngeal and tonsillar diphtheria is more severe because infection at the pharynx and tonsils is associated with substantial systemic absorption of toxin. Even more severe is laryngeal diphtheria, which can lead to airway obstruction, coma, and death. The extent of local disease and the amount of toxin produced are responsible for the severity and complications of diphtheria. The most frequent complications of diphtheria are myocarditis and diphtheric polyneuropathy (DP).

DP,[4] a dangerous and serious complication of diphtheria, manifests itself by bulbar, respiratory, and circulatory disturbances. The first symptoms of DP occur 3 to 5 weeks after the onset of diphtheria. Cranial nerve palsy, weakness of respiratory and abdominal muscles, quadriparesis and quadriplegia with areflexia and muscular hypotonia, peripheral sensory disturbances, pain syndrome in the arms and legs, and autonomic disturbances are the main clinical features. The cranial nerves are affected first with cranial nerve IX and X most severely disturbed, followed by quadriparesis and quadriplegia. A well-known characteristic of DP is the phenomenon of counterchanges of the neurologic symptoms where there is simultaneous recovery of the cranial nerves with aggravation of motor disturbances in the trunk and extremities.

Symptoms[2,4]

Localization site	Comment
Cranial nerves	***CN III–IV and VI:*** convergence disturbances, accommodation disturbance, diplopia, mydriasis, pupillary light reflex disturbance, anisocoria, and ptosis
	CN V: sensory and motor disturbances
	CN VII: facial weakness
	CN IX and X: dysphonia, dysphagia, respiratory disturbances and asphyxia, paralytic laryngospasm and laryngostenosis
	CN XI: paralysis of cranial nerve XI
	CN XII: paralysis of cranial nerve XII
Peripheral neuropathy	***Motor:*** proximal quadriparesis/quadriplegia, muscular atrophy
	Sensory: hypoesthesia and hyperesthesia, disturbances in point position sense, tactile discrimination and vibration
	Autonomic disturbance: sinus tachycardia, arterial hypotension, retention of urine, pronounced xeroderma and hyperkeratosis, and hyperemia and hyperhidrosis in the face, neck, and chest

Treatment Complications: Rare neurotoxic side effects of penicillin (e.g., seizures) or erythromycin class antibiotics.

References

1. Center for Disease Control and Prevention: Diphtheria. *Epidemiology and prevention of vaccine preventable diseases*, 13th ed. Atlanta, GA: Center for Disease Control and Prevention; 2015. pp. 107–118.
2. Sanghi V. Neurologic manifestations of diphtheria and pertussis. *Handb Clin Neurol*. 2014;12:1355–9.
3. Hadfield TL, McEvoy P, Polotsky Y, Tzinserling VA, Yakovlev AA. The pathology of diphtheria. *J Infect Dis*. 2000;181(Suppl 1):S116–20.
4. Piradov MA, Pirogov VN, Popova LM, Avdunina IA. Diphtheritic polyneuropathy. *Arch Neurol*. 2001;58:1438–42.

Diphtheria, Tetanus, and Pertussis Vaccine

Epidemiology and Demographics: The diphtheria, tetanus, and pertussis vaccine is routinely recommended for children, with a booster given to adults every 10 years.

Disorder Description: Two main versions of the vaccine are available: DTap (diphtheria, tetanus, and acellular pertussis) given to children and Tdap (tetanus toxoid, reduced diphtheria toxoid, and acellular pertussis) given as a booster to adults. Diphtheria and tetanus are caused by toxins secreted by bacteria. These toxins have different effects on the nervous system whereas pertussis does not have any effect on the nervous system.

Symptoms of disease

Localization site	Comment
Mental status and psychiatric aspects/ complications	Tetanus: irritability, restlessness
Cranial nerves	Diphtheria: paralysis locally caused by the pseudomembrane (paralysis of the soft palate and pharynx) and cranial neuropathies (cranial nerves III, VII, IX)
	Tetanus: cephalic form, involvement mainly of cranial nerve VII
Peripheral neuropathy	Diphtheria: peripheral neuritis, mild weakness to total paralysis
Muscle	Tetanus: painful tonic contractions and spasms (opisthotonus, trismus, risus sardonicus, dysphagia, apnea)

Secondary Complications: Anaphylaxis, generalized urticaria, angioedema, and neurologic complications.

Treatment Complications: Tetanus immunoglobulin can cause increased body temperatures, nephrotic syndrome, and anaphylaxis. Diphtheria antitoxin can cause serum sickness. Fever from pertussis vaccine reaction could induce seizures in susceptible populations.

Bibliography

Broder KR, Cortese MM, Iskander JK, et al. Preventing tetanus, diphtheria, and pertussis among adolescents: use of tetanus toxoid, reduced diphtheria toxoid and acellular pertussis vaccines: recommendations of the Advisory Committee on Immunization Practices (ACIP). *MMWR Recomm Rep*. 2006;55(RR-3):1–34.

Edwards N, Marshall M. Preventing and treating tetanus. *BMJ*. 2003;326:117–8.

McQuillan GM, Kruszon-Moran D, Deforest A, Chu SY, Wharton M. Serologic immunity to diphtheria and tetanus in the United States. *Ann Intern Med*. 2002;136(9):660–6.

Naiditch MJ, Bower AG. Diphtheria: a study of 1,433 cases observed during a ten-year period at the Los Angeles County Hospital. *Am J Med*. 1954;17(2):229–45.

Singleton JA, Greby SM, Wooten KG, Walker FJ, Strikas R. Influenza, pneumococcal, and tetanus toxoid vaccination of adults – United States, 1993–1997. *MMWR CDC Surveill Summ*. 2000;49(9):39–62.

Discitis

Epidemiology and Demographics: The incidence of discitis (also termed spinal osteomyelitis or vertebral osteomyelitis, or disc-space infection) ranges from 0.3 per 100,000 population among persons younger than 20 years of age to 6.5 per 100,000 among persons older than 70 years of age.[1]

Disorder Description: Discitis or vertebral osteomyelitis occurs as a result of hematogenous seeding, direct inoculation at the time of surgery, or contiguous spread from an infection in the adjacent soft tissue. The most common organisms implicated in discitis are *Staphylococcus aureus*, followed respectively by *Escherichia coli*, other gram-negative bacilli, coagulase-negative staphylococci, streptococci, and polymicrobial infection.[1] Coagulase-negative staphylococci and *Propionibacterium acnes* are the microorganisms most implicated in discitis after spinal surgery. The primary focus of infection in hematogenous discitis is the urinary tract, skin and subcutaneous tissues, infected vascular access sites, endocarditis, and bursitis or septic arthritis. Underlying medical diseases such as diabetes, coronary heart disease, immunosuppressive disorders, cancer, end-stage renal diseases, and use of intravenous drugs are often present in hematogenous discitis. Discitis can lead to paravertebral, epidural, and psoas abscesses by direct seeding in different compartments.

Discitis is most commonly located in the lumbar or lumbosacral spine, thoracic spine, and cervical spine, respectively. Neurologic complications such as motor weakness and paralysis occur in 38% of patients with discitis, with high rates among patients with cervical spine discitis.[2]

The clinical features of discitis include back pain, the most common initial symptom reported in 86% of cases, fever reported in 35–65% of cases, and neurologic impairment such as sensory loss, weakness, or radiculopathy reported in 30% of cases. The differential diagnosis of back pain in a patient with fever includes a viral syndrome, pyelonephritis, and pancreatitis.

Laboratory testing reveals an increased leukocyte count, increased erythrocyte sedimentation rate, and C-reactive protein. Blood cultures are key in evaluating discitis. A culture of a biopsy specimen obtained via CT guided or open technique has higher yield than a routine blood culture.

MRI is the most sensitive (93–96%) and specific (92.5–97%) modality for early detection of discitis. The diagnosis of discitis is often delayed, thus a high index of suspicion and prompt use of MRI avoid diagnostic delay.

Symptoms

Localization site	Comment
Spinal cord	Discitis can be complicated with spinal epidural abscess resulting in motor and sensory impairment[2]
Anterior horn cells	Weakness
Dorsal root ganglia	Radiculopathy and sensory impairment
Conus medullaris	Can be affected by epidural abscess
Cauda equina	Can be affected by epidural abscess
Specific spinal roots	Radiculopathy

Treatment Complications: Treatment involves antibiotic therapy and operative management consisting of drainage of abscesses, relief of compression of spinal cord, and spinal stabilization.[3]

Neurologic complications of antibiotics or of analgesics (e.g., cerebrovascular adverse events from NSAIDs) are rare.

References

1. Zimmerli W. Vertebral osteomyelitis. *N Eng J Med*. 2010;362:1022–9.
2. McHenry MC, Easley KA, Locker GA. Vertebral osteomyelitis: Long-term outcome for 253 patients from 7 Cleveland-Area Hospitals. *Clin Infect Dis*. 2002;34:1342–50.
3. Cebrian Parra JL, Martinez-Aedo ALU, Ivanez IS, Agreda E, Stern LP. Management of infectious discitis. Outcome in one hundred and eight patients in a University Hospital. *Int Orthop*. 2012;36:239–44.

Disruptive, Impulse-Control, and Conduct Disorders

Epidemiology and Demographics: More common in males and begin in childhood or adolescence.

Disorder Description: The DSM-5 uses this category to classify oppositional defiant disorder, intermittent explosive disorder, conduct disorder, antisocial personality disorder, pyromania, kleptomania, and other specified and unspecified disruptive, impulse-control, and conduct disorders. These disorders have in common an inability for an individual to control emotions or behaviors that results in trangression against the rights of others and/or break with societal expectations. When evaluating for these disorders, a person's phase of development and cultural norms must be considered. There is high comorbidity of these disorders with substance abuse and antisocial personality disorder.

Many of these disorders have been associated with neglectful, harsh, and/or abusive parenting. Some studies also show higher risk when a parent or sibling is affected. Difficult temperaments are also associated. Abnormal physiologic responses to fear have been noted in some of these disorders. Some studies have shown these disorders to be more prominent in Western cultures, while others demonstrate the same rates cross culturally.

Symptoms

Localization site	Comment
Cerebral hemispheres	Neuropsych testing: may have evidence of impaired frontal lobe functioning
Mental status and psychiatric aspects/ complications	Conduct disorder may have lower intellectual functioning (esp. verbal IQ)
	Intermittent explosive disorder: poorly controlled anger, aggression
	Some have increased risk for suicidal behavior
	May have comorbid attention deficit hyperactivity disorder symptoms and symptoms of substance abuse

Secondary Complications: Impairment in social and emotional functioning makes sustaining relationships difficult. Significant conflict across multiple settings, including school, occupation, and home. Run ins with the criminal justice system can be routine.

Bibliography

American Psychiatric Association. *Diagnostic and statistical manual of mental disorders: DSM-5.* 5th ed. Washington, DC: American Psychiatric Association; 2013.

Lorber MF. Psychophysiology of aggression, psychopathy, and conduct problems: a meta-analysis. *Psychol Bull.* 2004;130(4):531–52.

Nock MK, Hwang I, Sampson NA, Kessler RC. Mental disorders, comorbidity and suicidal behavior: results from the National Comorbidity Survey Replication. *Mol Psychiatry.* 2010;15(8):868–76.

Disruptive Mood Dysregulation Disorder

Epidemiology and Demographics: The 6-month to 1-year prevalence in children and adolescents is 2–5%, with male predominance.

Disorder Description: As per DSM-5, characterized by persistent irritable or angry mood, punctuated by temper outbursts occurring at least three times a week. Outbursts are marked by severe verbal or behavioral aggression, which appear as exaggerated response to the stimulus. The intervening irritability is pervasive and apparent enough to be noticed by others. Symptom onset must be prior to 10 years old and diagnosis must be made between 6 and 18 years old. Symptoms must be inappropriate for phase of development. Two or more areas of life settings must be affected, at least one of them severely. Duration must be at least 12 months without more than 3 consecutive months symptom-free.

Diagnosis cannot be made if there is any history of 1 day or longer of symptoms meeting criteria for manic episode. Another exclusion is if symptoms occur exclusively in the context of a depressive episode. There may be significant overlap with symptoms of bipolar syndrome and oppositional defiant disorder, warranting thoughtful evaluation.

To fit criteria, the condition must cause distress or impairment in several realms of functioning and is not better accounted for by effects of a substance, or another mental or medical condition. Comorbidities may include attention deficit hyperactivity disorder and depressive and/or anxiety disorders.

Symptoms

Localization site	Comment
Mental status and psychiatric aspects/ complications	Irritability, aggression, anger out of proportion to circumstances
	May have suicidal ideation
	May have symptoms of comorbid anxiety or depression

Secondary Complications: Can significantly impair relationships and function at home and school. There is also increased risk for hospitalization in the setting of aggressive, self-injurious, and/or suicidal behavior.

Bibliography

American Psychiatric Association. *Diagnostic and statistical manual of mental disorders: DSM-5.* 5th ed. Washington, DC: American Psychiatric Association; 2013.

Brotman MA, Schmajuk M, Rich BA, et al. Prevalence, clinical correlates, and longitudinal course of severe mood dysregulation in children. *Biol Psychiatry.* 2006;60(9):991–7.

Leibenluft E. Severe mood dysregulation, irritability, and the diagnostic boundaries of bipolar disorder in youth. *Am J Psychiatry.* 2011;168(2):129–42.

Dissociative Amnesia (Psychogenic Amnesia)

Dissociative amnesia is the inability to recall information, usually of a traumatic event, that is beyond ordinary forgetting.

Epidemiology and Demographics: Among adults, the annual prevalence of dissociative amnesia in the United States is approximately 1.8% (1.0% in males and 2.6% in females).

Disorder Description: As per the DSM-5, it is characterized by "an inability to recall important autobiographical information, usually of a traumatic or stressful nature, that is inconsistent with ordinary forgetting." Memory loss is due to difficulty with retrieval of information rather than encoding, therefore potentially reversible. This sets it apart from amnesia caused by cerebral structural injury or neurodegenerative process. There is a distinction between "localized" or "selective," in which memory for specific events is unable to be retrieved, and "generalized" amnesia in which one does not recall one's identity and/or personal history. Localized or selective amnesia is more common and typically assumes a slower time course than generalized. Insight into both is typically poor. To fit criteria, the condition must cause distress or impairment in several realms of functioning and is not better accounted for by effects of a substance, or another mental or medical condition. There is a specifier for dissociative fugue, which is amnesia associated with "apparently purposeful travel or bewildered wandering."

Environmental causes include exposure to trauma, such as that involved in combat, sexual assault, and childhood abuse. Risk of dissociative amnesia increases with frequency and severity of these experiences. It is seen across cultures, some cases with functional neurologic symptoms as comorbid features.

As specifically defined by the DSM-5, dissociative amnesia is:

A. An inability to recall important autobiographical information, usually of a traumatic or stressful nature, that is inconsistent with ordinary forgetting.

B. The symptoms cause clinically significant distress or impairment in social, occupational, or other important areas of functioning.

C. The disturbance is not attributable to the physiologic effects of a substance or a neurologic or other medical condition (e.g., partial complex seizures, transient global ischemia, sequelae of a closed heart injury/traumatic brain injury, other neurologic condition).

D. The disturbance is not better explained by dissociative identity disorder, posttraumatic stress disorder, acute stress disorder, somatic symptom disorder, or major or mild neurocognitive disorder.

Case Example: A 29-year-old nursing student is brought in for evaluation by her sister who reports "she is forgetting everything." Her sister reports that the patient received a failing grade in several classes and lost her part-time job the day before presentation. She initially appeared depressed and anxious but within hours seemed unusually calm. When seen, the patient reports the date as a year in the past, recalls episodes from popular shows from a year ago, and does not recall being in a part-time job or any information from the last year of nursing school. It is revealed that the patient also lost her grandmother within her amnestic period, and she says "I can't wait to see my grandmother after I leave the hospital."

Differential Diagnosis: The differential diagnosis of dissociative amnesia includes normal autobiographical memory, dissociative identity disorder, posttraumatic stress disorder, neurocognitive disorders, posttraumatic amnesia due to brain injury, seizure disorders, catatonic stupor, factitious disorder, and malingering.

In normal autobiographical memory, there is often amnesia to preverbal memories, fewer memories before age 5–6 years, amnesia for sleeping and dreaming, and a gradient for recall. In dissociative amnesia, recall is usually not a gradient, but rather a very specific amnesia with a distinct boundary of onset and offset (e.g., complete lack of memory of the winter of sophomore year, or all of fourth grade).

In dissociative identity disorder, there are discontinuities in sense of self and identity, and these are accompanied by many additional dissociative symptoms. The amnesias of those with dissociative amnesia are generally stable, whereas amnesias in dissociative identity disorder are more episodic, for example not remembering everyday events, fluctuations in skills and/or knowledge, and finding of unexplained possessions.

In posttraumatic stress disorder, there may be lack of recollection of a traumatic event. However, if amnesia spans beyond the immediate timeline of the trauma, a coexisting diagnosis of dissociative amnesia would be warranted.

In neurocognitive disorders, there can be memory loss for personal information, but this is usually in the context of decreasing intellectual and cognitive ability. In dissociative amnesia, memory deficits are for autobiographical information only, and do not present in the context of other neurocognitive decline.

In substance-related disorders, amnesic episodes occur only in the context of intoxication, and not in other situations. These diagnoses can be difficult to distinguish in the case of a patient who abuses substances and reports dissociative amnesia. A careful longitudinal history should be taken to ascertain whether symptoms occur outside of situations of intoxication. Prolonged substance abuse can lead to neurocognitive disorders, and these are characterized by a general neurocognitive decline (not a feature of dissociative amnesia).

In posttraumatic amnesia due to brain injury, there may be amnesia due to impact to the head or other mechanisms of rapid movement of the head and/or brain. Symptoms would present either immediately after the assault or immediately upon regaining consciousness.

In seizure disorders, patients may report amnesia during the seizure or postictally. Some report wandering during epileptic episodes – such wandering is usually without purpose and is limited to the timing of the seizure. Behavior in dissociative amnesia is generally purposeful and goal-oriented. Dissociative and epileptic amnesia may be co-occurring diagnoses.

In catatonic stupor, mutism may occur, but there is generally no failure of recall. Catatonic stupor is also characterized by coexisting symptoms including rigidity, posturing, and negativism.

There is no test to distinguish actual amnesia from feigned amnesia (malingering, factitious disorder). It has been noted that patients with factitious disorder and those malingering may continue to feign symptoms even during hypnosis. Many individuals who malinger confess spontaneously or during confrontation.

In normal and age-related memory changes, there is a more general neurocognitive decline than in a dissociative amnesia, in which there is often association with specific events.

Secondary Complications: In some cultures (Asia, Middle East, Latin America), non-epileptic seizures have been shown to accompany dissociative amnesia.

Dissociative amnesia ranges from mild, with virtually no functional consequences, to severe, in which an individual may have impairment in all aspects of functioning. Even after "re-learning" one's life history, he or she may continue to have severe interpersonal and vocational disability.

Suicide and other non-suicidal self-injurious behaviors are more common in dissociative amnesia than in the general population, and individuals are at particularly high risk if their amnesia suddenly remits and he or she becomes inundated with intolerable memories.

Many of those with dissociative amnesia have experienced physical or sexual abuse during childhood. Other psychologic outcomes associated with early life trauma include depression, suicidality, auditory hallucinations, post-traumatic stress disorder, anxiety, personality disorders, and eating disorders.

Psychologic, social, and occupational functioning is variable. Amnesia can resolve, resulting in the potential for significant impairment, self-harm, or suicidality with return of traumatic memories.

Treatment Complications: Dissociative amnesia management often includes psychotherapy, cognitive therapy, and hypnosis. Some do not recommend hypnosis in patients with dissociative disorders, as it may promote the formation of false memories. Pharmacotherapy is generally not used for dissociative amnesia. The hallmark of dissociative amnesia is an unconscious defense mechanism called repression. Given that it is unconscious, trying to confront the patient is not useful. Careful, composed, and empathic assessment may help the patient arrive at his/her own memories without causing trauma.

Bibliography

American Psychiatric Association. *Diagnostic and statistical manual of mental disorders: DSM-5.* 5th ed. Washington, DC: American Psychiatric Association; 2013.

Brand M, Eggers C, Reinhold N, et al. Functional brain imaging in 14 patients with dissociative amnesia reveals right inferolateral prefrontal hypometabolism. *Psychiatry Res.* 2009;174(1):32–9.

Cohen NJ, Squire LR. Preserved learning and retention of pattern-analyzing skill in amnesia: dissociation of knowing how and knowing that. *Science.* 1980;210(4466):207–10.

International Society for the Study of Trauma and Dissociation. Guidelines for treating dissociative identity disorder in adults, third revision. *J Trauma Dissociation.* 2011;12(2):115–87.

Johnson JG, Cohen P, Kasen S, Brook JS. Dissociative disorders among adults in the community, impaired functioning, and axis I and II comorbidity. *J Psychiatr Res.* 2006;40(2):131–40.

Kaszniak AW, Nussbaum PD, Berren MR, Santiago J. Amnesia as a consequence of male rape: a case report. *J Abnorm Psychol.* 1988;97(1):100–4.

Loewenstein RJ. Psychogenic amnesia and psychogenic fugue: a comprehensive review. In Tasman A, Goldfinger SM, eds. *The American Psychiatric Press Annual Review of Psychiatry*, Vol 10. Washington, DC: American Psychiatric Press; 1991. pp. 189–222.

Loewenstein RJ. Psychogenic amnesia and psychogenic fugue: a comprehensive review. In Spiegel D, ed. *Dissociative disorders: a clinical review.* Baltimore, MD: The Sidran Press; 1993. pp. 45–78.

Markowitsch HJ. Psychogenic amnesia. *Neuroimage.* 2003;20:S132–8.

Witztum E, Margalit H, van der Hart O. Combat-induced dissociative amnesia: review and case example of generalized dissociative amnesia. *J Trauma Dissociation.* 2002;3(2):35–55.

Dissociative Identity Disorder

Epidemiology and Demographics: In a community study of adults in the United States, prevalence of dissociative identity disorder (DID) was found to be 1.5% over 1 year, affecting males slightly more than females. It can present in childhood to late adulthood, though clinical manifestation differs based on phase of development.

Disorder Description: Formerly known as "multiple personality disorder," the DSM-5 describes DID as "disruption of identity characterized by two or more distinct personality states, which may be described in some cultures as an experience of possession." There are depersonalization symptoms, with detachment from the self and inability to control transition to alternate states. The states may vary in styles of thought, behavior, emotion, and other manners of functioning. One may have minimal insight into the characteristics of these altered states. Either the affected individual or another person may report these state changes. There are also recurrent episodes consistent with dissociative amnesia, in which personal information, routine life details, or stressful events are unable to be recalled. There may also be flashbacks of previous trauma. The condition must cause distress or impairment in one of several realms of functioning and is not better accounted for by effects of a substance, or another mental or medical condition.

In evaluating for the disorder, the role of cultural norms must be considered. When cultural practices can reasonably account for symptoms, this diagnosis is excluded.

Psychiatric comorbidities are common and include trauma and stressor-related mood and anxiety disorders, functional neurologic symptoms such as non-epileptic seizures, substance abuse, self-injurious behavior, and others.

The major risk factor, present in 90%, is childhood neglect, physical and sexual abuse. Recurrent forms of trauma are particularly associated with risk, including medical procedures, child prostitution, and military exposure.

Symptoms

Localization site	Comment
Mental status and psychiatric aspects/complications	Often limited or poor awareness of the features of altered identity states
	Loss of memory for autobiographical events or specific events or periods of time
	May have symptoms of psychiatric comorbidities, e.g., posttraumatic stress disorder, depression, anxiety

Secondary Complications: Levels of impairment are variable, from what may appear to be minimally impaired function to severe.

Bibliography

American Psychiatric Association. *Diagnostic and statistical manual of mental disorders: DSM-5.* 5th ed. Washington, DC: American Psychiatric Association; 2013.

Ellason JW, Ross CA, Fuchs DL. Lifetime Axis I and II comorbidity and childhood trauma history in dissociative identity disorder. *Psychiatry.* 1996;59(3):255–66.

Johnson JG, Cohen P, Kasen S, Brook JS. Dissociative disorders among adults in the community, impaired functioning, and axis I and II comorbidity. *J Psychiatr Res.* 2006;40(2):131–40.

Spiegel D, Loewenstein RJ, Lewis-Fernández R, et al. Dissociative disorders in DSM-5. *Depress Anxiety.* 2011;28(9):824–52. DOI:10.1002/da.20874

Distal Spinal Muscular Atrophy

Epidemiology and Demographics: Extremely rare.

Disorder Description: Distal spinal muscular atrophy (SMA) is within the group of rare SMAs that are not linked to mutations in chromosome 5. It is a rare genetic disorder that can present with recessive, dominant, or X-linked inheritance. The Muscular Dystrophy Association website highlights some gene types associated with distal SMA including UBA1, DYNC1H1, TRPV4, PLEKHG5, GARS, and FBXO38. Some distal SMA phenotypes overlap with Charcot–Marie–Tooth disease. Diagnosis depends on the degree of motor versus sensory symptoms.

Distal SMA more severely affects the muscles of the hands and feet. Prognosis is better than with other SMA forms.

Symptoms

Localization site	Comment
Spinal cord	Progressive loss of motor neurons in spinal cord
Muscle	Progressive muscular weakness of hands and feet

Secondary Complications: Respiratory impairments and associated secondary effects on the nervous system.

Treatment Complications: Treatment is mostly supportive including potential respiratory support.

Bibliography

Muscular Dystrophy Association. Spinal muscular atrophy. www.mda.org/disease/spinal-muscular-atrophy/types. Accessed May, 2017.

Muthukrishnan J, Varadarajulu R, Mehta SR, Singh AP. Distal muscular atrophy: Case report. *J Assoc Physicians India.* 2003;51:113–15.

Doose Syndrome (Myoclonic–Astatic Epilepsy or Epilepsy with Myoclonic–Atonic Seizures)

Epidemiology and Demographics: Occurs in 1/10,000 children and constitutes 1–2% of childhood epilepsies. Two-thirds of cases male. Onset ages 7 months to 6 years, with peak incidence between 3 and 4 years.

Disorder Description: Children developmentally normal prior to symptom onset. Seizures then begin, typically with intractable myoclonic and atonic seizures resulting in abrupt falls, and sometimes absence, tonic, or generalized tonic–clonic seizures. Syndrome appears to be genetic in etiology and has been linked to generalized epilepsy with febrile seizures plus (GEFS+) with mutations in the sodium channel (SCN1A and SCN1B), as well as mutations in the gamma-aminobutyric acid receptor (GABRG2) and solute carrier family 2 (SCL2A1/GLUT1) genes. Classically, there are no lesions or other organic causes for the seizures, though symptomatic lesions presenting with a similar phenotype have been described. Seizures may partially respond to corticosteroids or anticonvulsants such as ethosuximide, valproate, levetiracetam, topiramate, and zonisamide. The ketogenic diet may be most efficacious.

Symptoms

Localization site	Comment
Cerebral hemispheres	Myoclonic and atonic seizures
	Other generalized seizure types may be observed
	Myoclonic–astatic or atypical absence status epilepticus may occur

Localization site	Comment
	Interictal EEG with 2- to 5-Hz generalized spike/polyspike wave complexes, increased theta, and photosensitivity, with relative preservation of background rhythms. MRI usually normal or with generalized atrophy
Mental status and psychiatric aspects/ complications	Cognitive outcome favorable with appropriate treatment in the majority of patients. Attentional and behavioral issues have been described. Intractability, status epilepticus, tonic seizures, and abnormal EEG background associated with intellectual disability

Secondary Complications: Falls and traumatic injury.

Treatment Complications: The ketogenic diet is associated with anorexia, growth restriction, and metabolic acidosis. Antiepileptic drugs may be associated with a number of idiosyncratic reactions including mood changes and negative cognitive effects. Carbamazepine, phenytoin, and vigabatrin may dramatically worsen seizures and should be avoided. Lamotrigine may exacerbate myoclonic type seizures and is associated with a higher risk of rash. Duration of corticosteroid therapy is limited by systemic effects.

Bibliography

Kelley SA, Kossoff EH. Doose syndrome (myoclonic-astatic epilepsy): 40 years of progress. *Dev Med Child Neurol.* 2010;52(11):988–93.

Tang S, Pal DK. Dissecting the genetic basis of myoclonic-astatic epilepsy. *Epilepsia.* 2012;53(8):1303–13.

Dopa-Responsive Dystonia (DRD)

Epidemiology and Demographics: Dopa-responsive dystonia (DRD) is thought to affect 1 per million persons worldwide. DYT5a is the prototypical DRD and typically presents in children with a mean age of 11 years, although it may sometimes present in adults as well. The incidence is generally reported to be 2.5- to 4-fold greater in females than males. In males, the disease onset tends to be later and symptoms are often milder.

Disorder Description: The term DRD encompasses an array of clinically and genetically heterogeneous disorders that markedly improve with levodopa treatment. The typical phenotype is a childhood onset action dystonia, usually affecting the lower limb, which may progress to generalized dystonia. There is diurnal fluctuation and an excellent and sustained response to levodopa. The most well studied of these disorders is Segawa disease (DYT5a), which is an autosomal dominant deficiency of GTP cyclohydrolase1, involved in the production of an essential cofactor for the biosynthesis of monoamine neurotransmitters. DRD, however, may also result from deficiencies of other enzymes involved in the synthesis of dopamine and may be seen in other neurologic conditions.

Symptoms

Localization site	Comment
Mental status and psychiatric aspects/complications	Borderline intellectual functioning (rare) Depression, anxiety, obsessive-compulsive disorder
Unclear localization	Sleep disturbances with spontaneous arousals, excessive sleepiness

Secondary Complications: Scoliosis is commonly observed.

Treatment Complications: There is usually an excellent and sustained response to levodopa. However, there are rare reports of levodopa-induced dyskinesia requiring changes in treatment.

Bibliography

Lee WW, Jeon BS. Clinical spectrum of dopa-responsive dystonia and related disorders. *Curr Neurol Neurosci Rep.* 2014;14(7):1–13.

Segawa M. Dopa-responsive dystonia. *Handb Clin Neurol.* 2010;100:539–57.

Wijemanne S, Jankovic J. Dopa-responsive dystonia: clinical and genetic heterogeneity. *Nat Rev Neurol.* 2015;11(7):414–24.

Down Syndrome

Epidemiology and Demographics: Occurs in 1/691 US live births.[1] It is the most frequent live birth defect and chromosomal disorder[2] and the most common genetic cause of intellectual disabilities.[3] Equal distribution in males and females.

Disorder Description: Also known as trisomy 21, it is due to having a third copy in whole or part of chromosome 21. It is associated with characteristic facies (e.g., slanted eyes), intellectual disability, delayed and limited growth, and reduced life expectancy (usually no older than 60 years[4]).

Symptoms

Localization site	Comment
Cerebral hemispheres, mental status and psychiatric aspects/ complications	Intellectual disability typically to the level of an 8- to 9-year-old child. Speech impairments. Risks for autism. While demeanor is often positive, there is also elevated risk for developing depression, anxiety, or behavior impairments
	Alzheimer's dementia later in life
	Seizures with peak in infancy (e.g., infantile spasms), seizures in childhood or early adulthood, or as part of later stage Alzheimer's dementia
Cranial nerves	Hearing impairment from diverse anatomical causes, and otitis media is common
Spinal cord	Atlanto-axial instability in 15%[5] may cause myelopathy as evidenced by gait impairment, limb paresis, and sphincter dysfunction
Muscle	Decreased muscle tone

Secondary Complications: Obstructive sleep apnea, and its systemic complications, is common. Neurologic problems may result secondarily from other conditions that commonly occur including hypothyroidism, diabetes mellitus, cardiovascular disease, cancer such as leukemia, respiratory infections, and osteoporosis-related fractures.

References

1. Centers for Disease Control and Prevention. Birth defects: data and statistics in the United States. Updated April 30, 2018. Available from www.cdc.gov/NCBDDD/birthdefects/data.html. Accessed February 26, 2014.
2. Graber E, Chacko E, Regelmann MO, et al. Down syndrome and thyroid function. *Endocrinol Metab Clin North Am.* 2012;41:735–45.
3. Baumer N, Davidson EJ. Supporting a happy, healthy adolescence for young people with Down syndrome and other intellectual disabilities: recommendations for clinicians. *Curr Opin Pediatr.* 2014;26:428–34.
4. Yang Q, Rasmussen SA, Friedman JM. Mortality associated with Down's syndrome in the USA from 1983 to 1997: a population-based study. *Lancet.* 2002;359:1019–25.
5. Davidson MA. Primary care for children and adolescents with Down syndrome. *Pediatr Clin North Am.* 2008;55:1099–111.

Dravet Syndrome (DS) or Infantile Severe Myoclonic Epilepsy

Epidemiology and Demographics: Dravet syndrome (DS) has a prevalence of 1/20,000–40,000. Typically in the first year of life, peak age 5–8 months. Affects either sex equally except in PCDH19 mutation, which mainly affects girls.

Disorder Description: Type of epileptic encephalopathy characterized by early-onset, febrile or afebrile, unilateral clonic or generalized tonic–clonic seizures. Often presents as prolonged episodes of status epilepticus in an otherwise normally developing child. Myoclonus, atypical absences, and partial seizures can be observed later. In adulthood, seizures become somewhat less frequent and severe, and patients have mainly nocturnal generalized tonic–clonic seizures.

Mutations in SCN1A are the main genetic cause of DS (approximately 80%); other gene mutations (PCDH19, GABRA1, GABRG2) account for a small proportion of cases.

Interictal EEG usually normal early in disease and then may show generalized and multifocal epileptiform abnormalities. Photosensitivity common.

Refractory to antiepileptic drugs. Treatment options include stiripentol combined with sodium valproate or clobazam, cannabadiol, and ketogenic diet.

Symptoms

Localization site	Comment
Cerebral hemispheres	Hemiclonic seizures
	Generalized tonic–clonic seizures
	Status epilepticus
	Focal, myoclonic, or absence seizures
	Nocturnal convulsive seizures

Localization site	Comment
Mental status and psychiatric aspects/ complications	Mild to severe developmental delay, behavioral disturbances, and intellectual disability. Cognitive issues typically present during the second year of life or later with progressive decline. Studies suggest cognitive impairment may have stronger relation to gene mutation than epileptic factors
Cerebellum	Ataxia, dysarthria, intention tremor

Secondary Complications: Symptoms of epileptic encephalopathy in the neonate may include emesis, abdominal distention, apnea, irritability, sleeplessness, and abnormal eye movements. Hypoglycemia and lactic acidosis have been described. Kyphosis, scoliosis, flat feet, or claw feet often occur, impairing ambulation. Higher reported incidence of sudden unexpected death in epilepsy in patients with DS.

Treatment Complications: Inappropriate selection of antiepileptic drugs, such as carbamazepine (for generalized seizure types) and lamotrigine (for myoclonus), can worsen seizures. Adverse events of stiripentol are drowsiness, ataxia, nausea, abdominal pain, and loss of appetite. Cytochrome P450 enzyme inhibition may increase plasma concentrations of valproate and clobazam. Asymptomatic neutropenia is occasionally observed. Valproate side effects include weight gain, hyperactivity, transaminitis, thrombocytopenia, and pancreatitis. The ketogenic diet is associated with anorexia, growth restriction, and metabolic acidosis.

Bibliography

Auvin S, Cilio MR, Vezzani A. Current understanding and neurobiology of epileptic encephalopathies. *Neurobiol Dis.* 2016;92(Pt A):72–89.

Brigo F, Igwe SC. Antiepileptic drugs for the treatment of infants with severe myoclonic epilepsy. *Cochrane Database Syst Rev.* 2015(10):CD010483.

Brunklaus A, Zuberi SM. Dravet syndrome: from epileptic encephalopathy to channelopathy. *Epilepsia.* 2014;55(7):979–84.

McTague A, Howell KB, Cross JH, Kurian MA, Scheffer IE. The genetic landscape of the epileptic encephalopathies of infancy and childhood. *Lancet Neurol.* 2016;15(3):304–16.

Drop Attacks in Elderly Women

Epidemiology and Demographics: A drop attack can be defined as a sudden unprovoked fall without loss of consciousness. The most essential thing about drop attacks is to exclude the more common causes of falls in the elderly, i.e., syncope, seizures, and cardiac arrhythmias. These are more common in the elderly and in women. The reason and prognosis is unclear and variable.

Disorder Description: The classic description is of an elderly woman who, without any exacerbating factors (exertion, neck turning, tight collar, tripping or slipping), suddenly falls to the ground. This is not usually associated with loss of consciousness or any cephalic sensation (vertigo, dizziness, headache). They usually return to normal immediately but some patients can have variable weakness especially of proximal lower limb and back muscles that eventually recovers in minutes to hours.

Symptoms

Localization site	Comment
Cerebral hemispheres	Spaced out or feeling hazy after the episode
Muscle	Proximal lower limb and back muscle weakness causing difficulty in standing up

Secondary Complications: Subdural hematoma from head trauma causing confusion, delirium. Fractures due to fall.

Bibliography

Sheldon JH. Drop attacks in the elderly: a request for information. *J Coll Gen Pract.* 1962;5(1):107–9.

Stevens DL, Matthews WB. Cryptogenic drop attacks: an affliction of women. *Br Med J.* 1973;1(5851):439–42.

Drug-Induced Tremors

Epidemiology and Demographics: Drug-induced tremors occur more commonly in the elderly than in the young. They may be due to an enhancement of a physiologic tremor, a direct effect of the drug, or a side effect of the drug compounded with a multitude of comorbidities. Besides advanced age, patients with metabolic derangements, renal or liver failure, or various neurologic conditions are susceptible to drug-induced or drug-exacerbated tremors.[1-4]

Disorder Description: The disorder is defined as rhythmic, sinusoidal movements of a body part caused by regular contractions of reciprocally innervated muscles caused by taking certain drugs. Postural and intentional tremors are the most common type of tremors that occur, but enhanced physiologic tremor is also common. Resting tremors can occur and may be induced by medications that affect the extrapyramidal motor system, such as the antiemetic agent metoclopramide or the neuroleptic agents (i.e., typical antipsychotics).[1,4,5]

Determining that the condition is a drug-induced tremor can be a diagnostic challenge. Several considerations may be helpful to aid in the diagnosis. The temporal relationship between the tremor and initiation of the drug should be established. Other medical conditions including metabolic abnormalities must be excluded. The clinician should be aware that the class III anti-arrhythmic amiodarone may induce hyperthyroidism, which can subsequently cause tremors.[1] Additionally, understanding drug dynamics and kinetics will help differentiate between disease-induced tremor and drug-induced tremor. It should be noted that the interaction among drugs can lead to raised serum concentrations of one tremor-inducing drug, or may lead to additive effects of two tremor-inducing drugs. Most drugs are eliminated by the kidneys. Therefore, patients with renal failure may be more susceptible to higher drug concentrations and tremor induction.[1-6]

The drug classes that may cause tremor or exacerbate a pre-existing tremor are as follows:

Anti-arrhythmics[1]
Antimicrobials[1]
Antidepressants and mood stabilizers[6]
Antiepileptic drugs[1]
Beta-adrenergic agonists
Chemotherapeutic agents[1]
Substance abuse drugs[1]
Antiemetics[5]
Hormones[1]
Immunosuppressants[1]

Methylxanthines[1]
Neuroleptics[4,6]

The withdrawal of certain agents including benzodiazepines and alcohol may also induce an enhanced tremor.[1]

Symptoms

Localization site	Comment
Mental status and psychiatric aspects/ complications	The degree of tremor may influence the individual's social interactions and daily functioning, which may negatively impair their mood
Cerebellum	The chemotherapeutic agent cytarabine may damage cerebellar Purkinje cells in the lateral hemispheres.[1] Alcohol-induced cerebellar degeneration may induce postural tremor

Secondary Complications: Most drug-induced tremors are less disabling than drug-induced dystonia and parkinsonism. The mental health aspect of drug-induced tremor should be monitored as it can affect the patient's quality of life. The tremor may also be an indication that the drug is above the therapeutic dose, which may warrant further investigation.[1]

Treatment Complications: Once this disorder is diagnosed, the decision to treat must be made. As many of the drug-induced tremors are dose dependent, reduction of the dose is an option, aside from total discontinuation. The primary reasoning behind the use of the drug should be recalled. The antidepressants and antipsychotics are treating underlying psychiatric disease, making discontinuation an unfavorable option.[1,3]

References

1. Morgan JC, Sethi KD. Drug-induced tremors. *Lancet Neurol*. 2005;4(12):866–76.
2. Goetz CG, Dysken MW, Klawans HL. Assessment and treatment of drug-induced tremor. *J Clin Psychiatry*. 1980;41(9):310–5.
3. Gabellini AS, Martinelli P, Coccagna G. Drug-induced tremor of the tongue. *Ital J Neurol Sci*. 1989;10(1):89–91.

4. Caroff SN, Hurford I, Lybrand J, Campbell EC. Movement disorders induced by antipsychotic drugs: implications of the CATIE schizophrenia trial. *Neurol Clin.* 2011;29(1):127–48, viii.
5. Tarsy D, Indorf G. Tardive tremor due to metoclopramide. *Mov Disord.* 2002;17(3):620–1.
6. Arnold G, Trenkwalder C, Schwarz J, Oertel WH. Zotepine reversibly induces akinesia and rigidity in Parkinson's disease patients with resting tremor or drug-induced psychosis. *Mov Disord.* 1994;9(2):238–40.

Duchenne Muscular Dystrophy

Epidemiology and Demographics: Duchenne muscular dystrophy (DMD) is an X-linked disease that affects 1/3600–6000 live male births worldwide. DMD generally affects males, but may rarely occur in females. Boys often present between 3 and 5 years of age because of delayed motor milestones and falls. Mean lifespan in DMD has increased from 19 years to more than 25 years. There is no geographic predominance.

Disorder Description: DMD occurs as a result of mutations (mainly deletions) in the dystrophin gene *DMD*. Mutations lead to an absence of or defect in the protein dystrophin, which results in progressive muscle degeneration. Variable phenotypic expression relates mainly to the type of mutation and its effect on the production of dystrophin. The diagnosis is through DNA analysis. Advancements in gene therapy for DMD are promising, and recently the first FDA-approved medication was released (Eteplirsen) for patients who have a confirmed mutation of the dystrophin gene amenable to exon 51 skipping, which affects about 13% of the population with DMD.

DMD is an X-linked disorder due to defects in the *DMD* gene located at Xp21.

Symptoms

Localization site	Comment
Cerebral hemispheres	Cognitive involvement is common in DMD. Of patients with DMD, 30% have intellectual disability. The average patient's IQ is 85, one standard deviation below the mean. Verbal IQ is more affected than performance IQ, and delayed language development is common. Attention deficit hyperactivity disorder (10 to 15%), autism spectrum disorder (3 to 6%), and obsessive-compulsive disorder (5%) are also more prevalent in DMD
Muscles	Delayed motor milestones and falls, along with difficulty running and jumping starting at age 3–5 years. By convention at 12 years of age stop walking. Typically, examination reveals calf hypertrophy, mildly lordotic posture, waddling of gait, and poor hip excursion during running. Pulmonary function declines continuously and tracheostomy and mechanical ventilation is a choice made by some patients and their families later in disease
Spinal cord	Spinal cord compression due to severe kyphoscoliosis

Secondary Complications: Joint contractures occur in the ankles even while walking, and follow in the hips, knees, elbows, and wrists. Kyphoscoliosis accelerates when ambulation ceases and sometimes requires spinal fusion for optimal respiratory function. Cardiac involvement should be followed via ECG, Holter monitor, and echocardiography. Sinus tachycardia is common. Atrial and ventricular arrhythmias may follow, associated with cardiac fibrosis and a dilated cardiomyopathy.

Treatment Complications: Corticosteroids are the mainstay of treatment and should be offered to all boys with DMD. They are typically offered to boys older than 4 years of age with plateauing or declining motor function. Otherwise, management is supportive and requires a multidisciplinary health care team.

Patients can develop complications related to steroid therapy such as hyperglycemia, osteoporosis, cataracts, infections, weight gain, and steroid-induced myopathy.

Bibliography

Bushby K. Diagnosis and management of Duchenne muscular dystrophy, part 1: diagnosis, and pharmacological and psychosocial management. *Lancet Neurol.* 2010;9:77–93.

Hendriksen JG, Vles JS. Neuropsychiatric disorders in males with Duchenne muscular dystrophy: frequency rate of attention-deficit hyperactivity disorder (ADHD), autism spectrum disorder, and obsessive-compulsive disorder. *J Child Neurol.* 2008;23(5):477–81.

Dystonic Reaction

Epidemiology and Demographics: Most commonly occurs in young men during first time treatment with a typical neuroleptic drug. Reported prevalence of a dystonic reaction was as high as 60% for first time treatment of an acute psychotic episode. Prior studies report a 5% prevalence in all individuals who have taken dopamine receptor-blocking agents.

Disorder Description: Dystonic reaction is an acute condition characterized by involuntary, repetitive, simultaneous contraction of agonist and antagonist muscle groups, typically affecting the cranial and cervical musculature. It occurs in the first 7 days after exposure to dopamine receptor-blocking agents, including typical antipsychotics/neuroleptics (haloperidol), antiemetics (metoclopramide, prochlorperazine), antidepressants (selective serotonin reuptake inhibitors), drugs of abuse (cocaine, ecstasy), inhaled anesthetics, and tetrabenazine. Second generation antipsychotics have lower incidences of dystonic reaction. It is thought to occur during a transient period when dopamine is increased in the synaptic cleft and dopamine receptors have increased sensitivity. Symptoms are dramatic and include oculogyric crisis, blepharospasm, masseter spasm, trismus, mouth opening, torticollis, retrocollis, opisthotonus, and laryngospasm, which can be fatal. The extremities are less commonly affected. Risk factors include younger age (greater than 60% risk before 20 years, and near zero risk at 40 years), male sex, prior or current cocaine use, treatment with high-potency antipsychotics, prior dystonic reaction, and concurrent HIV infection.

Symptoms

Localization site	Comment
Cerebral hemispheres	Subcortical; abnormal dopaminergic activity increases efferent signals from the putamen, leading to inappropriate sensorimotor coordination in the cerebral cortex. Affects cranial nerves (oculogyric crisis, etc.) and muscles (opisthotonus and laryngospasm)
Mental status and psychiatric aspects/ complications	Often preceded by anxiety; unclear if it acts as trigger or is a prodromal symptom
	Can be mistaken for functional neurologic symptom disorder or malingering

Secondary Complications: Laryngospasm may require intubation and may lead to hypoxic brain injury or death if not treated appropriately.

Treatment Complications: Prophylaxis with anticholinergic agents is important in patients being given intramuscular haloperidol, particularly those naïve to antipsychotics. Patients whose condition necessitates isolation require prophylaxis to prevent laryngospasm.

Avoid prolonged use of prophylactic agents given their potential for abuse and anticholinergic side effects, which may be compounded in psychotic patients. Constipation may cause a bowel obstruction. Dry mouth in psychotic patients may be exacerbated and cause oral candidiasis in the setting of poor hygiene.

Bibliography

Ayd FJ Jr. A survey of drug-induced extrapyramidal reactions. *JAMA*. 1961;175:1054–60.

Chaudhuri KR, Ondo WG, Logishetty K, Redyy P, Sherman R. Other movement disorders. In Chaudhuri KR, Ondo WG, eds. *Handbook of movement disorders*. London: Current Medicine Group; 2009. pp. 89–92.

Greene PE. Tardive and neuroleptic-induced emergencies. In Frucht SJ, ed. *Movement disorder emergencies: diagnosis and treatment*. 2nd ed. New York: Springer; 2013. pp. 141–49.

Horn S. Drug induced movement disorders. *Continuum (Minneap Minn)*. 2004;10(3):142–53.

Rosebush PI, Mazurek MF. Acute drug induced dystonia. In Factor S, Lang A, Weiner W, eds. *Drug induced movement disorders*. 2nd ed. Malden, MA: Wiley-Blackwell; 2008. pp. 72–102.

Early Myoclonic Encephalopathy (EME)

Epidemiology and Demographics: Early myoclonic encephalopathy (EME) is rare. Onset either in the neonatal period or the first months of life. Affects both sexes equally.

Disorder Description: Essential clinical features are neonatal encephalopathy associated with erratic and fragmentary myoclonus, usually involving the face or extremities. Can be limited to a finger, the eyebrows, or lips occurring in the same muscle group and then migrating elsewhere in an asynchronous and asymmetric manner. May occur as soon as a few hours after birth. Other types of seizures can occur, including subtle focal seizures, massive myoclonia, and later, tonic spasms.

Etiology believed to be multifactorial, mainly due to metabolic abnormalities (non-ketotic hyperglycinemia, d-glyceric acidemia, propionic aciduria, molybdenum cofactor deficiency, pyridoxine deficiency, methylmalonic acidemia, sulfite oxidase deficiency, Menkes disease, and Zellweger syndrome). Genes associated with EME are ErbB4, PIGA, SETBP1, SIK1, and SLC25A22.

EEG is characterized by burst-suppression with bursts of spikes, sharp waves, and slow waves, disrupted by periods of electrical silence. More distinct during sleep. Myoclonia may not show EEG correlation. After 3–5 months of life, pattern generally evolves into atypical hypsarrhythmia or multifocal epileptiform abnormalities.

Prognosis poor. More than half die within weeks or months of onset. Patients with non-ketotic hyperglycinemia may benefit from a ketogenic diet.

Symptoms

Localization site	Comment
Cerebral hemispheres	Erratic, fragmentary, or massive myoclonus. Focal seizures, tonic spasms
Mental status and psychiatric aspects/complications	Severe delay in psychomotor acquisitions, disturbed alertness, vegetative state
Peripheral neuropathy	Peripheral neuropathy (rare)
Muscle	Marked hypotonia

Secondary Complications: Symptoms of epileptic encephalopathy in the neonate may include emesis, abdominal distention, apnea, irritability, sleeplessness, and abnormal eye movements. Hypoglycemia and lactic acidosis have been described. Nutritional deficiencies due to inability to eat, requiring tube feeding.

Treatment Complications: The ketogenic diet is associated with anorexia, growth restriction, and metabolic acidosis.

Bibliography

Beal JC, Cherian K, Moshe SL. Early-onset epileptic encephalopathies: Ohtahara syndrome and early myoclonic encephalopathy. *Pediatr Neurol.* 2012;47(5):317–23.

Khan S, Al Baradie R. Epileptic encephalopathies: an overview. *Epilepsy Res Treat.* 2012;2012:403592.

McTague A, Howell KB, Cross JH, Kurian MA, Scheffer IE. The genetic landscape of the epileptic encephalopathies of infancy and childhood. *Lancet Neurol.* 2016;15(3):304–16.

Eastern Equine Encephalitis Virus (EEE)

Epidemiology and Demographics: Eastern equine encephalitis (EEE) is generally more prevalent in the southeastern United States but has recently extended further north on the eastern US coast (New Hampshire, Maine) and into Canada.[1,2] According to the US Centers for Disease Control and Prevention, from 1964 to 2004 there were 220 confirmed human cases of EEE.

Disorder Description: EEE is a mosquito-borne arboviral infection and is probably the most virulent of the encephalitic alphaviruses, with a mortality rate of 50–70%. EEE virus transmission occurs most commonly in and around freshwater hardwood swamps and between birds and mosquitoes (*Culiseta melanura*). The principal arthropod vectors for EEE transmission to humans or to horses are *Aedes*, *Coquillettidia*, and *Culex* species, which tend to feed on both birds and mammals.[1] Transmission of the virus occurs from summer to early fall and depends on weather conditions of the specific forested swamp habitat where the main mosquito vector resides. MRI is highly sensitive for the central nervous system manifestations of EEE, with a predilection for early involvement of the basal ganglia, thalami, and brainstem. Lesions are best demonstrated on T2-weighted images, appearing as areas of increased signal intensity and on fluid-attenuated inversion recovery images.[3] The diagnosis of EEE requires specific serologic findings or the demonstration of the virus in cerebrospinal fluid or brain tissue. High initial white cell counts in cerebrospinal fluid and the development of severe hyponatremia during hospitalization prognosticate a poor outcome.

Symptoms[4]

Localization site	Comment
Cerebral hemispheres	Fever, headache, somnolence, confusion, seizures, stupor, coma, and focal weakness
	Site of anatomic abnormality: basal ganglia, thalamus, brainstem, cortex, periventricular area, meninges, hydrocephalus
Mental status and psychiatric aspects/ complications	Altered mental state
Cranial nerves	Oculomotor, cranial nerves VII and XII

Secondary Complications: Hyponatremia prognosticates a poor outcome[3] and may be associated with its own central nervous system complications such as altered mentation.

Treatment Complications: Treatment is mostly supportive and involves managing individual specific symptoms.

References

1. Zacks MA, Paessler S. Encephalitic alphaviruses. *Vet Microbiol.* 2010;140:1–9.
2. Amstrong PM, Andrealis TG. Eastern equine encephalitis virus: old enemy, new threat. *N Engl J Med.* 2013;368:1670–3.
3. Deresiewicz RL, Thaler SJ, HSU L, Zamani AA. Clinical and neuroradiographic manifestations of Eastern equine encephalitis. *N Engl J Med.* 1997;336:1867–74.
4. Hirsh MS, DeMara A, Schaefer PW, Branda JA. Case 22–2008: a 52-year-old woman with fever and confusion. *N Engl J Med.* 2008;359: 294–303.

Echinococcosis

Epidemiology and Demographics: Echinococcosis is highly endemic in pastoral communities in South America, the Mediterranean, Eastern Europe, the Near and Middle East, East Africa, Central Asia, China, and Russia. It is an important public health concern in parts of central and Eastern Europe, the Near East, Russia, China, and Northern Japan according to the World Heath Organization. In the United States, most infections are diagnosed in immigrants from endemic countries, although sporadic indigenous transmission has been found in Alaska, California, Utah, Arizona, and New Mexico.[1]

Disorder Description: Echinococcosis is a parasitic zoonosis caused by larval forms of *Echinococcus* (E) tapeworms. Among the six species of E identified, *E. granulosus* and *E. multilocularis*, which cause cystic echinococcosis (CE) and alveolar echinococcosis (AE), respectively, are of major clinical significance.[1–3]

Cystic echinococcosis. CE cysts occur in liver and lung, or both organs in more than 90% of the cases; the kidney, spleen, heart, bone, and central nervous system are less often involved. Small cysts are often asymptomatic, and due to the slow growth of the parasite, most cases are diagnosed in adults. Clinical features of CE depend on the infected organs, the size and position of the cysts, their effects on the organ and adjacent tissues, and complications arising from the rupture of the cysts inducing systemic immunologic reactions. Hepatic echinococcosis causes hepatic enlargement, right epigastric pain, nausea, and vomiting. When cysts rupture in the liver, mild or fatal anaphylaxis occurs. When cysts rupture in the lung, the membranes can serve as a nidus for bacterial or fungal infections.

Alveolar echinococcosis. AE occurs as a result of infection by the larval form of *E. multilocularis* from contact with dogs that have eaten infected rodents. The liver is the primary location in humans with local extension of the lesion and metastases to lungs and brain. Symptoms may be initially vague and then progress to epigastric pain with hepatomegaly, obstructive jaundice, and hepatic failure. Invasion to contiguous structures and metastases to the brain may occur.

Diagnosis of both CE and AE is based on clinical findings and imaging, including ultrasonography, CT scan, MRI, and serology.

Symptoms[4-6]

Localization site	Comment
Cerebral hemispheres	Increased intracranial pressure with a slowly growing mass, changes in level of consciousness, headache, vomiting, papilledema, hemiparesis, visual changes, aphasia, tremor, sensory changes, and meningeal signs
Brainstem	Cranial nerve palsies
Cranial nerves	Cranial nerve palsies
Spinal cord	Spinal cord involvement secondary to extension of the vertebral body disease and invasion into the spinal canal. Radicular pain, motor and sensory deficits, and changes in bladder function are the primary findings
Basal skull	Intraocular and intraorbital cysts are rare and present with pain, exophthalmos

Treatment Complications: Treatment options include surgery, percutaneous sterilization, drugs, and observation.[1-3] Benzimidazoles may cause dizziness and very rarely seizures, headache, or mood changes.

References

1. Moro P, Schantz PM. Echinococcosis: a review. *Int J Infect Dis*. 2009;13:125–33.
2. McManus DP, Gray DJ, Zhand W, Yang Y. Diagnosis, treatment, and management of echinococcosis. *BMJ*. 2012;344(1):13.
3. Brunetti E, Kern P, Vuitton DA. Expert consensus for the diagnosis and treatment of cystic and alveolar echinococcosis in humans. *Acta Tropica*. 2010;114: 1–16.
4. Kammerer WS. Echinococcosis affecting the central nervous system. *Semin Neurol*. 1993;13(2):144–7.
5. Neumayr A, Tamarozzi F, Goblirsch S, Blum J, Brunetti E. Spinal cystic echinococcosis – A systematic analysis and review of the literature: Part 1. Epidemiology and Anatomy. *PLoS Negl Trop Dis*. 2013:7(9):e2450. DOI:10.1371/journal.pntd.0002450.
6. Neumayr A, Tamarozzi F, Goblirsch S, Blum J, Brunetti E. Spinal cystic echinococcosis – A systematic analysis and review of the literature: Part 2. Treatment, follow-up and outcome. *PLoS Negl Trop Dis*. 2013;7(9):e2458. DOI:10.1371/journal.pntd.0002458.

Echovirus

Epidemiology and Demographics: Echovirus infections occur worldwide with peak incidence in the summer and fall in temperate climates and throughout the year in subtropical and tropical regions. Children are predominantly affected. The risk factors are lower socioeconomic status, large household size, crowded living conditions, and residency in urban areas or areas with poor sanitation.

Disorder Description: Echoviruses (ECHO: enteric cytopathogenic human organ) belong to the genus *Enterovirus* of the family Picornaviridae. They are small, non-enveloped viruses with a single-stranded positive-sense RNA genome. Transmission occurs via the fecal–oral route and less frequently via respiratory droplets, and the incubation period ranges from 2 to 10 days.[1] Most echovirus infections are asymptomatic, and the most common clinical presentation is an acute nonspecific febrile illness. Other clinical syndromes include respiratory disease, diarrhea, hepatic disturbance, exanthems and enanthems, conjunctivitis, pericarditis, myocarditis, aseptic meningitis, and encephalitis. Echoviruses are a major cause of aseptic meningitis in infants and young children. In a recent study, **echoviruses E9, E11, and E30** accounted for 60 out of the 92 cases of enteroviral aseptic meningitis; while in another study 163 out of 170 samples were identified as belonging to **species B enteroviruses consisting of echoviruses and coxsackievirus B.**[2] Echovirus 30 alone was responsible for 25.3% of the cases. Echoviruses 4, 5, 9, 11, 19, and 30 were identified as the causative organism in many cases of encephalitis.

Symptoms[3,4]

Localization site	Comment
Cerebral hemispheres	Aseptic meningitis: fever, neck stiffness, irritation
	Encephalitis: lethargy, altered sensorium, coma
Mental status and psychiatric aspects/complications	Altered sensorium, coma, lethargy
Brainstem	Ataxia, tremor, myoclonic jerks, oculomotor (nystagmus, strabismus, gaze paresis)

Localization site	Comment
	Bulbar palsy (dysphagia, dysarthria, dysphonia, and facial weakness)
Cerebellum	Tremor and ataxia
Cranial nerves	Oculomotor problems and bulbar palsy

Secondary Complications: Brainstem encephalitis caused by enteroviruses including echovirus can trigger rapidly progressive sympathetic hyperactivity, pulmonary edema and/or pulmonary hemorrhage, and cardiopulmonary collapse. Early recognition and aggressive supportive care including ventilation and fluid management are essential for survival.

References

1. Pathogen Regulation Directorate, Public Health Agency of Canada. Echovirus; 2011. www.canada.ca/en/public-health/services/laboratory-biosafety-biosecurity/pathogen-safety-data-sheets-risk-assessment/echovirus-pathogen-safety-data-sheet.html. Accessed Aug 15, 2018.
2. Holmes CW, Koo SSF, Osman H, et al. Predominance of enterovirus B and echovirus 30 as cause of viral meningitis in a UK population. *J Clin Virol*. 2016;81:90–3.
3. Jain S, Patel B, Bhatt GC. Enterovirus encephalitis in children: clinical features, pathophysiology, and treatment advances. *Pathog Glob Health*. 2014;108:216–22.
4. Dalwai A, Ahmad S, Al-Nakib W. Echoviruses are a major cause of aseptic meningitis in infants and young children in Kuwait. *Virol J*. 2010;7:236–41.

Eclampsia

Epidemiology and Demographics: Eclampsia is defined as generalized convulsions in women with pre-eclampsia. Thought to be the end-stage progression of pre-eclampsia. Occurs in 1–3/1000 women. The maternal mortality rate for eclampsia is 2–3 cases/10,000 births in Europe and North America and 16–69 cases/10,000 births in developing countries. Pregnant women over 35 years or younger than 17 years are at greater risk for eclampsia.

Predisposing factors are the same as for pre-eclampsia. The strongest risk factors are pre-existing vascular diseases. Antiphospholipid antibody syndrome carries the highest risk with 17% of affected women developing pre-eclampsia during pregnancy. Other strong risk factors in order of impact include pre-eclampsia in previous pregnancies, which increases the risk seven-fold from expected, pre-existing chronic hypertension, obesity, vascular disorders (such as renal disease) or gestational diabetes, multifetal pregnancy, older age at pregnancy, family history of pre-eclampsia, and nulliparity.

Disorder Description: Pre-eclampsia is a necessary prerequisite to eclampsia. The progression to eclampsia cannot be reliably predicted and occurs in 1/200 pre-eclampsia patients. Unaddressed pre-eclampsia may be present for a variable time, then may suddenly progress to eclampsia. Untreated eclampsia is usually fatal.

The brain injury in eclampsia is associated with cerebral edema and characteristic white matter changes of reversible posterior leukoencephalopathy syndrome, which is similar to findings noted in hypertensive encephalopathy. In addition to clinical findings, brain MRI should be undertaken to rule out hemorrhage or stroke in addition to edema. (See entry for *Pre-eclampsia* for more details regarding pathophysiology.)

Headache and visual disturbances with occipital lobe edema are common symptoms of eclamptic encephalopathy. The subcortical white matter of the occipital lobes is the most involved site for hyperperfusion and edema of eclampsia, although gray matter and anterior circulation may be involved with progressive severity. Seizure type may be focal or generalized. Other non-seizure neurologic symptoms can be decreased level of consciousness, confusion, or focal cognitive deficits such as aphasia.

Symptoms

Localization site	Comment
Neuromuscular junction	Hyperreflexia
Cerebral vasculature	Headaches, blurred vision, confused or altered mental status

Secondary Complications: Cerebrovascular complications, including stroke and cerebral hemorrhage, are responsible for the majority of eclampsia-related deaths.

Treatment Complications: Management of the neurologic symptoms of eclampsia includes rapid lowering of blood pressure, administration of magnesium sulfate ($MgSO_4$), and delivery of the fetus. $MgSO_4$ is the most effective treatment for eclampsia and for prevention of eclampsia in patients with severe pre-eclampsia. $MgSO_4$ is given as a 4-g dose, followed by a maintenance infusion of 1–2 g/hour by controlled infusion pump, with a maximum dose of approximately 23 g or until patellar reflexes are lost. Treatment with standard antiseizure medications should be undertaken if seizures persist.

Adverse effects of magnesium sulfate include nausea, diarrhea or vomiting, low blood pressure, irregular heartbeat, headache, and muscle aches. Magnesium exposure in utero is associated with low muscle tone and relatively lower than expected Apgar scores in newborns; however, there is no evident effect on longer term outcomes (see entry for *Pre-eclampsia*).

Bibliography

Cipolla MJ, Kraig RP. Seizures in women with preeclampsia: mechanisms and management. *Fetal Matern Med Rev.* 2011; 22(2):91–108.

Duley L. The global impact of pre-eclampsia and eclampsia. *Semin Perinatol.* 2009;33(3): 130–7.

Sibai BM. Diagnosis, prevention, and management of eclampsia. *Obstet Gynecol.* 2005;105(2):402–10.

Ecstasy (methylenedioxymethamphetamine, MDMA)

Disorder Description: Users of this amphetamine derivate drug experience a sense of euphoria, loss of inhibition, a feeling of closeness and/or empathy, and increased sensuality. Common recreational drug used in raves, bars, and clubs around the world; also known by the street name "molly."

Epidemiology and Demographics: White males are predominant users. Majority of users are 16–24 years old. There are rare cases of use in people in their fifth and sixth decades.

Symptoms

Localization site	Comment
Cerebral hemispheres	Cerebral atrophy (chronic)
	Cerebral ischemia (acute)
	Cerebral hemorrhage (acute)
	Cerebral venous thrombosis (acute)
	Seizures (acute)
Mental status and psychiatric aspects/ complications	Increase in impulsivity with poor decision making (acute and chronic)
	Depression (chronic)
	Hallucinations (acute)
	Anxiety (acute)
	Paranoia (acute)
	Panic attacks (acute)
	Coma (acute)
Brainstem	Dyresgulation
Cerebellum	Gait ataxia (acute)
Anterior horn cells	Hypertonia (acute)
Muscle	Rhabdomyolysis (acute)
	Chorea (acute)
	Hypertonia (acute)
Neuromuscular junction	Increase in dopamine and serotonin toxicity (risk for serotonin syndrome) (acute and chronic)

Secondary Complications: Indirectly:
- **Cardiovascular effects:** Dysregulation of heart rate and blood pressure, and dysrhythmias can result in strokes.
- **Hepatic complications:**
  - Acute liver failure may result in brain edema, amplified by hypoglycemia, hypoxia, and seizures.
  - Severe fatigue, cognitive dysfunction, and mood disorder.
- **Hematologic complications** – Disseminated intravascular coagulation leading to cerebral infarction.

- **Endocrinological complications:**
  - MDMA-induced syndrome of inappropriate antidiuretic hormone secretion leads to increase in cerebral edema with subsequent neurologic complications.
  - Hyperthermia dysregulation can lead to rhabdomyolysis.

Bibliography

Hahn I-H. MDMA toxicity. *Medscape*. Updated Dec 20, 2017. http://emedicine.medscape.com/article/821572-overview#a6. Accessed Aug 7, 2018.

Holland J, ed. *Ecstasy: The complete guide: A comprehensive look at the risks and benefits of MDMA*. Rochester, VT: Inner Traditions/Bear; 2001.

Quednow BB, Kühn K-U, Hoppe C, et al. Elevated impulsivity and impaired decision-making cognition in heavy users of MDMA ("Ecstasy"). *Psychopharmacology*. 2007;189:517. https://doi.org/10.1007/s00213-005-0256-4.

Wiegand T, Thai D, Benowitz N. Medical consequences of the use of hallucinogens: LSD, mescaline, PCP, and MDMA ("Ecstasy"). In Brick J, ed. *Handbook of the medical consequences of alcohol and drug abuse*. 2nd ed. New York: Routledge; 2008. p. 461.

Ehler–Danlos Syndrome (EDS)

Epidemiology and Demographics: Ehler–Danlos syndrome (EDS) is a group of relatively rare genetic disorders of connective tissue. Overall frequency is 1/5000.

Disorder Description: EDS is characterized by hyperextensible skin, joint hypermobility, and tissue fragility. The collagen disorder predisposes to extracranial artery dissections.

Symptoms

Localization site	Comment
Cerebral hemispheres	Thunderclap headache (associated with aneurysmal subarachnoid hemorrhage); seizure, hemiparesis, hemisensory loss, hemianopia related to intracranial or cervical dissection
Mental status and psychiatric aspects/complications	Altered level of consciousness or focal cognitive deficits in subarachnoid hemorrhage and intracerebral hemorrhage

Localization site	Comment
Cerebellum	Ataxia
Cranial nerves	Optic atrophy, deafness, Horner's syndrome (in the setting of carotid dissection)
Spinal cord	Weakness, numbness, gait difficulties, bowel and bladder incontinence (Kyphoscoliosis)
Peripheral neuropathy	Numbness and weakness
Muscle	Myotonia

Bibliography

Caplan LR, Van Gijn J. Clinical manifestations and diagnosis of Ehler-Danlos syndrome. UpToDate. Updated Jun 13, 2018. www.uptodate.com/contents/clinical-manifestations-and-diagnosis-of-ehlers-danlos-syndromes. Accessed Aug 15, 2018.

Ehrlichiosis

Epidemiology and Demographics: The incidence of human monocytotropic ehrlichiosis (HME) caused by *Ehrlichia chaffeensis* in the United States is estimated at 0.7 cases per million population with a geographic distribution in the Southeast, South Central, and Midwest states. The vector is the lone star tick, *Amblyomma*.

Human granulocytic anaplasmosis (HGA), previously known as human granulocytic ehrlichiosis (HGE), has an estimated incidence of 1.6 cases per million in the United States with a geographic distribution in Northern California, and Northeastern and North Central States. It is caused by *Anaplasma phagocytophilum*, and the vector is *Ixodes*.

The epidemiology of human ewingii ehrlichiosis (HEE) is poorly defined with geographic distributions in Southeast, South Central, and Midwestern United States. Its vector is the lone star tick *Amblyomma*. HEE infections are reported in patients with the human immunodeficiency virus or organ transplantation.

The median age of both HGE and HGA is 51 years, with more than 95% of cases reported in Caucasians and a slight male predominance.[1]

Disorder Description: HME is a severe acute febrile tick-borne disease caused by *Ehrlichia chaffeensis*, an obligate intracellular bacterial pathogen with gram-negative cell wall structure. HME can manifest as a multisystem disease resembling toxic or septic shock syndrome, cardiovascular failure, aseptic meningitis, hemorrhage, hepatic failure, and adult respiratory distress syndrome. Central nervous system (CNS) involvement occurs in 20% of HME patients, manifesting as meningitis or encephalitis, seizures, and coma.

HGA caused by *Anaplasma phagocytophilum* is a less severe illness than HME, although severe complications may include acute respiratory distress syndrome, acute renal failure, and hemodynamic collapse. Meningoencephalitis is the most common CNS involvement but is reported in only 1% of cases. Peripheral neuropathies, including brachial plexopathy, demyelinating polyneuropathy, and bilateral facial nerve palsy, have been reported in 10% of cases.

HEE occurs mainly in immunocompromised hosts, and its clinical manifestation is milder than that for HME and HGA. It has been associated with meningitis. Headache is a frequent symptom. Neurologic manifestation is not well defined.

Diagnosis of HME and HGA is based primarily on clinical suspicion. PCR is not available for rapid diagnosis, and detection of antibody does not occur at the time of presentation. Empirical therapy with doxycycline once suspected, otherwise prognosis worsens. Diagnosis can be confirmed by serologic detection of specific antibodies, detection of ehrlichial DNA by PCR, detection of morulae in peripheral blood or CSF, and isolation of bacteria. PCR is the only definitive diagnostic test for HEE because the bacteria are unculturable.[1]

Symptoms[2]

Localization site	Comment
Cerebral hemispheres	Meningitis or meningoencephalitis occurs in nearly 20% of patients with HME
	Seizures and coma can occur in HME
	Rare cases of meningitis with HGA
Mental status and psychiatric aspects/ complications	Cognitive delays have been reported in children with HME
Brainstem	Cranial nerve palsy complications rare

Localization site	Comment
Cranial nerves	Cranial nerve palsies with HGA
Plexus	Brachial plexopathy in HGA
Peripheral neuropathy	Demyelinating polyneuropathy with HGA

Secondary Complications: Both HME and HGA are multisystem diseases resembling septic shock syndrome. Cardiovascular failure, hemorrhage, hepatic failure, and adult respiratory distress syndrome occur, especially in HME. Meningitis or meningoencephalitis and other neurologic complications occur in 20% of patients with HME, while peripheral neuropathies occur more in HGA.[1]

Treatment Complications: Doxycycline may cause headache.

References

1. Ismail N, Bloch K, McBride JW. Human ehrlichiosis and anaplasmosis. *Clin Lab Med.* 2010;30:261–92.
2. Ratnasamy N, Everett ED, Roland WE, McDonald G, Caldwell C. Central nervous system manifestations of human ehrlichiosis. *Clin Infect Dis.* 1996;23:314–9.

Electrical Status Epilepticus in Sleep (ESES, CSWS)

Epidemiology and Demographics: Electrical status epilepticus in sleep (ESES) is uncommon, accounting for approximately 0.5–1% of childhood epilepsies. Onset in early to mid childhood, with improvements in seizures and plateauing of neuropsychologic decline sometimes occurring near puberty.

Disorder Description: Nearly continuous slow spike and wave discharges emerging in non-REM sleep, resulting in an epileptic encephalopathy associated with seizures and neuropsychologic regression. Symptoms of varying severity along a spectrum, with continuous spikes and waves during sleep (CSWS) syndrome being the more severe, but features that may overlap with Landau–Kleffner syndrome (see entry for *Landau–Kleffner Syndrome*) occurring with more focal symptoms involving language. CSWS is associated with more widespread or multifocal epileptiform discharges, frequent seizures, and global developmental regression. Early developmental lesions, including thalamic lesions or polymigrogyria, may be an important etiological factor though idiopathic forms have been described.

Antiepileptic drugs (such as valproate, ethosuximide, levetiracetam), high-dose benzodiazepines (diazepam, clonazepam, clobazam), and immunomodulatory therapy with steroids and intravenous immunoglobulin are commonly used. Surgery has been done for cases associated with focal epileptiform abnormalities, and early developmental lesions.

Longer duration ESES and early developmental lesions typically associated with a more severe prognosis.

Symptoms

Localization site	Comment
Cerebral hemispheres	Seizures of varying severity and type (partial motor, absence, generalized tonic–clonic seizures). Tonic seizures unusual. EEG centrotemporal or frontal maximal spikes during wakefulness with more broadly distributed sleep potentiated 1.5- to 3-Hz slow spike and wave activity. Deterioration of gross and fine motor skills may occur
Mental status and psychiatric aspects/ complications	Intellectual decline of varying severity, with global regression. May include progressive and fluctuant aphasia, inattention, short-term memory issues, emotional lability, anxiety and depression, reductions in IQ. Learning disorders, visuospatial impairments are also common
Cerebellum	Ataxia, incoordination

Secondary Complications: Behavioral and cognitive deterioration with developmental regression is common.

Treatment Complications: Antiepileptic drugs (AEDs) may be associated with a number of idiosyncratic reactions including multiorgan dysfunction, mood changes, and negative cognitive effects. AEDs such as phenytoin, carbamazepine, oxcarbazepine, and phenobarbital may exacerbate ESES and are typically avoided. Benzodiazepines are associated with sedation, respiratory depression, and confusion. Steroids are associated with an increased risk for mood lability, psychosis, peptic ulceration, avascular necrosis, and infection. IVIG may be associated with flu-like symptoms during infusion and rarely anaphylaxis.

Bibliography

Hughes JR. A review of the relationships between Landau-Kleffner syndrome, electrical status epilepticus during sleep, and continuous spike-waves during sleep. *Epilepsy Behav.* 2011;20(2):247–53.

Sanchez Fernandez I, Loddenkemper T, Peters JM, Kothare SV. Electrical status epilepticus in sleep: clinical presentation and pathophysiology. *Pediatr Neurol.* 2012;47(6):390–410.

Electroconvulsive Therapy (ECT)

Epidemiology and Demographics: A survey of US practices indicated use of electroconvulsive therapy (ECT) on 100,000 patients per year between 1988 and 1989, although use has declined since then. ECT is used worldwide; however, one study showed a trend toward use for older women with depression in Western cultures and younger men with schizophrenia in Asia.

Description: ECT is a procedure that uses delivery of localized electrical current to the brain to produce seizure activity. ECT is used to treat medication-resistant depression, bipolar disorder, schizophrenia, neuroleptic malignant syndrome, and catatonia. Exact mechanism for its benefit in these conditions is unknown. Patients must have a pre-procedure medical evaluation to determine the presence of comorbid cardiopulmonary and neurologic conditions, which may be affected by the hemodynamic changes caused by seizures.

Symptoms

Localization site	Comment
Cerebral hemispheres	Iatrogenically produced generalized seizure activity (cortex)
Mental status and psychiatric aspects/ complications	Improves symptoms of depression, mania, psychosis, catatonia, neuroleptic malignant disorder Adverse effects: acute confusion, anterograde or retrograde memory loss

Secondary Complications: Headache, nausea, and myalgias are common. Muscle relaxation with medications such as succinylcholine is important to prevent fractures, particularly in those with osteoporosis. Acute post-procedure confusion and both anterograde and retrograde memory loss can also occur. These are transient and most resolve within days but can last up to 2 weeks following treatment. The use of lithium can worsen cognitive side effects, therefore is contraindicated.

Bibliography

Hermann RC, Dorwart RA, Hoover CW, Brody J. Variation in ECT use in the United States. *Am J Psychiatry*. 1995;152:869.

Leiknes KA, Jarosh-von Schweder L, Høie B. Contemporary use and practice of electroconvulsive therapy worldwide. *Brain Behav*. 2012;2(3):283–344. DOI:10.1002/brb3.37.

Semkovska M, McLoughlin DM. Objective cognitive performance associated with electroconvulsive therapy for depression: a systematic review and meta-analysis. *Biol Psychiatry*. 2010;68:568.

Empty Sella Syndrome

Epidemiology and Demographics: True frequency is unknown as the condition may be undiagnosed due to its asymptomatic nature. Seen mostly in middle-aged women who are obese and hypertensive.[1] In children empty sella is more likely to be associated with clinical symptoms and endocrinopathies.[2]

Disorder Description: In this disorder the sella turcica is partially or completely filled with cerebrospinal fluid. Primary empty sella syndrome occurs as a result of pressure on the pituitary gland causing it to flatten or shrink. Secondary empty sella syndrome occurs as a result of intrinsic injury to the pituitary gland. Many individuals are asymptomatic.

Symptoms

Localization site	Comment
Cerebral hemispheres	Chronic headaches, unclear if due to empty sella syndrome or a coincidental finding. Many individuals with pseudotumor cerebri have an empty sella
Cranial nerves	Papilledema and decreased visual acuity
Pituitary gland	Decreased function

Treatment Complications: Treatment may not be required. If treatment is indicated, adverse effects may be associated with the specific hormone replacement that is administered.

References

1. National Organization for Rare Disorders. Empty sella syndrome. Available from http://rarediseases.org/rare-diseases/empty-sella-syndrome/. Accessed Dec 17, 2015.
2. Lenz AM, Root AW. Empty sella syndrome. *Pediatr Endocrinol Rev*. 2012;9(4):710–15. Review.

Encephalitis

Epidemiology and Demographics: Worldwide, the incidence of encephalitis varies from 0.07 to 12.6 cases per 100,000 with decreasing incidence over time. Encephalitis affects patients of all ages and in all parts of the world.[1]

Disorder Description: Encephalitis is a severe neurologic syndrome involving inflammation of the brain manifested by current or recent febrile illness with altered behavior, cognition, personality or consciousness, new onset seizures, or new focal neurologic signs.[1]

Four subclinical syndromes represent the encephalitic syndrome etiologically:

1. Unspecified encephalitis/meningoencephalitis;
2. Infectious encephalitis (viral or bacterial);
3. Immune-mediated encephalitis;
4. Infectious and immune-mediated encephalitis.

More than 50% of patients belonging to the unspecified encephalitis/meningoencephalitis category have no known cause. However, it is suspected that most are either secondary to unidentified viral or bacterial infections or to immune-mediated encephalitis. The most common global causes of infectious encephalitis (viral or bacterial) are herpes simplex virus (HSV), varicella zoster virus (VZV), enteroviruses, measles, mumps, Japanese encephalitis virus, influenza, adenovirus, *Mycoplasma*, and other less common agents.

Immune-mediated encephalitis[2,3] is characterized by antibodies against intracellular antigens (HU[ANNA1, Ma2, GAD]), antibodies against synaptic receptors (NMDA receptors, AMPA receptor, GABA receptor, mGluR5, dopamine 2 receptor), and antibodies against ion channel and other cell-surface proteins (LGI1, CASPR2, DPPX, and MOG). Immune-mediated encephalitis should be suspected when all three of the following criteria are met:

1. Subacute onset of working memory deficits, altered mental status, or psychiatric symptoms.

2. At least one of the following:
   a. New focal central nervous system (CNS) findings;
   b. Seizures not explained by a previously known seizure disorder;
   c. Cerebrospinal fluid (CSF) pleocytosis;
   d. MRI features suggestive of encephalitis.
3. Reasonable exclusion of viral and bacterial encephalitis.

Infectious and immune-mediated encephalitis have been grouped under the rubric of acute disseminated encephalomyelitis (ADEM). It is thought to be a final common pathway of autoimmune CNS injury triggered by viral agents such as enteroviruses, Epstein–Barr virus, human herpesvirus-6, parainfluenza, and bacteria such as *Mycoplasma pneumoniae*. Fifty percent to 70% of ADEM cases had a preceding history of infection manifested by fever, malaise, headache, and nausea.

All patients with encephalitis should undergo lumbar puncture and CSF investigations including opening pressure, total and differential white cell count, red cell count, culture and sensitivities for bacteria, protein and glucose. CT scan is not initially needed unless increased intracranial pressure is suspected.[4]

All patients with suspected encephalitis should undergo CSF PCR for HSV 1, VZV, and enteroviruses and further testing directed toward specific pathogens as guided by the clinical features, travel history, and animal and insect contact. MRI of the brain is the preferred imaging modality and should be performed as soon as possible especially if the diagnosis is uncertain. EEG can be performed to seek encephalitic changes and if subtle motor or non-convulsive seizures are suspected. Brain biopsy has no place in the initial evaluation of suspected acute viral encephalitis. Intravenous acyclovir should be started within 6 hours of admission if the initial CSF and/or imaging findings suggest viral encephalitis. Further workup for immune-mediated encephalitis should move forward if the infectious etiologies are ruled out. Corticosteroid (IV solumedrol) and intravenous immunoglobulin may be started if strongly suspected.

Symptoms

Localization site	Comment
Cerebral hemispheres	Altered mental status ranging from confusion, frank psychosis, or somnolence to stupor or coma
	Personality changes
	Seizures, speech dysfunction
	Movement disorder, dyskinesias
	Decreased level of consciousness
	Autonomic dysfunction or central hypoperfusion
Mental status and psychiatric aspects/ complications	Abnormal psychiatric behavior or cognitive deficits, memory loss
Brainstem	Bilateral external ophthalmoplegia
Cerebellum	Ataxia

Secondary Complications[5]: Cerebral edema is a strong predictor of mortality; however, a trend toward reduced death rates was observed in patients receiving ICP monitoring and hyperosmolar therapy. Status epilepticus and the presence of thrombocytopenia were strong markers of increased mortality in patients. Acyclovir is associated with nephrotoxicity. Kidney function is monitored, and hydration may prevent renal damage.

References

1. Granerod J, Tam CC, Crowcroft NS, et al. Challenge of the unknown: a systematic review of acute encephalitis in non-outbreak situations. *Neurology.* 2010;75:924–32.
2. Armangue T, Leypoldt F, Dalmau J. Auto-immune encephalitis as differential diagnosis of infectious encephalitis. *Curr Opin Neurol.* 2014;27(3):361–8.
3. Graus F, Titulaer MJ, Balu R, et al. A clinical approach to diagnosis of autoimmune encephalitis. *Lancet Neurol.* 2016;15(4):391–404.
4. Solomon T, Michael BD, Smith PE, et al. Management of suspected viral encephalitis in adults: Association of British Neurologists and British infection Association Guidelines. *J Infect.* 2012;64(4):347–73.
5. Thakur KT, Motta M, Asemota AO, et al. Predictor of outcome in acute encephalitis. *Neurology.* 2013;8(9):793–800.

Encephalitis Lethargica

Epidemiology and Demographics: Since the last epidemic in the 1920s, most cases of encephalitis lethargica (EL) have been sporadic. In a compilation of 20 new cases (9 females, 11 males), the age of onset ranged from 2 to 69 years old.[1]

Disorder Description: No known cause for EL has been found, although immune-mediated mechanisms have attracted wide interest. Anti-basal ganglia antibodies were found in 19 out of 20 cases in one study. The onset of the disease is acute to subacute to chronic. The main clinical features of EL may appear within hours or days. In some cases EL begins with general malaise, asthenia, subtle cranial nerve abnormalities, and behavioral changes for weeks and months before more obvious symptoms appear. More than half of the patients had upper respiratory tract infection and tonsillitis.

The predominant clinical features are sleep disturbance and lethargy, parkinsonism, dyskinesia, and psychiatric disturbance. Other features include profound reduction in consciousness, ocular abnormalities including ophthalmoplegia, ptosis, optic neuritis, seizures and memory loss, headache, meningism, incontinence, and limb pains.[1,2]

Symptoms[1,2]

Localization site	Comment
Cerebral hemispheres	Sleep disturbance and lethargy, profound reduction in consciousness, parkinsonism, dyskinesias, seizures
Mental status and psychiatric aspects/ complications	Psychiatric symptoms ranging from mutism, emotional disorders, depression, obsessive-compulsive disorder, anxiety, apathy and catatonia, feeling of euphoria, increased sexual drive
Brainstem	Ocular abnormalities ranging from ophthalmoplegia, ptosis, optic neuritis

Secondary Complications: Seventy percent of patients who recover from EL develop postencephalitic symptoms, which include parkinsonism, oculogyric crises, severe emotional changes, compulsive thoughts, other extrapyramidal disorders – dystonia, chorea, athetosis, myoclonus and disturbances of posture, and respiratory disturbances.[1]

References

1. Dale RC, Church AJ, Surtees RAH, et al. Encephalitis lethargica syndrome: 20 new cases and evidence of basal ganglia autoimmunity: *Brain*. 2004;127:21–33.
2. Cheyette SR, Cummings JL. Encephalitis lethargica: lessons for contemporary neuropsychiatry. *J Neuropsychiatry*. 1995;7:125–34.

Encopresis

Epidemiology and Demographics: Prevalence is 1–3% in ages 4–5 years. Male predominance.

Disorder Description: Encopresis is a type of elimination disorder characterized in the DSM-5 by the repeated inappropriate passage of feces in individuals of chronologic age 4 years or older (or corresponding developmental age). It consists of either voluntary or unintentional defecating in nondesignated places such as clothing or floor. Per criteria, the behavior must occur at least once a month for 3 months. The behavior is not better accounted for by a substance or medical condition other than constipation. Additional specification is made as to whether the behavior occurs in setting of constipation and overflow incontinence.

Encopresis is further described as primary (no previous achievement of fecal continence) versus secondary (regression to incontinence after a period of fecal continence). Risk factors include conditions that predispose to constipation.

Secondary Complications: Encopresis can affect a child's self-esteem and emotional well-being. Punishment by caregivers can further compound these issues.

Treatment Complications: Treatment involves evacuating the colon when constipation is a factor, behavioral interventions, and supportive therapy. No complications reported.

Bibliography

American Psychiatric Association. *Diagnostic and statistical manual of mental disorders: DSM-5.* 5th ed. Washington, DC: American Psychiatric Association; 2013.

Endocrine Myopathies

Epidemiology and Demographics: The age of presentation could be any time during the course of the endocrinopathy. Incidence, prevalence, and frequency are unknown due to the heterogeneous nature of the disease. Predominant age and sex depend on the specific cause of the endocrinopathy.

Disorder Description: Muscle may become affected at any time during the course of many endocrinopathies. The most common causes of endocrine myopathy are related to disturbance in thyroid, glucocorticoid, aldosterol, parathyroid, and insulin regulation with corticosteroid myopathy being the most common.

Symptoms

Localization site	Comment
Cerebral hemispheres	Poor cognition and ataxia may be present in hypoadrenalism while symptoms of increased intracranial pressure may be present in hyperadrenalism and hyperparathyroidism
Muscle	Commonly proximal muscle weakness and occasionally atrophy
	Bulbar and respiratory muscle weakness may occur with certain endocrinopathies
	Muscle stretch reflexes may be depressed yet present

Bibliography

Benvenga S, Toscano A, Rodolico C, et al. Endocrine evaluation for muscle pain. *J R Soc Med.* 2001;94(8):405–7.

Rodolico C, Toscano A, Benvenga S, et al. Myopathy as the persistently isolated symptomatology of primary autoimmune hypothyroidism. *Thyroid.* 1998;8(11):1033–8.

Ruff RL. Endocrine myopathies. In Engel AG, Banker BQ, eds. *Myology.* New York: McGraw Hill; 1986. p. 1871.

Siafakas NM, Alexopoulou C, Bouros D. Respiratory muscle function in endocrine diseases. *Monaldi Arch Chest Dis.* 1999;54(2):154–9.

Yu J. Endocrine disorders and the neurologic manifestations. *Ann Pediatr Endocrinol Metab.* 2014;19(4):184–90.

Endometriosis Ectopic Tissue

Epidemiology and Demographics: This is a rare disorder. The incidence is highest during the third and fourth decades, and it is usually seen in women who have fewer children and experience infertility.

Disorder Description: Endometriosis is presence of active ectopic endometrial glands and stroma outside of the uterus. The tissue may be present in the ovaries, pelvic peritoneum, appendix, colon, lungs, and, rarely, brain. Catamenial mononeuropathy and radiculopathy are a result of ectopic endometrial tissue causing compression on the peripheral nerves, most commonly the sciatic nerve. Patients present with cyclical neuropathic pain during menses. It is usually diagnosed radiologically and biopsy is required for confirmatory diagnosis. Treatment includes leuprolide acetate injections and oral contraceptives; however, pain may return upon stopping the medications. Laser ablation has also been curative. Extreme cases may require hysterectomy and oophorectomy.

Symptoms

Localization site	Comment
Specific spinal roots	May affect any spinal nerve roots, but most common is sciatic nerve compression
Plexus	Brachial or lumbosacral plexopathy
Peripheral neuropathy	Mainly due to compression. Cyclical bleeding may result in peripheral nerve damage

Secondary Complications: Endometriosis ectopic tissue may also be present in ovaries, pelvic peritoneum, appendix, and, rarely, in lung and brain. Symptoms are result of local tissue compression and bleeding complications.

Treatment Complications: Complications include hormonal side effects from medication use. If surgical treatment required, then surgical risk factors will also need to be considered including, but not limited to, infection at surgical site, bleeding, and associated anesthesia risk.

Bibliography

Zager J, Peeifer S, Brown MJ, Torosian MH, Hackney DB. Catamenial mononeuropathy and radiculopathy: a treatable neuropathic disorder. *J Neurosurg.* 1998;88;827–30.

Enterobacteriaceae

Epidemiology and Demographics: Enterobacteriaceae are common inhabitants of the intestinal microbiota of most animals and humans. They are found in water, soil, and decaying vegetation and are the most common gram-negative enteric pathogens of humans. They can breach the skin or mucous membranes and evade the immune system to cause disease and death in humans. In patients hospitalized in intensive care units (ICUs), the Enterobacteriaceae account for approximately one-third of all cases of ICU-acquired pneumonia, one-third of all cases of ICU-acquired urinary tract infection, and 10–15% of ICU-acquired bloodstream infections.

Disorder Description: The bacterial family Enterobacteriaceae has 53 genera, of which 26 are known to cause infections in humans. They are small gram-negative, nonsporing straight rods. Among the most medically important species of Enterobacteriaceae are *E. coli* and *Plesiomonas shigelloides*, and species of *Klebsiella, Enterobacter, Citrobacter, Proteus, Serratia, Shigella, Hafnia, Morganella,* and *Providencia*.[1] They are common causes of both community-acquired and hospital-acquired infections, including urinary tract, blood stream, and lower respiratory tract infections.[2] The primary therapeutic choice for the Enterobacteriaceae are β-lactam drugs and carbapenems, specifically used as antibiotics of last resort; however, the Enterobacteriaceae can develop multiple antibiotic resistance by acquiring genes that encode extended spectrum β-lactamases and carbapenemases, making these drugs ineffective. Antimicrobial resistance is a global health security threat as recognized by the World Health Organization. Not only is the mortality rate twice as high in patients with carbapenem-resistant Enterobacteriaceae bacteremia, but also the Centers for Disease Control and Prevention has estimated that antimicrobial resistance costs the United States $55 billion a year in direct healthcare costs and loss of productivity. Antimicrobial resistance among gram-negative bacteria has spread worldwide leaving clinicians with few therapeutic options. Understanding the mechanism of β-lactam and carbapenem resistance of gram-negative bacilli is of utmost importance to appreciate the epidemiology, treatment, and infection control. The Amber Classification categorizes the β-lactamases into four groups, and each group produces specific enzymes that inactivate the β-lactams. The carbapenem-resistant Enterobacteriaceae belong to three of the four groups of the Amber classification and produce carbapenemases that inactivate the carbapenems.[3] The risk factors for acquiring resistant gram-negative bacilli include prior and recent antibiotic use, residence in long-term facilities, admission into an ICU, presence of indwelling medical devices or wounds, **increased age**, solid organ or stem cell transplant, and travel to endemic areas. The optimal strategy is to take a proactive approach by combating antimicrobial resistance through infection, to detect resistant Enterobacteriaceae early through bacterial identification and susceptibility testing, to avoid careless use of antibiotics, and to treat the resistant Enterobacteriaceae through a combination of antibiotics.[4]

Symptoms[5]

Localization site	Comment
Cerebral hemispheres	Meningitis. Seizure, encephalopathy

Secondary Complications: Encephalopathy can occur in patients with urinary tract infections, pneumonia, and blood stream infections caused by the Enterobacteriaceae, especially in those who already have an underlying neurologic disorder.

Treatment Complications: Rare neurotoxicity (e.g., seizures or encephalopathy) of β-lactams.

References

1. Public Health England. Identification of Enterobacteriaceae. UK Standards forMicrobiology Investigations. ID 16, Issue 4. 2015. www.gov.uk/uk-standards-for-microbiology-investigations-smi-quality-and-consistency-in-clinical-laboratories.
2. Van Duin D, Doi Y. The global epidemiology of carbapenemase-producing Enterobacteriaceae. *Virulence.* 2017;8(4):460–9.
3. Vasoo S, Barreto JN, Tosh PK. Emerging issues in Gram-negative bacteria resistance: an update for the practicing clinician. *Mayo Clin Proc.* 2015;90:395–403.
4. Viale P, Giannella M, Tedeshi S, Lewis R. Treatment of MDR-Gram negative infections in the 21st century: a never ending threat for clinicians. *Curr Opin Pharmacol.* 2015;24:30–7.

5. Chang WN, Huang CR, Lu CH, Chien CC. Adult Klebsiella pneumoniae meningitis in Taiwan: an overview. *Acta Neurol Taiwan*. 2012;21:87–96.

Enteroviruses

Epidemiology and Demographics: Enteroviruses, some of the most common human viruses, infect an estimated 50 million people annually in the United States and more than a billion annually worldwide. Most infections are asymptomatic; however, enterovirus infections result in 30,000 to 50,000 hospitalizations per year in the United States.

Disorder Description: Enteroviruses are members of the Picornavirus family, a group of small nonenveloped viruses with a simple message sense RNA genome. The current taxonomy of the human enteroviruses consists of:

1. enterovirus-A(EV-A) group, which includes:
   a. coxsackievirus 6 (CVA6)
   b. coxsackievirus A16 (CVA16)
   c. enterovirus A71(EV-A71)
2. enterovirus-B (EV-B) group, which includes:
   a. coxsackievirus B1–B6 and 50 other serotypes
3. enterovirus-C (EV-C) group, which includes:
   a. three polioviruses and 20 other serotypes
4. enterovirus-D (EV-D) group, which includes:
   a. enterovirus D68, D70, D94, D111, D120.

Hand, foot, and mouth disease is caused by many enteroviruses, but most often by several of the EV-A species including CVA6 and CVA16, and EV-A71. There have been several outbreaks of EV-A71 where patients not only developed the hand, foot, and mouth disease, but also brainstem encephalitis and noncardiogenic pulmonary edema with a high mortality rate. Patients with EV-A71 who survived developed neurologic and neuropsychiatric sequelae.

Severe neonatal disease is caused by a recent outbreak of coxsackievirus B, a member of the EV-B species.

Acute flaccid myelitis is caused by EV-C105, a member of the EV-C. EV-D68, a member of the EV-D, was linked to clusters of severe respiratory illness and was also detected in a few patients with acute flaccid myelitis and in some patients with aseptic meningitis or encephalitis, and cranial nerve dysfunction.

Poliomyelitis results from destruction of motor neurons during infection with one of the three poliovirus serotypes. It occurs in about 1% of individuals infected with poliovirus. More commonly, polioviruses cause aseptic meningitis or mild nonspecific symptoms. Live-attenuated and inactivated poliovirus vaccines have almost eliminated the disease and provided immunity, except in very few areas of the world.

Aseptic meningitis is caused by enterovirus, which is its most common causative organism. It occurs mainly in the summer and fall in temperate climates and perennially in subtropical and tropical areas of the world. Its clinical course is usually benign. It is most common among infants under 3 months of age and presents with fever and irritability.

Encephalitis is a rare presentation of enterovirus infection although the prevalence can reach 21 to 22% in endemic regions or when the enterovirus is an aggressive neurotropic serotype. EV71 has been recognized as a causative organism in fatal brainstem encephalitis in Southeast Asian countries.

Symptoms

Localization site	Comment
Cerebral hemispheres	Aseptic meningitis, encephalitis, or meningoencephalitis
Mental status and psychiatric aspects/ complications	Visual hallucinations, changes in mental status, lethargy mostly secondary to encephalitis
Brainstem	Brainstem encephalitis; myoclonus
Cranial nerves	Cranial nerve dysfunction
Spinal cord	Acute flaccid myelitis
Anterior horn cells	Acute flaccid myelitis

Secondary Complications: Brainstem encephalitis caused by enterovirus can trigger rapidly progressive sympathetic hyperactivity, pulmonary edema and/or pulmonary hemorrhage, and cardiopulmonary collapse. Early recognition and aggressive supportive care including ventilation and fluid management are essential for survival.

Bibliography

Huang CC, Liu CC, Chang YC, et al. Neurologic complications in children with Enterovirus 71. *Infection*. 1999;41(13):936–42.

Jain S, Patel B, Bhatt GC. Enterovirus encephalitis in children: clinical features, pathophysiology, and treatment advances. *Pathog Glob Health.* 2014;108:216–22.

Lugo D, Krogstad P. Enteroviruses in the early 21st century: new manifestations and challenges. *Curr Opin Pediatr.* 2016;28:107–13.

Ooi MH, Wang S, Lewthwaite P, Cardosa MJ, Solomon T. Clinical features, diagnosis, and management of enterovirus 71. *Lancet Neurol.* 2010;9:1097–105.

Palacios G, Oberste MS. Enteroviruses as agents of emerging infectious diseases. *J Neurovirol.* 2005;11:424–33.

Enuresis

Epidemiology and Demographics: Bladder control is typically accomplished by 2–4 years of age. Prevalence of enuresis is variable based on criteria used. Prevalence for 5- to 7-year-olds is less than 10%, 10-year-olds less than 5%, and 15-year-olds or older 1%. High concordance multi-culturally. Most common in male gender.

Disorder Description: Enuresis is a type of elimination disorder characterized in the DSM-5 by the repeated inappropriate voiding of urine in individuals of chronologic age 5 years or older (or corresponding developmental age). Consists of either voluntary or unintentional voiding in non-designated places such as clothing or bed. Per criteria, the behavior must occur at least twice a week for 3 consecutive months. Alternatively, the behavior must occur in the context of clinically significant distress or functional impairment. The behavior is not better accounted for by a substance or medical condition. Additional specification is made as to whether the behavior occurs during sleep (most common), wakefulness, or both.

Further described as primary (no previous achievement of continence) versus secondary (regression to incontinence after a period of continence). It has a heritable, autosomal dominant predisposition and can be linked to disorders of sleep arousal, abnormalities in antidiuretic hormone secretion and receptor sensitivity, nocturnal polyuria, and low bladder capacity.

Symptoms

Localization site	Comment
Cerebral hemispheres	Abnormally low secretion of anti-diuretic hormone from hypothalamus may play a role
Mental status and psychiatric aspects/complications	Most are developmentally normal; however, subset with developmental delays in learning, motor skills, and/or language
Brainstem	Pons, reticular activating system, locus coeruleus may play role in disorders of sleep arousal in nocturia

Secondary Complications: Enuresis can affect a child's self-esteem and limit ability to engage in social activities including sleeping away from home. Punishment by caregivers, including abuse triggered by enuresis, further impacts child well-being.

Treatment Complications: Treatment involves behavioral interventions, including bed-wetting alarms. Pharmacotherapy includes use of desmopressin, with rare complications of water intoxication and seizures.

Bibliography

American Psychiatric Association. *Diagnostic and statistical manual of mental disorders: DSM-5.* 5th ed. Washington, DC: American Psychiatric Association; 2013.

Robson WL. Clinical practice. Evaluation and management of enuresis. *N Engl J Med.* 2009;360(14):1429–36.

Roson WL, Leung AK. Side effects and complications of treatment with desmopressin for enuresis. *J Natl Med Assoc.* 1994;86(10):775–7.

Ependymoma

Epidemiology and Demographics

- Overall rare, 2–3% of all primary brain tumors. Third most common brain tumor in pediatrics.
- Ependymomas account for 6–12% of brain tumors in children less than 18 years of age, but 30% of brain tumors in children less than 3 years of age.
- Adult cases, 60% are in spinal cord; pediatric cases, 90% are in the brain with majority in posterior fossa.

Disorder Description: Ependymoma arises from cells that line the ventricles in the central nervous system and central canal of the spinal cord.

- Ependymomas are typically found in three major locations: the posterior fossa (the area of the brain below the tentorium, containing the cerebellum and the brainstem), the supratentorium (the area of the brain above the tentorium containing the cerebral hemispheres), and the spinal cord.
- In adults, >75% of ependymomas arise within the spinal canal, but in children, about 90% arise within the brain in the posterior fossa, in or around the fourth ventricle, and only 10% arise within the spinal cord.

Symptoms

Localization site	Comment
Cerebral hemispheres	• In posterior fossa can lead to obstruction of cerebrospinal fluid flow; can develop signs and symptoms of increased intracranial pressure (headache, vomiting, head tilt, double vision). Specific localized symptoms can also occur • Tumors that arise on the floor of the fourth ventricle are associated with torticollis (wry neck with head tilted and twisted) and ataxia (loss of balance) • Those arising to the side of the fourth ventricle are associated with cranial nerve dysfunction including impaired hearing, dysarthria (problems with speech articulation), dysphagia (difficulty swallowing), and dysmetria (unsteady, clumsy movements) • Those arising on the roof of the fourth ventricle are associated with ataxia
Pituitary gland	Poor growth
Spinal cord	Spinal cord lesions can be associated with low back pain, sciatica, extremity weakness, leg length discrepancy, and scoliosis

Treatment Complications

- Surgery, especially infratentorial, may result in the development or worsening of balance, speech, or swallowing problems. Most of these changes will improve over several weeks or months. CSF leakage.
- Children experience some degree of decreased intellect and learning problems following radiation to large areas of the brain, which is correlated with location and size of area irradiated and is inversely related to the age of the patient. Significant reading, math, and short-term memory problems have

been reported with radiation to the upper part of the brain.
- Radiation: Poor growth may be a consequence of damage to the hypothalamus or pituitary gland. Weakening of the muscles in proximity to the spine and/or short stature may be a side effect of spine radiation.
- Platinum-based drugs often cause hearing loss, as can radiation therapy delivered near the ears.
- Some chemotherapy can cause infertility.

Bibliography

American Brain Tumor Association. Ependymoma. (n.d.). www.abta.org/tumor_types/ependymoma/. Accessed Oct 11, 2016.

CERN Foundation. Ependymoma clinical trials. (n.d.). www.cern-foundation.org/. Accessed Oct 11, 2016.

National Cancer Institute. Childhood ependymoma treatment. Updated July 6, 2018. Available from www.cancer.gov/types/brain/patient/child-ependymoma-treatment-pdq. Accessed Aug 3, 2018.

Ephedra and Ephedrine

Epidemiology and Demographics: There is no age, gender, race predilection.

Disorder Description: Ephedra and ephedrine are derived from the plant *Ephedra sinica*. Ephedrine is a sympathomimetic drug that stimulates both α- and β-adrenergic receptors.

Symptoms

Localization site	Comment
Cerebral hemispheres	Seizures (acute) Hemorrhagic and ischemic stroke (acute) Posterior reversible encephalopathy syndrome (PRES), seizures, mental status changes, and visual disturbances with hypertensive emergency
Mental status and psychiatric aspects/ complications	Paranoid schizophrenia (chronic) Psychomotor retardation (chronic use) Memory difficulties (chronic) Slowed speech (chronic) Blunted affect (chronic)

Localization site	Comment
Cranial nerves	PRES characterized by headache, confusion, seizures, and visual loss (acute)
Muscle	Rhabdomyolysis (acute)

Secondary Complications: Indirectly affects central nervous system.

- Cardiovascular effects – hypertensive vasculopathy causing an increased risk for stroke.
- Hematologic effects – coagulopathy in blood predisposing patient to risk of stroke.

Bibliography

Moawad FJ, Hartzell JD, Biega TJ, Lettieri CJ. Transient blindness due to posterior reversible encephalopathy syndrome following ephedra overdose. *Southern Medical Journal*, May, 2006. p. 511. *Academic OneFile*. Available from http://go.galegroup.com/ps/anonymous?id=GALE%7CA146844361&sid=googleScholar&v=2.1&it=r&linkaccess=fulltext&issn=00384348&p=AONE&sw=w&authCount=1&isAnonymousEntry=true. Accessed Aug 3, 2018.

Wiegand T, Thai D, Benowitz N. Medical consequences of the use of hallucinogens: LSD, mescaline, PCP, and MDMA ("Ecstasy"). In Brick J, ed. *Handbook of the medical consequences of alcohol and drug abuse.* 2nd ed. New York: Routledge; 2008. p. 461.

Epicondylitis

Epidemiology and Demographics: Annual incidence is 1–3% of the US population. It is more prevalent in current or past smokers.

Disorder Description: Repetitive strain injury that leads to tendonitis. There are two forms: lateral epicondylitis, referred to as tennis elbow, and medial epicondylitis, referred to as golfer's elbow. Lateral epicondylitis is more common than medial epicondylitis.

Symptoms

Localization site	Comment
Lateral elbow	Pain on the outside (lateral) of the upper forearm below the elbow; pain is exacerbated by lifting the arm or lifting an object, bending arm, attempting to write, grip objects, make a fist, or shake a person's hand. The pain also occurs when the hand is raised or on attempting to straighten wrist and twisting of forearms. There is a feeling of generalized weakness in the forearm
Medial elbow	Pain in the elbow/forearm when swinging golf club. Difficulty and pain when shaking hands is noted. Pain when flexing wrist is present; pain and difficulty in squeezing hands into a fist, throwing an object, or turning a door knob is reported. Pain while lifting weights is also reported

Treatment Complications: Nonsteroidal anti-inflammatories may cause rare vascular complications. Other treatments include rest, physical therapy/occupational therapy, work adjustments, forearm bracing, corticosteroid injections, and if needed, surgery. Surgery may uncommonly be associated with unanticipated new deficits.

Bibliography

Bisset L, Beller E, Jull G, et al. Mobilization with movement and exercise, corticosteroid injection or wait and see for tennis elbow: randomized trial. *BMJ*. 2006;333(7575):939.

Epidermoid

Epidemiology and Demographics

- Slow growing, presentation age ranges between 20s and late 50s.
- Approximately 1% of all primary intracranial tumors.
- Occurs equally in both sexes.

Disorder Description: Epidermoid or "pearly" tumors were described by Cruveilhier and designated the "most beautiful tumors of the body" by Dandy. They are slow-growing congenital or acquired lesions of ectodermal origin.

In general, there are several ways to acquire this tumor:

1. By skin cells that are deposited in the wrong place during neural tube closure causing "ectodermal elements" to be trapped.
2. Skin cell penetration, for example from a fall, infection, or puncture such as a spinal tap.
3. Radiation exposure.

Symptoms

Localization site	Comment
Mental status and psychiatric aspects/ complications	Vary from mild to severe; short-term memory loss, confusion, difficulty concentrating, decreased reasoning, impaired judgment, anger/rage, depression, or other emotions exaggerated or inappropriate for situation, sleepiness/fatigue
Cerebellum	Cerebellum compression symptoms
Vestibular system (and non-specific dizziness)	Dizziness or difficulty with balance and walking, unsteadiness, vertigo
Spinal cord	Motor disturbances, pain, sensory disturbances, and bowel or bladder dysfunction may be present
Cranial nerves	Hearing loss, tinnitus; vision problems such as blurred, double vision, etc.; swallowing and speech problems; trigeminal neuralgia, hemifacial spasm, other cranial nerves can be involved
Pituitary gland	Symptoms such as those resulting from endocrine abnormalities
Dorsal root ganglia	Loss of sensation in the arms, legs, or face
Brainstem	Symptoms due to compression; varies by location
Unclear localization	Epidermoid cysts can rupture and result in a meningitis-type reaction from inflammation; Loss of movement in the arms, legs, or face

Treatment Complications: Transient mild focal deficit impairments resulting from affectation of the nervous structure over a wide area. Higher rate of surgical complications with fourth ventricle and mesencephalic extended cerebellopontine angle tumors.

Bibliography

Chowdhury FH, Haque MR, Sarker MH. Intracranial epidermoid tumor; microneurosurgical management: an experience of 23 cases. *Asian J Neurosurg.* 2013;8(1):21–8. Available from http://doi.org/10.4103/1793-5482.110276

Dornelles C, da Costa SS, Meurer L, Schweiger C. Some considerations about acquired adult and pediatric cholesteatomas. *Braz J Otorhinolaryngol.* 2005;71(4):536–46. DOI: 10.1590/s0034-72992005000400023.

Isaacson G. Diagnosis of pediatric cholesteatoma. *Pediatrics.* 2007;120(3):603–8. DOI: 10.1542/peds.2007-0120.

Semaan MT., Megerian CA. The pathophysiology of cholesteatoma. *Otolaryngol Clin North Am.* 2006;39(6):1143–59. DOI: 10.1016/j.otc.2006.08.003.

Epidural Hematoma

Epidemiology and Demographics

- The most common cause of intracranial epidural hematoma (EDH) is traumatic, although spontaneous hemorrhage is known to occur: commonly from acceleration–deceleration trauma and transverse forces, blow to the side of the head, and on very rare occasions can be due to a contrecoup injury.
- The majority of bleeds originate from meningeal arteries, particularly in the temporal region.
- Ten percent of epidural bleeds may be venous, due to shearing injury from rotational forces.
- Only 20 to 30% of EDHs occur outside the region of the temporal bone.

Disorder Description: An epidural hematoma, also known as extradural hematoma, is bleeding between the inside of the skull and the outer covering of the brain (called the "dura"). An epidural hematoma is often caused by a skull fracture during childhood or adolescence. This type of bleeding is more common in young people because the membrane covering the brain is not as firmly attached to the skull as it is in older people. An epidural hematoma occurs when there is a rupture of a blood vessel, usually an artery. The blood vessel then bleeds into the space between the "dura mater" and the skull. The affected vessels are often torn by skull fractures. The fractures are most often the result of a severe head injury, such as those caused by motorcycle or automobile accidents. Epidural hematomas can be caused by bleeding from a vein (venous bleeding) in young children.

Rapid bleeding causes a collection of blood (hematoma) that presses on the brain. The pressure inside the head (intracranial pressure) increases quickly. This pressure may result in additional brain injury.

An extradural hemorrhage is an emergency. It may lead to permanent brain damage or death if left untreated. It may get worse very quickly, progressing from drowsiness to coma and death within minutes to hours.

Symptoms

Localization site	Comment
Cerebral hemispheres	EDHs are generally unilateral in more than 95% of cases; however, bilateral or multiple EDHs have been reported
	>95% are supratentorial
	A. temporoparietal: 60%
	B. frontal: 20%
	C. parieto-occipital: 20%
	<5% are located infratentorially in posterior fossa

	Special locations to consider, particularly those related to venous bleeding, include:
	 • vertex EDH (which displaces the superior sagittal sinus)
	 • anterior middle cranial fossa
	   • likely venous bleeding (sphenoparietal sinus)
	   • do not cause midline shift or herniation
	   • rarely grow

	Can be managed conservatively
Mental status and psychiatric aspects/ complications	Confusion Dizziness Drowsiness Varying levels of alertness Severe headache Nausea Vomiting Seizures Enlarged pupil in one eye

Localization site	Comment
	Weakness on one side of the body, typically on the side opposite the enlarged pupil Bruises around the eyes Bruises behind the ears Clear fluid draining from the nose or ears Shortness of breath or other changes in breathing patterns
Cranial nerves	Expanding high-volume EDHs can produce a midline shift and subfalcine herniation of the brain. Compressed cerebral tissue can impinge on the third cranial nerve, resulting in ipsilateral pupillary dilation and contralateral hemiparesis or extensor motor response
Pituitary gland	Dysfunction occurs in sub-acute stage: develops within first year after traumatic brain injury
Spinal cord	Symptoms begin with local or radicular back pain and percussion tenderness; they are often severe. Spinal cord compression may develop; compression of lumbar spinal roots may cause cauda equina syndrome and lower extremity paresis. Deficits progress over minutes to hours
Unclear localization	Hypermetabolism or increased metabolic rate: muscle wasting; pulmonary dysfunction: neurogenic pulmonary edema, aspiration pneumonia, fat and blood clots in lungs; blunt trauma to chest/ abdomen: CV dysfunction, GI symptoms such as erosive gastritis

Secondary Complications: Problems with *cognition* (thinking, memory, and reasoning) and behavior or mental health (depression, anxiety, personality changes, aggression, acting out, and social inappropriateness) are among the most frequent sequelae after traumatic brain injury (TBI). There has been a strong link with severe TBI and long-term cognitive impairments. Seizures vary with severity of TBI.

Neurodegenerative disorders such as dementia of the Alzheimer's type and parkinsonism are related to mild and moderate TBI. Language and communication problems are also common in TBI patients: Aphasia may occur in 19%, dysarthria in 30%, and dysphagia in 17%. Another prolonged effect of EDHs is called a post-concussion syndrome, which is characterized by dizziness, headache, vertigo, poor concentration, sleepiness, and emotional lability.

Bibliography

Besenski N. Traumatic injuries: imaging of head injuries. *Eur Radiol.* 2002;12:1237.

Bullock MR, Chesnut R, Ghajar J, et al. Surgical management of acute epidural hematomas. *Neurosurgery.* 2006; 58:S7.

Matsumoto K, Akagi K, Abekura M, Tasaki O. Vertex epidural hematoma associated with traumatic arteriovenous fistula of the middle meningeal artery: a case report. *Surg Neurol.* 2001;55:302.

Mayer S, Rowland L. Head injury. In Rowland L, ed. *Merritt's neurology.* Philadelphia: Lippincott Williams & Wilkins; 2000. p. 401.

McIver JI, Scheithauer BW, Rydberg CH, Atkinson JL. Metastatic hepatocellular carcinoma presenting as epidural hematoma: case report. *Neurosurgery.* 2001;49:447.

Ng WH, Yeo TT, Seow WT. Non-traumatic spontaneous acute epidural haematoma – report of two cases and review of the literature. *J Clin Neurosci.* 2004;11:791.

Safaz I, Alaca R, Yasar E, Tok F, Yilmaz B. Medical complications, physical function and communication skills in patients with traumatic brain injury: a single centre 5-year experience. *Brain Inj.* 2008;22:733–9.

Epidural Neoplasm; Spinal Cord Metastasis

Epidemiology and Demographics

- Between 5 and 10% of all cancer patients develop spinal metastases.
- Spinal epidural metastases (SEM) are diagnosed in 1 to 5% of patients with systemic cancer: 70% are in the thoracic, 20% in the lumbosacral, and 10% in the cervical part of the spine.
- Spinal epidural metastases are reported to be multiple in 17 to 30% of patients.

Disorder Description

- Systemic cancers that tend to metastasize to spine are: breast, prostate, lung, renal, lymphoma, sarcoma, and multiple myeloma. GI and pelvic malignancies are more likely to affect the lumbosacral spine, and lung and breast cancer affect the thoracic spine more.

- Causes 85% of cases of neoplastic spinal cord compression. In almost half the patients, breast or lung cancer is the primary tumor.

Symptoms

Localization site	Comment
Spinal cord	A Brown–Séquard syndrome may occur and is more common among patients with intramedullary rather than epidural metastases. Cord compression symptoms and other sensory and motor symptoms: paraplegia and bowel or bladder disturbances (e.g., constipation, urinary hesitancy, retention, incontinence) are usually late findings, except in conus medullaris syndrome, in which sphincter dysfunction and saddle anesthesia may emerge
Unclear localization	Pain often precedes other symptoms associated with spinal cord compression by 2–4 months

Treatment Complications: After treatment, 67 to 100% of patients with SEM who are ambulant at presentation can still walk; 30 to 40% of patients with paraparesis may regain ambulation with adequate treatment compared with only 10% or fewer patients with paraplegia. Unfortunately, more recent studies indicate that more than 20% of patients are unable to walk at the time of diagnosis.

Bibliography

Barron KD, Hirano A, Araki S, Terry RD. Experiences with metastatic neoplasms involving the spinal cord. *Neurology.* 1959;9:91–106.

Grant R, Papadopoulos SM, Sandler HM, Greenberg HS. Metastatic epidural spinal cord compression: current concepts and treatment. *J Neurooncol.* 1994;19:79–92.

Portenoy RK, Galer BS, Salamon O, et al. Identification of epidural neoplasm: radiography and bone scintigraphy in the symptomatic and asymptomatic spine. *Cancer.* 1989;64(11):2207–13.

Schiff D. Clinical features and diagnosis of neoplastic epidural spinal cord compression, including cauda equina syndrome. Available from www.uptodate.com/contents/clinical-features-and-diagnosis-of-neoplastic-epidural-spinal-cord-compression-including-cauda-equina-syndrome. Accessed Oct 11, 2016.

Epilepsy

Epidemiology and Demographics: About 150,000 new cases each year in the United States, with 1/26 people developing epilepsy in their lifetime. The age of seizure onset is bimodal with the majority beginning in childhood and incidence increasing again after age 60 years.

Disorder Description: Considered a disease defined as two unprovoked seizures >24 hours apart or one unprovoked seizure with high probability of further seizures (at least 60%). Wide range of causes including genetic or metabolic disorders, developmental disorders, structural abnormalities (tumor, stroke), infectious diseases (encephalitis), and other progressive neurologic illnesses. Epilepsy syndromic diagnosis is based on the constellation of seizure type, EEG findings, age at onset, mode of inheritance, provoking factors, and associated neurologic symptoms. This has implications with regard to medication selection, surgical options, and prognosis. Typically characterized as either symptomatic (associated with identifiable lesion or organic cause) or non-symptomatic (due to more isolated genetic factors), and either focal or generalized in nature.

Symptoms

Localization site	Comment
Cerebral hemisphere	Seizures characterized as generalized or bilaterally synchronous in onset versus focal in onset depending on syndrome. Both nonconvulsive and convulsive seizure types are described
Mental status and psychiatric aspects/ complications	High comorbidities with depression, anxiety, psychoses, and cognitive dysfunction

Secondary Complications: Injuries related to seizure occurrence including car accidents, drowning, or falling. Approximately 35% of people with epilepsy are affected by comorbid psychiatric disorders, with a two- to five-fold increased risk of suicidality. Likely multifactorial due to the damaging effects of seizures on the brain, effects of medication use, and psychosocial consequences of living with the disorder. Psychosis or depressive episodes may even occur in patients who reach remission with treatment-resistant seizure disorders. Sudden unexpected death in epilepsy (SUDEP) is more highly associated with chronic uncontrolled convulsions and polypharmacy.

Treatment Complications: Antiepileptic drugs (AEDs) may be associated with a number of idiosyncratic reactions, including multi-organ issues, and possible cognitive or psychiatric effects. Common side effects for AEDs include dizziness, fatigue, blurred vision, and gastrointestinal symptoms. Other reactions include rash, blood count abnormalities, liver toxicity, cognitive or mood complaints. There may be an increased risk of suicidality associated with AED use. Drug interactions are common. Antidepressants such as selective serotonin reuptake inhibitors appear to have a relatively low risk of exacerbating seizures, and should be considered in patients with epilepsy if indicated.

Bibliography

England MJ, Liverman CT, Schultz AM, Strawbridge LM. Epilepsy across the spectrum: promoting health and understanding. A summary of the Institute of Medicine report. *Epilepsy Behav.* 2012;25(2):266–76.

Fisher RS, Acevedo C, Arzimanoglou A, et al. ILAE official report: a practical clinical definition of epilepsy. *Epilepsia*, 2014;55(4):475–82.

Jones NC, O'Brien TJ. Stress, epilepsy, and psychiatric comorbidity: how can animal models inform the clinic? *Epilepsy Behav.* 2013;26(3):363–9.

Kanner AM. Management of psychiatric and neurological comorbidities in epilepsy. *Nat Rev Neurol.* 2016;12(2):106–16.

Epilepsy and Pregnancy

Epidemiology and Demographics: Seizures affect up to 10% of the population in their lifetime. Seizure frequency may either increase (17%) or decrease (16%) during pregnancy; pregnancy generally does not alter the frequency of seizures. Epilepsy is more prevalent in older population.

Disorder Description: Seizures are caused by excessive synchronous neuron activity in the brain, which is measured on the EEG. Epilepsy is the diagnosis of two unprovoked seizures separated by 24 hours or one unprovoked seizure wherein the practitioner estimates the chance of seizure recurrence within 10 years is at least 60%, in the case of brain structural lesions or an epilepsy syndrome for example.

Any injury can make the brain more susceptible to abnormal neuron activity. The most common etiologies in adult epilepsy are cerebrovascular disease, traumatic brain injury, and brain tumors.

Symptoms

Localization site	Comment
Cerebral hemispheres	Epilepsy: • There are many types of seizures, including simple partial seizures, complex partial seizures, and generalized seizures • Clinical manifestation depends on the seizure foci. For example, occipital seizures present as flashing lights, while left frontal seizures present as rhythmic jerking of the right arm and leg • Generalized tonic–clonic seizure is the most common type of generalized seizure, characterized by an initial choking cry, stiffening of the muscles, followed by jerking movements. There is alteration of consciousness • Partial seizures with altered awareness and generalized seizures are typically followed by a post-ictal period of confusion • Tongue bite, urinary and bowel incontinence are suggestive of generalized seizures

Secondary Complications: Maternal mortality is significantly higher than in the general population, with an odds ratio of approximately 10. The higher risk is possibly related to SUDEP (sudden unexpected death in epilepsy). Other complications, such as pre-eclampsia, prematurity, low birth weight, peripartum hemorrhage, and fetal mortality are slightly increased (OR about 1.5).

Seizures that occur during pregnancy do not seem to have many adverse effects on the fetus, except in cases of maternal trauma. Fetal bradycardia has been documented during maternal seizures, but there is little information on its long-term impact. Two studies have demonstrated that seizures during pregnancy may lead to a lower IQ of the child and low birth weight.

There is also a higher prevalence of peripartum depression among women with epilepsy, even when compared with other women with chronic illness.

Treatment Complications: It is a fine balance to treat the patient with epilepsy and her concerns for teratogenic effects on the fetus. Ideally, conversations with the patient should take place prior to conception and the epilepsy and medication history reviewed. For example, if epilepsy is not well controlled, the risk of drug withdrawal or cross-titration should be carefully weighed against the risk of teratogenicity. For some women, withdrawal of antiepileptic drugs (AEDs) prior to pregnancy may be considered based on appropriate clinical criteria. Serum AED levels should be obtained at baseline prior to pregnancy and monitored regularly during pregnancy.

AED choice should be based on seizure semiology. Some of the newer AEDs like lamotrigine and levetiracetam are felt to be safer during pregnancy, but there is little supporting data. The most effective AED for the patient should probably be continued, with the exception of valproate. Monotherapy with lamotrigine or oxcarbazapine has a higher rate of breakthrough seizures.

Patients should be monitored closely for any seizure activity, and should also follow up with an obstetrics and gynecology specialist. Fetal ultrasound can be conducted at 14–18 weeks to visualize fetal anatomy. AED levels should be checked on a regular basis (monthly) if possible, especially lamotrigine and oxcarbazepine. These drugs are metabolized by glucuronidation, which is induced in pregnancy, and this mechanism results in marked decline in levels of lamotrigine and oxcarbazepine. Other drug levels including topiramate, valproate, phenytoin, levetiracetam, and phenobarbital may also decrease, but to a lesser degree. Hyperemesis gravidarum may cause decreased absorption of AEDs and should be monitored clinically.

Patients should be supplemented with at least 1 mg folic acid daily prior to conception and throughout pregnancy. Vitamin K 10–20 mg per day is often supplemented during the last month of pregnancy due to increased risk of hemorrhagic disease of the newborn with carbamazepine, phenytoin, and phenobarbital use.

After delivery, AED dosage can be titrated down if there was an increase during pregnancy. Breastfeeding is generally safe except when the mother is taking phenobarbital, which poses a risk of sedation in the infant. Patients should avoid sleep deprivation as it lowers seizure threshold.

Finally, a seizure event during pregnancy in a woman with known epilepsy should not exclude the diagnoses of eclampsia, and appropriate workup should be implemented to rule out this potentially life-threatening diagnosis.

The risk of teratogenesis is three times higher with valproate than in untreated women with epilepsy. Neural tube defects, specifically spina bifida, develop in 2% of fetuses exposed to valproate, 10 times higher than in the general population. Intrauterine valproate is also associated with a lower IQ and an increased risk of autism. The effects of valproate are dose-dependent.

Phenytoin, topiramate, and phenobarbital have been associated with high rates of fetal malformation as well. Topiramate exposure in the first trimester is linked to orofacial clefts (10-fold greater than in general population). There is a very small association between carbamazepine and spina bifida (80% less than valproate).

In addition, polytherapy carries a higher risk of fetal malformations.

In patients who had a major congenital malformation in their first pregnancy, the risk of another major congenital malformation in the second pregnancy is significantly higher (35% vs 3%).

Bibliography

Baker GA, Bromley RL, Briggs M, et al. IQ at 6 years after in utero exposure to antiepileptic drugs. *Neurology*. 2015;84(4):382–90.

Bangar S, Shastri A, El-Sayeh H, Cavanna AE. Women with epilepsy: clinically relevant issues. *Funct Neurol*. 2016;31(3):127–34.

Borgelt LM, Hart FM, Bainbridge JL. Epilepsy during pregnancy: focus on management strategies. *Int J Womens Health*. 2016;19(8):505–17.

Harden CL. Pregnancy and epilepsy. *Continuum (Minneap Minn)*. 2014;20:60–79.

Kinney MO, Craig JJ. Pregnancy and epilepsy; meeting the challenges over the last 25 years: The rise of the pregnancy registries. *Seizure*. 2017;44:162–8.

Epilepsy Partialis Continua (EPC)

Epidemiology and Demographics: Epilepsy partialis continua (EPC) is estimated at <1 case per million. Incidence slightly higher in males.

Disorder Description: Medically refractory focal motor status epilepticus. Unremitting rhythmic clonic movements of one muscle group (face, arm, or leg)

lasting hours, days, or weeks. Typically with preserved mentation. Usually due to an underlying lesion, though sometimes undetectable on imaging. Etiologies include: cortical malformations, tumors, encephalitis, stroke, demyelinative lesions, metabolic abnormalities (hyperosmolarity), and degenerative conditions. Frequently observed in Rasmussen encephalitis. EEG may show focal repetitive slow-wave abnormalities or periodic spike and wave discharges over the central areas of the contralateral hemisphere. Prognosis and treatment dependent on underlying cause. The majority of cases require polytherapy with antiepileptic drugs (AEDs) due to their refractory nature.

Symptoms

Localization site	Comment
Cerebral hemispheres	Persistent focal seizures with motor manifestations. May be associated with progressive paresis of the limbs or face
	Focal lesions on MRI, focal repetitive discharges on EEG
Mental status and psychiatric aspects/ complications	Progressive aphasia and cognitive decline may occur in Rasmussen syndrome

Secondary Complications: Neurologic decline such as progressive motor or cognitive dysfunction has been observed, depending on etiology. EPC due to more acute or transient lesions may have a better prognosis.

Treatment Complications: AEDs may be associated with a number of idiosyncratic reactions, including multiorgan issues, and possible cognitive or psychologic effects. Benzodiazepines may be associated with excessive sedation, hypotension, or respiratory depression. Other treatments, such as immunosuppression, may be utilized depending on etiology and may be associated with other serious potential side effects.

Bibliography

Cockerell OC, Rothwell J, Thompson PD, Marsden CD, Shorvon SD. Clinical and physiological features of epilepsia partialis continua: cases ascertained in the UK. *Brain*. 1996;119(2):393–407.

Eggers C, Burghaus L, Fink GR, Dohmen C. Epilepsia partialis continua responsive to intravenous levetiracetam. *Seizure.* 2009;18(10):716–8.

Pandian JD, Thomas SV, Santoshkumar B. Epilepsia partialis continua: a clinical and electroencephalography study. *Seizure.* 2002;11(7):437–41.

Sinha S, Satishchandra P. Epilepsia partialis continua over last 14 years: experience from a tertiary care center from south India. *Epilepsy Res.* 2007;74(1):55–9.

Epstein–Barr Virus

Epidemiology and Demographics: Seroprevalence of Epstein–Barr virus (EBV) varies from 100% in developing countries by age 4 to up to 89% of the population infected by age 19 in higher socioeconomic groups in industrialized nations. Two strains of EBV exist in humans: EBV1, more common in United States and Europe, and EBV1 and EBV2, equally prevalent in Africa and New Guinea.

Disorder Description: EBV is a member of the herpesvirus family. The EBV genome, consisting of a linear DNA and encoding nearly 100 viral proteins, is encased within a nucleocapsid surrounded by a viral envelope. Infection of humans by EBV occurs by contact with oral secretions, and the virus infects both epithelial and B cells. B cell infection results in immortalization of the cells, which begets the persistence of EBV within the body.

EBV[1–3] is the causative agent of infectious mononucleosis (IM), which is characterized by fever, eruption, atypical lymphocytes in the peripheral blood, tonsillar and lymph node swelling, and liver dysfunction. IM can be complicated in 1 to 18% of patients by central nervous system complications including encephalitis, meningitis, cerebellitis, polyradiculomyelitis, transverse myelitis, cranial and peripheral neuropathies including Guillain–Barré syndrome, and psychiatric abnormalities. The spectrum of EBV-related disorders includes chronic active EBV infection, Burkitt's lymphoma, and central nervous system (CNS) lymphoma as well as CNS infections such as demyelinating disease, acute encephalitis, acute cerebellar ataxia, myelitis, or meningitis.

Symptoms[3,4]

Localization site	Comment
Cerebral hemispheres	Altered consciousness, somnolence, coma, encephalitis, meningitis, acute demyelinating encephalomyelitis, CNS lymphoma
Mental status and psychiatric aspects/ complications	Alice in Wonderland syndrome[5]: illusory changes in the size, distance, or position of stationary objects in the subject's visual field; illusory feelings of levitation; and illusory alterations in the sense of the passage of time
Brainstem	Cranial neuritis
Cerebellum	Cerebellitis
Cranial nerves	Hypoglossal palsy, facial palsy, and cranial neuritis
Spinal cord	Transverse myelitis
Peripheral neuropathy	Guillain–Barré syndrome

Secondary Complications: Chronic EBV infection and related lymphoproliferative disease as well as EBV-related tumors including nasopharyngeal carcinoma, Burkitt's lymphoma, Hodgkin's disease.

References

1. Cohen JI. Epstein-Barr virus infection. *New Engl J Med.* 2000;343:481–92.
2. Fujimoto H, Asaoka K, Amatzumi T, et al. Epstein Barr virus infections of the central nervous system. *Intern Med.* 2003;42:33–40.
3. Hausler M, Ramaekers VT, Doenges M, et al. Neurologic complications of acute of persistent Epstein-Barr virus infection in Paediatric patients. *J Med Virol.* 2002;68:253–63.
4. Martelius T, Lappalainen M, PaloMaki M, Antilla, VJ. Clinical characterisistics of patients with Epstein Barr virus in cerebrospinal fluid. *BMC Infect Dis.* 2011;11:281.
5. Todd J. The syndrome of Alice in Wonderland. *Canad Med Assoc J.* 1995;73:701–4.

Erectile Disorder

Epidemiology and Demographics: Overall prevalence is unknown; however, prevalence and incidence increase with age. Affects 2% of men younger than 40–50 years old and 40–50% of men 60–70 years old.

Disorder Description: As per DSM-5, marked by at least one of the following on all or at least 75% of sexual encounters: (1) difficulty obtaining erection, (2) difficulty maintaining erection through completion, or (3) decrease in erectile rigidity. Must persist for 6 months and cause significant distress. It is not better accounted for by another mental or medical disorder, substances, or secondary to severe distress in relationship.

The disorder can be lifelong, acquired, generalized, or situational. Lifelong course is most associated with psychologic factors, and acquired with biological factors (e.g., age, smoking history, diabetes, and sedentary lifestyle). Diagnostic procedures exist to help clinicians discriminate between these factors. Common comorbidities include major depressive disorder and other sexual diagnoses, as well as disorders involving endocrine, neurologic, and vascular systems. There is variable cultural representation.

Special consideration of factors related to the partner, relationship, individual vulnerability, associated psychiatric illness, culture, or medical condition can help elucidate cause and guide intervention.

Symptoms

Localization site	Comment
Mental status and psychiatric aspects/complications	Depressed mood, low self-esteem, anxiety

Secondary Complications: Low self-esteem, avoidance of sexual activity and/or intimacy, depressed mood. Impaired romantic relationships.

Treatment Complications: Psychotherapy can be helpful for psychogenic causes, along with treatment of any comorbid mental disorder. Medications directly targeting erectile dysfunction work by enhancing nitric oxide effect. Therefore caution required to prevent hemodynamic changes, particularly in patients with comorbid cardiac disease. Avoid in those with severe kidney or liver dysfunction.

Bibliography

American Psychiatric Association. *Diagnostic and statistical manual of mental disorders: DSM-5.* 5th ed. Washington, DC: American Psychiatric Association; 2013.

Beutel ME, Weidner W, Brähler E. Epidemiology of sexual dysfunction in the male population. *Andrologia.* 2006;38(4):115–21.

Prins J, Blanker MH, Bohnen AM, et al. Prevalence of erectile dysfunction: a systematic review of population-based studies. *Int J Impot Res.* 2002;14(6):422–32.

Essential Chorea

Epidemiology and Demographics: Essential chorea, also commonly known as benign hereditary chorea (BHC), is a rare autosomal dominant movement disorder characterized by a non-progressive form of chorea.[1] Symptoms begin to arise in children before they reach the age of 5 (median age 2.5–3 years).[2] Its prevalence is approximately 2/1,000,000. Although there is variation in penetrance with 100% in men and 75% in women,[3] large cohort studies have suggested that females are more commonly affected than males (0.64:0.46).[4,5]

Disorder Description: Chorea, derived from the Greek word "choros" meaning "dance," is a continuous flow of random, brief, involuntary muscle contractions.[1] First described in 1966, the disorder was identified in a child with chorea who as an infant experienced hypotonia and gross motor delays. The jerky movements in BHC are often generalized, affecting all body parts, not aggravated by voluntary movements, but worsening with stress or excitement.[2] It is often described as "nervous fidgeting." The disorder was first genetically linked in 2000 to the deletion of a gene that encodes thyroid transcription factor-1 (TITF1), or NKX2-1, after identifying the condition in a family with four generations of BHC.[4,6] The gene is associated with organogenesis of the basal ganglia, thyroid, and lungs. Since the discovery of the causative gene, the phenotype has expanded to include diseases of the lung, such as recurrent infections, and thyroid disorders. It is now referred to as the "brain–lung–thyroid" spectrum disorder.[2,4] Besides choreiform movements, other neurologic deficits such as gait impairment, intentional tremor, myoclonic jerks, or drop attacks may be present. Neuroimaging studies do not reveal causative lesions. In contrast to Huntington's disease, those with BHC tend to have normal or slightly below normal intelligence and chorea that is non-progressive.[2] The "benign" nature of the disease describes the improvement of chorea in late childhood to early adulthood. Despite this, there have been cases where choreiform movements have persisted throughout adulthood.

Symptoms

Localization site	Comment
Mental status and psychiatric aspects/ complications	Distress in the form of social embarrassment is common in younger age. Mild intellectual disabilities or attention deficit hyperactivity disorder can be present concurrently
Muscle	Unclear localization

Secondary Complications: BHC has varying phenotypic presentations. The classic BHC patient may improve over time and present without secondary complications. In contrast, complications have been observed in patients with "brain–lung–thyroid" involvement. They may experience severe respiratory conditions, including recurrent infections. Hypothyroidism is a common combined feature seen in patients. Lung, thyroid, and brain cancer has been seen in patients with BHC, alluding to a possible association with cancer.[6]

Treatment Complications: In classic BHC, not all symptomatic patients necessitate treatment given the benign nature of the disease. In more complex phenotypes, treatment may be sought. Unfortunately, there has been limited pharmacologic success for this condition. Gras et al.[4] described the successful use of oral tetrabenazine, and others have attempted to utilize levodopa; however, the results have been controversial.

References

1. Cardoso F, Seppi K, Mair KM, Wenning GK, Poewe W. Seminar on choreas. *Lancet Neurol.* 2006;5:589–602.
2. Peall KJ, Kurian MA. Benign hereditary chorea: an update. *Tremor Other Hyperkinet Mov (NY).* 2015;5:314.
3. Harper PS. Benign hereditary chorea: clinical and genetic aspects. *Clin Genet.* 1978;13(1):85–95.
4. Gras D, Jonard L, Roze E, et al. Benign hereditary chorea: phenotype, prognosis, therapeutic outcome and long term follow-up in a large series with new mutations in the TITF1/NKX2-1 gene. *J Neurol Neurosurg Psychiatry.* 2012;83(10):956–62.
5. Peall KJ, Lumsden D, Kneen R, et al. Benign hereditary chorea related to NKX2.1: expansion of the genotypic and phenotypic spectrum. *Dev Med Child Neurol.* 2014;56(7):642–8.
6. Inzelberg R, Weinberger M, Gak E. Benign hereditary chorea: an update. *Parkinsonism Relat Disord.* 2011;17(5):301–7.

Essential Myoclonus

Epidemiology and Demographics: The lifetime prevalence of myoclonus, as of 1990, was 8.6 cases per 100,000, essential myoclonus accounting for 11%. Prevalence of myoclonus–dystonia syndrome in Europe reported to be 2/1,000,000.

Disorder Description: Sudden, involuntary intermittent jerking of a muscle or group of muscles that occurs in the absence of epilepsy or other underlying disorder. Can be hereditary or sporadic in origin. It is non-progressive and usually multifocal in distribution. Cognition is normal. Hereditary essential myoclonus is autosomal dominant with variable severity. Symptoms start before the age of 20. Dystonia (typically cervical) is common among these patients, comprising the myoclonus–dystonia syndrome. Mutations in the ε-sarcoglycan gene have had the strongest association with this syndrome. Unknown function of this gene, localized to chromosome 7q21-q31. Recommended medications for treatment are clonazepam, valproic acid.

Symptoms

Localization site	Comment
Mental status and psychiatric aspects/ complications	Obsessive-compulsive disorder, anxiety disorders, and mild cognitive slowing have been variably associated with ε-sarcoglycan mutation in myoclonus–dystonia syndrome
Muscle	Sudden jerks, shakes, or spasms of muscles

Secondary Complications: Anxiety disorders appear to be more frequently observed in this syndrome.

Treatment Complications: Clonazepam can cause drowsiness and ataxia. Abrupt reductions and withdrawals can result in a marked deterioration in myoclonus and withdrawal seizures. Side effects of valproic acid include hair loss, tremor, hepatotoxicity, and drowsiness.

Bibliography

Caviness JN, Brown P. Myoclonus: current concepts and recent advances. *Lancet Neurol.* 2004;3(10):598–607.

Marechal L, Raux G, Dumanchin C, et al. Severe myoclonus-dystonia syndrome associated with a novel epsilon-sarcoglycan gene truncating mutation. *Am J Med Genet B Neuropsychiatr Genet.* 2003;119B(1):114–7.

Essential Thrombocythemia

Epidemiology and Demographics: Diagnosed in older adults, with a female predominance. Estimated prevalence of 24/100,000 in the United States.

Disorder Description: Diagnosis of exclusion for a myeloproliferative disorder with platelet count greater than 600,000 cells/μL and megakaryocytic hyperplasia on bone marrow biopsy; other etiologies for reactive thrombocytosis usually require thorough investigation. Majority but not all have *JAK2* mutation. Patients with elevated platelet counts are often asymptomatic. Symptoms are primarily attributed to vasomotor dysfunction causing features such as livedo reticularis.

Symptoms

Localization site	Comment
Cerebral hemispheres	Transient ischemic attack-like symptoms of hemiparesis or monocular vision loss without alternative explanation. Syndrome often accompanied by headache and migraine-like visual scintillations.[1] More rarely can cause thrombotic events such as small vessel stroke[2]
Unclear localization	Hard to localize spells of unstable gait or lightheadedness

Secondary Complications: Well-known complication of erythromelalgia (burning pain in hands or feet with warmth and redness). Can also cause more generalized rash, atypical pain syndromes, or systemic thrombosis.

Treatment Complications: Symptoms usually treated with aspirin, which can cause bleeding complications. Treatment with hydroxyurea carries risk of mucocutaneous toxicity.

References

1. Michiels JJ, Koudstaal PJ, Mulder AH, van Vliet HH. Transient neurologic and ocular manifestations in primary thrombocythemia. *Neurology.* 1993;43:1107–10.
2. Pósfai É, Marton I, Szőke A, et al. Stroke in essential thrombocythemia. *J Neurol Sci.* 2014;336: 260–2.

Essential Tremor

Epidemiology and Demographics: Essential tremor (ET) is the second most common movement disorder, behind restless leg, affecting up to 5% of the world's population and approximately 7 million Americans. Incidence and prevalence both increase with age, particularly above age 40 years. Peak onset of age is 70–79 years. Familial ET accounts for half of all cases, and 5–15% of those patients may present in childhood.

Disorder Description: ET is an 8- to 12-Hz predominately kinetic, postural bilateral tremor. Fifty percent of cases have an intention tremor. It may affect the arms, head, voice, neck, trunk, and legs. Symptoms include sloppy, large, and irregular handwriting. There may be difficulty with fine motor tasks (using a screwdriver, shaving), using utensils, and pouring liquids. Patients can have difficulty with tandem gait. It is exacerbated by stress, exercise, fatigue, strong emotions, extreme temperatures, and caffeine. It improves with alcohol and subsides during sleep.

Symptoms

Localization site	Comment
Cerebral hemispheres	Pathology likely involves a circuit between the primary motor cortex, thalamus, and cerebellum. Surgical ablation and deep brain stimulation target the thalamus
Mental status and psychiatric aspects/ complications	Anxiety and depression, difficulties with visual perception, encoding, verbal fluency, and working memory. Increased risk for mild cognitive impairment
Brainstem	Brainstem Lewy bodies discovered in 8 out of 33 ET patients postmortem but the clinical significance is controversial
Cerebellum	Postmortem studies found Purkinje cell body and axonal loss. Patients may demonstrate slight ataxia such as difficulty with tandem walking

Secondary Complications: Medications used to treat ET may be associated with side effects. Propranolol is relatively contraindicated in patients with asthma, diabetes, or cardiac arrhythmias. Primidone can cause an acute toxic reaction with the first dose, leading to sedation, vertiginous symptoms, nausea, malaise, and confusion. This is often so severe patients will refuse to take the drug again. Topiramate may cause weight loss, paresthesias, anxiety, confusion, sedation, and nephrolithiasis. Complications associated with thalamic deep brain stimulation include paresthesias, dysarthria, dystonia, ataxia, and limb weakness. Gamma knife thalamotomy may cause thalamic bleeds, paresthesias, transient dyskinesias of the foot, transient or permanent hemiparesis, and dysarthria. Laryngeal botulinum toxin may cause dysphagia, a weak voice, and coughing.

Bibliography

Benito-León J, Louis ED, Mitchell AJ, Bermejo-Pareja F. Elderly-onset essential tremor and mild cognitive impairment: a population-based study (NEDICES). *J Alzheimers Dis.* 2011;23:727–35.

Bhalsing KS, Saini J, Pal PK. Understanding the pathophysiology of essential tremor through advanced neuroimaging: a review. *J Neurol Sci.* 2013;335(1–2):9–13.

Brust JC. Substance abuse and movement disorders. *Mov Disord.* 2010;25(13):2010–20.

Chandran V, Pal PK, Reddy JY, et al. Non-motor features in essential tremor. *Acta Neurol Scand.* 2012;125(5):332–7.

Deuschl G, Raethjen J, Hellriegel H, Elble R. Treatment of patients with essential tremor. *Lancet Neurol.* 2011;10(2):148–61. DOI:10.1016/S1474-4422(10)70322-7.

Elble RJ. Diagnostic criteria for essential tremor and differential diagnosis. *Neurology.* 2000;54(11 Suppl 4):S2–6.

Fernandez, H, Machado A, Pandya M. *Practical approach to movement disorders: diagnosis and management.* 2nd ed. New York: Demos Medical; 2014.

Louis ED. The primary type of tremor in essential tremor is kinetic rather than postural: cross-sectional observation of tremor phenomenology in 369 cases. *Eur J Neurol.* 2013;20(4):725–7.

Louis ED. From neurons to neuron neighborhoods: the rewiring of the cerebellar cortex in essential tremor. *Cerebellum.* 2014;13(4):501–12.

Louis ED, Ottman R How many people in the USA have essential tremor? Deriving a population estimate based on epidemiological data. *Tremor Other Hyperkinet Mov (N Y).* 2014;4:259.

Rana, AQ, Hedera P. Essential tremor. In *Differential diagnosis of movement disorders in clinical practice.* New York, NY: Springer; 2014. pp. 6–19.

Young RF, Li F, Vermeulen S, Meier R. Gamma knife thalamotomy for treatment of essential tremor: long-term results *J Neurosurg.* 2010;112:1311–17.

Ethylene Oxide

Epidemiology and Demographics: Ethylene oxide is a gas used in sterilizing hospital equipment and supplies, and toxicity is commonly seen in nurses and health care workers that frequent the OR. Mechanism of nerve injury is from the toxic byproduct (ethylene chlorohydrin), which may be directly absorbed through the skin, or transmitted by blood or inhalation.

Disorder Description: Patients present primarily with dermatologic complaints at the site of exposure (rash with sensory neuropathy, most commonly decreased vibratory sense). Treatment is to reduce exposure to the neurotoxin.

Symptoms: Other neurologic sequela (confusion, seizures, and headaches). Prolonged exposure is associated with peripheral neuropathy and memory dysfunction.

Secondary Complications: Few retrospective studies have been performed, but studies suspect CNS involvement given that long-term sequelae involve neuropsychologic and mild cerebral atrophy.

Bibliography

Brashear A, Unverzagt FW, Farber MO, et al. Ethylene oxide neurotoxicity: a cluster of 12 nurses with peripheral and central nervous system toxicity. *Neurology.* 1996;46(4):992–8.

Eyelid Retraction

Epidemiology and Demographics: Eyelid retraction may affect any age group without sex predilection.

Disorder Description: The normal upper eyelid normally rests 1 mm lower than the upper limbus (peripheral pupil border), while the lower eyelid normally rests at the lower limbus. Eyelid retraction is seen when the upper eyelid rests higher than normal and/or the lower eyelid rests lower than normal. The most common pathologic process to cause eyelid retraction is thyroid eye disease, but a number of other conditions may also be the cause.

Symptoms

Localization site	Comment
Brainstem	Dorsal midbrain syndrome may be caused by midbrain tumor, demyelination, or stroke. The main clinical findings include eyelid retraction, paralysis of upgaze, convergence retraction nystagmus, light near dissociation, and skew deviation
Basal ganglia	Progressive supranuclear palsy is classically associated with supranuclear vertical gaze paresis that is worse in down- than upgaze. However, these patients may also have characteristic facies with eyelid retraction and neurologic symptoms of parkinsonism
Cranial nerves	Marcus Gunn jaw wink syndrome is a congenital aberrant connection between cranial nerves V and III. In this syndrome, when the patient moves his or her jaw, usually laterally, this also activates the levator muscle via the third cranial nerve, causing it to elevate and appear retracted
	Facial nerve paresis may present with eyelid retraction on the paretic side due to unopposed action of the levator muscle
Unclear localization	Graves' disease is the most common cause of eyelid retraction, thought to be due to fibrosis of the levator muscle and/or proptosis, which causes the globe to protrude abnormally beyond the eyelids, thus making them appear retracted. Other ocular findings include proptosis, ophthalmoplegia with diplopia, and compressive optic neuropathy with vision loss
	Hering's phenomenon is seen in patients with asymmetric ptosis. To compensate for the ptotic side, a patient may elevate both eyelids so that the non-ptotic side appears retracted while the ptotic side appears normal. This phenomenon may confuse the clinician to think the retracted side is abnormal and initiate a workup for eyelid retraction when contralateral ptosis is the real problem

Secondary Complications: Eyelid retraction may lead to exposure keratopathy, corneal ulceration, and perforation.

Treatment Complications: Surgical overcorrection of eyelid retraction may cause ptosis, while undercorrection may leave the patient with retraction, necessitating additional surgery.

Bibliography

Bartley GB. The differential diagnosis and classification of eyelid retraction. *Ophthalmology*. 1996;103:168–76.

Guimaraes FC, Cruz AAV. Palpebral fissure height and downgaze in patients with Graves upper eyelid retraction and congenital blepharoptosis. *Ophthalmology*. 1995;102:1218–22.

Stout AU, Borchert M. Etiology of eyelid retraction in children: a retrospective study. *J Pediatr Ophthalmol Strabismus*. 1993;30:96–9.

Fabry Disease (Fabry's; Fabry–Anderson, Anderson–Fabry Disease, α-Galactosidase A Deficiency)

Epidemiology and Demographics: Fabry disease is an X-linked condition, and as such, males are predominantly affected. Females may be asymptomatic carriers, have milder symptoms at a later age of onset, or can be as symptomatic as classic males. Males with classic presentations present as younger children while milder forms of the disease present later in life.

The overall incidence of Fabry disease is 1/50,000 males; however, an active database shows that the number of people affected may be underestimated, particularly in those with milder phenotypes. The international databases (Fabry Registry and the Fabry Outcome Survey [FOS]) allow for natural history data and the effect of enzyme replacement therapy on the disease course.

Disorder Description: Fabry disease is caused by a deficiency of the enzyme α-galactosidase (α-Gal A); lack of this enzyme results in the progressive accumulation of globotriaosylceramide in lysosomes (GL-3).

The classic form occurs in childhood in males with <1% enzyme activity. Common symptoms include pain crises in hands and feet (acroparesthesias), angiokeratomas, abnormal sweating, opacities of the cornea and lens, protein in the urine, with progressive kidney dysfunction and end-stage renal disease by the third to fifth decade. As adults, patients develop cardiac and/or cerebrovascular disease with strokes, leading to higher morbidity and mortality.

The milder form occurs in males with higher enzyme activity (>1%), with late-onset cardiac disease (left ventricular hypertrophy, cardiomyopathy, mitral valve insufficiency) and protein in the urine. Another variant exists that is renal involvement only, without angiokeratomas or pain crises.

While all ethnic, racial, and demographic groups are affected, there is a higher prevalence among the Taiwan Chinese who have primarily cardiac symptoms.

Symptoms

Localization site	Comment
Cerebral hemispheres	Stroke due to multifocal small vessel involvement: thrombosis, transient ischemic attacks (TIA), cerebral hemorrhage
Mental status and psychiatric aspects/complications	Depression, anxiety, severe fatigue, and other psychosocial manifestations Excessive guilt, fatigue, occupational difficulty, suicidal ideation, and depression have been noted in heterozygotes The pain of Fabry disease may be mistaken for malingering or conversion disorder. Pain is usually seen with a low-grade fever, but misdiagnosis is common
Brainstem	Basilar artery ischemia and aneurysm
Vestibular system (and non-specific dizziness)	Labyrinthine disorders due to stroke
Cranial nerves	Cranial nerve VIII involvement. High-frequency hearing loss, tinnitus, and dizziness have been reported
Peripheral neuropathy	Acroparesthesias are due to peripheral nerve involvement from accumulation of storage material in blood vessels and subsequent vasospasm

Secondary Complications: The secondary complications of Fabry disease include end-stage renal failure, ischemic heart disease, cerebrovascular disease, and strokes.

Treatment Complications: For renal involvement, hemodialysis and renal transplant may be indicated and these treatments have associated complications, including encephalopathy from chronic renal failure.

Bibliography

Cole AL, Lee PJ, Hughes DA, et al. Depression in adults with Fabry disease: a common and under-diagnosed problem. *J Inherit Metab Dis.* 2007;30:943–51.

Desnick RJ, Ioannou YA, Eng CM. Alpha-galactosidase A deficiency: Fabry disease. In Scriver CR, Beaudet AL, Sly WS, et al., eds.

The metabolic and molecular bases of inherited diseases. 8th ed. New York: McGraw-Hill; 2001. pp. 3733–74.

Eng CM, Fletcher J, Wilcox WR, et al. Fabry disease: baseline medical characteristics of a cohort of 1765 males and females in the Fabry Registry. *J Inherit Metab Dis.* 2007;30:184–92.

Mehta A, Hughes DA. Fabry disease. Aug 5, 2002 [Updated Oct 17, 2013]. In Pagon RA, Adam MP, Ardinger HH, et al., eds. *GeneReviews®* [Internet]. Seattle, WA: University of Washington; 1993–2016. Available from www.ncbi.nlm.nih.gov/books/NBK1292/. Accessed Aug 6, 2018.

Mehta A, Ricci R, Widmer U, et al. Fabry disease defined: baseline clinical manifestations of 366 patients in the Fabry Outcome Survey. *Eur J Clin Invest.* 2004;34:236–42.

Sadek J, Shellhaas R, Camfield CS, Camfield PR, Burley J. Psychiatric findings in four female carriers of Fabry disease. *Psychiatr Genet.* 2004;14:199–201.

Facial Myoclonus

Epidemiology and Demographics: There are no specific data about facial myoclonus alone. Approximately 15% of cases of myoclonus are epileptic, and the remainder are secondary.

Disorder Description: Facial myoclonus is a focal myoclonus that may be induced by action or external stimuli. It may be epileptic and occur in myoclonic epilepsies (juvenile myoclonic epilepsy, benign rolandic epilepsy), myoclonic encephalopathies (Rasmussen syndrome), or may be hereditary as seen in PRICKLE1-related progressive myoclonus epilepsy with ataxia. Secondary causes include olivopontocerebellar degeneration, postanoxic myoclonus, secondary palatal myoclonus, hyperekplexia (startle reflex), metabolic derangements (although rarely isolated to the face alone), or drug induced. Facial myoclonus can be differentiated from tics, fasciculations, and myokymia by electrophysiologic studies. Functional neurologic symptom disorders demonstrate a Bereitschaftspotential on EEG, indicating the movement was subconsciously or consciously planned, which is absent in myoclonus. Premonitory urges associated with facial tics are absent.

Symptoms

Localization site	Comment
Cerebral hemispheres	Focal seizures involving the motor cortex (cortical)
	Myoclonic encephalopathies (cortical)
	Benign rolandic epilepsy (cortical)
	Striatal lesions may allow for increased cortical excitability (subcortical)
Mental status and psychiatric aspects/ complications	Dementia (neurodegenerative disorders)
Brainstem	Olivopontocerebellar atrophy
	Hyperekplexia/startle reflex
	Secondary palatal myoclonus due to a lesion within the Guillain–Mollaret triangle may also cause focal facial myoclonus
	Post hypoxic/Lance Adams syndrome
Cranial nerves	Hemifacial spasm secondary to compression of the facial nerve, often by a vascular malformation
Cerebellum	Cerebellar lesions may play a role in increased cortical excitability found in pure cortical epilepsy
Muscle	Ragged red fibers found in myoclonic epilepsy with ragged red fibers

Secondary Complications: Depakote can exacerbate carnitine deficiency in patients with MERRF and should be supplemented with L-carnitine. Phenytoin, carbamazepine, and lamotrigine may worsen cortical epilepsy in patients with progressive myoclonic encephalopathy.

Bibliography

Caviness JN, Brown P. Myoclonus: current concepts and recent advances. *Lancet Neurol.* 2004;3(10): 598–607.

Espay AJ, Chen R. Myoclonus. *Continuum (Minneap Minn).* 2013;19:1264–86.

Factor S, Lang A, Weiner W, eds. *Drug induced movement disorders.* 2nd ed. Malden, MA: Wiley-Blackwell; 2008.

Fahn S, Jankovic J. Myoclonus phenomenology, etiology, physiology, and treatment. *Principles and Practice of Movement Disorders.* 2nd ed. Philadelphia: Saunders; 2011. p. 447.

Gálvez-Jiménez N, Tuite P, eds. *Uncommon causes of movement disorders.* Cambridge, UK: Cambridge University Press; 2011.

Jau-Shin L, Valls-SolÃ J, Toro C, Hallett M. Facial action myoclonus in patients with olivopontocerebellar atrophy. *Mov Disord.* 2004;9(2): 223–6.

Facial Nerve Neoplasm

Epidemiology and Demographics: Epidemiology depends on the type of tumors. For example, facial nerve schwannomas tend to present in the 5th decade of life and do not have a side preponderance. Malignant peripheral nerve sheath tumor involving the facial nerve typically occurs between 20 and 50 years of age.

Disorder Description: Facial nerve neoplasms can be benign (e.g., schwannoma and hemangioma) or primary malignant as well as metastatic from breast and kidney. Schwannoma and hemangiomas are the two most common neoplasms. Secondary malignant tumors spread in a hematogenous manner from the breast, lung, and kidney.

Symptoms

Localization site	Comment
Cranial nerves	Facial palsy that is slowly progressive (over 2–3 weeks) either isolated or along with hearing loss and tinnitus
	Recurrent facial palsy
	Hemangiomas at the geniculate ganglion in addition causes hemifacial spasm

Treatment Complications:

Craniotomies: Cerebrospinal fistula, seizures, hydrocephalus, and infection.

Mastoid or translabyrinthine approach: Hearing loss, tinnitus, vertigo, and infection.

Bibliography

Marcos-Salazar S, Prim-Espada MP, De Diego-Sastre JI, et al. [Facial nerve tumours]. *Rev Neurol.* 2004;39(12):1120–2.

Shirazi MA, Leonetti JP, Marzo SJ, Anderson DE. Surgical management of facial neuromas: lessons learned. *Otol Neurotol.* 2007;28(7):958–63.

Szudek J. Intratemporal tumors of the facial nerve. Updated March 11, 2016. Medscape. https://emedicine.medscape.com/article/846352-overview. Accessed Aug 15, 2016.

Facial Nerve Palsy

Epidemiology and Demographics: First described by Sir Charles Bell in the early 1800s, described as facial palsy related trauma to the peripheral branches of the facial nerve. Bell's palsy or "idiopathic facial paralysis" has an annual incidence of 13–34/100,000. No race, geographic, or gender predilection. There is an increased risk in patients with diabetes and during pregnancy (especially during the 3rd trimester or 1st week postpartum). The cause of facial palsy remains unknown, but suspected to be associated with Lyme disease, herpes simplex virus (HSV), herpes zoster virus, intranasal flu vaccine, genetics, or ischemia to the facial nerve.

Disorder Description: The facial nerve is a mixed nerve containing motor axons that innervate the face, parasympathetic fibers innervating the lacrimal, submandibular and sublingual salivary glands, afferent fibers responsible for the sensation of taste in the anterior two-thirds of the tongue, and somatic sensation in the external auditory canal and pinna. Facial nerve palsy has a prodrome of pain in the ear or occipital area and sensation of facial numbness. Followed by acute and sudden onset of unilateral facial paralysis including the forehead, eyebrow, inability to close the eye, drooping of the mouth. Associated with decreased tearing, hyperacusis, loss of taste on the affected side. The diagnosis is a clinical one, and neuroimaging and further evaluation if no improvement of symptoms over 3–4 months, slow progression beyond 3 weeks, multiple cranial nerve dysfunction. Differential diagnosis for facial palsy is wide and includes Lyme disease, Guillain–Barré syndrome, HIV, sarcoidosis, mass lesions, stroke, otitis media, herpes zoster oticus (Ramsay Hunt syndrome type II), and HSV infection. Facial palsy is generally self-limiting, and prognosis is favorable. Recovery is usually seen within the first 21 days from onset. Treatment involves initiation of oral glucocorticoids within 3 days of symptom onset, and an anti-viral agent is indicated as the possibility of a concurrent HSV infection is higher. Supportive care with natural tears, eye patching, and lubricating drops at bedtime. Electromyography/nerve conduction studies and blink study may be performed to assess for the integrity of the facial nerve.

Symptoms: Site of involvement is the facial nerve throughout its course to the facial muscles.

Secondary Complications: Dysarthria, trouble chewing, corneal dryness, abrasions or infection. Severe residual facial weakness may require plastic surgery.

Treatment Complications: Adverse effects from steroids.

Bibliography

Ronthal M. Bell's palsy: Pathogenesis, clinical features, and diagnosis in adults. *UpToDate*. Feb 2015. Waltham, MA. Available from www.uptodate.com/home.

Ronthal M. Bell's palsy: Prognosis and treatment in adults. *UpToDate*. Dec 2015. Waltham, MA. Availabe from http://uptodate.com/home

Facial Nerve Trauma

Epidemiology and Demographics: Sport injuries account for the majority of facial injuries among young adults. Other causes include motor vehicle accidents, domestic violence, falls, and animal bites. Injuries often are blunt force trauma, penetrating, or more commonly both.

Disorder Description: Facial nerves innervate the most anterior muscle layers of the face. Facial nerves travel through the temporal bone and are highly vulnerable to injury when the bone is fractured.

Symptoms: Facial injuries should be evaluated as well as the extent of the facial injuries (is the face symmetric, are there discrepancies in motor function, etc.).

Secondary Complications: Facial nerve trauma should be evaluated with trauma basics (primary survey). Once the patient is stabilized, the secondary survey can be conducted to further evaluate facial injuries. Airway compromise is commonly associated with facial trauma, especially in the setting of dysphonia, edema of the oropharynx, stridor, heavy bleeding, etc.

Bibliography

Mayersak R. Facial trauma in adults. *UpToDate*. Dec 2015. Waltham, MA. Available from http://uptodate.com/home

Facial Tics

Epidemiology and Demographics: Tics are common; however, epidemiological data are varied and contingent upon the methodology used. Twenty to 30% of children exhibit tics before the age of 18. Three percent of children develop some features of Tourette's syndrome (TS). TS is more common in boys than in girls. Ninety percent of patients with Tourette's syndrome carry comorbid psychiatric diagnoses.

Disorder Description: Facial tics are unwanted brief purposeless movements of facial muscles with premonitory sensations. They are suppressible to some extent and have stereotyped patterns with respect to the individual, although they vary greatly from person to person. They may be transient or chronic (>1 year), primary or secondary. Primary tics are more common, the most common of which are from Tourette's syndrome. Secondary causes are numerous and include neurodevelopmental disorders (autism spectrum disorder, Rett syndrome, Fragile X disorder, tuberous sclerosis, neurofibromatosis), neurodegenerative disorders (Huntington disease, neuroacanthocytosis, brain iron accumulation), systemic diseases (antiphospholipid syndrome), drug induced (stimulants, D2 blockers, anticonvulsants, levodopa), and structural lesions (posttraumatic, vascular, postinfectious), although these are uncommon.

Symptoms

Localization site	Comment
Cerebral hemispheres	Tourette syndrome is associated with structural and functional changes in the cortico-striatal-thalamo-cortical (CSTC) loop. The somatosensory and posterior parietal cortical regions, putamen, and amygdala/hippocampus complex demonstrate increased activity in spontaneous tics, while the anterior cingulate cortex and the caudate demonstrate decreased activity
Mental status and psychiatric aspects/complications	Obsessive-compulsive disorder, attention deficit hyperactivity disorder, impulse control disorder (self-injurious behavior), rage. Tics increase in frequency with stress, decrease when engaged in tasks. Tics associated with Tourette syndrome may also be associated with echophenomenon, pali phenomenon, and corpro phenomenon
Cranial nerves	Unintentional weakness from botulinum toxin
Muscle	Unintentional weakness from botulinum toxin

Treatment Complications: Hypotension, irritability, and disrupted sleep may occur with treatment with α-2 agonists. First generation antipsychotics may exacerbate anxiety and lead to dysphoria, gynecomastia, galactorrhea, irregular menses, sexual dysfunction, prolonged corrected QT interval/electrocardiogram changes, and weight gain. Sulpiride (used in Europe) may cause sedation. Tetrabenazine may cause depression, drowsiness, nausea, and fatigue. Botulinum toxin can cause temporary unintentional muscle weakness.

Bibliography

Fahn S, Jankovic J. Tics and Tourette syndrome. In *Principles and practice of movement disorders.* 2nd ed. Philadelphia: Saunders; 2011. pp. 350–79.

Martino D, Espay AJ, Fasano A, Morgante F. Tics. In *Disorders of movement: a guide to diagnosis and treatment.* New York: Springer; 2016. pp. 97–118.

Martino D, Mink JW. Tic disorders. *CONTINUUM (Minneap Minn).* 2013;19:1287–311.

Münchau A. Tics. In Brandt VC, ed. *Neuropsychiatric symptoms of movement disorders.* New York: Springer International; 2015. pp. 223–59.

Facioscapulohumeral Muscular Dystrophy (FSHD)

Epidemiology and Demographics: Prevalence of facioscapulohumeral muscular dystrophy (FSHD) is estimated at 7/100,000; however, it can surpass 13/100,000 due to unrecognized cases. FSHD is the third most common type of muscular dystrophy, behind Duchenne and Becker muscular dystrophies. There is no sex predominance. About 90% of patients show signs of disease by 20 years of age. There is no major geographic predominance.

Disorder Description: The facial, periscapular, biceps, triceps, pectoral, and leg muscles are the most affected. The deltoid muscles tend to be spared. Weakness spreads rostro-caudally, and asymmetric involvement is common. The physical exam usually reveals scapular winging, reversal of the anterior axillary folds, triple-hump sign, weak abdominal muscle, and foot drop. Hearing loss is reported in 75% of patients with FSHD, retinal vascular abnormalities in 60%, and 20% of patients eventually require wheelchair use. Dysphagia only in late stages of disease.

FSHD is an autosomal dominant disorder and up to 30% of cases are sporadic. While exact mechanism and etiology are unclear, it is thought to be an inappropriate expression of the double homeobox protein 4 gene (DUX4) on 4q35 region.

On diagnostic testing, CK levels range from normal to 1000 U/L. EMG reveals myopathic motor units with or without muscle membrane instability. The definitive diagnosis is based on genetic analysis.

Symptoms

Localization site	Comment
Cranial nerves	Retinal vascular abnormalities in 60% Hearing loss
Muscle	Involvement of facial, periscapular, biceps, triceps, pectoral, and leg muscles. Weakness spreads rostro-caudally, and proximal muscles more involved than distal

Secondary Complications: Patients can develop contractures, pain, wheelchair requirement in 20% of cases, and neurogenic dysphagia in late stages of disease. Cardiac arrhythmias are present in a slightly higher proportion of FSHD patients than control.

Treatment Complications: There is no current treatment at this time. Management is supportive and requires a multidisciplinary approach.

Bibliography

Orrell RW. Facioscapulohumeral dystrophy and scapuloperoneal syndromes. *Handb Clin Neurol.* 2011;101:167–80.

Factitious Disorder

Epidemiology and Demographics: Overall prevalence unclear, but present in estimated 1% of hospital population. Gender predominance is unknown. Onset is often in early adulthood, frequently after a hospitalization.

Disorder Description: Characterized by intentional misrepresentation of physical or psychologic symptoms in the absence of overt external reward (i.e., not referable to "secondary gain"). In order to meet DSM-5 criteria, an individual must present self as ill, impaired, or injured. Evidence for deception must be established and the behavior is not better explained by another mental disorder. Can appear as single episode or recurrent. Another variation is factitious disorder imposed on another (formerly known as Munchausen syndrome by proxy), which involves falsification of symptoms in another, also in setting of identified deception and absence of external reward.

These disorders are distinct from malingering, in which secondary gain is established. They are also not to be confused with other disorders in the classification of somatic symptom disorder, in which symptoms occur in absence of external reward, but in context of "primary gain," with absence of evidence of deception.

Risk factors include childhood trauma, including receiving significant attention for mental or physical issues in childhood, prior hospitalization, and certain personality disorders such as narcissistic, borderline, and antisocial. Individual may be employed in healthcare profession.

Symptoms

Localization site	Comment
Mental status and psychiatric aspects/ complications	History may be vague, false information given, fluctuating course of symptoms, symptoms may occur only when watched, usually sophisticated knowledge of medical terminology, attention-seeking behavior, may have evidence of multiple surgeries and/or procedures

Secondary Complications: Frequent healthcare utilization, intermittent reinforcement of maladaptive behaviors in medical settings, leading to intractability. Potential for iatrogenic complications from medication, procedures, and surgeries. Potential legal implications with factitious disorder imposed on another.

Treatment Complications: Patients often resistant to accepting therapy; however, supportive psychotherapy found to be helpful, as well as treatment of psychiatric comorbidity when present.

Bibliography

American Psychiatric Association. *Diagnostic and statistical manual of mental disorders: DSM-5.* 5th ed. Washington, DC: American Psychiatric Association; 2013.

McEwen DR. Recognizing Munchausen's syndrome. *AORN J.* 1998;67:206–11.

Reich P, Gottfried LA. Factitious disorders in a teaching hospital. *Ann Intern Med.* 1983;99(2):240–7.

Factitious Disorder (Imposed on Self or Imposed on Another) (Munchausen's Syndrome, and Munchausen's Syndrome by Proxy), Additional Facts

Epidemiology and Demographics: Factitious disorder involves a conscious act of simulating medical conditions in order to be in the sick role. Among hospitalized patients, approximately 1% have presentations that meet the criteria for factitious disorder. Factitious disorder is a diagnosis of exclusion. Since psychiatric comorbidity such as depression and personality disorders are common, a detailed psychiatric assessment should be performed in these patients.

Disorder Description: Based on DSM-5, factitious disorder is further subdivided into "imposed on self" and "imposed on another":

A. Conscious falsification of physical or psychologic signs or symptoms, or induction of injury or disease in oneself or another individual (victim).

B. The individual presents him/herself or the victim to others as ill, impaired, or injured.

C. The behavior is evident even in the absence of obvious external rewards, since the reward, to obtain the sick role, is unconscious to the patient.

D. The behavior is not better explained by another mental disorder, such as delusional disorder or another psychotic disorder.

Munchausen syndrome (and Munchausen syndrome by proxy) are terms used to describe factitious disorder in which there are predominant physical signs and symptoms.

Differential Diagnosis: Differential diagnosis should include somatic symptom disorder, malingering, conversion disorder, borderline personality disorder, and medical condition or mental disorder not associated with intentional symptom falsification.

In somatic symptom disorder, there may be perceived medical concerns, but the individual is not purposely falsifying information or being deceptive. Hence, both the motive and the act are unconscious to the patient.

In malingering, the falsification of symptoms is for personal gain (e.g., money or time off from work, drugs). In factitious disorder, there is an absence of external rewards. In malingering, both the act and the motive are conscious to the patient.

In conversion disorder (functional neurologic symptom disorder), neurologic symptoms may be inconsistent with neurologic pathophysiology. In conversion, both the motive and the act are unconscious to the patient.

In borderline personality disorder, there may be deliberate self-harm in the absence of suicidal intent. Factitious disorder can be distinguished because it requires that such self-harm occur with deceptive intent and usually is linked with falsification of medical symptoms.

The presence of factitious disorder does not exclude a medical condition or mental disorder not associated with intentional symptom falsification. For example, someone who manipulated blood sugar levels to produce symptoms may also have diabetes. Hence, it is doubly important to rule out or treat the co-occurring medical illness.

Secondary Complications: In cases wherein symptoms are produced through modes of self-harm (e.g., insulin injections, swallowing dangerous objects), a variety of medical complications may arise and should be assessed.

Treatment Complications: Psychotherapy to address specific behaviors such as self harm and the incessant need for the sick role would be the treatment of choice.

Selective serotonin reuptake inhibitors (SSRIs) have been shown to be effective in managing underlying problems in factitious disorder since anxiety and depression are commonly comorbid.

SSRI side effects include nausea, diarrhea, insomnia, headache, anorexia, weight loss, sexual dysfunction, restlessness (akathisia-like), serotonin syndrome (fever diaphoresis, tachycardia, hypertension, delirium, neuromuscular excitability), hyponatremia, seizures (0.2%).

If factitious disorder is imposed on another and if the victim is a child, involvement of the local child protective agencies is warranted.

Bibliography

American Psychiatric Association. *Diagnostic and statistical manual of mental disorders: DSM-5.* 5th ed. Washington, DC: American Psychiatric Association; 2013.

Krahn LE, Li H, O'Connor MK. Patients who strive to be ill: factitious disorder with physical symptoms. *Am J Psychiatry.* 2003;160(6):1163–8.

Sutherland AJ, Rodin GM. Factitious disorders in a general hospital setting: clinical features and a review of the literature. *Psychosomatics.* 1990;31(4):392–9.

Factor V Leiden Mutation

Epidemiology and Demographics: Most common inherited form of thrombophilia. Complicated frequency statistics with different rates among varying populations and heterozygosity versus homozygosity.

Disorder Description: Factor V activation by APC (activated protein C) is an essential step in the breakdown of Factor VIIIa. A mutation in Factor V leads to it becoming resistant to APC cleavage, which, in turn, results in reduced degradation of Factor VIIIa. This leaves the person thrombophilic with the potential for cerebral vein or dural sinus thrombosis (CVT).

Symptoms

Localization site	Comment
Cerebral hemispheres	Headache, thunderclap headache (in CVT), aphasia, hemiparesis, hemisensory loss, seizures, intracranial hemorrhage (in CVT), embolic stroke due to paradoxical embolism from deep vein thrombosis through a patent foramen ovale
Mental status and psychiatric aspects/ complications	Altered mental status/coma (in CVT)

Secondary Complications: Deep vein thrombosis of lower extremity or pelvic vein can embolize through a patent foramen ovale causing ischemic stroke.

Treatment Complications: Anticoagulation can cause intracranial hemorrhage or systemic bleeding with blood loss, both of which can lead to altered mental status.

Bibliography

Biffi A, Greenberg SM. Cerebral amyloid angiopathy: a systematic review. *J Clin Neurol.* 2011;7(1):1–9.

Caplan LR. Factor V Leiden: clinical manifestations and diagnosis. In Bogousslavsky K, ed. *Uncommon causes of stroke.* 2nd ed. Cambridge, UK: Cambridge University Press; 2008. Chapter 6.

Familial Cerebral Amyloid Angiopathy

Epidemiology and Demographics: Hereditary Aβ amyloid angiopathy is a group of cerebral amyloid angiopathies (CCAs) classified on the basis of where they were first described. Most of the familial CAAs are caused by a mutation in one of several genes, including: APP gene on chromosome 21 (Danish, Flemish, Italian, Iowa); Cystatin C on chromosome 20 (Icelandic); BRI gene on chromosome 13 (British, Danish).

There is also an atypical form of familial oculoleptomeningeal CAA (transthyretin CAA).

Disorder Description: The syndrome of cerebral amyloid angiopathy is usually recognized when a patient over 65 years old presents with a lobar hemorrhage that ruptures into the ventricular system. Microhemorrhages identified on susceptibility weighted MRI sequences serve to establish the diagnosis, although there is overlap with patients having severe, uncontrolled hypertension. Patients are also at risk for small vessel ischemic disease with lacunar strokes or vascular dementia.

Symptoms

Localization site	Comment
Cerebral hemispheres	Hemiparesis, aphasia, hemisensory loss, and hemianiopia may result from intracerebral hemorrhage (ICH), ischemic stroke, transient ischemic attack, or focal seizures
Mental status and psychiatric aspects/ complications	Loss of working and intermediate memory (dementia), altered mental status after ICH
Cerebellum	Ataxia (British type, Danish type)
Cranial nerves	Cataracts, deafness (Danish type), vision loss (transthyretin CAA)
Peripheral neuropathy	Painful neuropathy with dizziness, erectile dysfunction due to autonomic involvement (transthyretin CAA)

Secondary Complications: Falls causing subdural hematoma with altered mental status. Dementia can cause acute delirium in hospital setting.

Treatment Complications: Antipsychotics used to treat delirium in dementia patients are associated with increased mortality. Anticoagulation or use of dual antiplatelet agents should generally be avoided as bleeding risk is high.

Bibliography

Caplan LR, ed. *Uncommon causes of stroke.* 2nd ed. Cambridge, UK: Cambridge University Press; 2010.

Familial Hemiplegic Migraine

Epidemiology and Demographics: In one study of the population in Denmark, the prevalence of hemiplegic migraine is estimated at 0.01%. Attacks can occur as early as age 5–7 years and mean onset is at age 12–17 years. This type of headache usually ceases after the age of 50 years, but there are few reports of some patients who continue to have these headaches. Hemiplegic migraines affect women more than men at a ratio of 2.5–4.3:1.

Disorder Description: This condition involves a migraine headache associated with scintillating scotoma, hemianopsia, aphasia, lethargy, confusion, positive or negative hemisensory symptoms, hemiparesis, fever, coma, status epilepticus, and even death. These patients also endure migraine headaches with aura attacks. Some cases present with acute neurologic signs that are initially indistinguishable from ischemic strokes. One percent of hemiplegic migraine patients do not experience actual headaches. The presence of motor weakness that is reversible as part of aura is a necessary component for diagnosis of this condition. For familial hemiplegic migraine diagnosis, the patient must have at least one first- or second-degree relative with similar attacks.

Symptoms

Localization site	Comment
Cerebral hemispheres	Involvement of CACNA1A gene that encodes P/Q calcium channels that are expressed in the brain

Secondary Complications: Some presentations of this condition can mimic acute ischemic stroke. In these patients, imaging will be required as these symptoms can persist for days.

Treatment Complications: There are no abortive therapies that have been studied with randomized and controlled trials. However, verapamil has been used successfully as a prophylactic treatment for seizures. Additionally, acetazolamide has been used with some success. Intranasal ketamine has also been used successfully. No extensive studies have been performed with these medications to enlist known side effects or complications with these treatments.

Bibliography

Black DF. Sporadic and familial hemiplegic migraine: diagnosis and treatment. *Semin Neurol.* 2006;26:208–16.

Bradshaw P, Parsons M. Hemiplegic migraine, a clinical study. *Q J Med.* 1965;34:65–86.

Thomsen LL, Eriksen MK, Roemer SF, et al. An epidemiological survey of hemiplegic migraine. *Cephalalgia.* 2002;22:361–75.

Whitty CWM. Familial hemiplegic migraine. *J Neurol Neurosurg Psychiatry.* 1953;16:172–7.

Familial Idiopathic Basal Ganglia Calcification (FIBGC)

Epidemiology and Demographics: Familial idiopathic basal ganglia calcification (FIBGC) is a rare neurodegenerative disease. Its true prevalence is unknown as it has been reported in only a few family case series and individual case reports. There may be a male predominance in families studied. The age of onset is variable but commonly occurs in the fourth or fifth decades.

Disorder Description: FIBCG is a neurodegenerative disease characterized by calcifications in the basal ganglia with or without other brain regions, not attributed to any known etiology. Patients typically present with progressive movement disorders, changes in cognition, and psychiatric states. Onset is insidious. An akinetic-rigid syndrome with or without tremor is the most common presenting symptom. Hyperkinetic movement disorders are rarer. FIBCG is typically inherited in an autosomal dominant fashion but sporadic cases have been reported. Mutations in the SLC20A2, PDGFRB, and PDGFB genes have been identified to be causative in some patients. However, there is both significant genetic and clinical variability. Pathophysiology is unclear and may involve abnormal calcium and phosphate homeostasis with disruption of the blood–brain barrier.

Symptoms

Localization site	Comment
Cerebral hemispheres	Calcifications are most commonly found in the globus pallidus. They are also seen in the striatum, cerebral cortex and white matter, the internal capsule, and thalamus
	Parkinsonism
	Gait disorder
	Chorea
	Tremor
	Dystonia
	Athetosis
	Orofacial dyskinesia
	Seizure
	Paresis and stroke-like event
Mental status and psychiatric aspects/ complications	Cognitive impairment
	Depression
	Psychosis with both hallucinations and delusions
	Schizophrenia-like symptoms
	Bipolar disorder-like symptoms with mania and depression
	Anxiety
	Catatonia
	Aggression and irritability
	Personality changes
Cerebellum	Calcifications found in the cerebellar hemispheres, dentate nucleus
	Dysarthria
	Ataxia
Vestibular system (and non-specific dizziness)	Vertigo
Unclear localization	Migraine with and without aura
	Orthostatic hypotension
	Syncope

Bibliography

Keller A, et al. Mutations in the gene encoding PDGF-B cause brain calcifications in humans and mice. *Nat Genet.* 2013;45(9):1077–82.

Manyam BV, et al. Bilateral striopallidodentate calcinosis: clinical characteristics of patients seen in a registry. *Mov Disord.* 2001;16(2):258–64.

Nicolas G, et al. Mutation of the PDGFRB gene as a cause of idiopathic basal ganglia calcification. *Neurology.* 2013;80(2):181–7.

Nicolas G, et al. Phenotypic spectrum of probable and genetically-confirmed idiopathic basal ganglia calcification. *Brain.* 2013;136(11): 3395–407.

Wang C, Li Y, Shi L, et al. Mutations in SLC20A2 link familial idiopathic basal ganglia calcification with phosphate homeostasis. *Nature Genet.* 2012;44(3):254–6.

Familial Vestibulocerebellar Syndrome (aka Vestibulocerebellar Ataxia)

Epidemiology and Demographics: Very rare autosomal dominant inherited disorder traced to the pedigree of three families with ties to North Carolina.

Disorder Description: At childhood, affected individuals may develop a combination of ocular abnormalities including poor smooth pursuit, diplopia, oscillopsia, and abnormalities in the vestibule-ocular reflex resulting in gaze-paretic nystagmus and rebound nystagmus. Periodic attacks of vertigo and tinnitus following sudden head movements or fatigue may also be a presenting sign. Older individuals may exhibit motor dysfunction with episodic attacks of ataxia not associated with dysarthria or loss of limb motor control. This syndrome is caused by a failure of function of the flocculus in the vestibulocerebellum.

Symptoms

Localization site	Comment
Inner ear	Unaffected, in the classical case
Cranial nerves	The cochleovestibular nerve is not affected
Central nervous system	Dysfunction of the flocculonodular lobe of the cerebellum

Secondary Complications: Vertigo attacks can result in falls for these patients. A form of progressive ataxia may occur, rendering afflicted individuals incapacitated.

Treatment Complications: Treatment is supportive – lying down, closing eyes following an attack. Acetazolamide and antihistamines have demonstrated some benefit. Vestibular suppressants may cause drowsiness and anticholinergic effects. Acetazolamide can cause paresthesias and anorexia.

Bibliography

Harris CM, Walker J, Shawkat F, Wilson J, Russell-Eggitt I. Eye movements in a familial vestibulocerebellar disorder. *Neuropediatrics.* 1993;3:177–22.

Theunissen EJ, Huygen PL, Verhagen WI. Familial vestibulocerebellar dysfunction: a new syndrome? *J Neurol Sci.* 1989;89:49–155.

Fasciitis

Epidemiology and Demographics: Plantar fasciitis is the most common reason for heel pain, which is seen in 80% of cases. It is more common in women, military recruits, older athletes, obese individuals, and young male athletes.

Disorder Description: Plantar fasciitis refers to pain in the heel and bottom of leg. Pain is more severe with first step of the day or following rest. The pain increases with exercise and obesity.

An inflammation of the connective tissue that may be caused by streptococcal or other types of infection, an injury, or an autoimmune reaction. There are several types:

1. Necrotizing fasciitis is a fulminating group A streptococcal infection beginning with severe or extensive cellulitis that spreads to involve the superficial and deep fascia, leading to thrombosis of the subcutaneous vessels and gangrene of the underlying tissue.
2. Nodular fasciitis is a reactive proliferation of fibroblasts in the subcutaneous tissue. It is usually seen in deep fascia.
3. Pseudosarcomatous fasciitis is a benign soft tissue tumor occurring subcutaneously and occasionally from deep muscle and fascia.
4. Eosinophilic fasciitis is an inflammation of fascia of the lymphatic system, eosinophilia, edema, and swelling, usually after strenuous exercise.

5. Proliferative fasciitis is a benign reactive proliferation of the fibroblasts in subcutaneous tissues resembling nodular fasciitis. Basilar joint cells are seen. They occur in skeletal muscles in older patients.

Symptoms

Localization site	Comment
Heels	Pain in heel and bottom of feet, one-third can be bilateral
Site of infection of necrotizing fasciitis	Increasing pain, erythema, and swelling in excess of what would be expected. Fever, chills, skin, ulceration, bullae and blister formation, necrotic scar, gas formation in tissue is noted, sepsis can occur with this
Eosinophilic fasciitis	Hardening of the area, redness, warmth of the skin surface are noted

Treatment Complications: Treatments include nonsteroidal anti-inflammatories, rest, heat, ice, exercises. Extracorporeal shock wave therapy can also be used. Iontophoresis surgery, dry needling, and Botox can also be considered. Necrotizing fasciitis will require IV antibiotics, debridement of necrotic tissue, prednisone, methotrexate, cyclophosphamide, mycophenolate mofetil (CellCept) and rituximab (Rituxan). For nodular fasciitis, excisional biopsy should be done.

Corticosteroid therapy could result in plantar fascia rupture.

Bibliography

CDC. Acting fast is key with necrotizing fasciitis. June 15, 2016. www.cdc.gov/features/necrotizingfasciitis/index.html. Accessed Aug 15, 2019.

Lareau CR, Sawyer GA, Wang JH, Digiovanni CW. Plantar and medial heel pain: diagnosis and management. *J Am Acad Orthoped Surg.* 2014;22(6) 372–80.

Fascioliasis

Epidemiology and Demographics: It is estimated that there are 2.4 million and perhaps as many as 17 million affected people[1,2] in many countries including the Americas, Europe, Africa, and Asia. These rates may be even higher, depending on unknown prevalence rates in Asia and Africa.

Disorder Description: Fascioliasis, a foodborne and waterborne zoonotic disease, is caused by two parasite species, the liver flukes *Fasciola hepatica* and *F. gigantica*. *F. hepatica* and *F. gigantica* are parasites of the large biliary passages and the gallbladder of ruminants, mainly sheep, goats, and cattle. Human infections usually occur after the ingestion of aquatic plants that contain encysted organisms or by consumption of contaminated water. The parasite has a special tropism for the liver and also affects many other organ systems. It manifests itself into an acute form consisting of prolonged fever, hepatomegaly, and abdominal pain; and a chronic form consisting of symptoms of biliary obstruction, frank cholangitis, or pancreatitis.

Blood eosinophilia and the ingestion of watercress or any freshwater plants are suggestive of a fascioliasis diagnosis. The definitive diagnosis is made by the presence of *Fasciola* eggs in a stool or gallbladder sample, or on a positive serologic test plus radiologic findings indicating fascioliasis.[3]

Triclabendazole is the drug of choice. The alternative is nitazoxanide. No significant side effects have been reported to date.

Symptoms[4]

Localization site	Comment
Cerebral hemispheres	Cephalgia, meningeal syndrome, focal symptoms, and seizures
Mental status and psychiatric aspects/ complications	Altered intellectual functioning

References

1. Ashrafi K, Bargues MD, O'Neill S, Mas-Coma S. Fascioliasis: a worldwide parasitic disease of importance in travel medicine. *Travel Med Infect Dis.* 2014;12:636–49.
2. Mas-Coma MS, Esteban JG, Bargues MD. Epidemiology of human fascioliasis: a review and proposed new classification. *Bull World Health Organ.* 1999;77:340–6.
3. Saba R, Korkmaz M, Inan D, et al. Human fascioliasis. *Clin Microbiol Infect.* 2004;10:385–7.
4. Arjona R, Riancho JA, Aguado JM, Salesa R, Gonzalez-Macias J. Fascioliasis in developed countries: a review of classic aberrant forms of the disease. *Medicine.* 1995;74:13–23.

Fatal Familial Insomnia

Epidemiology and Demographics: Fatal familial insomnia (FFI) has been identified in rare familial clusters but sporadic cases have been described. Onset occurs in adulthood, usually between 35 and 60 years old.

It is inherited as an autosomal dominant disease and results from a missense mutation at the codon 178 of the *PRNP* gene located on chromosome 20p13. The clinical syndrome varies by M129V genotype with manifestation of disease in homozygous individuals at a younger age and with a shorter course versus heterozygous individuals.

Disorder Description: FFI is a prion disease that is rapidly fatal. It is characterized by progressive insomnia and loss of normal circadian sleep–wake pattern. During waking hours, a confusional dream-like state may occur with behavioral changes including inattention, impaired memory, confusion, and hallucinations. In more advanced stages, motor symptoms manifest such as myoclonus, ataxia, spasticity, dysarthria, and dysphagia. Dysautonomia and endocrine disturbances can also occur, which among the prion diseases are differentiating features of FFI.

Diagnosis is difficult, as routine laboratory testing, CT, MRI, and CSF studies are unremarkable. Fluorodeoxyglucose PET may show reduced glucose utilization in the thalamus, and these changes can be seen early in the disease course. Polysomnography will show reduction in total sleep time and abnormal sleep architecture.

Symptoms

Localization site	Comment
Forebrain	Thalamic degeneration of anterior and dorsomedial thalamic nuclei with reactive gliosis. Spongiform changes in cortical layers have been described
	Deposition of proteinase K-resistant prion protein type 2 in the gray matter but not white matter
	Somatomotor symptoms manifest as dysarthria, dysphagia, tremor, myoclonus (spontaneous or reflex), ataxia, and positive Babinski sign
Mental status and psychiatric aspects/ complications	Initially symptoms of difficulty initiating and maintaining sleep that progresses to spontaneous lapses into sleep with enacted sleep (oneiric stupor). Difficulty concentrating, memory impairments, and hallucinations are common
	Cognitive function is maintained until the final stages of disease that are characterized by an inability to identify any distinct sleep stages, stupor, coma, and death

In the early stages of disease, EEG shows periods of relaxed wakefulness alternating with EEG desynchronization and rapid eye movement (REM) bursts. There is also a loss of antigravity muscle tone and irregular tremor-like and myoclonic limb muscle activities associated with vivid dreams, which is termed oneiric stupor.

As the disease progresses there is a paucity of sleep spindles and a loss of the features of slow wave sleep.

Loss of circadian rhythms including body temperature, blood pressure, respiratory and heart rate, as well as endocrine rhythms of hormone secretion (i.e., growth hormone, adrenocorticotrophic hormone, prolactin, luteinizing hormone, and follicular-stimulating hormone).

Secondary Complications: Autonomic dysregulation, dysphagia with increased risk of food aspiration, and skin breakdown from immobility in later stages of disease. Infections (usually respiratory or genitourinary) are common and often the cause of death in patients.

Treatment Complications: There is no effective treatment for FFI and the disorder is universally fatal within 8 to 72 months.

Bibliography

American Academy of Sleep Medicine. *The international classification of sleep disorders*. 3rd ed. Chicago, IL; American Academy of Sleep Medicine; 2014.

Krasnianski A, Bartl M, Sanchez Juan PJ, et al. Fatal familial insomnia: Clinical features and early identification. *Ann Neurol*. 2008;63(5):658.

Manetto V, Medori R, Cortelli P, et al. Fatal familial insomnia: clinical and pathologic study of five new cases. *Neurology*. 1992;42(2):312.

Mastrianni JA, Nixon R, Layzer R, et al. Prion protein conformation in a patient with sporadic fatal insomnia. *New Engl J Med*. 1999;340:1630–8.

Peng B, Zhang S, Dong H, Lu Z. Clinical, histopathological and genetic studies in a case of fatal familial insomnia with review of the literature. *Int J Clin Exp Pathol*. 2015;8:10171–7.

Fat Embolism

Epidemiology and Demographics: Fat embolism occurs mostly after trauma (95%) involving long bone fractures. Other non-trauma-related causes (5%)

are liposuction, bone marrow transplant, sickle cell, lipid infusions, and osteomyelitis.

Disorder Description: Emboli from adipose tissue and bone marrow enter the blood stream and by direct mechanical as well as toxic intermediates cause the various clinical manifestations of fat embolism syndrome.

Symptoms

Localization site	Comment
Cerebral hemispheres	Hemiplegia, aphasia, apraxia, seizures, embolic strokes (often reversible)
Mental status and psychiatric aspects/complications	Altered mental status, initially with restlessness and irritability
Unclear localization	Tachycardia, tachypnea

Secondary Complications: Hypoxia due to lung emboli and acute respiratory distress syndrome causing altered mental status.

Treatment Complications: Corticosteroids (sometimes given) can cause psychosis.

Bibliography

Gupta A, Riley CS. Fat embolism. *Contin Educ Anaesth Crit Care Pain.* 2007;7(5):148–51. DOI: 10.1093/bjaceaccp/mkm027.

Febrile Convulsions and Temporal Lobe Epilepsy with Digenic Inheritance

Epidemiology and Demographics: In 2001, the condition was described in a single French family. Mean age of epilepsy onset was 9 years old. Genes associated were 1q25-q31 and 18qter.

Disorder Description: A number of individual genes have independently been associated with the development of febrile seizures (FS). Although the majority of children with FS do not develop temporal lobe epilepsy (TLE), the former has been well established as a risk factor for the latter. At least in some cases, the occurrence of TLE following infantile FS is due to a digenic mechanism. The single family described with this condition had normal MRI findings in patients with TLE. There were nine affected family members over four generations. Multiple family members were clinically unaffected, with a single gene mutation.

The variety of TLE in these patients was relatively mild (all patients except one were seizure-free off medication by age 24 years). EEG data were limited.

Symptoms

Localization site	Comment
Cerebral hemispheres	No hippocampal structural abnormalities. Seizures possibly temporal neocortical in origin
Mental status and psychiatric aspects/complications	One case report of associated personality problems and mild intellectual impairment

Treatment Complications: Antiepileptic drugs are the primary treatment for TLE. These may be associated with cognitive impairment, ataxia, dizziness, and more rarely severe allergic reactions, liver failure, or pancreatitis. Surgical resection of the temporal lobe commonly causes a visual field cut and rarely has more severe complications including stroke.

Bibliography

Baulac S, et al. Evidence for digenic inheritance in a family with both febrile convulsions and temporal lobe epilepsy implicating chromosomes 18qter and 1q25-q31. *Ann Neurol.* 2001;49(6):786–92.

Febrile Seizures (FS)

Epidemiology and Demographics: Febrile seizures (FS) are the most common form of childhood seizures, occurring in 2–5% of children, with increased incidence in those with affected first-degree relatives. Peak incidence around 18 months of age.

Disorder Description: Defined as a seizure occurring with a febrile illness in a child over 1 month of age without history of afebrile seizures. Occurs in absence of central nervous system infection or acute metabolic abnormality. Onset of fever can be after seizure occurrence. Any bacterial or viral illness (rarely an immunization) may be the precipitant of the fever, e.g., HHV6. Etiology appears to be genetic in origin, with multiple gene mutations described in association with FS. Simple FS: most common, generalized convulsions that last <15 minutes and do not occur again within 24 hours. Complex FS: seizure with focal features, lasting longer than 15 minutes or occurring more than once within 24 hours. There is increased risk of occurrence in children with two of the following factors: a history of febrile seizures in a first- or second-degree relative, a neonatal nursery stay of more than 30 days, developmental delay, or attendance at daycare. Primary treatment is to treat underlying cause for fever. Rescue medications such as benzodiazepines may be considered.

Symptoms

Localization site	Comment
Cerebral hemispheres	Generalized tonic–clonic seizure with fever
	Febrile status epilepticus may occur

Secondary Complications: Respiratory complication may occur due to prolonged seizures. Risk of later developing epilepsy near 1 in 40 cases. Increased risk of history of complex FS.

Treatment Complications: Acetaminophen may be associated with liver dysfunction at high doses. Benzodiazepines may be associated with excessive sedation, hypotension, or respiratory depression.

Bibliography

Ashwal S, Swaiman KF. *Swaiman's pediatric neurology.* 5th ed. Edinburgh: Saunders; 2012.

Patel N, et al. Febrile seizures. *BMJ.* 2015;351:h4240.

Female Sexual Interest/Arousal Disorder

Epidemiology and Demographics: Overall prevalence is unknown. In general, prevalence of diminished sexual desire is higher than distress about sexual functioning among women.

Disorder Description: Defined in DSM-5 as low or lack of interest in sexual activity or arousal associated with at least three of the following: (1) no or low interest in sex, (2) no or infrequent thoughts about sex, (3) no or infrequent initiation of sex and lack of response to partner initiation, (4) no or low pleasure or excitement in all or over 75% of sexual encounters, (5) no or low sexual interest or arousal with internal or external erotic cues, and/or (6) no or low genital or nongenital sensations during sexual activity in all or over 75% of sexual encounters. Symptoms present at least 6 months and cause significant distress.

Symptoms are not better accounted for by another mental or medical disorder, substances, or secondary to severe distress in relationship. The disorder can be classified as lifelong, acquired, generalized, or situational. Special consideration of factors related to the partner, relationship, individual vulnerability (including history of prior sexual abuse), associated psychiatric illness, culture, or medical condition (e.g., diabetes and thyroid disease) can help elucidate cause and guide intervention. There is a high association with other sexual difficulties and depression. There may be a genetic predisposition.

Low sexual desire may be more prominent in women of East Asian culture than European and Canadian cultures as per one study. There is significant cultural variability, some of which may reflect differences in cultural norms of behavior.

Symptoms

Localization site	Comment
Mental status and psychiatric aspects/complications	Depressed mood, anxiety

Secondary Complications: Dissatisfaction with sex life, impaired romantic relationships.

Treatment Complications: Filbanserin, FDA approved for this condition, may be accompanied by side effects of hypotension with alcohol use, insomnia, sedation, dizziness, and/or nausea.

Bibliography

American Psychiatric Association. *Diagnostic and statistical manual of mental disorders: DSM-5.* 5th ed. Washington, DC: American Psychiatric Association; 2013.

Bancroft J, Loftus J, Long JS. Distress about sex: a national survey of women in heterosexual relationships. *Arch Sex Behav.* 2003;32(3):193–208.

Woo JS, Brotto LA, Gorzalka BB. The relationship between sex guilt and sexual desire in a community sample of Chinese and Euro-Canadian women. *J Sex Res.* 2012;49(2–3):290–8.

Femoral Neuropathy

Epidemiology and Demographics: The femoral nerve is the largest branch of the lumbosacral plexus, formed from the L1–L4 nerve roots. It is responsible for knee extension and anterior thigh sensation.

It courses beneath the inguinal ligament and has a pure sensory branch, the saphenous nerve, that extends down to the medial calf and into the foot.

Disorder Description: Femoral nerve is commonly injured from compression secondary to hip or pelvic fractures or masses within the iliacus such as hematomas. Saphenous nerve injuries can be seen with mild trauma to the knee or after knee operations. Femoral nerve injuries have been associated with diabetic neuropathies, hip replacement procedures, abdominal and pelvic surgeries, inguinal lymph node biopsies, femoral nerve blocks, prolonged lithotomy positioning, and femoral artery punctures.

Commonly present with isolated quadriceps weakness with hip adduction intact (innervated by obturator nerve). Associated with sensory loss over the anterior and medial thigh extending to the medial calf and foot. Patellar reflexes are diminished or absent.

Electromyography/nerve conduction velocity is helpful in confirming the presence of femoral neuropathy, ruling out a lumbar radiculopathy, and prognosticates by determining the degree of axonal loss. Management of femoral nerve injuries is generally supportive (including managing pain and physical therapy), surgical management by relieving compression and draining compressive hematomas, or nerve repair/grafting in transection or ligation injuries.

Symptoms: Weakness of the femoral nerve innervated muscles and sensory changes in the distribution of the sensory fibers.

Bibliography

Rutkove S. Overview of lower extremity peripheral nerve syndromes. Dec 2014. *Uptodate.* Availabe from www.uptodate.com/contents/overview-of-upper-extremity-peripheral-nerve-syndromes?topicRef=5278&source=see_link

Fibromuscular Dysplasia

Epidemiology and Demographics: Fibromuscular dysplasia involving the craniocervical arteries occurs in approximately 0.02% population. Whites are affected more than the black population, women more than men. It is seen in young to middle-aged adults.

Disorder Description: Angiopathy affects medium size arteries. Young women of childbearing age are susceptible. Renal involvement is noted in 60–75% of patients; cerebrovascular involvement is seen in 25–30% of patients. Visceral involvement in 9% and limb involvement in 5%.

Symptoms

Localization site	Comment
Cerebral hemisphere	Headache, lightheadedness, vertigo, tinnitus, speech disturbance, neck pain, or carotidynia
Face	Transient or permanent neurologic deficits of face
Extremities	Transient or permanent neurologic deficits of extremities. Intermittent leg claudication due to extremity artery involvement reported
Eyes	Visual changes
Cerebral vasculature	Aneurysms, which may rupture
Renal	Hypertension
Mesenteric or visceral artery involvement	Abdominal pain due to ischemic bowel

Treatment Complications: Stroke associated with this disorder is treated with tissue plasminogen activator, which carries potential bleeding complications. Hypertension is treated if there is aneurysmal rupture based on angiography. Surgery might be required. Dissection warrants anticoagulation.

Bibliography

Luscher TF, Lie JT, Stanson AW, et al. Arterial fibromuscular dysplasia. *Mayo Clin Proc.* 1987;62(10):931–52.

Flavivirus

Epidemiology and Demographics: The flaviviruses[1,2] are arthropod-borne or arboviruses and are transmitted by either mosquitoes or ticks. The genus contains more than 70 viruses, of which dengue virus, Japanese encephalitis virus (JEV), West Nile virus (WNV), and tick-borne encephalitis are the most important human pathogenic flaviviruses that are neuroinvasive. Each species of flavivirus has distinct geographic distribution.

Dengue is the second most common mosquito-borne disease affecting humans after malaria and causes 100 to 200 million infections with more than 20,000 deaths annually.

Japanese encephalitis virus is endemic in Southeast Asia and causes severe encephalitis in 50,000 cases with 25 to 30% fatality each year.

West Nile virus was known to be endemic in parts of Africa, Europe, Asia, and Australia but has emerged recently on the East Coast of the United States and has spread to North America, Central America, and South America.

Tick-borne encephalitis virus is found in many parts of Europe and Central and Eastern Asia and accounts for more than 10,000 cases per year of central nervous system (CNS) infection in adults.

Disorder Description: Flaviviruses are single-stranded, positive-sense RNA viruses; transmission cycles consist of vertebrate hosts and insect vectors. Humans are dead-end hosts. Flavivirus infections in humans range from relatively mild fever and arthralgia to severe hemorrhagic and encephalitic manifestations. Neuroinvasive infections[3,4] occur frequently with JEV, WNV, dengue virus, and tick-borne encephalitis viruses.

Dengue infection follows only malaria as the most common etiology of fever in individuals returning from the developing world, and symptomatic infections can present from aspecific or mild febrile disease to dengue hemorrhagic fever or dengue shock syndromes. In addition encephalopathy may result from the consequences of systemic infections. Dengue encephalitis is significantly underreported. CNS manifestations include non-specific alterations of consciousness, seizures, headache, meningeal signs, and paralytic and parkinsonian syndrome.

Japanese encephalitis virus infection presents as a febrile syndrome that commonly progresses to neurologic symptoms, which include alterations of consciousness, seizures, parkinsonian movement disorder, and dystonia. Seventy percent of symptomatic infections manifest as encephalitis while 10% present as meningitis. Another 5–20% of patients will develop multifocal paralysis or paresis. Fifty percent of survivors manifest persistent cognitive and movement disorders.

West Nile virus has become the leading cause of arboviral encephalitis in the United States. Eighty percent of infections are asymptomatic and the symptomatic infections give rise to a self-limited febrile syndrome. It is estimated that 1 in 150 patients develop CNS complications, mainly among the elderly and immunocompromised. Meningitis, encephalitis, and acute flaccid paralysis are the three main clinical syndromes.

Tick-borne encephalitis virus mostly affects the elderly and is the most common cause of arboviral encephalitis in Europe. Neurologic manifestations consist of meningitis in 50% and encephalitis in the other 50% of symptomatic cases.

Symptoms[1,3]

Localization site	Comment
Cerebral hemispheres	JEV: alteration of consciousness, seizures, parkinsonian movement disorder
	WNV: temporal lobe, basal ganglia, and thalamus are affected
	Dengue virus: infiltration of both gray and white matter with DENV-positive microphage in close proximity to neurons
	Tick-borne encephalitis: diffuse inflammatory infiltrates in combination with astrogliosis in the basal ganglia
Mental status and psychiatric aspects/complications	JEV: alteration of consciousness. Permanent sequelae of cognitive or movement disoders
Brainstem	JEV: autopsy studies have identified lesions in anterior horns of the medulla
	WNV: predilection for gray matter areas of the brainstem
	Tick-borne encephalitis: diffuse inflammatory infiltrates in combination with astrogliosis
Cerebellum	WNV: affects cerebellar Purkinje cells
	Tick-borne encephalitis: diffuse inflammatory infiltrates in combination with astrogliosis
Spinal cord	JEV: autopsy studies have identified lesions in cervical spinal cord
	WNV: affects neurons, mostly pyramidal motor neurons of the anterior horns

References

1. Gregorius J, Sips GJ, Wilschut J, Smit JM. Neuroinvasive flavivirus infections. *Rev Med Virol.* 2012;22: 69–87.
2. Mackenzie JS, Gubler DJ, Petersen LR. Emerging flaviviruses: the spread and resurgence of Japanese encephalitis, West Nile and dengue viruses. *Nature Med.* 2004;10: S98–S109.
3. Solomon T. Flavivirus encephalitis. *New Engl J Med.* 2004;351:370–8.
4. Reiman CA, Hayes EB, Diguiseppi C, et al. Epidemiology of neuroinvasive arboviral disease in the United States, 1999–2007. *Am J Trop Med Hyg.* 2008;79:974–9.

Folinic Acid-Responsive Seizures

Epidemiology and Demographics: Rarely encountered, though possibly under-recognized. Typically occurring in infancy.

Disorder Description: Neonatal epileptic encephalopathy with highly intractable seizures. Early diagnosis and treatment are important to potentially improve neurologic outcomes, as rates of mortality and developmental morbidity are high for this condition. The molecular basis for the disease is not well understood. Recent findings point towards mutations in the same gene (ALDH7A1) that cause pyridoxine-dependent epilepsy (see entry for *Pyridoxine-Dependent Seizures*). Mutations in the antiquitin gene result in α–aminoadipic semialdehyde (AASA) dehydrogenase deficiency and abnormal lysine catabolism. AASA and pipecolic acid are increased in the CSF, along with other monoamine metabolites. Given the association with pyridoxine-dependent epilepsy, pyridoxine supplementation in addition to folinic acid, and dietary treatments such as lysine restriction or arginine supplementation, should be administered. Of note, cerebral folate deficiency may be associated with folinic acid-responsive seizures and may occur in the setting of other genetic and metabolic disorders.

Symptoms

Localization site	Comment
Cerebral hemispheres	Medically refractory spasms, clonic or myoclonic seizures, and epileptic encephalopathy are typical
	Interictal EEG abnormalities may include slowing and discontinuity, generalized or multifocal spike and wave discharges. Cortical atrophy and white matter lesions have been described on MRI
	Central deafness has been described
Mental status and psychiatric aspects/ complications	Subsequent developmental delay and chronic cognitive disabilities are common. Motor delays and spastic quadraparesis may result
Cranial nerves	Optic atrophy may occur

Secondary Complications: Symptoms of epileptic encephalopathy in the neonate may include emesis, abdominal distention, apnea, irritability, sleeplessness, and abnormal eye movements. Hypoglycemia and lactic acidosis have been described.

Treatment Complications: Pyridoxine infusion may be associated with apnea and should be done in a monitored setting. Oral supplementation is associated with gastrointestinal symptoms and may be associated with peripheral sensory neuropathy at high doses. Pyridoxal phosphate (PLP) may be associated with liver enzyme abnormalities. Lysine restriction and arginine supplementation require monitoring of diet, caloric intake, and amino acid levels. High doses of pyridoxine, PLP, and folinic acid have been associated with increased seizures in some patients but later testing showed these not to be indicated.

Bibliography

Gallagher RC, et al. Folinic acid-responsive seizures are identical to pyridoxine-dependent epilepsy. *Ann Neurol.* 2009;65(5):550–6.

Tabarki B, Thabet F. [Vitamin-responsive epilepsies: an update]. *Arch Pediatr.* 2013;20(11):1236–41.

Fragile X Syndrome

Epidemiology and Demographics: Fragile X syndrome (FXS) is an X-linked disorder. Therefore, the frequency is increased in males compared with females.

In very young children, including infants, symptoms may include low muscle tone (hypotonia), GERD (gastroesophageal reflux), and recurrent otitis media.[1]

In the first few years of life into later childhood, symptoms include intellectual disability, developmental delays (gross motor, speech), and autism spectrum disorder as well as dysmorphic features including large protruding ears, large testes, long face, macrocephaly, and prominent forehead and chin, which may become more obvious with age. Other neurobehavioral symptoms include hyperactivity, temper tantrums, self-mutilatory behavior, and stereotypies (hand flapping).

Post-puberty, symptoms include autistic tendencies such as poor eye contact, perseverative speech, attention difficulties, and impulsivity, and a diagnosis of autism is made in at least 25%.[2] Other symptoms may include strabismus and joint hyperextensibility.

Recent prevalence among males with intellectual disability and genetic confirmation of FXS is 16–25/100,000[3] or 1:5164.[4] African American males have a higher reported prevalence of 39/100,000.[6]

The prevalence among females is about 1/2500, with many females unaffected.

Disorder Description: FXS is the most common form of inherited intellectual disability. Over 50% of patients with FXS also have autism spectrum disorder.

The fragile X mutation is located on the *FMR1* (FRAXA) gene on the long arm of the X chromosome. The gene, a trinucleotide repeat sequence (CGG), has a length of 10 to 50 CGG repeats in unaffected individuals. Patients with fragile X syndrome have more than 200 CGG repeats. Unaffected individuals may have intermediate repeats (46–60) or carry a premutation status of 55–200 CGG repeats.

Potential downstream effects of the FMR1 trinucleotide repeat mutations include the metabotropic glutamate receptor (mGluR) theory of fragile X intellectual disability, which hypothesizes that mGluR-dependent protein synthesis is unopposed and therefore overexpressed, due to absence of FMRP, which normally represses mRNA translation.[5] Other hypotheses include overactivation of specific pathways due to absence of the normal FMR protein, including the PI3K/ERK pathway and/or the BMPR2/LIMK1 pathway.

Symptoms

Localization site	Comment
Cerebral hemispheres	Periventricular heterotopia[7]
Mental status and psychiatric aspects/ complications	Intellectual disability (IQ 30–50) Concentration/attention problems Impulsivity Anxiety, obsessive-compulsive disorder aggression Depression Autism

Secondary Complications: FXS leads to many secondary complications including global developmental delays, behavioral problems (ADHD, anxiety, OCD, depression, aggression, autism), intellectual disability, and epilepsy.

Treatment Complications: Behavioral management may involve pharmaceutical interventions, each with their own side effects.

Bibliography

OMIM. Fragile X mental retardation syndrome (300624). 2006. www.omim.org/entry/300624. Accessed Aug 7, 2018.

Saul RA, Tarleton JC. FMR1-related disorders. In Pagon RA, Adam MP, Ardinger HH, et al., eds. *GeneReviews®* [Internet]. Seattle, WA: University of Washington, Seattle; 1993–2016. Available from www.ncbi.nlm.nih.gov/books/NBK1384/. Accessed Aug 7, 2018.

References

1. Hagerman RJ, Hagerman PJ. The fragile X premutation: into the phenotypic fold. *Curr Opin Genet Dev.* 2002;12:278–83.
2. Hatton DD, Sideris J, Skinner M, et al. Autistic behavior in children with fragile X syndrome: prevalence, stability, and the impact of FMRP. *Am J Med Genet A.* 2006;140A:1804–13.
3. de Vries BB, van den Ouweland AM, Mohkamsing S, et al. Screening and diagnosis for the fragile X syndrome among the mentally retarded: an epidemiological and psychological survey. Collaborative Fragile X Study Group. *Am J Hum Genet.* 1997;61:660–7.

4. Coffee B, Keith K, Albizua I, et al. Incidence of fragile X syndrome by newborn screening for methylated FMR1 DNA. *Am J Hum Genet.* 2009;85:503–14.

5. Bear MF, Huber KM, Warren ST. The mGluR theory of fragile X mental retardation. *Trends Neurosci.* 2004;27:370–7.

6. Crawford DC, Meadows KL, Newman JL, et al. Prevalence of the fragile X syndrome in African-Americans. *Am J Med Genet.* 2002;110:226–33.

7. Moro F, Pisano T, Bernardina BD, et al. Periventricular heterotopia in fragile X syndrome. *Neurology.* 2006;67:713–5.

Fragile X Tremor Ataxia Syndrome (FXTAS)

Epidemiology and Demographics: Fragile X tremor ataxia syndrome (FXTAS) presents predominantly in men, with a mean age of 60 years. The age of onset correlates with the number of enlarged CGG repeats in pre-mutation carriers. Females occasionally present with clinical and pathologic features of FXTAS but symptoms are almost always milder. In the general population 1/259 females and 1/813 males are pre-mutation carriers making FXTAS one of the most common late-onset progressive neurodegenerative disorders in men associated with a single gene mutation.

Disorder Description: FXTAS is a late-onset neurodegenerative disease characterized by intention tremor and cerebellar ataxia. Other features include parkinsonism and cognitive changes. FXTAS occurs predominantly in carriers of a moderate CGG trinucleotide expansion (pre-mutation range 55–200 repeats) within the fragile X mental retardation 1 (FMR1) gene. However, there are rare reports that expansions within the gray zone (45–54 repeats) and full mutations (>200 repeats) may also present with FXTAS clinically. The pathologic mechanism is related to overexpression and toxicity of FMR1 mRNA leading to possible dysfunction of nuclear proteins.

Symptoms

Localization site	Comment
Cerebral hemispheres	Diffuse cerebral atrophy, non-specific white matter changes, migraine
Mental status and psychiatric aspects/ complications	Dysexecutive symptoms, dementia, disinhibition and personality change, developmental disorders, autism spectrum disorders, depression, anxiety
Brainstem	Brainstem atrophy Autonomic dysfunction: orthostatic hypotension, sexual dysfunction, loss of bowel and bladder control have been reported
Cerebellum	Cerebellar volume loss The middle cerebellar peduncle sign may be seen in 60% of cases
Vestibular system	Vertigo, dizziness
Peripheral neuropathy	Decreased vibration sense, hypoactive deep tendon reflexes
Unclear localization	Chronic pain syndrome, fibromyalgia

Bibliography

Berry-Kravis E, et al. Fragile X-associated tremor/ataxia syndrome: clinical features, genetics, and testing guidelines. *Mov Disord.* 2007;22(14): 2018–30.

Hagerman PJ, Hagerman RJ. Fragile X-associated tremor/ataxia syndrome. *Ann. NY Acad Sci.* 2015;1338:58–70. DOI:10.1111/nyas.12693

Jacquemont S, et al. Fragile X premutation tremor/ataxia syndrome: molecular, clinical, and neuroimaging correlates. *Am J Hum Genet.* 2003;72(4):869–78.

Friedrich's Ataxia (Friedreich Ataxia, FA, FRDA)

Epidemiology and Demographics: The mean age of onset of Friedrich's ataxia (FRDA) symptoms is between 10 and 15 years,[1] usually before age 25. Symptoms may appear in early childhood (as early as age 2), typically with gait ataxia followed by dysarthria and dysmetria. Symptoms may appear in early adulthood and as late as the eighth decade. FRDA is an autosomal recessive disorder and both sexes are affected. The prevalence of FRDA is 2/100,000 to 4/100,000.[2]

Disorder Description: FRDA is an autosomal recessive neurodegenerative disorder caused by trinucleotide repeat mutations in the *FXN* gene located on chromosome 9q. The most common mutation is an expanded GAA triplet repeat in intron 1 on both alleles of *FXN*. Unaffected individuals can have 5–30 GAA repeats, but people affected by FA have 70–1000 repeats.[3] Within the intermediate zone of repeats, there is potential for being an asymptomatic carrier or exhibiting symptoms later in life.

The trinucleotide repeat expansion mutations lead to decreased frataxin production, causing a disruption of iron homeostasis within the mitochondria, resulting in increased free iron and reactive oxygen species. Free oxygen radicals cause cellular damage in the heart and central nervous system.

FRDA is a progressive multisystemic disorder with cerebellar symptoms (ataxia, dysarthria, dysphagia), muscle weakness, spasticity, areflexia (in 75%), neuropathy (with loss of proprioception), scoliosis, bladder dysfunction (urinary frequency and urgency), hypertrophic cardiomyopathy, diabetes mellitus, optic nerve atrophy, and deafness. Progression from symptom onset to being unable to walk is about 10 years, with death in the 3rd decade.[4] Death is attributed to cardiac causes in more than half of the patient population, with pneumonia being the second common cause.[5]

FRDA is seen in Europe, the Middle East, South Asia (Indian subcontinent), and North Africa and is the most common inherited ataxia in these areas. It is seen with lower prevalence in Mexico. FRDA has not been seen in Southeast Asia, in sub-Saharan Africa, or among Native Americans. A lower than average prevalence of FRDA is noted in Mexico.

Symptoms

Localization site	Comment
Cerebral hemispheres	Progressive degeneration of corticospinal tracts
Mental status and psychiatric aspects/ complications	Slowing of motor planning and mental reaction times. Concrete thinking, poor concept formation, poor visuospatial reasoning, reduced speed of information processing.[6] Poor attention and working memory have also been demonstrated[7]
Brainstem	Symmetric volume loss in the dorsal medulla; progressive degeneration of corticospinal tracts
Cerebellum	Progressive degeneration; atrophy of the cerebellum (hemispheres, vermis, and dentate nuclei); atrophy of the superior cerebellar peduncle
Cranial nerves	CN II: optic atrophy, reduced visual acuity CN VIII: sensorineural hearing loss

Localization site	Comment
Spinal cord	Progressive degeneration of posterior columns, corticospinal tracts and dorsal spinocerebellar tracts; atrophy of the cervical spinal cord
Dorsal root ganglia	Progressive degeneration
Peripheral neuropathy	Sensory and motor neurons; mixed axonal peripheral neuropathy; delayed motor nerve conduction velocity; reduced or absent sensory nerve action potential with an absent H reflex
Syndromes with combined spinal cord and peripheral nerve lesions	Progressive degeneration of posterior columns and peripheral nerves

For psychiatric symptoms/disorders, focus on neurologic manifestations and what neurologic condition the psychiatric symptoms can be mistaken for.

Secondary Complications: The secondary complications of FRDA include: cardiomyopathy, gait disturbance (ataxia), hearing loss, depression, spasticity, and dysautonomia.

Treatment Complications: Medications for the secondary complications have specific side effects. See specific topic entries such as antidepressants under the entry *Major Depressive Disorder* or in the medication section of the text.

References

1. Delatycki MB, Paris DB, Gardner RJ, et al. Clinical and genetic study of Friedreich ataxia in an Australian population. *Am J Med Genet.* 1999;87:168–74.

2. Bidichandani SI, Delatycki MB. Friedreich ataxia. In Pagon RA, Adam MP, Ardinger HH, et al., eds. *GeneReviews®* [Internet]. Seattle, WA: University of Washington, Seattle; 1993–2016. Available from www.ncbi.nlm.nih.gov/books/NBK1281/

3. Al-Mahdawi S, Pinto RM, Varshney D, et al. GAA repeat expansion mutation mouse models of Friedreich ataxia exhibit oxidative stress leading to progressive neuronal and cardiac pathology. *Genomics.* 2006;88(5):580–90.

4. Delatycki MB, Knight M, Koenig M, et al. G130V, a common FRDA point mutation, appears to have arisen from a common founder. *Hum Genet.* 1999;105:343–6.

5. Tsou AY, Paulsen EK, Lagedrost SJ, et al. Mortality in Friedreich ataxia. *J Neurol Sci.* 2011;307:46–9.

6. Mantovan MC, Martinuzzi A, Squarzanti F, et al. Exploring mental status in Friedreich's ataxia: a combined neuropsychological, behavioral and neuroimaging study. *Eur J Neurol.* 2006;13:827–35.

7. Klopper F, Delatycki MB, Corben LA, et al. The test of everyday attention reveals significant sustained volitional attention and working memory deficits in Friedreich ataxia. *J Int Neuropsychol Soc.* 2011;17:196–200.

Suggested Reading

Lynch DR, Farmer JM, Tsou AY, et al. Measuring Friedreich ataxia: complementary features of examination and performance measures. *Neurology.* 2006;66:1711–6.

Lynch DR, Perlman SL, Meier T. A phase 3, double-blind, placebo-controlled trial of idebenone in Friedreich ataxia. *Arch Neurol.* 2010;67:941–7.

Lynch DR, Regner SR, Schadt KA, et al. Management and therapy for cardiomyopathy in Friedreich's ataxia. *Expert Rev Cardiovasc Ther.* 2012;10:767–77.

Lynch DR, Willi SM, Wilson RB, et al. A0001 in Friedreich ataxia: biochemical characterization and effects in a clinical trial. *Mov Disord.* 2012;27:1026–33.

Frontal Lobe Epilepsy (FLE)

Epidemiology and Demographics: Frontal lobe epilepsy (FLE) accounts for 20–30% of all focal epilepsies. Second most frequent type after temporal lobe epilepsy (TLE). Nearly 20–30% of operative procedures are for intractable epilepsy.

Disorder Description: Semiology of events based on anatomical region of frontal lobe involved. Classically FLE includes unilateral clonic seizures, asymmetric tonic seizures, and hypermotor seizures. Seizures are short, tend to cluster, and are often nocturnal. May present with stereotypical posturing, vocalizations, odd complex behaviors, and appear bizarre. Postictal effects may be absent or of short duration. Ictal and interictal EEG may not be reliable, localizing in less than one-third of patients.

FLE associated with neuropsychiatric symptoms, including changes in sleep disturbances, cognition, mood, thought process and content.

Underlying structural causes are trauma, neoplasia, vascular malformations, encephalitis, and cortical dysplasia. Autosomal dominant nocturnal FLE (ADNFLE) associated with mutations in nicotinic acetylcholine receptor genes (nAChR α4 and β2 subunits).

Antiepileptic drugs (AEDs) such as carbamazepine and its derivatives may be more effective for ADNFLE. Refractory cases should be referred for surgical evaluation.

Symptoms

Localization site	Comment
Cerebral hemispheres	Seizure semiology dependent on localization: • Orbitofrontal – staring, alteration of consciousness, vigorous complex automatisms. Olfactory hallucinations. Autonomic manifestations • Frontopolar – early head version with associated loss of consciousness, speech, or motor arrest • Dorsolateral frontal lobe – unspecific auras of dizziness or fear, followed by head and eye version and contralateral tonic or clonic activity • Primary motor cortex – focal motor clonus with Jacksonian march, dystonia, tonic stiffening. Speech disruption • Supplementary sensorimotor area – bilateral asymmetric tonic or dystonic posturing. Vocalization/speech arrest • Opercular – epigastic aura, mastication, salivation, and swallowing symptoms. Autonomic features • Cingulate – loss of awareness, oral and upper extremity automatisms, fear, behavioral alterations, and autonomic manifestations
Mental status and psychiatric aspects/complications	Psychosis, mood, anxiety, and personality changes (ictal or postictal) may occur. Attentional issues, mild memory deficits, and problems with encoding. Trouble with linguistic skills, visual–perceptual reasoning, working memory, and planning abilities worse in patients with refractory seizures
	Neurocognitive deficits at onset of epilepsy in children – demonstrated by consistently lower normal IQ scores at diagnosis

Secondary Complications: Potential complications include status epilepticus, accidental injury, neuropsychiatric dysfunction. Misdiagnosis and confusion with psychogenic nonepileptic seizures may occur due to peculiarity of presenting symptoms.

Treatment Complications: AEDs may be associated with a number of idiosyncratic reactions. Carbamazepine may cause rash or abnormalities in blood cell counts, hyponatremia, hepatic dysfunction, and accelerated bone loss.[1–3]

References

1. Gold JA, Sher Y, Maldonado JR. Frontal lobe epilepsy: a primer for psychiatrists and a systematic review of psychiatric manifestations. *Psychosomatics.* 2016;57:445–64.
2. Matricardi S, Deleo F, Ragona F, et al. Neuropsychological profiles and outcomes in children with new onset frontal lobe epilepsy. *Epilepsy Behav.* 2016;55:79–83.
3. Bagla R, Skidmore CT. Frontal lobe seizures. *Neurologist.* 2011;17(3):125–35.

Frontotemporal Dementia (FTD)

Epidemiology and Demographics: Frontotemporal dementia (FTD) is a leading cause of early-onset dementia (before age 65), with a prevalence of 15–22/100,000 in persons 45 to 64 years old. About 20,000 to 30,000 persons are affected in the United States.[1] This number is likely an underestimate, as FTD can be mistaken for psychiatric illness or Alzheimer's disease (AD). Age of onset is between 45 and 64 years in 60%, older than 64 years in 30%, and less than 45 years in 10% of FTD patients.[2]

Disorder Description: FTD refers to a clinical syndrome of frontal and/or temporal lobe dysfunction, arising from a heterogeneous array of pathologies, and commonly categorized into several distinct clinical variants. These include behavioral variant FTD (bvFTD), two variants of primary progressive aphasia (PPA), semantic variant or agrammatic variant (svPPA or agPPA), and FTD associated with motor neuron disease (FTD-MND). The most common variant of FTD in the United States is bvFTD.[2]

bvFTD presents with a striking change in personality, including apathy for previously valued activities, new onset of impulsive behavior, socially inappropriate remarks, and/or loss of empathy for family and friends. Apathy can manifest as reduced interest in work or social activities, and can initially be mistaken for depression. Patients may engage in careless spending, gambling, or sometimes criminal activities. Hyperorality is also observed, and patients may binge on sweets or alcohol. Individuals who were previously reserved may start to over-share information with strangers, or make tactless, embarrassing remarks in public.[2,3] Loss of empathy can result in a disregard for others. For example, one patient prioritized going to the grocery store over attending the funeral of his spouse's parent.[2] Perhaps unsurprisingly, patients with bvFTD perform poorly on tests of social cognition, such as recognition of facial expressions, and theory of mind tasks.[3]

PPA presents with early, prominent language impairment (see entry for *Primary Progressive Aphasia*). agPPA is characterized by non-fluent, effortful speech in short phrases, with omissions of words lacking semantic meaning (grammatical morphemes) such as "the" or "not." Patients have difficulty understanding grammatically complex sentences. SvPPA is characterized by prominent deficits in naming and single-word comprehension, with relative preservation of other language domains. Patients may also have difficulty reading and writing words with irregular spellings (e.g., chamois).[4] As the disease progresses, the clinical picture converges for all three variants, as patients develop global cognitive impairment, become bed-bound, and eventually succumb, commonly from infection.[2] Average survival varies, with the shortest time for FTD-MND (around 2 to 3 years), about 9 to 10 years for bvFTD and agPPA, and the longest time for svPPA (around 12 years).[3]

Most pathologically confirmed cases of FTD show abnormal accumulations of either tau or TDP-43 (transactive response DNA-binding protein 43 kDa), while a minority of cases demonstrate FUS (the RNA-binding protein Fused In Sarcoma) inclusions. MRI typically shows atrophy of the right frontal or right temporal lobe in bvFTD. If structural imaging is inconclusive, FDG-PET may show hypometabolism of the right temporal, right frontal, or bifrontal lobes. Amyloid PET scan can also be done, which typically shows low levels of amyloid binding in bvFTD, in contrast to high levels of amyloid binding in AD. Left inferior frontal lobe atrophy is found in agPPA, and left anterior temporal lobe atrophy is observed in svPPA.[3]

FTD symptoms occur in 30% of ALS patients.[3] Conversely, 12.5% of bvFTD patients develop motor neuron disease.[2] C9orf72 noncoding repeat expansions (in reading frame 72) on chromosome 9 are the most common genetic cause for both FTD and familial ALS, accounting for 25.9% and 34.2% of cases, respectively.[5] Psychosis is a characteristic feature in patients with C9orf72 repeat expansions.[2]

About 60% of FTD is sporadic, and 40% is autosomal dominant. Genetic variants of FTD commonly present as bvFTD or agPPA. SvPPA is almost always sporadic. Mutations in three genes – C9ORF72, GRN (progranulin), and MAPT (microtubule-associated protein tau) – account for the majority of cases of genetic FTD. A genetic mutation for FTD can be found in 6% of patients without a positive family history, and genetic counseling is important for all patients presenting with FTD.

Symptoms

Localization site	Comment
Cerebral hemispheres	Disproportionate frontotemporal atrophy is found, with involvement of the right frontotemporal lobe in bvFTD, left inferior frontal lobe in agPPA, and left anterior temporal lobe in svPPA[3]

Secondary Complications: Impulsive behavior can lead to reckless spending and financial ruin. Disinhibited, socially inappropriate behavior can cause ostracism and social isolation. Hyperorality can lead to binge eating and significant weight gain.

Treatment Complications: There are currently no approved treatments for FTD, though selective serotonin reuptake inhibitors are commonly used off-label for symptomatic management of agitation, obsessive-compulsive behaviors, and hyperphagia.[3]

References

1. Knopman DS, Roberts RO. Estimating the number of persons with frontotemporal lobar degeneration in the US population. *J Mol Neurosci.* 2011:45:330–5.

2. Bang J, Spina S, Miller BL. Frontotemporal dementia. *Lancet.* 2015;386:1672–82.

3. Finger EC. Frontotemporal dementias. *Continuum (Minneap Minn).* 2016;22:464–89.

4. Gorno-Tempini ML, Hillis AE, Weintraub S, et al. Classification of primary progressive aphasia and its variants. *Neurology.* 2011;76:1006–14.

5. van Blitterswijk M, DeJesus-Hernandez M, Rademakers R. How do C9ORF72 repeat expansions cause amyotrophic lateral sclerosis and frontotemporal dementia: can we learn from other noncoding repeat expansion disorders? *Curr Opin Neurol.* 2012;25:689–700.

Functional Neurologic Symptom Disorder (FND; Conversion Disorder)

Epidemiology and Demographics: Prevalence of functional neurologic symptom disorder (FND) in the community is up to 0.05% and in clinical settings is 2–6%. Predisposition toward female gender, with most cases presenting between 10 and 35 years old.

Disorder Description: As defined in DSM-5, FND consists of one or more symptoms of altered voluntary motor or sensory function, with evidence of incompatibility between symptoms and established neurologic or medical conditions. It is not better accounted for by another medical or mental disorder. There is clinically significant distress or impairment in functioning as result. Additional specification is made for specific symptom types such as weakness or paralysis, abnormal movement or attacks/seizures, and others. Further classification is made as to whether symptoms are acute (less than 6 months) or persistent (6 months or greater) and whether there is an identifiable stressor. There is a high rate of comorbidity with other psychiatric disorders such as depressive and anxiety disorders.

Symptoms

Localization site	Comment
Mental status and psychiatric aspects/ complications	High comorbidity with anxiety and depressive disorders. Signs include functional speech deficits, motor weakness, abnormal movements, transient attacks of seizure-like activity with or without altered awareness, visual and sensory disturbances

Secondary Complications: Individuals can become more avoidant of environments that trigger functional symptoms, therefore risk isolation. Physical injury can result from falls. Patients may face stigma within the medical community and misdiagnosis as malingering, resulting in feelings of hopelessness and invalidation.

Treatment Complications: Treatment consists of delivery of diagnosis in validating and reassuring manner, cognitive-behavioral therapy and/or dynamic therapy, and pharmacotherapy for comorbid psychiatric conditions. No reported complications.

Bibliography

American Psychiatric Association. *Diagnostic and statistical manual of mental disorders: DSM-5.* 5th ed. Washington, DC: American Psychiatric Association; 2013.

LaFrance WC, et al. *Treating nonepileptic seizures.* New York: Oxford University Press; 2015.

Functional Vision Loss (Non-physiologic Vision Loss, Hysteria, Psychogenic Vision Loss, Non-organic Vision Loss)

Epidemiology and Demographics: Though functional vision loss can affect any race/ethnicity of either sex at any age, conversion disorder is most common in children and women, sometimes in association with psychosocial stress. Malingering is associated with pursuit of financial gain through insurance or legal channels.

Disorder Description: Functional vision loss is the experience of a subjective loss of vision that cannot be accounted for by known lesions in the visual pathway. This is typically identified through inconsistencies in performance or findings on testing or examination such that the examiner can confirm that visual function is better than reported. It often occurs in association with known visual pathway lesions, in which case the etiology of vision loss may be multifactorial (i.e., the functional vision loss is an exaggeration).

Symptoms

Localization site	Comment
Mental status and psychiatric aspects/ complications	Malingering is diagnosed when patient gives deliberate history and feigns exam findings for the purposes of secondary gain. This is associated with pursuit of financial gain through insurance or legal channels. Patients are often confrontational with the physician
	Factitious disorder is diagnosed when the patient is consciously creating the symptoms for the purposes of assuming a sick role
	Conversion disorder is the non-intentional experience of physical symptoms that are not accounted for by disease in the organ system in which the symptom localizes

Bibliography

Bruce BB, Newman NJ. Functional visual loss. *Neurol Clin North Am.* 2010;28(3):789–802.

Lim SA, Siatkowski RM, Farris BJ. Functional visual loss in adults and children. *Ophthalmology.* 2005;112:1821–8.

Fungal Meningitis

Epidemiology and Demographics: Fungal infections of the central nervous system (CNS)[1-3] are rare clinical diseases and evolve due to interaction between the host's immune system and the fungal virulence factors. With the advent of human immunodeficiency virus (HIV) infections, growing number of organ transplants, and the use of chemotherapeutic agents, the incidence of fungal infections is increasing, mainly among immunocompromised hosts.

Disorder Description: Common presentations to all CNS fungal infections are basal meningitis, space-occupying lesions (abscess and granulomas), and hydrocephalus. The fungal infections of the CNS can be grouped into distinctive neurologic clinical syndromes[1-3]:

1. Meningitis, meningoencephalitis, and hydrocephalus
2. Intracranial fungal space-occupying lesions
3. Orbito-rhino-cerebral and skull base syndrome

The clinical features of the syndrome of meningitis, meningo-encephalitis, and hydrocephalus caused by fungi are headache, nausea, vomiting, visual impairment, papilledema, neck stiffness with fever, personality changes, seizures, deterioration in sensorium, cranial nerve palsies, and hydrocephalus. Cryptococcosis usually presents with typical features of meningitis and is one of the most common CNS fungal infections in immunocompromised patients. *Coccidioides* cause the most virulent of the human fungal infections, causing meningeal inflammation with accumulation of exudates, opacification of leptomeninges, and obliteration of sulci with caseous granulomatous lesions at the base of the brain and in the cervical region. Obstructive hydrocephalus is the result of extensive fibrosis and multiple aneuryms are the result of invasion of blood vessels. Disseminated candidiasis, a complication of the infection, can result spontaneously in candidal meningitis, which can also occur as a complication of an infected wound or ventriculostomy via direct inoculation of the organism into the CNS. Intracranial hypertension with and without hydrocephalus is the result of obliteration of intracranial subarachnoid spaces caused by the basal fungal meningitis.

The intracranial fungal space-occupying lesions[1-3] are mostly due to candidiasis, aspergillosis, cryptococcosis, cladosporiosis, and mucormycosis. Infection is disseminated hematogenously from an extracranial site and causes multiple areas of infection within the brain. These multiple areas of infection result in meningo-encephalitis with vasculitis–thrombosis and late hemorrhagic cerebral infarction and then abscess formation. The fungi responsible for aspergillosis, histoplasmosis, blastomycosis, paracoccidioidomycosis, cladosporiosis, mucormycosis, and cryptococcosis produce CNS fungal granulomas. Clinical symptoms depend on the fungal infection at the primary location and the site of brain lesion as well as associated meningitis, edema, and mass effect.

The orbito-rhino-cerebral and skull base syndrome is the result of fungal infections involving the nasal cavities, paranasal sinuses, orbits, and cranial bones, extending to cranial and intracranial structures especially the basifrontal and basitemporal areas. The initial presenting features are nasal discharge or blockage with periorbital pains, recurrent headache, proptosis, impaired ocular movements, progressive visual loss, sensory impairment in ophthalmic and maxillar divisions of the trigeminal nerve, chemosis progressing to ophthalmoplegia, blindness, and periorbital-facial swelling. Direct cerebral involvement and invasion of vascular structures at the skull base–internal carotids and vertebrobasilar systems cause headache, confusion, irritability, seizures, speech disturbances, and focal signs and indicate a poor prognosis. Diabetic ketoacidosis is the most common predisposing factor. Invasive fungi such as *Aspergillus*, *Cladosporium*, and Zygomycetes as well as fungi-like bacteria such as Actinomycetes and *Nocardia* are the most common causes.

Spinal fungal infections are relatively rare, occur predominantly in immunocompromised patients, and may present as intradural, extradural, and/or vertebral lesions. They can present as radiculopathy, myeloradiculopathy, myelitis, granulomas, and intramedullary abscess causing progressive myelopathy.

Symptoms[1-3]

Localization site	Comment
Cerebral hemispheres	Headache, confusion, irritability, seizures, speech disturbances, and stroke
Mental status and psychiatric aspects/ complications	Confusion, irritability, and speech disturbances
Base of skull	Basal meningitis
Cranial nerves	Progressive visual loss, ophthalmoplegia, blindness, sensory impairment in ophthalmic and maxillary divisions of the trigeminal nerve
Spinal cord	Progressive myelopathy due to mass effect from granulomas and intramedullary abscess

Treatment Complications: Fungal meningitis, especially due to *Cryptococcus* and *Candida*, usually responds well to intravenous amphotericin B therapy with or without flucytosine. Flucanazole is used as a maintenance therapy in cryptococcal meningitis in AIDS patients. Aggressive antifungal medications are used for small fungal space-occupying lesions while conventional, stereotactic, or ultrasound-guided surgical interventions are used for large lesions. The prognosis is poor for patients with CNS fungal infections presenting with acute stroke. Amphotericin may cause headaches and rarely can induce seizures or encephalopathy. Intrathecal meningitis may rarely cause a chemical meningitis.

References

1. Sharma RR. Fungal infections of the nervous system: Current perspective and controversies in management: *Int J Surg.* 2010;8:591–601.
2. Gavito-Higuera J, Mullins CB, Ramos-Duran L, et al. Fungal infections of the central nervous system: a pictorial review. *J Clin Imaging Sci.* 2016;6:24.
3. Mathur M, Johnson CE, Sze G. Fungal infections of the central nervous system. *Neuroimag Clin N Am.* 2012;22(4):609–32.

Fusobacterium

Epidemiology and Demographics: The annual incidence of *Fusobacterium* bacteremia varies from 0.55 to 0.99 per 100,000 population in multiple studies.

Fusobacterium necrophorum causes infection in mostly healthy young adults up to 40 years of age, while the incidence of *F. nucleatum* increases with age (median age of 53.5 years).[1–3]

Disorder Description: *Fusobacterium* is a genus of anaerobic, non-spore-forming gram-negative bacilli containing 13 heterogeneous species. *F. necrophorum* and *F. nucleatum*, although rare, cause the majority of serious human infections. *F. necrophorum* was identified as the causal agent of Lemierre syndrome, consisting of oropharyngeal infection followed by septic thrombophlebitis of the internal jugular vein with sepsis and metastatic disease to the lung.[3,4] It is also a frequent primary cause of infection in the head and neck and plays a major role in the pathogenesis of tonsillitis, paratonsilar abscess, post-anginal cervical lymphadenitis, and otitis media in children and sinusitis in adults.[5] *F. nucleatum*, a common member of the human oropharyngeal flora, is an agent of gingival and periodontal disease, and is among the oral anaerobes that are most likely to metastasize to the liver, joints, heart valves, and brain. It is associated with periodontitis, obstetric infections, brain abscess complicating periodontal disease, and bacteremia during prolonged neutropenia. Most patients infected with *F. nucleatum* are older individuals with underlying comorbidities including dialysis and malignancy. Both *F. necrophorum* and *F. nucleatum* can cause brain abscess, albeit more common with *F. nucleatum*.[5]

Treatment Complications: Metronidazole may cause peripheral neuropathy.

References

1. Citron DM. Update on the taxonomy and clinical aspects of the genus Fusobacterium. *Clin Infect Dis.* 2002;35(Suppl 1):S22–7.

2. Afra K, Laupland K, Leal J, Lloyd T, Gregson D. Incidence, risk factors, and outcomes of Fusobacterium species bacteraemia. *BCM Infect Dis.* 2013;13:264.

3. Huggan PJ, Murdoch DR. Fusobacterial infections: clinical spectrum and incidence of invasive disease. *J Infect.* 2008;57:283–9.

4. Nohrström E, Mattila T, Pettilä V, et al. Clinical spectrum of bacteraemic Fusobacterium infections: from septic shock to nosocomial bacteraemia. *Scand J Infect Dis.* 2011;43(6–7):463–70. DOI: 10.3109/00365548.2011.565071.

5. Hsieh MJ, Chang WN, Lui CC, et al. Clinical characteristics of fusobacterial brain abscess. *Jpn J Infect Dis.* 2007;60:40–4.

6. Olson KR, Freitag SK, Johnson JM, Branda JA. Case 36–2014: an 18 year-old woman with fever, pharyngitis, and double vision. *N Engl J Med.* 2014;371:2018–27. DOI:10.1056/NEJMcpc131001.

Symptoms[5,6]

Localization site	Comment
Cerebral hemispheres	Rare cases of meningitis reported
	Brain abscess with focal neurologic signs depending on the localization with clinical features of headache, fever, seizure, visual disturbances, hemiparesis, consciousness disturbances
	Cerebral thrombosis not rare
Cranial nerves	Horizontal diplopia reported

GABA Transaminase Deficiency

Epidemiology and Demographics: Rare with only three published cases.

Disorder Description: GABA transaminase metabolizes GABA into succinic semialdehyde, which is metabolized to succinic acid and then enters the tricarboxylic acid cycle. GABA transaminase deficiency results in excessive GABA activity.

This autosomal recessive disorder is characterized by severe neonatal encephalopathy, epilepsy, and growth acceleration. The latter is likely related to GABA-induced stimulation of growth hormone. Encephalopathy may be directly related to high central nervous system levels of GABA and beta-alanine. Death in early childhood.

Diagnosed by detection of elevated GABA using magnetic resonance spectroscopy or measured in serum and CSF. Confirmation by enzymatic activity or molecular analysis is available. Neuropathology is inconsistent and may depend upon particularities of gene defect.

Symptoms

Localization site	Comment
Cerebral hemispheres	Seizures, hypotonia, and spasticity
	One case had severe ventricular enlargement and increased cisternal and sulcal spaces and a spongiform quality of the white matter in cerebral hemispheres, cerebellum, and brainstem; with poor or absent myelination in the white matter of the gyri
	In another only mild delay in myelination with restricted diffusion in the internal and external capsules and the subcortical white matter was present
Mental status and psychiatric aspects/complications	Encephalopathy
Other	Growth acceleration

Treatment Complications: Antiepileptic drugs associated with a number of idiosyncratic reactions, including multi-organ issues, and possible cognitive or psychiatric effects. Medication interactions are common.

Bibliography

Parviz M, et al. Disorders of GABA metabolism: SSADH and GABA-transaminase deficiencies. *J Pediatr Epilepsy.* 2014;3(4):217–27.

Tsuji M, et al. A new case of GABA transaminase deficiency facilitated by proton MR spectroscopy. *J Inherit Metab Dis.* 2010;33(1):85–90.

GALOP Syndrome: Gait Disorder Autoantibody Late-Age Onset Polyneuropathy

Epidemiology and Demographics: Classic presentation is late onset in elderly individuals 60–85 years old with history of progressive unsteady gait and frequent falls over months to years. Caused by an autoimmune IgM to sulfatide (a neuronal protein associated with myelin-related inhibition of axonal outgrowth).

Disorder Description: Mild symmetric distal sensory loss in the arms and legs associated with weakness. Electromyography/nerve conduction studies show axonal sensorimotor polyneuropathy with occasional demyelinating features. Diagnosed by the presence of IgM to sulfatide in serum and on nerve biopsy. Immunomodulating treatments with intravenous immunoglobulin (IVIG) or cyclophosphamide may result in functional improvement.

Symptoms: Distal sensory nerves in the foot/lower leg and at later stages, the hands/forearm are potential sites of involvement.

Secondary Complications: Complications from falls and injuries in the elderly.

Treatment Complications: Adverse effects from IVIG, plasmapheresis, or cyclophosphamide.

Bibliography

Katirji B, et al. *Neuromuscular disorders in clinical practice.* 2nd ed. New York: Springer; 2014. DOI: 10.1007/978-1-4614-6567-6.

Ganglioglioma

Epidemiology and Demographics: Ganglioglioma is the most frequent type of glioneuronal tumor, constituting 4–6% of primary brain tumors in children; 80% of the cases occur in patients less than 30 years old, with a slight male predominance.

Disorder Description: Ganglioglioma is a well-differentiated, slowly growing neuroepithelial tumor, composed of neoplastic, mature ganglion cells and neoplastic glial cells. It is usually a benign tumor but rarely can transform to the malignant form – anaplastic ganglioglioma.

Symptoms

Localization site	Comment
Cerebral hemispheres	New onset seizures and refractory epilepsy are the most common presentations. (Complex partial seizures are common as tumor typically occurs in medial temporal lobe – 85%.) Hemiparesis
Mental status and psychiatric aspects/complications	Memory disturbances and psychiatric symptoms
Brainstem	Loss of gag reflex and horizontal nystagmus (rare)
Cerebellum	Ataxia
Cranial nerves	Hearing loss, intractable facial pain
Spinal cord	Progressive myelopathy (commonly cervical cord)
Unclear localization	Increased intracranial pressure

Treatment complications: Surgical resection can lead to memory problems if lesion is in the temporal lobe.

Radiotherapy (gamma knife radiotherapy) has minimal side effects including nausea, dizziness, and hair loss.

Bibliography

Safavi-Abbasi S, Di Rocco F, Chantra K, et al. Posterior cranial fossa gangliogliomas. *Skull Base.* 2007;17(4):253–64.

Song JY, Kim JH, Cho YH, Kim CJ, Lee EJ. Treatment and outcomes for gangliogliomas: a single-center review of 16 patients. *Brain Tumor Res Treat.* 2014;2(2):49–55.

Zentner J, Wolf HK, Ostertun B, et al. Gangliogliomas: clinical, radiological, and histopathological

findings in 51 patients. *J Neurol Neurosurg Psychiatr.* 1994;57(12):1497–502.

Ganglion Cyst

Epidemiology and Dermographics: More common in women than in men; 70% of cases occur between 20 and 40 years of age. Seen rarely in children younger than 10 years. Most common soft tissue tumor of the hand and wrist.

Disorder Description: Ganglion cyst, also known as synovial cyst, Gideon's disease, and bible cyst, is a non-neoplastic soft tissue mass that may occur in any joint, but more commonly seen around joints and tendons in the hands or feet. It could be due to irritation or chronic damage causing cystic space formation.

Symptoms

Localization site	Comment
Dorsal wrist	Joint instability, weakness, limitation of movement
Carpal tunnel	Compression of median nerve causing pain and numbness
Ulnar side of the wrist	Ulnar nerve compression within the tunnel of Guyon causing paresthesias and pain

Treatment Complications: Treatment includes orthoscopic resection, open excision, corticosteroid injection with aspiration, or aspiration alone.

Complications include wrist stiffness or neurovascular injury, particularly with radial artery laceration. Infection can occur. Decreased motion and ligament instability with open excision can be seen.

Bibliography

The American Society for Surgery of the Hand. E-Hand.com (The electronic textbook of hand surgery). The American Society for Surgery of the Hand. www.eatonhand.com/. Accessed Aug 7, 2018.

Gastrointestinal Cancers

Epidemiology and Demographics: The incidence of brain metastases is <4% in esophageal and colorectal cancer and <1% in pancreatic and gastric cancer.

Disorder Description: Gastrointestinal tumors are more likely to metastasize to the posterior fossa than to the supratentorial region. They involve cerebellum more than other tumors and more often will be solitary lesions. Gastric tumors are more likely to have leptomeningeal metastasis, while paraneoplastic features and spinal cord compression are rare compared with lung and breast carcinoma.

Symptoms

Localization site	Comment
Cerebral hemispheres	Solitary or multiple lesions causing seizures, headache, nausea, vomiting, and hemiparesis (most commonly from colorectal cancer)
Mental status and psychiatric aspects/complications	Leptomeningeal spread: headaches, nausea, vomiting, cognitive changes, and occasionally seizures
Cerebellum	Unsteadiness, headache, and nausea. (Solitary mass; rarely paraneoplastic cerebellar degeneration)
Cranial nerves	Leptomeningeal spread: paresis of third, fourth, and sixth nerves is most common; rarely facial weakness, decreased hearing, and involvement of the optic, trigeminal, and hypoglossal nerves
Pituitary gland	Diabetes insipidus and pituitary apoplexy (rare)
Spinal cord	Progressive myelopathy (93%), Brown–Séquard syndrome (22.5%), or pseudo or partial Brown–Séquard syndrome (Intramedullary spread in colorectal cancer)
Specific spinal roots	Leptomeningeal spread: pain, weakness, and paresthesias (lumbosacral region)
Plexus	Lumbosacral plexopathy: prominent pain radiating into the lumbar fossa, hip and buttocks, and leg weakness

Special mention: Turcot's syndrome: colorectal cancer with central nervous system neoplasms.

Secondary Complications: Paraneoplastic syndrome of inappropriate antidiuretic hormone secretion (SIADH), Cushing's syndrome, acanthosis nigricans.

Treatment Complications: Gastrectomy can result in pernicious anemia due to deficiency of intrinsic factor thereby causing vitamin B12 deficiency, which can lead to weakness and loss of proprioception and vibration due to subacute combined deficiency.

5 Fluorouracil in combination with levamisole produces multifocal inflammatory leukoencephalopathy. The combination is not used anymore.

Bibliography

Lee JL, Kang YK, Kim TW, et al. Leptomeningeal carcinomatosis in gastric cancer. *J Neurooncol.* 2004;66(1-2):167–74.

Lisenko Y, Kumar AJ, Yao J, Ajani J, Ho L. Leptomeningeal carcinomatosis originating from gastric cancer: report of eight cases and review of the literature. *Am J Clin Oncol.* 2003;26(2): 165–70.

Schiff D, O'Neill BP, Suman VJ. Spinal epidural metastasis as the initial manifestation of malignancy: clinical features and diagnostic approach. *Neurology.* 1997;49(2):452–6.

Gender Dysphoria

Epidemiology and Demographics: Onset is as early as 2–4 years old, into adulthood. Estimates of prevalence are likely low due to only a limited number of individuals seeking medical healthcare services. For adults born biologically male, estimates range from 0.005 to 0.014%. For females, the range is 0.002 to 0.003%. In children, male-to-female gender distribution range is 2:1 to 4.5:1.

Disorder Description: Characterized in the DSM-5 as "distress that may accompany the incongruence between one's experienced or expressed gender and one's assigned gender." Duration is at least 6 months. As per DSM, in adolescents and adults, must be associated with at least two of the following features: (1) conflict between one's gender identity and his/her biologic sex characteristics, (2) strong desire for biologic sex characteristics to either not develop or be eliminated, (3) strong desire for the biologic sex characteristics congruent with one's gender identity, (4) strong desire to be another gender, (5) strong desire to be treated as another gender, and (6) belief that one has the internal experience of another gender. There is significant distress and impairment in several realms of function. There are specifiers for disorder of sex development or post-transition to the desired gender. There is a separate set of criteria for children that are based more on behavioral manifestations.

During development, individuals often make efforts to conceal emergent secondary sex characteristics, seek hormone treatments and/or surgery.

Genetic factors likely play a role, as seen with twin studies. Atypical gender behaviors in childhood help predict gender dysphoria. It is seen across many cultures. Comorbidities in children often include the disruptive, impulse-control, anxiety, depressive, and autism spectrum disorders. In adults, they are mostly depressive and anxiety disorders.

Symptoms

Localization site	Comment
Mental status and psychiatric aspects/complications	May have higher rates of suicidal ideation May have symptoms of comorbid disorders: disruptive, impulse-control, anxiety, depressive, and autism spectrum disorders

Secondary Complications: Due to nonconformity of social norms, there is increased risk for stigmatization and victimization. School and work functioning can be impacted. There can be isolation and challenges in relationships, emotionally and sexually. There is a high rate of suicide attempts.

Treatment complications: Hormone treatments and sexual reassignment surgery carry their own respective risks of adverse effects.

Bibliography

American Psychiatric Association. *Diagnostic and statistical manual of mental disorders: DSM-5.* 5th ed. Washington, DC: American Psychiatric Association; 2013.

Haas AP, Rodgers PL, Herman J. *Suicide attempts among transgender and gender non-conforming adults: findings of the national transgender discrimination survey.* New York/Los Angeles: American Foundation for Suicide Prevention/The Williams Institute; 2014.

Heylens G, De Cuypere G, Zucker K, et al. (2012). Gender identity disorder in twins: a review of the case report literature. *J Sex Med.* 2012;8(3):751–7.

Generalized Anxiety Disorder

Epidemiology and Demographics: Nearly twice as common in females, with cultural variability. Most common phase of life affected is middle adulthood. In the United States, 1-year prevalence is 0.9% in adolescents and 3.1% in adults. It more commonly affects those of European descent.

Disorder Description: Characterized in the DSM-5 by "excessive anxiety or worry (apprehensive expectation)" that occurs with regards to several areas of life and is difficult to control. It affects most days per week over at least a 6-month period of time. It can be pervasive and without specific triggers. To meet DSM criteria, the anxiety or worry must be accompanied by three or more of the following: restlessness, easy fatigue, difficulty concentrating, irritability, muscle tension, and/or sleep disturbance. Symptoms must cause significant distress and not be better accounted for by the effects of a substance or another mental or medical condition.

Risk factors are genetic and trait-based, including tendency toward harm avoidance and negative affect states. Environmental factors such as early adversity or overprotective parenting may also play a role.

Symptoms

Localization site	Comment
Mental status and psychiatric aspects/complications	Anxiety, irritability, difficulty concentrating, poor working memory, restlessness, fatigue

Secondary Complications: Associated difficulties with sleep, concentration, and fatigue can contribute to challenges with efficiency and effectiveness in multiple realms.

Treatment complications: Selective serotonin reuptake inhibitors carry potential side effects such as insomnia, headache, gastrointestinal distress, and sexual dysfunction.

Bibliography

American Psychiatric Association. *Diagnostic and statistical manual of mental disorders: DSM-5.* 5th ed. Washington, DC: American Psychiatric Association; 2013.

Beesdo K, Pine DS, Lieb R, Wittchen HU. Incidence and risk patterns of anxiety and depressive disorders and categorization of generalized anxiety disorder. *Arch Gen Psychiatry.* 2010;67(1):47–57.

Kessler RC, Petukhova M, Sampson NA, et al. Twelve-month and lifetime prevalence and lifetime morbid risk of anxiety and mood disorders in the US. *Int J Methods Psychiatr Res.* 2012;21(3):169–84.

Lewis-Fernández R, Hinton DE, Laria AJ, et al. Culture and the anxiety disorders: recommendations for DSM-V. *Depress Anxiety.* 2010;27(2):212–29.

Generalized Tonic–Clonic Seizures (GTCS)

Epidemiology and Demographics: Generalized tonic–clonic seizures (GTCS) are the most common seizure type, constituting about 50% of seizures in adults.

Disorder Description: Can manifest as primary or secondary GTCS. When primary, seizures begin abruptly with bilateral tonic contraction of limbs, loss of consciousness, jaw clenching, upward eye deviation, eyelid and mouth opening. May involve respiratory muscles producing forced expiration and an "epileptic cry." Gradually transitions to clonic activity. Initially, rhythmic jerking may be high frequency and low amplitude and evolves to have lower frequency and transiently higher amplitude movements before cessation. Event followed by a post-ictal period. Secondarily GTCS are of focal onset with seizure activity that spreads to the bilateral hemispheres. Focal clinical features at onset and asymmetric or asynchronous motor activity are more common. Idiopathic causes are typically genetic in origin. Symptomatic causes include developmental abnormalities, trauma, infection, stroke, and tumor.

Symptoms

Localization site	Comment
Cerebral hemispheres	Full body stiffening and rhythmic jerking, loss of awareness
Mental status and psychiatric aspects/ complications	Altered level of consciousness acutely, post-ictal obtundation, confusion, lethargy, agitation. Post-ictal psychiatric symptoms including depression, anxiety, and psychosis may occur in the days following a convulsion

Secondary Complications: Serious injuries can occur including: head trauma, fractures, dislocations, dental damage, and burns. Cardiopulmonary compromise less common. Uncontrolled GTCS the strongest risk factor for sudden unexpected death in epilepsy (SUDEP).

Treatment Complications: Primary GTCS may respond well only to broad-spectrum antiepileptic drugs (AEDs), whereas narrow-spectrum agents such as carbamazepine or gabapentin may exacerbate seizures. AEDs are associated with a number of idiosyncratic reactions, including multi-organ issues, and possible cognitive or psychiatric effects. Common side effects for AEDs include dizziness, fatigue, blurred vision, and gastrointestinal symptoms. Other reactions include rash, blood count abnormalities, liver toxicity, cognitive or mood complaints. There may be an increased risk of suicidality associated with AED use. Drug interactions are common.

Bibliography

Hauser WA, Annegers JF, Kurland LT. Incidence of epilepsy and unprovoked seizures in Rochester, Minnesota: 1935–1984. *Epilepsia.* 1993;34(3):453–68.

Ropper A., et al. *Adams and Victor's principles of neurology.* 9th ed. New York: McGraw-Hill Medical; 2009.

Germ Cell Tumors

Epidemiology and Demographics: Germ cell tumors are a heterogeneous group of lesions that may occur in the ovary, testicles, or extragonadally, including intracranially.

Ovarian germ cell tumors account for 20–25% of ovarian neoplasms overall, but only 5% of all malignant ovarian neoplasms. Malignant ovarian germ cell tumors are more frequent among Asian/Pacific Islanders and Hispanic women than Caucasians. They arise typically in young women between 10 and 30 years old.

Testicular germ cell tumors account for 95% of testicular cancers, commonly affecting males between 15 and 35 years, and are more common in males of Japanese/Asian descent. Overall incidence of testicular germ cell tumors among American men was about 5/100,000 per data around the turn of the century and is rising, as opposed to the incidence of ovarian germ cell tumors, which appears to have declined.

Extragonadal germ cell tumors occur in different sites depending on age, with sacrococcygeal and intracranial germ cell tumors common in young children, and tumors in anterior mediastinum, retroperitoneum, and intracranially, particularly pineal and suprasellar regions, common in adults. There is an annual incidence of 0.5/100,000 (found in a Norwegian study). There is a 5- to 8-fold increased incidence of intracranial germ cell tumors in Japan. Males are twice as likely as females to develop intracranial germ cell tumors. The only known risk factor for extragonadal germ cell tumors is Klinefelter syndrome (47XXY), which is associated with mediastinal nonseminomatous germ cell tumors.

Disorder Description: Germ cell tumors consist of multiple histologic types, carrying a prognosis and treatment strategy depending on their type, location, and patient's age and gender. They are classified as follows:

Teratomas
    Benign cystic mature teratomas
    Immature teratomas
Dysgerminomas or germinomas in females/seminomas in males
Yolk sac tumors
Mixed germ cell tumors: combinations of teratoma with yolk sac, dysgerminoma, and/or embryonal carcinoma
Rare ovarian germ cell tumors (OGCTs): pure embryonal carcinomas, nongestational choriocarcinomas, pure polyembryoma, gonadoblastoma

Most germ cell tumors produce hormones that function as tumor markers, which can aid in diagnosis as well as monitoring, such as the beta subunit of human chorionic gonadotropin (hCG), alpha fetoprotein, or lactate dehydrogenase (LDH).

Ovarian germ cell tumors are derived from primordial germ cells of the ovary and may be malignant or benign. They are less common than epithelial ovarian neoplasms, but grow more rapidly. Patients typically present with abdominal enlargement, abdominal pain, precocious puberty, abnormal vaginal bleeding, or symptoms of pregnancy.

Testicular germ cell tumors are grouped into seminomas or non-seminomatous tumors and typically present as a nodule or painless swelling of the testicle. Please see the entry for *Testicular Cancer* for additional information on testicular germ cell tumors.

Extragonal germ tell tumors, without primary tumors in the ovaries or testes, tend to occur in the midline. Intracranial germinonas tend to be very sensitive to radiation therapy, whereas intracranial nongerminomatous tumors characteristically are not.

Symptoms

Localization site	Comment
Cerebral hemispheres	**Ovarian:** nongestational choriocarcinomas are likely to metastasize to brain via hematogenous spread, highly prone to hemorrhage. Predilection for the posterior fossa. May also form neoplastic aneurysms via tumor embolization to the brain presenting with subarachnoid hemorrhage or intracranial hemorrhage **Testicular:** may metastasize to cerebral hemispheres **Extragonadal:** intracranial germ cell tumors (often germinomas) typically occur in pineal or suprasellar region, less commonly surrounding fourth ventricle, basal ganglia, thalamus. Pineal or fourth ventricle germ cell tumors may cause obstructive hydrocephalus
Spinal cord	**Testicular:** metastases to spinal cord, which can result in motor deficits, sensory deficits, bowel/bladder dysfunction, gait imbalance depending on location within cord
Mental status	**Ovarian:** anti-N-methyl-D-aspartate (NMDA) receptor autoimmune encephalitis can rarely be produced by mature or immature ovarian teratomas presenting with psychiatric symptoms (hallucinations, emotional lability, behavioral changes, altered level of consciousness, seizures, central hypoventilation) and autonomic dysregulation **Extragonadal:** pineal/fourth ventricle tumors causing obstructive hydrocephalus leading to headache, lethargy, somnolence, ataxia, behavioral changes
Lumbosacral plexopathy	**Ovarian:** local compression by pelvic masses leading to local or radicular pain, sensory loss to anterior thigh and foot, weakness or knee flexion, ankle dorsiflexion or ankle inversion **Testicular:** Retroperitoneal metastases

Secondary Complications

Ovarian germ cell tumors:
    Endocrinopathies – precocious puberty, abnormal vaginal bleeding, symptoms of pregnancy related to tumor hormonal hCG production

Testicular germ cell tumors:
    Endocrinopathies – paraneoplastic hyperthyroidism, gynecomastia (associated with hCG production)
    Lumbar back pain – due to retroperitoneal metastases to the psoas muscle
    Bone pain – due to skeletal metastases
    Lower extremity swelling – due to iliac or caval venous obstruction or thrombosis

Extragonadal germ cell tumors:
    Endocrinopathies – most commonly diabetes insipidus although precocious puberty or delayed puberty, growth hormone deficiency, hypothyroidism, and adrenal insufficiency can also be seen, especially if tumor in suprasellar location
    Decreased visual acuity – occasionally with bitemporal hemianopsia if in a suprasellar location
    Obstructive hydrocephalus associated with pineal/fourth ventricle tumors causing altered mental status, lethargy, changes in academic performance and behavior
    Headaches

Treatment Complications

Peripheral nerve injury: secondary to pelvic surgery. Femoral is the most commonly injured nerve, but lumbosacral plexus injury may also occur. Ilioinguinal or iliohypogastric nerve injuries may occur due to post-operative scars or adhesions.

Peripheral neuropathy: secondary to chemotherapy agents, typically cis-platinum or paclitaxel. Cis-platinum typically produces a large fiber neuropathy with loss of position and vibratory sensation.

Paclitaxel more commonly affects all sensory nerve fibers and may also cause a proximal motor neuropathy.

Encephalopathy: secondary to ifosfamide aklylating chemotherapy agent, with alterations in consciousness (somnolence vs delirium vs coma), as well as possible hallucinations, seizures, cerebellar dysfunction. The encephalopathy is usually reversible in 3–4 days.

Bibliography

Abrey LE. Neurologic complications of female reproductive tract cancer. In Schiff D, Kesari S, Wen PY, eds. *Current Clinical Oncology: Cancer Neurology in Clinical Cancer*. Totowa, NJ: Humana Press; 2008. pp. 449–58.

Bosl GJ, Motzer RJ. Testicular germ-cell cancer. *N Engl J Med*. 1997;337:242.

Packer RJ, Cohen BH, Coney K. Intracranial germ cell tumors. *Oncologist*. 2000;5:312–20.

Rosenfeld MR, Dalmau J. Update on paraneoplastic neurologic disorders. *Oncologist*. 2010;15: 603–17.

Giant Cell Tumor of Bone

Epidemiology and Demographics: Giant cell tumors comprise approximately 5% of all skeletal tumors and 21% of benign tumors. About 1% occur in the skull and most common location is sphenoid and temporal bone. There is a female preponderance in the incidence.

Disorder Description: Giant cell tumors are benign lesions that typically occur at the epiphyses of long bones. Metastatic disease is found in approximately 1–9% of patients. Pulmonary metastases are the most common, though skull and spinal cord metastases have been reported.

Symptoms

Localization site	Comment
Cerebral hemispheres	Headaches and hemiparesis (Cortical or subcortical metastasis to brain)
Mental status and psychiatric aspects/complications	Confusion
Cranial nerves	Visual field defects, blindness, and diplopia (involvement of sphenoid bone) Abducens palsy (clivus involvement)
Spinal cord	Progressive hemiparesis (intramedullary thoracic metastasis)

Treatment Complications: Denosumab may cause osteonecrosis of jaw and increased susceptibility to infections.

Bibliography

Jain S, Sam A, Yohannan DI, et al. Giant cell tumor of the temporal bone: an unusual presentation. *Clin Neurol Neurosurg.* 2013;115(5):646–8.

Wong RH, Thakral B, Watkin WG, et al. Intracranial, intra-axial metastatic giant cell tumor of bone: case report and review of literature. *Clin Neurol Neurosurg.* 2014;117:40–3.

Glaucoma

Epidemiology and Demographics: Glaucoma is the second leading cause of blindness worldwide, affecting about 60 to 70 million people. It is the leading cause of irreversible blindness. There are two major forms of glaucoma: primary angle closure glaucoma (PACG) in which the outflow structures of aqueous humor in the eye are obstructed; and primary open angle glaucoma (POAG) in which these outflow structures are freely accessible to aqueous humor. The epidemiology and demographics of the two forms are distinct. PACG is most common in Eskimos and East Asian individuals. The incidence also increases with age. Women are more likely to have PACG. Family history is also a risk factor. No systemic factors are known to contribute to PACG. POAG is more prevalent in individuals of African and Hispanic descent than in Caucasians. The incidence of POAG increases significantly with age. Family history is an important risk factor, with studies reporting that an individual has a two- to fourfold increased risk of glaucoma if he or she has an affected first-degree relative. There is no difference in prevalence among males and females.

Disorder Description: Glaucoma is a broad term to describe a diverse group of eye conditions that share the common feature of progressive optic neuropathy with visual field loss and corresponding structural changes to the optic nerve. Any description of glaucoma requires a basic understanding of the pathway of aqueous humor flow in the eye. Aqueous humor is a fluid made in the anterior part of the eye by the ciliary body behind the iris. This fluid maintains eye shape and provides nutrients to structures in the eye. It exits the eye through the trabecular meshwork located in the "angle" created by the intersection of the cornea and the iris, then into Schlemm's canal and into the blood circulation. Although intraocular pressure is not included in the definition of glaucoma, elevated intraocular pressure is associated with most forms of glaucoma and is typically associated with resistance to aqueous humor outflow from the eye.

PACG is associated with an identifiable mechanical obstruction of the trabecular meshwork. This may present acutely, subacutely (intermittent angle closure), or chronically. It can also be categorized as primary (anatomic predisposition typically due to a shallow anterior chamber) or secondary angle closure (angle closure secondary to another pathologic process in the eye). In POAG there is no macroscopically identifiable obstruction to the outflow structures in the eye, but trabecular meshwork dysfunction leads to aqueous backup and chronically elevated pressures in the eye. These chronically elevated pressures ultimately lead to the death of retinal ganglion cells and their axons by cellular mechanisms that are poorly understood. Besides POAG and PACG, there are rarer secondary glaucomas in which glaucoma develops secondary to other identified ocular or systemic conditions such as trauma, intraocular inflammation, and ischemic processes.

Symptoms: Chronic forms of glaucoma (e.g., POAG) are insidious in nature. Patients remain asymptomatic with slow elevation of intraocular pressure and progressive loss of peripheral visual field. Central visual acuity remains intact even in severe forms of the disease. Hence, as many as 50% of patients in the developed world with glaucoma are unaware of their disease. Acute symptoms of angle-closure glaucoma include severe eye pain, blurred vision, photophobia, halos around lights, even headache, nausea and vomiting. This constellation of symptoms overlaps with that of migraine. The most common forms of glaucoma, POAG and PACG, are not associated with neurologic symptoms.

Localization site	Comment
Cerebral hemispheres	**Neurofibromatosis I** is a genetic syndrome characterized by skin changes, optic nerve gliomas, iris nodules, bony dysplasia, and neurofibromas or other solid central nervous system tumors. NF1 is a rare cause of secondary glaucoma due to abnormalities of the angle structures

Localization site	Comment
	Juvenile xanthogranuloma (JXG) is an uncommon proliferative disorder of histiocytes that typically manifests with skin lesions. Systemic JXG is rare but has been associated with intracranial lesions. JXG is a rare cause of unilateral glaucoma. Vascular lesions of the iris (the most commonly affected structure in the eye) can form. These vascular lesions can bleed spontaneously leading to hyphema (blood in the anterior chamber) and secondary glaucoma
	Elevated episcleral venous pressure can cause open-angle glaucoma by obstructing the outflow of aqueous humor into the venous drainage system. Conditions that can cause this include **carotid–cavernous fistula and dural–cavernous fistula**
	Sturge–Weber syndrome (SWS) is a sporadic neurocutaneous disorder. Seizures are the most common neurologic abnormality. The condition is also characteristically associated with leptomeningeal hemangiomatosis ipsilateral to the skin findings. SWS patients develop multifactorial glaucoma from developmental abnormalities in the angle structures and/or secondary to vascular anomalies of the episcleral and conjunctiva. These anomalies create outflow obstruction, elevated episcleral venous pressure, and ultimately elevated intraocular pressure
Cranial nerves	**Neurofibromatosis I** (see above) is associated with glaucoma and optic nerve gliomas
Plexus	**Neurofibromatosis I** (see above) is associated with glaucoma and plexiform neurofibromas

Secondary Complications: Glaucoma is a progressive disease that can result in irreversible loss of vision despite treatment. Studies show that over 20 years, 9% of treated patients with adequate IOPs will develop bilateral blindness. As the visual field constriction progresses, glaucoma patients report increasing difficulties with a broad range of activities such as walking, reading, and driving. Patients severely impaired by glaucoma may also experience adverse mental health effects such as anxiety and depression.

Treatment Complications: Intraocular pressure is the only modifiable risk factor that can slow glaucoma progression. Pressure-lowering drops are typically the first line of treatment, and there are five major classes of medications. As all pressure-lowering drops are used chronically, they can become toxic to the ocular surface. Prostaglandin analogs cause local pigmentary changes in the iris and eyelid and eyelash growth. Pilocarpine is associated with headache. Systemic absorption of eye drops such as beta blockers can lead to cardiovascular and pulmonary side effects. Carbonic anhydrase inhibitors can be prescribed systemically to lower intraocular pressure. These are associated with parasthesias, altered taste, and fatigue.

Laser or incisional surgery is considered when other modalities do not adequately control the intraocular pressure. Complications can arise from surgically related infections, bleeding, failure of surgery to create a successful aqueous outflow tract, and hypotony (very low eye pressure) from excessive aqueous outflow.

Bibliography

Kass MA, Heuer DK, Higginbotham EJ, et al. The Ocular Hypertension Treatment Study: a randomized trial determines that topical ocular hypotensive medication delays or prevents the onset of primary open-angle glaucoma. *Arch Ophthalmol.* 2002:120(6):701–13; discussion 829–30.

Tielsch JM, Katz J, Sommer A, Quigley HA, Javitt JC. Hypertension, perfusion pressure, and primary open-angle glaucoma: a population-based assessment. *Arch Ophthalmol.* 1995:113(2):216–21.

Gliomatosis Cerebri

Epidemiology and Demographics: Due to the rarity of the condition, no reliable estimates are available on the incidence of gliomatosis cerebri. There is a slight male predominance, and the age of presentation is around 40 years.

Disorder Description: Rare primary brain tumor in which there is a diffuse infiltration of the brain with neoplastic glial cells that can affect multiple cerebral lobes. World Health Organization defines it as a diffusely infiltrating glial neoplasm affecting at least three cerebral lobes, usually with bilateral involvement of the cerebral hemispheres and/or deep gray matter. Spinal cord, optic nerve, and brainstem involvement has also been reported.

Symptoms

Localization site	Comment
Cerebral hemispheres	Seizures; hemiparesis (interruption of the corticospinal pathways); atypical parkinsonism (basal ganglia)
Mental status and psychiatric aspects/complications	Apathy and impaired executive functions (bifrontal location of the tumor)
Cranial nerves	Blurry vision (tumor involvement of the optic nerve)
Spinal cord	Progressive sensory loss and paraparesis (intramedullary location)
Specific spinal roots	Decreased sensation in the dermatomal distribution
Unclear localization	Headache, nausea, vomiting, papilledema (increased intracranial pressure)

Treatment Complications: Temozolamide can cause nausea, vomiting, diarrhea, transaminitis, pancytopenia, infertility. Radiation can cause anorexia, pancytopenia, bleeding diathesis, infection, fatigue, weakness, weight loss.

Bibliography

Artigas J, Cervos-navarro J, Iglesias JR, Ebhardt G. Gliomatosis cerebri: clinical and histological findings. *Clin Neuropathol.* 1985;4(4):135–48.

Grisold W, Soffietti R, eds. *Neuro-Oncology: Part I.* Vol 104. 1st ed. Amsterdam: Elsevier; 2012.

Kim DG, Yang HJ, Park IA, et al. Gliomatosis cerebri: clinical features, treatment, and prognosis. *Acta Neurochir (Wien).* 1998;140(8):755–62.

Glomus Jugulare Tumor

Epidemiology and Demographics: Estimated annual incidence is 1 case per 1.3 million people. Occurs predominantly in women in the fifth and sixth decades of life.

Disorder Description: Slow-growing, hyper-vascular tumor that arises within the jugular foramen of the temporal bone. The tumor is locally invasive. Catecholamines,

norepinephrine, or dopamine excreted by the tumor causing headache and tachycardia can be the first or leading symptoms in about 2–4% of cases.

Symptoms

Localization site	Comment
Base of skull	Erosion and invasion of skull base
Cranial nerves	Conductive hearing loss and pulsatile tinnitus (most common); **jugular foramen syndrome** or **Vernet's syndrome** paresis of 9th–11th (with or without 12th) cranial nerves
Unclear localization	Headache, hydrocephalus, and elevated intracranial pressure may be produced by intracranial extension of the tumor

Treatment Complications: Complications of surgery include death, cranial nerve palsies, bleeding, cerebrospinal fluid (CSF) leak, meningitis, uncontrollable hypotension/hypertension, and tumor regrowth.

Complications of radiation include internal carotid artery thrombosis, secondary tumor development, pituitary–hypothalamic insufficiency, CSF leak, tumor growth, and radiation necrosis of bone, brain, or dura.

Bibliography

Kumar K, Ahmed R, Bajantri B, et al. Tumors presenting as multiple cranial nerve palsies. *Case Rep Neurol.* 2017;9(1):54–61.

Larner JM, Hahn SS, Spaulding CA, Constable WC. Glomus jugulare tumors: long-term control by radiation therapy. *Cancer.* 1992;69(7):1813–7.

Glossopharyngeal Neuralgia

Epidemiology and Demographics: There are limited case reports on this condition and no large population-based studies to estimate incidence or prevalence. This condition is rare. By its very nature, glossopharyngeal neuralgia is considered to be strongly associated with facial pain syndromes. One estimate suggests that glossopharyngeal neuralgia occurs in 0.2–1.3% of facial pain sydromes.

Disorder Description: A rare facial pain syndrome characterized by paroxysmal severe pain in the sensory distribution of cranial nerves IX and X. Pain is described as stabbing in nature; patients often refer to pain as occurring on one side of throat near the tonsils and sometimes radiating to the ear. These events are associated with syncope, convulsions, asystole, and bradycardia. In the event there is an association, the condition is called vagoglossopharyngeal neuralgia. There are two variants as described by the International Headache Society: classic type versus symptomatic type. The classic type has the same characterization of pain as symptomatic but is episodic in nature. By contrast, the symptomatic type exhibits persistent aching pain between acute exacerbations.

Symptoms

Localization site	Comment
Cranial nerves	Some studies suggest a role of demyelination along cranial nerves IX and X. Other studies suggest an association with compressive neuropathy secondary to tumors, vasculature, abscess, post-surgical disturbances, Eagle syndrome

Secondary Complications: This condition is often mistaken for trigeminal neuralgia; however, treatments for either trigeminal neuralgia or glossopharyngeal neuralgia are similar.

Treatment Complications: If there is an association with syncope or other cardiac problem in glossopharyngeal neuralgia, strong consideration should be taken to stabilize the patient hemodynamically first before pursuing treatment of the pain. Conventional medications to treat this condition include carbamazepine, gabapentin, phenytoin, oxcarbazepine, or pregabalin. Outside of listed side effects to these medications, no known complications specifically associated with glossopharyngeal neuralgia have been reported. Occasionally, pharmacologic intervention will fail and surgical intervention is needed, specifically nerve blocks and decompression. Known complications from this surgery include deficits associated with the cranial nerves such as vocal cord paralysis and dysphagia.

Bibliography

Blumenfeld A, Nikolskaya G. Glossopharyngeal neuralgia. *Curr Pain Headache Rep.* 2013;17:343.

Elias J, Kuniyoshi R, Carloni WV, et al. Glossopharyngeal neuralgia associated with cardiac syncope. *Arq Bras Cardiol.* 2002;78(5):510–9.

Rey-Dios R, Cohen-Gadol AA. Current neurosurgical management of glossopharyngeal neuralgia and technical nuances for microvascular decompression surgery. *Neurosurg Focus.* 2013;43(3):E8.

Singleton AO. Glossopharyngeal neuralgia and its surgical relief. *Ann Surg.* 1926;83(3):338–44.

Glue-Sniffing Neuropathy

Epidemiology and Demographics: Volatile substance abuse is most common in teenagers. It is also more common in the lower socioeconomic classes.

Disorder Description: Caused by intentional inhalation of the volatile vapors of various adhesive substances. One example of volatile substance abuse that also includes gasoline, typewriter correction fluid, and others. The chemical composition of glue may include n-hexane, toluene, benzene, phenol, chloroform, and methyl ketone. Multiple chemicals in glue can cause neurologic symptoms with acute euphoria, sedation, hallucinations, and seizures. With repeated exposure, peripheral neuropathy develops, which is primarily related to hexacarbons. With very high-level acute exposure, acute neuropathy mimicking Guillain–Barré syndrome may be seen.

Symptoms

Localization site	Comment
Cerebral hemispheres	Seizures may occur
Mental status and psychiatric aspects/complications	Euphoria, confusion, lethargy, and hallucinations
Vestibular system (and non-specific dizziness)	Dizziness
Peripheral neuropathy	Acute neuropathy mimicking Guillain–Barré syndrome after massive intentional inhalation. Low-level chronic abuse leads to central–peripheral distal axonopathy
Syndromes with combined upper and lower motor neuron deficits	Distal portions of corticospinal tract axons damaged with central peripheral distal axonopathy resulting from chronic low-level exposure

Bibliography

Djurendic-Brenesel M, Stojiljkovic G, Pilija V. Fatal intoxication with toluene due to inhalation of glue. *J Forensic Sci*. 2016;61(3):875–8. PMID: 27122437.

Smith AG, Albers JW. n-Hexane neuropathy due to rubber cement sniffing. *Muscle Nerve*. 1997;20(11):1445–50. PMID:9342162.

Glutamic Acid Decarboxylase Antibody (GAD Ab) Syndromes

Epidemiology and Demographics: Glutamic acid decarboxylase antibody syndromes (GAD Abs) have been described in association with stiff person syndrome (SPS), cerebellar ataxia, limbic encephalitis, palatal or branchial myoclonus, thyroid disorders, and type 1 diabetes (T1D). GAD Abs are also of interest in patients with chronic medically refractory epilepsy in and out of association with other neurologic syndromes and T1D. GAD Abs reported in 60 to 88% of patients presenting with SPS. GAD Abs are also observed in up to 80% of patients with T1D.

Disorder Description: GAD is involved in enzymatic conversion of L-glutamic acid to GABA and is present in GABA-ergic neuronal cytoplasm and secretory vesicles. GAD is also present in pancreatic beta islet cells where it may regulate insulin secretion. The 65.4-kDa isoform (GAD65) is encoded by a gene located on chromosome 2, while the gene for the 66.6 kDa isoform (GAD67) is located on chromosome 10. Both isoforms have been observed in the central nervous system, but differ in subcellular localization, membrane interaction, and mode of GABA release.

In neurons, GAD Abs may impair conversion of glutamate to GABA, thus reducing the release of GABA, decreasing inhibitory synaptic transmission, and increasing neuronal hyperexcitability in a widespread manner. Variations in clinical phenotype remain unaccounted for at this time. GAD Abs may recognize different epitopes specific to neurologic syndromes, distinct from those in T1D. Higher GAD Ab titers are observed in association with neurologic syndromes than in T1D. Other autoantibodies may co-occur with GAD Abs, such as those against GABA, amphiphysin, or glycine receptors. Infrequently associated with thymic or lung cancers.

GAD Abs may be implicated in patients who develop both T1D and primary generalized epilepsy, given higher than expected rates of concurrence. GAD Abs have also been reported to be associated with other forms of epilepsy, including focal syndromes.

Treatment for SPS may involve baclofen and benzodiazepines, such as diazepam. Antiepileptic medications may be indicated for seizures or myoclonus. Symptoms of SPS or limbic encephalitis may resolve via immunotherapy with high-dose steroids, intravenous immunoglobulins (IVIG), and plasma exchange (PE), corresponding with reduction in absolute GAD Ab titers. Rituxamab has also been utilized with some benefit.

Symptoms

Localization site	Comment
Cerebral hemispheres	Seizures, generalized or focal in onset, myoclonus, encephalitis
Mental status and psychiatric aspects/complications	Encephalopathy, confusion, delirium
Brainstem	Neuronal hyperexcitability resulting in limb stiffness in SPS. Oculomotor abnormalities, nystagmus. Palatal myoclonus
Cerebellum	Ataxia and progressive degeneration
Spinal cord	Neuronal hyperexcitability in SPS resulting in truncal or limb stiffness. Myelitis has been described
Anterior horn cells	EMG may show continuous motor-unit activity in SPS
Muscle	Stiffness, rigidity, spasms, aches, rhabdomyolysis in SPS. EMG may show continuous motor-unit activity

Secondary Complications: Respiratory failure and rhabdomyolysis due to SPS. Complications of seizures include, among others, aspiration, respiratory complications, psychiatric symptoms, cognitive deficits, and accidental injury.

Treatment Complications: Benzodiazepines are associated with sedation, respiratory depression, and confusion. Baclofen associated with sedation and a lowered threshold for seizures. IV hydration requires monitoring of fluid balance and serum electrolytes. Steroids associated with an increased risk for mood lability, psychosis, peptic ulceration, avascular necrosis, and infection. IVIG may be associated with flu-like symptoms during infusion, and rarely anaphylaxis.

Bibliography

Arino H, et al. Paraneoplastic neurological syndromes and glutamic acid decarboxylase antibodies. *JAMA Neurol.* 2015;72(8):874–81.

Baizabal-Carvallo JF, Jankovic J. Stiff-person syndrome: insights into a complex autoimmune disorder. *J Neurol Neurosurg Psychiatry.* 2015;86(8):840–8.

Ryvlin P, et al. *From first unprovoked seizure to newly diagnosed epilepsy.* Progress in epileptic disorders series. Montrouge: John Libbey Eurotex; 2007.

Glut1 Deficiency Syndrome

Epidemiology and Demographics: Wide range of age of onset. The "classic" syndrome presents within the first few months of life.

Disorder Description: Typically caused by heterozygous mutation in the gene encoding the GLUT1 transporter (SLC2A1) on chromosome 1p35-p31.3. Deficits are due to malfunction of the central nervous system secondary to impaired transport of glucose across the blood–brain barrier. CSF glucose less than 40 mg/dL and low CSF lactate are generally diagnostic. Genetic testing may also be performed.

The presentation is variable. The most severe is the classic phenotype consisting of infantile-onset intellectual disabilities, microcephaly, motor incoordination, spasticity, seizures, non-epileptic paroxysmal events including exercise-induced dyskinesia, and generalized seizures.

Ketogenic diet is the treatment of choice.

Symptoms

Localization site	Comment
Cerebral hemispheres	Seizures, incoordination, spasticity, dyskinesias
Mental status and psychiatric aspects/complications	Intellectual disability

Treatment Complications: Risks of the ketogenic diet include kidney stones, elevated blood lipids, growth restriction, and weight loss. Antiepileptic drugs may be associated with psychiatric symptoms, cognitive impairment, ataxia, dizziness, and more rarely, severe allergic reactions, liver failure, or pancreatitis.

Bibliography

Gras D, et al. GLUT1 deficiency syndrome: an update. *Rev Neurol (Paris).* 2014;170(2):91–9.

Gradenigo Syndrome

Epidemiology and Demographics: Rare but life-threatening complication of acute otitis media, most commonly seen in children. Also known as petrous apicitis; originally described in 1907 by Guiseppe Grandenigo. Infection spreads through Dorello's canal from the mastoid air cells to the petrous apex. Commonly caused by aerobic bacteria, but anaerobic bacteria have also been reported in the literature.

Disorder Description: Classic triad of otitis media, deep facial pain (involving the V1/V2 trigeminal distribution), and ipsilateral abducens palsy. Average interval between onset of otic symptoms and 6th CN involvement was 9.6 days. Diagnosed commonly on MRI. Treatment is with beta-lactam antibiotics plus metronidazole or clindamycin. Patients with thrombus will require anticoagulation. Outcome is generally favorable though there is reported residual abducens palsy.

Symptoms: Potential localized inflammatory reaction of the nearby vessels (especially in the cavernous sinus and internal carotid artery).

Secondary Complications: Vascular complications include sinus venous thrombosis, cavernous sinus and internal carotid artery thrombosis.

Treatment Complications: Adverse effects from antibiotics and anticoagulation.

Bibliography

Heshin-Bekenstein M, et al. Gradenigo's syndrome: Is *Fusobacterium* different? Two cases and review of literature. *Int J Pediatr Otorhinolaryngol.* 2014;78(1):166–9.

Granulomatosis with Polyangiitis (Wegener's Granulomatosis)

Epidemiology and Demographics: Onset of granulomatosis with polyangiitis (GPA) may occur at any age, although patients typically present at 35–55 years. Extremely rare in childhood. In European populations, this condition is slightly more common in men, with a male-to-female ratio of 1.5:1. More common in individuals of northern European descent (approximately 90%). Extremely rare in African American and Japanese populations. The prevalence of this condition in the United States is estimated to be 3/100,000 people.

Disorder Description: GPA is part of a larger group of vasculitic syndromes called systemic vasculitides or necrotizing vasculopathies, all of which feature an autoimmune attack by an abnormal type of circulating antibodies termed ANCAs (antineutrophil cytoplasmic antibodies) against small and medium-size blood vessels. Central nervous system manifestations include vasculitis of the small and medium-sized blood vessels of the brain or spinal cord, and granulomatous masses of the orbit, optic nerve, meninges, and the brain. Furthermore, peripheral nervous system involvement has been seen in 67% of patients with this condition. Peripheral system manifestations occur late in the disease and include mononeuritis multiplex, sensorimotor polyneuropathy, and cranial nerve palsies.

Potential causes include:

Diffuse-staining cytoplasmic ANCA (C-ANCA) that is directed against serine proteinase 3 antigen (PR3-ANCA)

Defective allele for alpha-1 antitrypsin, polymorphism of CTLA-4, presence of PTPN22*620W allele, carrying the DPB1*0401 allele, Fcγ receptor IIIb on surface of neutrophils and monocytes/macrophages

Staphylococcus aureus, which has been associated with relapses of this disease process

Exposure to solvents and silica

Risk factors include:

Male gender between ages 35 and 55

Northern European descent (Caucasians)

History of farming

History of drug/environmental allergies

History of exposure to silica or solvents

No specific regions are known to have higher proclivity for GPA.

Symptoms

Localization site	Comment
Central nervous system: brain and spinal cord, small and medium-sized blood vessels, orbit, orbit–optic nerve, meninges	Stroke
	Seizures
	Vision deficits
	Headache
	Uveitis/episcleritis
	Hearing loss secondary to serous otitis media
	Granulomatous masses of orbit, optic nerve, meninges, brain
	Cranial nerve palsies
Peripheral nervous system	Mononeuritis multiplex
	Sensorimotor polyneuropathy

Secondary Complications

1. Hearing loss
2. Vision loss
3. Cranial nerve palsies
4. Peripheral neuropathy with resultant weakness and/or numbness
5. Residual weakness/numbness as a result of stroke
6. Diabetes insipidus (involvement of granulomatous disease of the infundibulum)
7. Diminished higher intellectual functioning in those suffering from seizures

Treatment Complications

Immunosuppressants: Rituximab and cyclophosphamide are commonly used to treat this condition. Rituximab is a monoclonal antibody medication that carries the risk of cardiac arrest, tumor lysis syndrome, progressive multifocal leukoencephalopathy (PML), immunotoxicity, cytokine release syndrome, pulmonary toxicity, and bowel obstruction/perforation. It has also been known to reactivate hepatitis B infection and other viral infections. Cyclophosphamide has been known to cause hemorrhagic cystitis, neutropenia or lymphoma, premature menopause, and infertility in men and women. Cyclophosphamide is carcinogenic and therefore increases the risk for developing lymphomas, leukemia, skin cancer, transitional cell carcinoma of the bladder, and multiple myeloma. Hematopoietic complications with methotrexate are seen in patients not supplemented with folic acid. Furthermore, medications such as azathio-prine and methotrexate are teratogenic, and hence careful avoidance of such drugs during pregnancy is advised. Methotrexate can cause patients to develop ulcerative stomatitis, aplastic anemia, agranulo-cytosis, leukoencephalopathy, seizures, Stevens–Johnson syndrome, among other complications. Azathioprine can cause patients to develop progres-sive multifocal leukoencephalopathy, lymphoma, and possibly other malignancies.

Steroids: Methylprednisolone is commonly used concurrently with immunosuppressants to treat this condition. Methylprednisolone can cause an increased risk of infection, hyperglycemia, avascu-lar necrosis of the hip, psychosis, Cushing's disease, and osteoporosis.

Bibliography

Holle JU, Gross WL. Neurological involvement in Wegener's granulomatosis. *Curr Opin Rheumatol.* 2011;23(1):7–11.

Kubaisi B, Samra KA, Foster CS. Granulomatosis with polyangiitis (Wegener's disease): An updated review of ocular disease manifestations. *Intractable Rare Dis Res.* 2016;5(2):61–9.

Guanidinoacetate Methyltransferase (GAMT) Deficiency

Epidemiology and Demographics: Guanidinoacetate methyltransferase (GAMT) deficiency is rare; approximately 110 affected individuals reported. One-third are of Portuguese origin. Age of onset is 3 months to 3 years.

Disorder Description: Inherited in an autosomal recessive pattern. GAMT is used in the synthesis of creatine from glycine, arginine, and methionine. The effects of GAMT are most severe in organs and tissue requir-ing large amounts of energy, especially the brain.

Cerebral creatine deficiency may be apparent by brain MR spectroscopy. The diagnosis may be fur-ther confirmed by measurement of guanidinoac-etate (GAA), creatine, and creatinine in urine and plasma; and molecular genetic testing. If molecular genetic test results are inconclusive, GAMT enzyme activity may be directly assayed.

Early treatment is highly recommended, and treatment of newborn siblings of affected individu-als has been shown to prevent disease manifestation.

Symptoms

Localization site	Comment
Cerebral hemispheres	Seizures, severity and semiology have wide variation
Mental status and psychiatric aspects/complication	Autism. Intellectual disability may be mild to severe
Basal ganglia	Patients with or without movement disorders may have abnormal MRI signal in the basal ganglia. Approximately 30% will have chorea, athetosis, dystonia, or gait disorder
Cerebellum	Ataxia may occur

Treatment Complications: Treatment includes oral cre-atine monohydrate, as well as supplementation of ornithine and dietary restriction of arginine or protein. Treatment appears to be safe. Antiepileptic drugs for seizures may have a variety of side effects.

Bibliography

Mercimek-Mahmutoglu S, Salomons GS. Creatine deficiency syndromes. In Pagon RA, Adam MP, Ardinger HH, et al., eds. *GeneReviews®* [Internet]. Seattle, WA: University of Washington, Seattle; 1993.

Gynecologic Cancer

Epidemiology and Demographics: Neurologic complica-tions can occur in about 25% of gynecologic tumors.

Disorder Description: Gynecologic cancers cause neuro-logic symptoms predominantly by local invasion. They are also associated with well-defined para-neoplastic syndromes.

Symptoms

Localization site	Comment
Cerebral hemispheres	Headache, seizure, and hemiparesis (rare to have cerebral metastasis). Choriocarcinoma is most common and can also hemorrhage
Mental status and psychiatric aspects/ complications	Confusion, memory loss, seizures, irritability, and depression (paraneoplastic limbic encephalitis)

Localization site	Comment
	NMDA encephalitis: Behavioral changes, memory deficits, and psychosis. Dyskinesia of the face and limbs, autonomic dysfunction, status epilepticus, and catatonia (associated with ovarian teratoma)
Cerebellum	Truncal ataxia, nystagmus, dizziness, and dysarthria (paraneoplastic cerebellar degeneration anti-Yo and anti-Ri antibodies)
Spinal cord	Low back pain and paraplegia (epidural metastasis causing compression or intramedullary metastasis – spread through Baton's venous plexus)
Conus medullaris	Paraplegia and bladder/bowel dysfunction (compression of conus medullaris)
Plexus	Lumbosacral or pelvic pain (direct invasion and local spread)

Treatment Complications

Vincristine: Sensorimotor peripheral polyneuropathy
Femoral neuropathy: prolonged immobilization during surgery
Radiotherapy: Lumbosacral plexopathy

Bibliography

Kouhen F, Afif M, El Kabous M, et al. [Brain metastasis of endometrial cancer: report of a case and review of literature]. *Pan Afr Med J.* 2015;20:68.

Lesniak MS, Olivi A. Brain metastases from gynecologic cancers. In *Intracranial metastases: current management strategies*. Chichester: Wiley;2008. pp. 331–50.

Ogawa K, Yoshii Y, Aoki Y, et al. Treatment and prognosis of brain metastases from gynecological cancers. *Neurol Med Chir (Tokyo)*. 2008;48(2):57–62.

Haemophilus Influenzae Type B

Epidemiology and Demographics: *Haemophilus influenzae* type B (Hib) disease occurs worldwide. In the early 1980s, approximately 20,000 cases occurred annually in the United States, predominantly among children younger than 5 years of age. With widespread use of vaccines, the incidence of Hib has declined by more than 99%. In 2011, only 14 cases of invasive disease due to Hib were reported in the United States among children younger than 5 years.[1]

Disorder Description: *Haemophilus influenzae*[2] (Hi) is a gram-negative coccobacillus and is generally aerobic with the ability to grow as a facultative anaerobe. Hib is categorized into two main strains, one composed of a polysaccharide capsule and the other an unencapsulated strain. The capsule forms the basis of a sero-typing scheme, six serotypes (a–f) consisting of six antigenically and biochemically distinct types, and plays an important role in virulence and immunity. In the prevaccine era, type b strains (Hib) dominated and accounted for 95% of invasive Hib disease. The major risk factors for invasive Hib disease are household crowding, large household size, childcare attendance, low socioeconomic status, low parental education, school-aged siblings, and chronic disease (sickle cell disease, antibody deficiency, and malignancies especially during chemotherapy). The most common types of invasive disease caused by Hib are meningitis, epiglottitis, pneumonia, arthritis, and cellulitis.[3]

Diagnosis is based on Gram staining of an infected body fluid, which demonstrates small gram-negative coccobacilli. A positive culture on appropriate media for Hib confirms the diagnosis. Serotype-specific real-time PCR is available for detection of the specific target gene of each Hi serotype.

Symptoms[1,2]

Localization site	Comment
Cerebral hemispheres	Meningitis: fever, decreased mental status, and stiff neck
	Neurologic sequelae in 15–30% of survivors
Cranial nerves	Hearing loss in 15 to 30% of survivors

Treatment Complications: Antimicrobial therapy with an effective third-generation cephalosporin or chloramphenicol in combination with ampicillin is used. Penicillin-class drugs may rarely induce seizures or lower seizure threshold as well as cause encephalopathy.

The case fatality rate is 3–6% despite appropriate antimicrobial therapy.

References

1. Livorsi, DJ, MacNeil JR, Cohn AC, et al. Invasive *Haemophilus influenzae* in the United States, 1999–2008: epidemiology and outcomes. *J Infect.* 2012;65:496–504.
2. Centers for Disease Control and Prevention. *Haemophilus influenzae* type B. In *Epidemiology and prevention of vaccine-preventable diseases*. 13th ed. Atlanta, GA: Centers for Disease Control and Prevention; 2015. pp. 119–33.
3. Agrawal A, Murphy TF. *Haemophilus influenzae* infections in the *H. influenzae* type b conjugate vaccine era. *J Clin Microbiol*. 2011;49:3728–32.

Hand–Schuller–Christian Disease (HSC)

Epidemiology and Demographics: Hand–Schuller–Christian (HSC) disease is one of the three components included in histiocytosis X, the other two being eosinophilic granuloma and Letterer–Siwe disease. HSC disease is primarily seen in infants and children and is rarely seen in adults.

Disorder Description: The classical triad of HSC disease – exophthalmos, diabetes insipidus, and calvarial lytic lesions – is seen in only one-third of patients.

Symptoms

Localization site	Comment
Cerebral hemispheres	Seizures, increased intracranial pressure, hemiparesis
Mental status and psychiatric aspects/complications	Intellectual disabilities and tremors
Brainstem	Tetraparesis and respiratory depression (due to medulla oblongata compression – rare)
Cranial nerves	Hearing loss
Pituitary gland	Diabetes insipidus, delay in sexual maturity and bone development

Secondary Complications: Diabetes insipidus, vertebral fracture and spinal cord compression.

Treatment Complications: Complications of surgery include cosmetic deformities, orthopedic deformities, or loss of function. Complications of radiation include fractures and bone weakness. Side effects of methotrexate, vinblastine, etoposide, and mercaptopurine include neuropathy, cytopenia, vomiting, hair loss, and leukoencephalopathy.

Bibliography

Cugati G, Singh M, Pande A, Ramamurthi R, Vasudevan MC. Hand Schuller Christian disease. *Indian J Med Paediatr Oncol.* 2011;32(3):183–4.

Jacquet G, Plouvier E, Billerey C, Godard J, Steimle R. [Hand-Schüller-Christian disease with tumor localization in the posterior fossa]. *Presse Med.* 1988;17(17):855–7.

Khristov V, Manov A, Apostolov P, Kolebinov N, Nachev S. [Long-term observation of a case of Hand-Schüller-Christian disease]. *Vutr Boles.* 1989;28(5):87–91.

Hashimoto's Thyroiditis

Epidemiology and Demographics: Hashimoto's thyroiditis is the most common autoimmune thyroid disorder. It is the most common cause for hypothyroidism in iodine sufficient countries. Prevalence is greater in women than in men (7:1), and this ratio increases with age. A genetic susceptibility has been confirmed in twin studies.[1]

Disorder Description: Destruction of the thyroid gland occurs due to lymphocytic infiltration. Autoantibodies to the thyroid gland are prevalent in those affected.[1] Symptoms may be insidious and the diagnosis is often missed.

Symptoms

Localization site	Comment
Cerebral hemispheres	Acute to subacute altered mental status/confusion. Headaches may occur. Sleep disturbances. Seizures present in 60%. May progress to coma
Mental status and psychiatric aspects/ complications	Poor memory and concentration. Personality changes including psychotic delusions and paranoia

Localization site	Comment
Cerebellum	Ataxia and speech difficulties
Cranial nerves	Diplopia
Peripheral neuropathy	Paresthesias
Muscle	Myalgias, myoclonus, tremor

Treatment Complications: If Hashimoto's thyroiditis leads to thyroid hormone insufficiency, thyroid hormone supplementation may be indicated. Careful monitoring is required as excess dosage may lead to symptoms of hyperthyroidism.

Reference

1. Zaletel K, Gaberšček S. Hashimoto's thyroiditis: from genes to the disease. *Curr Genom.* 2011;12(8):576–88.

Suggested Reading

Ju C, Zhang L. Diplopia in a patient with Hashimoto's thyroiditis: a case report and literature review. *Medicine (Baltimore).* 2017;96(26):e7330.

Mocellin R, Walterfang M, Velakoulis D. Hashimoto's encephalopathy: epidemiology, pathogenesis and management. *CNS Drugs.* 2007;21(10):799–811.

Souza PV, Bortholin T, Pinto WB, Santos AJ. Progressive hearing loss and cerebellar ataxia in anti-Ma2-associated autoimmune encephalitis. *Arq Neuropsiquiatr.* 2017;75(1):74–5. https://dx.doi.org/10.1590/0004-282x20160169

Headache and Pregnancy

Epidemiology and Demographics: Headaches are common in reproductive women; about 60% of women under age 40 report experiencing at least one headache in the previous year. Ten percent of primary headaches are first diagnosed during pregnancy. The most common primary headaches in this population are migraine (17% annual prevalence in women) and tension headache (more than 80% life time prevalence) followed by medication overuse headache.

Cluster headache is rare. Sixty to 70% of migraine and tension headaches tend to improve during pregnancy, especially if there was a menstrual association.

Common secondary causes of headache are sinus thrombosis, reversible cerebral vasoconstriction syndrome (RCVS), and pre-eclampsia/eclampsia, which are discussed separately in this book. The secondary headaches that will be discussed here are pituitary apoplexy, idiopathic intracranial hypertension (IIH), and post-lumbar puncture headache; pituitary apoplexy is a rare phenomenon. The annual incidence of IIH is about 1/100,000, but increases to 20 per 100,000 in women who are 20% over their ideal weight. Post lumbar puncture (LP) headache affects up to one-third of patients who undergo spinal anesthesia. Most common between 30 and 39 years.

The female sex is a risk factor for migraine and tension headache; only cluster headache is more common in men. There are several genes linked to the predisposition for migraines with a complex inheritance pattern that is still currently not well understood.

The pituitary gland tends to enlarge during pregnancy. A preexisting pituitary adenoma can enlarge during pregnancy and become more prone to hemorrhage. Obesity and excessive weight gain during pregnancy are associated with an increased risk of IIH. Women who receive spinal anesthesia during delivery are at risk for post-LP headache. Another risk factor of post-LP headache is bevel orientation perpendicular to the dura during the procedure.

Disorder Description: Migraines were once thought to be related to cerebral vasodilation. However, the cortical spreading depression theory is more widely accepted now. It hypothesizes that migraine and migraine aura are due to neuronal and glial depolarization and subsequent activation of nociceptive trigeminal afferents located around the pia. Tension headache has a similar proposed pathophysiology that involves the activation of myofascial nociceptors.

IIH is due to increased intracranial pressure from excessive cerebrospinal fluid (CSF), while post-LP headache is due to decreased intracranial pressure from a CSF leak through a tract created by the puncture needle.

Symptoms

Localization site	Comment
Cerebral hemispheres	Migraine • Severe unilateral throbbing headache lasting 4–72 hours, with photophonophobia and nausea, with or without aura Tension type headache • Bilateral non-throbbing headache that is mild to moderate in severity, without photo-phonophobia or nausea • Typical descriptors include "dull," "band-like," and "heavy"
Pituitary gland	Pituitary apoplexy • Thunderclap headache, decreased level of consciousness, and visual disturbances (visual loss or diplopia) • Hypopituitarism, including hypotension from corticosteroid deficiency
Ventricular system	Idiopathic intracranial hypertension • Diffuse headache worse with lying down, coughing, and straining (activities that increase intracranial pressure). Other symptoms are transient visual loss, tinnitus, and diplopia • On physical exam, there may be papilledema, an enlarged blind spot, visual field defect, and cranial nerve VI palsy Post-LP headache • Postural headache that typically develops within 5 days of procedure. There may be associated dizziness and neck stiffness

Secondary Complications: Disabling headaches are a source of emotional stress. Lost time and physical burden due to the illness can negatively impact a person's mental health. Mood disorders are more prevalent in patients suffering from migraines, possibly linked to a genetic predisposition as well.

Migraine is associated with an increased risk of thrombosis, pre-eclampsia, and gestational hypertension. In the hypercoagulable pregnant state, patients should be monitored carefully for signs and symptoms suggestive of these comorbid conditions.

Treatment Complications: Non-pharmacologic treatments are worth trying as many medications used in headache are FDA category C, D, and even X (valproic acid). Women should be encouraged to stay well hydrated, exercise regularly, keep a regular sleep schedule, reduce stress level, and avoid excessive intake or withdrawal of caffeinated products. Magnesium and CoQ10 can be used as migraine prophylaxis. Vitamin D deficiency is associated with an increased risk of migraine and should be supplemented. Breastfeeding helps prolong the protective effects of pregnancy against headaches.

Analgesics like acetaminophen and NSAIDs, and opiates for very severe pain are relatively safe if used with discretion. A short course of steroids may be used for emergent treatment of headache but should not be used chronically. Triptans are FDA category C but adverse effects have not been reported and are deemed to be generally safe to use in pregnancy if other treatments are ineffective. Ergots are contraindicated. For prophylactic treatment, low dose beta-blockers and tricyclic antidepressants are probably safe. Antiepilectics (topiramate and valproic acid), calcium channel blockers, and lithium must be avoided if possible.

Pituitary surgery is often necessary in pituitary apoplexy with visual symptoms, followed by hormonal and corticosteroid supplementation.

Acetazolamide, a carbonic anhydrase inhibitor, is first-line in IHH treatment. Other diuretics and even surgical intervention such as optic nerve sheath fenestration and shunting have been pursued in refractory cases.

Post-LP headaches are treated conservatively first with bed rest, caffeine, and oral analgesics. If symptoms do not improve, an epidural blood patch is the definitive treatment.

Symptomatic Treatment: NSAIDs have been associated with an increased risk of bleeding and premature closure of the fetal ductus arteriosus. Chronic opiate use may cause neonatal withdrawal symptoms. Ergots increase the risk of miscarriage.

Prophylactic treatment: beta-blockers may cause fetal bradycardia and decrease uterine contraction when used peripartum. Calcium channel blockers also have a tocolytic (delivery-delaying) effect. Topiramate is associated with increased risk of oral clefts and valproic acid with neural tube defects, decreased IQ, and atrial septal defect among others. Lithium is teratogenic as well and has been shown to cause fetal cardiac defects. Botulinum toxin, which is now increasingly used for chronic migraine, still lacks data on its effect on pregnancy and lactation.

Bibliography

Piantanida E, Gallo D, Lombardi V, et al. Pituitary apoplexy during pregnancy: a rare, but dangerous headache. *J Endocrinol Invest*. 2014;37(9):789–97.

Schoen JC, Campbell RL, Sadosty AT. Headache in pregnancy: an approach to emergency department evaluation and management. *West J Emerg Med*. 2015;16(2):291–301.

Vetvik KG, MacGregor EA. Sex differences in the epidemiology, clinical features, and pathophysiology of migraine. *Lancet Neurol*. 2017;16(1):76–87.

Von Wald T, Walling AD. Headache during pregnancy. *Obstet & Gyn Survey*. 2002;57(3):179–85.

Hemangioblastoma

Epidemiology and Demographics: Hemangioblastomas are rare intracranial neoplasms, but the most common primary adult intraaxial tumor of the posterior fossa. They occur either sporadically or as a component in von Hippel–Lindau disease (VHLD). Sporadic form presents in the fourth and fifth decade while in VHLD, it presents in the second and third decade.

Disorder Description: Hemangioblastomas are slow-growing, benign vascular tumors predominantly occurring in the posterior fossa. Sporadic forms are in general solitary while in VHLD, they are multiple.

Symptoms

Localization site	Comment
Cerebral hemispheres	Headache (increased ICP)
Brainstem	Nystagmus
Cerebellum	Headache, ataxia, nausea, and vomiting
Cranial nerves	Loss of vision (optic nerve hemangioblastoma)
Spinal cord	Focal back or neck pain and sensory loss or weakness. 60% of spinal hemangioblastomas are intramedullary, associated with syrinx
Specific spinal roots	Radiculopathy (21% of spinal tumors)
Peripheral neuropathy	Mononeuropathy, e.g., ulnar nerve

Secondary Complications: Polycythemia (paraneoplastic erythropoietin production).

Treatment Complications: Complications of surgery include CSF leakage, pseudomeningocele, brainstem injury leading to cranial nerve palsy and hemiparesis.

Complications of bevacizumab include thrombotic microangiopathy, stroke, intracerebral hemorrhage, GI perforations, vomiting, nausea, diarrhea, and headache.

Radiation can cause leukoencephalopathy and radionecrosis.

Bibliography

Acikalin MF, Oner U, Tel N, Paşaoğlu O, Altinel F. Supratentorial hemangioblastoma: a case report and review of the literature. *Arch Pathol Lab Med.* 2003;127(9):e382–4.

Lonser RR, Butman JA, Huntoon K, et al. Prospective natural history study of central nervous system hemangioblastomas in von Hippel-Lindau disease. *J Neurosurg.* 2014;120(5):1055–62.

Na JH, Kim HS, Eoh W, et al. Spinal cord hemangioblastoma: diagnosis and clinical outcome after surgical treatment. *J Korean Neurosurg Soc.* 2007;42(6):436–40.

Hematomyelia/Syringomyelia

Epidemiology and Demographics: This condition is seen in 8.4 cases per 100,000 population. It is more common in men than in women. It is seen most commonly in the third to fourth decades of life.

Disorder Description: Development of a fluid-filled cavity or syrinx within the spinal cord. More than 10% communicate with fourth ventricle, 50% due to blockage of cerebrospinal fluid circulation. The blockage of CSF circulation is the most common form. It could be due to Arnold–Chiari malformation. Other causes include spinal trauma, radiation necrosis, or hemorrhage (from aneurysm rupture, arteriovenous malformation, or tumor). Some are idiopathic.

Symptoms

Localization site	Comment
Spinal cord	Myelopathy, root irritation with pain, mild-to-severe gait abnormality, loss of position sense and vibration sense, dysesthesias

Secondary Complications: Include recurrent pneumonia, paraplegia or quadriplegia, decubitus ulcers, bowel and urinary dysfunction, Charcot joints, and acute painful enlargement of the shoulders.

Bibliography

Williams B. Prognosis and syringomyelia. *Neurol Res.* 1986;8(3):130–45.

Hemiballism

Epidemiology and Demographics: If occurring following stroke, the incidence in men and women is equal, with an average age of between 63.3 and 70 years. If occurring in relation to hyperglycemia, a higher incidence has been reported in older women of Asian origin

Disorder Description: Hemiballism (HB) is characterized by large-amplitude, violent, arrhythmic involuntary movements of a limb from a proximal joint. Common etiologies include hyperglycemia, occlusive or hemorrhagic strokes, lesions related to tumor, or demyelinating plaques in multiple sclerosis.

Symptoms

Localization site	Comment
Brainstem	Hemiballism +/– chorea

Secondary Complications: HB may result in falls, if involving the lower limbs.

Treatment Complications: Treatment options include both typical and atypical anti-dopaminergic agents, catecholamine-depleting agents, and benzodiazepines. Side effects of the above include sedation, severe depression, hypotension, and parkinsonism.

Bibliography

Alarcon F, Zijlmans JC, Duenas G, Cevallos N. Post-stroke movement disorders: report of 56 patients. *J Neurol Neurosurg Psychiatry.* 2004;75:1568–74.

Ching LP, Chin KP, Wah ESA. Hyperglycemia-associated hemichorea-hemiballism: the spectrum of clinical presentation. *Intern Med.* 2015;54(15):1881–4.

Ghika-Schmid F, Ghika J, Regli F, Bogousslavsky J. Hyperkinetic movement disorders during and after acute stroke: the Lausanne Stroke Registry. *J Neurol Sci.* 1997;146:109–16.

Handley A, Medcalf P, Hellier K, Dutta D. Movement disorders after stroke. *Age Ageing.* 2009;38: 260–66.

Kim JS. Delayed onset mixed involuntary movements after thalamic stroke. Clinical, radiological and pathophysiological findings. *Brain.* 2001;124:299–309.

Hemicrania Continua

Epidemiology and Demographics: Incidence and prevalence of hemicrania continua is unknown as this condition has not been studied extensively. From limited studies, the age range is 10 to 67 years, with mean onset at 30 years. One case report noted that women were more likely to have hemicrania continua than men at a 5:1 ratio; more recent studies have reduced that bias to 1.8:1 suggesting that there is a small female preponderance for this condition.

Disorder Description: This condition is described as a unilateral and continuous headache without side shift. The pain has to be continuous without pain-free periods for at least 3 months. At least one ipsilateral cranial autonomic symptom should be present: conjunctival injection, lacrimation, nasal blockage, rhinorrhea, ptosis, or miosis. Some case reports have shown that side shifting can occur; other case reports have shown the presence of photophobia and phonophobia (unilateral) during headache exacerbation. More than half of these patients have sensitivity to movement and show signs of agitation or restlessness.

Symptoms

Localization site	Comment
Cerebral hemispheres	Unilateral headache that is continuous for at least 3 months
Brainstem	Involvement of posterior hypothalamus, dorsal rostral pons, ventrolateral midbrain, and pontomedullary junction on imaging studies
Cranial nerves	Associated with trigeminal autonomic cephalalgias

Secondary Complications : Severe headache pain can be associated with irritation and agitation.

Treatment Complications: Indomethacin is the essential management of hemicrania continua. Complications of indomethacin use include peptic ulcer disease.

Bibliography

Bordini C, Antonaci F, Stovner LJ, Schrader H, Sjaastad O. "Hemicrania continua": a clinical review. *Headache.* 1991;31:20–6.

Cittadini E, Goadsby PJ. Update on hemicrania continua. *Curr Pain Headache Rep.* 2011;15:51–6.

Medina JL, Diamond S. Cluster headache variant: spectrum of a new headache syndrome. *Arch Neurol.* 1981;38:705–9.

Wheeler S. Clinical spectrum of hemicrania continua. *Neurology.* 2000;54:422.

Hemifacial Spasm

Epidemiology and Demographics: Presents between 40 and 50 years of age; male-to-female ratio is 2:1. More common in Asians.

Disorder Description: Tonic and clonic contractions of the facial muscles innervated by the ipsilateral facial nerve. Initial site of onset: orbicularis oculi muscle in 90%, cheek in 11%, and perioral region in <10%. Spasms spread gradually to other muscles innervated by the ipsilateral facial nerve in a synchronous manner. Bilateral involvement uncommon at <0.5% prevalence. Facial spasms are spontaneous and may persist during sleep. Symptoms are frequently aggravated by stress, fatigue, anxiety, and voluntary facial movements. Localizes most commonly to peripheral injury of the facial nerve by trauma, compression of the facial nerve at the cerebellopontine angle (CPA), or reverberant activity in the facial motonucleus centrally. Associated with symptoms of tinnitus, hearing loss, trigeminal neuralgia (uncommon).

Most commonly caused by a vascular compression of the facial nerve by vasculature (anterior or posterior cerebellar artery or the vertebral artery) or intracranial tumors at CPA. Diagnosed with MRI/MRA and using electrophysiologic evidence of compression at the facial nerve root exit.

Differential diagnosis includes facial myokymia, psychogenic facial spasm, blepharospasm, Meige syndrome, tics, and tardive dyskinesia.

Spontaneous resolution in <10% of patients. Botulinum toxin is the treatment of choice, which is effective for several months. Most common surgical procedure is microvascular decompression of the facial nerve at the CPA.

Symptoms: Facial nerve along its course is a potential site of involvement.

Secondary Complications: Facial weakness may be seen in long-standing cases.

Treatment Complications: Adverse effects from Botox include transient dry eyes, ptosis, eyelid and facial weakness, diplopia, and excessive tearing. If surgery is performed, hearing loss is the most common adverse effect.

Bibliography

Tan NC, et al. Hemifacial spasm and involuntary facial movements. *QJM.* 2002;95(8):493–500.

Hemimasticatory Spasm

Epidemiology and Demographics: Rare. Onset ranges from 15 to 57 years (mean age of 31), with female predominance.

Disorder Description: Characterized by paroxysmal unilateral involuntary contraction of jaw-closing muscles. The pathophysiology is unclear, but may be due to ephaptic transmission at nerve entry zone. It is described to be associated with localized scleroderma and facial hemiatrophy. Electrodiagnostic studies are suggestive of demyelination of trigeminal peripheral motor pathway. The characteristic findings on needle electromyography are irregular bursts of motor unit action potentials, correlating with the involuntary movement.

Symptoms

Localization site	Comment
Cranial nerve	Trigeminal peripheral motor pathway: neurologic examination is normal, except for hypertrophy of involved muscle. Sensation is spared

Secondary Complications: Pain due to spasm and hypertrophy of involved muscle.

Treatment Complications: Botulinum toxin injection and microvascular decompression were reported to be successful in treatment for hemimasticatory spasm. Botulinum toxin injection may cause weakness.

Bibliography

Kim HJ, Jeon BS, Lee KW. Hemimasticatory spasm associated with localized scleroderma and facial hemiatrophy. *Arch Neurol.* 2000;57(4):576–80.

Hemiparkinsonism–Hemiatrophy Syndrome (HPHA)

Epidemiology and Demographics: Hemiparkinsonism–hemiatrophy syndrome (HPHA) is a rare condition, and its true prevalence is unknown as it has been reported only in a few case series and case reports. Men and women seem to be equally affected. Hemiatrophy occurs early in childhood but may not be noticeable to some. Hemiparkinsonism usually develops later in life with mean ages ranging from 38 to 49 years.

Disorder Description: HPHA is a heterogeneous disorder associated with early somatic hemiatrophy commonly affecting the hands. The face, feet, and other body areas may also be affected. Hemiatrophy is thought to be due to a failure of growth rather than atrophy occurring later in life. Focal dystonia of the hemiatrophic side is a common presenting symptom. Patients may then develop bradykinesia, stiffness, tremor, and gait abnormalities. Symptoms are slowly progressive but may also develop on the other side of the body over time. The exact pathophysiology of HPHA is unknown but may be related to pre/perinatal and early brain injury with selective vulnerability of affected neurons at different stages of development.

Symptoms

Localization site	Comment
Cerebral hemispheres	Neuroimaging is variable: a third of imaging may reveal focal or hemicerebral atrophy with ventricular enlargement of the affected side; another third may have normal imaging and the remainder may reveal incidental changes or focal lesions within the basal ganglia including cystic lesions, calcifications, and rarefaction
Mental status and psychiatric aspects/ complications	Early developmental delay with learning disabilities requiring special education
Brainstem	Midbrain atrophy and focal lesions on imaging
Muscle	Variable somatic hemiatrophy

Secondary Complications: HPHA is often associated with scoliosis and joint and musculoskeletal abnormalities including striatal hands and feet.

Treatment Complications: Response to treatment is variable but most respond to levodopa. Rarely, some patients develop motor fluctuations with dyskinesia and "OFF time." Thalamotomy seems to provide only short-term benefit for tremor. Deep brain stimulation (DBS) with subthalamic (STN) and thalamic targets has been described. STN DBS was reported to be effective for dyskinesia and prolonging "ON time."

Bibliography

Buchman AS, Goetz CG, Klawans HL. Hemiparkinsonism with hemiatrophy. *Neurology.* 1988;38: 527–30.

Giladi N, Burke RE, Kostic V, et al. Hemiparkinsonism-hemiatrophy syndrome: clinical and neuroradiologic features. *Neurology.* 1990;40(11):1731–4.

Klawans HL. Hemiparkinsonism as a late complication of hemiatrophy: a new syndrome. *Neurology.* 1981;31:625–8.

Wijemanne S, Jankovic J. Hemiparkinsonism-hemiatrophy syndrome. *Neurology.* 2007;69(16): 1585–94.

Hemolytic–Uremic Syndrome

Epidemiology and Demographics: Two different etiologies and epidemiologies for hemolytic–uremic syndrome (HUS). In children, usually post-infectious, affecting young children with incidence of about 2/100,000 per year. In adults (and about 10% of children), related to genetic mutations in genes expressing proteins in the complement cascade.

Disorder Description: Defined clinically by triad of non-immune (negative Coombs test) hemolytic anemia with schizocytes, thrombocytopenia, and renal impairment. HUS is a thrombotic microangiopathy distinguished from thrombotic thrombocytopenia purpura (TTP) by normal ADAMTS13 protein activity (abnormally low in TTP). Majority of cases in children associated with Shiga toxin-producing *Escherichia coli* infection. Cases have also been described following *Streptococcus pneumoniae* infection. Adult cases more likely to be from genetic disorders affecting components of alternative complement pathway resulting in unregulated complement activation. These patients often have positive family history.[1] HUS usually *but not always* primarily affects the renal vasculature (cerebrovascular disease is the most common extra-renal site).

Symptoms

Localization site	Comment
Cerebral hemispheres	Can cause multifocal primarily posterior lesions by the syndrome of posterior reversible encephalopathy syndrome (PRES) in association with hypertension and renal insufficiency. HUS can also affect cerebrovasculature causing multifocal deep and superficial lesions[2]
Mental status and psychiatric aspects/complications	Symptoms of PRES can vary but commonly include drowsiness, confusion, cortical visual abnormalities, and seizures. Multifocal small vessel strokes often cause focal deficits and confusion. If renal failure progresses, uremic encephalopathy may also result

Secondary Complications: Renal insufficiency requiring dialysis. With renal failure, there can be associated hyperkalemia, acidosis, and volume overload. Infrequently, HUS may also cause myocardial injury and ischemic injury in other vascular distributions.

Treatment Complications: Usually treated supportively in children. For inherited mutations, may be treated with plasma exchange or ecluzimab (monoclonal antibody to C5), which increases the risk of life-threatening meningococcal infections.

References

1. Noris M, Remuzzi G. Hemolytic uremic syndrome. *J Am Soc Nephrol JASN.* 2005;16: 1035–50.
2. Loirat C, Frémeaux-Bacchi V. Atypical hemolytic uremic syndrome. *Orphanet J Rare Dis.* 2011;6:60.

Hemorrhage into Abscess

Epidemiology and Demographics: Hemorrhage into pyogenic brain abscess is a rare clinical condition. Exact epidemiology has not been studied or published.

Disorder Description: Most of the case reports regarding hemorrhage into brain abscess share a single dominant clinical feature, which is a dramatic alteration in the patient's mental status. Most patients already had symptoms of infection (e.g., fever, nuchal rigidity) as well as symptoms of a space-occupying lesion (e.g., headache, nausea and vomiting, seizures) before the sudden change of mental status occurred.

Symptoms

Localization site	Comment
Cerebral hemispheres	If patient already has cortical symptom from existing brain abscess, hemorrhage into it may worsen already existing symptom or produce new cortical symptom on the top of it
Mental status and psychiatric aspects/ complications	As noted, the most common symptom of hemorrhage into brain abscess is a sudden change in mental status due to increased size of space-occupying lesion. This results in increased intracranial pressure and risk of brain herniation
Cerebellum	Hemorrhage into a cerebellar abscess may result in compression of the 4th ventricle with resulting acute non-communicating hydrocephalus and risk of immediate herniation
Cranial nerves	Increase in intracranial pressure may cause transtentorial or uncal herniation, which can induce cranial nerve deficits, typically a CN III palsy producing a "blown pupil"

Secondary Complications: Seizures and increasing focal neurologic deficit may accompany the alteration of consciousness, which is typical of hemorrhage into an abscess.

Treatment Complications: Treatment plan for brain abscess usually requires combination of surgical drainage and antibiotics. Neurosurgical procedures always slightly increase risk of infection or tissue injury near surgical site. If an extraventricular drain is placed, that further increases the risk of ventriculitis.

Bibliography

Inamasu J, Nakamura Y, Saito R, et al. Hemorrhagic brain abscess in infective endocarditis. *Emerg Radiol.* 2001;8:308. https://doi.org/10.1007/PL00011929.

Thamburaj K, Agarwal AK, Sabat SB, Nguyen DT. Hemorrhage in the wall of pyogenic brain abscess on susceptibility weighted MR sequence: a report of 3 cases. *Case Rep Radiol.* 2014: Article ID 907584. https://doi.org/10.1155/2014/907584.

Hemorrhage into Stroke

Epidemiology and Demographics: Incidence of hemorrhage into stroke, frequently referred to as hemorrhagic transformation (HT), ranges from 38 to 71% in autopsy studies, whereas the incidence of symptomatic HT is from 0.6 to 20%.

Disorder Description: HT is a spectrum of ischemia-related brain hemorrhage and is a frequent complication of ischemic stroke, especially after thrombolytic therapy. There are several risk factors, such as age, blood glucose level, thrombolytic agent used, size of the infarction, location of infarction, and time window allowed for the initiation of the therapy. HT can be further sub-divided into hemorrhagic infarction (HI) and parenchymal hematoma (PH). HI is a heterogeneous hyperdensity occupying a portion of the ischemic infarct zone on CT scan. PH is a more homogeneous, dense hematoma with mass effect. Only large PHs (>30% of infarcted area) with space-occupying effect independently cause clinical deterioration and impair prognosis.

Symptoms

Localization site	Comment
Cerebral hemispheres	Large PHs can produce multiple cortical symptoms related to space-occupying effect, such as new headache that is often posture-related, nausea, vomiting, and seizures. New focal findings can be seen as well
Mental status and psychiatric aspects/ complications	Increased intracranial pressure secondary to hematoma-induced mass effect can worsen the patient's mental status
Brainstem	HT into a brainstem infarct is very rare but can happen. Once it occurs, compression of the medulla may lead to respiratory failure. Compression of the 4th ventricle can produce acute non-communicating hydrocephalus and risk of immediate herniation

Localization site	Comment
Cerebellum	HT in cerebellar infarct can happen. Patient will complain of worsening of the cerebellar symptoms, such as ataxia or vertigo. The effects of compression of the 4th ventricle or medulla would be similar to the brainstem
Vestibular system (and non-specific dizziness)	Rare HT into a pontine infarct may develop vestibular symptoms, especially if the vestibular nucleus is involved
Cranial nerves	HT in the brainstem can induce various cranial nerve findings by affecting cranial nerve nuclei in the brainstem

Secondary Complications: Cortical compression by hematoma-related mass effect can induce epilepsy. In the setting of non-convulsive status epilepticus, patient may fail to arouse after control of seizures without clear etiology.

Treatment Complications: Mainstay of the HT treatment is supportive, including blood pressure control, glucose control, and avoiding antiplatelet or antico-agulative agents. Avoiding anti-thrombotic agents leaves the patient at risk for recurrent ischemic events. Fortunately, this is uncommon. Because deep vein thrombosis prophylaxis is usually restricted to physical means only for the first 48 hours, the risk of DVT increases.

Bibliography

Berger C, et al. Hemorrhagic transformation of ischemic brain tissue: asymptomatic or symptomatic? *Stroke.* 2001;32:1330–5.

Zhang J, et al. Hemorrhagic transformation after cerebral infarction: current concepts and challenges. *Ann Transl Med.* 2014;2(8):81.

Hemorrhage into Tumor

Epidemiology and Demographics: Hemorrhage occurs in 2–3% of brain tumors. Both primary as well metastatic tumors can hemorrhage, and the frequency varies widely among different tumor types. About 14% of metastatic tumors bleed; metastatic malignant melanoma, choriocarcinoma, thyroid carcinoma, hepatocellular carcinoma, and those of lung and breast are the common metastatic tumors that hemorrhage.

Disorder Description: Hemorrhage can occur in any intracranial neoplasm, and the frequency varies widely among different tumor types. Likely pathogenesis is due to rupture of an irregular and fragile vascular architecture in fast-growing and highly vascularized neoplasms.

Symptoms

Localization site	Comment
Cerebral hemispheres	Seizures, change in mental status, hemiparesis, and homonymous hemianopia
Mental status and psychiatric aspects/ complications	Drowsiness, comatose, pathologic posturing, and even herniation leading to death
Cranial nerves	Oculomotor palsy (cranial nerves 3, 4, 6)

Bibliography

Kondziolka D, Bernstein M, Resch L, et al. Significance of hemorrhage into brain tumors: clinicopathological study. *J Neurosurg.* 1987;67(6):852–7.

Lieu AS, Hwang SL, Howng SL, Chai CY. Brain tumors with hemorrhage. *J Formos Med Assoc.* 1999;98(5):365–7.

Wakai S, Yamakawa K, Manaka S, Takakura K. Spontaneous intracranial hemorrhage caused by brain tumor: its incidence and clinical significance. *Neurosurgery.* 1982;10(4):437–44.

Henoch–Schönlein Purpura

Epidemiology and Demographics: Henoch–Schonlein purpura (HSP) is a small vessel vasculitis commonly affecting children. The condition also affects adults but much less commonly. The incidence is around 10 per 10,000 population.

Disorder Description: HSP is a small vessel leukocytoclastic vasculitis caused by IgA deposition in vessel walls of skin, gut, kidneys, and other organs.

Symptoms

Localization site	Comment
Cerebral hemispheres	Seizures, cortical blindness (see entry for *Posterior Reversible Encephalopathy Syndrome [PRES]*), intracerebral hemorrhage, ischemic strokes
Mental status and psychiatric aspects/complications	Encephalopathy
Cranial nerves	Cranial neuropathies are rare but facial palsies can occur
Mononeuropathy or mononeuropathy multiplex	Guillain–Barré syndrome, brachial plexopathy, or mononeuritis multiplex involving posterior tibial, femoral, or ulnar nerve
Polyneuropathy	Persistent polyneuropathy has been described but is rare

Secondary Complications: Kidney failure leading to uremic encephalopathy. Electrolyte abnormalities leading to seizures or encephalopathy.

Treatment Complications: Steroids can cause psychosis and myopathy. Immunosuppressive therapy increases the risk of opportunistic infections, including those involving the central nervous system.

Bibliography

Bérubé MD, Blais N, Lanthier S. Neurological manifestations of Henoch-Schonlein purpura. *Handb Clin Neurol.* 2014;120:1101–11. DOI: 10.1016/B978-0-7020-4087-0.00074-7.

Caplan LR, ed. *Uncommon causes of stroke.* 2nd ed. Cambridge, UK: Cambridge University Press; 2010.

Garzoni L, et al. Nervous system dysfunction in Henoch-Schonlein syndrome: systematic review of the literature. *Rheum (Oxford).* 2009;48(12):1524–9.

Heparin-Induced Thrombocytopenia (HIT)

Epidemiology and Demographics: Incidence of heparin-induced thrombocytopenia (HIT) is 1–3% in patients using unfractionated heparin and <1% in patients using low-molecular-weight heparin. Many (30–50%) HIT patients experience thrombotic events, but hemorrhagic complications are very rare.

Disorder Description: HIT is an immune-mediated drug reaction to heparin. Formatted antibodies bind to a platelet surface protein, which leads to platelet activation and initiates blood clot formation and thrombocytopenia. Because of this, the risk of a major thrombosis is high in HIT despite the very low platelet count. HIT usually occurs between 5 and 14 days from the commencement of heparin.

Symptoms

Localization site	Comment
Cerebral hemispheres	Due to high risk of thrombosis, patients are at risk for thromboembolic ischemic stroke (e.g., major vessel occlusion or multifocal punctate infarcts in more than two vascular territories)
Mental status and psychiatric aspects/complications	In the setting of large vessel occlusion (e.g., proximal middle cerebral artery occlusion), the patient's mental status may change significantly
Brainstem	Brainstem infarction can happen from posterior vessel occlusion, such as posterior inferior cerebellar artery. This usually occurs with cerebellar infarction. Brainstem localized symptoms will be seen, such as cranial nerve dysfunction or crossed paresis (facial weakness contralateral to limbs)
Cerebellum	Cerebellar ischemic stroke can also happen from thromboembolic events secondary to HIT. Cerebellar localized symptoms will be seen, such as ataxia, vertigo, or oscillopsia, accompanied by perpendicular tremors and nystagmus
Cranial nerves	Cranial nerve symptoms can occur when brainstem is involved (e.g., ophthalmoparesis, bulbar symptoms)

Secondary Complications: Venous thrombosis such as deep vein thrombosis (DVT) or pulmonary embolus occurs much more commonly than arterial (ratio 4:1). In patients with patent foramen ovale, DVT can also produce ischemic stroke by paradoxical thrombosis.

Treatment Complications: Mainstay of treatment is discontinuation of heparin and replacing it with a newer anticoagulant, such as argatroban or lepirudin. Similar to classic anticoagulants (e.g., warfarin), newer anticoagulants increase risk of intracranial bleeding or GI bleeding, although incidence rate is lower than with classic anticoagulants.

Bibliography

Alving BM. How I treat heparin-induced thrombocytopenia and thrombosis. *Blood*. 2003;101:31–7.

Hepatic Failure, Acute

Epidemiology and Demographics: Acute liver failure or fulminant hepatic encephalopathy is an uncommon disorder that accounts for approximately 6% of liver-related deaths in the United States and about 7% of liver transplant cases. Acetaminophen toxicity is the most common cause, which accounts for about 40% of the cases, with other idiosyncratic drug reactions, viral infections, toxins such as mushroom toxicity, acute fatty liver of pregnancy, Budd–Chiari syndrome, and autoimmune hepatitis being accountable for the majority of other cases.

Disorder Description: Acute liver failure is characterized by rapid and fulminant destruction of hepatocytes in a previously healthy liver. Clinically, patients initially experience non-specific symptoms such as nausea and vomiting and malaise, followed by jaundice, coagulopathy, gastrointestinal bleeding, and encephalopathy. The onset of symptoms to the development of encephalopathy takes less than 8 weeks. Encephalopathy is presumably caused by conversion of urea to glutamine by astrocytes. Mortality is about 40% despite advances in critical care and liver transplant.

Symptoms

Localization site	Comment
Cerebral hemispheres	Hepatic encephalopathy
	Seizures (focal, generalized, subclinical)
	Cerebral edema and increased intracranial pressure
Mental status and psychiatric aspects	Ranges from impaired attention and concentration in early stages to coma in severe cases
Brainstem	Compression of brainstem due to herniation
Spinal cord	Multifocal myoclonus

Secondary Complications: Coagulopathy might lead to intracerebral hemorrhage. Compressive neuropathies can occur as a result of hematomas. Rapid changes in concentration of sodium can cause central pontine myelinolysis.

Treatment Complications: Prolonged ICU stay and infections put patients at risk for critical illness myopathy/neuropathy. Immunosuppressive medications that are used after the liver transplant increase the risk of central nervous system infections and malignancies such as lymphoma. Cyclosporine toxicity can cause syndrome of posterior reversible encephalopathy, seizures, and confusional state. Tacrolimus toxicity can also cause altered mental status and seizure. Haloperidol, which is often used to control agitation, can cause drug-induced extrapyramidal symptoms and rarely neuroleptic malignant syndrome.

Bibliography

Datar S, Wijdicks EF. Neurologic manifestations of acute liver failure. *Handb Clin Neurol*. 2014;120:645–59.

Fridman V, Galetta SL, Pruitt AA, Levine JM. MRI findings associated with acute liver failure. *Neurology*. 2009;72(24):2130–1.

White H. Neurologic manifestations of acute and chronic liver disease. *Continuum (Minneap Minn)*. 2014;20(3 Neurology of Systemic Disease):670–80.

Wijdicks EF, Hocker SE. Neurologic complications of liver transplantation. *Handb Clin Neurol*. 2014;121:1257–66.

Wijdicks EF, Plevak DJ, Wiesner RH, Steers JL. Causes and outcome of seizures in liver transplant recipients. *Neurology*. 1996;47(6):1523–30.

Hepatic Failure, Chronic

Epidemiology and Demographics: Chronic liver failure and cirrhosis is one of the leading causes of death in the United States. Alcoholic liver disease, chronic viral hepatitis, non-alcoholic steatohepatitis (NASH), and autoimmune hepatitis are among the leading causes of chronic liver failure.

Disorder Description: Manifestations of chronic liver failure depend on the level of compensated liver function. Some patients have stable and well-compensated liver function and therefore minimal symptoms, while others might have decompensated liver function and be very symptomatic. Symptoms include non-specific symptoms such as malaise, nausea, anorexia, and abdominal pain.

More advanced cases might present with ascites, edema, and complications of portal hypertension such as gastrointestinal bleeding, jaundice, and encephalopathy.

Symptoms

Localization site	Comment
Cerebral hemispheres	Hepatic encephalopathy
	Cerebral edema
	Seizures
	Parkinsonism
Mental status and psychiatric aspects/complications	Depression
	Impaired attention and concentration
	Behavioral changes
	Hepatic encephalopathy
Cerebellum	Ataxia
Spinal cord	Hepatic myelopathy
Peripheral neuropathy	Hepatic neuropathy

Secondary Complications: Secondary complications are similar to acute liver failure. Coagulopathy might lead to intracerebral hemorrhage. Compressive neuropathies can occur as a result of hematomas. Rapid changes in concentration of sodium can cause central pontine myelinolysis.

Treatment Complications: Metronidazole, which is sometimes used to treat the gut flora and reduce the endogenous production of ammonia for treatment of hepatic encephalopathy, can cause neuropathy. Immunosuppressive medications that are used after the liver transplant increase the risk of central nervous system infections and malignancies such as lymphoma. Cyclosporine toxicity can cause syndrome of posterior reversible encephalopathy, seizures, and confusional state. Tacrolimus toxicity can also cause altered mental status and seizure. Haloperidol, which is often used to control agitation, can cause drug-induced extrapyramidal symptoms and rarely neuroleptic malignant syndrome.

Bibliography

Cocito D, Maule S, Paolasso I, et al. High prevalence of neuropathies in patients with end-stage liver disease. *Acta Neurol Scand.* 2010;122(1):36–40.

Ferro JM, Oliveira S. Neurologic manifestations of gastrointestinal and liver diseases. *Curr Neurol Neurosci Rep.* 2014;14(10):487.

Sureka B, Bansal K, Patidar Y, et al. Neurologic manifestations of chronic liver disease and liver cirrhosis. *Curr Probl Diagn Radiol.* 2015;44(5):449–61.

Utku U, Asil T, Balci K, et al. Hepatic myelopathy with spastic paraparesis. *Clin Neurol Neurosurg.* 2005;107(6):514–16.

White H. Neurologic manifestations of acute and chronic liver disease. *Continuum (Minneap Minn).* 2014;20(3 Neurology of Systemic Disease):670–80.

Wijdicks EF, Hocker SE. Neurologic complications of liver transplantation. *Handb Clin Neurol.* 2014;121:1257–66.

Hepatitis, Acute

Epidemiology and Demographics: Acute hepatitis is the rapid onset of inflammation of the liver. Viral hepatitis is the most common cause of this condition. Hepatitis B is a very common condition, and it has been estimated that up to one-third of the world's population are exposed to it. Hepatitis C affects about 170 million people around the world, with this number increasing by about 4 million a year.

Disorder Description: Acute hepatitis is defined by presence of the symptoms for less than 6 months. Symptoms can range from mild and nonspecific to fulminant and life threatening. Malaise, fatigue, arthralgia, myalgia, nausea, vomiting, and loss of appetite are the initial symptoms. Jaundice, pruritus, diarrhea, abdominal pain can follow. Acute hepatitis can resolve spontaneously or with treatment or can lead to chronic hepatitis.

Symptoms

Localization site	Comment
Cerebral hemispheres	Aseptic meningitis (Hep A)
	Encephalitis (Hep A [rare], Hep E)
	Acute disseminated encephalomyelitis (Hep B)
	Seizure (Hep E)

Localization site	Comment
Cranial nerves	Optic neuritis (Hep A)
	Bell's palsy (Hep E)
Spinal cord	Transverse myelitis (Hep B)
Plexus	Brachial plexopathy (Hep E, 2 cases)
Mononeuropathy or mononeuropathy multiplex	Mononeuritis multiplex (Hep C, Hep B)
Peripheral neuropathy	Guillain–Barré syndrome (GBS) (Hep A [rare], Hep B, Hep E, Hep C)
Muscle	Myopathy (Hep B)

Localization site	Comment
Mental status and psychiatric aspects/complications	Depression (Hep C)
Cranial nerves	Optic neuropathy (Hep C)
Spinal cord	Myelopathy (Hep C)
Mononeuropathy or mononeuropathy multiplex	PAN-associated vasculitic neuropathy (Hep B)
	Cryoglobulinemia-associated vasculitic neuropathy (Hep C)
Peripheral neuropathy	Distal symmetric axonal neuropathy (Hep C)
Muscle	Inflammatory myopathy (Hep C)

Treatment Complications: Clevudine, used for treatment of Hep B, can cause myopathy. Interferons can cause depression, irritability, GBS, demyelinating disease of central nervous system, dystonia, and optic neuropathy.

Bibliography

Sellner J, Steiner I. Neurologic complications of hepatic viruses. *Handb Clin Neurol.* 2014;123:647–61.

Hepatitis, Chronic

Epidemiology and Demographics: Hepatitis B can become chronic in about 10% of cases; the rate of chronic hepatitis is much higher in hepatitis C, and without treatment up to 80% of the cases can turn into chronic hepatitis. Other less common causes of chronic hepatitis include autoimmune hepatitis, alcoholic liver disease, and non-alcoholic steatohepatitis (NASH).

Disorder Description: Chronic hepatitis is defined by presence of hepatitis for more than 6 months. Symptoms vary based on level of activity of the disease and can range from symptoms of hepatitis, such as malaise, abdominal pain, nausea and vomiting, and jaundice, to development of cirrhosis and symptoms associated with it.

Symptoms

Localization site	Comment
Cerebral hemispheres	Vasculitis (polyarteritis nodosa [PAN], Hep B; cryoglobulinemia, Hep C)
	Ischemic and hemorrhagic strokes (Hep B)
	Encephalitis (Hep C)

Bibliography

Acharya JN, Pacheco VH. Neurologic complications of hepatitis C. *Neurologist.* 2008;14(3):151–6.

Sellner J, Steiner I. Neurologic complications of hepatic viruses. *Handb Clin Neurol.* 2014;123:647–61.

Thames AD, Castellon SA, Singer EJ, et al. Neuroimaging abnormalities, neurocognitive function, and fatigue in patients with hepatitis C. *Neurol Neuroimmunol Neuroinflamm.* 2015;2(1):e59.

Hepatitis A Virus Infection (HAV)

Epidemiology and Demographics: Hepatitis A virus (HAV) is present in a worldwide distribution with the highest prevalence of infection occurring in regions of poor sanitation. There are approximately 1.4 million clinical cases of HAV reported annually. HAV is transmitted via the fecal–oral route or by contaminated water and food.[1]

Disorder Description: HAV is a member of the single-stranded RNA family Picornaviridae and is a major international cause of epidemic hepatitis. Liver cell damage is caused by a cell-mediated immune response. Extrahepatic manifestations in hepatitis A are rare. A number of neurologic syndromes have been reported in patients infected with hepatitis A, including encephalitis, meningoencephalitis, meningitis, transverse myelitis, Guillain–Barré syndrome, sensory neuropathy, mononeuropathy simplex and multiplex, myasthenia gravis, myopathy, and polymyositis.

Hepatitis A encephalitis[2]: The involvement of the nervous system is rare. Encephalitis is manifested by neck stiffness and a clouding of consciousness accompanied by CSF abnormalities, which differentiate it from encephalopathy.

Hepatitis A meningoencephalitis[3,4]: A few cases have been reported where the patient has acute viral hepatitis proven by liver biopsy and IGM-specific hepatitis A. One patient developed increased obtundation, fever, nuchal rigidity, and bilateral Babinski responses and coma. It was attributed to hepatic encephalopathy due to fulminant hepatitis; however, CSF pleocytosis and elevated protein level support the diagnosis of meningoencephalitis. The other patient, in addition to having fulminant hepatitis A, developed an episode of convulsion, severe headache, vomiting, confusion, and nuchal rigidity. Neurologic examination was significant for brisk reflexes and extensor plantar reflexes bilaterally. Magnetic resonance imaging (MRI) indicated meningeal enhancement in the left temporo-parieto-occipital region. An electroencephalogram revealed sharp and slow wave discharges from the left temporoparietal region. CSF analysis demonstrated lymphocytic pleocytosis (7 cells/mL), with mildly elevated proteins.

Hepatitis A transverse myelitis (TM)[5]: TM is a rare complication of hepatitis A and usually occurs in acute hepatitis A with a protracted course. Patient presented with acute hepatitis A diagnosed with AntiHAVIgM, then developed paresthesia and progressive weakness of both lower extremities, but preserved urination and defecation. Examination revealed motor power of 3/5 bilaterally, diminished pain sensation below C6 dermatone, impaired proprioception on both feet, hyperreflexia, and positive Babinski's. Laboratory testing revealed elevated liver enzymes. MRI of the cervical spine demonstrated increased signal intensity of the cervical spinal cord at C4–6 level in T2-weighted images. Cerebrospinal fluid analysis showed WBC 10 and elevated protein and was negative on PCR for cytomegalovirus, varicella zoster, herpes zoster, and Ebstein–Barr virus. Patient was treated with intravenous pulse of methylprednisone 1 g/day for 5 days and continued with oral prednisolone 60 mg/day tapered over a week. The patient recovered fully and antiHAV IgG was positive 6 months later. The pathogenesis of TM from hepatitis A remains unclear; however, an autoimmune process has been proposed.

Hepatis A Guillain–Barré syndrome (GBS)[6]: GBS is commonly associated with other viral infections. The association of hepatitis A with GBS is based on the temporal sequence of events and absence of other trigger events. Most patients suffered clinical evidence of hepatitis with jaundice before the onset of neurologic symptoms. The symptoms included limb paresis, bulbar paresis, dyspnea requiring ventilator support, sensory ataxia, and pharyngo-cervical-brachial variants of GBS. Electrodiagnostic studies revealed demyelinating polyradiculoneuropathy with a few cases of dominant axonal involvement. CSF tests positive for anti-HAV-IgM antibodies. It is unnecessary to test patients with GBS for HAV because the association is rare, and HAV-infected patients have clinical evidence of hepatitis before the onset of GBS.

Hepatitis A sensory neuropathy: An association between neuropathy and HAV is based on the temporal sequence of events without another detectable trigger for the neuropathy.

Hepatitis A mononeuropathy simplex and multiplex[6]: A rare association exits between acute HAV infection and mononeuropathy and mononeuropathy multiplex and is established on the temporal sequence of events and the absence of another cause of mononeuropathy. There are reports of mononeuropathy multiplex of the oculomotor and facial nerves as well as ulnar and lateral cutaneous nerves in patients with acute HAV infection.

Symptoms

Localization site	Comment
Cerebral hemispheres	Seizure, headache, confusion, stupor, and coma
Mental status and psychiatric aspects/complications	Confusion and altered mental state
Vestibular system (and non-specific dizziness)	Positional vertigo and sudden, profound, irreversible, unilateral hearing loss due to mononeuropathy – rare
Cranial nerves	Oculomotor palsy, facial palsy, trigeminal sensory neuropathy
Spinal cord	Sensory level, proprioception abnormality, limb weakness, hyperreflexia with bilateral Babinski response – symptoms of transverse myelitis

Localization site	Comment
Mononeuropathy or mononeuropathy multiplex	Oculomotor palsy, facial palsy, trigeminal sensory neuropathy, ulnar neuropathy, and lateral cutaneous neuropathy
Peripheral neuropathy	Sensory neuropathy and GBS

References

1. Yong HT, Son R. Hepatitis A virus: a general overview. *Int Food Res J.* 2009;16:455–67.
2. Lee JJ, Kang K, Park JM, Kwon O, Kim BK. Encephalitis associated with acute hepatitis A. *J Epilepsy Res.* 2011;1:27–8.
3. Bromberg K, NewHall DN, Peter G. Hepatitis A and meningoencephalitis. *JAMA.* 1982;247:815.
4. Mathew T, Aroor S, Nadig R, Sarma G. Focal meningoencephalitis of hepatitis A: a clinico-radiologic picture. *Pediatr Neurol.* 2012;47:222–3.
5. Chonmaitree P, Methawasin K. Transverse myelitis in acute hepatitis A infection: the rare co-occurrence of hepatology and neurology. *Case Rep Gastroenterol.* 2016;10:44–9.
6. Stubgen JP. Neuromuscular complications of hepatitis A virus infection and vaccines. *J Neurol. Sci.* 2011;300:2–8.

Hepatitis B Virus Infection (HBV)

Epidemiology and Demographics: Hepatitis B virus (HBV),[1] a DNA virus transmitted percutaneously, sexually, and perinatally, affects 1.25 million persons in the United States and 350 to 400 million persons worldwide. HBV infection accounts annually for 4000 to 5500 deaths in the United States and 1 million deaths worldwide from cirrhosis, liver failure, and hepatocellular carcinoma. In the Far East, most HBV infections are acquired perinatally while in the West, most acute HBV infections occur during adolescence and early adulthood through sexual activity, injection drug use, and occupational exposure.

Disorder Description: Besides fulminant hepatic failure, cirrhosis, liver failure, and hepatocellular carcinoma, HBV causes many extrahepatic manifestations throughout the body through mainly immune complexes and cell-mediated immunity against HbsAg. Neurologic manifestations of hepatitis B infection include polyarteritis nodosa, neuropathy, Guillain–Barré syndrome (GBS), chronic neuropathies, mononeuropathy, myopathy, dermatomyositis, and subclinical hepatic encephalopathy in cirrhosis.

Polyarteritis nodosa (PAN) is a systemic necrotizing vasculitis.[2,3] HBV infection can cause a vasculitis that almost always takes the form of PAN, characterized by hepatitis B surface antigen positivity. PAN occurs in only 1% or less of the total population of patients who are HBsAG+. Circulating immune complexes containing viral proteins are involved in the pathogenesis of hepatitis B virus related to PAN. The clinical features of PAN are weight loss in 80.5% of patients, peripheral neuropathy both motor and sensory in 83%, and multiple nerve involvement in 68.2% in addition to other systemic involvement (renal, urologic, abdominal, arterial hypertension, and cardiac failure). Clinical parameters associated with increased risk of death include age greater than 65 years, recent onset of hypertension, and/or gastrointestinal manifestations requiring surgery at diagnosis. Outcomes in PAN patients have improved due to step-by-step identification of a more effective treatment protocol involving a combination of plasma exchanges and a short course of corticosteroid and antiviral agents.

Neuropathy associated with hepatitis B virus infection[4,5]: Results from a multicenter French study of 190 patients infected with HBV reported clinical evidence of sensorimotor neuropathy in 5% of cases. The pathogenesis involves deposition of immune complexes in nerves or blood vessel walls.

Guillain–Barré syndrome: The association between GBS and acute viral hepatitis is rare (1% of GBS). GBS recurred during viral relapse after an asymptomatic interval of up to 2 years and at times with evidence of a viral relapse.

Chronic neuropathies related to HBV include chronic relapsing polyneuropathy, chronic relapsing polyradiculoneuropathy with cranial nerve and respiratory muscle involvement, mononeuritis multiplex, and chronic relapsing demyelinating polyneuropathy.

Polymyositis and dermatomyositis[6,7] have been reported in both acute and chronic HBV infection. In particular, manifestations of dermatomyositis occurred during HBV-related hepatocellular carcinoma.

Noninflammatory myopathy[6,7] was reported in a 23-year-old woman with a painful myopathy following acute HBV hepatitis. Muscle biopsy showed many intermyofibrillar microvacuoles filled with neutral lipid, without evidence of inflammation.

Subclinical hepatic encephalopathy (SHE)[8] has been found in between 30 and 84% of patients with cirrhosis. Neuropsychiatric manifestations include a number of quantifiable neuropsychiatric defects using psychometric and electrophysiologic assessment; however, the mental and neurologic status on examination are normal.

Symptoms[2–8]

Localization site	Comment
Cerebral hemispheres	Encephalopathy and rare central nervous system vasculitis
Mental status and psychiatric aspects/complication, suicidal ideation	Neuropsychiatric defects on psychometric assessment with normal mental and neurologic examination
Specific spinal roots	Rare cause of GBS
Mononeuropathy or mononeuropathy multiplex	Up to 83% in PAN
Peripheral neuropathy	5% of 190 HBV positive patients in French study
Muscle	Rare case of polymyositis and dermatomyositis, one case of noninflammatory myopathy

Treatment Complications: Treatment of hepatitis B infection and extrahepatic disease consists of plasma exchange and short course of corticosteroid and antiviral agents. Seven drugs are licensed in the United States: interferon alfa, pegylated interferon alfa-2a, lamivudine, adefovir, entecavir, telbivudine, and tenofir. Flu-like symptoms, marrow suppression, depression and anxiety, and autoimmune disorders, especially autoimmune thyroiditis are the side effects of interferon. Close monitoring and medical supervision are essential. Adefovir and tenofovir may cause nephrotoxic effects, which require periodic monitoring of renal function. Myopathy and neuropathy have been associated with nucleoside analog therapy for hepatitis B.

References

1. Dienstag JL. Hepatitis B virus infection. *N Eng J Med.* 2008;359:486–500.
2. Guillevin L, Lhote F, Cohen P, et al. Polyarteritis nodosa related to hepatitis B virus. A prospective study of long term observation of 41 patients. *Medicine.* 1995;74:238–53.
3. Guillevin L, Mahr A, Callard P, et al. Hepatitis B virus-associated polyarteritis nodosa: clinical characteristics, outcome and impact of treatment in 115 patients. *Medicine.* 2005;84:313–22.
4. Wada Y, Yanagihara C, Nishimura Y, Oka N. Hepatitis B virus-related vasculitis manifesting as severe neuropathy following influenza vaccination. *Clin Neurol Neurosurg.* 2008;110:750–2.
5. Verma R, Lalla R, Babu S. Mononeuritis multiplex and painful ulcers as the initial manifestation of hepatitis B infection. *BMJ Case Rep.* 2013:1–4. DOI:10.1136/bcr-2013-009666
6. Fleischer RD, Lok ASF. Myopathy and neuropathy with nucleo(t)ide analog therapy for hepatitis B. *J Hepatol.* 2009;51:787–91.
7. Stubgen JP. Neuromuscular disorders associated with hepatitis B virus infection. *J Clin Neuromusc Dis.* 2011;13:26–34.
8. Baig S, Alamgir M. The extrahepatic manifestation of hepatitis B virus. *J Coll Physicians Surg Pak.* 2008;18:451–7.

Hepatitis C Virus Infection (HCV)

Epidemiology and Demographics: Hepatitis C virus (HCV) has a prevalence rate of 2.8% worldwide and affects around 185 million people.[1]

Disorder Description: HCV causes severe hepatitis, cirrhosis, and hepatocellular carcinoma. It is a systemic disease with extrahepatic complications involving various organs including the eye, gut, thyroid, cardiovascular system, dermatome, and nervous system. Chronic HCV infections are characterized by hepatic and systemic inflammations inducing immunologic response and metabolic imbalance. HCV-related neurologic syndromes include autoimmune disorders, peripheral neuropathy, cerebrovascular events, myelitis, encephalopathy, encephalomyelitis, cognitive impairment, and psychiatric disorders including anxiety, depression, and fatigue. Many such neurologic conditions are associated with the presence of mixed cryoglobulinemia.

Symptoms[1–3]

Localization site	Comment
Cerebral hemispheres	Stroke, transient ischemic attack, lacunar syndromes, and central nervous system vasculitis
	Acute encephalopathic forms: confusion, altered consciousness, incontinence
	Leukoencephalopathy: multifocal signs and symptoms, cognitive dysfunction, tetraparesis, aphasia
Mental status and psychiatric aspects/ complications	Cognitive/neuropsychiatric: sensation of physical and mental exhaustion, depression, anxiety, alterations in verbal recall, working memory, sustained attention, concentration, and learning skills
Spinal cord	Myelitis: sensory ataxia, spastic paraplegia
Mononeuropathy or mononeuropathy multiplex	Mononeuropathy: deep aching pain, truncal deficits
	Mononeuropathy multiplex: stocking–glove asymmetric neuropathy
Peripheral neuropathy	Sensorimotor axonal polyneuropathies: sensory loss and distal weakness
	Large fibers sensory neuropathies: reduced touch and proprioception sensations, sensory ataxia
	Small fibers sensory neuropathies: burning feet, pain, and restless legs syndrome
	Motor axonal polyneuropathies: distal weakness
Muscle	Noninflammatory myopathy: progressive proximal and generalized weakness, atrophy
	Inflammatory myopathy: progressive symmetric proximal weakness, atrophy, dysphagia, interstitial lung disease

Treatment Complications: Standard of care for HCV treatment includes pegylated interferon plus ribavirin in addition to viral protease inhibitors such as boceprevir and telaprevir. Interferon is known to cause neuropsychiatric side effects[1–3] including headache, fatigue, cognitive impairment, and confusional state as well as mood alteration.

References

1. Mathew S, Faheem M, Ibrahim SM, et al. Hepatitis C virus and neurological damage. *World J Hepatol.* 2016;8:545–56.

2. Adinolfi LE, Nevola R, Lus G, et al. Chronic hepatitis C virus infection and neurological and psychiatric disorders: An overview. *World J Gastroenterol.* 2015;21:2269–80.

3. Monaco S, Ferrari S, Gajofatto A, Zanusso G, Mariotto S. HCV-related nervous system disorders. *Clin Developmental Immunol.* 2012;2012:236148. DOI:10.1155/236148.

Hepatitis Neuropathy

Epidemiology and Demographics: In patients with hepatitis C virus (HCV) infection, peripheral neuropathy occurs in about 10%, and most cases are associated with mixed cryoglobulinemia. Peripheral neuropathy develops in about 5% of patients with hepatitis B virus (HBV) infection, and most cases are associated with vasculitis and polyarteritis nodosa (PAN).

Disorder Description: HCV and HBV may be associated with a mild peripheral polyneuropathy. However, when mixed cryoglobulinemia in HCV infection and polyarteritis nodosa in HBV infection occur, the risk of developing a prominent neuropathy increases significantly.

Symptoms

Localization site	Comment
Peripheral neuropathy (HCV)	Mixed cryoglobulinemia is associated with HCV infection in about 80% of patients. Up to 90% of patients with mixed cryoglobulinemia have neuropathy. Sensory or sensorimotor axonal polyneuropathy is the most common presentation, followed by mononeuropathy multiplex with a predilection for the radial nerves
Peripheral neuropathy (HBV)	Mononeuropathy multiplex is the most common neuropathy and is due to HBV-related polyarteritis nodosa or vasculitis without classical PAN. HBV infection without PAN tends to have a mild axonal polyneuropathy

Secondary Complications: Untreated neuropathy leads to loss of motor function, neuropathic ulceration, and neuropathic pain.

Treatment Complications: Mainly due to side effects from medication for hepatitis viral infection.

Bibliography

Hehir MK 2nd, Logigian EL. Infectious neuropathies. *Continuum (Minneap Minn)*. 2014;20(5 Peripheral Nervous System Disorders):1274–92.

Stubgen JP. Neuromuscular disorders associated with hepatitis B virus infection. *J Clin Neuromuscul Dis*. 2011;13(1):26–37.

Stubgen JP. Neuromuscular diseases associated with chronic hepatitis C virus infection. *J Clin Neuromuscul Dis*. 2011;13(1):14–25.

Hereditary Motor Sensory Neuropathy Type 1 (Charcot–Marie–Tooth [CMT1] Disease: Hereditary Sensorimotor Neuropathy)

Epidemiology and Demographics: Prevalence of Charcot–Marie–Tooth (CMT) disease is 1/2500 to 1/10,000; about 50% of cases are CMT1. Age of onset of symptoms ranges typically between 5 and 25 years of age. Males and females are equally affected, except for the X-linked type, which is much more common in males.

Disorder Description: CMT1 is a subtype of CMT, which is a heterogeneous group of hereditary diseases of the peripheral nerve for which several genes have been recognized. It is characterized by pes cavus, hammer toes, and slowly progressive more distal than proximal weakness with steppage gait. Nerve conduction velocities are slow (less than 35 m/s in forearms).

CMT1 specifically is demyelinating. Inheritance pattern is autosomal dominant mostly and rarely X-linked recessive forms, the most common gene being PMP22 point mutation (CMT1A). Other common genetic causes include MPZ (CMT1B) and NEFL mutations. De novo mutations should be sought for if negative family history.

Symptoms

Localization site	Comment
Cerebral hemispheres	CMTX: unilateral or bilateral white matter changes mimicking central nervous system demyelinating disease (rare) CMT1B: deafness and dysphagia (rare)
Peripheral neuropathy	Chronic uniform demyelinating peripheral polyneuropathy resulting in foot deformities, slowly progressive weakness, sensory loss, and disability
Muscle	Secondary neurogenic atrophy is seen from chronic demyelination and secondary axonal loss

Secondary Complications: Complications of CMT1 include disability from slowly progressive weakness needing braces and assistive walking devices. These patients are more prone to compressive neuropathies with prolonged malpositioning, such as during surgery. They are also more prone to worsening polyneuropathy when exposed to neurotoxins such as chemotherapeutic agents (e.g., vincristine). Pain is common. Respiratory insufficiency is rare.

Bibliography

Katirji B, Kaminski HJ, Ruff RL. *Neuromuscular disorders in clinical practice*. 2nd ed. New York: Springer-Verlag New York; 2014.

Mathis S, Goizet C, Tazir M, et al. Charcot-Marie-Tooth diseases: an update and some new proposals for the classification. *J Med Genet*. 2015;52(10):681–90.

Miller LJ, Saporta AS, Sottile SL, et al. Strategy for genetic testing in Charcot-Marie-disease. *Acta Myol*. 2011;30(2):109–16.

Hereditary Motor Sensory Neuropathy Type 3 (Dejerine–Sottas Disease; Also Called Hypertrophic Polyneuropathy)

Epidemiology and Demographics: Characterized by onset in infancy or early childhood. Equal gender involvement.

Disorder Description: Dejerine–Sottas disease is a severe subtype of Charcot–Marie–Tooth disease, a hereditary neuropathy. It is caused by mutations in different genes, including MPZ, PMP22, EGR2, and PRX, with autosomal dominant or autosomal recessive inheritance patterns. It is characterized by early-onset, progressive, severe, distal sensory loss with ataxia, pes cavus, distal weakness, palpable hypertrophied nerves, pain, and severe gait disturbance. Nerve conduction studies are characterized by very slow NCV (<10 m/s in forearms).

Symptoms

Localization site	Comment
Cranial nerves	Nystagmus, hearing loss, restriction in extraocular movements can be seen (rare)
Peripheral neuropathy	Chronic demyelinating peripheral polyneuropathy resulting in progressive disability at an earlier age
Muscle	Secondary effect on muscle from neurogenic process

Secondary Complications: Complications include disability at a young age from progressive weakness needing braces and assistive walking devices. These patients are more prone to compressive neuropathies with prolonged malpositioning, such as during surgery. Pain is common. Respiratory insufficiency is rare.

Bibliography

Plante-Bordeneuve V, Said G. Dejerine-Sottas disease and hereditary demyelinating polyneuropathy of infancy. *Muscle Nerve.* 2002;26(5):608–21.

Hereditary Motor Sensory Neuropathy Type 4 (Refsum Disease)

Epidemiology and Demographics: Prevalence of disease is unknown. Predominantly seen in late childhood or adolescence, occasionally seen later in life.

Disorder Description: Refsum disease is an autosomal recessive disorder of either the *PHYH* gene or the *PEX7* gene resulting in defective alpha oxidation of phytanic acid, which is a branched chain fatty acid, resulting in accumulation of phytanic acid in blood, fat, and nerves. Neurologic manifestations include a demyelinating neuropathy, pes cavus, cerebellar ataxia, retinitis pigmentosa, hearing loss, and scaly skin.

Symptoms

Localization site	Comment
Cerebellum	Cerebellar ataxia
Vestibular system (and non-specific dizziness)	Sensorineural hearing loss

Localization site	Comment
Cranial nerves	Retinitis pigmentosa leading to loss of night vision Anosmia
Peripheral neuropathy	Motor and sensory demyelinating polyneuropathy leading to weakness and sensory ataxia

Secondary Complications: Cardiac involvement (conduction abnormalities and cardiomyopathy), occasionally with premature death. Epiphyseal dysplasia results in syndactyly and a characteristic shortening of the fourth toe.

Bibliography

US Department of Health and Human Services. Genetics Home Reference. Refsum disease. 2016. Available from https://ghr.nlm.nih.gov/condition/refsum-disease. Accessed Aug 24, 2018.

Wills AJ, Manning NJ, Reilly MM. Refsum's disease. *QJM.* 2001;94(8):403–6.

Hereditary Spastic Paraplegia

Epidemiology and Demographics: There are fewer than 10,000 cases in the United States. Ten percent of people with hereditary spastic paraplegia have complicated hereditary spastic paraplegia. In Europe 1–9 cases per 100,000 are noted. Manifests in second to fourth decades of life.

Disorder Description: Group of inherited diseases whose main features are progressive stiffness and spasticity in the lower limbs. Progressive weakness of the affected person's legs is noted. It can be an autosomal dominant, autosomal recessive, or X-linked recessive trait. There are more than 40 genetic loci, that is, SPG1 through SPG48 have been identified. Some patients may have only spasticity in the lower extremities, known as pure hereditary spastic paraplegia, or it may be associated with other symptoms.

It is a clinically and genetically heterogeneous neurologic disorder that manifests with slowly progressive spastic paraparesis. Most common form is pure spastic paraparesis. Complicated form can have other neurologic involvement, including optic atrophy, bulbar dysfunction, neuropathy, extrapyramidal deficit, cerebellar atrophy, and behavioral problems.

Symptoms

Localization site	Comment
Cerebral hemispheres	Intellectual disabilities, dementia, epilepsy
Cranial nerves	Optic neuropathy, visual or hearing dysfunction, retinopathy
Subcortical dysfunction	Extrapyramidal symptoms
Adrenal gland	Adrenal insufficiency, skin ichthyosis
Spinal cord	Paraplegia often developing progressively and slowly from a paraparesis, spasticity, back and knee pain, fatigue, urinary urgency, abnormal gait. There can also be decreased sense of balance. Gastrocnemius–soleus contracture
Psychiatric	Stress and depression
Peripheral nerves	Peripheral neuropathy

Secondary Complications: Skeletal deformities such as pes cavus and joint contractures. Cardiac involvement (conduction abnormalities and cardiomyopathy), occasionally with premature death. Epiphyseal dysplasia results in syndactyly and a characteristic shortening of the fourth toe.

Treatment Complications: Treatments may include physical therapy, range of motion and muscle strengthening exercises, and aerobic conditioning of the cardiovascular system. Antispasticity agents, e.g., tizanidine, and baclofen can lead to sedation.

Bibliography

Fink JK. Hereditary spastic paraplegia: clinical principles and genetic advances. *Semin Neurol.* 2014;34(3):293–305.

Katirji B, Kaminski HJ, Ruff RL. *Neuromuscular disorders in clinical practice.* 2nd ed. New York: Springer-Verlag New York; 2014.

Reid E. Pure hereditary spastic paraplegia. *J Med Genet.* 1997;34(6):499–503.

Salinas S, Provkakis C, Crosby A, Warner TT. Hereditary spastic paraplegia: Clinical features and pathogenetic mechanisms. *Lancet Neurol.* 2008;7(12):1127–38.

Herniated Nucleus Pulposus – Cervical

Epidemiology and Demographics: Herniated nucleus pulposus in asymptomatic patients is seen on MRI in 10% of the population younger than 40 years and 5% of individuals over age 40 years. True incidence and prevalence are unknown. It is seen equally in men and woman.

Disorder Description: Herniated nucleus pulposus is an abnormality of the intravertebral disc, which occurs when the inner core of the intravertebral disc bulges out through the outermost fibrous layer that surrounds the disc.

Symptoms

Localization site	Comment
C5	Weakness of shoulder abduction, external rotation, elbow flexion, and supination of the wrist Sensory loss on the shoulder may or may not be present. Biceps, brachii, and brachioradialis deep tendon reflexes can be diminished
C6	Above plus extension of elbow (triceps, pronation and extension of the wrist) (C7). Pain or sensory symptoms radiating down the arm into the middle digit, weakness of elbow extension and wrist flexion, finger extension and reduced triceps reflex can be noted
C8–T1	Sensory disturbance affecting the medial aspect of the hand and forearm along with hand weakness

Treatment Complications: Symptomatic decompressive surgery can be offered. Tricyclic antidepressants help. Narcotics can be used in acute phase. Analgesics may cause sedation and addiction among other many potential complications. Surgically induced neurologic deficits may occur.

Bibliography

Windsor RE. Frequency of asymptomatic cervical disc protrusion. Cervical disc injuries. eMedicine; 2006. https://emedicine.medscape.com/article/93635-overview. Accessed Aug 14, 2018.

Herniated Nucleus Pulposus – Lumbar

Epidemiology and Demographics: Increased prevalence in patients aged 30–50 years, with a 2:1 ratio of males to females.

Disorder Description: It is the most common cause of low back pain. Herniated nucleus pulposus of the lumbar spine is defined as nuclear material that is displaced into the spinal canal.

Symptoms

Localization site	Comment
Nerve root L2	Thigh flexion loss of cremasteric reflex, anterior thigh sensory loss can be noted
Nerve root L3	Leg extension, weakness, hip flexion, and adduction weakness. Medial knee sensory loss is noted. Quadriceps reflex loss is noted
Nerve root L4	Leg extension, hip flexion, and adduction weakness can be seen. Medial leg sensory loss can be seen. Quadriceps reflex can be diminished
Nerve root L5	Great toe dorsiflexion, dorsiflexion of digits 2 through 5 and foot weakness, ankle inversion and eversion weakness, knee flexion, and hip abduction weakness. Sensory loss on the great toe, dorsum of foot, and distal and lateral leg can be noted
S1 nerve root	Foot plantar flexion weakness, toe and knee flexion, and hip extension. Sensory loss in the digits 4 and 5. Lateral foot and heel as well as plantar surface sensory loss can be seen. Achilles reflex can be lost

Secondary Complications: Cauda equina syndrome can occur with urinary, bowel, and sexual dysfunction. This may warrant urgent decompression.

Treatment Complications: Recommendations include to continue activity, avoid heavy lifting, repetitive actions or prolonged sitting. Short-term corticosteroids sometimes help. Other interventions include nonsteroidal anti-inflammatories, narcotics, and surgery. Narcotics can cause sedation, addiction, etc.

Bibliography

Sahrakar K. Lumbar disc disease. Medscape. Updated Dec 12, 2017. https://emedicine.medscape.com/article/249113-overview. Accessed Aug 24, 2018.

Heroin Toxicity

Epidemiology and Demographics: The common user is male aged 20 years and older. There is no race or ethnicity predilection. In the United States, 0.2% of the population uses or has used heroin.

Disorder Description: Heroin is an opioid drug synthesized from morphine derived from the opium plant; it has several modalities of absorption into the human body, and ultimately is converted to morphine as it enters the brain. Heroin toxicity affects the body in many ways as indicated below.

Symptoms

Localization site	Comment
Cerebral hemispheres	Epileptic seizures (acute)
	Stroke (acute)
	Toxic spongiform leukoencephalopathy – progressive damage to the white matter
	Delayed post-anoxic encephalopathy – person usually experiences a brief hypoxic episode and will eventually develop a relapse characterized by apathy, confusion, agitation, and/or progressive neurologic deficits
Mental status and psychiatric aspects/ complications	Euphoria (acute)
	Coma (acute)
	Apathy (acute)
	Abulia (acute)
	Bradyphrenia (acute)
Brainstem	Dysregulation of body autonomic function
Cerebellum	Cerebellum ataxia
Cranial nerves	Toxic amblyopia – reaction involving optic nerve that results in visual loss (acute)
	Miosis (acute)
Pituitary gland	Dysregulation of hypothalamus–pituitary–adrenal axis
Spinal cord	Transverse myelopathy (acute)
Anterior horn cells	Transverse myelopathy (acute)
Dorsal root ganglia	Transverse myelopathy (acute)
Cauda equina	Transverse myelitis (acute)
Specific spinal roots	Transverse myelitis (acute)

Localization site	Comment
Plexus	Plexopathy (acute) symptoms of pain, loss of motor control, and sensory deficits specifically affecting brachial and lumbar region
Mononeuropathy or mononeuropathy multiplex	Mononeuropathy Compartment syndrome (acute) – elevated pressures in a confined body space
Peripheral neuropathy	Acute inflammatory demyelinating polyradiculoneuropathy (acute) – autoimmune process involving areflexic weakness and sensory changes
Spinal cord	Transverse myelopathy (acute) – acute motor, sensory, and autonomic dysfunction of the spinal cord
Muscle	Rhabdomyolysis syndrome – breakdown of muscle fibers into bloodstream Compartment syndrome (acute) – elevated pressures in a confined body space Fibrosing myopathy Acute bacterial myopathy – muscle damage induced by transmission of bacteria
Syndromes with combined upper and lower motor neuron deficits	Heroin induced leukoencephalopathy (acute–chronic) consisting of stage of progressive neurologic degeneration such as cerebral ataxia, extrapyramidal symptoms, chorea, athetosis, hyperactive reflexia to hypoactive reflexia leading to death
Syndromes with combined spinal cord and peripheral nerve lesions	Transverse myelopathy (acute) Acute inflammatory demyelinating polyradiculoneuropathy (acute) – autoimmune process with areflexic weakness and sensory changes

Secondary Complications: Cardiac arrest leads to anoxic–ischemic cerebral injury. Respiratory failure leads to cerebral white matter damage.

Treatment Complications: Complications of detoxification are those of opiate withdrawal described in the entry *Heroin Withdrawal*. Methadone may acutely cause sedation, euphoria, a "drug high," or insomnia. Longer term use has been associated with impaired cognition.

Buprenorphine may cause sedation and other potential opiate-related symptoms. The opioid naltrexone may cause mood changes, hallucinations, insomnia, anxiety, and other opiate withdrawal symptoms.

Clonidine, which can be used to treat anxiety and agitation associated with heroin abuse, may cause sedation or rarely induces altered mentation and hallucinations.

Bibliography

Enevoldson T. Recreational drugs and their neurological consequences. *J Neurol Neurosurg Psychiatry*. 2004;75:iii9–iii15. DOI:10.1136/jnnp.2004.045732.

Habal R. Heroin toxicity. Medscape. Updated Dec 26, 2017. http://emedicine.medscape.com/article/166464-overview#a6. Accessed Aug 14, 2018.

Kulkantrakorn K. Heroin brachial plexopathy. *Neurol Asia*. 2011;16(1):85–7.

Neuromuscular Disease Center. Myotoxic myopathy. http://neuromuscular.wustl.edu/mother/myotox.htm. Accessed Aug 14, 2018.

Pascual Calvet J, Pou A, Pedro-Botet J, Gutiérrez Cebollada J. [Non-infective neurologic complications associated to heroin use.] *Arch Neurobiol (Madr)*. 1989;52(Suppl 1):155–61.

The Discovery House. The truth about marijuana abuse vs. heroin addiction. April 20, 2015. www.linkedin.com/pulse/truth-marijuana-abuse-vs-heroin-addiction-the-discovery-house. Accessed Aug 14, 2018.

Heroin Withdrawal

Epidemiology and Demographics: Predominant users are males 18–24 years of age. No race predilection.

Disorder Description: Heroin is a diamorphine drug. Symptoms of withdrawal typically start after 6–12 hours and can last for months.

Heroin withdrawal symptoms include:
- Abdominal pain
- Sweating
- Shaking
- Nervousness
- Agitation
- Depression
- Muscle spasms
- Cravings for drugs
- Relapse

Symptoms

Localization site	Comment
Cerebral hemispheres	Cerebral atrophy (chronic)
Mental status and psychiatric aspects/complications	Depression (chronic)
	Cogntive difficulties (acute)
	Agitation (acute)
	Substance abuse disorder (chronic)
	Apathy (chronic)
Cranial nerves	Mydriasis (acute)
Muscle	Myalgia (acute)
	Tremors (chronic)

Treatment Complications: Methadone may acutely cause sedation, euphoria, a "drug high," or insomnia. Longer term use has been associated with impaired cognition.

Buprenorphone may cause sedation and other potential opiate-related symptoms. The opioid naltrexone may cause mood changes, hallucinations, insomnia, anxiety, and other opiate withdrawal symptoms.

Clonidine, which can be used to treat anxiety and agitation associated with opiate withdrawal, may cause sedation or rarely induce altered mentation and hallucinations.

Bibliography

American Addiction Centers. Heroin withdrawal timeline, symptoms and treatment.http:// americanaddictioncenters.org/withdrawal-timelines-treatments/heroin/. Accessed Aug 8, 2018.

Options Behavioral Health System. Heroin abuse & addiction treatment. 2018. www.optionsbehavioral healthsystem.com/addiction/heroin. Accessed Aug 24, 2018.

Herpes Simplex Virus 1

Epidemiology and Demographics: The seroprevalence of herpes simplex virus 1 (HSV-1) is estimated at 54% in the United States according to a 2005–10 survey among Americans aged between 14 and 49 years. The incidence of HSV-1 encephalitis worldwide as well as in the United States is between 2 and 4 cases /1,000,000, and HSV-1 is responsible for 90% or more of HSV encephalitis in adults and children. Bimodal distribution exists with peak incidence in the very young (3 years old or younger) and in adults aged >50 years. There is no gender predisposition in the majority of adults aged >50 years.[1]

Disorder Description: HSV-1 is one the eight human herpes viruses, which are large double-stranded DNA viruses that cause lifelong infection in humans.[2] The most likely routes of infection are retrograde transport through the olfactory or trigeminal nerve and possibly hematogenous dissemination. HSV-1 encephalitis is the most common sporadic and treatable encephalitis in the world. Early recognition and treatment lead to improving outcome and can be lifesaving. As most encephalitic syndromes, HSV presents with altered mental status and features of brain parenchymal inflammation, which include fever, new seizures, focal neurologic signs, cerebrospinal fluid pleocytosis, and abnormalities on MRI and EEG.

The clinical manifestations of HSV-1 encephalitis[2,3] are similar to other etiologies of encephalitis; thus, the differential diagnosis can be classified into four broad categories:

1. Unspecified encephalitis/meningoencephalitis
2. Infectious encephalitis (viral or bacterial)
3. Immune-mediated encephalitis
4. Infectious and immune-mediated encephalitis

Among the most common treatable mimics are other infections (viral, bacterial, mycobacterial, and fungal) and the immune-mediated encephalitis.

Early recognition and treatment lead to improved outcomes not only for herpes simplex virus encephalitis (HSVE), but also for other causes of infectious encephalitis and immune-mediated encephalitis, therefore rapid and effective evaluation is necessary. The advent of MRI and the availability of HSV PCR have greatly improved the ability to diagnose HSVE. Lumbar puncture is not only necessary for HSV PCR, but also to rule out other central nervous system infections as well as the other immune-mediated encephalitis associated with anti-NMDA receptor (NMDAR) and voltage-gated potassium channel antibodies.

Symptoms[2,3]

Localization site	Comment
Cerebral hemispheres	Seizures, loss of consciousness, aphasia, and memory impairment
Mental status and psychiatric aspects/complications	Abnormal behavior, confusion, and disorientation

Secondary Complications: The infectious process and the host immune response cause cytotoxic and vasogenic edema, which lead to focal and global mass effect and increased intracranial pressure (ICP) in HSVE. ICP monitoring and prompt management of herniation show a trend toward improved outcome. Seizures are a common presentation in encephalitis and during the course of the illness 15% develop status epilepticus. Antiepileptic medications are strongly recommended to all patients with seizures and encephalitis to prevent further brain injury in case of recurrent seizures.

Treatment Complications: Intravenous acyclovir 10 mg/kg q8h for HSVE as well as antimicrobials for bacterial meningoencephalitis should be initiated promptly. The latter should also be included because it cannot be excluded merely on clinical grounds. Acyclovir may cause depressed consciousness and encephalopathy.

References

1. Bradley H, Markowitz LE, Gibson T, McGuillan GM. Seroprevalence of herpes virus type 1 and 2 – United States, 1999–2010. *J Infect Dis.* 2014;209(3):325–33.
2. Bradshaw MJ, Venkatesan A. Herpes simplex virus-1 encephalitis in adults: pathophysiology, diagnosis, and management. *Neurotherapeutics.* 2016;13(3):493–508.
3. Singh TD, Fugate JE, Rabinstein AA. The spectrum of acute encephalitis: causes, management, and predictors of outcome. *Neurology.* 2015;84:359–66.

Herpes Simplex Virus 2

Epidemiology and Demographics: The seroprevalence[1] of herpes simplex type 2 (HSV-2) is estimated at 15.7% in the United States according to a survey from 2005 to 2010 among Americans aged between 14 and 49 years. HSV-2 infection is transmitted mainly, although not exclusively, through sexual activity, and it is delayed until adolescence and early adulthood with the advent of sexual activity. The seroprevalence of HSV-2 increases with the number of sexual partners, the age of sexual activity, and the presence of other sexually transmitted diseases including HIV. It is more common in Blacks and Hispanics. Primary HSV-2 infection is usually asymptomatic in immunocompetent adolescents and adults although primary HSV-2 infection causing genital ulcers facilitates the transmission of HIV. HSV-2 causes a multitude of neurologic diseases, which may result from primary or reactivation of latent HSV-2. The most common site of HSV-2 latency is the sacral ganglia although polymerase chain reaction (PCR) techniques have shown HSV-2 latency in ganglia throughout the central nervous system.

Disorder Description: HSV-2 is one the eight human herpes viruses, which are double-stranded DNA viruses that cause lifelong infection in human. HSV-2 associated neurologic diseases[2] include neonatal herpes simplex encephalitis, acute septic meningitis in adults, recurrent aseptic meningitis, adult HSV-2 encephalitis, HSV-2 ascending myelitis, HSV-2 radiculopathy, cranial neuropathy, acute retinal necrosis, and HSV-2 in the setting of HIV infection.

Neonatal herpes encephalitis is a devastating neurologic disease found in neonates born to mothers infected with HSV-2 especially in the third trimester. Focal and generalized seizures are the presenting symptoms and dissemination of the virus into the central nervous system occurs in 70% of all infected neonates.

Aseptic meningitis occurs in 36% of women with primary HSV-2 genital lesions and in 13% of men. Hospitalization occurs in 6.4% of infected women and 1.6% of infected men. Headache, neck stiffness, and low-grade fever occur during the prodrome of genital herpes and the herpetic eruption.

Recurrent aseptic meningitis due to HSV-2 manifests as headache, neck stiffness, and low-grade fever. Confusion, focal neurologic signs, and cranial neuropathies may also be present. Before the advent of PCR, many were diagnosed as Mollaret meningitis, which should now be restricted to recurrent meningitis without an identifiable cause.

Adult HSV-2 encephalitis is much less common than HSV-1 encephalitis. Both HSV-1 and HSV-2 affect the mesial temporal or orbitofrontal lobes; HSV-2 has a predilection for the brainstem and manifests as altered level of consciousness, cranial neuropathies, hemiparesis, and hemisensory loss.

HSV-2 ascending myelitis, affecting the thoracic and lumbosacral region, is seen almost exclusively in immunocompromised patients, particularly those with HIV infection. Pain, often anogenital or radicular, limb numbness, paresthesia, and weakness are the characteristic clinical presentation. Herpetic skin lesions may be present. MRI of the spine reveals enlargement of the lower cord or conus medullaris with increased signal on T2-weighted images and contrast enhancement of adjacent nerve roots.

HSV-2 radiculopathy is often misdiagnosed unless it occurs simultaneously with the genital herpes. History of recurrent genital herpes outbreak accompanied by radicular symptoms is useful diagnostically. It affects the lumbar or sacral nerve roots. Paresthesia, urinary retention, constipation, anogenital discomfort, and leg weakness may accompany the radicular pain. Nerve root and lower spinal cord edema, enlargement, and hyperintensity and contrast enhancement may be shown on T2-weighted MRI.

Cranial neuropathy including Bell's palsy is an extremely rare result of HSV-2, although Bell's palsy has been reported after acyclovir discontinuation in a patient treated for HSV-2 encephalitis.

HSV-2 in the setting of HIV infection: Synergism occurs between HSV-2 and HIV. HSV-2 facilitates HIV transmission by two- to four-fold. Neurologic diseases associated with HSV-2 appear early and are severe in the presence of HIV/AIDs.

CSF PCR for HSV-2 is highly sensitive and highly specific for the diagnosis of HSV-2-associated neurologic disease. Acyclovir is the standard therapy.

Symptoms[2]

Localization site	Comment
Cerebral hemispheres	Affects the mesial temporal or orbitofrontal lobe less often than HSV-1
Mental status and psychiatric aspects/ complications	Altered consciousness, confusion, and disorientation may occur
Brainstem	HSV-2 encephalitis has a prediction for the brainstem
Cranial nerves	Bell's palsy although extremely rare
Spinal cord	HSV-2 myelitis characterized by pain, often anogenital or radicular, with associated limb numbness, paresthesia, and weakness

Localization site	Comment
Anterior horn cells	Limb weakness
Dorsal root ganglia	Limb numbness
Conus medullaris	Radicular pain, paresthesia, urinary retention, and constipation occur in HSV-2. Radiculopathy with enlargement of the lower cord or conus medullaris on T2-weighted MRI
Cauda equina	Radicular pain, paresthesia, urinary retention, and constipation occur in HSV-2. Radiculopathy with enlargement of the lower cord or conus medullaris on T2-weighted MRI

Secondary Complications: As with HSV-1 encephalitis, cytogenic and vasogenic edema may occur in HSV-2 encephalitis as a result of the infectious process and host immune response. Cytogenic and vasogenic edema may lead to focal and global mass effect and increased intracranial pressure. Similarly, seizures and status epilepticus may develop. Three cases of ischemic stroke have been reported following HSV-2 meningitis/encephalitis.[3]

Treatment Complications: Intravenous acyclovir for severe cases may cause depressed consciousness and encephalopathy.

References

1. Bradley H, Markowitz LE, Gibson T, McGuillan GM. Seroprevalence of herpes virus type 1 and 2 – United States, 1999–2010. *J Infect Dis.* 2014;209(3):325–33.
2. Berger RJ, Houff S. Neurologic complications of herpes simplex virus type 2 infection. *Arch Neurol.* 2008;65:596–600.
3. Zis P, Stritsou P, Angelidakis P, Tavernarakis A. Herpes simplex virus type 2 encephalitis as a cause of ischemic stroke: case report and systematic review of the literature. *J Stroke Cerebrovasc Dis.* 2016;25(2):335–9.

Herpes Zoster Myelitis

Epidemiology and Demographics: Herpes zoster is primarily a disease of the elderly and immunocompromised. The incidence in the United States is approximately 4 cases/1000 persons annually.

Neurologic complications occur in approximately 1/2000 cases of primary varicella among children. Five percent to 20% of patients with zoster will develop postherpetic neuralgia after zoster. Transverse myelitis is seen in about 0.3% of patients post varicella infection.

Disorder Description: The main neurologic syndromes related to primary acute varicella infections are meningitis, encephalitis, acute cerebellar ataxia, and myelitis. Myelitis may also be seen due to reactivation of the virus (herpes zoster). Presence of the rash prior to the myelopathic clinical features is a useful clue to diagnosis (although the rash may not always precede it). There is a high frequency of thoracic dermatomal involvement. Although myelitis has typically been described in immunocompromised patients, it has also occurred in immunocompetent patients. The pathogenesis is likely similar to that of encephalitis with small vessel vasculopathy with or without demyelination and necrosis. Diagnosis of varicella zoster virus (VZV) myelitis is based on clinical and radiologic features (transverse myelitis pattern, may involve multiple levels presenting as a longitudinally enhancing transverse myelitis, restricted diffusion if spinal cord infarction) and is supported by the detection of VZV DNA by PCR or the production of VZV IgG in the cerebrospinal fluid.

Symptoms

Localization site	Comment
Cerebral hemispheres	Encephalitis frequently accompanies myelitis VZV infection can produce stroke syndromes secondary to infection of cerebral arteries
Mental status and psychiatric aspects/complications	Encephalitis frequently accompanies myelitis
Cranial nerves	Cranial neuropathies may be associated – herpes zoster ophthalmicus, ophthalmoplegia (cranial nerves III, IV, VI), and Ramsay–Hunt syndrome (herpes zoster oticus). This painful fluid-filled blistering shingles rash can affect cranial nerves VII and VIII and therefore can result in facial palsy and hearing loss

Localization site	Comment
Spinal cord	Myelitis is seen a few days after the rash (presumed to spread into the spinal cord directly from the roots). It characteristically presents with upper motor neuron signs, including weakness, hyperreflexia, and positive Babinski sign. Seen often as a complication of zoster in HIV patients
Anterior horn cells	Segmental motor paresis develops in approximately 3% of patients with zoster, felt to result from spread of VZV from the dorsal root ganglia to the anterior root/horn
Specific spinal roots	Dermatomal involvement typically involves thoracic segments, typically single dermatome. In the immunocompromised, multiple dermatomes are likely to be involved. Post-herpetic neuralgia is a complication Acute inflammatory demyelinating polyneuropathy has been described rarely independent of the myelitis with progressive, symmetric muscle weakness and loss of deep-tendon reflexes over days to a week after symptom onset. Presentation severity can vary leading to weakness of respiratory, facial, and bulbar muscles

Secondary Complications: Disseminated VZV in immunocompromised patients (HIV, post-transplant status).

Treatment Complications: Intravenous (IV) acyclovir (10 mg/kg every 8 hours for 14 days) in conjunction with IV methylprednisolone (1 g IV for 5 days) are used to treat herpes zoster myelitis. Prehydration and slow infusion of the acyclovir prevents renal toxicity and deposition of acyclovir crystals in the tubules. Neurotoxicity is seen with acyclovir in patients with renal failure and may present with agitation, tremors, delirium, hallucinations, and myoclonus as well as delirium.

Bibliography

Gilden D, Nagel M, Cohrs R, Mahalingam R, Baird N. Varicella zoster virus in the nervous system. *F1000Res* 2015a;4. PMID 26918131

Whitley RJ. Varicella-zoster virus. In Mandell GL, Bennett JE, Dolin R, eds. *Principles and practice of infectious diseases*. 4th ed. New York: Churchill-Livingstone; 1995. pp. 1345–51.

Hexane (n-Hexane) Exposure

Disorder Description: Single episodes of high-level acute hexane exposure cause central nervous system depression and narcosis. However, with repeated massive exposure (i.e., glue sniffing), a subacute, predominately motor neuropathy with cranial nerve dysfunction develops that may be confused with Guillain–Barré syndrome. This neuropathy may be associated with autonomic dysfunction including impotence, hyper- or anhidrosis, and vasomotor instability. Occupational or recreational exposure to lower doses over a longer time period results in a slowly developing central–peripheral axonopathy affecting the sensory and motor systems in a length-dependent fashion.

- Hexacarbons are present in many solvents and glues, and exposure is most commonly occupational.
- The neuropathy associated with hexacarbon exposure results in giant axonal swellings and distal slowing of conduction velocity.
- Hexacarbon neuropathy may continue to worsen for some time after cessation of exposure (coasting).

Symptoms

Localization site	Comment
Cerebral hemispheres	Sedation, euphoria acutely
Mental status and psychiatric aspects/ complications	Sedation, euphoria acutely. Disinhibition, visual and auditory hallucinations. With repeated abuse, dysphoria and depression with suicidal ideation
Brainstem	Dizziness
Cerebellum	Ataxia
Cranial nerves	Deafness reported with abuse
Peripheral neuropathy	The neuropathy associated with hexacarbon exposure results in giant axonal swellings and distal slowing of conduction velocity. The neuropathy may continue to worsen for some time after cessation of exposure (coasting)
Syndromes with combined upper and lower motor neuron deficits	Distal portions of corticospinal tract axons damaged with central–peripheral distal axonopathy resulting from chronic low-level exposure

Bibliography

Agency for Toxic Substances and Disease Registry. Public Health Statement for n-Hexane. Jan 21, 2015. Available from: www.atsdr.cdc.gov/phs/phs .asp?id=391&tid=68. Accessed Aug 30, 2018.

Committee on Acute Exposure Guideline Levels; Committee on Toxicology; Board on Environmental Studies and Toxicology; Division on Earth and Life Studies; National Research Council. Acute Exposure Guideline Levels for Selected Airborne Chemicals: Hexane: acute exposure guideline levels. Vol 14. Washington, DC: National Academies Press (US); Apr 26, 2013. Available from: www.ncbi.nlm.nih .gov/books/NBK201488/. Accessed Aug 30, 2018.

Hip Pathology and Surgical Procedures

Epidemiology and Demographics: Hip dislocation and hip surgery are associated with sciatic neuropathy, usually peroneal division, due to its proximity to hip joint. Prevalence of sciatic neuropathy in hip dislocation is 10% in adults and 5% in children. The overall prevalence of nerve injury during hip surgery is approximately 1%, with sciatic nerve being the most common. Perioperative superior gluteal, obturator, and femoral nerve injuries have also been reported.

Disorder Description: In patients with hip dislocation, sciatic nerve can be lacerated, stretched, or compressed. Reported etiologies for perioperative nerve injury include significant leg lengthening, improper retractor placement, cement extravasation, cement-related thermal damage, patient positioning, and postoperative hematoma.

Symptoms

Localization site	Comment
Mononeuropathy	Sciatic mononeuropathy with greater involvement of peroneal division. Prominent foot drop in mild cases. Flail foot seen in severe cases

Secondary Complications: Partial recovery occurs in 60–70% of patients with hip dislocation. Among patients with perioperative sciatic nerve injury, 41% have complete recovery, 41% have mild deficit, while 15% have limitation of ambulation and/or persistent dysesthesia. Joint contracture with equinus foot may develop.

Bibliography

Brown GD, Swanson EA, Nercessian OA. Neurologic injuries after total hip arthroplasty. *Am J Orthop (Belle Mead NJ)*. 2008;37(4):191–7.

Schmalzried TP, Noordin S, Amstutz HC. Update on nerve palsy associated with total hip replacement. *Clin Orthop Relat Res*. 1997;344:188–206.

Histoplasma capsulatum/Darling's disease

Epidemiology and Demographics: *Histoplasma capsulatum* is a dimorphic fungus with two variants, *Histoplasma capsulatum* variety *capsulatum* (United States and the tropics) and variety *duboisii* (Africa). Infection is endemic to certain areas of the United States, including the Mississippi and Ohio River Valleys, as well as parts of Central America, South America, Africa, and Southeast Asia. The organism is commonly found in soil contaminated with bat and bird excrement that increase its sporulation. Individuals working in construction sites have an increased risk of exposure. Inhalation of spores causes infection, which primarily involves the lungs. Immunocompromised individuals (HIV, post-transplant patients) and those at extremes of age are at an increased risk for disseminated infection.

Of the documented histoplasmosis infections in immunocompetent individuals, 50 to 90% are asymptomatic, and of the symptomatic infections, 80% require no therapy and are self-resolving. Three to 5% of AIDS patients within endemic areas of North America develop disseminated histoplasmosis. Of these 3–5% infected immunocompromised patients, 90% have infections that advance into progressive disseminated histoplasmosis. Of this 90%, central nervous system involvement is clinically recognized in 10 to 20%.

Disorder Description: Central nervous system (CNS) involvement can occur in both disseminated disease and in isolation (rare). There is a report of CNS involvement occurring in 25% of disseminated cases of which 25% have neurologic involvement. Clinical syndromes include subacute and chronic meningitis (most common manifestation), encephalitis, cerebritis, cerebral abscess, and focal brain and spinal cord lesions (histoplasmomas) as well as stroke syndromes. Isolated CNS histoplasmosis in immunocompetent hosts has been described in the setting of ventriculoperitoneal shunt. These patients present with idiopathic hydrocephalus. CNS histoplasmosis presents similarly to CNS tuberculosis and is a close differential diagnosis.

The diagnostic workup for patients with suspected disseminated histoplasmosis includes urine and serum antigen *Histoplasma capsulatum* polysaccharide antigen (HPA) testing as well as blood cultures. Serology testing in HIV positive patients is often falsely negative in the setting of active infection. Antigen detection in CSF culture has a sensitivity of 38% and a specificity of 98%. Culturing of the cerebrospinal fluid or CNS parenchymal tissue is the gold standard for diagnosis of CNS histoplasmosis.

Symptoms

Localization site	Comment
Cerebral hemispheres	Histoplasma meningitis/encephalitis/cerebritis presents with mental status changes, headaches, fever, seizures, confusion, and cranial nerve palsies, especially involving the oculomotor, abducens, and facial nerves. In subacute or chronic meningitis, MRI shows leptomeningeal thickening within the basilar meninges. Meningeal enhancement with multiple enhancing nonspecific lesions in the brain suggests histoplasmosis
	Focal brain lesions (histoplasmomas) can cause seizures, motor weakness, and ataxia. Localized brain lesions occur in one-third of those with CNS involvement. They are hypodense on noncontrast CT, and appear as enhancing, ring-like structures on contrast CT. Ring-enhancing lesions are also evident on MRI, with a low signal intensity on T1 sequences and increased signal intensity on T2 sequences
	Stroke syndromes can occur as a result of emboli from *Histoplasma* endocarditis or arteritis from infection within Virchow–Robin spaces, although these syndromes are less common
	Hemichorea has been described with HIV-associated CNS histoplasmosis
	Hydrocephalus may be seen in patients with CNS histoplasmosis. (Detected on CT or MRI.) May be diagnosed even prior to the meningitis

Localization site	Comment
Mental status and psychiatric aspects/ complications	Mental status changes may be seen in patients with encephalitis and cerebritis
Brainstem	Involvement as a result of encephalitis or cerebritis
Cerebellum	Involvement as a result of encephalitis or focal brain lesions
Base of skull	Often commonly involved and may result in "basal meningitis" with multiple cranial neuropathies
Cranial nerves	Multiple cranial neuropathies as a result of basal meningitis – cranial nerves 3, 6, and 7 typically are involved
Spinal cord	Focal spinal cord lesions, intramedullary granulomas of the spinal cord (rare), and spinal meningitis (rare) occur Typically, slowly progressive weakness in the lower extremities, numbness below the mid-thoracic area, urinary incontinence is seen clinically. Meningeal enhancement with multiple enhancing nonspecific lesions in the brain or spinal cord suggests histoplasmosis
Mononeuropathy or mononeuropathy multiplex	Unusual presentation includes peroneal nerve dysfunction

Secondary Treatment Complications: In HIV patients, initiation of highly active antiretroviral therapy (HAART) can cause an immune reconstitution inflammatory syndrome (IRIS), with new symptoms or worsening of previous symptoms associated with histoplasmosis, along with increased CD4 count – hypothesized due to paradoxical reaction to antigens or unmasking of undetected active infection.

With treatment, patients with central nervous system (CNS) infection have a mortality rate of 20 to 40%. Additionally, approximately 50% of those who respond to antifungal treatment relapse after discontinuation of their drug.

In immunocompetent patients, or if focal brain lesions, liposomal amphotericin B, 3 to 5 mg/kg/day, is recommended for 2 to 4 weeks followed by itraconazole or fluconozale for a year to prevent relapse. Urine HPA is tested in follow up.

In immunosuppressed patients with disseminated *Histoplasma*, treatment is prolonged. Liposomal amphotericin B (5.0 mg/kg, for a total dose of 100 to 150 mg/kg given over 6 to 12 weeks) is preferred over the standard formulation, as the liposomal form has greater CNS penetration and lower toxicity. Treatment is continued with itraconazole, 200 mg 2 or 3 times a day for 1 year, or fluconazole, 600 to 800 mg once a day for 1 year (lifelong if immunosuppressed state is irreversible).

If an immune reconstitution inflammatory syndrome occurs, continuation of highly active antiretroviral therapy and starting or continuation of antifungal therapy is recommended.

Bibliography

Hariri OR, Minasian T, Quadri SA, et al. Histoplasmosis with deep CNS involvement: case presentation with discussion and literature review. *J Neurol Surg Rep*. 2015;76(1):e167–72. DOI:10.1055/s-0035-1554932.

Harris EA, Roos KL. Medlink Neurology. Histoplasmosis of the nervous system. Originally released Aug 11, 2005; last updated Jan 4, 2016. www.medlink.com/article/histoplasmosis_of_the_nervous_system. Accessed Aug 30, 2018.

HIV and AIDS

Epidemiology and Demographics: Since the start of the human immunodeficiency virus (HIV) epidemic, more than 70 million people have been infected with the virus, and 35 million have died from complications of HIV. At the end of 2015, 36.7 million people were living with HIV infection globally. Although approximately 0.8% of adults between 15 and 49 years of age worldwide are infected with HIV, the burden of the epidemic is concentrated in Sub-Saharan Africa, where nearly 1 in 25 adults is living with HIV. The incidence of opportunistic infections declined from 13.1/1000 in 1996–1997 to 1/1000 in 2006–2007, and since 1999, the worldwide annual incidence has declined by 19%.

Disorder Description: The vast majority of prevalent cases of HIV infection are caused by HIV-1, a retrovirus. HIV damages neurons not by direct infection, but rather by the release of neurotoxic viral proteins from infected cells. Neurologic manifestations can occur at every stage of the disease. Neurologic manifestations of acute HIV are less common than in chronic disease but occur in 17% to 24% of cases.

Symptoms

Localization site	Comment
Cerebral hemispheres	Aseptic meningitis is the most common neurologic presentation of acute HIV infection. Severe cases of meningoencephalitis also occur **Ischemic stroke** HIV-associated vasculopathy (abnormality of the cerebral blood vessels as a direct or indirect result of HIV infection, but excluding opportunistic infection vasculitis): • Associated with aneurysm formation (either intracranial or extracranial) • Vasculitis (as a direct result of HIV infection, excluding opportunistic infection) • Accelerated atherosclerosis (also related to HAART therapy) Opportunistic infection or neoplasia: • Opportunistic infection causing stroke (e.g., tuberculous meningitis, varicella zoster virus vasculitis, meningovascular syphilis) • Neoplasia, such as lymphoma involving cerebral blood vessels Cardioembolism: • Bacterial endocarditis • Marantic endocarditis • HIV-associated cardiac dysfunction • Ischemic heart disease Other established cause: • Coagulopathy (e.g., antiphospholipid syndrome) • HIV-associated hyperviscosity **Hemorrhagic stroke** • HIV-associated vasculopathy (aneurysm or vasculitis-associated) • HIV-associated thrombocytopenia • Mycotic aneurysm (secondary to bacterial endocarditis)
Mental status and psychiatric aspects/ complications	HIV-associated neurocognitive disorder (HAND) comprises 3 entities: • *Asymptomatic neurocognitive impairment* – poor performance in 2 or more domains on neuropsychologic testing in HIV patient who is otherwise asymptomatic • *Mild neurocognitive disorder* – impaired performance on neuropsychologic testing with impairments in daily functioning not attributable to pre-existing head injury or prior central nervous system (CNS) opportunistic disease. May have a coexisting movement disorder (e.g., tremor, gait disturbance, loss of dexterity) • *HIV dementia* – severe neurocognitive impairment (greater than 2 standard deviations below the mean in at least 2 domains) Combination antiretroviral therapy is the mainstay of treatment for HIV-associated neurocognitive disorder

Localization site	Comment
Brainstem	Stroke, CNS infection, lymphoma is less common
Cerebellum	Stroke, CNS infection
Spinal cord	HIV vacuolar myelopathy: most common myelopathy in AIDS, 30% in autopsy series. Presentation is with asymmetric leg weakness, spasticity, dorsal column sensory loss, urinary frequency, and erectile dysfunction Other myelopathies seen in HIV include HTLV-1 associated (subacute) or compressive myelopathies in the setting of lymphomatous metastasis, tuberculous or bacterial spinal abscess
Specific spinal roots	Rarely may develop either acute inflammatory demyelinating polyneuropathy (Guillain–Barré syndrome), or chronic inflammatory demyelinating polyneuropathy. Symmetric ascending weakness, areflexia, and CSF albuminocytological dissociation are classic Progressive lumbosacral polyradiculopathy due to cytomegalovirus infection is important to recognize because, unlike many other neurologic complications of AIDS, this serious disorder can be effectively treated if appropriately diagnosed. Occurs in patients with CD4 <50/µL
Mononeuropathy or mononeuropathy multiplex	Mononeuropathy multiplex typically occurs uncommonly in patients with symptomatic HIV-1 infection. Presentation is with asymmetric weakness and lower motor neuron signs
Peripheral neuropathy	Distal, symmetric, mixed small and large fiber polyneuropathy, typically affects the feet. Pain is the most common complaint. Some specific combination antiretroviral therapy medications themselves can contribute to the neuropathy
Muscle	A polymyositis-like syndrome can occur with HIV infection rarely Mitochondrial myopathy with lactic acidosis associated with the use of nucleoside reverse transcriptase inhibitors (NRTIs), including AZT, d4T, ddl, and 3TC

Secondary Complications: Secondary complications are primarily related to opportunistic infections, malignancies, and treatment related.

Primary CNS lymphoma (PCNSL): Confusion, lethargy, memory loss, hemiparesis, aphasia, and/or seizures. In addition, constitutional symptoms, such as fever, night sweats, and weight loss.

Solitary (>4 cm) and multiple mass lesions occur with approximately equal frequency. Lesions that involve the corpus callosum or the periventricular or periependymal areas are more likely to be due to PCNSL. Enhancement pattern may be a ring-enhancing pattern or may be irregular and patchy.

CNS opportunistic infections:

Toxoplasmosis. Fever, headache, altered mental status, and focal neurologic complaints or seizures. Presence of *Toxoplasma* antibodies and advanced immunosuppression with CD4 counts <100 cells/μL support the diagnosis. Lesions tend to be multifocal involving the frontal and parietal lobes, thalamus or basal ganglia, and the corticomedullary junctions. Ninety percent of the lesions tend to be ring enhancing. Solitary lesions tend to be less than 4 cm.

Neurocysticercosis or tuberculosis can present as single or multiple mass lesions. Tuberculomas can present as a focal lesion without evidence of systemic illness or meningeal infection.

Cytomegalovirus encephalitis. Results from reactivation in patients with CD4 cell counts below 50 cells/μL. Patients present with delirium, confusion, and focal neurologic abnormalities. MRI shows diffuse micronodular encephalitis in the basal ganglia, brainstem, and cerebellum, or ventriculoencephalitis.

Cryptococcosis presents as a subacute meningitis. Clinical manifestations can be remarkably benign, with vague malaise but more commonly headache and fever are the presenting features as well as cranial nerve palsies. Lesions are along the basal ganglia. CSF cryptococcal antigen testing is highly sensitive and specific.

Neurosyphillis. Meningitis, cerebral arteritis, and cerebritis, as well as optic neuropathy and deafness. Evaluation of HIV-infected patients with a positive serum treponemal antibody test is diagnostic for late latent syphilis or a positive CSF VDRL in the setting of abnormal spinal fluid establishes the diagnosis of latent neurosyphilis. Unfortunately, the sensitivity of the CSF VDRL in the setting of HIV disease is estimated at only 70% at best.

Progressive multifocal leukoencephalopathy. Opportunistic demyelinating disease caused by the JC (John Cunningham) virus, which gets reactivated in the setting of severe immunosuppression. Patients present with rapidly progressive focal neurologic deficits including hemiparesis, visual field deficits, ataxia, aphasia, and cognitive impairment. Progressive multifocal leukoencephalopathy lesions are multifocal, noncontrast enhancing bilateral, asymmetric, and localized preferentially to the periventricular areas and the subcortical white matter. Mass effect on surrounding structures is absent. CSF JCV PCR is highly specific but sensitivity is about 55% at best with HAART therapy.

Treatment Complications: NRTIs as a class are associated to variable degrees with osteomalacia, bone marrow suppression, increased risk of myocardial infarction, insulin resistance, dyslipidemia, hepatic effects, lipodystrophy, lactic acidosis, myopathy (zidovudine), peripheral neuropathy, and urolithiasis. Non-nucleoside reverse transcriptase inhibitors are associated with hepatotoxicity, dyslipidemia, rash, and neuropsychiatric effects. Protease inhibitors are associated with spontaneous bleeding, myocardial infarcts, chronic kidney disease, cholelithiasis, nephrolithiasis, rash, and diarrhea. Integrase strand transferase inhibitors are associated with insomnia, depression, gastrointestinal side effects, and dyslipidemia.

Entry inhibitors can cause hepatotoxicity.

Immune reconstitution inflammatory syndrome (IRIS) occurs due to an abnormally exuberant response of the recovering immune system to residual pathogen antigens in the CNS; typically, these are due to opportunistic pathogens, such as *Cryptococcus*, *Mycobacterium tuberculosis*, and JC virus and less commonly due to HIV itself. The best predictors of developing IRIS are a very low CD4 cell count nadir, presence of an opportunistic infection, and a rapid rate of immune recovery, which may be indirectly related to the drop in viral load.

Bibliography

Benjamin LA. HIV infection and stroke: current perspectives and future directions. *Lancet Neurol.* 2012;11(10):878–90.

Maartens G, et al. HIV infection: epidemiology, pathogenesis, treatment, and prevention. *Lancet.* 2014;384(9939):258–71.

NIH. Guidelines for the use of antiretroviral agents in adults and adolescents living with HIV. Updated Oct 17, 2017. https://aidsinfo.nih.gov/guidelines/html/1/adult-and-adolescent-arv-guidelines/31/adverse-effects-of-arv. Accessed Aug 16, 2018.

World Health Organization. HIV. 2018. www.who.int/
hiv/. Accessed Aug 16, 2018.

Hoarding Disorder

Epidemiology and Demographics: Point prevalence estimates range from 2 to 6% in the United States and
Europe as measured by community surveys, but
lower when strict DSM-5 criteria were employed.
Symptoms may start as early as teen years and
become more clinically apparent over time, with
older adults most predominantly affected.

Disorder Description: As per the DSM-5, this disorder is
characterized by "persistent difficulty discarding or
parting with possessions, regardless of their value,
due to a perceived need to save these items and distress associated with discarding them." If a third
party does not intervene, subsequent accumulation
of items can occur to the degree that obstructs living
areas and interferes with their use. This causes significant distress in important areas of functioning.
Symptoms are not better accounted for by the effects
of a substance or another mental or medical condition. There are specifiers for excessive acquisition
and levels of insight.

   Hoarding has a genetic basis, with up to 50% having a family member with the same affliction. Other
risk factors include a trait of indecisiveness and history of stress or trauma. It is seen cross-culturally. A
majority of individuals have comorbidity of mood
or anxiety disorder.

Symptoms

Localization site	Comment
Mental status and psychiatric aspects/complications	May have symptoms of comorbid depression or anxiety

Secondary Complications: When hoarding is severe,
there can be risks to physical health and safety,
including increased risk of fire and falls.
Behaviors can also negatively impact work and
relationships and lead to legal consequences such
as eviction.

Treatment Complications: First-line is cognitive behavioral therapy. Refractory cases treated with selective
serotonin reuptake inhibitors, which carry potential
side effects such as insomnia, headache, gastrointestinal distress, and sexual dysfunction.

Bibliography

American Psychiatric Association. *Diagnostic and
statistical manual of mental disorders: DSM-5.*
5th ed. Washington, DC: American Psychiatric
Association; 2013.

Grisham JR, Frost RO, Steketee G, et al. Age of
onset of compulsive hoarding. *J Anxiety Disord.*
2006;20(5):675–86.

Landau D, Iervolino AC, Pertusa A, et al. Stressful
life events and material deprivation in hoarding
disorder. *J Anxiety Disord.* 2011;25(2):192–202.

Nordsletten AE, Reichenberg A, Hatch SL, et al.
Epidemiology of hoarding disorder. *Br J
Psychiatry.* 2013;203:445.

Pertusa A, Frost RO, Fullana MA, et al. Refining the
diagnostic boundaries of compulsive hoarding: a
critical review. *Clin Psychol Rev.* 2010;30(4):371–86.

Samuels J, Bienvenu OJ 3rd, Pinto A, et al. Hoarding
in obsessive-compulsive disorder: results from
the OCD Collaborative Genetics Study. *Behav Res
Ther.* 2007;45(4):673–86.

Homocysteinemia

Epidemiology and Demographics: Homocysteinemia is a
rare disease, the exact incidence of which is unknown.

Disorder Description: Homocysteine, a nonproteogenic
amino acid, is derived from the demethylation of dietary methionine. Homocysteine can be remethylated
to form methionine or undergo trans-sulfuration
to form cysteine. Genetic deficiency in the enzymes
needed for these processes, deficiency of vitamin
cofactors (B6, B12, folate), or certain medications
and medical conditions can interfere with these pathways, leading to homocysteinemia. A mutation of
the methylene tetrahydrofolate reductase (MTHFR)
gene is the most common genetically inherited form
of homocysteinemia. High levels of homocysteine
increase the risk for atherosclerosis and stroke.

Symptoms

Localization site	Comment
Cerebral hemispheres	Cerebral infarct – focal neurologic signs
Mental status and psychiatric aspects/complications	Dementia, depression
Brainstem	Cerebral infarct – focal neurologic signs

Secondary Complications: Homocystinuria can be seen in patients with homocysteinemia (see entry for *Homocystinuria*).

Treatment Complications: Treatment includes B-vitamin and folate supplementation with no known complications. Patients with history of infarct can be treated with antithrombotic therapy, which increases the risk of bleeding.

Bibliography

Bahatia P, Singh N. Homocysteine excess: delineating the possible mechanism of neurotoxicity and depression. *Fundam Clin Pharmacol*. 2015;29(6):522–8.

Kang SS, Wong PW, Susmano A, et al. Thermolabile methylenetetrahydrofolate reductase: an inherited risk factor for coronary artery disease. *Am J Hum Genet*. 1991;48(3):536–45.

Yoo JH, Chung CS, Kang SS. Relation of plasma homocysteine to cerebral infarction and cerebral atherosclerosis. *Stroke*. 1998;29(12):2478–83.

Homocystinuria

Epidemiology and Demographics: Homocystinuria is a rare disease with an incidence of about 1/100,000 in the United States.

Disorder Description: Homocysteine, a nonproteogenic amino acid, is derived from the demethylation of dietary methionine. Homocysteine can be remethylated to form methionine or undergo trans-sulfuration to form cysteine. An autosomal recessive inherited deficiency in the enzymes needed for these processes can interfere with these pathways, leading to homocysteinemia and homocystinuria. Symptoms can appear in early infancy or later in childhood and can include intellectual disabilities, skeletal abnormalities, downward lens dislocation, and increased risk of thrombotic episodes.

Symptoms

Localization site	Comment
Cerebral hemispheres	Cerebral infarct – focal neurologic signs Seizures
Mental status and psychiatric aspects/complications	Intellectual disabilities
Brainstem	Cerebral infarct – focal neurologic signs

Secondary Complications: Thrombotic complications of end organs leading to organ failure.

Treatment Complications: Treatment includes B-vitamin and folate supplementation with no major complications. Patients may be treated with antithrombotic therapy which increases the risk of hemorrhage.

Bibliography

Bahatia P, Singh N. Homocysteine excess: delineating the possible mechanism of neurotoxicity and depression. *Fundam Clin Pharmacol*. 2015;29(6):522–8.

Walter J, Jahnke N. Newborn screen for homocystinuria. *Cochrane Database System Rev*. Oct 2015. DOI: 10.1002/14651858.CD008840.pub4.

Yoo JH, Chung CS, Kang SS. Relation of plasma homocysteine to cerebral infarction and cerebral atherosclerosis. *Stroke*. 1998;29(12):2478–83.

Hopkins Syndrome (Acute Postasthmatic Amyotrophy)

Epidemiology and Demographics: Hopkins syndrome is a very rare condition. It occurs mostly in children younger than 13 years of age. A few cases post-puberty have also been reported.

Disorder Description: A sudden onset of a flaccid paralysis of one or more extremity occurs approximately 1 week after an acute asthmatic attack. The etiology is unknown, but it is presumed to be due to an infectious or immunologic mechanism.

Symptoms

Localization site	Comment
Anterior horn cells	Flaccid weakness of either an arm or a leg without sensory dysfunction

Secondary Complications: Poor recovery has been reported. Disuse atrophy and joint contracture may develop.

Treatment Complications: Standard treatment has not been established. Steroids and intravenous immunoglobulin (IVIG) were used as a treatment trial. Steroids may cause hyperglycemia and gastric ulcer. IVIG may lead to anaphylactoid reaction in IgA-deficiency patients, as well as thromboembolic event.

Bibliography

Liedholm LJ, Eeg-Olofsson O, Ekenberg BE, Nicolaysen RB, Torbergsen T. Acute postasthmatic amyotrophy (Hopkins' syndrome). *Muscle Nerve.* 1994;17(7):769–72.

HTLV-1-Associated Myelopathy (HAM)/ Tropical Spastic Paraparesis

Epidemiology and Demographics: HTLV-1-associated myelopathy (HAM) is essentially a disease of persons of Caribbean and Japanese origins, but through horizontal transmission more Caucasians are affected as well as Canadian Natives of the Northwest Pacific, Equatorial and southern Africa, Melanesia, and immigrants from Eastern Iran and West Indies. It affects females more often than males (ratio 3:2). Only about 1 in 400 people infected with HTLV-1 goes on to develop a neurologic disease. HTLV-1 is transmitted by bodily secretions and blood.

Disorder Description: HAM is a retroviral disease specific to certain ethnic groups and transmitted in a manner similar to HIV. Clinically it looks like spinal cord primary progressive multiple sclerosis and is a close differential diagnosis. Spinal cord MRI with serology and PCR in the cerebrospinal fluid (CSF) will make the diagnosis.

The thoracic spinal cord bears the brunt of the disease, which eventually becomes atrophic (seen on MRI in 50–74% of patients). The thoracic cord is primarily affected based on the hypothesis that cell extravasation from the blood stream to the spinal cord is increased in this area where blood flow is slower. In areas where HTLV-1 is not endemic, the likelihood of exposure and the finding of a positive serology should be sufficient for diagnosis in the presence of an inflammatory myelopathy. The diagnosis of inflammatory myelopathy is made when there is a progressive myelopathy with CSF lymphocytosis, and increased synthesis of CSF IgG and oligoclonal bands, and if the MRI rules out anatomic causes. CSF serology for HTLV-1 and polymerase chain reaction can be used to confirm the diagnosis.

Symptoms start insidiously with painful burning sensations occurring symmetrically in the legs in an ascending pattern and dysesthesia in the lower back in band-like fashion. Bladder dysfunction is manifested by chronic urinary retention or urinary urgency with incontinence. Spasticity sets in within months to years and evolves towards pronounced extensor spasms and scissoring. Spasticity is out of proportion to the milder muscle weakness. There is sparing of the arms for a long time, and weakness involves distal muscles predominantly.

Symptoms

Localization site	Comment
Cerebral hemispheres	Cerebral white matter lesions were found in of 85% of HTLV-I carriers and 80% of HAM/TSP patients. Cognitive function is found to be lower but does not correlate with the number of lesions
Peripheral neuropathy	A peripheral neuropathy that can be found in carriers and HAM/TSP patients has been reported. It may be multifactorial, as demyelination, inflammatory infiltrates, and axonal degeneration have been found on biopsies. Neuropathic pain associated with HAM/TSP may be indicative of neuritis/peripheral neuropathy
Muscle	Polymyositis is directly due to the HTLV-1 virus and is associated with infiltration of muscle by CD8+ cells. It remains clinically silent, and is recognized by increased creatine phosphokinase and by biopsy. It is present among patients with HAM/TSP but not in carriers. When proximal muscle weakness occurs in TSP, polymyositis should be suspected
Syndromes with combined upper and lower motor neuron deficits	An HTLV-1-associated amyotrophic lateral sclerosis-like syndrome is rarely seen. There are cases described with upper extremity weakness, atrophy, and fasciculations confirmed by EMG and accompanied by up-going toes, fulfilling ALS criteria for diagnosis. The distinguishing factor was the bladder involvement in patients with HTLV-1
Syndromes with combined spinal cord and peripheral nerve lesions	HAM/TSP may be associated with peripheral neuropathy

Secondary Complications: Other disease associations include Sjögren's syndrome, sarcoidosis, monoclonal gammopathy, and idiopathic thrombocytopenic purpura. HTLV-1-associated myelopathy is a progressive disorder leading to triple flexion/extension paralysis, decubitus ulcers, urinary sepsis, and death in 2 to 3 decades.

Treatment Complications: There is no recognized effective treatment for HTLV-1-associated myelopathy. Symptomatic treatment of spasticity (baclofen 30 to 60 mg/day or tizanidine 2 to 12 mg/day) can result in hypotonia (2 to 35%), drowsiness (6 to 21%), and confusion (1 to 11%).

Repeated treatments with methylprednisolone (1000 mg IV monthly) may be of help in reducing spasticity. Steroids can cause acute reactions such as insomnia and psychosis, in addition to hyperglycemia and hypertension. Long-term use of steroids can lead to osteoporosis, higher infection risk, bruising, weight gain, and cataract among others.

Bladder care (anticholinergic agents such as oxybutynin chloride 5 to 30 mg/day or tolterodine tartrate 2 to 8 mg/day) can cause confusion/cognitive impairment and further retention of urine in patients with poor appreciation of bladder fullness. Clean self-catheterization is helpful but may be complicated by urinary tract infection if improperly performed.

Interferon beta-1a doses up to 60 µg twice weekly did not reduce the proviral DNA load, but reduced spontaneous lymphoproliferation and the frequency of HTLV-1-specific CD8+cells. Headache (58 to 70%), fatigue (33 to 41%), depression (18 to 25%), altered liver enzymes, injection site reactions, fever, flu-like symptoms, and thyroid disease are some of the adverse effects associated with interferon beta-1a use.

Bibliography

Matsuzaki T, Nakagawa M, Nagai M, et al. HTLV-I-associated myelopathy (HAM)/tropical spastic paraparesis (TSP) with amyotrophic lateral sclerosis-like manifestations. *J Neurovirol.* 2000;6(6):544–8.

Oger J, Reder AT. HTLV-1 associated myelopathy. Medlink Neurology. Originally released April 3, 2001; last updated June 9, 2016. www.medlink.com/article/htlv-1_associated_myelopathy. Accessed Aug 16, 2018.

Olindo S, Cabre P, Lezin A, et al. Natural history of human T-lymphotropic virus 1-associated myelopathy: a 14-year follow-up study. *Arch Neurol.* 2006;63(11):1560–6. PMID 17101824.

Human Herpes Virus 6 (HHV-6)

Epidemiology and Demographics: Human herpes virus 6 (HHV-6) has a worldwide distribution. In HIV-1 endemic regions (sub-Saharan Africa), the predominant form in infant infections was found to be HHV-6A. In Europe and the United States, HHV-6B is the agent mainly responsible infections.

Disorder Description: HHV-6 infection most commonly occurs after maternal antibodies have waned, usually between the ages of 6 months and 3 years (average, 9 months). The virus is shed in and probably spread through saliva of asymptomatic seropositive children. Primary HHV-6 infection is rare in adults. However, reactivation can occur at any age. The majority of human herpesvirus 6 (HHV-6) transmission events are thought to occur via shared saliva early in life.

HHV-6 causes roseola, a mild illness, in children who are immunocompetent. In some rare cases, patients who are immunocompetent may develop additional symptoms, including respiratory distress, multiorgan involvement, and seizures.

In adults who are immunosuppressed, HHV-6A can cause disseminated organ involvement, accelerated organ rejection (post-transplant), and death. Examples of immunosuppressed conditions include hematopoietic cell (allogenic especially major histocompatibility complex mismatched hematopoietic cell transplantation [HCT] more than autologous HCT) and solid organ post-transplant status, or AIDS.

In adults who are immunocompetent, primary infection or reactivation with HHV-6 can produce a mononucleosis-like illness and, more rarely, severe disease, including encephalitis.

Symptoms

Localization site	Comment
Cerebral hemispheres	Roseola in infants: febrile with erythematous maculopapular rash, with irritability, febrile seizures (10–15%), bulging fontanelle, meningoencephalitis features with otitis, upper respiratory tract infections, hepatitis
	In immunocompetent adults: fever with lymphadenopathy, a mononucleosis-like disease (with negative EBV), encephalitis, and hepatitis. Clinical presentations have included altered level of consciousness, seizures, psychosis, acute cerebellar ataxia, and focal neurologic signs (i.e., cranial nerve deficits or hemiparesis)
	In transplant recipients "post-transplant acute limbic encephalitis" has been described as a distinct syndrome of anterograde amnesia, syndrome of inappropriate antidiuretic hormone, mild CSF pleocytosis, temporal EEG abnormality often reflecting clinical or subclinical seizures, and MRI hyperintensities in the limbic system
	HHV-6 has been associated with mesial temporal lobe epilepsy (MTLE)
	HHV-6 has been implicated in both acute and chronic inflammatory demyelinating diseases
Mental status and psychiatric aspects/ complications	Psychosis may be seen as a manifestation of encephalitis
	Delirium may be seen (described in post-HCT) independent of encephalitis
Brainstem	As a manifestation of encephalitis, the brainstem may be affected leading to alterations in level of consciousness and cranial nerve deficits
Cerebellum	Acute cerebellar ataxia as a manifestation of encephalitis
Vestibular system (and nonspecific dizziness)	Hearing loss may be seen as a complication of encephalitis
Spinal cord	HHV-6 myelitis is seen in post-transplant patients
Peripheral nerves	Rare cases of peripheral neuropathy
Non-localizable	Chronic fatigue syndrome

Secondary Complications: In immunocompetent patients, encephalitis, multi-organ dysfunction, hepatitis, and rarely fatal.

Following HCT, complications include encephalitis (limbic encephalitis) and bone marrow suppression, also possibly graft-versus-host disease, cytomegalovirus reactivation, pneumonitis, and death.

Treatment Complications: No FDA approved agent available for treatment. Foscarnet (60 mg/kg IV every 8 hours or 90 mg/kg IV every 12 hours) is associated with electrolyte depletion, which can lower the seizure threshold, as well as nephrotoxicity and genital ulcers. Prehydration before each dose of foscarnet is used to protect the kidneys. Ganciclovir (5 mg/kg IV every 12 hours) causes bone marrow suppression, which is of concern in HCT recipients.

Bibliography

Agut H. Deciphering the clinical impact of acute human herpesvirus 6 (HHV-6) infections. *J Clin Virol*. 2011;52(3):164–71.

Pellett PE, Ablashi DV, Ambros PF, et al. Chromosomally integrated human herpesvirus 6: questions and answers. *Rev Med Virol*. 2012;22(3):144–55.

Humeral Fracture

Epidemiology and Demographics: A third of proximal humeral fractures are associated with nerve injury. Axillary nerve injury is the most common. Suprascapular, radial, and musculocutaneous nerves may also be affected in proximal humeral fracture. Approximately 18% of humeral shaft fractures have associated radial nerve injury, and more commonly in distal third humeral fracture. Supracondylar fracture is more common in children. Up to 50% of supracondylar fractures result in median nerve injury.

Disorder Description: The humerus bone has close proximity to neurovascular bundle, and humeral fracture commonly results in mononeuropathy. Affected nerve depends on site of the fracture.

Symptoms

Localization site	Comment
Mononeuropathy	• Proximal humeral fracture: axillary mononeuropathy • Humeral shaft fracture: radial mononeuropathy • Medial epicondyle fracture: ulnar mononeuropathy • Supracondylar fracture: median mononeuropathy

Secondary Complications: Neuropathic pain, numbness, and residual weakness leading to joint contracture may occur.

Bibliography

Wheeless CR. *Wheeless' textbook of orthopaedics.* [Internet] Duke University Medical Center's Division of Orthopedic Surgery and Data Trace Internet Publishing, LLC; 2015. Available from www.wheelessonline.com/. Accessed Aug 30, 2018.

Huntington's Chorea

Epidemiology and Demographics: The worldwide prevalence of Huntington's chorea (HD) is estimated to be 2.71/100,000. There is a higher prevalence of this disease in Europe, North America, and Australia: 5.70/100,000 vs 0.4/100,000 in Asia.

Disorder Description: HD is an autosomal dominant, neurodegenerative disorder, characterized by trinucleotide repeat of equal or greater than 40 CAG repeats within the Huntington gene (HTT). The symptoms are described in three categories of motor, cognitive, and psychiatric. The motor symptoms are progressive in nature and present as involuntary movements of chorea. These symptoms in the initial phases may present as restlessness. The cognitive symptoms often start with deficits in executive functioning and decision making, goal-directed activity and multitasking, eventually leading to a more global dementia in later stages. The psychiatric symptoms, due to frontal lobe involvement, can range from disinhibition and emotional dysregulation to apathy, abulia, or depression. In the early stages of the disease, family members of the patient might report noticeable personality changes.

Symptoms

Localization site	Comment
Caudate	Rapid, involuntary, non-repetitive movement of face, trunk, and limbs (chorea) are seen
Eye movement	Eye movement abnormality is a prominent feature, which involves delays in initiation of volitional saccades, and decrease in saccade velocity
Frontal lobe	Typical frontal lobe disinhibition leading to irritability, impulsivity, and mood dysregulation. Fontal abulic constellation involving apathy, loss of initiative, creativity, and curiosity can also be seen

Localization site	Comment
Corticostriatal pathway	The deficit in this pathway leads to executive functioning difficulties such as problems with decision making, planning, and multi-tasking
Psychiatric symptoms (diffuse)	These symptoms include irritability, anxiety, depression, obsessive-compulsive disorder, delusions, and hallucinations. These symptoms can occur at any stage of the disease

Secondary Complications: Patients often report depression in early phases of the disease, and there is an increased risk of suicidality. The natural progression of HD leads to a subcortical dementia involving the cortico-striatal pathway.

Treatment Complications: Since there is no cure or disease-modifying treatment available, HD management is symptom-based and is often challenging. Typical or atypical neuroleptics, as well as tetrabenazine, can be used to treat the patient's chorea. Underlying mood/anxiety symptoms should be treated appropriately with pharmacologic regimens such as selective serotonin reuptake inhibitors. Non-pharmacologic management can include physiotherapy, occupational therapy, and speech therapy as well as high calorie diet due to high metabolic demand.

Bibliography

Hout P, Levesque M, Parent A. The fate of striatal dopaminergic neurons in Parkinson's disease and Huntington's chorea. *Brain.* 2007;130(1):222–32.

Nopoulos PC, Aylward EH, Ross CA, et al. Cerebral cortex structure in prodromal Huntington disease. 2010;40(3):544–54.

Pringsheim T, Wiltshire K, Day L, et al. The incidence and prevalence of Huntington's disease: a systematic review and meta-analysis. *Mov Disord.* 2012;27(9):1083–91.

Walker FO. Huntington's disease. *The Lancet.* 2007;369(9557):218–28.

Hyperadrenalism

Epidemiology and Demographics: Hypercortisolism (see entry for *Cushing Disease*) affects about 10–15 per million people with a female predominance usually in the 20–50 years age range. Hyperaldosteronism has a female preponderance and is more frequently discovered in adults. The incidence of pheochromocytoma is about 2–8/1,000,000 occurring most commonly in the 4th to 5th decade of life.

Disorder Description: Caused by excessive levels of adrenal hormones in the body including aldosterone, corticosteroids, androgenic steroids, epinephrine, and norepinephrine.

Symptoms

Localization site	Comment
Cerebral hemispheres	Episodic and chronic headache. Stroke and hypertensive encephalopathy. Visual blurring and papilledema
Mental status and psychiatric aspects/ complications	Cognitive deficits, behavioral disturbances. Depression, anxiety and irritability, insomnia, decreased libido, hallucinations
Muscle	Muscle weakness. Spasms. Tremor

Secondary Complications: Hypertension from primary aldosteronism and pheochromocytoma may cause hypertension, which increases the risk for ischemic or hemorrhagic strokes and posterior reversible encephalopathy syndrome.

Treatment Complications: Treatment is dependent on the specific excess hormone produced and associated specific etiologies. Treatment may involve specific medications (e.g., those that reduce cortisol production, such as metyrapone or pasireotide) or sometimes surgical removal of an adrenal gland.

Bibliography

Fardella CE, Mosso L. Primary aldosteronism. *Clin Lab*. 2002;48(3–4):181–90.

Salpietro V, Polizzi A, Di Rosa G, et al. Adrenal disorders and the paediatric brain: pathophysiological considerations and clinical implications. *Int J Endocrinol*. 2014;2014:282489.

Sharma V, Borah P, Basumatary LJ, et al. Myopathies of endocrine disorders: a prospective clinical and biochemical study. *Ann Indian Acad Neurol*. 2014;17:298–302.

Sweeney AT, Griffing, GT. Pheochromocytoma. eMedicine. August 2, 2011. Available from https://emedicine.medscape.com/article/124059-overview. Accessed Aug 30, 2018.

Hyperammonemia

Epidemiology and Demographics: Statistical data on hyperammonemia are limited, though the prevalence of urea cycle disorders is approximately 1/40,000 births, globally.

Disorder Description: Dangerous metabolic condition marked by elevated levels of ammonia in the blood. Neurotoxicity may result from ammonia crossing the blood–brain barrier, altering the neurotransmitter system, as well as modifying water and electrolyte homeostasis in the brain. Early onset hyperammonemia may be caused by autosomal recessively inherited congenital urea cycle disorders or X-linked ornithine transcarbamoylase deficiency. Onset later in life may result from acquired liver disease of diverse potential causes, alcohol abuse, or medications or substance abuse, that overwhelms hepatic metabolic processes.

Symptoms

Localization site	Comment
Cerebral hemispheres	Altered level of consciousness, coma, intellectual impairment, headache, seizures
Mental status and psychiatric aspects/complications	Hyperactivity, sleep disturbance, agitation, mania, psychosis
Cerebellum	Ataxia

Secondary Complications: Encephalopathy, depressed consciousness leading to death.

Treatment Complications: Treating seizures with valproic acid increases ammonia levels and may worsen the condition. Osmotic demyelination syndrome may result from cellular fluid shifts, particularly in ornithine transcarbamylase deficiency. Low protein diets should be replaced with sufficient calories to avoid malnutrition.

Bibliography

Bachmann C. Mechanisms of hyperammonemia. *Clin Chem Lab Med*. 2002;20(7):653–62.

DeWolfe JL, Knowlton RC, Beasley MT, et al. Hyperammonemia following intravenous valproate loading. *Epilepsy Res*. 2009;85(1):65–71.

Haeberle J, Boddaert N, Burlina A, et al. Suggested guidelines for the diagnosis and management of urea cycle disorders. *Orphanet J Rare Dis*. 2012;7(1):32.

Lichter-Konecki U, Mangin JM, Gordish-Dressman H, Hoffman EP, Gallo V. Gene expression profiling of astrocytes from hyperammonemic mice reveals altered pathways for water and potassium homeostasis in vivo. *Glia*. 2008;56(4):365–77.

Hypercarbia

Epidemiology and Demographics: Hypercarbia severe enough to cause neurologic complications is mainly seen in hospitalized patients. Since the etiology of hypercarbia varies from patient to patient, the exact overall incidence of hypercarbia in the population is not known.

Disorder Description: There are many medical causes of hypercarbia. It can be caused by sedative use, primary lung disorders, or cardiac dysfunction, and can cause many neurologic signs and symptoms. Chronically elevated levels of carbon dioxide can be secondary to chronic pulmonary insufficiency.

Symptoms

Localization site	Comment
Cerebral hemispheres	Encephalopathy, seizures, headache, papilledema, asterixis, myoclonus
Mental status and psychiatric aspects/complications	Confusion, lethargy, anxiety, coma

Secondary Complications: Hypercarbia can depress mental status, leading to poor ventilation and hypoxemia. The need for possible ventilatory support can lead to many complications including infection and death.

Treatment Complications: Worsening of hypercarbia with oxygen administration.

Bibliography

Durrington HJ, Flubacher M. Initial oxygen management in patients with an exacerbation of chronic obstructive pulmonary disease. *QJM*. 2005;98(7):499–504.

Pal P, Chen R. Breathing and the nervous system. In Aminoff MJ, Josephson SA, eds. *Aminoff's neurology and general medicine*. London, UK: Elsevier; 2014. pp. 3–23.

Hypereosinophilic Syndrome

Epidemiology and Demographics: Rare disorder with incidence of 0.035/100,000 per year in the United States, usually in adults.

Disorder Description: Generally defined as sustained peripheral blood eosinophil count greater than 1500 cells/μL measured 1 month apart or pathologic confirmation of eosinophilic infiltration of tissue. The disorder can be neoplastic, secondary to other provoking factors such as parasitic helminthic infection, idiopathic (75% of cases of hypereosinophilia), or hereditary. Clinical symptoms are from tissue infiltration and injury from eosinophil infiltration most commonly in the lung and skin and less commonly affecting cardiac and neurologic function. Eosinophilic myocarditis often precedes cardioembolism causing strokes.[1]

Symptoms

Localization site	Comment
Cerebral hemispheres	Central nervous system neurologic symptoms most commonly caused by strokes affecting focal regions. Can also cause more diffuse injury and altered cognition from meningoencephalitis or demyelination. Can infrequently cause venous sinus thrombosis[2]
Mental status and psychiatric aspects/complications	Multifocal injury from strokes or by meningoencephalitis can present as non-specific encephalopathy
Peripheral neuropathy	Symmetric or asymmetric sensorimotor neuropathy

Secondary Complications: Extensive eosinophilic cardiac injury can lead to endomyocardial fibrosis and restrictive heart failure. Chronic lung injury usually associated with dry cough but can progress to restrictive lung disease. Endovascular injury from hypereosinophilia may cause thrombotic complications. Eosinophils can also infiltrate gastrointestinal tract resulting in abdominal pain, diarrhea, or nausea/vomiting.

Treatment Complications: Traditional treatment of idiopathic hypereosinophilia with corticosteroids and hydroxycarbamide is often poorly tolerated with hematologic and gastrointestinal toxicity.

References

1. Roufosse FE, Goldman M, Cogan E. Hypereosinophilic syndromes. *Orphanet J Rare Dis*. 2007;2:37.
2. Lee D, Ahn T-B. Central nervous system involvement of hypereosinophilic syndrome: a report of 10 cases and a literature review. *J Neurol Sci*. 2014;347:281–7.

Hyperglycemia

Epidemiology and Demographics: In 2014, estimated global prevalence of diabetes was 9% in adults. Approximately 50% of diabetic patients have polyneuropathies associated with both type 1 and type 2 diabetes mellitus (DM.)

Disorder Description: Elevated blood sugar levels strongly associated with DM type 1 or type 2. Duration and severity of hyperglycemia may lead to neuropsychiatric manifestations from a complex interplay of metabolic, vascular, and hormonal factors. Type 1 diabetes is due to a lack of insulin from an autoimmune destruction of islet cells in the pancreas. Type 2 diabetes is due to insulin resistance associated with sedentary lifestyle, poor diet, obesity, and genetic predisposition.

Symptoms

Localization site	Comment
Cerebral hemispheres	Seizures
Mental status and psychiatric aspects/ complications	Confusion, cognitive decline, major depression, anxiety, eating disorders
Cranial nerves	Oculomotor neuropathy: diplopia, ptosis, eye pain. Bell's palsy
Spinal roots	Intercostal radiculopathy: aching pain, paresthesias, electric pain
Plexus	Brachial/lumbosacral plexopathy: deep muscular pain
Mononeuropathy	Carpal tunnel syndrome, ulnar neuropathy, meralgia paresthetica

Localization site	Comment
Peripheral neuropathy	Symmetric "stocking and glove" distribution neuropathy: paresthesias, burning, pain, itching, numbness. Dysautonomia: orthostatic dizziness, postural orthostatic tachycardia syndrome, arrhythmia, abnormal sweating/anhidrosis. Erectile dysfunction. Gastrointestinal neuropathy: satiety, nausea, dysphagia, diarrhea, constipation/ incontinence. Neurogenic bladder
Muscle	Wasting secondary to late diabetic polyneuropathy, loss of deep tendon reflexes

Secondary Complications: Acute hyperglycemia in the diabetic patient may lead to diabetic ketoacidosis or hyperglycemic hyperosmolar nonketotic coma. Diabetes may lead to increased risk of Alzheimer's dementia, stroke, heart disease, diabetic retinopathy, diabetic nephropathy, infection, and poor wound healing.

Treatment Complications: Over-administration of insulin may cause hypoglycemia and related complications, including coma and death. See entry for *Hypoglycemia*.

Bibliography

Ducat L, Philipson LH, Anderson BJ. The mental health comorbidities of diabetes. *JAMA*. 2014;312(7):691–2.

Dyck PJ, Kratz KM, Karnes JL, et al. The prevalence by staged severity of various types of diabetic neuropathy, retinopathy, and nephropathy in a population-based cohort: The Rochester Diabetic Neuropathy Study. *Neurology*. 1993;43:817.

Edwards JL, Vincent AM, Cheng HT, Feldman EL. Diabetic neuropathy: mechanisms to management. *Pharmacol Ther*. 2008;120(1):1.

Ewing DJ. Recent advances in the non-invasive investigation of diabetic autonomic neuropathy. In Bannister R, ed. *Autonomic failure*. Oxford: Oxford University Press; 1988. p. 667.

Wilbourn AJ. Diabetic entrapment and compression neuropathies. In Dyck PJ, Thomas PK, eds. *Diabetic neuropathy*, 2nd ed. Toronto: WB Saunders; 1999. p. 481.

World Health Organization. *Global status report on noncommunicable diseases 2014*. Geneva: World Health Organization; 2014.

Hyperhomocysteinemia

Epidemiology and Demographics: Severe hyperhomocysteinemia with homocystinuria is a rare autosomal recessive disease with developmental delay, premature atherosclerosis, and other defects. Mild elevation in homocysteine levels present in up to 7% of population.

Disorder Description: Elevated levels of homocysteine are independently associated with stroke and atherosclerosis including carotid artery stenosis. Homocysteinemia can occur from deficiency of pyridoxine (vitamin B6), folate, or vitamin B12.

Symptoms

Localization site	Comment
Cerebral hemispheres	Associated with arterial ischemic strokes resulting in focal deficits

Secondary Complications: Associated with coronary artery disease. May also increase risk of venous thromboembolism.

Treatment Complications: Lowering homocysteine levels with vitamin supplementation in patients with diabetes or vascular disease did not decrease risk of cardiovascular outcomes. There are insufficient data to guide vitamin supplementation for secondary prevention of stroke in patients with mild to moderately elevated homocysteine.

Bibliography

Lonn E, Yusuf S, Arnold MJ, et al. Homocysteine lowering with folic acid and B vitamins in vascular disease. *N Engl J Med.* 2006;354:1567–77.

Wierzbicki AS. Homocysteine and cardiovascular disease: a review of the evidence. *Diab Vasc Dis Res.* 2007;4:143–50.

Hyperkalemic Periodic Paralysis

Epidemiology and Demographics: Onset is in childhood and usually occurs by adolescence. The estimated prevalence is 1/200,000. There is high penetrance in both sexes.

Disorder Description: Autosomal dominant disorder characterized by episodic weakness that is precipitated by hyperkalemia. Linked to the sodium channel mutation SCN4A. Weakness is usually mild but can lead to flaccid paralysis. Attacks can vary in frequency from several episodes daily to several episodes yearly. The duration is usually brief lasting 15–60 minutes, but episodes may last days. It is differentiated from hypokalemic periodic paralysis by the presence of myotonia (delayed muscle relaxation after contraction), which occurs between attacks (either spontaneously or after muscle percussion). Serum potassium concentration is usually normal between and during attacks. Episodes are normally triggered by rest after vigorous exercise, stress, fatigue, or foods high in potassium.

Symptoms

Localization site	Comment
Peripheral neuropathy	Paresthesia
Muscle	Episodic weakness, muscle tension. Flaccid quadriparesis. Progressive myopathy. Prominent paradoxical myotonia of the eyelids during attacks

Secondary Complications: Precaution should be taken for patients requiring anesthesia for surgical procedures because it may result in paralysis, lasting hours. Medications such as opioids or depolarizing agents may complicate intubation and ventilation because they may cause a myotonic reaction in these patients. Muscle relaxants should also be avoided. It is important to perform an EKG to rule out Anderson syndrome, where a prolonged QT interval may be evident.

Treatment Complications: Thiazide or loop diuretics could cause hypokalemia, which may lead to cardiac arrhythmias (supraventricular or ventricular tachyarrhythmia), respiratory failure, paralytic ileus, and muscle paralysis. Other complications of hypokalemia include nephrogenic diabetes insipidus and glucose intolerance.

Bibliography

Goldman L, Schafer A. Muscle diseases. In *Goldman's Cecil medicine.* 24th ed. Philadelphia, PA: Saunders; 2011. Chapter 429.

Kerchner G, Ptacek L. Channelopathies: episodic and electrical disorders of the nervous system. In Daroff RB, et al., eds. *Bradley's Neurology in Clinical Practice.* 6th ed. Philadelphia, PA: Saunders; 2012. Chapter 64.

Moxley R, Heatwole C. Channelopathies. In Swaiman KF, ed. *Swaiman's pediatric neurology: principles and practice.* Philadelphia, PA: Saunders; 2012. pp. 1667–89.

Riggs J. Neurologic complications of electrolytes disturbances. In Aminoff MJ, Josephson SA, eds. *Aminoff's neurology and general medicine.* 5th ed. London, UK: Elsevier; 2014. pp. 317–26.

Hyperlordosis

Disorder Description: Lordosis refers to the normal inward lordotic curvature of the lumbar and cervical region of the spine. Excessive lordotic curvature is called lumbar hyperlordosis. It can be associated with Ehlers–Danlos syndrome. It can be seen in dancers. True epidemiological numbers are not known. Treatments include conservative exercise maneuvers like hamstring stretches or use of the Boston brace.

Symptoms

Localization site	Comment
Ruptured disc	Radiculopathy, weak iliopsoas, swayed back

Bibliography

Hay O, Dar G, Abbas J, et al. The lumbar lordosis in males and females, revisited. *Plos One.* Aug 24, 2015. https://doi.org/10.1371/journal.pone .0133685.

Hypermagnesemia

Epidemiology and Demographics: Rare disorder mainly seen in renal failure patients given high amounts of magnesium. There is no difference in the prevalence between men and women. It is seen more commonly in the elderly population.

Disorder Description: Magnesium is required for the activation of many intracellular enzymes and has a key role in synaptic transmission throughout the nervous system. High serum levels of magnesium can be seen with magnesium supplementation in patients who cannot properly excrete the electrolyte (renal failure patients).

Symptoms

Localization site	Comment
Cerebral hemispheres	Seizures
Mental status and psychiatric aspects/complications	Confusion, somnolence, and lethargy
Neuromuscular junction and muscle	Loss of deep tendon reflexes and paralysis

Secondary Complications: Weakness can lead to failure of the respiratory muscles. This can lead to apnea, increased carbon dioxide concentrations, coma, and possible death.

Treatment Complications: Hypermagnesemia is treated by holding magnesium supplementation, which can rarely lead to hypomagnesemia. Treatment in severe renal failure may also require dialysis and all the associated complications.

Bibliography

Riggs J. Neurologic manifestations of electrolyte disturbances. *Neurol Clin.* 2002;20:227–39.

Riggs J. Neurologic complications of electrolyte disturbances. In Aminoff MJ, Josephson SA, eds. *Aminoff's neurology and general medicine.* London, UK: Elsevier; 2014. pp. 317–26.

Hypernatremia

Epidemiology and Demographics: Most often seen in infants or the elderly populations.

Disorder Description: Neurologic symptoms of hypernatremia are not usually seen until sodium concentrations elevate above 160 mEq/L. The usual cause is dehydration, either from decreased fluid uptake or increase in fluid loss (sweat, urine, feces). However, it can also occur secondary to iatrogenic causes of administration of hypertonic solution or rarely hypothalamic lesions.

Symptoms

Localization site	Comment
Cerebral hemispheres	Seizures, coma, tremor, myoclonus
Mental status and psychiatric aspects/complications	Confusion, somnolence and lethargy; can proceed to coma
Neuromuscular	Weakness, rhabdomyolysis

Treatment Complications: Overcorrecting the hypernatremia can lead to both fluid overload and hyponatremia.

Bibliography

Riggs J. Neurologic manifestations of electrolyte disturbances. *Neurol Clin*. 2002;20:227–39.

Riggs J. Neurologic complications of electrolyte disturbances. In Aminoff MJ, Josephson SA, eds. *Aminoff's neurology and general medicine*. London, UK: Elsevier; 2014. pp. 317–26.

Hyperparathyroidism

Epidemiology and Demographics: Primary hyperparathyroidism is common and is seen in 1/500–1000 adults. It is more common in females with a female-to-male ratio of 3:1 under the age of 40 years, and 5:1 in those older than 75 years of age. The prevalence increases with age and is estimated to be 2/1000 in females older than 60 years of age. The highest incidence is seen in postmenopausal women.

Secondary hyperparathyroidism occurs in patients with dialysis-dependent chronic kidney disease and may progress to tertiary hyperparathyroidism. Children in poor and developing countries may develop nutritional rickets, a form of secondary hyperparathyroidism. Risk factors include genetic predisposition to hyperparathyroidism and childhood exposure to external neck irradiation.

Disorder Description: Solitary parathyroid adenoma is the most common cause of primary hyperparathyroidism (85%) and results from the oversecretion of parathyroid hormone. Other causes include multiple parathyroid adenoma, parathyroid hyperplasia, and ectopic parathyroid glands. It also rarely arises secondary to parathyroid cancer, radiation therapy, and multiple endocrine neoplasia (MEN-1 or MEN-2). Secondary hyperparathyroidism is seen in chronic kidney disease and vitamin D deficiency and results from the compensatory oversecretion of parathyroid hormone secondary to abnormalities in calcium metabolism. Other less common causes include pseudohypoparathyroidism, metastatic prostate cancer, cholestatic liver or biliary disease, malabsorption, and medications (lithium, anticonvulsants, ketoconazole, rifampin, leucovorin).

Symptoms

Localization site	Comment
Cerebral hemispheres	Headaches, seizures, and dystonia. Extrapyramidal signs including choreathetosis and parkinsonism (increased motor tone and tremors)
Mental status and psychiatric aspects/complications	Encephalopathy, fatigue, lethargy, irritability, difficulty concentrating, memory deficits, and dementia
	Depression, affective disorders, personality changes, delirium, decreased social interactions, and psychosis (elderly population is particularly vulnerable)
Cerebellum	Ataxia. Calcium deposits in cerebellum
Base of skull	Subperiosteal bone resorption
Spinal cord	Myelopathy secondary to compression by discrete lytic bone lesions in osteitis fibrosa cystica
Anterior horn cells	Motor neuron disease
Mononeuropathy or mononeuropathy multiplex	Chvostek or Trousseau sign
Peripheral neuropathy	Paresthesia
Muscle	Proximal weakness, muscle pain, and stiffness
Syndromes with combined upper and lower motor neuron deficits	May mimic amyotrophic lateral sclerosis

Secondary Complications: Hypercalcemia and nephrolithiasis are commonly seen. Nephrocalcinosis also occurs but less commonly. Chrondrocalcinosis, fractures, osteoporosis (from progressive bone loss), and episodes of acute gout can occur in patients with primary hyperparathyroidism. Osteitis fibrosa cystica (subperiosteal bone resorption in the distal phalanges and skull) can be seen in patients with secondary hyperparathyroidism, secondary to renal failure. Acute or subacute monoarticular inflammatory arthritis may develop from calcium pyrophosphate dihydrate crystal arthropathy. Joint laxity, ectopic calcifications, and ruptures of tendon are also seen. Some studies suggest that these patients may be insulin resistant and at greater risk for cardiovascular events.

Treatment Complications: Parathyroidectomy is the only curative treatment but complications include recurrent laryngeal nerve damage, postoperative hypocalcemia, and permanent hypoparathyroidism. Cinacalcet is used to lower serum calcium levels but it does not normalize parathyroid hormones or prevent future bone loss.

Bibliography

Brown R, Fischman A, Showalter C. Primary hyperparathyroidism, hypercalcemia, paranoid deluisons, homicide and attempted murder. *J Foren Sci.* 1987;32(4):1460–3.

Fuleihan G, Silverberg S. Primary hyperparathyroidism: Clinical manifestations. UpToDate. 2015. Available from www.uptodate.com/contents/primary-hyperparathyroidism-clinical-manifestations. Accessed Aug 16, 2018.

Lockwood A. Toxic and metabolic encephalopathies. In Daroff RB, et al., eds. *Bradley's neurology in clinical practice.* 6th ed. Philadelphia, PA: Saunders; 2012. Chapter 56.

Schipper H, Jay C, Abrams G. Sex hormone, pituitary, parathyroid, and adrenal disorders and the nervous system. In Aminoff MJ, Josephson SA, eds. *Aminoff's neurology and general medicine.* 5th ed. London, UK: Elsevier; 2014. pp. 369–397.

Wysolmerski J, Insogna K. The parathyroid glands, hypercalcemia, and hypocalcemia. In *Goldman's Cecil medicine.* 24th ed. Philadelphia, PA: Saunders; 2011. Chapter 253.

Hyperprolactinemia

Epidemiology and Demographics: Prolactinomas are the most common cause of hyperprolactinemia, and they occur most frequently in females aged 20–50 years. Other less common causes of hyperprolactinemia include decreased dopamine inhibition of prolaction secretion, hypothalamic or pituitary disorders, and drug induced (mainly antipsychotics). Symptoms present earlier in women as compared with men.

Disorder Description: Prolactin is a hormone, mainly secreted by the lactotroph cells of the anterior pituitary gland. Hyperprolactinemia leads to amenorrhea, infertility, and galactorrhea in women and decreased libido and impotence in men. Neurologic deficits are mainly due to mass effect.

Symptoms

Localization site	Comment
Cerebral hemispheres	Headache due to mass effect
Mental status and psychiatric aspects/complications	Anxiety and depression may occur independent of comorbid psychiatric illness or treatment with antipsychotics
	Mass effect causing visual and olfactory hallucinations due to perceptual disturbances as well as episodes of "losing time," and apathy have been reported
Cranial nerves	Visual complaints due to mass effect
Pituitary gland	Hypopituitarism in men due to delayed diagnosis

Treatment Complications: Dopamine agonist treatment for prolactinomas may induce or exacerbate psychotic symptoms.

References

Catli G, Abaci A, Altincik A. Hyperprolactinemia in children: clinical features and long-term results. *J Pediatr Endocrinol Metab.* 2012;25(11–12):1123–8. DOI: 10.1515/jpem-2012-0130.

Ou H-Y, Hsiao S-H, Yu EH, Wu T-J. Etiologies and clinical manifestations of hyperprolactinemia in a medical center in Southern Taiwan. Department of Internal Medicine, Department of Pharmacy National Cheng Kung University Hospital, Tainan, Taiwan.

Wong A, Eloy JA, Couldwell WT, Liu JK. Update on prolactinomas. Part 1: Clinical manifestations and diagnostic challenges. *J Clin Neurosci.* 2015;22(10):1562–7. DOI: 10.1016/j.jocn.2015.03.058.

Zahajszky J, Quinn DK, Smith FA, et al. Cognitive and perceptual disturbances in a young man. *Prim Care Companion J Clin Psychiatry.* 2007;9:59–63. [PMC free article][PubMed].

Hypertension, Chronic

Epidemiology and Demographics: Approximately 30% of US adults have chronic hypertension (29% of Caucasians, 33.5% of African Americans).

Disorder Description: Systolic blood pressure >130 mmHg or diastolic blood pressure >80 mmHg defines hypertension. In 95% is essential hypertension and in 5% is secondary hypertension. Long-standing uncontrolled hypertension induces lipohyalinosis in small vessels that leads to end-organ ischemic damage. Hypertension can also increase risk of bleeding by persistently loading pressure to weak points of small vessel walls. Chronic hypertension may also increase risk of cerebral aneurysm. See entry for *Lacunar Strokes*.

Symptoms

Localization site	Comment
Cerebral hemispheres	Chronic hypertension is classical risk factor for stroke and transient ischemic attack, especially lacunar strokes. Chronic hypertension also increases risk of intraparenchymal hemorrhage, usually in deep brain areas. Subarachnoid hemorrhage occurs secondary to aneurysmal rupture
Mental status and psychiatric aspects/ complications	Large intraparenchymal or subarachnoid hemorrhage commonly induces mental status deterioration. If patients are awake, they usually complain of sudden onset severe headache
Brainstem	Chronic hypertension increases risk of brainstem lacunar infarct and hemorrhage
Cerebellum	Risk of cerebellar lacunar infarct and hemorrhage is also increased. In case of large cerebellar hemorrhage, expansion to 4th ventricle is common and risk of cerebral aqueduct occlusion is high
Cranial nerves	Cranial symptoms usually present as a part of brainstem infarction or hemorrhage

Secondary Complications: Cardiovascular complications of hypertension (e.g., coronary artery disease, congestive heart failure, aortic dissection) increase risk of thromboembolism, which can cause multifocal small cerebral infarcts or large vessel occlusion.

Treatment Complications: Supratherapeutic antihypertensive medication dosing can cause decreased cerebral blood flow, which leads to depressed mentation.

Bibliography

Biller J. *The interface of neurology and internal medicine*. Philadephia, PA: Wolters Kluwer. 2007.

Hypertensive Crisis

Epidemiology and Demographics: One percent to 5% of patients with hypertension will develop a hypertensive crisis in their lifetime. Incidence is higher in older adults, African-Americans, and men. It is commonly caused by sudden escalation of chronic essential hypertension, drug interaction, or withdrawal from antihypertensive drugs.

Disorder Description: "Hypertensive crisis" contains two concepts: hypertensive urgency and emergency. SBP>180 or DBP>120 mmHg is defined as hypertensive urgency. If acute symptomatic end-organ ischemic damage occurs with hypertensive urgency, it is called hypertensive emergency. The brain is one of the most sensitive end organs and is frequently affected.

Symptoms

Localization site	Comment
Cerebral hemispheres	Both ischemic and hemorrhagic stroke can be caused by hypertensive crisis. These result in acute onset of focal cortical symptoms, such as hemiparesis, aphasia, or hemiparesthesia. Acute onset of headache and confusion or lethargy are common with hemorrhages
Mental status and psychiatric aspects/ complications	If diffuse, higher cortical symptoms are seen in hypertensive crisis, which is called hypertensive encephalopathy. Various cortical symptoms can be seen, including headache, confusion, restlessness, altered consciousness, and seizures. Nausea and vomiting are also common
	Posterior reversible encephalopathy syndrome is a radiographic finding that is present in severe hypertensive encephalopathy, typically involving the posterior cerebral hemispheres on MRI or CT
Brainstem	Brainstem hemorrhage can be caused by hypertensive crisis
Cerebellum	Cerebellar hemorrhage can be caused by hypertensive crisis
Cranial nerves	Multiple cranial nerve dysfunctions can happen as a part of brainstem hemorrhage, but isolated optic nerve injury can also happen. Blurry vision is common, and patient usually has papilledema. Retinal hemorrhages can be induced by hypertensive crisis as well

Secondary Complications: The liver and kidney can be damaged by hypertensive crisis as well, with secondary superimposed metabolic derangements and even encephalopathy. Sudden onset of congestive heart failure may occur because of the extremely high afterload.

Treatment Complications: Intravenous antihypertensive agents are the choice of treatment for hypertensive emergency. It is important not to drop the mean arterial pressure by more than 25% during the first 24 hours to avoid hypoperfusion brain injury such as watershed infarct. This 25% rule may apply for several days so that careful clinical follow-up is essential on further lowering of blood pressure.

Bibliography

Biller J. *The interface of neurology and internal medicine.* Philadephia, PA: Wolters Kluwer. 2007.

Hyperthyroidism

Epidemiology and Demographics: More common in women than men (5:1 ratio).[1] Prevalence is between 0.5 and 2% in women. Higher incidence in smokers.[2]

Disorder Description: Most common causes of hyperthyroidism are Graves' disease followed by toxic multinodular goiter and autonomously functioning thyroid adenoma. More commonly occurring in iodine-replete communities.

Symptoms

Localization site	Comment
Cerebral hemispheres	Encephalopathy and seizure activity with thyroid storm.[3] If untreated, may progress to agitated delirium and coma
	Cardioembolic strokes from thyrotoxic induced atrial fibrillation
Mental status and psychiatric aspects/ complications	Overactivity of the adrenergic system is thought to cause anxiety, emotional lability, depression, and problems with sleep and rarely acute psychotic episodes and delirium.[4] These behavioral manifestations can be accompanied by impaired concentration, confusion, poor orientation and immediate recall, amnesia, and constructional difficulties[5]

Localization site	Comment
Peripheral neuropathy	Axonal sensory polyneuropathy and rarely demyelinating polyneuropathy
	Basedow paraplegia acutely in the hyperthyroid state[6] characterized by weakness and areflexia
	Carpel tunnel syndrome in thyrotoxicosis
Muscle	High-frequency low-amplitude tremor and hyperreflexia with thyrotoxicosis due to stimulation of the beta adrenergic system. Chorea is a rare complication due to dopamine modulation[7]
	Myalgias. Proximal muscle weakness with normal creatine kinase levels

Secondary Complications: Stroke as a result of thyrotoxic atrial fibrillation. Cerebral venous thrombosis as a result of an induced hypercoagulable state due to hyperthyroidism may occur.

Treatment Complications: Antithyroid medications propylthiouracil and methimazole may cause arthralgia or myalgia. Other treatments include radioactive iodine and total or partial thyroidectomy. Adverse effects of these therapies include hypothyroidism that often warrants thyroid hormone supplementation.

References

1. Hollowell JG, Staehling NW, Flanders WD, et al. Serum TSH, T(4), and thyroid antibodies in the United States population (1988 to 1994): National Health and Nutrition Examination Survey (NHANES III). *J Clin Endocrinol Metab.* 2002;87(2):489–99.
2. Asvold BO, Bjøro T, Nilsen TI, Vatten LJ. Tobacco smoking and thyroid function: a population-based study. *Arch Intern Med.* 2007;167(13):1428–32. DOI:10.1001/archinte.167.13.1428.
3. Aiello DP, DuPlessis AJ, Pattishall EG 3rd, Kulin HE. Thyroid storm. Presenting with coma and seizures in a 3-year-old girl. *Clin Pediatr (Phila).* 1989;28:571–4.
4. Awad AG. The thyroid and the mind and emotions/thyroid dysfunction and mental disorders. Thyroid Foundation of Canada. 2000. Available from https://thyroid.ca/resource-material/articles/e-10-f/. Accessed Aug 16, 2018.
5. Martin FI, Deam DR. Hyperthyroidism in elderly hospitalised patients. Clinical features and treatment outcomes. *Med J Aust.* 1996;164:200.

6. Charcot J. Nouveaux signes de la maladie de basedow. *Bull Med.* 1889;3:147–9.

7. Seeherunvong T, Diamantopoulos S, Berkovitz GD. A nine year old girl with thyrotoxicosis, ataxia, and chorea. *Brain Dev.* 2007;29:660–1.

Hypertrophic Cardiomyopathy

Epidemiology and Demographics: The prevalence of hypertrophic cardiomyopathy (HCM) worldwide is approximately 0.2%, and it occurs equally in men and women as it is an autosomal dominant genetic disorder. Clinical symptoms of HCM may present at any age throughout life.

Disorder Description: HCM is an autosomal dominant disorder that has been linked to mutations of at least 11 genes that encode proteins of the sarcomere. These mutations result in a thickened (hypertrophied) yet nondilated left ventricle and irregularities of the mitral valve, which in many cases leads to an outflow tract obstruction.

Symptoms

Localization site	Comment
Cerebral hemispheres	Cerebral hypoperfusion resulting in symptoms of presyncope and/or syncope as a result of outflow tract obstruction if present. In addition, secondary arrhythmias may also provoke similar hypoperfusion with presyncope/syncope and potentially sudden death
Mental status and psychiatric aspects/complications	Dizziness, lightheadedness, and confusion along with impairment of consciousness plus syncope and presyncope
Brainstem	Same as above
Cerebellum	Same as above
Vestibular system (and non-specific dizziness)	Same as above
Base of skull	Same as above

Secondary Complications: Atrial fibrillation and its associated complications, progressive heart failure, and sudden death may all result from HCM.

Treatment Complications: A treatment used for patients with severe symptoms is surgical myectomy whose risks include infection, arrhythmias, myocardial infarction, stroke, and death. An alternative procedure is alcohol septal ablation, which carries similar risks of morbidity and mortality. An implantable defibrillator may be used for patients with high risk of sudden death; in addition common medications include beta blockers and calcium channel blockers.

Bibliography

Cleveland Clinic. Septal myectomy. June, 2009. Available from http://my.clevelandclinic.org/services/heart/disorders/septal_myectomy Accessed June 22, 2015.

Maron BJ, Olivotto I. Hypertrophic cardiomyopathy. In Mann DL, Zipes D, Libby P, Bonow RO, Braunwald E, eds. *Braunwald's heart disease: A textbook of cardiovascular medicine.* 10th ed. Philadelphia, PA: Elsevier/Saunders; 2015. pp. 1574–86.

Mayo Clinic Staff. Hypertrophic cardiomyopathy. Feb 18, 2015. Available from www.mayoclinic.org/diseases-conditions/hypertrophic-cardiomyopathy/home/ovc-20122102. Accessed June 22, 2015.

Hyperventilation Syndrome

Epidemiology and Demographics: In those with an anxiety disorder, studies show a wide range of prevalence from 25 to 83%. Prevalence outside the context of anxiety is unclear. It is more common in women. Affects teens to elderly.

Disorder Description: A syndrome in which an individual breathes at a volume and/or rate above that which is required for metabolic needs, resulting in a decrease in arterial pCO_2. There is no consensus for standardized criteria. It occurs intermittently, typically lasts minutes to hours and resolves on its own. It is often accompanied by symptoms of dyspnea, dizziness, palpitations, chest tightness, paresthesias, and/or carpopedal spasm. There may or may not be insight into the fact that one is hyperventilating.

It is commonly associated with panic disorder, but which process is primary or secondary is unclear. When associated with distressing psychologic processes, symptoms include the feeling that one is not getting enough air, shallow and irregular breathing patterns, and frequent sighing. Increased physiologic fear sensitivity has been theorized to be associated with hyperventilation that is associated with psychiatric disorders. Other neurologic and pulmonary factors may also play a role.

Many disorders can present with hyperventilation, but a diagnosis of hyperventilation syndrome implies there is no known underlying cardiac, pulmonary, metabolic, or other medical etiology.

Symptoms

Localization site	Comment
Cerebral hemispheres	Differential diagnosis: central hyperventilation syndrome (pontine lesion), post-ictal hyperventilation
Mental status and psychiatric aspects/complications	Anxiety, fear, and panic
Vestibular system (and non-specific dizziness)	Dizziness
Peripheral neuropathy	Paresthesias, carpopedal spasm

Secondary Complications: Emergency department presentation, which may be recurrent.

Treatment Complications: First line is reassurance and cognitive behavioral techniques. Beta blockers and benzodiazepines are also used for refractory cases, with associated side effects of potential worsening of asthma and dependence/tolerance, respectively.

Bibliography

Cowley DS, Roy-Byrne PP. Hyperventilation and panic disorder. *Am J Med*. 1987;83:929.

Lewis RA, Howell JB. Definition of the hyperventilation syndrome. *Bull Eur Physiopathol Respir*. 1986;22:201.

Pfortmueller CA, Pauchard-Neuwerth SE, Leichtle AB, et al. Primary hyperventilation in the emergency department: a first overview. *PLoS One*. 2015;10:e0129562.

Saisch SG, Wessely S, Gardner WN. Patients with acute hyperventilation presenting to an inner-city emergency department. *Chest*. 1996;110:952.

Hyperviscosity Syndrome

Epidemiology and Demographics: Hyperviscosity syndrome usually occurs from Waldenström macroglobulinemia (85%) and less frequently from multiple myeloma or disorders with elevated blood counts such as leukemia or polycythemia. White blood cell counts are generally over 100,000/µL in leukemias, while in polycythemia, the hemoglobin level is usually greater than 18 g/dL.

Disorder Description: Red blood cells typically determine blood viscosity in healthy individuals. In hyperviscosity syndrome with paraproteinemia, excess protein forms aggregates increasing resistance to flow. Serum viscosity is generally greater than 4 centipoise in symptomatic patients. In disorders with elevated blood counts, there is leukostasis resulting in sluggish flow.

Symptoms

Localization site	Comment
Cerebral hemispheres	Diffuse localization causing headache, confusion, and somnolence. Focal stroke from thrombosis can also occur
Cerebellum	Vertigo, nystagmus, and ataxia
Cranial nerves	Blurred vision, retinal hemorrhages, or central retinal vein thrombosis

Secondary Complications: Mucosal bleeding and purpura are common. Other clinical effects include heart failure, kidney injury, and pulmonary edema.

Treatment Complications: Usual treatment with daily plasmapheresis carries risk of thrombosis and infection in often immunocompromised individuals.

Bibliography

Lewis MA, Hendrickson AW, Moynihan TJ. Oncologic emergencies: Pathophysiology, presentation, diagnosis, and treatment. *CA Cancer J Clin*. 2011;61:287–314.

Stone MJ, Bogen SA. Evidence-based focused review of management of hyperviscosity syndrome. *Blood*. 2012;119:2205–8.

Hypocalcemia

Epidemiology and Demographics: Relatively rare condition that is seen mainly in neonates or in patients with renal failure. It occurs in all age groups, especially those with genetic predisposition for pseudohypoparathyroidism, vitamin D receptor abnormalities, and hypoparathyroidism.

Disorder Description: It is defined as a serum ionized calcium less than 4.65 mg/dL or a total serum calcium less than 8.5 mg/dL. Patients usually become symptomatic when serum calcium concentrations fall below 7.5 mg/dL. It is seen in conditions associated with hypoparathyroidism (primary or secondary), pseudohypoparathyroidism (parathyroid hormone-resistant syndromes), vitamin D deficiency, acute pancreatitis, or malabsorption syndromes. Severe acute hypocalcemia commonly occurs following thyroid or parathyroid surgery. Other causes of hypocalcemia include hypomagnesemia from alcohol use, vomiting, or poor oral intake. Hyperphosphatemia secondary to excessive oral or parenteral phosphate, tumor lysis syndrome, and rhabdomyolysis-induced acute renal failure can also lead to hypocalcemia. Medications such anticonvulsants and antimicrobials (foscarnet, pentamidine, and ketoconazole) can cause hypocalcemia. Risk factors include acute pancreatitis, hypoparathyroidism, vitamin D deficiency, and chronic kidney disease.

Symptoms

Localization site	Comment
Cerebral hemispheres	Seizures (focal or generalized) nonresponsive to anticonvulsants, and pseudotumor cerebri
	Chronic hypocalcemia may result in headaches (secondary to increased intracranial pressure) and chorea or parkinsonism
Mental status and psychiatric aspects/ complications	Irritability, confusion, agitation, mental dullness and intellectual disabilities, anxiety, delirium, delusions, hallucinations, psychosis, depression, and dementia
Spinal cord	Myelopathy secondary to vertebral lamina overgrowth
Peripheral neuropathy	Perioral paresthesia. Limb paresthesia (distal then spread proximally)
Muscle	Tetanic muscle contraction, which may progress to opisthotonos if truncal spasms occur. Laryngeal spasms. Carpopedal spasm

Secondary Complications: Cataracts and papilledema. Cardiac arrhythmias and abnormal EKG findings (prolonged QT interval and ST flattening). Basal ganglia calcifications in chronic hypoparathyroidism. Osteopetrosis, dental abnormalities, dry skin, coarse hair, and psoriasis in chronic untreated cases.

Treatment Complications: Overcorrection of calcium and magnesium may lead to EKG changes and careful monitoring is warranted. Magnesium toxicity may lead to diminished deep tendon reflexes and intravenous calcium gluconate can be used as a useful antidote.

Bibliography

Fong J, Khan A. Hypocalcemia: updates in diagnosis and management for primary care. *Canad Fam Physician*. 2012;58(2):158–62.

Lockwood A. Toxic and metabolic encephalopathies. In Daroff RB, et al., eds. *Bradley's neurology in clinical practice*. 6th ed. Philadelphia, PA: Saunders; 2012. Chapter 56.

Riggs J. Neurologic complications of electrolyte disturbances. In Aminoff MJ, Josephson SA, eds. *Aminoff's neurology and general medicine*. London, UK: Elsevier; 2014. pp. 317–26.

Wysolmerski J, Insogna K. The parathyroid glands, hypercalcemia, and hypocalcemia. In *Goldman's Cecil medicine*. 24th ed. Philadelphia, PA: Saunders; 2011. Chapter 253.

Hypoglossal Nerve Palsy

Epidemiology and Demographics: Prevalence is unknown.

Disorder Description: The twelfth or hypoglossal nerve is a purely motor nerve controlling the extrinsic and intrinsic muscles of the tongue (except palatoglossus). Peripheral lesion could be due to head and neck tumor, internal carotid artery aneurysm or dissection, trauma, retropharyngeal abscess, or radiation therapy. Iatrogenic cases may follow internal jugular vein cannulation, carotid endarterectomy, and glomus jugulare resection. Motor neuron diseases, syringobulbia, tumor, and stroke may cause lesion to hypoglossal nucleus.

Symptoms

Localization site	Comment
Cranial nerves or cranial nerve nuclei	Ipsilateral tongue atrophy with tongue deviation toward the side of lesion. Difficulty in swallowing and talking, particularly in bilateral lesion

Secondary Complications: Aspiration and malnutrition due to swallowing problem.

Treatment Complications: Complication varies with treatment for each underlying cause.

Bibliography

Lin HC, Barkhaus PE. Cranial nerve XII: the hypoglossal nerve. *Semin Neurol.* 2009;29(1):45–52.

Hypoglycemia

Epidemiology and Demographics: Hypoglycemia can occur in any age group. It is seen in 10–30% per year of patients with type 1 diabetes mellitus and 1.2% per year in patients with type 2 diabetes mellitus.

Disorder Description: The brain is very vulnerable to hypoglycemia because of the normally low concentration of glucose in the brain and its high cerebral metabolic rate. There are many causes of hypoglycemia secondary to the complexity of glucose homeostasis (insulin release, glycogen breakdown, and gluconeogenesis). It can result from conditions causing *fasting hypoglycemia* such as exogenous insulin, oral hypoglycemics, glucose overuse, elevated insulin levels, ketotic hypoglycemia, hypermetabolic state (sepsis), normal to low insulin levels, antibodies to endogenous insulin, excessive islet cell function (prediabetes, obesity), islet cell disorders (adenoma, cancer, nesidioblastosis), extrapancreatic tumors, and carnitine deficiency. It can also result from conditions causing *postprandial hypoglycemia* such as postoperative rapid gastric emptying, fructose intolerance, galactosemia, and leucine intolerance. Medications inducing hypoglycemia, severe malnutrition, alcohol abuse, hormone deficiencies (growth hormone, glucagon, and hypoadrenalism), disorders of metabolism, and liver disease can also increase the risk of hypoglycemia.

Symptoms

Localization site	Comment
Cerebral hemispheres	Alternating hemiparesis, seizures; permanent and irreversible injury to the cortex, basal ganglia, and dentate gyrus
Mental status and psychiatric aspects/ complications	Acute symptoms: feelings of detachment from the environment, restlessness, and anxiety, leading to panic and ataxia
	Subacute symptoms: inattention, confusion, drowsiness, altered consciousness, disorientation, clumsiness, and amnesia of episode
	Chronic: personality, behavior and memory changes, which may mimic dementia
	Coma in severe cases, with tremor and myoclonus sometimes preceding coma

Secondary Complications: There is significant morbidity associated with hypoglycemia such as injuries, convulsions, and mortality. Hypoglycemic unawareness is a condition seen in diabetic patients, especially those with type 1 diabetes. It is related to both alteration in neuroendocrine responses that are involved in the regulation of blood glucose levels and dysfunction in the central nervous system affecting counterregulatory hormonal responses. It is challenging because if prolonged and not recognized, it can lead to irreversible neuronal injury.

Treatment Complications: Treatment can lead to hyperglycemia (see entry for *Hyperglycemia*). Of note, beta blockers can mask premonitory systemic symptoms such as perspiration, anxiety, tachycardia, nausea, and tremors.

Bibliography

Goldman L, Schafer A. Hypoglycemia. In *Goldman's Cecil medicine.* 24th ed. Philadelphia, PA: Saunders; 2011. pp. 237–8.

Lockwood A. Toxic and metabolic encephalopathies. In Daroff RB, et al., eds. *Bradley's neurology in clinical practice.* 6th ed. Philadelphia, PA: Saunders; 2012. Chapter 56.

Sircar M, Bhatia A, Munshi M. Review of hypoglycemia in the older adult: clinical implications and management. *Can J Diabetes.* 2016;40(1):66–72. DOI: 10.1016/j.jcjd.2015.10.004. Epub Dec 29, 2015.

Zochodne D, Toth C. Diabetes and the nervous system. In Aminoff MJ, Josephson SA, eds. *Aminoff's neurology and general medicine.* London, UK: Elsevier; 2014. pp. 351–68.

Hypokalemic Periodic Paralysis

Epidemiology and Demographics: Hypokalemic periodic paralysis is the most common primary periodic paralysis. Onset is usually during adolescence, and 60% are affected by the age of 16 years. The prevalence is approximately 1/100,000, and symptoms are more severe in males. Attacks usually become less frequent and may cease during the fourth and fifth decades of life.

Disorder Description: It is an autosomal dominant disorder characterized by limb weakness in the setting of hypokalemia. It is caused by a mutation in the gene CACNA1S on chromosome 1q (70% of cases) and 10–20% of families have mutations in the gene SCN4A on chromosome 17q. The attacks commonly occur in the morning and are triggered by rest following strenuous exercise or are precipitated after ingestion of a carbohydrate load and high salt diet the previous night. Serum potassium concentrations are usually low during an attack. The attacks usually last several hours but may vary from minutes to days. Patient usually makes a full recovery but mild weakness may persist for several days and rarely may result in permanent weakness. It is important to consider secondary causes of hypokalemic weakness such as hypothyroidism, excessive insulin, barium poisoning, poor potassium intake, excessive potassium excretion, and renal loss of potassium.

Symptoms

Localization site	Comment
Peripheral neuropathy	Paresthesia
Muscle	Diurnal fluctuation with proximal weakness of the limbs, muscle cramps. Progressive myopathy

Secondary Complications: Cardiac arrhythmias can be seen as a complication of hypokalemia. Oliguria or anuria may develop during major attacks, and patient may be constipated. Hypokalemia also could potentially lead to glucose intolerance, secondary to decreased insulin secretion, increasing risk of stroke. Some patients may have permanent weakness with recurrent attacks.

Treatment Complications: Acetazolamide may worsen symptoms in patients with hypokalemic periodic paralysis caused by sodium channel mutations. It is important not to overestimate the replacement of intravenous potassium because it can lead to hyperkalemia. Hyperkalemia can result in cardiac arrest and lead to EKG changes; it could also cause ascending muscle paralysis.

Bibliography

Goldman L, Schafer A. Muscle diseases. In *Goldman's Cecil medicine*. 24th ed. Philadelphia, PA: Saunders; 2011. Chapter 429.

Kerchner G, Ptacek L. Channelopathies: episodic and electrical disorders of the nervous system. In Daroff RB, et al., eds. *Bradley's neurology in clinical practice*. 6th ed. Philadelphia, PA: Saunders; 2012. Chapter 64.

Moxley R, Heatwole C. Channelopathies. In Swaiman KF, ed. *Swaiman's pediatric neurology: principles and practice*. Philadelphia, PA: Saunders; 2012. pp. 1667–89.

Riggs J. Neurologic complications of electrolytes disturbances. In Aminoff MJ, Josephson SA, eds. *Aminoff's neurology and general medicine*. London, UK: Elsevier; 2014. pp. 317–26.

Hypomagnesemia

Epidemiology and Demographics: Hypomagnesemia is seen in approximately 12% of hospitalized patients and is seen most commonly in critical care illness. There is no difference in the prevalence between men and women.

Disorder Description: Magnesium is required for the activation of many intracellular enzymes and has a key role in synaptic transmission throughout the nervous system. Low serum levels of magnesium can be seen with decreased intake or gastrointestinal absorption or with increased renal loss. It is also seen in patients on cisplatin or with a history of a cardioskeletal mitochondrial myopathy.

Symptoms

Localization site	Comment
Cerebral hemispheres	Seizures
Mental status and psychiatric aspects/complications	Agitation, irritability, and confusion
Peripheral nerves, neuromuscular junction, and muscle	Tetany, hyperreflexia, Trousseau and Chvostek signs, muscle spasms, and cramps

Secondary Complications: Hypocalcemia or hypomagnesemia can be worsened by hypomagnesemia causing decreased parathyroid hormone release or increased resistance to the action of parathyroid hormone throughout the body.

Treatment Complications: Intravenous magnesium must be given slowly with calcium gluconate available at bedside in case administration leads to hypermagnesemia, which can cause failure of the respiratory muscles.

Bibliography

Agus ZS. Hypomagnesemia. *J Am Soc Nephrol.* 1999;10:1666–22.

Riggs J. Neurologic complications of electrolytes disturbances. In Aminoff MJ, Josephson SA, eds. *Aminoff's neurology and general medicine.* London, UK: Elsevier; 2014. pp. 317–26.

Hyponatremia

Epidemiology and Demographics: Most common electrolyte abnormality in hospitalized patients; 15–20% have a serum sodium level <135 mEq/L.

Disorder Description: Electrolyte abnormality characterized by serum sodium less than 135 mEq/L or, in severe cases, serum sodium less than 125 mEq/L. Classification breaks down to normal osmolarity (rare), hyperosmolarity (usually from hyperglycemia), and hypo-osmolarity (most common.) Hypo-osmolar hyponatremia can be further classified into low, normal, and high extracellular volume status.

Hyponatremia may be caused by relatively high free water concentrations from polydipsia, to the syndrome of inappropriate antidiuretic hormone secretion (SIADH) seen in *euvolemic hypo-osmolar hyponatremia.* SIADH can be observed following strokes, head traumas, subarachnoid hemorrhage, and pituitary surgery. Medications may also cause hyponatremia – particularly antiepileptic agents carbamazepine and oxcarbazepine, as well as chemotherapeutic agents, antidepressants, and diuretics. Associated neurologic conditions often depend on the rapidity of electrolyte disturbance.

Symptoms

Localization site	Comment
Cerebral hemispheres	Related to cerebral edema: headaches, dizziness, nystagmus, nausea, seizures (in severe cases serum sodium <120 mEq/L). Unilateral focal signs: aphasia, hemiparesis, may be secondary to aggravated underlying lesions
Mental status and psychiatric aspects/complications	Confusion, delirium
Muscle	Muscle cramping

Secondary Complications: Hyponatremia can cause nausea and vomiting, which can lead to other electrolyte disorders.

Treatment Complications: Rapid correction of serum sodium to >10–12 mEq/L per day may cause osmotic demyelination syndrome (formerly central pontine myelinolysis) – demyelination of the central nervous system, causing spastic quadriparesis and bulbar palsy.

Bibliography

Decaux G, Soupart A. Treatment of symptomatic hyponatremia. *Am J Med Sci.* 2003;326(1):25–30.

Spasovaski G, Vanholder R, Allolio B, et al. Clinical practice guideline on diagnosis and treatment of hyponatremia. *Nephrol Dial Transplant.* 2014;170(3):G1–47.

Sterns RH, Riggs JE, Schochet SS. Osmotic demyelination syndrome following correction of hyponatremia. *N Engl J Med.* 1986;314:1535.

Hypoparathyroidism

Epidemiology and Demographics: In the United States, the prevalence of hypoparathyroidism is estimated to be 37/100,000 person-years. Age of onset depends on the etiology. Found equally in men and women.

Disorder Description: Can be transient or more sustained, inherited, or acquired. The most common cause is secondary to surgical removal or autoimmune destruction of the parathyroid glands. Hypoparathyroidism is characterized by hypocalcemia, hyperphosphatemia, and low levels of parathyroid hormone.

Symptoms

Localization site	Comment
Cerebral hemispheres	Seizures, increased intracranial pressure. Cerebral calcifications
Mental status and psychiatric aspects/ complications	Irritability. Memory loss. Psychosis
Brainstem	Basal ganglia calcifications. Thalamic infarcts. Ectrapyramidal disorders due to chronic hypocalcemia
Cerebellum	Cerebellar calcifications
Muscle	Carpopedal spasms as noted by one study to be the most common presenting symptom. Chorea. Fasciculations. Dystonia
Unclear localization	Gait instability

Treatment Complications: Some reported side effects of calcium, vitamin D, and uncommonly parathyroid hormone supplementation include dizziness and leg cramps. Uncommonly, excessively high or low calcium may result in extrapyramidal symptoms, mood changes, or seizures.

Bibliography

Al-Azem H, Khan AA; Hypoparathyroidism. *Best Pract Res Clin Endocrinol Metab.* 2012;26(4):517–22. DOI: 10.1016/j.beem.2012.01.004.

Bhadada SK, Bhansali A, Upreti V, Subbiah S, Khandelwal N. Spectrum of neurological manifestations of idiopathic hypoparathyroidism and pseudohypoparathyroidism. *Neurol India.* 2011;59:586–9.

Clarke BL, Brown EM, Collins MT, et al. Epidemiology and diagnosis of hypoparathyroidism. *J Clin Endocrinol Metab.* 2016;101(6):2284–99. DOI: 10.1210/jc.2015-3908.

Fonseca OA, Calverley JR. Neurological manifestations of hypoparathyroidism. *Arch Intern Med.* 1967;120(2):202–6. DOI:10.1001/archinte.1967.00300020074009.

Hypophosphatemia

Epidemiology and Demographics: Hypophosphatemia can be seen in approximately 5% of hospitalized patients and is much more common in patients with a history of alcoholism, sepsis, or with other critical illness.

Disorder Description: There are many medical causes of hypophosphatemia. It can be caused by a shift of phosphate into the cells (insulin administration, respiratory alkalosis), decreased absorption or intake (starvation, alcoholism, phosphate binders, malabsorption), renal dysfunction, and parathyroid dysfunction.

Symptoms

Localization site	Comment
Cerebral hemispheres	Seizures
Mental status and psychiatric aspects/complications	Confusion, lethargy, irritability, delirium
Muscle	Myopathy with weakness, rhabdomyolysis

Secondary Complications: Weakness can lead to failure of the respiratory muscles. This can lead to apnea, increased carbon dioxide concentrations, coma, and possible death.

Treatment Complications: High intravenous doses of phosphate can lead to hyperphosphatemia that can cause renal injury, hypocalcemia, and cardiac arrhythmia.

Bibliography

Felsenfeld A, Levine B. Approach to treatment of hypophosphatemia. *Am J Kidney Dis.* 2012;60(4):655–61.

Subramanian R, Khardori R. Severe hypophosphatemia: pathophysiologic implications, clinical presentations, and treatment. *Medicine.* 2009;79(1):1–8.

Hypoxia

Epidemiology and Demographics: Incidence and prevalence of hypoxia vary and are linked to a multitude of cardiopulmonary and toxic disorders. Given its broad association, the specific incidence in gender, ethnicity, or region is difficult to define.

Disorder Description: Hypoxia is literally defined as deficiency in oxygen, which can be further broken down into generalized hypoxia or local tissue hypoxia. Generalized hypoxia can occur in cases of insufficient alveolar oxygen such as high altitude. Generalized hypoxia can also be seen in a multitude of respiratory conditions such as cases of disrupted or compromised blood supply. Among the most prevalent causes of hypoxia (chronic obstructive pulmonary disease, acute respiratory distress syndrome [ARDS], obstructive sleep apnea), it has been well documented that cognitive impairment is the most common detrimental effect. In ARDS, profound hypoxemia is seen acutely with high associated mortality rates. Alveolar microvascular injury and associated fluid leakage leads to large alveolar–arterial gradient and perfusion defect. Patients with a diagnosis of ARDS are often found to have cognitive dysfunction up to 1 to 2 years following discharge. In fact one case noted ongoing cognitive deficits up to 6 years after discharge, which further supports cognitive dysfunction as the most common effect of hypoxia and hypoxemia.

Symptoms

Localization site	Comment
Cerebral hemispheres	Hypoxia, cellular dysfunction prominent at prefrontal cortex, choreoathetosis, and coma
Mental status and psychiatric aspects/complications	Cognitive dysfunction, memory impairment, poor verbal fluency, and depression
Cerebellum	Cerebellar ataxia
Muscle	Poor fine motor skills, myoclonus

Secondary Complications: Profound hypoxia from conditions such as altitude sickness can lead to cerebral edema. Hypoxia and hypoxemia if severe can lead to programed cell death in highly metabolic tissues such as cardiac myocytes.

Treatment Complications: Since treatment of hypoxia and hypoxemia often involves supplemental O_2, detrimental effects from high fraction of inspired oxygen (FiO_2) are seen. Prolonged exposure to increased FiO_2 allows formation of reactive oxygen species and further tissue damage, especially in those tissues previously hypoxic.

Bibliography

Alchanatis M, Zias N, Deligiorgis N, et al. Sleep apnea-related cognitive deficits and intelligence: an implication of cognitive reserve theory. *J Sleep Res.* 2005;14, 69–75.

Bruce AS, Aloia MS, Ancoli-Israel S. *Neuropsychological assessment of neuropsychiatric and neuromedical disorders.* Oxford: Oxford University Press; 2009.

Kozora E, Filley C, Julian L, Cullum C. Cognitive functioning in patients with chronic obstructive pulmonary disease and mild hypoxemia compared with patients with mild Alzheimer disease and controls. *J Neuropsychiatry Neuropsychol Behav Neurol.* 1999;12:178–83.

Martin DS, Grocott M. Oxygen therapy in critical illness. *Crit Care Med.* 2013;41(2):423–32.

Rothenhausler HB, Ehrentraut S, Stoll C, Schelling G, Kapfammer HP. The relationship between cognitive performance and employment and health status in long-term survivors of the acute respiratory distress syndrome: Results of an exploratory study. *Gen Hosp Psychiatry.* 2001;23(2):90–6.

Ice Pick Headache

Epidemiology and Demographics: Some studies estimate a prevalence of 2–35% in the general population. This condition affects mostly women at a ratio of 1.46–2.6:1 One study performed in Sweden demonstrated an incidence of 2%. Another study done in Norway showed an incidence of up to 35%.

Disorder Description: Ice pick headache is also called idiopathic or primary stabbing headache. The condition is characterized by paroxysmal, ultra-short stabs of pain in the head that can be unilateral or bilateral. For proper diagnosis, this condition must not be secondary to any disease in the surrounding structures of the brain. The International Headache Consortium defines this condition as a single stab or series of stabs occurring in the V1 distribution of the trigeminal nerve. However, studies reveal that this stabbing attack does not always follow the V1 dermatome. This stabbing pain can last up to 3 seconds and occur multiple times during the day; stabbing pain of longer duration have been reported. There are no associated cranial autonomic features; however, this condition is associated with nausea, vomiting, photophobia, phonophobia, and dizziness. The presentation of this condition can change with each attack. Diagnosis is made based on clinical presentation only.

Symptoms

Localization site	Comment
Cerebral hemispheres	Can present unilaterally or bilaterally
Cranial nerves	Formal criteria list V1 trigeminal dermatome as affected area but subsequent reports reveal that this is not always the case

Secondary Complications: The presentation of ice pick headache should always be concerning for alternative etiologies before arriving at diagnosis of this condition. Specifically, patients who are male and older presenting with this symptom should warrant additional imaging work up and consideration for alternative pathology.

Treatment Complications: Indomethacin is considered to be first line treatment for this condition; however, up to 40% of patients with this condition do not respond to treatment, have side effects to this treatment, or harbor contraindications. Alternative treatments have been found like external hand warming.

Bibliography

Chua AL, Nahas S. Ice pick headache. *Curr Pain Headache Rep*. 2016;20:30.

Fuh JL, Kuo KH, Wang SJ. Primary stabbing headache in a headache clinic. *Cephalalgia*. 2007;27(9):1005–9.

Mathew NT. Indomethacin responsive headache syndromes. *Headache*. 1981;21(4):147–50.

Raskin NH, Schwartz RK. Ice pick-like pain. *Neurology*. 1980;3: 203–5.

Idiopathic Hypersomnia

Epidemiology and Demographics: Prevalence and incidence are not known. May be more common in women. Frequently develops in adolescence.

Disorder Description: Idiopathic hypersomnia is characterized by an irrepressible need to sleep or falling asleep during the daytime, daily for at least 3 months. There must be an absence of cataplexy symptoms. A Multiple Sleep Latency Test (MSLT) performed must show fewer than two or no sleep onset REM periods with a sleep onset latency of less than or equal to 8 minutes, which is consistent with hypersomnolence. Insufficient sleep syndrome must be ruled out and the findings of hypersomnolence on MSLT are not better explained by another sleep disorder such as sleep apnea, medical or psychiatric disorder, or the use of medications or recreational drugs. Supportive features include symptoms of sleep inertia (prolonged difficulty waking up with repeated returns to sleep, irritability, and confusion) and long naps of greater than or equal to 1 hour that are not refreshing.

Symptoms: Unknown pathophysiology and neurobiology. CSF hypocretin-1 levels as well as other neurotransmitters have been studied and found to be normal in this group of patients. Recent evidence, although still investigational, suggests a possible endogenous GABA receptor ligand of unclear etiology in idiopathic hypersomnia.

Secondary Complications: Prolonged sleep inertia with associated symptoms of headache, orthostatic disturbance, perception of temperature dysregulation, and peripheral vascular complaints. These symptoms may be related to a dysfunction of the autonomic nervous system.

Treatment Complications: Treatment focuses on improvement of excessive daytime somnolence. Options include modafinil, armodafinil, methylphenidate, and amphetamines.

Stimulants can cause and/or worsen systemic hypertension as well as cause symptoms of anxiety and dysphoria, tachycardia, headaches, and hepatitis. Amphetamines may be rarely linked to pulmonary hypertension.

Bibliography

Ali M, Auger RR, Slocumb NL, Morganthaler TI. Idiopathic hypersomnia: clinical features and response to treatment. *J Clin Sleep Med.* 2009;5:562–8.

American Academy of Sleep Medicine. *International classification of sleep disorders.* 3rd ed. Darien, IL: American Academy of Sleep Medicine; 2014.

Anderson KN, Pilsworth S, Sharples RD, Smith IE, Shneerson JM. Idiopathic hypersomnia: a study of 77 cases. *Sleep.* 2007;30:1274–81.

Mayer G, Benes H, Young P, Bitterlich M, Rodenbeck A. Modafinil in the treatment of idiopathic hypersomnia without long sleep time: a randomized, double-blind, placebo-controlled study. *J Sleep Res.* 2015;24:74–81.

Rye DB, Bliwise DL, Parker K, et al. Modulation of vigilance in the primary hypersomnias by endogenous enhancement of GABAA receptors. *Sci Trans Med.* 2012;21:161.

Idiopathic Intracranial Hypertension (Pseudotumor Cerebri)

Epidemiology and Demographics: Idiopathic intracranial hypertension (IIH), also known as pseudotumor cerebri, is a disease mainly of obese women of reproductive age. It occurs rarely in individuals of normal weight, children, and male patients. There are about 0.5 to 2 cases per 100,000 people per year in the general population, but between 12 and 20 cases per 100,000 in obese women aged 20 to 44 years.

Disorder Description: IIH occurs when there are symptoms of elevated intracranial pressure without clear etiology (i.e., not due to mass, tumor, or other secondary cause). It presents classically with headache, sometimes worsened with Valsalva maneuvers. Other reported symptoms include transient visual obscurations (blackening or dimming of vision lasting under 60 seconds, often with changes in posture), pulsatile tinnitus, back or neck pain, and sometimes vision loss.

When suspected, neuroimaging with contrast – preferably MRI brain with and without contrast – is usually obtained. As young female patients are also at risk of venous sinus thrombosis, a venogram study, such as magnetic resonance venography, is also often obtained. Formal visual field testing should also be obtained promptly to assess the patient's baseline and to monitor improvement.

Once a secondary cause of raised intracranial pressure has been ruled out (such as a mass lesion or venous sinus thrombosis), the following criteria help to refine the diagnosis, as per 2013 revised diagnostic criteria:

A. Papilledema
B. Normal neurologic exam (except cranial nerve abnormalities)
C. Neuroimaging with normal brain parenchyma, no hydrocephalus, mass or other structural lesion, and no abnormal meningeal enhancement or venous sinus thrombosis with appropriate cerebral venous imaging
D. Normal CSF composition
E. Elevated opening pressure on lumbar puncture (>25 cmH$_2$O in the lateral decubitus position)

A diagnosis can also be made if no papilledema is detected, but there is a sixth neve palsy and criteria B–E are met. Finally, in the absence of papilledema and sixth nerve palsy, a suspected diagnosis can be made with certain radiographic features (flattening of the posterior globe, empty sella, perioptic subarachnoid space distention with or without optic nerve tortuosity, and transverse venous stenosis).

Recently, optical coherence tomography, with an increased thickness of the retinal fiber layer detected in patients with papilledema, has been used to aid diagnosis.

IIH can lead to permanent visual field loss, loss of visual acuity, and in rare cases, blindness. And despite successful treatment, even with improvement in vision, persistent headache remains a common complaint.

Symptoms

Localization site	Comment
Psychiatric aspects/complications	Occasional cognitive disturbances, manifesting with increased reaction time and increased processing speed
Vestibular system	Dizziness, pulsatile tinnitus
Cranial nerves	Sixth nerve palsy (third, fourth, and other cranial nerve palsies have also been reported)
	Diplopia
	Transient visual obscurations
	Vision loss, including an enlarging blind spot, visual field constriction, or loss of nasal visual field
	Low frequency hearing loss
	Papilledema
Spinal cord	Neck or back pain, often with radicular features
Unclear localization	Headache: with or without nausea, vomiting, photophobia, phonophobia

Secondary Complications: Spontaneous cerebrospinal fluid leaks have been reported with IIH, and this can result in bacterial meningitis.

Treatment Complications: In cases of mild visual field loss, conservative management is recommended, with weight loss and the carbonic anhydrase inhibitor acetazolamide, titrated up to 4 g per day.

The landmark Idiopathic Intracranial Hypertension Treatment Trial studied lifestyle modification (including weight loss) in patients with mild vision loss assigned to either treatment with acetazolamide versus placebo. The trial demonstrated that the treatment group (i.e., lifestyle modification and acetazolamide) demonstrated a greater improvement in follow-up visual field testing and other parameters, such as improvement in grade of papilledema and visual quality of life measures, as compared to the placebo group. Other potential pharmacologic treatments include furosemide or topiramate, but efficacy is less well established for these agents.

Treatment complications or negative side effects of acetazolamide use include dysgeusia, nausea, vomiting, fatigue, and paresthesias.

Surgical interventions are sought for cases of rapid vision loss or those refractory to conservative treatment measures. Surgical interventions carry their own risks and treatment complications. Optic nerve sheath fenestration, for example, can cause traumatic optic neuropathy or retinal vascular occlusion. CSF diversion with ventriculoperitoneal or lumboperitoneal shunting can lead to shunt failure (up to 75% at 2 years), infection, or intracranial hypotension. Venous sinus stenting is another potential intervention, but carries risks of stent thrombosis, stent migration, or vessel perforation.

Bibliography

Friedman DI. Papilledema and idiopathic intracranial hypertension. *Continuum (Minneap Minn)*. 2014;20(4):857–76.

Markey K, Mollan S, Jensen R, Sinclair A. Understanding idiopathic intracranial hypertension: mechanisms, management and future directions. *Lancet Neurol.* 2016;15(1):78–91.

Pérez MA, Bialer OY, Bruce BB, Newman NJ, Biousse V. Primary spontaneous cerebrospinal fluid leaks and idiopathic intracranial hypertension. *J Neuroophthalmol.* 2013;33(4):330–7.

Wall M, Kupersmith MJ, Kieburtz KD, et al. The idiopathic intracranial hypertension treatment trial: clinical profile at baseline. *JAMA Neurol.* 2014;71(6):693–701.

Idiopathic Thrombocytopenic Purpura (ITP)

Epidemiology and Demographics: Idiopathic thrombocytopenic purpura (ITP) occurs in 5/100,000 children per year. Spontaneous recovery is typical. Intracranial hemorrhage occurs in 0.5–1.0% of affected children, and half are fatal. The incidence in adults is 2/100,000 and spontaneous remission rate varies between 5 to 11%.

Disorder Description: Primary ITP involves isolated thrombocytopenia due to idiopathic immune platelet destruction. Secondary ITP is associated with infections, systemic lupus erythematosus, lymphoproliferative diseases, and drugs, including heparin. Patients usually present with insidious onset of mucocutaneous bleeding, such as easy bruising or purpura. On CBC, decreased number of platelets is found while the other cell lines are within normal range. Peripheral blood smear shows large platelets.

Symptoms

Localization site	Comment
Cerebral hemispheres	Thrombocytopenia increases the risk of intracranial hemorrhage, either spontaneous or traumatic. Based on the site where hemorrhage occurs, various neurologic symptoms can be seen. Commonly, patient complains of sudden onset headache with neurologic symptoms. (See also entries for *Intracranial Hemorrhage*, *Subdural Hematoma*, and *Subarachnoid Hemorrhage*)
Mental status and psychiatric aspects/ complications	If the hemorrhage is large, especially when it produces midline shift, this can suppress cerebral cortex broadly and lead to altered mental status. Thalamic or brainstem hemorrhage can also cause mental status change regardless of the hematoma size
Brainstem	Brainstem hemorrhage occurs rarely, but is usually fatal. Patients typically show highly localized cranial nerve symptoms such as diplopia, facial weakness, or vertigo, with change in mental status. If it expands to medulla, respiratory failure will occur
Cerebellum	Cerebellar hemorrhage can occasionally happen and produces localized symptoms such as ataxia, vertigo, or oscillopsia. If the hemorrhage is big enough to compress the 4th ventricle, it leads to acute non-communicating hydrocephalus with high risk of hernation
Cranial nerves	Cranial nerve dysfunctions can be seen as a part of brainstem hemorrhage but rarely in isolation

Treatment Complications: Steroid therapy is used as first-line treatment in ITP. Long-standing use of steroid can induce myopathy. Intravenous immunoglobulin (IVIG) is also chosen frequently for ITP treatment. IVIG may increase risk of venous thrombosis, including dural sinus thrombosis.

Bibliography

Fogarty PF, Segal JB. The epidemiology of immune thrombocytopenic purpura. *Curr Opin Hematol.* 2007;14(5):515–9.

Marie I, Maurey G, Hervé F, Hellot MF, Levesque H. Intravenous immunoglobulin-associated arterial and venous thrombosis: report of a series and review of the literature. *Br J Dermatol.* 2006;155(4):714–21.

Illness Anxiety Disorder (Hypochondriasis)

Epidemiology and Demographics: Occurs at rate of 3 million per year in United States. Prevalence in community setting is 1.8–10% with equal predominance in males and females. Onset is typically in early to mid adulthood.

Disorder Description: Marked by excessive preoccupation around having or getting an illness. As per DSM-5 criteria, physical symptoms, when present, are often mild. If there is an existing underlying medical condition or risk of one, the preoccupation is disproportionately higher than expected. There is high anxiety about health, often manifesting as frequent health-related behaviors (such as repeatedly examining self or researching disorders) or avoidance of medical care. Must be present for 6 months and not better explained by another psychiatric disorder.

Risk factors may include history of childhood abuse, significant illness as a child, threat of serious illness that did not end up manifesting, and family member with serious illness. Course tends to be chronic and relapsing. Rates similar cross-culturally.

Symptoms

Localization site	Comment
Mental status and psychiatric aspects/ complications	Anxiety, excessive worry, or rumination. When comorbid with depressive, anxiety, or somatic symptom disorder, may have clinical features of those illnesses

Secondary Complications: Excessive health care utilization (or avoidance of care) with potential desensitization by providers. Iatrogenic complications from repeated testing and procedures. Impairment in social and occupational realms.

Treatment Complications: Supportive psychotherapy and cognitive behavioral therapy found to be helpful, as well as treatment of psychiatric comorbidity when present.

Bibliography

American Psychiatric Association. *Diagnostic and statistical manual of mental disorders: DSM-5.* 5th ed. Washington, DC: American Psychiatric Association; 2013.

Noyes R Jr, Stuart S, Langbehn DR, et al. Childhood antecedents of hypochondriasis. *Psychosomatics.* 2002;43(4):282–9.

Noyes R Jr, Carney CP, Hillis SL, et al. Prevalence and correlates of illness worry in the general population. *Psychosomatics.* 2005;46(6):529–39.

Infantile Spasms

Epidemiology and Demographics: Majority of cases are between 3 and 7 months of age, ranging from a few weeks old to >3 years of age. Incidence about 1/2000–4000 live births.

Disorder Description: Seizure type described as sudden, bilateral, and symmetric contractions of neck, trunk, and extremity muscles. Seizures often occur in clusters and may be subtle enough to cause delay in diagnosis. Ictal EEG during spasms shows a high-amplitude slow wave correlating with the spasm, then a diffuse electrodecremental response. Infantile spasms with hypsarrhythmia and psychomotor delay is known as West syndrome. Hypsarrhythmia is a disorganized interictal EEG pattern with high-voltage multifocal spike wave discharges.

Symptomatic etiologies include: hypoxic ischemic encephalopathy, stroke, cortical dysplasia, tuberous sclerosis, meningoencephalitis, TORCH (Toxoplasmosis, Other [syphilis, varicella-zoster, parvovirus B19], Rubella, Cytomegalovirus [CMV], and Herpes infections) infections, trauma, chromosomal abnormalities (Down syndrome), or metabolic causes. Idiopathic cases occur, with better long-term prognosis. Treatments include adrenocorticotropic hormone (ACTH) and vigabatrin.

Symptoms

Localization site	Comment
Cerebral hemispheres	Ictal spasms with abrupt flexor or extensor contraction of the axial muscles and limbs
	EEG with interictal hypsarrhythmia, and high-amplitude slow wave with electrodecremental response during spasms
	MRI abnormalities depend on underlying etiology

Localization site	Comment
Mental status and psychiatric aspects/ complications	Developmental regression
	Neurocognitive impairments in up to 70–90% of patients. Prognosis better for earlier treated infants with good response to therapy and no delays prior to onset
Cranial nerves	Auditory or visual abnormalities in up to 33–50% of patients

Secondary Complications: Neurodevelopmental delays and evolution to Lennox–Gastaut syndrome are common. Death in a third of patients by age 3 years.

Treatment Complications: ACTH may have side effects of hypertension, immune suppression, electrolyte imbalance, gastrointestinal disturbances, ocular opacities, hypertrophic cardiomyopathy, cerebral atrophy, growth impairment, and rarely, death. Vigabatrin treatment may cause irreversible retinal dysfunction and concentric visual field constriction.

Bibliography

Go CY, et al. Evidence-based guideline update: medical treatment of infantile spasms. Report of the Guideline Development Subcommittee of the American Academy of Neurology and the Practice Committee of the Child Neurology Society. *Neurology.* 2012;78(24): 1974–80.

Taghdiri MM, Nemati H. Infantile spasm: a review article. *Iran J Child Neurol.* 2014;8(3): 1–5.

Werz MA, Pita-Garcia IL. *Epilepsy syndromes.* Philadelphia, PA: Saunders/Elsevier; 2010.

Infective Endocarditis

Epidemiology and Demographics: The incidence of infective endocarditis (IE) is less than 10 cases per 100,000 person-years, and males are more likely to be seen with IE than women.

Disorder Description: Many pathogenic bacteria and fungi may cause infective endocarditis, an infection of the heart tissue, but gram-positive cocci bacteria are the most common pathogens involved. IE is seen most often in the mitral valve and aortic valve, and a regurgitant valve is more susceptible to infections than a stenotic valve. Further circumstances that contribute to a risk of IE include congenital heart disease (excluding bicuspid aortic valve disease), a history of IE, history of intravenous drug abuse, diabetes mellitus, immunosuppressive therapy, and history of invasive dental procedures. Patients with artificial heart valves are also more prone to IE as pathogens are more likely to attach to a prosthetic heart valve.

Symptoms

Localization site	Comment
Cerebral hemispheres	Embolic/microembolic cerebral infarction may occur, which may impair cortical and subcortical function. In addition, endocarditis may result in patients with aortic regurgitation/stenosis (see entries for *Aortic Regurgitation* and *Aortic Stenosis* for their specific nervous system sequelae)
Mental status and psychiatric aspects/ complications	May result in focal lesions as well as diffuse microemboli resulting in significant nervous system deficits including effects on speech and movement, disorientation, and dementia
Brainstem	Same as above
Cerebellum	Same as above
Vestibular system (and non-specific dizziness)	Same as above
Base of skull	Same as above

Secondary Complications: Destruction of the valves with worsening regurgitation, heart failure, valvular abscess of the infection, and embolic events are often seen early in the natural history of IE.

Treatment Complications: High risk of embolic event, and persistent and unresolved infection despite treatment with antibiotics. Surgical interventions include excision of infected area and reconstruction of damaged structure/valve, and replacement of a prosthetic valve may be necessary.

Bibliography

Baddour LM, Freeman WK, Suri RM, Wilson WR. Cardiovascular infections. In Mann DL, Zipes D, Libby P, Bonow RO, Braunwald E, eds. *Braunwald's heart disease: A textbook of cardiovascular medicine.* 10th ed. Philadelphia, PA: Elsevier/Saunders; 2015. pp. 1524–43.

Mayo Clinic Staff. Endocarditis. June 14, 2014. Available from www.mayoclinic.org/diseases-conditions/endocarditis/basics/definition/con-20022403. Accessed June 21, 2015.

Influenza

Epidemiology and Demographics: Influenza is an acute respiratory illness caused by influenza A or B viruses that occurs in outbreaks and epidemics worldwide, mainly during the winter season (which is different in the Southern and Northern Hemispheres). Dry air may dehydrate mucous membranes, preventing effective expulsion of the virus and cold temperature promote longer survival of the virus. Increased travel and increased indoor stay may promote the transmission of the virus in the colder season.

Disorder Description: The most common symptoms include high fever, runny nose, sore throat, muscle pains, headache, coughing, and fatigue. These symptoms typically begin a couple of days after exposure to the virus and most last less than a week. Infection can be transmitted via droplets through sneezing and coughing. Older adult patients may not have the typical symptoms, fever may be absent, and general symptoms such as anorexia, malaise, weakness, and dizziness may predominate. Gastrointestinal illness, such as vomiting and diarrhea, is usually not part of influenza infections in adults but can occur in 10–20% of influenza infections in children. Pneumonia is the most common complication of influenza. Central nervous system (CNS) complications include encephalopathy, encephalitis, Guillain–Barré syndrome, transverse myelitis, and aseptic meningitis. Other complications include myositis and rhabdomyolysis. Specifically, in children certain CNS complications such as acute necrotizing encephalopathy, febrile seizures, and Reye's syndrome have been described.

Rapid influenza diagnostic tests (RIDTs) are immunoassays that can identify the presence of influenza A and B viral nucleoprotein antigens in respiratory specimens, and display the result in a qualitative way. Molecular assays such as RT-PCR are recommended for testing hospitalized patients.

Symptoms

Localization site	Comment
Cerebral hemispheres	Encephalopathy/encephalitis may be seen as a complication of influenza usually affecting children younger than 5 years, with neurologic deterioration occurring 1–3 days after onset of influenza symptoms. The most common clinical findings of encephalitis are high fever, seizures, intracranial hypertension, altered consciousness, and coma. Neuroimaging results in influenza-associated encephalopathy might be normal, but in severe cases, abnormalities can include diffuse cerebral edema and bilateral thalamic lesions. Mortality can be as high as 30%. There is a report that novel influenza H1N1 is associated with increased risk of encephalopathy syndromes
	Reye's syndrome is not as common with the diminished use of aspirin in children with influenza
	Acute necrotizing encephalopathy is a fulminant type of encephalopathy characterized by multiple and symmetric brain lesions, affecting the bilateral thalami, and by the involvement of systemic organs leading to disseminated intravascular coagulation or multiorgan failure in the severest cases. It is associated with certain genetic predispositions
	Acute encephalopathy with biphasic seizures and late reduced diffusion (AESD) is associated with febrile convulsions and status epilepticus
	Mild encephalitis/encephalopathy with a reversible splenial lesion (MERS) characterized by neurologic symptoms, such as delirium, stupor, and seizures, and by the typical MRI finding of a lesion in the splenium of the corpus callosum. More common in children between 3 and 8 years of age. Outcome is good in most cases
Mental status and psychiatric aspects/ complications	Febrile delirium is a common but ill-defined syndrome prevalent among young children with acute febrile diseases. Clinically, this condition is a mild impairment of consciousness, manifested with fear, anxiety, disorientation, and hallucination, lasting for several minutes or hours
Cerebellum	Acute cerebellitis may be seen in children with influenza. It has a good prognosis
Muscle	Elevated creatine kinase was seen in about 50% of children and 25% of adults with myalgia
	In about 5.5 to 33.9% of children, a specific syndrome referred to as "benign acute childhood myositis," presenting with sudden-onset calf pain and difficulty walking, with tenderness, swelling of gastrocnemius muscles, soleus, or other muscles
	Rhabdomyolysis is a rare, potentially fatal syndrome due to the breakdown of skeletal muscle with the rapid release of large quantities of potassium, calcium, organic acids, and myoglobin, which can lead to renal tubular toxicity and acute renal failure as well as cardiac arrhythmias and compartment syndrome. A review of 300 cases of influenza-associated myositis found that only 3% developed rhabdomyolysis; however, among all viruses that cause rhabdomyolysis, influenza virus is the most common (42%)
Specific spinal roots	Guillain–Barré syndrome

Secondary Complications: Adults at high risk for complications of influenza include residents of nursing homes, age more than 65 years, pregnant women, patients with diabetes and hemoglobinopathies.

Post-encephalitis morbidity, neurologic sequelae, and mortality are high especially with the acute necrotizing variant. Death is ascribed to cerebral edema/seizures or multiorgan failure.

Kleine–Levin syndrome (rare and complex neurologic disorder characterized by recurring periods of excessive amounts of sleep and altered behavior) is described in association with influenza infection.

Treatment Complications: Vaccination is an important prophylaxis against influenza, decreasing the infection rate and preventing severe complications. Vaccines are associated with the rare complication of Guillain–Barré syndrome.

Neuraminidase inhibitors (oseltamivir, peramivir, and zanamivir) have activity against influenza A and B viruses (including H1N1), and are recommended for use preferably within the first 24 to 48 hours of symptom onset. Adverse effects include potential bronchospasm with inhaled zanamivir, and nausea, vomiting, and headache from oseltamivir. Diarrhea is the most common side effect of peramivir.

Neurologic complications are treated symptomatically – anti-seizure medications for seizures, steroids for cerebral edema, and plasma exchange or intravenous immunoglobulin for Guillain–Barré syndrome.

Bibliography

Ekstrand JJ. Neurologic complications of influenza. *Semin Pediatr Neurol.* 2012;19(3):96–100.

Mizuguchi M. Influenza encephalopathy and related neuropsychiatric syndromes. *Influenza Other Respir Viruses.* 2013; 7(Suppl. 3):67–71.

Insomnia, Chronic

Epidemiology and Demographics: Chronic insomnia occurs in approximately 10% of the population. It is more common in females and older adults. It occurs more commonly in those with medical or psychiatric disorders, substance use disorders, and of lower socioeconomic status.

A history of prior transient episodes of poor sleep, difficulty sleeping during stressful times, and those who report being light sleepers are predisposed to developing chronic insomnia. Anxiety and depression as well as restless legs syndrome, gastroesophageal reflux, and chronic pain can all be predisposing factors to chronic insomnia. Precipitators include major life events such as death of a loved one, divorce, job stress, and employment loss.

A familial pattern to chronic insomnia is not well documented though the prevalence is higher in first-degree relatives and between mothers and daughters.

Disorder Description: Chronic insomnia is characterized by difficulty initiating or maintaining sleep. For diagnosis, symptoms must be present for at least 3 months and occur at least 3 times a week. Often there are complaints of early wake ups, with termination of sleep at least 30 minutes before the desired waking time and reduced total sleep time. In children there may be resistance to going to sleep and difficulty sleeping without caregiver intervention. The degree of sleep disturbance is dependent on the subjective sleep complaints by the individual. In general, sleep onset latency and periods of wakefulness after sleep onset are considered to be clinically significant when >20 minutes in children and young adults and >30 minutes in adults.

There must be an adequate opportunity to sleep in an appropriate environment (i.e., quiet, dark, and comfortable).

These disruptions to sleep initiation and sleep maintenance must result in daytime consequences such as sleepiness, fatigue, or functional impairment.

The sleep/wake difficulty cannot better be explained by another sleep disorder. A polysomnogram is not indicated in the routine evaluation of insomnia though it is helpful in evaluating for other sleep disorders. Chronic insomnia can occur in isolation or in relation to a mental disorder, medical condition, or substance use.

Symptoms

Localization site	Comment
Mental status and psychiatric aspects/ complications	Physiologic hyperarousal during sleep and wakefulness – increased heart rate, increased cortisol and adrenocorticotropin levels, and altered heart rate variability. Increased body temperature during NREM sleep
	Daytime fatigue with lack of energy, reduced concentration, attention and motivation, memory impairment, and irritability

Secondary Complications: Daytime fatigue with lack of energy, reduced concentration, attention and motivation, memory impairment, and irritability may all be associated with insomnia. Individuals may report reduced performance at work or school and impaired social functioning. There is an increased risk of depression, hypertension, work disability, and prolonged use of prescription hypnotics and over-the-counter sleep aids.

Treatment Complications: Initial approach to treatment includes behavioral therapy with counseling on sleep hygiene and stimulus control. Behavioral therapies including sleep restriction therapy and cognitive behavioral therapy should be considered. Treatment of underlying medical conditions, pain, or psychiatric disorders that may be contributing to insomnia is also imperative.

Medications such as hypnotics (nonbenzodiazepine BZ-receptor agonists zolpidem, zaleplon, and eszopiclone; orexin receptor antagonist suvorexant; melatonin receptor agonist ramelteon; benzodiazepine hypnotic temazepam) and sedating antidepressants (trazadone, mirtazepine) may be used alone or in combination with behavioral therapies.

All hypnotics may cause residual daytime somnolence with morning performance impairment and rebound insomnia after discontinuation. Respiratory suppression may also occur with some hypnotics and can worsen obstructive sleep apnea and hypoventilation. Complex sleep-related behaviors such as somnambulism, driving, and sleep eating can occur as well. Combination with alcohol or another central nervous system depressant can lead to overdose and respiratory depression.

Multiple observational studies have found an association between long-term use of hypnotics and all-cause mortality, although causality has not been established. As many patients who use hypnotic drugs also have other medical and psychiatric disorders, there are likely multiple confounders to these findings. There has yet to be a prospective study examining the effects and long-term risk of hypnotic use versus placebo or behavioral therapy.

Bibliography

American Academy of Sleep Medicine. *International classification of sleep disorders*, 3rd ed. Darien, IL: American Academy of Sleep Medicine, 2014.

Bonnet MH, Arand DL. Consequences of insomnia. *Sleep Med Clin*. 2006;1:351.

Bonnet MH, Arand DL, Javaheri S. Cardiovascular implications of poor sleep. *Sleep Med Clin*. 2007;2:529.

Buscemi N, Vendermeer B, Friesen C, et al. The efficacy and safety of drug treatments for chronic insomnia in adults: a meta-analysis of RCTs. *J Gen Intern Med*. 2007;22:1335.

Kripke DF, Langer RD, Kline LE. Hypnotics' association with mortality or cancer: a matched cohort study. *BMJ Open*. 2012;2:e000850.

LeBlanc M, Merette C, Savard J, et al. Incidence and risk factors of insomnia in a population-base sample. *Sleep*. 2009;32:1027.

Vgontzas AN, Liao D, Bixler EO, Chrousos GP, Vela-Bueno A. Insomnia with objective short sleep duration is associated with a high risk for hypertension. *Sleep*. 2009;32:491.

Insomnia, Short-Term

Epidemiology and Demographics: Short-term insomnia has a 1-year prevalence of 15–20%. It is more common in females and older adults. It occurs more commonly in those with medical or psychiatric disorders, substance use disorders, and of lower socioeconomic status.

Predisposing Factors: A history of prior transient episodes of poor sleep, difficulty sleeping during stressful times, and those who report being light sleepers predisposes to development of insomnia. Precipitators include major life events such as death of a loved one, divorce, job stress, and employment loss.

Disorder Description: Short-term insomnia is characterized by difficulty initiating or maintaining sleep. For diagnosis, symptoms must be present for less than 3 months and less than 3 nights a week. Often there are complaints of early wake ups, with termination of sleep at least 30 minutes before the desired waking time and reduced total sleep time. The degree of sleep disturbance is dependent on the subjective sleep complaints by the individual. In general, sleep onset latency and periods of wakefulness after sleep onset are considered to be clinically significant when >20 minutes in children and young adults and >30 minutes in adults. There must be an adequate opportunity to sleep in an appropriate environment (i.e., quiet, dark, comfortable).

These disruptions to sleep initiation and sleep maintenance must result in daytime consequences such as sleepiness, fatigue, or functional impairment.

The sleep/wake difficulty cannot better be explained by another sleep disorder.

Symptoms

Localization site	Comment
Brainstem, cerebral cortex	Increased metabolic activity in the pontine tegmentum and in thalamocortical networks in a frontal, anterior temporal, and anterior cingulate distribution
Mental status and psychiatric aspects/ complications	Physiologic hyperarousal during sleep and wakefulness – increased heart rate, increased cortisol and adrenocorticotropin levels, and altered heart rate variability. Increased body temperature during NREM sleep
	Daytime fatigue with lack of energy, reduced concentration, attention and motivation, memory impairment, and irritability

Secondary Complications: Daytime fatigue with lack of energy, reduced concentration, attention and motivation, memory impairment, and irritability may all be associated with insomnia. Individuals may report reduced performance at work or school and impaired social functioning. There is an increased risk of depression, hypertension, work disability, and use of prescription hypnotics and over-the-counter sleep aids.

Treatment Complications: Initial approach to treatment includes behavioral therapy with counseling on sleep hygiene and stimulus control. Treatment of underlying medical conditions, pain, or psychiatric disorders that may be contributing to insomnia is also imperative.

Short-term use of hypnotic medications such as nonbenzodiazepine BZ-receptor agonists zolpidem, zaleplon, and eszopiclone, orexin receptor antagonist suvorexant, melatonin receptor angonist ramelteon, and benzodiazepine hypnotic temazepam may be used alone or in combination with behavioral therapies. Over-the-counter hypnotics such as antihistamines may be considered.

All hypnotics may cause residual daytime somnolence with morning performance impairment and rebound insomnia after discontinuation. Respiratory suppression may also occur with some hypnotics and can worsen obstructive sleep apnea and hypoventilation. Complex sleep-related behaviors such as somnambulism, driving, and sleep eating can occur as well. Combination with alcohol or another central nervous system depressant can lead to overdose and respiratory depression.

Multiple observational studies have found an association between long-term use of hypnotics and all-cause mortality, although causality has not been established. As many patients who use hypnotic drugs also have other medical and psychiatric disorders, there are likely multiple confounders to these findings. There has yet to be a prospective study examining the effects and long-term risk of hypnotic use versus placebo or behavioral therapy.

Bibliography

American Academy of Sleep Medicine. *International classification of sleep disorders*. 3rd ed. Darien, IL: American Academy of Sleep Medicine; 2014.

Ellis JG, Gehrman P, Espie CA, et al. Acute insomnia: Current conceptualizations and future directions. *Sleep Med Rev*. 2012;16:5–14.

Nofzinger EA, Nissen C, Germain A, et al. Regional cerebral metabolic correlates of WASO during sleep in insomnia. *J Clin Sleep Med*. 2006;2:316–22.

Insufficient Sleep Syndrome

Epidemiology and Demographics: All ages and both sexes are affected. A higher frequency occurs in adolescents who have increased sleep requirements, but due to a tendency toward delayed sleep time and societal pressure for early wake up times, will obtain inadequate sleep. No familial pattern is known.

Disorder Description: Patient's sleep time as determined by history, sleep logs, and/or actigraphy is usually shorter than expected for age. This results in excessive daytime somnolence. Extension of total sleep time results in resolution of these symptoms.

Associated symptoms include irritability, deficits in concentration, reduced vigilance, dysphoria, malaise, and anergia.

Symptoms

Localization site	Comment
Mental status and psychiatric aspects/ complications	Irritability, deficits in concentration, reduced vigilance, dysphoria, and anergia

Secondary Complications: Increased daytime sleepiness, inability to concentrate, and low energy levels may lead to social dysfunction and impact employment and school performance. Stimulant abuse, motor vehicle accidents, and injuries may occur.

Insufficient sleep has been associated with increased prevalence of obesity, diabetes, and hypertension.

Treatment Complications: Treatment goal is to increase total sleep time.

Bibliography

American Academy of Sleep Medicine. *The international classification of sleep disorders*. 3rd ed. Chicago, IL: American Academy of Sleep Medicine; 2014.

Knutson KL. Sleep duration and cardiometabolic risk: a review of the epidemiologic evidence. *Best Pract Res Clin Endocrinol Metab*. 2010;24:731–43.

Tucker AM, Whitney P, Belenky G, Hinson JM, Van Dongen HPA. Effects of sleep deprivation on dissociated components of executive functioning. *Sleep*. 2010;33:45–57.

Intensive Care Unit (ICU) Psychosis (and Postoperative Psychosis)

Epidemiology and Demographics: The prevalence of delirium in medical and surgical intensive care unit (ICU) settings has varied from 20 to 80% in studies.

Disorder Description: See also entry for *Delirium*.

DSM-5 describes delirium as a disturbance in attention and cognition over a short period of time. ICU psychosis is a phrase used by many clinicians to describe delirium in the context of an acutely ill patient, often in a medical or surgical ICU setting. The American Psychiatric Association and many experts recommend that the term "delirium" be used uniformly to describe this disturbance, regardless of setting. Factors that are believed to play a part in this are: sensory deprivation (being placed in a room without windows, and away from friends/family), sensory overload (machines that create noise day and night), pain (uncontrolled specifically), sleep deprivation, disruption of the normal day–night rhythm, pre-existing cognitive impairment, advanced age, psychoactive drugs (such as opiates), prolonged immobilization, and loss of control over their lives that patients feel while in ICU. One patient in every three who spends more than 5 days in an ICU experiences some form of psychotic reaction. More recently, it was shown that 40% of older ICU patients had ongoing delirium during the post-ICU period and that almost 20% of elderly patients had delirium at the time of admission to subacute facilities.

Differential Diagnosis: See entry for *Delirium*.

Secondary Complications: In medical ICU patients, delirium is associated with adverse outcomes and hospital stay complications, increased healthcare costs, and mortality. Self-extubation, removal of catheters, and failed extubation are more common in ICU patients with delirium. Delirium in ICU patients was also predictive of neurocognitive decline 1–3 years after hospital discharge.

Treatment Complications: Typical and atypical antipsychotics including haloperidol and olanzapine have been successful in treatment studies of delirium in the ICU setting, albeit lacking placebo control groups. Side effects of typical antipsychotics include the extrapyramidal side effects including parkinsonism (mask-like facies, bradykinesia, cogwheel rigidity, pill-rolling tremor), akathisia, and dystonia. Other side effects include hyperprolactinemia, and sedation, weight gain, orthostatic hypotension, cardiac abnormalities, sexual dysfunction, anticholinergic side effects (dry mouth, tachycardia, urinary retention, blurry vision, constipation, worsening of narrow-angle glaucoma), tardive dyskinesia, and neuroleptic malignant syndrome. Atypical antipsychotic side effects are similar, but more frequently and to a larger extent include metabolic syndrome, weight gain, hyperlipidemia, and hyperglycemia. Melatonin has also been shown to be useful, to restore the normal sleep cycle and circadian rhythm. This has been helpful to reduce "sundowning" in patients (being more confused at night as part of the delirium).

Besides anti-psychotic medication, some non-pharmacologic interventions are helpful. These are frequent re-orientation by the staff, keeping the lights on during the daytime, and having the clock visible to the patient. These interventions in addition to pharmacologic therapy can decrease the length of delirium.

Bibliography

Al-Aama T, Brymer C, Gutmanis I, et al. Melatonin decreases delirium in elderly patients: A randomized, placebo-controlled trial. *Int J Geriatr Psychiatry*. 2011;26(7):687–94.

American Psychiatric Association. *Diagnostic and statistical manual of mental disorders: DSM-5*. 5th ed. Washington, DC: American Psychiatric Association; 2013.

Cavallazzi R, Saad M, Marik PE. Delirium in the ICU: an overview. *Ann Intens Care*. 2012; 2(1):1.

Ely E, Gautam S, Margolin R, et al. The impact of delirium in the intensive care unit on hospital length of stay. *Intensive Care Med*. 2001;27(12):1892–1900.

Ely EW, Shintani A, Truman B, et al. Delirium as a predictor of mortality in mechanically ventilated patients in the intensive care unit. *JAMA*. 2004;291(14):1753–62.

Girard TD, Pandharipande PP, Ely EW. Delirium in the intensive care unit. *Crit Care*. 2008;12(Suppl 3):S3.

Inouye SK, Bogardus ST Jr, Charpentier PA, et al. A multicomponent intervention to prevent delirium in hospitalized older patients. *New Engl J Med*. 1999; 340(9):669–76.

Intermittent Explosive Disorder

Epidemiology and Demographics: Intermittent explosive disorder (IED) has an annual prevalence in the US population of approximately 2.7%. It is more prevalent among younger individuals (<40 years) and those with a high school education or less. Some studies have shown increased prevalence among males, but others have shown no difference between genders. IED is an impulse control disorder and the hallmark of IED is "reactive aggression" as opposed to "proactive aggression." Reactive aggression is when the individual acts out impulsively when faced with a situation that induces anger or frustration, e.g., a teenager who is angry with his teacher for setting limits "blows up" and throws a chair at the teacher. His impulsivity keeps him from acknowledging the consequences of this action.

It is important to note that irritability is a frequent indicator of mood disorders such as depression and bipolar disorder. Especially in children and the elderly, anger and irritability is a common presenting symptom of depression. It is essential to rule out comorbid psychiatric conditions through a thorough psychiatric assessment.

Disorder Description: As per DSM-5, IED can be defined as:

A. Recurrent behavioral outbursts representing a failure to control aggressive impulses as manifested by either of the following:
   i. Verbal aggression (e.g., temper tantrums, tirades, verbal arguments), physical aggression toward property, animals, or other individuals, occurring twice weekly, on average, for a period of 3 months. The physical aggression does not result in damage or destruction of property and does not result in physical injury to animals or other individuals.
   ii. Three behavioral outbursts involving damage or destruction of property and/or physical assault involving physical injury against animals or other individuals occurring within a 12-month period.

B. The magnitude of aggressiveness expressed during the recurrent outbursts is grossly out of proportion to the provocation or to any precipitating psychosocial stressors.

C. The recurrent aggressive outbursts cause either marked distress in the individual or impairment in occupational or interpersonal functioning, or are associated with financial or legal consequences.

D. Chronologic age is **at least 6 years** (or equivalent developmental level).

E. The recurrent aggressive outbursts are not better explained by another mental disorder (e.g., major depressive disorder, bipolar disorder, disruptive mood dysregulation disorder, a psychotic disorder, antisocial personality disorder, borderline personality disorder) and are not attributable to another medical condition (e.g., head trauma, Alzheimer's disease) or to the physiologic effects of a substance (e.g., a drug of abuse, a medication). For children aged 6–18 years, aggressive behavior that occurs as part of an adjustment disorder should not be considered for this diagnosis.

Differential Diagnosis: Differential diagnosis should include disruptive mood regulation disorder, antisocial personality disorder, delirium, major neurocognitive disorder, and personality change due to another medical condition (aggressive type), attention-deficit hyperactivity disorder (ADHD), conduct disorder, oppositional defiant disorder, and autism spectrum disorder.

In contrast to intermittent explosive disorder, disruptive mood dysregulation disorder is characterized by a persistently negative mood state most of the day nearly every day in between explosive outbursts.

In antisocial personality disorder any impulsive or aggressive outbursts tend to be much lower in intensity and severity than in intermittent explosive disorder. The hallmark of antisocial personality disorder is proactive aggression where acts are planned, contemplated, and executed.

In delirium, major neurocognitive disorder, and personality changes due to another medical condition, there may be aggressive or impulsive outbursts. However, these outbursts are secondary to the other mental condition. The aggression usually resolves when the underlying medical cause is addressed.

In substance or medication intoxication or withdrawal, impulsive or aggressive outbursts occur secondary to intoxication or withdrawal from a substance. Such substances include alcohol, phencyclidine (PCP), cocaine and other stimulants, barbiturates, and inhalants among many others. The onus is on the clinician to stay up to date on the latest drugs on the streets, for example, K2 or bath salts.

Websites such as www.Erowid.org can help one to stay abreast with the latest substances in use.

In ADHD, conduct disorder, oppositional defiant disorder, and autism spectrum disorder, individuals may also have impulsive or aggressive outbursts. Individuals with ADHD are typically impulsive, and may thus exhibit impulsive aggressive outbursts. Aggression associated with ADHD typically remits with ADHD treatment. Individuals with conduct disorder may also exhibit impulsive aggressive outbursts, but the form of aggression, as in antisocial personality disorder, is proactive and predatory. Aggression in oppositional defiant disorder is typically characterized by temper tantrums and arguments with authoritative figures, whereas outbursts in IED occur in a much broader context.

Secondary Complications: IED can lead to social, financial, occupational, and legal problems. Depressive disorders, anxiety disorders, and substance use disorders are frequently comorbid with intermittent explosive disorder.

Treatment Complications: Treatment usually consists of psychotherapy and/or medications.

Psychotherapy may utilize a cognitive-behavioral approach. If legal issues are frequent, the patient may require mandated treatment.

Commonly used medications include selective serotonin reuptake inhibitors (SSRIs) and anticonvulsant mood-stabilizers in refractory cases. Antipsychotic medications may also be efficacious. In emergency settings, high-potency antipsychotics such as haloperidol are usually combined with benzodiazepines such as lorazepam for the treatment of acute agitation.

SSRI side effects include nausea, diarrhea, insomnia, headache, anorexia, weight loss, sexual dysfunction, restlessness (akathisia-like), serotonin syndrome (fever diaphoresis, tachycardia, hypertension, delirium, neuromuscular excitability), hyponatremia, and seizures (0.2%).

Anticonvulsant mood stabilizers may be used in the treatment of IED that is refractory to SSRIs. Valproic acid, oxcarbazepine, or carbamazepine may be utilized. Levetiracetam should be avoided in patients with aggression, mood disorders, or suicidality.

Bibliography

American Psychiatric Association. *Diagnostic and statistical manual of mental disorders: DSM-5.* 5th ed. Washington, DC: American Psychiatric Association; 2013.

Best M, Williams JM, Coccaro EF. Evidence for a dysfunctional prefrontal circuit in patients with an impulsive aggressive disorder. *Proc Nat Acad Sci.* 2002;99(12):8448–53.

Coccaro EF. Intermittent explosive disorder. *Curr Psychiatry Rep.* 2000;2(1):67–71.

Coccaro EF, Lee EF, Kavoussi RJ. A double-blind, randomized, placebo-controlled trial of fluoxetine in patients with intermittent explosive disorder. *J Clin Psychiatry.* 2009;70(5):653–62.

Davanzo P, Yue K, Thomas MA, et al. Proton magnetic resonance spectroscopy of bipolar disorder versus intermittent explosive disorder in children and adolescents. *Am J Psychiatry.* 2003;160(8):1442–52.

Jones RM, Arlidge J, Gillham R, et al. Efficacy of mood stabilisers in the treatment of impulsive or repetitive aggression: systematic review and meta-analysis. *Br J Psychiatry.* 2011;198(2):93–8.

Kant R, Chalansani R, Chengappa KR, Dieringer MF. The off-label use of clozapine in adolescents with bipolar disorder, intermittent explosive disorder, or posttraumatic stress disorder. *J Child Adolesc Psychopharmacol.* 2004; 14(1):57–63.

McCloskey MS, Noblett KL, Deffenbacher JL, Gollan JK, Coccaro EF. Cognitive-behavioral therapy for intermittent explosive disorder: a pilot randomized clinical trial. *J Consult Clin Psychol.* 2008;76(5):876.

Murray-Close D, Ostrov JM, Nelson DA, Crick NR, Coccaro EF. Proactive, reactive, and romantic relational aggression in adulthood: Measurement, predictive validity, gender differences, and association with Intermittent Explosive Disorder. *J Psychiatr Res.* 2010;44(6):393–404.

Olvera RL. Intermittent explosive disorder. *CNS Drugs.* 2002;16(8):517–26.

Internal Iliac Artery Ischemia

Epidemiology and Demographics: Internal iliac artery ischemia is caused by internal iliac artery stenosis (IIAS). Incidence and prevalence of IIAS have not been established in the general population. IIAS is often associated with common iliac artery stenosis. The major etiology is atherosclerosis. The internal iliac artery may be ligated intentionally to control severe pelvic bleeding.

Disorder Description: The main symptom of IIAS is claudication at lower back, hip, buttock, or thigh, which is called proximal claudication (or buttock claudication). As a vascular claudication, symptoms are typically induced by ambulation and rapidly fade with rest, but it can be variable and mimic non-vascular claudication. Pain may appear when IIAS is severe.

Symptoms

Localization site	Comment
Plexus	Acute lumbosacral plexopathies have been reported after surgical internal iliac artery clamping, especially in older patients with known vascular disease. Acute burning pain in the affected limb with multiple peripheral neuropathies is more common than isolated mononeuropathy
Muscle	Ischemic myopathy may occur to the muscles served by the internal iliac artery (iliopsoas and quadratus lumborum). Patients may experience weakened hip flexion on the affected side

Secondary Complications: No clear secondary complications have been reported.

Treatment Complications: Endovascular angioplasty and stenting is the treatment of choice. The most common procedural complication is a small dissection near the internal iliac artery. Although there is a theoretical risk of thrombosis, no severe neurologic complications have been reported.

Bibliography

Mahé G, Kaladji A, Le Faucheur A, Jaquinandi V. Internal iliac artery stenosis: diagnosis and how to manage it in 2015. *Front Cardiovasc Med.* 2015;2:33. DOI: 10.3389/fcvm.2015.00033.

Shin RK, Stecker MM, Imbesi SG. Peripheral nerve ischaemia after internal iliac artery ligation. *J Neurol Neurosurg Psychiatry* 2001;70:411–12. DOI:10.1136/jnnp.70.3.411.

Intra-arterial Injections

Epidemiology and Demographics: Most drugs are delivered intravenously. Rarely, intra-arterial injections may occur inadvertently, most commonly in the antecubital fossa, where branches of ulnar and brachial arteries are superficial and easily entered.

There are no clear epidemiologic data on intra-arterial injection.

Disorder Description: The initial symptom of an intra-arterial injection is an immediate severe burning pain radiating distally from the injection site. Thereafter, various peripheral sensory and motor dysfunctions follow. Pathophysiologic mechanism remains unclear. Several theories have been proposed, such as endothelial inflammation, thrombosis, high osmolality, and norepinephrine-induced vasoconstriction. All proposed mechanisms involve tissue ischemia distal to the injection site.

Symptoms

Localization site	Comment
Peripheral neuropathy	Ischemic polyneuropathy can be induced, especially distal to the injection site. Uncomfortable paresthesias occur immediately after injection. Further pain will develop as a part of compartment syndrome
Muscle	Ischemic myopathy can occur due to occlusion of distal arteries from injection-induced thrombosis. Muscle weakness and involuntary muscle contracture have been reported

Secondary Complications: Few data are available on secondary complications.

Treatment Complications: Because of the incomplete understanding of the pathophysiology, specific treatment algorithms have not been developed. Removal of the intra-arterial catheter and anticoagulation is commonly proposed treatment. However, anticoagulation can increase the risk of hemorrhage, especially for the patients who already have had a large acute stroke.

Bibliography

Sen S, et al. Complications after unintentional intra-arterial injection of drugs: risks, outcomes, and management strategies. *Mayo Clin Proc.* 2005;80(6):783–95.

Intracranial Atherosclerosis

Epidemiology and Demographics: Intracranial atherosclerosis is one of the major etiologies of ischemic stroke. In the United States, it causes 50,000 strokes annually. Non-Caucasians have higher rates of intracranial atherosclerosis than Caucasians. Conversely, Caucasians have higher rates of extracranial atherosclerosis. The prevalence of strokes in intracranial atherosclerosis is 3, 13, and 15 per 100,000 for Caucasians, Hispanics, and African-Americans, respectively.

Disorder Description: Atherosclerosis is a narrowing and hardening of the arteries, caused by a plaque build-up around the arterial walls, especially around bifurcations. Over time, the build-up can reduce or block blood flow, which leads to tissue ischemia. Contributing risk factors include smoking, hypertension, diabetes, hypercholesterolemia, and obesity (the metabolic syndrome).

Symptoms

Localization site	Comment
Cerebral hemispheres	Intracranial atherosclerosis is a major cause of ischemic stroke. This more commonly affects large arteries than small arterioles. Transient blood flow reduction due to high-grade stenosis or platelet plugging can cause transient ischemic attack. Complete occlusion of major vessels causes highly localized neurologic symptoms related to the occluded vascular territory. (See other stroke-related entries in this book)
Mental status and psychiatric aspects/ complications	Major vessel occlusion, especially middle cerebral artery, can easily put patients in altered mental status. Complete posterior cerebral artery (PCA) infarct can also cause severe mental status change, by involving thalami. (See entry for *Middle Cerebral Artery Occlusion*)
Brainstem	Brainstem infarct is associated with intracranial atherosclerosis, especially of the vertebral or basilar arteries. If the basilar artery is involved, this can lead to ischemic stroke of bilateral PCA, superior cerebellar artery (SCA), and anterior inferior cerebellar artery (AICA) territory
Cerebellum	Again, if the basilar artery is occluded, the SCA or AICA territory is at risk of infarction, including the upper and middle portions of the cerebellum
Cranial nerves	Cranial nerve symptoms usually occur as a part of brainstem stroke

Secondary Complications: Atherosclerosis can also occur in extracranial arteries. If proximal extracranial vessels (e.g., ICA) have narrowed and the patient experiences a sudden drop in blood pressure, this can induce watershed infarcts ipsilaterally. These patients have higher risk of ischemic heart disease and peripheral arterial disease.

Treatment Complications: Mainstay of atherosclerosis treatment is daily low-dose aspirin, cholesterol-lowering medications (statins), and lifestyle modification. Long-term usage of statins may increase risk of statin-induced myopathy. Aspirin may increase the risk of mucocutaneous bleeding slightly.

Bibliography

Jeng J-S, et al. Epidemiology, diagnosis and management of intracranial atherosclerotic disease. *Expert Rev Cardiovasc Ther*. 2010; 8(10):1423–32.

Arenillas JF. Intracranial atherosclerosis: current concepts. *Stroke*. 2011;42:S20–3.

Intravascular Malignant Lymphomatosis

Epidemiology and Demographics: It is a rare malignancy and hence the true incidence is unknown. Most of the literature is from case series and case reports. Median age at diagnosis is in the sixth to seventh decades; there is no sex predilection.

Disorder Description: Intravascular lymphomatosis is a rare neoplastic disorder due to malignant proliferation of lymphocytes occurring exclusively in the vessels. Central nervous system and skin involvement are common. There are multiple small- and large-vessel occlusions by neoplastic cells.

Symptoms

Localization site	Comment
Cerebral hemispheres	Seizures and stroke-like episodes, gait disturbance with asymmetric lower limb weakness (left > right), urinary retention, and diffuse headache
Mental status and psychiatric aspects/ complications	Dementia (most common symptom) and delirium
Cerebellum	Ataxia (cerebellar infarctions)
Spinal cord	Progressive urinary retention and weakness (spinal cord infarction due to occlusion of vessels with large lymphoma cells)

Localization site	Comment
Dorsal root ganglia	Dysesthesia (occlusion of parenchymal small vessels of dorsal root ganglia with large lymphoma cells)
Specific spinal roots	Polyradiculopathy (occlusion of parenchymal small vessels of spinal roots with large lymphoma cells)
Muscle	Lower motor neuron (LMN) type of weakness (tumor cells were also identified at targets in between nerve roots and muscles)

Treatment Complications: R-CHOP regimen (rituximab, cyclophosphamide, doxorubicin, vincristine, and prednisone) is used for treatment. This can result in cardiomyopathy, neuropathy, and pulmonary complications such as *Pneumocystis jirovecii* pneumonia, drug-induced interstitial fibrosis, and pulmonary tuberculosis.

Bibliography

Beristain X, Azzarelli B. The neurological masquerade of intravascular lymphomatosis. *Arch Neurol.* 2002;59(3):439–43.

Fonkem E, Dayawansa S, Stroberg E, et al. Neurological presentations of intravascular lymphoma (IVL): meta-analysis of 654 patients. *BMC Neurol.* 2016;16:9.

Mihaljevic B, Sternic N, Skender Gazibara M, et al. Intravascular large B-cell lymphoma of central nervous system: a report of two cases and literature review. *Clin Neuropathol.* 2010;29(4):233–8.

Intraventricular Hemorrhage (IVH)

Epidemiology and Demographics: Primary intraventricular hemorrhage (IVH) is uncommon, accounting for 3% of all spontaneous hemorrhages. Secondary IVH, which is an extension of blood from intracerebral hemorrhage (ICH) or subarachnoid hemorrhage (SAH), is more common. Incidence of secondary IVH lies between 19.1% and 55.26% among 12 retrospective and prospective trials.

Disorder Description: IVH is an extension of intracranial hemorrhage into the ventricles and can happen early or late in the sequence of events. Data demonstrate that the amount of blood in the ventricles relates directly to the clinical outcome. Patients always have symptoms of SAH or ICH with the symptoms described below.

Symptoms

Localization site	Comment
Mental status and psychiatric aspects/ complications	Blood in the ventricles may clot and obstruct CSF outflow. This can lead to hydrocephalus and increased intracranial pressure, which produces disorientation, confusion, headache, nausea, and vomiting
Brainstem	Blood in the ventricles circulates with CSF, and tends to clot and obstruct CSF outflow. If it occludes the foramen of Magendie or Luschka, the aqueduct of Sylvius, or the 4th ventricle, the hematoma can compress the brainstem, leading to cranial neuropathies, altered consciousness, and respiratory compromise
Cerebellum	Cerebellum can be compressed by hematoma in 4th ventricle with symptoms such as ataxia, dysmetria, or oscillopsia
Cranial nerves	Isolated cranial nerve abnormalities are uncommon. CN III and VI are the most commonly affected nerves, due to stretching across the basilar skull surface. These are important "false localizing" signs

Secondary Complications: Most patients become bedbound for a long time, which can increase risk of deep vein thrombosis, pneumonia, urinary tract infections, and muscular atrophy.

Treatment Complications: Classical ventriculostomy is the treatment of choice if obstructive hydrocephalus occurs secondary to IVH. Similar to other neurosurgical procedures, this can mildly increase risk of intracranial hemorrhage or infection and, less commonly, injury to the neural tissues near the surgical site.

Bibliography

Hanley DF. Intraventricular hemorrhage: severity factor and treatment target in spontaneous intracerebral hemorrhage. *Stroke.* 2009;40:1533–8.

Iron Deficiency

Epidemiology and Demographics: Iron deficiency anemia is present in 1–2% in the United States. In developed countries, iron deficiency *without* anemia is more common, occurring in as many as 10% of women.

Disorder Description: Primary cause of iron deficiency in developed countries is blood loss. Decreased iron intake is a more common cause in developing regions. Decreased iron absorption is an uncommon cause but can occur in malabsorption syndromes. Iron is used not only in hemoglobin formation but also is essential in multiple cellular processes, hence deficiency results in neurologic symptoms. In non-inflamed states, total body iron stores are best measured by serum ferritin levels rather than absolute blood iron levels.[1]

Symptoms

Localization site	Comment
Unclear localization	Pica – appetite for non-food items such as ice, dirt, or paper. Restless leg syndrome characterized by discomfort in legs at rest resolved with movement. Fatigue and difficulty concentrating are common. Unusual eating behaviors of pregnancy may be related to relative iron deficiency

Secondary Complications: Increased risk of preterm labor during pregnancy. Iron deficiency may be associated with worsening heart failure.

Treatment Complications: The benefit of treating asymptomatic iron deficiency for fatigue is unclear. In areas with endemic malaria, iron supplementation may increase susceptibility to malaria (the *Plasmodium* parasite is less efficient at infecting iron-deficient erythrocytes).

Reference

1. Camaschella C. Iron-deficiency anemia. *N Engl J Med.* 2015;372:1832–43.

Irregular Sleep–Wake Rhythm Disorder

Epidemiology and Demographics: There is no known sex predominance. The disorder may occur at any age. Compared with the general population, irregular sleep–wake rhythm disorder (ISWRD) is commonly observed in patients with neurodegenerative disorders, psychiatric disorders, and in children with developmental disorders. Patients with Alzheimer's disease, Parkinson's disease, and Huntington's disease, children with developmental disorders such as autism, Asperger's syndrome, or pervasive developmental disorders not otherwise specified, and patients with schizophrenia are the most commonly reported to have ISWRD. Poor sleep hygiene and lack of exposure to zeitgebers may predispose to the development of ISWRD.

Disorder Description: Patients with ISWRD lack a defined circadian rhythm of sleep and wake. They tend to have fragmented sleep with the longest bouts of sleep being 2–4 hours in duration. Often these patients take multiple naps throughout the daytime to make up for decreased sleep time at night. Symptoms may include insomnia and excessive sleepiness; however, this will vary based upon their particular sleep–wake pattern. Patients present with complaints of difficulty initiating sleep, trouble awakening in the morning, and excessive daytime sleepiness. The abnormalities of ISWRD are thought to be multifactorial in origin, including decreased visual input to the suprachiasmatic nuclei and lack of a strong day–night rhythm in the institutionalized environment.

Diagnosis of irregular sleep–wake rhythm disorder is made if the patient meets the following criteria: (1) there is a chronic or recurrent pattern of irregular sleep and wake episodes throughout the 24-hour period with symptoms of insomnia during the scheduled sleep period or excessive daytime sleepiness or both; (2) the symptoms are present for ≥3 months; (3) sleep log and when possible actigraphy for ≥7 days demonstrates no major sleep period and ≥3 irregular sleep bouts during a 24-hour period; and (4) the sleep disturbance is not better explained by another disorder or medication.

Sleep logs and actigraphy are key instruments and 7–14 days of data are needed to ensure that working and non-working days are included. Although not necessary, biologic markers of endogenous circadian timing such as salivary or plasma dim light melatonin onset can provide important information.

Symptoms

Localization site	Comment
Cerebral hemispheres	The main site of the endogenous circadian rhythm is in the suprachiasmatic nuclei
Mental status and psychiatric aspects/complications	In adolescents may present with school absences, chronic tardiness, and academic failure

Secondary Complications: In the elderly there is an increased risk of nocturnal wandering and falls.

Treatment Complications: The approach to patients with ISWRD must be individualized and different approaches should be taken in the population of elderly adults with dementia compared with children and adolescents with neurologic disorders. For the elderly with dementia, studies involving light therapy in the morning to consolidate sleep and improve behavior have had mixed results. The American Academy of Sleep Medicine (AASM) recommends against the use of sleep-promoting medications, melatonin or melatonin agonists, and combination treatments in this population. For children and adolescents with neurologic disorders, the ASSM recommends timed oral administration of melatonin or melatonin agonists.

Bibliography

Abbott SM, Zee PC. Irregular sleep-wake rhythm disorder. *Sleep Med Clin.* 2015;10:517–22.

Ancoli-Israel S, Gehrman P, Martin JL, et al. Increased light exposure consolidates sleep and strengthens circadian rhythms in severe Alzheimer's disease patients. *Behav Sleep Med.* 2003;1:22–36.

Auger RR, Burgess HJ, Emens JS, et al. Clinical practice guideline for the treatment of intrinsic circadian rhythm sleep-wake disorders: Advanced sleep-wake phase disorder (ASWPD), delayed sleep-wake phase disorder (DSWPD), non-24-hour sleep-wake rhythm disorder (N24SWD), and irregular sleep-wake rhythm disorder (ISWRD). An update for 2015: An American Academy of Sleep Medicine Clinical Practice Guideline. *J Clin Sleep Med.* 2015;11:1199–236.

Bjorvatn B, Pallesen S. A practical approach to circadian rhythm sleep disorders. *Sleep Med Rev.* 2009;13:47–60.

Sack RL, Auckley D, Auger RR, et al. Circadian rhythm sleep disorders: Part II, Advanced sleep phase disorder, delayed sleep phase disorder, free-running disorder, and irregular sleep-wake rhythm. *Sleep.* 2007;30:1484–501.

Sateia M, Berry RB, Bornemann MC, et al. *International classification of sleep disorders.* 3rd ed. Darien, IL: American Academy of Sleep Medicine; 2014.

Ischemic Demyelination

Epidemiology and Demographics: Ischemic white matter lesions are present in Binswanger disease, migraine, and CADASIL (cerebral autosomal dominant arteriopathy with subcortical infarcts and leukoencephalopathy). Ischemic white matter lesions also have an association with intracerebral hemorrhage.

Prevalence of Binswanger disease is 1.2–4.2% in patients over the age of 65. There are no consistent data on gender predilection.

Migraine is most common between the ages of 30 and 39. Prevalence is 24% in women and 7% in men.

The prevalence of CADASIL is 2/100,000. The age of onset is typically adulthood, and men and women are equally affected.

Prevalence of amyloid angiopathy is 2.3% for 65–74, 8% for 75–84, and 12.1% for more than 85 years old. There is no strong predilection for gender.

Disorder Description: Binswanger disease, also known as subcortical arteriosclerotic encephalopathy, is associated with extensive microvascular ischemic changes or white matter lesions due to hypertension. It is associated with cognitive decline and cortical release signs may be found on exam. CADASIL is an autosomal dominant neurologic disorder. It is characterized by stroke-like symptoms, migraine, white matter angiopathy in subcortical and periventricular areas, and dementia as the disease progresses. It is diagnosed by genetic testing, which shows a mutation in the Notch3 gene, or by skin biopsy, which reveals granular osmiophilic material. Patients with migraine can have white matter ischemic changes on MRI with no other risk factors. Finally, lobar hemorrhage and amyloid angiopathy are associated with white matter ischemic change and cognitive decline.

Symptoms

Localization site	Comment
Cerebral hemispheres	Subcortical infarcts, intracerebral hemorrhage, amyloid angiopathy, migraine
Mental status and psychiatric aspects/ complications	Cognitive decline, encephalopathy, dementia

Secondary Complications: Dependency and disability due to focal neurologic deficit from intracerebral hemorrhage or infarct and from cognitive decline due to dementia and amyloid angiopathy.

Bibliography

Greenberg SM, Vonsattel JP. Diagnosis of cerebral amyloid angiopathy. Sensitivity and specificity of cortical biopsy. *Stroke*. 1997;28:1418.

Hébert R, Brayne C. Epidemiology of vascular dementia. *Neuroepidemiology*. 1995;14:240.

Kelley RE. Ischemic demyelination. *Neurol Res*. 2006;28(3):334–40.

Lipton RB, Bigal ME, Diamond M, et al. Migraine prevalence, disease burden, and the need for preventive therapy. *Neurology*. 2007;68:343.

Ischemic Monomelic Neuropathy (IMN)

Epidemiology and Demographics: Ischemic monomelic neuropathy (IMN) is a rare condition, although the exact incidence is unclear due to lack of adequate study.

Disorder Description: IMN involves multiple distal mononeuropathies owing to acute arterial occlusion or low blood perfusion to an extremity. Both sensory and motor nerves are affected. This condition is usually axonal. The nerves in the distal limb are most affected. It is most commonly associated with recent surgical procedures, typically arteriovenous fistula or dialysis graft formation, arterial catheterization, abdominal aneurysm repair, or use of intra-aortic balloon pump (IABP). Hypercoagulable states, trauma or laceration, intra-arterial injection, cellulitis, and peripheral vascular disease are also possible causes.

Symptoms

Localization site	Comment
Mononeuropathy or mononeuropathy multiplex	Although symptoms can vary depending on the location of ischemia, patients usually present with acute pain and weakness of the distal upper or lower extremities. Variable sensorimotor deficits are seen as well. Weakness and paresthesias occur along the several different peripheral nerve distributions

Secondary Complications: Decreased sensation to distal extremities can increase the frequency of injury, especially burns and infections, at the affected site.

Particularly in diabetic patients, this can lead to uncontrolled infections and sepsis.

Treatment Complications: There is no standard treatment algorithm proposed and, therefore, no specific neurologic complications of treatment. When ischemic neuropathy is associated with identifiable systemic vasculitis or connective tissue disease, immunosuppressive therapy can be tried.

Bibliography

Rodriguez V, Shah D, Gover V, et al. Ischemic monomelic neuropathy: a disguised diabetic neuropathy. *Pract Neurol*. March/April 2013. http://practicalneurology.com/2013/04/ischemic-monomelic-neuropathy-a-disguised-diabetic-neuropathy/. Accessed Aug 30, 2018.

Sheetal S, Byju P, Manoj P. Ischemic monomelic neuropathy. *J Postgrad Med*. 2017;63(1):42–3. DOI:10.4103/0022-3859.194221.

Ischemic Myelopathy (Secondary to Surgery or Traumatic Laceration of Aorta)

Epidemiology and Demographics: Spinal cord infarctions represent 1% of all strokes and 5% to 8% of acute myelopathies, but their precise incidence is unclear, and the likelihood of their occurrence varies greatly with the clinical situation. There is no sex predominance. The peak incidence of spinal cord infarction is between the sixth and seventh decades. There is no major geographic distribution.

Disorder Description: The spinal cord is supplied by three main longitudinal arteries: the anterior spinal artery and the two smaller posterior spinal arteries. Ischemia typically affects the anterior spinal artery territory. The most common location of spinal cord infarction is the lower thoracic cord, and the most frequently encountered sensory level is at T10. Typically seen after trauma, centrospinal infarction can be partially reversible, with recovery of leg strength and persistent weakness of the arms, in a pattern often referred to as man-in-the-barrel syndrome.

Spinal cord infarctions can have multiple causes, but aortic surgery is by far the most common. Trauma is another common cause.

The diagnosis of spinal cord infarction is primarily clinical. Spinal cord MRI T2-weighted and fluid-attenuated inversion recovery sequences will show an infarction that takes the appearance of "owl eyes," reflecting the preferential involvement of the ventral gray matter.

Symptoms

Localization site	Comment
Spinal cord	Most common location of spinal cord infarction is the lower thoracic cord
	Flaccid weakness below the lesion (paraplegia or quadriplegia). Anesthesia or hypoesthesia to pain and temperature below the lesion. Urinary retention (atonic bladder). Constipation (paralytic ileus). Areflexia below the lesion. Absent rectal tone. Preservation of proprioception and vibration (usually). Respiratory failure (with rare midcervical and upper cervical infarctions)
Anterior horn cells	Muscular atrophy, fasciculation, and areflexia
Specific spinal roots	Back or radicular pain at the level of the lesion

Secondary Complications: Respiratory failure (with rare midcervical and upper cervical infarctions). Patients with spinal cord infarction are at high risk of secondary systemic complications, especially venous thromboembolism, urosepsis, and pressure ulcers. Aspiration pneumonia and autonomic dysreflexia are additional threats for patients with cervical spinal cord infarction.

Treatment Complications: The treatment of spinal cord infarction consists of trying to improve cord perfusion through collateral flow. This can sometimes be achieved by the combination of hemodynamic augmentation and lumbar drainage. No recanalization therapy has been formally tested in spinal cord infarction.

Complications of hemodynamic augmentation are largely fluid overload and are primarily a risk for patients with comorbid heart failure.

Bibliography

Rabinstein AJ. Vascular myelopathies. *Continuum (Minneap Minn)*. 2015;21(1):67–83.

Ullery BW, Cheung AT, Fairman RM, et al. Risk factors, outcomes, and clinical manifestations of spinal cord ischemia following thoracic endovascular aortic repair. *J Vasc Surg*. 2011;54(3):677–84.

Japanese Encephalitis

Epidemiology and Demographics: Japanese encephalitis (JE) virus is a flavivirus spread by *Culex* mosquitoes. It is the leading cause of vaccine-preventable encephalitis in Asia and the western Pacific, with an estimated 68,000 new cases each year. Annual incidence of clinical disease within endemic countries ranges from <1 to >10 per 100,000 population. Twenty-four countries in the World Health Organization South-East Asia and Western Pacific regions have endemic Japanese encephalitis transmission, exposing more than 3 billion people to risk of infection. Children are more frequently and severely affected. Thirty percent of those affected by the virus are adults; males are more frequently affected than females.

The case-fatality rate can be as high as 30%. Permanent neurologic or psychiatric sequelae can occur in 30% to 50% of patients. TLR3 gene polymorphism might confer host genetic susceptibility to Japanese encephalitis in the Indian population. In temperate areas, the virus spreads during the warmer months; in tropical areas it spreads during the rainy season and pre-harvest period in rice cultivation regions.

Disorder Description: Most JEV infections are mild (fever, diarrhea, coryza, rigors, and headache) or without apparent symptoms, but approximately 1 in 250 infections results in severe clinical illness. Severe disease is characterized by rapid onset of high fever, headache, neck stiffness, disorientation, coma, seizures, spastic paralysis, and ultimately death. In a proportion of patients, recovery is rapid and spontaneous ("abortive encephalitis"). The thalamus, basal ganglia, midbrain, cerebellum, and anterior horns of the spinal cord are heavily affected, providing anatomical correlates for the tremor, dystonias, and flaccid paralysis that characterize the disease. Diagnostic tests include lumbar puncture, neuroimaging, and serology. CSF shows pleocytosis of 10 to 100 cells per cubic millimeter, with predominant lymphocytes, mildly elevated protein (50 to 200 mg%), and a normal glucose ratio. MRI shows bilateral thalamic lesions with or without hemorrhagic changes as well as in the substantia nigra, medial temporal lobes, cerebellum, cerebral cortex, and white matter. Serologic tests include IgM ELISA testing of Japanese encephalitis virus-specific IgM antibody in serum or CSF, Japanese encephalitis virus antigens in tissue by immunohistochemistry, Japanese encephalitis virus genome in serum, plasma, blood, cerebrospinal fluid, or tissue by reverse transcriptase polymerase chain reaction, or isolation of the virus in serum, CSF, or tissue.

Symptoms

Localization site	Comment
Cerebral hemispheres	Aseptic meningitis – without encephalopathic features
	Classical description of Japanese encephalitis includes a dull, flat "mask-like" face with wide unblinking eyes, tremor, generalized hypertonia, and cogwheel rigidity. Rigidity spasms, particularly on stimulation, occur in about 15% of patients and are associated with a poor prognosis. There may be other extrapyramidal features including head nodding and pill-rolling movements, facial grimacing, lip-smacking, opisthotonus, and choreoathetosis
	Seizures may occur as a manifestation in up to 8% of children and 10% of adults
Mental status and psychiatric aspects/ complications	Cognitive impairment may be seen as a sequela
Brainstem	Brainstem encephalitis may occur and present with opsoclonus, gaze palsies, and pupillary changes with waxing and waning character
Cerebellum	Cerebellar signs are distinctly absent
Spinal cord	Transverse myelitis in association with JE virus has been reported
Anterior horn cells	Polio-like acute flaccid paralysis: weakness occurred more frequently in the legs than the arms and was usually asymmetric. 30% of such patients subsequently developed encephalitis, with reduced level of consciousness and upper motor neuron signs, but in the majority, acute flaccid paralysis was the only feature. Presence of flaccid paralysis is a poor prognostic factor

Secondary Complications: Twenty percent of patients have severe cognitive and language impairment (most with motor impairment too) and 20% have further convulsions. Children have a higher rate of sequelae than adults. Some patients may have subtle sequelae such as learning difficulties, behavioral problems, and subtle neurologic signs. Coinfection of neurocysticercosis and Japanese encephalitis has frequently been noted in the endemic regions, often resulting in poor outcome.

Treatment Complications: There is currently no specific antiviral treatment for Japanese encephalitis. Patients are treated symptomatically for seizures, fever, and cerebral edema. WHO recommends JE immunization in all regions where the disease is a recognized public health priority.

Bibliography

Garg RK, Greenlee JE. Japanese encephalitis. Medlink Neurology. Originally released August 17, 2000; last updated July 21, 2017. Available from www.medlink.com/article/japanese_encephalitis. Accessed Aug 20, 2018.

Solomon T. Current concepts: Flavivirus encephalitis. *New Engl J Med.* 2004;351:370–8. PMID 15269317.

Solomon T, Cardosa MJ. Emerging arboviral encephalitis. *BMJ.* 2000;321:1484–5. PMID 11118162.

Jet Lag Sleep Disorder

Epidemiology and Demographics: Jet lag sleep disorder affects all age, sex, and racial groups. The prevalence is unknown.

Predisposing factors include disturbed sleep and reduced amount of sleep prior to and during the travel. Stress, caffeine, and alcohol consumption may worsen symptoms of insomnia and impaired daytime function.

Disorder Description: The disorder is defined by a misalignment of the sleep and wake cycle generated by the individual's circadian rhythm and that of the new time zone. At least two time zones must have been traveled. Symptoms of disturbed sleep with a reduction of total sleep time, daytime fatigue, and sleepiness are all characteristic of jet lag sleep disorder. The severity and duration of symptoms are dependent on the number of time zones traveled, the direction of travel, ability to sleep during travel, and exposure to circadian cues. It is typically more difficult to travel east than west.

Symptoms

Localization site	Comment
Midbrain	Suprachiasmatic nucleus of the hypothalamus (circadian clock alteration)
Mental status and psychiatric aspects/ complications	Impaired daytime function, general malaise, sleepiness with difficulty concentrating, and memory difficulties

Secondary Complications: Impaired daytime function, general malaise, sleepiness with difficulty concentrating, and memory difficulties.

Treatment Complications: Treatment should focus on preparing prior to travel with phase shifting sleep in accordance with the direction in which the individual is traveling (phase advancing bedtime and wake time for eastward travel, phase delay for westward travel). The individual should be well rested prior to travel to decrease sleep debt. During travel, staying hydrated and avoiding alcohol and caffeine is important, as either one may promote insomnia. Upon arrival, the appropriately timed exposure to light is important; for eastward travel, minimize morning light and maximize afternoon light. On westward flights, stay awake while it is light out. The administration of melatonin before bedtime and sleep scheduling are also important to the realignment of the individual's circadian rhythm and their environment.

The use of short-acting nonbenzodiazepine non-BZ receptor agonist hypnotics such as zolpidem and zaleplon can be effective to help initiate sleep but has been associated with amnesia, nausea, and somnabulism. To help counteract the symptoms of daytime sleepiness, modafinil or armodafinil may be considered. However, there are limited data on efficacy and the adverse effects of headaches, nausea, and palpitations may outweigh the benefits of therapy. Caffeine consumption in the earlier part of the day may help with maintaining wakefulness, but it should be judiciously consumed in those prone to insomnia.

Treatment Complications: Melatonin has been associated with sleepiness, dizziness, and headache; however, it is unclear if this is a medication side effect or the effect of jet lag.

Short-acting nonbenzodiazepine non-BZ receptor agonist hypnotics such as zolpidem and zaleplon have been associated with amnesia, nausea, and sleepwalking.

Modafinil or armodafinil may be considered, but there are limited data on efficacy and the adverse effects of headaches, nausea, and palpitations may outweigh the benefits of therapy. Caffeine consumption may cause sleep disruption in those prone to insomnia.

Bibliography

American Academy of Sleep Medicine. *International classification of sleep disorders*, 3rd ed. Darien, IL: American Academy of Sleep Medicine; 2014.

Burgess HJ, Crowley SJ, Gazda CJ, et al. Preflight adjustment to eastward travel: 3 days of advancing sleep with and without morning bright light. *J Biol Rhythms*. 2003;18:318.

Herxheimer A, Petrie KJ. Melatonin for the prevention and treatment of jet lag. *Cochrane Database Syst Rev*. 2002;2:CD001520.

Jamieson AO, Zammit GK, Rosenberg RS, et al. Zolpidem reduces the sleep disturbance of jet lag. *Sleep Med*. 2001;2:423.

Morris HH 3rd, Estes ML. Traveler's amnesia. Transient global amnesia secondary to triazolam. *JAMA*. 1987;258:945.

Rosenberg RP, Bogan RK, Tiller JM, et al. A phase 3, double-blind, randomized, placebo-controlled study of armodafinil for excessive sleepiness associated with jet lag disorder. *Mayo Clin Proc*. 2010;85:630.

Sack RL. Clinical practice. Jet lag. *N Engl J Med*. 2010;362:440–6.

Sack RL, Auckley D, Auger RR, et al. Circadian rhythm sleep disorders: Part I, basic principles, shift work and jet lag disorders. *Sleep*. 2007;30:1460–83.

Juvenile Absence Epilepsy

Epidemiology and Demographics: Age of onset 8–16 years, peak occurrence between 10 and 12 years. Incidence and prevalence are not known. Family history of epilepsy in 11%. Males and females affected equally.

Disorder Description: Type of idiopathic generalized epilepsy syndrome, predominantly composed of absence seizures, though generalized tonic–clonic seizures (GTCS) and myoclonic seizures may occur. Genetic factors appear to play a major role, with mutations identified in genes encoding the voltage-gated sodium and potassium channels, as well as the GABA receptor.

Impairment of consciousness milder than in childhood absence epilepsy (CAE) and may occur once per day or in clusters after wakening. GTCS and age of onset help distinguish from CAE. Interictal EEG generally normal. Absence seizures on EEG similar to those in CAE; however, frequency often faster than 3 Hz (3.5–4.0 Hz). AEDs usually required lifelong.

Symptoms

Localization site	Comment
Cerebral hemispheres	Absence seizures, GTCS, myoclonic seizures
	EEG with 3.5–4 Hz generalized spike and wave activity
	MRI normal
Mental status and psychiatric aspects/ complications	Attention deficit hyperactivity disorder (ADHD), learning difficulties

Secondary Complications: ADHD and learning difficulties have been described. Increased risk of accidental injury, risks associated with driving or operating heavy machinery.

Treatment Complications: An inappropriate selection of antiepileptic drugs, such as vigabatrin, gabapentin, phenytoin, phenobarbital, or carbamazepine and its derivatives, can worsen seizures. Ethosuximide may be associated with headache or rash, and less commonly with a lupus-like syndrome, blood dyscrasias, and psychosis. Valproate side effects include hyperactivity, weight gain, transaminitis, thrombocytopenia, pancreatitis, and known teratogenic effects.

Bibliography

Asadi-Pooya AA, Farazdaghi M. Seizure outcome in patients with juvenile absence epilepsy. *Neurol Sci*. 2016;37(2):289–92.

Trinka E, et al. Long-term prognosis for childhood and juvenile absence epilepsy. *J Neurol*. 2004;251(10):1235–41.

Werz MA, Pita-Garcia IL. *Epilepsy syndromes*. Philadelphia, PA: Saunders/Elsevier; 2010. p. ix, 216.

Juvenile Myoclonic Epilepsy (JME)

Epidemiology and Demographics: Juvenile myoclonic epilepsy (JME) accounts for 26% of idiopathic generalized epilepsy and up to 10% of all cases of epilepsy. Onset after puberty; mean age 15 years.

Disorder Description: An idiopathic generalized epilepsy syndrome characterized by myoclonic seizures, generalized tonic–clonic seizures (GTCS), and less frequently, absence seizures. Myoclonic seizures are most frequent in the morning within the first hour after awakening, and may present as isolated jerks involving one or both arms, sometimes as subtle as a finger twitch. EEG findings include generalized 4–6 Hz polyspike-and-wave (in 61%) or 3–4 Hz spike-and-wave discharges (in 14%), with otherwise normal background activity. Photosensitivity described in a third of patients. JME appears to be a heritable syndrome but with several different susceptibility genes indentified. Seizures typically well controlled on broad-spectrum antiepileptic drugs (AEDs), but requiring lifelong treatment.

Symptoms

Localization site	Comment
Cerebral hemispheres	Myoclonic seizures, GTCS, absence seizures EEG with 4–6 Hz generalized spike and wave activity MRI normal
Mental status and psychiatric aspects/ complications	Increased incidence of psychiatric comorbidity in about a third of patients, and frequently observed subtle cognitive deficits and learning difficulties. Neuropsychologic profiles are suggestive of frontal lobar dysfunction

Secondary Complications: Increased risk of accidental injury; risks associated with driving or operating heavy machinery secondary to seizures.

Treatment Complications: An inappropriate selection of AEDs such as vigabatrin, gabapentin, phenytoin, or carbamazepine and its derivatives can worsen seizures. Valproate considered first line; however, may lead to weight gain, hyperactivity, transaminitis, thrombocytopenia, and pancreatitis. Valproate has the greatest risk of teratogenicity among the AEDs. Other broad-spectrum AEDs may be effective such as levetiracetam, topiramate, zonisamide, and lamotrigine (may exacerbate myoclonus).

Bibliography

de Araujo Filho GM, Yacubian EM. Juvenile myoclonic epilepsy: psychiatric comorbidity and impact on outcome. *Epilepsy Behav.* 2013;28(Suppl 1):S74–80.

Swaiman KF. *Pediatric neurology: principles and practice.* 5th ed. Edinburgh: Elsevier Saunders; 2012.

Wolf P, et al. Juvenile myoclonic epilepsy: A system disorder of the brain. *Epilepsy Res.* 2015;114:2–12.

Keratitis

Epidemiology and Demographics. Keratitis can affect any age group without sex predilection.

Disorder Description: Keratitis refers to inflammation of the cornea due to exposure, infection, or inflammation. Corneal exposure, from poor eyelid closure, is a major risk factor for corneal infective keratitis. This exposure keratitis may start innocuously with punctate epithelial erosions, which are tiny defects in the corneal epithelium. If the exposure is not corrected, these erosions may coalesce into a larger epithelial defect called an abrasion. Without the protective corneal epithelium, the underlying corneal stroma is at risk for infection and corneal ulceration. An untreated corneal ulcer may quickly progress to perforation.

Symptoms

Localization site	Comment
Cranial nerves	**Trigeminal neuropathy**: The ophthalmic branch of the trigeminal nerve provides sensation to the cornea. Corneal sensation is important to detect foreign bodies, exposure, or dryness that elicit a normal blink reflex to clear them. Without normal sensation, neurotrophic keratopathy may result, potentially leading to corneal infection, ulceration, and perforation. Common causes include herpetic infection and diabetes
	Facial nerve paresis may result in various degrees of flaccid paralysis of the ipsilateral muscles of facial expression. Paralysis of the orbicularis oculi muscle results in an inability to close the eye and exposure of the cornea, which may lead to exposure keratitis, ulceration, or perforation
Autonomic nervous system	**Riley–Day syndrome**, or familial dysautonomia, is a hereditary sensory neuropathy that can lead to neurotrophic keratopathy

Secondary Complications: Corneal perforation is the most feared complication of keratitis. Perforation may lead to endophthalmitis, vision loss, or complete loss of the eye. Corneal ulcers may result in scarring of the cornea, which can compromise vision. Some corneal scars can be treated with corneal transplantation.

Treatment Complications: Exposure keratitis in facial paralysis may be treated with a number of surgical procedures to help close the eyelids. Tarsorrhaphy is the placement of one or more sutures to hold the eyelids closed. These sutures may be the full width of the eyelid or partial. If the sutures are not placed correctly, they may make contact with the corneal surface causing an abrasion. An eyelid weight (made of gold or platinum) or spring (made of nickel alloy) can be implanted into the upper eyelid to assist in closure of the eyelid. Both of these devices may extrude through the skin. The weights only work with the force of gravity. When patients are supine, they may not close the eyelid at all. The spring works independently of gravity, and one of its advantages over an eyelid weight is that it works regardless of patient positioning.

Bibliography

Shaheen B, Bakir M, Jain S. Corneal nerves in health and disease. *Surv Ophthalmol.* 2014;59(3):263–85.

Kernicterus

Epidemiology and Demographics: One in 50,000 to 100,000 live births will have abnormal neurologic outcomes as a result of extreme hyperbilirubinemia (>25 mg/dL). It is less common in black infants and females. The prevalence of kernicterus has remained unchanged in the last 30 years, thought to be attributed to increasingly earlier discharge of term infants. Risk factors include hemolytic disease, particularly Rh incompatibility between mother and baby, and a family history of RBC abnormalities (i.e., G6PD deficiency, hereditary spherocytosis). Polycythemia and the breakdown of extravasated blood (e.g., severe cephalhematoma, subgaleal hemorrhage) may also be a significant source of bilirubin, whilst hypoalbuminemic states and hepatic dysfunction will reduce bilirubin-conjugating abilities. Certain cultural postnatal practices, such as salting babies in Middle Eastern cultures, may cause hypernatremia, exacerbating the effects of hyperbilirubinemia.

Disorder Description: Kernicterus is a neurologic condition in the neonate, characterized by cerebral deposition of unconjugated bilirubin. While historically a pathologic entity, the term kernicterus (lit. "yellow kern" in Latin, describing the yellow staining of the deep nuclei of the brain) is used clinically to describe the associated clinical finding of bilirubin-induced neurologic dysfunction (BIND). This clinical entity is composed of movement disorder, hearing loss, and visuomotor abnormalities secondary to hyper-bilirubinemia. Cognitive function is usually spared.

The clinical expression of BIND varies with location, severity, and time of assessment, and is influenced by the amount, duration, and developmental age of exposure to the excessive unbound bilirubin. Clinical findings include:

a. Acute bilirubin encephalopathy – three stages:
   1. First few days: Non-specific – decreased alertness, hyptonia, poor feeding.
   2. Variable onset and duration: hypertonia of extensor muscles, with retrocollis (backward arching of neck), and opisthotonus. Progression to this phase indicates the development of long-term neurodisability.
   3. >1 week: hypotonia.
b. Chronic bilirubin encephalopathy.

Symptoms and signs evolve slowly, characterized by hypotonia and delayed acquisition of motor milestones. Tonic neck reflex can still be observed in children older than 1 year. In those older than 1 year, abnormalities are characterized by a tetrad of movement disorder (usually extrapyramidal), auditory dysfunction, oculomotor impairments (especially upgaze), and dental enamel hypoplasia of deciduous teeth. Dental dysplasia affects only deciduous (baby) teeth.

Pathophysiology. Laboratory investigations have demonstrated that bilirubin is neurotoxic at a cellular level, and acute bilirubin toxicity appears to occur in the first few days of life of term infants. Preterm infants may be at higher risk of toxicity for slightly longer than a few days, with factors such as acidosis and infection affecting the permeability of the blood–brain barrier. Bilirubin staining can be noted in the basal ganglia (especially globus pallidus and subthalamic nucleus), brainstem nuclei – especially auditory (cochlear nucleus, inferior colliculus, superior olivary complex), and oculomotor and vestibular nuclei. Other susceptible areas include the cerebellum (especially Purkinje cells) and hippocampus (CA2 sector). Neuronal necrosis is necessary to lead to the clinical findings in chronic bilirubin encephalopathy.

Different patterns of expression may relate to amount and duration of exposure, variability in the susceptibility of the developing nervous system, and whether surviving neurons become functionally normal or are more susceptible to other stressors.

Symptoms

Localization site	Comment
Cerebral hemispheres	Deep nuclei:
	Globus pallidus interna, subthalamic nucleus – initial hypotonia, developing into athetosis and dystonia, but may also include spasticity. Upper extremities usually more affected than lower limbs. Bulbar function can be impacted
	Cognitive deficits:
	Relatively spared – often mistakenly considered to have intellectual disabilities because of their choreoathetoid movement disorder and hearing deficits
Cerebellum	Truncal tone and postural abnormalities
Brainstem	Auditory brainstem nuclei – sensorineural high-frequency hearing loss, auditory neuropathy, auditory dys-synchrony – abnormal auditory brainstem response with normal inner ear function. CN VIII (auditory nerve) may be directly affected
	Oculomotor nuclei – impaired upgaze (may improve with age). Other gaze abnormalities may coexist

Treatment Complications: Treatment of acute hyperbilirubinemia is via exchange transfusion, to mechanically remove already formed bilirubin from the blood.

Bibliography

American Academy of Pediatrics Clinical Practice Guideline Subcommittee on Hyperbilirubinemia. Management of hyperbilirubinemia in the newborn infant 35 or more weeks of gestation. *Pediatrics*. 2004;114:297–316.

Bhutani VK, Johnson L. Review: kernicterus in the 21st century: frequently asked questions. *J Perinatol*. 2009;29:S20–4.

Shapiro SM. Definition of the clinical spectrum of kernicterus and bilirubin-induced neurologic dysfunction (BIND). *J Perinatol*. 2005;25:54–9.

Ketamine Abuse

Epidemiology and Demographics: Typical abusers of ketamine are adolescents or young adults, with ages ranging from 13 to 60 years.

Disorder Description: Ketamine is an arylcycloalkylamine that is structurally related to phencyclidine (PCP). Ketamine is a dissociative anesthetic and hallucinogen. It also possesses opioid receptor activity and sympathomimetic properties.

Symptoms

Localization site	Comment
Cerebral hemispheres	Coma (acute)
	Cortical atrophy: frontal, parietal, occipital, para hippocampal (chronic)
	Petit mal seizure activity (acute)
Mental status and psychiatric aspects/complications	Depressed mental status (acute)
	Phobia (acute)
	Agitation (acute)
	Euphoria (acute)
	Hallucinations (acute)
	Schizophrenic psychosis/behavior (acute)
Brainstem	Hypersomnia (chronic)
	Brainstem degeneration (chronic)
Cerebellum	Ataxia (acute)
	Cerebellar degeneration (chronic)
Cranial nerves	Nystagmus: rotatory, vertical, or horizontal (acute)
	Mydriasis (acute)
Spinal cord	Analgesic effects (acute)
Anterior horn cells	Analgesic effects (acute)
Dorsal root ganglia	Analgesic effect (disrupting sodium channels) (acute)
Specific spinal roots	Analgesic effects (acute)
Plexus	Analgesic effects (acute)
Mononeuropathy or mononeuropathy multiplex	Analgesic effects (acute)
Peripheral neuropathy	Analgesic effects (acute)
Muscle	Tremors (chronic)
	Hypertonia (acute)
Neuromuscular junction	Blocks glutamate receptors (acute)

Secondary Complications: Indirectly affects nervous system via:

- **Respiratory complications** – respiratory depression/apnea can result in cerebral ischemia.
- **Cardiovascular complications** – sympathomimetic effect of and increases in blood pressure increase risk for stroke.

Treatment Complications: The use of benzodiazepines for treatment of agitation episodes increases risk of addictive behavior for patients.

Bibliography

Hoffman RJ. Ketamine poisoning. UpToDate. Updated Aug 15, 2017. www.uptodate.com/contents/ketamine poisoning?source=search_result&search=Ketamine%20abuse&selectedTitle=1~150. Accessed Aug 20, 2018.

Wang C, Zheng D, Xu J, Lam W, Yew DT. Brain damages in ketamine addicts as revealed by magnetic resonance imaging. *Front Neuroanat.* July 17, 2013. http://journal.frontiersin.org/article/10.3389/fnana.2013.00023/full

Zhou Z-S, Zhao ZQ. Ketamine blockage of both tetrodotoxin (TTX)-sensitive and TTX-resistant sodium channels of rat dorsal root ganglion neurons. *Brain Res Bull.* 2000;52(5):427–33.

Kleine–Levin Syndrome

Epidemiology and Demographics: This is a rare disorder, with an estimated prevalence of 1 to 2 cases per million. Onset typically occurs in the second decade of life with a male gender predominance of 2:1. A higher prevalence has been reported in Ashkenazi Jews.

Family patterns have been reported in up to 5% of patients. HLA DQBI*02 has been shown to be increased in one large retrospective study in patients with Kleine–Levine syndrome; however, this was not confirmed in a large prospective study.

Flu-like illness and an upper respiratory tract infection have been reported to precede some cases, with other less common triggers including alcohol intoxication, head trauma, and anesthesia.

Disorder Description: The disorder is characterized by recurrent episodes of prolonged hypersomnolence with associated alterations in sensorium and memory as well as behavioral disturbances. Periods of hypersomnolence with generalized psychomotor slowing are often accompanied by hypersexuality, hyperphagia or anorexia, and altered perception of the environment, known as derealization. The first episode is typically triggered by an infection or alcohol intake and lasts a median of 10 days. These recurrent episodes usually occur more than once a year.

In between episodes, patients are in their normal state of sleep, cognition, mood, and eating. The disease typically resolves after approximately a decade; however, adult-onset cases may be prolonged.

Menstrual-related Kleine–Levin syndrome is a variant with episodes of hypersomnolence occurring just before or during menstruation with associated compulsive eating, depressed mood, and sexual disinhibition.

Electroencephalogram findings of general slowing of brain activity with brief 0.5- to 2-second bursts of generalized 5- to 7-Hz waves. Computed tomography and magnetic resonance imaging are normal.

Symptoms

Localization site	Comment
Forebrain	Brain functional imaging is typically abnormal with hypoperfusion of the thalamus, hypothalamus, temporal–parietal junction, and frontal lobes
	Possible autoimmune etiology
	HLA DQBI*0201 increased allele frequency has been identified in one study
Mental status and psychiatric aspects/ complications	Hypersomnolence, cognitive slowing, hypersexuality, hyperphagia or anorexia, derealization, social dysfunction

Secondary Complications: Social and occupational impairment is a common phenomenon during disease episodes. Physical safety of the patient and caregiver is of utmost importance during these episodes. Patients are at increased risk of motor vehicle accidents.

Treatment Complications: Treatment is mainly supportive and includes education of family members and caregivers on keeping patients safe and allowing them to sleep while waiting for the episode to end. Symptom-based pharmacologic therapies may be considered such as stimulants and nonamphetamine

wakefulness-promoting agents. Antipsychotics have also been used. However, pharmacologic therapy is based on case series and retrospective series and therefore is not generally recommended.

Menstrual-related Kleine–Levin syndrome has been treated with estrogen-containing contraceptives with a variable response.

Modafinil and armodafinil are hepatically metabolized and inducers of the cytochrome P450 enzyme system, which may affect the metabolism of other drugs. Methylphenidate and amphetamines are both central nervous system stimulants and can cause systemic hypertension and psychiatric events such as psychosis, anorexia, and anxiety.

Bibliography

American Academy of Sleep Medicine. *The international classification of sleep disorders*. 3rd ed. Chicago, IL: American Academy of Sleep Medicine; 2014.

Arnulf I. Kleine-Levin syndrome. *Sleep Med Clinics*. 2015;10(2):151–61.

Arnulf I, Lin I, Gadoth N, et al. Kleine-Levin syndrome: a systematic study of 108 patients. *Ann Neurol*. 2008;63:482–93.

Billiard M, Jaussent I, Dauvilliers Y, Besset A. Recurrent hypersomnia: a review of 339 cases. *Sleep Med Rev*. 2011;15:247–57.

Dauvilliers Y, Mayer G, Lecendreux M, et al. Kleine-Levin syndrome. An autoimmune hypothesis based on clinical and genetic analyses. *Neurology*. 2002;59:1739–45.

Klinefelter Syndrome

Epidemiology and Demographics: Klinefelter syndrome (KS) is limited to males. It is one of the most common genetic causes of male infertility, with estimated frequencies ranging between 1:500 and 1:1000 men overall, and with rates of 0.1–0.2% in newborn male infants, 3–4% among infertile males, and 10–12% in azoospermic males. It is present at birth, with a broad spectrum of presentation depending on the expressed phenotype. There is some evidence that it is increasing in frequency, potentially due to more common paternal meiotic errors. However, due to the frequency of mild phenotypes, it can often go undiagnosed. There is no specific geographic distribution.

Disorder Description: KS is a disease of genetic aneuploidy with a wide and varied presentation, with mosaics presenting with less severe symptoms. Because of this wide variety, and frequency of mild phenotypes, it can often go undiagnosed. It is a disease based on abnormal chromosomal counts, most commonly 47, XXY karyotype (80–90%), while the remaining 10–20% are a mixture of aneuploidies with 46–48 chromosomes, potentially in mosaic form with or without chromosomal structural abnormalities. It can occur due to nondisjunction or inconsistent X chromosome loss (for mosaics). Risk factors include advanced maternal, and possibly paternal, age at conception, such that reports have shown a >fourfold increase in KS where mothers >40 vs <24.

KS is first clinically suspected, then confirmed through karyotyping. However, clinical suspicion is frequently followed by investigating serum levels of gonadotropins (follicle-stimulating hormone and luteinizing hormone), evaluation of sperm counts (for azoospermia), or, for pre-natal diagnoses (about 10%), via chorionic villus sampling or amniocentesis.

Symptoms

Localization site	Comment
Mental status and psychiatric aspects/ complications	Normal to slightly decreased verbal intelligence (language learning or reading impairment), frequent deficits in executive functions, and there may also be delays in motor development
Outside central nervous system (CNS)	Infertility (azoospermia: inability to produce sperm, oligospermia with hyalinization and fibrosis of the seminiferous tubule), sparse facial and body hair, small testes, tall stature, gynecomastia (enlarged breasts) in late puberty, gynoid aspect of hips (broad hips), signs of androgen deficiency and low serum testosterone coupled with elevated gonadotropins

Secondary Complications: Secondary complications are primarily related to the hypogonadism, and result in the aforementioned extra-CNS symptoms.

Treatment Complications: Treatment is largely hormone supplementation with testosterone. Supportive psychologic and physical therapy can be helpful. In certain cases, surgical options to remedy psychologic issues can be done (e.g., breast removal), but this is not standard of care.

There are minimal complications with optimal management, but complications are largely related to testosterone effects, such as cosmetic/dermatologic changes, emotional lability/irritability, and changes in smell sensation, but mostly endocrinologic (hyperlipidemia, increased thyroid-stimulating hormone, hypokalemia, etc.).

Bibliography

Bonomi M, Rochira V, Pasquali D, et al.; ItaliaN Group (KING). Klinefelter syndrome (KS): genetics, clinical phenotype and hypogonadism. *J Endocrinol Invest.* 2017;40(2):123–34.

Korsakoff Syndrome

Epidemiology and Demographics: Korsakoff syndrome refers to a chronic neurologic condition that usually occurs as a consequence of Wernicke encephalopathy.

Approximately 80% of alcoholics recovering from classic Wernicke encephalopathy develop the memory disturbance of Korsakoff syndrome. Korsakoff syndrome is seen less frequently in nonalcoholics.[1] It is believed that ethanol neurotoxicity is a contributing factor for development of Korsakoff syndrome.[2] Korsakoff syndrome has also been described in the literature in the absence of ethanol ingestion.[3–8]

Some alcohol abusers develop Korsakoff syndrome without a noticeable episode of Wernicke encephalopathy, but lesions of Wernicke encephalopathy are present at autopsy.[9–11] In these cases, Korsakoff syndrome may result from a series of subclinical or unrecognized episodes of Wernicke encephalopathy.

Disorder Description: Korsakoff syndrome was described by Russian psychiatrist Sergei Korsakoff. He described chronic amnestic syndrome in which memory was impaired out of proportion to other cognitive domains. In Korsakoff syndrome, patients develop anterograde amnesia (unable to recall new information) despite normal immediate memory, attention span, and level of consciousness. Memory for new events is seriously impaired, whereas memory prior to the illness remains relatively intact. Oxidative stress, glutamate-related excitotoxicity, and inflammation play a role in damaging memory processing centers of the limbic system, thalamus, and hypothalamus. Patients are confused, disoriented, and cannot store information for more than a few minutes. Patients may be conversant, engaging, and able to perform simple tasks and follow immediate commands. Confabulation is common, although not always present.[9,12,13] Mammillary body atrophy may be visible on MRI in the chronic phase.[12]

It is most commonly caused by severe thiamine (vitamin B1) deficiency.

Symptoms: Amnestic defect is related to lesions in the dorsal medial nuclei of the thalamus.[14] Confabulation is related to lesion, which interferes with parts of the frontal network.[12]

Neurologic diseases that give rise to an amnestic state include tumors (of the sphenoid wing, posterior corpus callosum, thalamus, or medial temporal lobe), infarctions (in the territories of the anterior or posterior cerebral arteries), head trauma, herpes simplex encephalitis, paraneoplastic limbic encephalitis, and degenerative dementias such as Alzheimer dementia and Pick disease.[12]

Korsakoff syndrome is believed to result from irreversible damage to the medial thalamic nuclei and mammillary bodies associated with previous thiamine deficiency.

Secondary Complications: There are few long-term studies but approximately 25% of patients fail to recover and may require institutionalization.

Treatment Complications: There are anecdotal reports that favor the use of acetylcholinesterase inhibitors and memantine leading to improvement in attention and memory.[15–17]

References

1. Freund G. Chronic central nervous system toxicity of alcohol. *Annu Rev Pharmacol.* 1973;13:217.

2. Gregory MC, Hammond ME, Brewer ED. Renal deposition of cytomegalovirus antigen in immunoglobulin-A nephropathy. *Lancet.* 1988;1:11.

3. Parkin AJ, Blunden J, Rees JE, Hunkin NM. Wernicke-Korsakoff syndrome of nonalcoholic origin. *Brain Cogn.* 1991;15:69.

4. Pittella JE, de Castro LP. Wernicke's encephalopathy manifested as Korsakoff's syndrome in a patient with promyelocytic leukemia. *South Med J.* 1990;83:570.

5. Engel PA, Grunnet M, Jacobs B. Wernicke-Korsakoff syndrome complicating T-cell lymphoma: unusual or unrecognized? *South Med J.* 1991;84:253.

6. Cruickshank EK. Wernicke's encephalopathy. *Q J Med.* 1950;19:327.

7. Becker JT, Furman JM, Panisset M, Smith C. Characteristics of the memory loss of a patient with Wernicke-Korsakoff's syndrome without alcoholism. *Neuropsychologia.* 1990;28:171.

8. Beatty WW, Bailly RC, Fisher L. Korsakoff-like amnesic syndrome in a patient with anorexia and vomiting. *Int J Clin Neuropsychol.* 1988;11:55.

9. Victor M, Adams RA, Collins GH. *The Wernicke-Korsakoff syndrome and related disorders due to alcoholism and malnutrition.* Philadelphia: F. A. Davis; 1989.

10. Harper C. The incidence of Wernicke's encephalopathy in Australia: a neuropathological study of 131 cases. *J Neurol Neurosurg Psychiatry.* 1983;46:593.

11. Blansjaar BA, Van Dijk JG. Korsakoff minus Wernicke syndrome. *Alcohol Alcohol.* 1992;27:435.

12. Kasper DL, Fauci AS, Hauser SL, et al., eds. *Harrison's principles of internal medicine.* 19th ed. New York: McGraw-Hill Education/Medical; 2015.

13. Eckardt MJ, Martin PR. Clinical assessment of cognition in alcoholism. *Alcohol Clin Exp Res.* 1986;10:123.

14. Harding A, Halliday G, Caine D, Kril J. Degeneration of anterior thalamic nuclei differentiates alcoholics with amnesia. *Brain.* 2000;123(Pt 1):141.

15. Phillips BK, Ingram MV, Grammer GG. Wernicke-Korsakoff syndrome and galantamine. *Psychosomatics.* 2004;45:366.

16. Cochrane M, Cochrane A, Jauhar P, Ashton E. Acetylcholinesterase inhibitors for the treatment of Wernicke-Korsakoff syndrome: three further cases show response to donepezil. *Alcohol Alcohol.* 2005;40:151.

17. Rustembegović A, Kundurović Z, Sapcanin A, Sofic E. A placebo-controlled study of memantine

(Ebixa) in dementia of Wernicke-Korsakoff syndrome. *Med Arh.* 2003;57:149.

Krabbe Disease

Epidemiology and Demographics: The prevalence of Krabbe disease is estimated at 1–9/100,000. Caused by a homozygous or compound heterozygous mutation in the galactosylceramidase gene (GALC) on chromosome 14q31.

Disorder Description: Krabbe disease is a rare autosomal recessive lysosomal disorder affecting the white matter of **both** the central and peripheral nervous systems.

There are multiple forms including an infantile "classic" (onset 6 months, death by 2 years), late-infantile (6 months to 3 years), juvenile (3 to 8 years), and adult form. Most patients (90%) present within the first 6 months of life with infantile classic disease manifesting as extreme irritability, spasticity, and developmental delay. There is severe motor and mental deterioration, with death by 2 years of age. Later-onset forms are variable, but generally less severe and more slow to progress. The adult onset form usually manifests with weakness, gait disturbance (spastic paraparesis or ataxia), burning paresthesia, hemiplegia, and visual loss with or without peripheral neuropathy. Cognitive regression is variable and often absent in adult forms. Disease severity is variable, even within families. Adult-onset patients can survive many years after symptom onset.

The GALC gene encodes a lysosomal enzyme, galactocerebrosidase, which catabolizes the hydrolysis of galactose from galactocerebroside, a normal constituent of myelin. The deficiency leads to the accumulation of cytotoxic psychosine within microglial cells. These cells become filled with the material and later become described as "globoid" cells. The apoptosis of oligodendrocytes leads to demyelination in both the central nervous system and peripheral nervous system.

Nerve conduction studies demonstrate involvement of the peripheral nervous system, while brain MRI appearance showing central periventricular white matter demyelination with subcortical U-fiber sparing is suggestive of the diagnosis. Definitive diagnosis is by enzyme activity in white cells, or mutation analysis.

Symptoms

Cerebral hemispheres	a. **Cognitive deficits** – cognitive regression (rare in adult form) b. Gait disturbance – white matter loss leads to spastic paraparesis or ataxia, hemiplegia MRI – T2 high signal periventricular demyelination with non-contrast enhancement (T1); centrum semiovale and deep gray matter; subcortical U-fiber sparing
Cranial nerves	CN II – optic neuropathy, visual loss
Peripheral nervous system	Peripheral neuropathy Burning paresthesia Peripheral neuropathy – motor and sensory

Treatment Complications: Stem cell transplantation has been shown to slow progression of disease in pre-symptomatic patients. Other treatment options (i.e., chaperone therapy, enzyme replacement therapy, gene therapy) are currently under investigation in animal models (see https://clinicaltrials.gov/ct2/results?cond=%22krabbe+disease%22).

Side effects of drugs used in immunosuppressive therapy for bone marrow transplantation include neurobehavioral disorders, neurocognitive dysfunction, including changes in attention and processing speed, PRES (posterior reversible encephalopathy syndrome), and peripheral neuropathies.

Bibliography

Gaillard F, Weerakkody Y. Krabbe disease. Radiopaedia.org. Available from http://radiopaedia.org/articles/krabbe-disease. Accessed Mar 30, 2016.

Tappino B, Biancheri R, Mort M, et al. Identification and characterization of 15 novel GALC gene mutations causing Krabbe disease. *Hum Mutat.* 2010;31:E1894–914.

Wenger DA. Krabbe disease. In: Pagon RA, Adam MP, Ardinger HH, et al., eds. *GeneReviews*® [Internet]. Seattle (WA): University of Washington, Seattle; 2000 [Updated Mar 31, 2011]. pp. 1993–2016.

Kyphosis

Epidemiology and Demographics: Kyphosis is seen in 12% of girls and 15.3% of boys.

Disorder Description: Kyphosis refers to the accentuation of the normal curvature of the thoracic and sacral spine.

Symptoms

Localization site	Comment
Cervical spine	Pain
Thoracic spine	Pain, myelopathy, hyperreflexia, restrictive lung disease
Lumbosacral spine	Pain

Secondary Complications: Discitis, vertebral osteomyelitis, and osteoporosis.

Treatment Complications: Narcotics can cause sedation and dependency. After surgery, atelectasis, blood loss, wound infection, and pseudoarthrosis can be seen.

Bibliography

Nitzschke E, Hildenbrand M. [Epidemiology of kyphosis in school children.] *Z Orthop Ihre Grenzgeb*. 1990;128(52):477–81.

Song KS, Chang BS, Yeom JS, et al. Surgical treatment of severe angular kyphosis with myelopathy, anterior and posterior approach with pedicle screw instrumentation. *Spine*. 2008;33(11):1229–35. DOI: 10.1097/BRS.0b013e31817152b3.

La Crosse Virus

Epidemiology and Demographics: La Crosse virus is the most pathogenic member of the California encephalitis serogroup. It is transmitted by the tree-hole mosquito, *Aedes triseriatus*, and causes the most prevalent arboviral infection in children in North America. Nevertheless, La Crosse encephalitis often goes unrecognized. Human infections occur in the central and eastern United States, mostly in school-aged children from July through September. Most infections are asymptomatic. A small percentage develop encephalitis of which 1–3% are fatal, and another 15% of patients have long-term nervous system problems.

Disorder Description: Symptomatic disease, after an incubation period of 3–7 days, presents with headache, fever, vomiting, and altered mentation. Seizures occur in about half the patients and focal neurologic abnormalities in about 20%. The virus typically cannot be recovered from cerebrospinal fluid, and the disease can masquerade as enteroviral meningitis when mild and as herpes simplex encephalitis when severe.

CSF shows pleocytosis with either neutrophilic or lymphocytic predominance. Electroencephalography is abnormal in two-thirds of patients, mainly with slowing or epileptiform discharges. The diagnosis of La Crosse encephalitis can be made by demonstration of IgM antibody by capture immunoassay of CSF, a fourfold rise in serum antibody titers against La Crosse virus, or isolation of virus from or demonstration of viral antigen or genomic sequences in tissue, blood, or CSF.

Symptoms

Localization site	Comment
Cerebral hemispheres	Aseptic meningitis alone, without evidence of encephalitis, occurred in 13%
	Severe cases mimic herpes simplex encephalitis with fever, altered mental status, seizures, and temporal lobe involvement
Mental status and psychiatric aspects/complications	Long-term sequelae of cognitive impairment in about 15% of encephalitis cases

Secondary Complications: Cerebral edema and seizures may be seen as a complication of the encephalitis specifically as temporal lobe involvement is seen. Mortality is 1–3% in patients with severe encephalitis. Neurologic sequelae occur in about 15% of the patients and include recurrent seizures, hemiparesis, and cognitive and neurobehavioral abnormalities.

Treatment Complications: Treatment is supportive, with emphasis on control of cerebral edema and seizures. Ribavirin has been used, but efficacy is unproven.

Bibliography

Centers for Disease Control and Prevention. La Crosse encephalitis. Apr 13, 2016. www.cdc.gov/lac/tech/symptoms.html. Accessed Aug 21, 2018.

McJunkin JE, et al. La Crosse encephalitis in children. *N Engl J Med.* 2001;344:801–7. DOI: 10.1056/NEJM200103153441103.

Lacunar Strokes

Epidemiology and Demographics: Lacunar strokes account for 30–40% of all ischemic strokes. While essential hypertension is by far the most common cause of chronic hypertension, chronic cocaine abuse or severe sleep apnea may cause elevated blood pressure (the latter two causes usually unrecognized since blood pressure is often unchecked in these circumstances). Typical atherosclerotic risk factors may accelerate the condition.

Disorder Description: Lacunar strokes occur in the terminal distribution of penetrating arteries of the brain. These small arteries and arterioles branch off larger vessels at right angles and are subject to narrowing of their orifice due to chronic hypertension. Because the vessels have few or no collaterals, occlusion virtually always produces infarction.

Symptoms

Localization site	Comment
Cerebral hemispheres	The typical lacunar stroke affects the basal ganglia, thalamus, internal capsule, or periventricular white matter, although the cortex may be affected. Because the lesions are typically small, less than 1.5 cm, the neurologic deficit is often very restricted. The classic syndromes are pure motor hemiparesis (including dysarthria – clumsy hand syndrome) or pure hemisensory loss. However, thalamic lesions may mimic nearly any syndrome of the cerebral hemisphere

Localization site	Comment
Mental status and psychiatric aspects/ complications	Larger thalamic lesions may alter consciousness or produce sensorimotor syndromes resembling a middle cerebral artery syndrome
Brainstem	Most brainstem strokes are lacunar in nature. Again, the small size of the involved vessel produces highly localized deficits such as diplopia, vertigo, dysarthria, a peripheral facial weakness, or isolated facial sensory syndromes. Involvement of the base of the pons produces hemiparesis, often including incoordination from involvement of cerebellar pathways. A treacherous lacunar syndrome to recognize occurs in the midline of the medulla, producing bilateral leg weakness and dysarthria. If untreated, it may progress to respiratory failure and intractable dysphagia
Cerebellum	The cerebellum is occasionally involved in lacunar strokes and produces localized syndromes such as ataxia of one limb, gait ataxia with veering to one side, vertigo or oscillopsia, which is the subjective symptom of nystagmus
Vestibular system (and nonspecific dizziness)	The vestibular system may be involved by lacunar strokes at the pontomedullary junction, producing vertigo accompanied by nausea and/or vomiting, often with gait ataxia. Because the blood supply of the inner ear derives from the basilar artery through penetrating blood vessels, the vertigo may appear to be "peripheral" on exam and may involve hearing loss when it does
Cranial nerves	True involvement of the cranial nerves outside of the brainstem due to a lacunar stroke is unusual

Secondary Complications: Lacunar strokes may cause dysphagia requiring feeding tubes or rarely respiratory compromise due to failure to protect the oropharyngeal airway. Diplopia may require eye patching. Facial weakness can produce ulceration of the cornea. Falls are common due to the associated weakness. Shoulder dislocations may occur. Cognitive decline or a parkinsonian syndrome occurs on occasion. Mortality rate is less than 5%.

Treatment Complications: The modern management of lacunar strokes is intravenous tissue plasminogen activator (tPA). The primary complication is intracerebral hemorrhage, which occurs in about 3% of patients, usually with severe consequences. Systemic hemorrhage occurs much less frequently. Patients who present beyond the therapeutic window for intravenous tPA (variously set at 3 or 4.5 hours) usually receive antiplatelet therapy. Systemic bleeding or intracranial hemorrhage, including subdural hematoma, can occur with chronic therapy in 2–5% of patients.

Bibliography

Agranoff AB. Lacunar stroke. Medscape. Updated May 23, 2017. https://emedicine.medscape .com/article/322992-overview. Accessed Aug 30, 2018.

Ropper AH, Samuels MA, Klein JP. *Adams and Victor's principles of neurology.* 10th ed. New York: McGraw-Hill Education/Medical; 2014. Chapter 34.

Lafora Disease

Epidemiology and Demographics: It can be found in any population, particularly those with consanguinity. It is rare, considered an orphan disease. Estimated prevalence is four per million individuals.

Normally has onset in adolescence (6–19 years is the reported range; late onset is 20 years). Presents initially as myoclonus, followed by visual, atonic, tonic–clonic, and absence seizures. There is also progressive cognitive decline, and death generally occurs within 10 years of onset.

Disorder Description: Autosomal recessive progressive myoclonic epilepsy. It is caused by mutations in the EPM2A and EPM2B genes, which regulate glycogen structure. Pathogenesis of the disease is characterized by accumulations of Laphora bodies (LBs), which are polyglucosans (malformed and insoluble glycogen molecules).

LBs accumulate in brain as well as in periportal hepatocytes of the liver, skeletal and cardiac myocytes, eccrine ducts (sweat glands), and apocrine myoepithelial cells. Diagnosis is made via skin biopsy. Genetic testing confirms diagnosis.

Antiepileptics have only partial effect on myoclonus and seizures and may be more effective initially; as the disease progresses, polytherapy is used. Differential diagnosis includes other progressive myoclonic epilepsy syndromes.

Symptoms

Localization site	Comment
Cerebral – diffuse	LBs found in brain, diffusely. EEG abnormalities often precede clinical presentation. MRI is usually normal at onset
Mental status and psychiatric considerations/ complications	Often present with **visual hallucinations as manifestation of focal visual seizures**. Not all visual hallucinations are epileptic. Behavioral changes, apathy, depression, psychosis, are often present. As disease progresses to intractable myoclonus, refractory seizures, psychosis, dementia, and dysarthria
	Visual hallucinations sometimes respond to antipsychotic medication
Cerebellum	Ataxia
Spinal cord	LBs are rare or absent in the anterior part of spinal cord
Muscle	Myoclonus remains asymmetric as disease progresses and becomes almost constant

Treatment Complications: Some antiepileptic medications can exacerbate myoclonus.

Bibliography

Turnbull J, et al. Lafora disease. *Epileptic Disord.* 2016;S2:S38–S62.

Lambert–Eaton Myasthenic Syndrome (LEMS)

Epidemiology and Demographics: The mean age of onset of Lambert–Eaton myasthenic syndrome (LEMS) is 50 years. Those patients with associated small cell lung cancer (SCLC) tend to develop symptoms later. The prevalence of LEMS among small cell lung cancer cases is approximately 1–3%.

Disorder Description: Presynaptic neuromuscular junction disorder due to antibody to P/Q type voltage-gated calcium channel on presynaptic membrane. As a result of low calcium in presynaptic nerve terminal, fewer acetylcholine vesicles are released. LEMS may be autoimmune or paraneoplastic. Small cell lung carcinoma is the most common associated malignancy in paraneoplastic cases.

Symptoms

Localization site	Comment
Neuromuscular junction	• Fatigable proximal muscle weakness (lower limbs worse than upper limbs) with decreased or absent deep tendon reflexes • Proximal lower extremity weakness without bulbar weakness and improving with repetitive activity, with recovery of tendon reflexes • Oculomotor or bulbar weakness • Dysautonomic manifestations: dry mouth, impotence, constipation
Unclear localization	• Dry mouth, chest pain, erectile dysfunction, hypotension, pain in weakened limb

Secondary Complications: Neuropathic pain, focal weakness, disability, insomnia, erectile dysfunction. Respiratory insufficiency may rarely occur in severe cases.

Treatment Complications: 3,4-Diaminopyridine (3,4-DAP) improves both neuromuscular and autonomic manifestations in 80% of patients with LEMS. The most serious adverse effect of 3,4-DAP is seizure. In addition, 3,4-DAP causes side effect of perioral or digital paresthesia. Concomitant use of 3,4-DAP and pyridostigmine may cause cramp, diarrhea, nausea, and vomiting. Immunosuppressants are used when 3,4-DAP is not effective and may cause leukopenia. Maintenance pulse intravenous immunoglobulin is also a useful treatment.

Bibliography

Bataller L, Dalmau J. Paraneoplastic disorders of the nervous system. *Continuum (Minneap Minn).* 2005;11(5, Neuro-Oncology):69–92. DOI: 10.1212/01.con.0000293680.24426.ae.

Katirji B, Kaminski HJ, Ruff RL. *Neuromuscular disorders in clinical practice.* 2nd ed. New York: Springer-Verlag; 2014.

Lancaster E. Paraneoplastic disorders. *Continuum (Minneap Minn).* 2015;21(2, Neuro-Oncology):452–75. DOI: 10.1212/01. CON.0000464180.89580.88.

Nicolle MW. Myasthenia gravis and Lambert-Eaton myasthenic syndrome. *Continuum (Minneap Minn).* 2016;22(6, Muscle and Neuromuscular Junction Disorders):1978–2005. DOI: 10.1212/ CON.0000000000000415.

Vernino S. Paraneoplastic disorders affecting the neuromuscular junction or anterior horn cell. *Continuum (Minneap Minn)*. 2009;15(1, Myasthenic Disorders and ALS):132–46. DOI: 10.1212/01.CON.0000300011.79845.eb.

Landau–Kleffner Syndrome (Progressive Epileptic Aphasia)

Epidemiology and Demographics: Rare. Onset in children aged usually between 3 and 8 years (range 2–14 years). Boys affected more frequently.

Disorder Description: An epileptic encephalopathy of childhood associated with a subacute progressive loss of language function associated with epileptic activity and seizures. EEG with frequent epileptiform discharges and nearly continuous fronto-, centro-, or posterior temporal maximal slow spike and wave activity in non-REM sleep. Formal neuropsychologic testing and speech therapy are indicated.

Diagnosis and early initiation of treatment associated with better outcomes. Antiepileptic drug (AED) therapy, such as valproate, is typically initiated first, but is infrequently associated with improvements in speech. Steroids and intravenous immunoglobulin may be effective for some individuals, suggesting an autoimmune or inflammatory component of this syndrome. Autoantibodies including those against brain-derived neurotrophic factor (BDNF) have been detected in some patients. Steroids are typically continued for several months. Multiple subpial transections have also been performed in severe cases with notable improvements.

Prognosis variable, with a third of patients despite therapy experiencing severe loss of language function, a third with moderate impairments, and a third with recovery of language function. Overt clinical seizures may be infrequent. EEG typically shows spontaneous improvement in puberty by age 15.

Symptoms

Localization site	Comment
Cerebral hemispheres	Seizures in 70–80% (absence, focal, or generalized tonic–clonic seizures). Progressive aphasia of variable severity EEG with typically unilateral peri-Sylvian 1.5- to 2.5-Hz spike wave discharges continuous in non-REM sleep

Localization site	Comment
Mental status and psychiatric aspects/ complications	Progressive loss of language skills. Verbal and auditory agnosia, word finding difficulty, expressive and receptive aphasia, mutism. Hypersensitivity to sound. Attention and short-term memory often impaired. Hyperactivity, disinhibition, emotional lability, anxiety, depression are common. Sleep disorders common

Secondary Complications: Psychiatric issues related to loss of speech: attention deficit hyperactivity disorder, anxiety, depression, sleep disorders.

Treatment Complications: AEDs such as phenytoin, carbamazepine, oxcarbazepine, and phenobarbital may exacerbate electrical status epilepticus in sleep and are typically avoided. Steroids are associated with an increased risk for mood lability, psychosis, peptic ulceration, avascular necrosis, and infection. Intravenous immunoglobulin may be associated with flu-like symptoms during infusion and rarely anaphylaxis.

Bibliography

Hughes JR. A review of the relationships between Landau–Kleffner syndrome, electrical status epilepticus during sleep, and continuous spike-waves during sleep. *Epilepsy Behav.* 2011;20(2):247–53.

Sanchez Fernandez I, et al. Electrical status epilepticus in sleep: clinical presentation and pathophysiology. *Pediatr Neurol.* 2012;47(6): 390–410.

Tuft M, et al. Landau–Kleffner syndrome. *Tidsskr Nor Laegeforen.* 2015;135(22):2061–4.

Lead Toxicity (Adults) Including Lead Neuropathy

Epidemiology and Demographics: Lead toxicity is rare in adults. Most cases have a clear exposure history and routine testing for lead or other heavy metals without any exposure in cases of neuropathy is not indicated.

Disorder Description: Lead intoxication as a result of working in indoor firing range, burning batteries for heat, or drinking moonshine made in automobile radiators causes encephalopathy commonly in children but rarely in adults, while the opposite is true regarding neuropathy. Anemia and GI disturbances are almost always present. The neuropathy is classically motor greater than sensory, but in a study evaluating workers with chronic low-level exposure there was predominant sensory involvement.

Symptoms

Localization site	Comment
Cerebral hemispheres	Seizures with acute high-level exposure only
Mental status and psychiatric aspects/complications	Encephalopathy in adults only with acute high-level exposure. Hallucinations may occur. Can progress to coma. Cognitive and behavioral changes may occur with chronic low-level exposure
Peripheral neuropathy	Classically motor predominant neuropathy but with chronic low-level exposure sensory involvement is more frequent

Bibliography

Rubens O, Logina I, Kravale I, Eglite M, Donaghy M. Peripheral neuropathy in chronic occupational inorganic lead exposure: a clinical and electrophysiologic study. *J Neurol Neurosurg Psychiatry.* 2001;71:200–4. PMID 11459892.

Spencer PS, Schaumburg HH. *Experimental and clinical neurotoxicology.* 2nd ed. Oxford, UK: Oxford University Press; 2000. pp. 315–17.

Leber's Hereditary Optic Atrophy

Epidemiology and Demographics: Affects males more than females. Age of onset is usually in late teens, but age of onset ranges from age 8 to 60 years.

Disorder Description: A subacute bilateral optic neuropathy caused by mutations in the mitochondrial genome. It is a result of mutations at 3460, 11778, and 11484 nucleotide positions. It presents with visual loss due to demyelination of the optic tracts and cell loss and gliosis of the geniculate bodies. It can also present with tremor, extrapyramidal symptoms, seizures, ataxia, spasticity, and intellectual disabilities. There is no current treatment.

Symptoms

Localization site	Comment
Cerebral hemispheres	Visual loss, seizures, spasticity
Mental status and psychiatric aspects/complications	Intellectual disabilities, extrapyramidal symptoms

Secondary Complications: Physical injury due to difficulty walking and loss of vision.

Bibliography

Brown MD, Sun F, Wallace DC. Clustering of Caucasian Leber hereditary optic neuropathy patients containing the 11778 or 14484 mutations on an mtDNA lineage. *Am J Hum Genet.* 1997;60:381.

Newman NJ, Lott MT, Wallace DC. The clinical characteristics of pedigrees of Leber's hereditary optic neuropathy with the 11778 mutation. *Am J Ophthalmol.* 1991;111:750.

Uemura A, Osame M, Nakagawa M, et al. Leber's hereditary optic neuropathy: mitochondrial and biochemical studies on muscle biopsies. *Br J Ophthalmol.* 1987;71:531.

Wallace DC, Singh G, Lott MT, et al. Mitochondrial DNA mutation associated with Leber's hereditary optic neuropathy. *Science.* 1988;242:1427.

Left Anterior Cerebral Artery (ACA) Infarction

Epidemiology and Demographics: Anterior cerebral artery (ACA) infarction is the least common large vessel stroke syndrome, accounting for ~1.3–3% of all strokes. African Americans and Hispanics are at higher risk for an ACA infarct.

Disorder Description: ACA infarction may occur as a result of cardiogenic emboli, emboli originating from the internal carotid artery, or in situ atherosclerosis. The ACA commonly supplies the parasagittal motor, sensory, prefrontal cortices, and the supplemental motor areas. Infarction to these areas may present with right-sided weakness and sensory loss (leg > arm). Other symptoms can include aphasia, abulia, and alien limb syndrome due to callosal disconnection. Patients with hypertension, hyperlipidemia, diabetes, atrial fibrillation, history of myocardial infarction, and smokers are at increased risk for ACA stroke.

Symptoms

Localization site	Comment
Cerebral hemispheres	Right hemiparesis and right-sided sensory loss (leg > arm), mutism, transcortical motor aphasia
Mental status and psychiatric aspects/complications	Acute confusional state, frontal lobe behavioral disorder

Secondary Complications: Increased intracranial pressure.

Treatment Complications: Complications of thrombolysis, i.e., intracerebral hemorrhage, systemic bleeding, and angioedema.

Bibliography

Bogousslavsky J, Regli F. Anterior cerebral artery territory infarction in the Lausanne Stroke Registry: clinical and etiologic patterns. *Arch Neurol.* 1990;47(2):144–50.

Gacs G, Fox AJ, Barnett HJ, Vinuela F. Occurrence and mechanisms of occlusion of the anterior cerebral artery. *Stroke.* 1983;14(6):952–9.

Kumral E, Bayulkem G, Evyapan D, Yunten N. Spectrum of anterior cerebral artery territory infarction: clinical and MRI findings. *Eur J Neurol.* 2002;9(6):615–24.

Leigh Disease/Subacute Necrotizing Encephalomyelopathy

Epidemiology and Demographics: Occurs by 1 year of age in more than 50% of patients, but may present as late as early adulthood. Occurs in 1/40,000 new borns, and occurs more commonly in Canada and the Faroe Islands.

Disorder Description: Mitochondrial neurodegenerative disorder with a wide range of clinical presentations. In infants or children it presents as loss of head control, vomiting, irritability, hypotonia, generalized seizures, myoclonic jerks, dysarthria, ataxia, tonic spasms, ophthalmoplegia, nystagmus, episodic hyperventilation, peripheral neuropathy, autonomic failure, or delay in walking. In adults it may present as progressive dementia. It can present episodically or progressively with exacerbations. It is usually exacerbated by viral illness or infection.

Symptoms

Localization site	Comment
Cerebral hemispheres	Generalized seizures, myoclonic jerks, tonic spasms, choreiform movements
Mental status and psychiatric aspects/complications	Dementia, psychomotor regression, developmental delay
Brainstem	Ataxia, dysarthria
Cerebellum	Ataxia
Cranial nerves	Nystagmus, ophthalmoplegia
Spinal cord	Myelopathy
Peripheral neuropathy	Areflexia, weakness, atrophy, slow conduction velocities on nerve testing

Secondary Complicatons: Respiratory issues associated with this disease including apnea, dyspnea, and dysphagia can lead to infections and eventual death.

Bibliography

Finsterer J. Leigh and Leigh-like syndrome in children and adults. *Pediatr Neurol.* 2008;39(4):223–35. DOI: 10.1016/j.pediatrneurol.2008.07.013.

Ropper AH, Samuels MA, Klein JP. Inherited metabolic diseases of the nervous system. In *Adams & Victor's principles of neurology*, 10th ed. New York, NY: McGraw-Hill; 2014. Chapter 37.

Lennox–Gastaut Syndrome (LGS)

Epidemiology and Demographics: Onset of Lennox–Gastaut syndrome (LGS) is between 2 and 6 years old. Incidence is unknown; estimated to comprise between 1% and 10% of all childhood epilepsies.

Disorder Description: LGS is characterized by multiple seizure types, cognitive delay, and characteristic EEG pattern. Symptomatic etiologies include genetic abnormalities, neurocutaneous syndromes, hypoxic–ischemic injury, and head injury. West syndrome may precede diagnosis in 30–65% of patients.

Generally poor prognosis, with medically intractable seizures and developmental delays. Treatment options include lamotrigine, topiramate, rufinamide, felbamate, clobazam, zonisamide, and valproate. Corpus callosotomy or vagal nerve stimulation may be palliative.

Symptoms

Localization site	Comment
Cerebral hemispheres	Seizure types include atonic, tonic, atypical absence seizures, and generalized tonic–clonic seizures. Focal onset seizures may occur as well
	EEG findings include slowing, disorganization, a slow spike and wave pattern at 1.5–2.5 Hz, and bursts of paroxysmal fast activity
Mental status and psychiatric aspects/complications	Psychomotor delay and intellectual impairment
	Attention deficit hyperactivity disorder, anxiety, aggressive behavior, psychosis, and depression
	Social dysfunction
	Sleep cycle disruption

Secondary Complications: Developmental delay, intellectual disability, and intractable seizures. Injuries and falls related to seizures leading to head trauma, dental injury, and fractures.

Treatment Complications: Felbamate carries a black box warning for aplastic anemia and hepatic failure, and is associated with anorexia and insomnia. Topiramate and zonisamide are associated with somnolence, anorexia, and nephrolithiasis. Lamotrigine is associated with risk for serious rash. Rufinamide is associated with gastrointestinal upset. Valproate is associated with liver dysfunction, thrombocytopenia, tremor, hair changes, and weight gain. Clobazam is associated with sedation, hypersecretion, constipation, paroxysmal agitation, and insomnia. Corpus callosotomy may be associated with surgical complications, a disconnection syndrome, and transient symptoms of frontal lobe dysfunction (paresis, akinetic-mutism). Vagal nerve stimulation is most commonly associated with hoarseness.

Bibliography

Arzimanoglou, A., et al. Lennox–Gastaut syndrome: a consensus approach on diagnosis, assessment, management, and trial methodology. *Lancet Neurol.* 2009;8(1):82–93.

Kerr M, Kluger G, Philip S. Evolution and management of Lennox–Gastaut syndrome through adolescence and into adulthood: are seizures always the primary issue? *Epileptic Disord.* 2011;13(Suppl 1):S15–26.

Montouris GD, Wheless JW, Glauser TA. The efficacy and tolerability of pharmacologic treatment options for Lennox–Gastaut syndrome. *Epilepsia.* 2014;55(Suppl 4):10–20.

Werz MA, Pita-Garcia IL. *Epilepsy syndromes.* Philadelphia, PA: Saunders/Elsevier; 2010. pp. ix, 216 p.

Lens Subluxation

Epidemiology and Demographics: Lens subluxation, or ectopia lentis, may be an autosomal dominant or recessive trait and may be isolated or associated with other ocular abnormalities. In a Danish national survey, 396 cases were identified, with equal male and female prevalence, with an estimated prevalence rate of 6.4/100,000 people. The majority of cases in the study had ectopia lentis as a manifestation of systemic disease with Marfan syndrome being the most common condition. Isolated ectopia lentis may present at any age, including being present at birth.

Disorder Description: The lens is a transparent structure that alters the refraction of light entering the eye. It is suspended behind the iris by zonular fibers that attach the lens to the surrounding ciliary body. The zonules can be broken by trauma or iatrogenically during intraocular surgery, causing the lens to decenter, or dislocate entirely. As mentioned above, the lens can also dislocate because of inherited disorders that affect zonular strength. The lens is displaced away from the area of weakened zonules. Visual acuity, refractive error, and intraocular pressure can all be affected by lens location and these need to be monitored regularly in affected patients.

Symptoms: Symptoms depend on the severity of lens subluxation. Patients with mild decentration, where the edge of the lens remains outside the visual axis, maintain the best correctable vision and may be asymptomatic. If the subluxation extends such that the lens is no longer in the visual axis, the patient becomes effectively aphakic. Patients may also complain of fluctuating vision as the lens moves from zonule instability.

Localization site	
Cerebral hemispheres	**Homocystinuria** is a multisystem disorder of metabolism resulting in elevated levels of homocysteine, which is associated with downward lens subluxation. Thromboembolic events and seizures are other neurologic complications if the condition is untreated
	Marfan syndrome, a connective tissue disorder, is associated with upward lens subluxation. Vascular complications such as dissection of cerebral arteries leading to stroke have been reported
Mental status and psychiatric aspects/ complications	**Homocystinuria** (see above) is associated with intellectual disabilities **Sulfite oxidase deficiency** is a rare disorder of lens subluxation associated with intellectual disability, attenuated growth of the brain, and seizures

Secondary Complications: Secondary complications include progression of lens subluxation, cataract formation, pupil block glaucoma, or retinal detachment. A subluxed lens can become cataractous even if it does not dislocate completely.

Treatment Complications: Many cases of lens subluxation can be managed medically, typically by correcting the refractive error with glasses or contact lenses. Surgery for a subluxated lens requires additional surgical planning to minimize the risk of complications such as dropped lens (when the lens dislocates completely and falls into the vitreous cavity) and vitreous prolapse (vitreous entering the anterior chamber). As with cataract surgery, treatment complications include vision loss, pain, and diplopia.

Bibliography

Chandra A, Charteris D. Molecular pathogenesis and management strategies of ectopia lentis. *Eye.* 2014;28(2):162–8.

Leprosy (Lepromatous Neuropathy)

Epidemiology and Demographics: About 200 new cases annually in the United States. More than 75% of cases were immigrants. Global prevalence is 175,000 in 2014. Most cases occur in developing countries including India, Brazil, and Indonesia. Male-to-female ratio is 1.5 to 1.

Disorder Description: Leprosy is caused by *Mycobacterium leprae* infections. *Mycobacterium leprae* can be transmitted by respiratory route or direct contact with armadillos. Depending on the host immune responses, clinical manifestation can be either tuberculoid (pauci-bacillary) or lepromatous (multi-bacillary). Skin and peripheral nerves are commonly affected. Patients with leprosy usually present with characteristic skin lesions, hair loss, sensory loss, neuropathic pain, claw hand, and foot drop.

Symptoms

Localization site	Comment
Cerebral hemispheres	Dementia
Peripheral nerves	Neuropathy of median nerve, ulnar nerve, common peroneal and posterior tibial nerve, facial nerve, radial cutaneous nerve, great auricular nerve. Segmental demyelination is thought to be the pathogenesis. Nerve enlargement often occurs
	Symmetric polyneuropathy has been reported

Secondary Complications: Systemic inflammatory response (immunologic reactions) can cause deformity and paralysis secondary to severe nerve injury.

Treatment Complications: Dapsone inhibits folic acid synthesis with subsequent peripheral neuropathy. Minocycline can cause dizziness and unsteadiness.

Bibliography

Lastória JC, de Abreu MAMM. Leprosy: review of the epidemiological, clinical, and etiopathogenic aspects – Part 1. *An Bras Dermatol.* 2014;89(2):205–18. http://doi.org/10.1590/abd1806-4841.20142450.

Su TW, Wu LL, Lin CP. The prevalence of dementia and depression in Taiwanese institutionalized leprosy patients, and the effectiveness evaluation of reminiscence therapy: a longitudinal, single-blind, randomized control study. *Int J Geriatr Psychiatry.* 2012;27(2):187–96.

Leptospirosis

Epidemiology and Demographics: The reported incidence of leptospirosis worldwide is 870,000 cases annually. Leptospirosis is more prevalent in tropical climates.

Disorder Description: Leptospirosis is a zoonotic disease caused by *Leptospira* spirochetes. Infected animal or environmental exposure is the main route of transmission. Patients with leptospirosis usually present with sudden-onset fever, myalgia, headache, and conjunctival suffusion. Hemorrhagic diathesis, hypokalemia/hyponatremia, and transaminitis are common laboratory abnormalities. Severe leptospirosis can lead to Weil syndrome (Weil's disease), which is characterized by jaundice, renal failure, and hemorrhagic manifestations.

Symptoms

Localization site	Comment
Cerebral hemispheres	Aseptic meningitis (most common), cerebral venous thrombosis, and intracranial hemorrhage
Cerebellum	Ataxia
Cranial nerves	Optic neuritis
Spinal cord	Myelitis
Peripheral nerves	Neuropathy

Secondary Complications: Hepatic failure and renal failure secondary to severe leptospirosis can lead to altered mental status.

Treatment Complications: Antimicrobial treatment of leptospirosis can lead to Jarisch–Herxheimer reaction, an acute inflammatory response to spirochete clearance. Common symptoms include fever, rigors, and low blood pressure.

Bibliography

Day N. Epidemiology, microbiology, clinical manifestations, and diagnosis of leptospirosis. In Post TW, ed. UpToDate. Waltham, MA. www.uptodate.com/contents/leptospirosis-epidemiology-microbiology-clinical-manifestations-and-diagnosis?search=Epidemiology,%20microbiology,%20clinical%20manifestations,%20and%20diagnosis%20of%20leptospirosis&source=search_result&selectedTitle=1~77&usage_type=default&display_rank=1. Accessed Aug 30, 2018.

Day N. Leptospirosis: treatment and prevention. In Post TW, ed. UpToDate. Waltham, MA. www.uptodate.com/contents/leptospirosis-treatment-and-prevention?topicRef=5527&source=see_link. Accessed Aug 30, 2018.

Singh R, et al. Cerebellar ataxia due to leptospirosis: a case report. *BMC Infect Dis.* 2016;16:748.

Vale TC, et al. Weil syndrome: a rare cause of cerebral venous thrombosis. *JAMA Neurol.* 2014;71(2):238–9.

Lesch–Nyhan Syndrome

Epidemiology and Demographics: Prevalence of Lesch–Nyhan syndrome (LNS) is 1/380,000, with similar frequency in all populations. The genetic defect is X-linked recessive, with males almost exclusively affected. The HPRT-1 gene encodes an enzyme responsible for purine metabolism, resulting in breakdown but not recycling of purines. This in turn results in abnormally high levels of uric acid. Low dopamine levels have also been noted, and may explain some of the neurobehavioral profile.

Disorder Description: LNS is a neurodevelopmental disease caused by deficiency of the hypoxanthine–guanine phosphoribosyl transferase (HPRT) enzyme. It is characterized by hyperuricemia, neurologic disability, and behavioral problems. Diagnosis is suggested by raised uric acid and a raised urinary urate to creatinine ratio greater than 2.0. Cell enzyme activity <1.5% is diagnostic. Symptoms begin from age 3–6 months, with hypotonia and developmental delay evident. Within the first few years, extrapyramidal (dystonia, chorea) and then pyramidal involvement is evident. Cognitive impairment and behavioral disturbances emerge between ages 2 and 3 years. Behavioral problems include intellectual disability, aggressive, impulsive behaviors, and obsessive self-injurious behavior, with persistent self-injurious behavior (biting fingers, hands, lips, and cheeks) being a hallmark of the syndrome. The deposition of "orange sand" in diapers of infants (urate crystals) may occur from the age of 6 months; urate nephrolithiasis may predispose to UTI and hematuria. In older children, uric acid deposition may manifest as gouty tophi in joints and ears.

There is a clinical spectrum of severity with partial syndromes being increasingly recognized. In these milder variants, self-injury may not occur, cognition may be normal, and dystonia may be mild or absent. Some patients may demonstrate renal effects of hyperuricemia alone.

Symptoms

Localization site	Comment
Cerebral hemispheres	Deep nuclei: – Extrapyramidal movement disorder – Hypotonia, then severe action dystonia, choreathetosis, ballismus, opisthotonus, resembling athetoid cerebral palsy Pyramidal involvement – spasticity, hyperreflexia, extensor plantar response: – Most children with classic LNS never walk Cognitive behavioral deficits: – Difficult to assess because of behavioral disturbance – Aggression, vomiting, spitting, coprolalia – Self-mutilation – biting of hands and lips MRI demonstrates nonspecific atrophy with reduced caudate nucleus volume
Skull base/cervical spine	Death may occur from atlantoaxial subluxation from forcible opisthotonus

Secondary Complications: Confusion secondary to urosepsis or endstage renal disease due to renal stones.

Treatment Complications: Management includes the use of allopurinol for renal complications, but has no effect on the neurobehavioral profile. Symptomatic treatment of dystonia and spasticity (baclofen, benzodiazepine), behavioral therapy, and protective equipment and restraints to reduce injury from self-harming behaviors. Deep brain stimulation (DBS) has been used with mixed results, and ecopipam, a D1/D5 dopamine antagonist, is currently being studied in phase III trials.

Potential treatment adverse effects:

Sedation may result from benzodiazepines, baclofen, and ecopipam.

Benzodiazepines in overdose can cause confusion and respiratory depression and coma.

Hypotonia, particularly axial hypotonia, may result from baclofen.

Seizures may result from a lowered seizure threshold (baclofen).

Mild emesis and anxiety from ecopipam.

Bibliography

European Medicines Agency. Public summary of opinion on orphan designation. Ecopipam for the treatment of Lesch–Nyhan disease. Mar 2, 2010. www.ema.europa.eu/docs/en_GB/document_library/Orphan_designation/2010/03/WC500075166.pdf. Accessed Aug 21, 2018.

Jinnah HA. Lesch–Nyhan disease: from mechanism to model and back again. *Dis Model Mech.* 2009;2:116–21; DOI: 10.1242/dmm.002543.

Nyhan WL, O'Neill JP, Jinnah HA, Harris JC. Lesch–Nyhan syndrome. In Pagon RA, Adam MP, Ardinger HH, et al., eds. Updated May 15, 2014. *Gene Reviews®*. Seattle (WA): University of Washington, Seattle; 1993–2016. Available from: www.ncbi.nlm.nih.gov/books/NBK1149/. Accessed Aug 21, 2018.

Leukemia

Epidemiology and Demographics: According to the National Cancer Institute, the incidence in the United States is nearly 14/100,000, with over 400,000 individuals diagnosed with leukemia in 2015. Lifetime risk of developing leukemia is believed to be 1.5% of the population.

Disorder Description: Leukemias are neoplasms characterized by malignant cells in the bloodstream with origin from granulocytic or lymphoid precursors. Neurologic involvement is most commonly due to meningeal metastasis. It can also be due to mass lesions (chloroma), direct parenchymal infiltration, conversion of chronic lymphocytic leukemia to a non-Hodgkin lymphoma (Richter syndrome), and side effects of treatment.

Symptoms

Localization site	Comment
Cerebral hemispheres	Hemorrhagic and nonhemorrhagic stroke due to septic emboli, nonseptic embolic disease (nonbacterial thrombotic endocarditis), or disseminated intravascular coagulation Hemiparesis, aphasia, visual disturbances, headache, abrupt loss of consciousness, or seizures
Mental status and psychiatric aspects/complications	Confusion and encephalopathy (along with seizures and blurry vision in **reversible posterior leukoencephalopathy**)

Localization site	Comment
Cerebellum	Ataxia due to mass (chloroma)
Base of skull	Skull-based chloroma: results in cranial or optic neuropathies
Spinal cord	**Paraneoplastic necrotizing myelopathy (no known antibody so far):** bilateral motor, sensory, and sphincter deficits (ascending, transverse cord dysfunction affecting both anterior and posterior horns of the spinal cord)
Peripheral nerves	**Paraneoplastic sensory neuropathy** (very rare anti-Hu antibodies and anti-CV2 antibodies): both upper and lower extremities are affected and can be either symmetric or asymmetric
Unclear localization	**Bacterial meningitis:** opportunistic infections

Treatment Complications: There are many chemotherapeutic drugs that can result in multiple complications, including:

Cisplatin: autonomic neuropathy, encephalopathy, cortical blindness, optic neuritis, ototoxicity, peripheral neuropathy

Cyclophosphamide: blurred vision, dizziness, encephalopathy, seizures

Ifosfamide: encephalopathy, extrapyramidal syndrome, peripheral neuropathy, seizures

L-asparaginase: venous sinus thrombosis

Radiotherapy used in treatment can result in leukoencephalopathy.

Bibliography

Armentrout SA, Ulrich RF. Neurological manifestations of acute granulocytic leukemia. *West J Med*. 1974;121(1):1–5.

Narayanaswamy AS, Prakash MP, Kakkar R. Neurological manifestations of leukemia: clinical and pathological findings. *J Assoc Physicians India*. 1992;40(11):740–2.

National Cancer Institute. Cancer stat facts: leukemia. https://seer.cancer.gov/statfacts/html/leuks.html. Accessed Aug 30, 2018.

Lewy Body Dementia (LBD)

Epidemiology and Demographics: Lewy body dementia (LBD) is an umbrella term encompassing both dementia with Lewy bodies (DLB) and Parkinson's disease dementia (PDD). LBD is the second most common neurodegenerative dementia after Alzheimer's disease (AD). Cognitive decline in DLB patients typically occurs after age 55 years. The incidence of dementia in Parkinson's disease increases with the duration of illness.[1]

Disorder Description: When dementia occurs before or within 1 year of the development of parkinsonian motor signs, DLB is the diagnosis. When motor signs present first and cognitive impairment develops later, PDD is the diagnosis. This distinction is somewhat arbitrary, and at autopsy, Lewy bodies are found in the brainstem and throughout the cortex and limbic system in both DLB and PDD. Similarly, loss of dopaminergic neurons in the midbrain and loss of cholinergic neurons in the ventral forebrain are found in both LBD and PDD. Amyloid plaques are found in both. It is not possible to distinguish the two entities reliably based solely on neuropathologic features.[1,2] Some speculate that DLB and PDD may represent different phenotypes of a similar underlying pathologic process. In DLB, the limbic system and basal forebrain are affected early on. In PDD, Lewy bodies initially deposit in the medulla (Braak stage 1), spreading up the brainstem to the midbrain including the substantia nigra (stages 2, 3), and later on involve diffuse regions of the cortex (stages 4 to 6).[3]

Clinical features of DLB include visual hallucinations, fluctuations in the level of alertness and/or wakefulness, and "soft" parkinsonian signs. Visual hallucinations occur early in DLB, whereas in AD and PDD, they are features of more severe disease. Visual hallucinations in DLB are typically well formed and often feature people or small animals. They can be either emotionally neutral or dysphoric. Fluctuations in arousal are another core feature of DLB. Patients can be lucid and coherent one moment, and confused or somnolent the next.[1]

Dementia occurs in a significant percentage of Parkinson's patients, with one study finding an 8-year prevalence rate of 78%.[4] Medications used to treat PD occasionally impair cognition and/or behavior. Dopamine agonists often precipitate hallucinations. Amantadine and anti-cholinergic drugs such as triphexyphenidyl can be associated with cognitive impairment.[1]

Cognitive impairment presents similarly in DLB and PDD. Executive dysfunction occurs in both.

Patients may also have problems with visuospatial orientation, and become lost. Impairment of recent memory is a common finding. Problems with memory retrieval with relatively preserved encoding (storage) distinguish patients with DLB from AD patients where storage problems predominate. For example, the DLB/PDD patient may have problems with free recall, but performance may improve when given category cues. Such cues are less helpful in patients with AD.[1]

Symptoms

Localization site	Comment
Cerebral hemispheres	Lewy body disease throughout the cortex and limbic system, loss of dopaminergic neurons in the midbrain, and loss of cholinergic neurons in the ventral forebrain all contribute to a global picture of cognitive impairment and neuropsychiatric symptoms
Brainstem/cranial nerves	LBD occurs initially in the brainstem in PD, subsequently ascending to the midbrain including the substantia nigra, presenting clinically with the cardinal features of PD

Secondary Complications: Late in the disease course, the individual becomes bedbound and susceptible to decubitus ulcers and assorted infections, as well as severe malnourishment. Decisions concerning the best ways to provide nutrition are challenging and require repeated discussion with family members over several visits. Referral to specialists such as social workers, family clergy, and support groups can be invaluable.

Treatment Complications: Cholinesterase inhibitors (for example, rivastigmine) can be used for cognitive impairment in both DLB and PDD, and may also improve psychotic symptoms (although in the authors' experience this effect is modest). Carbidopa/levodopa is the mainstay for treating motor features of PD. When motor features in DLB such as gait impairment warrant a therapeutic trial, carbidopa/levodopa is often ineffective and may worsen hallucinations and/or cognition. DLB patients are especially sensitive to neuroleptics that may exacerbate motor slowing and gait impairment, and can also cloud cognition further by impairing alertness. Neuroleptics should be used with caution in DLB. Nonetheless, hallucinations may be so frightening that pharmacologic therapy is needed.

Quetiapine, clozapine, and pimavanserin are reasonable choices as they exacerbate parkinsonism less than most other neuroleptics.[1]

Treating parkinsonian motor symptoms with dopaminergic drugs may worsen hallucinations or exacerbate cognitive dysfunction for patients with PDD. Treating psychosis in DLB with neuroleptics may precipitate clinical worsening, as DLB patients are highly sensitive to neuroleptics.

References

1. Gomperts SN. Lewy body dementias: dementia with Lewy bodies and Parkinson disease dementia. *Continuum (Minneap Minn)*. 2016;22:435–63.
2. Tsuboi Y, Dickson DW. Dementia with Lewy bodies and Parkinson's disease with dementia: are they different? *Parkinsonism Relat Disord*. 2005;11;S47–51.
3. Braak H, Del Tredici K, Rüb U, et al. Staging of brain pathology related to sporadic Parkinson's disease. *Neurobiol Aging*. 2003;24:197–211.
4. Aarsland D, Andersen K, Larsen JP, Lolk A, Kragh-Sørensen P. Prevalence and characteristics of dementia in Parkinson disease: an 8-year prospective study. *Arch Neurol*. 2003;60:387–92.

Lhermitte–Duclos Disease (LDD)

Epidemiology and Demographics: Lhermitte–Duclos disease (LDD) is a rare condition, usually affecting patients aged 30–50 years with no sex predilection. About 220 LDD cases have been reported in the literature so far.

Disorder Description: Lhermitte–Duclos disease, also known as dysplastic gangliocytoma of the cerebellum, is a rare benign cerebellar mass characterized by enlargement of the cerebellar folia; MRI typically shows "tiger striping" sign. It can be associated with Cowden's disease.

Symptoms

Localization site	Comment
Cerebellum	Falls and unsteady gait with cerebellar signs on examination
Unclear localization	Increased intracranial pressure due to obstructive hydrocephalus: headache, nausea, vomiting, papilledema

Treatment Complications: Surgical resection can cause ataxia.

Bibliography

Govindan A, Premkumar S, Alapatt JP. Lhermitte–Duclos disease (dysplastic gangliocytoma of the cerebellum) as a component of Cowden syndrome. *Indian J Pathol Microbiol.* 2012;55(1):107–8.

Nayil K, Wani M, Ramzan A, et al. Lhermitte–Duclos disease with syrinx: case report and literature review. *Turk Neurosurg.* 2011;21(4): 651–4.

Rivera M, Lara-Del Rio JA, Di Pasquale-Guadalupe L, Zequeira J. Silent presentation of a solid pseudopapillary neoplasm of the pancreas. *Am J Case Rep.* 2017;18:656–9.

Lightning Strike

Epidemiology and Demographics: Annual death rate less than 0.1 cases per million for the last 5 years. Direct strike injuries are seen in 3 to 5% of injuries. Lightning injuries are multisystem, primary neurologic injuries and widely variable injuries. Occasionally, a person may incur secondary injuries such as blunt trauma, burns, penetration by shrapnel or bits of an exploded tree.

Symptoms

Localization site	Comment
Cardiac	Cardiac arrest
Respiratory	Respiratory arrest
Autonomic nervous system	Hypertension, positive tilt table test, autonomic instability
Extremities	Chronic pain syndrome
Neurocognitive	Cognitive blunting, short-term memory problems, and working memory deficits, attention deficit, easy distractibility, decreased executive function, difficulty multitasking, dizziness, balance problems
Otologic system	Tinnitus, hearing loss, balance problems, and dizziness

Localization site	Comment
Cerebral hemisphere	Headache, nausea, vomiting, sleep disorder, atypical seizure disorder, hemiplegia, coma, secondary endocrine deficits, hypothalamic damage. Keraunoparalysis is defined as temporary paralysis, which may last minutes to hours
Pituitary	Secondary endocrine effects, hypothalamic damage
Ophthalmic	Cataracts, macular holes, corneal lesions, hyphema, iritis, vitreous hemorrhage, retinal detachment, and optic nerve injury

Secondary Complications: Hearing loss, cataracts, neurocognitive deficits, isolation, and depression.

Treatment Complications: Nonsteroidal anti-inflammatories can cause GI side effects; narcotics and tricyclic antidepressants can cause drowsiness. Narcotics can cause dependency.

Bibliography

Andrews CJ, Cooper MA, Darveniza M. *Lightening injuries: Electrical, medical, and legal aspects.* Boca Raton, FL: CRC Press; 1992.

Center for Disease Control and Prevention. Lightening associated deaths – United States, 1980–1995. *MMWR Morb Mortal Wkly Rep.* 1998;47(19):391–4.

Listeria monocytogenes

Epidemiology and Demographics: The annual incidence of *Listeria monocytogenes* infection is 0.29/100,000 persons. The incidence is significantly higher in immunocompromised individuals, including neonates, older adults (1.3/100,000), and pregnant women (3/100,000).

Disorder Description: *Listeria monocytogenes* is a short, gram-positive rod with tumbling activity that can cause self-limited gastroenteritis in immunocompetent individuals and invasive disease, including bacteremia and central nervous system (CNS) infection, in immunocompromised patients. Patients usually acquire infection from contaminated food. Severe fetal complications such as fetal death, premature birth, or newborn infection can occur in pregnancy-related listeriosis, although CNS infection during pregnancy is uncommon.

Symptoms

Localization site	Comment
Cerebral hemispheres	Meningoencephalitis is most common, and can present with fever, altered mental status, or event coma. Cerebritis, brain abscess with focal findings or seizures
Brainstem	Rhombencephalitis with fever, nausea, vomiting, headache, and later cranial nerve palsy and ataxia. Respiratory failure can occur
Cerebellum	Ataxia secondary to encephalitis
Cranial nerves	Cranial nerve palsy secondary to encephalitis, deafness

Secondary Complications: In previous studies, about 60% of survivors from either rhombencephalitis or brain abscess develop chronic neurologic sequelae. Highest mortality rate was found in patients with bacteremia, in whom 3-month mortality rate is more than 50%.

Treatment Complications: Ampicillin is used to treat listeria bacteremia. Ampicillin and gentamicin are the combination therapy for CNS listeria infection. If patient has penicillin allergy and is unable to be desensitized, trimethoprim–sulfamethoxazole or meropenem can be used. Gentamicin can lead to neuromuscular blockade and ototoxicity and meropenem can cause headache and seizure.

Bibliography

Charlier C, et al. Clinical features and prognostic factors of listeriosis: the MONALISA national prospective cohort study. *Lancet Infect Dis.* 2017;17(5):510–19.

de Noordhout CM, et al. The global burden of listeriosis: a systematic review and meta-analysis. *Lancet Infect Dis.* 14(11):1073–82.

Lobar Hemorrhages

Epidemiology and Demographics: Lobar hemorrhages result from ruptured vessels within the white matter or at the gray–white junction of the cerebral hemispheres. Chronic or severe acute hypertension and cerebral amyloid angiopathy are the most common causes by far. Acute hypertension may result from abuse of cocaine or other sympathomimetic drugs. Amyloid angiopathy, practically speaking, occurs after the age of 65 and the relative contribution to lobar hemorrhages of this disorder increases with age. Anticoagulation for atrial fibrillation or other cardiac or coagulapathic disorders is increasingly common as a cause. However, underlying lesions must always be excluded, especially primary or metastatic malignancies, and arteriovenous malformations.

Disorder Description: Lobar hemorrhage is a parenchymal hemorrhage that usually occurs suddenly and without warning. There is increased risk during Valsalva maneuver such as may occur during straining at a bowel movement or on lifting a heavy object. Focal symptoms are typically maximal at onset but level of consciousness can deteriorate with time as edema develops. Diagnosis is by CT and/or MRI.

Symptoms

Localization site	Comment
Cerebral hemispheres	Lobar hemorrhage can occur in the frontal, parietal, occipital, or temporal lobe and will produce focal findings appropriate to that lobe. Frontal lobe lesions tend to produce apathy with contralateral weakness. Parietal lesions produce neglect with sensory disturbance and apraxia. Temporal lesions produce memory disturbances and confusion as described below. Dominant hemisphere lesions also cause aphasia, typically Wernicke's type. Occipital lesions cause hemianopia
Mental status and psychiatric aspects/ complications	Lobar hemorrhages of the temporal lobe produce confusion and frequently agitation immediately. When speech disturbance occurs, the patient is often extremely frustrated, adding to their agitation. They are frequently misdiagnosed with an acute psychiatric disturbance. Lobar hemorrhages in any location can produce alteration of consciousness, from mild drowsiness to coma

Secondary Complications: Lobar hemorrhages may be associated with intraventricular extension of the hemorrhage (IVH). This is typical of amyloid angiopathy. In the setting of hypertension, this increases mortality risk. Hydrocephalus is common after IVH.

Seizures occur in up to 50% so that most patients with lobar intracerebral hemorrhage (ICH) receive a prophylactic antiepileptic drug. All of the usual complications associated with altered consciousness are common, including respiratory failure, ventilator-associated pneumonia, DVT, pulmonary embolus, and UTI.

Treatment Complications: When lobar hemorrhage occurs in patients taking antiplatelet agents or anticoagulants, it is routine to provide a dose of platelets or to reverse the anticoagulant. This exposes the patient to risk of the thrombotic event for which the agent had been prescribed. Hyperventilating patients to reduce elevated intracranial pressure exposes the patient to risk of global central nervous system ischemia if pCO_2 falls below 25 mmHg. After hypertensive ICH, lowering systolic blood pressure to 140 mmHg may yield a mean arterial pressure that is insufficient to support cerebral perfusion if their autoregulatory curve has shifted significantly to the right due to severe chronic hypertension. This may result in watershed infarcts in the cerebral hemispheres. In general, lowering the mean arterial pressure by more than 25% from baseline should be avoided. When an extraventricular drain is inserted, there is the risk of bleeding or of ventriculitis, especially if the drain is retained for more than 5 days. Craniectomy is often associated with a scaphoid appearance of the head overlying the large bone flap that is removed between the acute period and bone flap reinsertion. Skin breakdown may occur on the edges.

Bibliography

Aguilar MI, Freeman WD. Spontaneous intracerebral hemorrhage. *Semin Neurol.* 2010;30(5):555–64. DOI: 10.1055/s–0030–1268865. Epub 2011 Jan 4.

Locked-In Syndrome

Epidemiology and Dermographics: Locked-in syndrome nearly always results from thrombosis of the basilar artery, which is usually due to atherosclerosis or cardioembolus but can occur with any type of injury to the vertebrobasilar system, including dissection or operative complications. Locked-in syndrome is estimated to occur in less than 1% of strokes and is considered to be very rare. A transient syndrome similar to locked-in syndrome may result from neuromuscular paralysis from any cause.

Disorder Description: Locked-in syndrome is among the most catastrophic neurologic syndromes because the patient has normal consciousness but is paralyzed and virtually unable to communicate. The hallmark of the syndrome is the preserved ability to elevate the eyes on request. Locked-in syndrome must be tested for in all apparently comatose patients by seeking this sign, including while holding their eyelids open and requesting the patient to look up.

Symptoms

Localization site	Comment
Cerebral hemispheres	The patient is usually awake and has normal mentation
Mental status and psychiatric aspects/ complications	It is difficult to imagine the psychiatric reaction of patients with this disorder. Because communication is limited, even with the use of custom communicative devices, full expression is rarely achieved
Brainstem	The syndrome results from infarction of basis pontis and part of the pontine tegmentum so that all cranial nerve function is lost except that the patient may have preserved upgaze and eyelid opening, which permits identification of the syndrome and provides the only means of communication. Interruption of the corticospinal tracts in basis pontis produces complete bilateral hemiplegia

Secondary Complications: These patients are paralyzed and require ventilation so that they are at high risk for pulmonary, skin, and genitourinary tract infections as well as DVT and pulmonary emboli.

Treatment Complications: Because of the catastrophic nature of the established syndrome, intra-arterial thrombolysis is recommended for up to 24 hours after symptom onset. Aggressive efforts at the later times are associated with hemorrhagic complications within the brainstem and cerebellum. Systemic thrombolysis or anticoagulation carry risk of local or systemic bleeding.

Bibliography

Patterson JR, Grabois M. Locked-in syndrome: a review of 139 cases. *Stroke.* 1986;17:758–64.

Roussea M-C, et al. Quality of life in patients with locked-in syndrome: Evolution over a 6-year period. *Orphanet J Rare Dis.* 2015;10:88.

Loiasis

Epidemiology and Demographics: Loiasis is prevalent in west and central Africa. About 3–13 million people are estimated to have *Loa loa* infection worldwide. *Chrysops* species, biting deerflies, are the major vector transmitting *Loa loa*.

Disorder Description: Loiasis (African eye worm) is caused by the nematode *Loa loa*. Patients with loiasis are usually asymptomatic but can present with two characteristic symptoms: Calabar swelling (localized, transient swelling) and subconjunctival worm migration. Pathology is caused by hypersensitivity reaction to parasite or adult worm migration. Loiasis can be diagnosed by direct visualization or serologic testing and can be treated with antiparasite therapy including diethylcarbamazine, albendazole, or ivermectin.

Symptoms

Localization site	Comment
Cerebral hemispheres	Encephalitis is associated with high *Loa loa* microfilariae concentration in the blood; often occurs after treatment
Eye	Adult worm migrates underneath the conjunctiva, which can be visualized directly. Rarely, eye pain or intraocular inflammation can occur
Peripheral neuropathy	Compression, entrapment, or angioedema of peripheral nerves can occur as a consequence of Calabar swelling, a form of transient localized angioedema secondary to hypersensitivity reaction to parasite or microfilariae

Secondary Complications: Severe eosinophilia induced by the parasite can lead to endomyocardial fibrosis and subsequent cardiomyopathy. Renal failure was reported in some cases secondary to immune complex deposition.

Treatment Complications: Adverse effects from treatment are highly correlated with microfilariae blood counts. It is recommended to monitor patients in the first 3 days of treatment for hypersensitivity response and, more severely, encephalopathy. For patients with high microfilariae blood counts (>50,000 microfilariae/mL blood), apheresis or pretreatment with albendazole should be considered prior to diethylcarbamazine.

Bibliography

Klion AD. Loiasis (Loa loa infection). In Post TW, ed. *UpToDate*. Waltham, MA. Updated May 4, 2017.

Padgett JJ, Jacobsen KH. Loiasis: African eye worm. *Trans R Soc Trop Med Hyg*. 2008;102(10):983–9. DOI: 10.1016/j.trstmh.2008.03.022.

Lumbar Disc Degeneration

Epidemiology and Demographics: In the United States back pain is the second leading symptom that prompts a visit to a physician. Eighty percent of adults in the United States experience at least one episode of low back pain during their lifetime and 5% have chronic problems. It is much more prevalent in African Americans than the white population. It is equally seen in males and females.

Lumbar disc degeneration can be associated with mild to severe low back pain associated with aging due to decreased water and proteoglycan content in the discs combined with increased collagen. Risk factors include being overweight, obesity, and diminished physical and social functioning. Metabolic syndrome is four times more prevalent in patients with radiographic evidence of severe degenerative disc disease.

Symptoms

Localization site	Comment
Lumbosacral spine	Low back pain, which is increased with activity. It can also cause buttock pain

Secondary Complications: Can cause deep-seated spinal ache. Patients may describe extremity or perianal pain. Depression is common.

Treatment Complications: Narcotics and tricyclic antidepressants can cause dizziness and drowsiness. Dependency can be seen with the use of narcotics.

Bibliography

Kirkaldy-Willis WH, ed. The pathology and pathogenesis of low back pain. In *Managing low back pain*. New York, NY: Churchill Livingstone; 1988. p. 49.

Lumbar Spondylolisthesis

Epidemiology and Demographics: Prevalence of this condition is 5% from age 5 to 7 years, 6–7% by age 18 years. Seen more in males. It is more common in white population compared with black population.

Disorder Description: Spondylolisthesis is defined as a forward or backward slippage of one vertebra on an adjacent vertebra. Potential identifiable causes are trauma, degeneration, tumor, or congenital etiology.

Symptoms

Localization site	Comment
Lumbar spine	Pain in the affected thigh, hamstring tightness
Roots	Numbness and tingling in the legs. Cauda equina-related symptoms

Secondary Complications: Spondylolisthesis can lead to deformity of the spine as well as narrowing of the spinal canal (central spinal stenosis) or compression of the exiting nerve roots (foraminal stenosis).

Treatment Complications: Nonsteroidal anti-inflammatory drugs can cause gastrointestinal side effects or uncommonly vascular events.

Bibliography

Newman PH. Spondylolisthesis, its cause and effect. *Ann R Coll Surg Engl*. 1955;16(5):305–23. PMC 2377893.

Lumbar Spondylolysis

Epidemiology and Demographics: More common in males. Prevalence is 6.4% in white men, 2.8% in black men, 2.3% in white women, and 1.1% in black women.

Disorder Description: Lumbar spondylosis is a unilateral or bilateral defect of the pars interarticularis that affects one or more of the lumbar vertebrae. It is most common at L5. Most of the time it is asymptomatic.

Symptoms

Localization site	Comment
Lumbosacral spine	Pain with activity on the right

Bibliography

O'Neill TW, McCloskey VE, Kanis JA, et al. The distribution determinants and clinical correlates of vertebral osteophytosis: a population based survey. *J Rheumatol*. 1999;26(4):A42–8.

Lumbar Spondylosis

Epidemiology and Demographics: Lumbar spondylosis can be present in 27–30% of the asymptomatic population; 84% of men and 74% of women have vertebral osteophytes. It is most commonly seen at T9 to T10 level and L3 level. This condition is seen equally in men and women.

Disorder Description: Lumbar spondylosis is described as bony overgrowth with osteophytes, predominately those at the anterior, lateral, and less commonly posterior aspect of the superior and inferior margins of the vertebral body. The condition increases with age but is often asymptomatic.

Symptoms

Localization site	Comment
Lumbosacral spine	Sciatica, low back pain

Secondary Complications: Nerve compression from posterior osteophytes if neural foramina is reduced to less than 30% of normal.

Treatment Complications: Surgery is sometimes used with equivocal benefit for some. Post-surgical complications including pain or new deficits are possible.

Bibliography

O'Neill TW, McCloskey VE, Kanis JA, et al. The distribution determinants and clinical correlates of vertebral osteophytosis: a population based survey. *J Rheumatol*. 1999;26(4):A42–8.

Lumbar Sprain

Epidemiology and Demographics: Eighty percent of adults experience low back pain in their lifetime; 7–13% of all sports injuries in intercollegiate athletes are low back injuries, 60% of which are muscle sprains.

Disorder Description: Lumbar sprain is defined as musculoligamentous injury that arises when ligaments become ripped from their attachments.

Symptoms

Localization site	Comment
Lumbosacral spine	Low back pain radiating into the buttocks if condition progresses to radiculopathy. Pain increases with activity. Decreased range of motion will be noted

Secondary Complications: This condition may progress to root compression causing sciatica or radiculopathy. May cause bowel or bladder dysfunction if severe.

Bibliography

Keene JS, Albert MS, Springer SL, Drummond DS, Clancy WG Jr. Back injuries in college athletes. *J Spinal Disord.* 1989;2(3):190–5.

Lumbar Stenosis

Epidemiology and Demographics: Eighty percent of patients in the United States have low back pain. It is seen more frequently in men. Lumbar stenosis affects the middle-aged and elderly population.

Disorder Description: Entrapment of the cauda equina roots occurs due to hypertrophy of the osseous and soft tissue structures surrounding the lumbar spinal canal.

Symptoms

Localization site	Comment
Lumbosacral spine	Thighs, calves, back, rarely buttock pain increased by erect posture, ambulation, extension of the spine. Pain relieved by squatting, bending forward, and sitting

Secondary Complications: Cauda equina syndrome can occur due to compression of the nerve roots in the lumbosacral spine distal to the conus medullaris.

Treatment Complications: Surgery can uncommonly be complicated by wound infection, hematoma formation, dural tears with subsequent cerebral spinal fluid leaks, and risk of meningitis.

Bibliography

Lee SY, Kim T-H, Oh JK, Lee SJ, Park MS. Lumbar stenosis: a recent update by review of literature. *Asian Spine J.* 2015;9(5):818–28. DOI:10.4184/asj.2015.9.5.818.

Lumbosacral Plexopathy: Immune (Vasculopathy)

Epidemiology and Demographics: Immune lumbosacral plexopathy is rare. True incidence is unknown. It occurs in approximately 1% of diabetic patients. It usually presents in middle age (average 65 years), with no gender preference.

Disorder Description: Characterized by epineurial and perineurial microvasculitis resulting in multifocal ischemia of nerve, followed by axonal loss. Clinical entities include diabetic, idiopathic, and post-surgical lumbosacral plexopathy. There is association with significant weight loss of greater than 10 lbs. It is usually a monophasic illness.

Symptoms

Localization site	Comment
Lumbosacral plexus	Patients present with acute to subacute severe pain in legs, followed by weakness. Pain usually improves when patient presents with weakness. Disease starts focally then progresses to adjacent segment or contralateral side in an asymmetric distribution. Proximal leg is more involved than distal part. Course progresses over 6 months before improvement

Secondary Complications: Minority of patients have residual weakness. Seventeen percent of idiopathic cases have recurrence in the same or opposite lower limb.

Treatment Complications: Spontaneous recovery occurs. Intravenous methylprednisolone may hasten recovery, but not improve functional outcome. Steroid may cause hyperglycemia and gastric ulcer. Intravenous immunoglobulin (IVIG) in addition to steroid is considered in severe cases; however, there is no randomized controlled trial to support this. IVIG may lead to anaphylactoid reaction in IgA-deficiency patients, as well as thromboembolic event.

Bibliography

Dyck PJ, Norell JE, Dyck PJ. Non-diabetic lumbosacral radiculoplexus neuropathy: natural history, outcome and comparison with the diabetic variety. *Brain.* 2001;124(6):1197–207.

Katirji B, Kaminski HJ, Ruff RL. *Neuromuscular disorders in clinical practice.* 2nd ed. New York: Springer-Verlag; 2014.

Lumbosacral Plexopathy: Intra-arterial Injections

Epidemiology and Demographics: Rare. There is a limited number of case reports.

Disorder Description

1. Administration of cisplatin into internal iliac artery may be complicated by lumbosacral plexopathies. This is postulated to be due to a combination of small vessel injury leading to nerve infarct and direct toxicity from the chemotherapy.
2. Injections into buttock area could cause ischemic injury due to an accidental intra-arterial injection of vasoactive drugs, causing retrograde propagation of vasospasm and thrombosis.

Symptoms

Localization site	Comment
Lumbosacral plexus	Patients develop paresthesia, pain, and weakness in lumbosacral distribution after receiving medication. Symptoms develop after 12–48 hours in patients who received intra-arterial cisplatin, and within minutes to hours in buttock injection cases

Secondary Complications: In those who received injection to buttock area, skin discoloration and ischemia (embolia cutis medicamentosa) may be observed. This may be followed by skin necrosis.

Bibliography

Castellanos AM, Glass JP, Yung WK. Regional nerve injury after intra-arterial chemotherapy. *Neurology.* 1987;37(5):834–7.

Stohr M, Dichgans J, Dorstelmann D. Ischaemic neuropathy of the lumbosacral plexus following intragluteal injection. *J Neurol Neurosurg Psychiatry.* 1980;43(6):489–94.

Lumbosacral Plexopathy: Ischemic

Epidemiology and Demographics: Rare. True incidence is unknown. Most cases were reported in patients with atherosclerotic risk factors.

Disorder Description

1. Chronic ischemia: atherosclerotic stenosis of distal aorta or iliac arteries causing steal phenomenon during muscular exertion.
2. Acute ischemia:
   Ischemic monomelic neuropathy occurs from acute noncompressive occlusion of proximal arteries, e.g., emboli to aortoiliac arteries, intra-aortic balloon pump placement. Distal nerve is more vulnerable to ischemia; results in distal to proximal gradient symptoms, physical signs, and electrodiagnostic studies. The injury is axonal degeneration of nerves.
   Occlusion or damage to iliac artery during aortoiliac artery surgery or the use of intraaortic balloon pumps can also result in damage to entire lumbosacral plexus.

Symptoms

Localization site	Comment
Lumbosacral plexus and peripheral nerve	1. Chronic ischemia: pain in the gluteal region after exertion, followed by paresthesia and possible weakness. The sensory loss is not in dermatomal pattern, but has ascending involvement from distal to proximal segments. Minority of patients have sensory loss and weakness without pain. Symptoms resolve after rest and improve after revascularization 2. Acute ischemia: in ischemic monomelic neuropathy, deep, burning pain in feet is the most prominent symptom. Examination reveals impairment of all sensory modalities and weakness in intrinsic muscle of affected foot. Patient could be misdiagnosed, because pain is out of proportion to physical signs, and pain may persist after revascularization. In case of complete lumbosacral plexopathy, entire limb could be affected with variable degree of pain, sensory loss, and weakness. There was also report of associated skin ischemia

Bibliography

Wilbourn AJ, Furlan AJ, Hulley W, Ruschhaupt W. Ischemic monomelic neuropathy. *Neurology.* 1983;33(4):447–51.

Wohlgemuth WA, Rottach KG, Stoehr M. Intermittent claudication due to ischaemia of the lumbosacral plexus. *J Neurol Neurosurg Psychiatry.* 1999;67(6):793–5.

Lumbosacral Plexopathy: Obstetric–Gynecologic Complications

Epidemiology and Demographics: Often seen in primigravida mothers of short stature with relatively large fetus.

Disorder Description: Injury is a result of compression of fetal head on lumbosacral cord (trunk), formed mostly by the L5 root, over pelvic brim. The lesion is usually demyelinating.

Symptoms

Localization site	Comment
Lumbosacral plexus	Symptoms begin during second stage of labor. There may be sciatica or paresthesia in lateral side of leg and dorsum of foot. However, symptoms are more often noticeable when patients attempt to walk after delivery. Foot drop is the most common complaint. Neurologic finding mimics L5 radiculopathy with weak ankle dorsiflexion, inversion, eversion, and hip abduction

Secondary Complications: Prognosis is good with complete recovery within 3 months.

Bibliography

Katirji B, Kaminski HJ, Ruff RL. *Neuromuscular disorders in clinical practice.* 2nd ed. New York: Springer-Verlag; 2014.

Lumbosacral Plexopathy: Trauma-Induced

Epidemiology and Demographics: Unlike brachial plexus, traumatic lumbosacral plexopathy is relatively uncommon because it is protected in the pelvic bone. Incidence of lumbosacral plexopathy is 2.03% among patients with sacral fractures, and 0.7% among patients with pelvic and acetabular fractures.

Disorder Description: Most cases are associated with high impact injury with pelvic ring fracture. Other causes of traumatic plexopathy include gunshot wound, compression from associated retroperitoneal hematoma, and avulsion of nerves.

Symptoms

Localization site	Comment
Lumbosacral plexus	Weakness, more commonly affected muscles innervated by common peroneal and gluteal nerves than those innervated by tibial and femoral nerve. Sensory symptom is predominantly in sciatic and posterior femoral cutaneous nerve distribution. Electrodiagnostic study is helpful in prognosis. Conservative management is recommended, unless compression of nerve fiber is identified

Bibliography

Katirji B, Kaminski HJ, Ruff RL. *Neuromuscular disorders in clinical practice.* 2nd ed. New York: Springer-Verlag; 2014.

Lung Cancer

Epidemiology and Demographics: According to the American Cancer Society, approximately 234,000 new cases of lung cancer occurred in the United States in 2018, with comparable frequency in men and women. Lung tumors are one of the common tumors associated with brain metastases.

Disorder Description: Lung tumors commonly involve the cerebral hemispheres. They can homogeneously spread as well as produce paraneoplastic syndromes and affect any part of the nervous system. The neurologic manifestations can precede the tumor diagnosis in many cases.

Symptoms

Localization site	Comment
Cerebral hemispheres	Seizures, headaches, and focal neurologic deficits such as hemiparesis, heminumbness, aphasia, or hemianopia
Mental status and psychiatric aspects/ complications	Encephalitis with confusion, agitation, somnolence (paraneoplastic – syndrome of inappropriate antidiuretic hormone secretion [SIADH])
Cerebellum	Truncal ataxia and tremor (paraneoplastic)

Localization site	Comment
Cranial nerves	Diplopia (cranial nerve VI, III, and IV dysfunction) and visual blurring (optic nerve involvement). (All due to leptomeningeal spread)
Pituitary gland	Visual changes, polyuria, and polydipsia
Spinal cord	Pain and paraplegia (Due to epidural spinal cord compression)
Conus medullaris	Bowel and bladder dysfunction (epidural compression)
Specific spinal roots	Limb weakness, pain referable to the involved nerve roots (leptomeningeal spread)
Muscle	**Stiff person syndrome**: muscle rigidity that waxes and wanes with concurrent spasm (rare; paraneoplastic – amphiphysin antibodies)
Neuromuscular junction	**Lambert–Eaton myasthenic syndrome**: fluctuating weakness, fatigue, and autonomic dysfunction (paraneoplastic syndrome in small cell lung cancer with voltage-gated calcium channel [VGCC] antibodies)

Secondary Complications: Lambert–Eaton myasthenic syndrome (antibodies against VGCCs), limbic encephalitis (anti-Hu antibodies), cerebellar degeneration (anti-Hu and anti CV2 antibodies), SIADH, Cushing syndrome, and stroke (hypercoagulable).

Treatment Complications:

Radiation: Fatigue, loss of appetite, sore throat, dysphagia, skin irritation, lung fibrosis, cough, fever, dyspnea.

Chemotherapy: Carboplatin, cisplatin, doclitaxel, paclitaxel, pemetrexed, or vinorelbine can cause cytopenia, opportunistic infection, hair loss, nausea and vomiting, and peripheral neuropathy.

Avastin: stroke, intracerebral hemorrhage.

Erlotinib: rash, diarrhea.

Bibliography

Giglio P, Gilbert MR. Neurologic complications of cancer and its treatment. *Curr Oncol Rep.* 2010;12(1):50–9.

Höftberger R, Rosenfeld MR, Dalmau J. Update on neurological paraneoplastic syndromes. *Curr Opin Oncol.* 2015;27(6):489–95.

Lyme Disease

Epidemiology and Demographics: Lyme disease is the most common tick-borne disease in both the United States and Europe. The incidence in the United States is approximately 300,000 cases per year. The majority of cases (94%) occur in the northeast and selected states (Minnesota and Wisconsin) in the Midwest. Lyme disease affects all age groups but exhibits bimodal distribution in 5- to 10-year-old and 35- to 50-year-old age groups. About 53% of cases are in men. Due to climate changes, both the incidence and prevalence have been increasing recently.

Disorder Description: Lyme disease is caused by *Borrelia burgdorferi*, which is transmitted by *Ixodes* deer ticks. Eighty percent of patients with Lyme disease have skin manifestations, about 60% develop joint symptoms, and 10–15% have neurologic symptoms.

There are three clinical stages of Lyme disease. Early localized disease is featured by erythema migrans ("bull's eye"), and nonspecific symptoms that resemble viral infections develop within the first month of infection. Early disseminated disease usually occurs within weeks to months and is characterized by neurologic or cardiac symptoms. Late disseminated disease often develops months or years after the initial infection and is associated with arthritis involving one or more large joints, mild encephalopathy, or polyneuropathy.

Symptoms: The neurologic manifestation of Lyme disease (also called neuroborreliosis) is primarily a result of multifocal inflammatory axonal processes and only occurs during the disseminated stage of the disease. Classic triad of neuroborreliosis is meningitis, cranial neuritis, and radiculoneuritis.

Localization site	Comment
Cerebral hemispheres	Lymphocytic meningitis is the most common central nervous system involvement, with symptoms resembling viral meningitis and variable meningeal symptoms
	Cranial neuropathy and radiculoneuropathy often occur concurrently
	Elevated intracranial pressure
	"Pseudotumor-like" presentation often occurs in pediatric population presenting with headache and associated with visual symptoms or even blindness secondary to optic nerve compression
	Transient ischemic attack and ischemic stroke can occur as a result of Lyme vasculitis
Vestibular system (and nonspecific dizziness)	Involvement of CN VIII can lead to vestibular symptoms
Cranial nerves	Cranial neuropathies usually present suddenly early in the disease
	Facial nerve (CN VII) is the most common cranial nerve involved; in almost 80% of cranial neuropathies, however, all cranial nerves can be affected. Involvement can be unilateral or bilateral
Spinal cord	Lyme encephalomyelitis can have segmental spinal cord involvement at the same level as radiculopathy. Clinical symptoms and CSF findings can mimic multiple sclerosis
Specific spinal roots	Lyme radiculoneuritis is the most common missed diagnosis, with possible involvement of motor, sensory, or both. Usually first presents with radicular pain in one or several dermatomes. Constellation of painful radiculoneuritis is the hallmark of Garin–Bujadoux–Bannwarth syndrome (or Bannwarth syndrome)
Plexus	Plexopathy (brachial, lumbosacral) can occur early in infection
Mononeuropathy or mononeuropathy multiplex	Mononeuropathy, mononeuropathy multiplex, confluent mononeuropathy multiplex, and simulating diffuse polyneuropathy can occur later in infection
Peripheral neuropathy	Including cranial neuropathy, radiculopathy, mononeuropathy, mononeuropathy multiplex, and plexopathy

Secondary Complications: If left untreated, the majority of infected individuals will develop chronic neurologic sequelae including persistent numbness, weakness, or even paralysis, dysfunction of cranial nerves.

Treatment Complications: *Borrelia* infection usually responds very well to appropriate antibiotic treatment including doxycycline, amoxicillin, or ceftriaxone. The timing of treatment is the key. Identification of the neurologic symptoms of Lyme disease is crucial to minimize long-term neurologic complications.

Bibliography

Halperin JJ. *Nervous system Lyme disease*. In Post TW, ed. UpToDate. Waltham, MA. www.uptodate.com/contents/nervous-system-lyme-disease. Accessed May 18, 2017.

Koedel U, et al. Lyme neuroborreliosis: epidemiology, diagnosis and management. *Nat Rev Neurol*. 2015;11(8):446–56.

Schwenkenbecher P, Pul R, Wurster U, et al. Common and uncommon neurological manifestations of neuroborreliosis leading to hospitalization. *BMC Infect Dis*. 2017;17(1):90.

Steere AC. Lyme borreliosis. In Kasper DL, Fauci AS, Hauser SL, et al., eds. *Harrison's principles of internal medicine*. 19th ed. New York: McGraw-Hill Education/Medical; 2015. p. 1401.

Lymphocytic Choriomeningitis Virus (LCMV)

Epidemiology and Demographics: About 5% of mice are infected with lymphocytic choriomeningitis virus (LCMV) in the United States. Approximately 5% of American adults have positive antibodies to LCMV.

Disorder Description: LCMV is an arenavirus that infects humans via contact with secretions from infected rodents, inhalation of aerosolized virus, or infection through organ transplant. LCMV has strong neurotropism and leads to several neurologic disorders including meningitis, encephalitis, and neurologic birth defects. Patients with acquired LCMV infection usually present with "flu-like" symptoms, followed by temporary symptom relief. Symptoms involving central nervous system often develop after as a second phase with "meningitis like" symptoms. Diagnosis can be established by detecting virus in CSF. Supportive care is the treatment of choice.

Symptoms

Localization site	Comment
Cerebral hemispheres	Aseptic meningitis, encephalitis, hydrocephalus (congenital and acquired)
	Microencephaly, periventricular calcifications, gyral dysplasia, and focal cerebral destruction in congenital LCMV
Cerebellum	Cerebellar hypoplasia in congenital LCMV
Spinal cord	Transverse myelitis
Peripheral neuropathy	Guillain–Barré syndrome

Secondary Complications: Subsequent static encephalopathy, seizure, spastic weakness, and severe vision problems can occur after congenital LCMV infection. Post meningitis and ventriculitis, normal pressure hydrocephalus is a common complication requiring ventriculoperitoneal shunting for management.

Infections acquired by solid organ transplantation are always severe. Recipients of infected organs typically develop fever, leukopenia, and lethargy several weeks post-transplantation and then rapidly progress to multi-organ system failure and shock. Most of these cases are fatal.

Treatment Complications: No specific approved antiviral for use. Steroids are used for severe meningitis or encephalitis. Symptomatic treatment of spasticity and seizures. Complications of ventriculoperitoneal shunting include infections and shunt failure.

Bibliography

Bonthius DJ. Lymphocytic choriomeningitis virus: an underrecognized cause of neurologic disease in the fetus, child, and adult. *Semin Pediatr Neurol.* 2012;19(3):89–95.

Kunz S, Rojek JM, Roberts AJ, et al. Altered central nervous system gene expression caused by congenitally acquired persistent infection with lymphocytic choriomeningitis virus. *J Virol.* 2006;80:9082–92.

Lymphomatoid Granulomatosis

Epidemiology and Demographics: Lymphomatoid granulomatosis occurs more frequently in patients with immunosuppressive conditions and autoimmune conditions. It is common in fourth to sixth decades of life.

Disorder Description: Lymphomatoid granulomatosis is a rare Epstein–Barr virus (EBV)-associated systemic angiodestructive and lymphoproliferative disease. It is characterized by prominent pulmonary involvement but can also involve multiple extrapulmonary sites.

Symptoms

Localization site	Comment
Cerebral hemispheres	Headache, hemiparesis, involuntary movements, incontinence, and seizures
Mental status and psychiatric aspects/complications	Disorientation, memory loss
Brainstem	Diplopia, facial and abducens nerve palsy
Spinal cord	Spastic gait and paraplegia (thoracic and cervical cord)
Peripheral neuropathy	Distal sensory neuropathy or mononeuritis multiplex (due to vasculitis)

Treatment Complications: Rituximab can result in transfusion reactions, hepatitis B/C reactivation, and progressive multifocal leukoencephalopathy.

Bibliography

Cetin B, Benekli M, Akyurek N, et al. Isolated primary lymphomatoid granulomatosis of central nervous system. *Indian J Hematol Blood Transfus.* 2013;29(1):39–42.

Kermode AG, Robbins PD, Carroll WM. Cerebral lymphomatoid granulomatosis. *J Clin Neurosci.* 1996;3(4):346–53.

Olmes DG, Agaimy A, Kloska S, Linker RA. Fatal lymphomatoid granulomatosis with primary CNS involvement in an immunocompetent 80-year-old woman. *BMJ Case Rep.* 2014; DOI: 10.1136/bcr-2014-206825.

Lysergic Acid Diethylamide (LSD) abuse

Disorder Description: Lysergic acid diethylamide (LSD) is a hallucinogenic drug (also known as "acid") that alters perception, mood, and thought, and may have mild sympathomimetic effects that stem from the disruption of serotonin.

Epidemiology and Demographics: Young white males are predominant users.

Symptoms

Localization site	Comment
Cerebral hemispheres	Seizures (acute)
Mental status and psychiatric aspects/ complications	Anxiety (acute)
	Delusions (acute)
	Paranoia
	Panic attacks (acute)
	Strong correlation in development of schizophrenia schizoaffective disorder (chronic)
	Prolonged psychosis (chronic)
	Depression (chronic)
	Post-hallucinogen disorder (chronic)
	Hallucinations (acute)
	Comatose (acute)
Brainstem	Dysregulation of the sleep–wake cycle
Cerebellum	Gait ataxia (acute)
Cranial nerves	Mydriasis (acute)
Spinal cord	Hyperreflexia (acute)
Muscle	Rhabdomyolysis (acute)
Neuromuscular junction	5-HT2A dysregulation (chronic)
	Dopamine dysregulation (chronic)

Secondary Complications: Indirectly affects nervous system via:

Respiratory complications: respiratory arrest/acute respiratory distress syndrome, which leads to cerebral ischemia.

Coagulopathy complications: disseminated intravascular coagulopathy with secondary complication of stroke.

Hepatic complications: acute hepatic failure from hyperthermia resulting in mood/cognitive disorders.

Endocrinologic complications: hyperthermia resulting in psychomotor agitation, ataxia, delirium, seizures, and coma.

Bibliography

Wiegand T, Thai D, Benowitz N. Medical consequences of the use of hallucinogens: LSD, mescaline, PCP, and MDMA ("Ecstasy"). In Brick J, ed. *Handbook of the medical consequences of alcohol and drug abuse.* 2nd ed. New York: Routledge; 2008. p. 461.

Lysosomal Storage Disorders

Disorder Description: The lysosomal storage disorders are a heterogeneous group of more than 50 rare inherited disorders, characterized by the accumulation of macromolecules within storage organelles named lysosomes; ultimately resulting in cellular dysfunction and clinical abnormalities.

The disorders often result from abnormalities associated with the enzymes involved in metabolism within lysosomes (hydrolases), but also include enzymes which act as activator proteins, or intracellular trafficking proteins. Given varying distribution within organs in the body, they lead to accumulation within organ systems, including the skeleton, brain, skin, heart, and central nervous system. Age of onset and clinical manifestations may vary widely among patients with a given lysosomal storage disease, and significant phenotypic heterogeneity between family members is common.

Lysosomal storage diseases are generally classified by the accumulated substrate.

The lysosomal disorders with available specific treatments (enzyme replacement therapy – ERT) include:

- Gaucher's disease I, III
- Mucopolysaccharidosis types I, II, VI
- Acid maltase deficiency (glycogen storage disease type II, Pompe's disease)
- Fabry's disease

ERT has been successful in preventing progression of peripheral manifestations, but largely unsuccessful in improving central nervous system symptoms, presumably due to the inability of the enzyme to cross the blood–brain barrier.

Hunter – MPS II

Epidemiology and Demographics: Very rare cases of female presentations. Prevalence ~1/100,000, with no ethnic predisposition.

Disorder Description: The most common lysosomal storage diseases are the mucopolysaccharidoses (MPS), caused by a deficiency of lysosomal enzymes required for the degradation of mucopolysaccharides or glycosaminoglycans (GAGs). Eleven distinct single lysosomal enzyme deficiencies are known to cause seven different and recognized phenotypes of MPS. All of the MPS are inherited in an autosomal recessive fashion, except for Hunter syndrome, which is X-linked recessive.

Mutations of the gene Xq28 cause iduronate sulfatase deficiency (IDS), leading to accumulation of chondroitin sulfate B and heparan sulfate.

There is a varying clinical picture due to cell-line mosaicism. Initial symptoms between 18 months and 4 years of age. Features include distinctive coarse facies – thickening of lips and nostrils, enlarged and protruding tongue; macrocephaly due to overgrowth; frequent respiratory tract infections and otitis media; umbilical and inguinal hernias; bone dysplasia and short stature; cardiomyopathy; hepatosplenomegaly; sleep apnea, and behavioral problems.

Two subtypes exist: MPSIIA – a severe form with early psychomotor regression and mortality before age 25; and MPSIIB – an attenuated form without cognitive involvement and survival into adulthood up to 60 years of age.

Diagnosis is based on screening urinary glycosaminoglycans and confirmation by measuring I2S activity and analyzing *I2S* gene mutations.

Symptoms

Localization site	Comment
Cerebral hemispheres	Macrocephaly and hydrocephalus MRI – T2 hyperintense cystic perivascular lesions – accumulation of foam cells in Virchow–Robin spaces
Cranial nerves	Hearing and visual involvement
Peripheral nervous system	Carpal tunnel syndrome due to overgrowth

Secondary Complications

Macroglossia and adenotonsillar hypertrophy may predispose to obstructive sleep apnea and secondary cardiac and behavioral (attention deficit hyperactivity disorder) comorbidities – require sleep studies and continuous positive airway pressure (CPAP).

Cardiomegaly – yearly cardiac follow-up.

Atlantoaxial instability and cervicomedullary spinal stenosis due to overgrowth.

Dysostosis predisposes to hip pathology – requires orthopedic surveillance.

Hepatosplenomegaly.

Special risks associated with general anesthesia include:

ankylosis of the temporomandibular (TM) joint, which can restrict oral access to the airway; difficult intubation due to macroglossia.

Care must be taken to avoid hyperextension of the neck secondary to atlantoaxial instability.

Treatment Complications: Idursulfase (recombinant I2S) (Elaprase) enzyme replacement therapy (ERT) improves walking capacity and respiratory function, and reduces spleen and liver size and urinary glycosaminoglycan levels. Intrathecal ERT is under investigation. Treatment complications are pyrexia and headache in approximately two-thirds of cases, arthralgia, anxiety, and irritability.

Bibliography

Giugliani RV, Villareal MLS, Valdez C, et al. Guidelines for diagnosis and treatment of Hunter Syndrome for clinicians in Latin America. *Genet Mol Biol.* 2014;37(2):315–29. https://dx.doi.org/10.1590/S1415-47572014000300003.

Raluy-Callado M, Chen WH, Whiteman DA, Fang J, Wiklund I. The impact of Hunter syndrome (mucopolysaccharidosis type II) on health-related quality of life. *Orphanet J Rare Dis.* 2013;8:101. DOI: 10.1186/1750-1172-8-101.

Scarpa M, Almassy Z, Beck M, et al. Mucopolysaccharidosis type II: European recommendations for the diagnosis and multidisciplinary management of a rare disease. *Orphanet J Rare Dis.* 2011;6:72. DOI: 10.1186/1750-1172-6-72.

Macular Degeneration

Epidemiology and Demographics: Age-related macular degeneration (AMD) is a leading cause of vision loss in elderly individuals affecting 30 to 50 million people worldwide. Macular degeneration is rare before the age of 55 with the highest prevalence in individuals over 80. It is primarily seen in developed nations.

Disorder Description: AMD is a multifactorial degenerative disease of the macula (central part of the retina). Age, genetics, and ethnic environmental factors have all been shown to play a role in disease development. Smoking is consistently associated with all forms of AMD in epidemiologic studies. Early on in the disease, deposits known as drusen appear in the macula. Patients are generally asymptomatic at this stage. As the disease progresses, significant vision loss can occur through two major mechanisms. In what is referred to as the "dry" form of AMD, well-defined areas of atrophy of the retina appear. This is known as geographic atrophy. In the "wet" form of AMD, choroidal neovascularization (abnormal blood vessel growth under the retina) occurs leading to fluid accumulation in the retina, exudates, and hemorrhage. Dry AMD accounts for the majority of diagnosed cases but wet AMD is responsible for the majority of vision loss.

Symptoms

Localization site	Comment
Cerebral hemispheres	It is well accepted that genetics and inflammation play an important role in AMD. Many hypothesize that AMD is a local manifestation of systemic dysregulation of inflammation and lipid metabolism. AMD has also been theorized to be a vascular disorder. Epidemiologic studies linking AMD and cardiovascular risk (such as for stroke), however, are inconsistent

Localization site	Comment
Mental status and psychiatric aspects/complications	Visual release hallucinations (sometimes termed Charles Bonnet syndrome) may occur in patients with macular degeneration and severe vision loss. These patients will report seeing geometric shapes, small characters, or faces, but they have insight into the hallucinations and recognize that they are not real. These patients do not have psychiatric disease, but may be disturbed by the images, and afraid to admit that they see them for fear of being labelled with psychiatric disease

Secondary Complications: Late manifestations of AMD, geographic atrophy and choroidal neovascularization, are associated with central vision loss. The risk of disease progression is highly variable. Higher risk clinical features include large drusen and pigmentary changes, particularly if bilateral. When both eyes are affected by late stages of AMD, vision is markedly reduced, and tasks such as reading, driving and facial recognition are compromised. Peripheral vision is typically spared.

Treatment Complications: There are currently no treatments for the most common dry form of AMD. Antioxidant supplementation through vitamin pills, smoking cessation, and nutritional modification have been shown to slow the progression of disease. Treatments for neovascular AMD have been studied extensively. The current standard of care is intravitreal injections of the anti-vascular endothelial growth factor (VEGF) agents ranibuzumab, aflibercept, or bevacuzumab. Serious ocular side effects are rare but endophthalmitis (inflammation of ocular structures usually secondary to infection) and uveitis have been reported. Anti-VEGF agents administered systemically have been known to cause serious side effects including thromboembolic events and death. There is concern that repeated injections of anti-VEGF agents can result in clinically significant systemic levels of these agents but the exact systemic risks are unclear.

Bibliography

Age-Related Eye Disease Study Research Group. A randomized, placebo-controlled, clinical trial of high-dose supplementation with vitamins C and E, beta carotene, and zinc for age-related macular degeneration and vision loss. *Arch Ophthalmol.* 2001;119(10):1417–36.

Schadlu AP, Schadlu R, Shepherd JB. Charles Bonnet syndrome: a review. *Curr Opin Ophthalmol.* 2009:20(3):219–22.

Major Depressive Disorder

Epidemiology and Demographics: In the United States, the 12-month prevalence of major depressive disorder (MDD) is about 7%. Prevalence differs according to age with rates in 18- to 19-year-olds threefold higher than in those 60 years or older. Females have a 1.5- to 3-fold increased incidence of MDD relative to males. Depression should be screened for in patients who have neurologic disorders such as Parkinson's, stroke, and epilepsy. These rates are discussed under the appropriate headings below.

Disorder Description: As stated in the DSM-5, MDD can be defined as:

A. Five or more of the following symptoms have been present during the same 2-week period and represent a change from previous functioning; at least one of the symptoms is either (1) depressed mood or (2) loss of interest or pleasure.

    i. Depressed mood most of the day, nearly every day, as indicated by either subjective report (e.g., feels sad, empty, hopeless) or observation made by others (e.g., appears tearful). (In children and adolescents, this can manifest as irritability.)

    ii. Markedly diminished interest or pleasure in all, or almost all, activities most of the day, nearly every day (as indicated by either subjective account or observation).

    iii. Significant weight loss when not dieting or weight gain, or decrease or increase in appetite nearly every day.

    iv. Insomnia or hypersomnia nearly every day.

    v. Psychomotor agitation or retardation nearly every day (observed by others).

    vi. Fatigue or loss of energy nearly every day.

    vii. Feelings of worthlessness or excessive or inappropriate guilt (which may be delusional) nearly every day.

    viii. Diminished ability to think or concentrate, or indecisiveness, nearly every day.

    ix. Recurrent thoughts of death, recurrent suicidal ideation without a specific plan, or a suicide attempt or a specific plan for committing suicide.

B. The symptoms cause clinically significant distress or impairment in social, occupational, or other important areas of functioning.

C. The episode is not attributable to the physiologic effects of a substance or to another medical condition.

D. The occurrence of the major depressive episode is not better explained by schizoaffective disorder, schizophrenia, schizophreniform disorder, delusional disorder, or other specified and unspecified schizophrenia spectrum and other psychotic disorders.

E. There has never been a manic episode or hypomanic episode.

Differential Diagnosis: Differential diagnosis should include manic episodes with irritable mood or mixed episodes, mood disorder due to another medical condition, substance/medication-induced depressive or bipolar disorder, attention deficit hyperactivity disorder, adjustment disorder with depressed mood, sadness and grief. In grief, the predominant affect is feelings of emptiness and loss, while in MDD it is persistent depressed mood and inability to anticipate happiness and pleasure.

In manic disorders with irritable mood or mixed episodes, there is the presence of manic symptoms, thus patients with depressive symptoms should be carefully examined for past manic episodes. This can differentiate between unipolar and bipolar depressive episode.

In a mood disorder due to another medical condition, there is a direct pathophysiologic link between the medical condition and the mood occurrence.

Substance/medication-induced depressive or bipolar disorder is characterized by depression or mania caused by intoxication or withdrawal of a substance.

In attention deficit hyperactivity disorder, there may also be distractibility and low frustration tolerance (as in MDD). The two disorders are not mutually exclusive; if criteria are met for each, both disorders should be diagnosed.

In adjustment disorder with depressed mood, the full criteria for MDD are not met (five of nine symptoms, most of the day, nearly every day for at least 2 weeks).

Episodes of sadness are fundamental aspects of the human experience. These episodes should not be diagnosed as MDD, unless they meet the full criteria (five of nine symptoms, most of the day, nearly every day for at least 2 weeks, causing clinically significant distress or impairment).

MDD in stroke: Poststroke depression is common, although difficult to quantify precisely due to differences among studies. Depression at 3 months after stroke is correlated with a poor outcome at 1 year. Nonetheless, remission of depression is associated with better functional outcome at 3 and 6 months than continued depression. A 2008 systematic review of 12 pharmacotherapy trials with 1121 subjects found that antidepressant therapy is modestly beneficial for remission of poststroke depression. However, adverse events were significantly more common with antidepressants. There is no definitive evidence to guide specific choice of therapy for patients with poststroke depression. However, major depression (MDD) is a treatable illness that responds to a variety of therapeutic interventions, and it is likely that the standard approach to the treatment of depression in adults is generalizable to patients with poststroke depression. Also, fluoxetine has been looked at to see whether it can help early poststroke depression. It was deemed an efficacious and well-tolerated treatment; however, further research is needed.

MDD in seizure disorder: Mood disorders, particularly anxiety and depression, are common in patients with epilepsy; prevalence ranges from 13 to 35%. In a community survey, epilepsy was associated with 43% higher odds of depression after adjustment for other demographic factors. Epilepsy-related disability, including unemployment and activity restriction (e.g., driving), along with impaired social support, are risk factors for depression. Suicide risk is a particular concern in patients with epilepsy. A population-based study in Denmark saw a three times higher rate of suicide in patients with epilepsy compared with controls. In addition, antiseizure drugs have also been associated with increased risk of suicidality. Clinicians prescribing these drugs should identify a current or past history of depression, anxiety, and suicidal ideations or behavior in their patients. History of depression has been associated with onset of seizures, given that a history of depression increases the risk of developing a seizure.

MDD in Parkinson's disease: Depression is one of the most common psychiatric disturbances seen in patients with Parkinson's disease (PD). It has a negative impact on motor disability and decreased quality of life. There is no clear consensus regarding use of antidepressants for the treatment of depression in patients with PD. However, a review by the Academy of Neurology (AAN) of six small randomized controlled trials that evaluated pharmacologic intervention of depression in patients with PD found that in one of the trials, amitriptyline but not fluoxetine treatment was associated with significant improvement. Since the 2006 AAN report, a number of small randomized placebo-controlled trials have reported the following observations: desipramine and citalopram were equally effective, nortriptyline was efficacious while paroxetine controlled release was not, atomoxetine was not beneficial, and paroxetine and venlafaxine improved depression and did not worsen motor function. Ropinirole and pramipexole may improved depressive symptoms. In the absence of a clear first choice, it is reasonable to start with a selective serotonin reuptake inhibitor (SSRI) in most patients, as the likelihood of adverse events is lower with SSRIs than with tricyclic antidepressants. The anticholinergic side effects of tricylics, such as cognitive impairment and orthostatic hypotension, may be particularly problematic in a patient with PD. However, for patients who do not improve with an SSRI, a tricyclic antidepressant may work when tremor is the dominant symptom and potential benefits outweigh the risk. There are two potential concerns regarding SSRI use in PD patients: the possibility of aggravating motor symptoms and the possibility of an adverse interaction with selegiline (monoamine oxidase [MAO] B inhibitor) used to treat PD. Extrapyramidal symptoms such as dystonia, akathisia, tremor, and parkinsonism are associated with SSRIs. This is due to increased serotonin-mediated inhibition of dopamine release in the substantia nigra. Fluoxetine and paroxetine have been the SSRIs most commonly associated with increased parkinsonism, while sertraline has been associated with relatively few cases.

Serotonin syndrome: Serotonin syndrome is a potentially severe condition associated with increased serotonergic activity in the central nervous system and severely disturbed mental, motor, and autonomic function. The MAO B inhibitors selegiline and rasagiline should be used only at recommended doses and with caution when combined with other anti-depressants, because of the risk of causing serotonin syndrome. Also, at higher than recommended doses (10 mg daily for selegiline and 1 mg daily for rasagiline), the MAO B inhibitors may also inhibit MAO A, and when given with antidepressants, carry the risk of tyramine cheese reaction, also called hypertensive crisis.

Secondary Complications: Impairment secondary to MDD can be severe. In some cases, the individual may exhibit complete incapacity to care for him or herself, or is mute or catatonic. At that time, electroconvulsive therapy can be considered as a treatment. These individuals may also have more pain and physical illness and greater decreases in physical, social, and role functioning. The possibility of suicide exists throughout major depressive episodes. The most frequently described risk factor is a past history of suicide attempts or threats. Additional risk factors include male sex, being single or living alone, and having prominent feelings of hopelessness.

Treatment Complications: First-line treatment for MDD usually consists of SSRIs. This can be followed by tricyclic antidepressants (TCAs) and MAOIs, and possible an atypical antipsychotic adjuvant. SSRIs have black box warnings for risk of increased suicidal thoughts.

SSRI side effects include nausea, diarrhea, insomnia, headache, anorexia, weight loss, sexual dysfunction, restlessness (akathisia-like), serotonin syndrome (fever diaphoresis, tachycardia, hypertension, delirium, neuromuscular excitability), hyponatremia, and seizures (0.2%).

Treatment with antidepressants has been controversial given the propensity of some antidepressants to increase risk of seizure. However, risk of seizure with most antidepressants is quite small when these agents are used at standard doses. Citalopram, setraline, venlafaxine, and transcortical stimulation have all been used successfully in patients with epilepsy without significantly worsening the underlying seizure disorder.

TCAs are highly protein bound and lipid soluble and thus have many drug interactions. They have antihistaminic properties including sedation and weight gain; anti-adrenergic properties including orthostatic hypotension, dizziness, reflex tachycardia, arrhythmias; and anti-muscarinic effects including dry mouth, constipation, urinary retention, blurry vision, tachycardia, and exacerbation of narrow angle glaucoma. TCAs are lethal in overdose and thus suicide risk should be carefully assessed. Symptoms of overdose include agitation, tremors, ataxia, arrhythmias, delirium, hypoventilation (secondary to central nervous system depression), myoclonus, hyperreflexia, seizures, and coma. Serotonergic effects are also seen in TCAs including erectile/ejaculatory dysfunction in males and anorgasmia in females.

MAOI side effects include serotonin syndrome (usually when taken in combination with SSRIs). Serotonin syndrome first consists of lethargy, restlessness, confusion, flushing, diaphoresis, tremor, and myoclonic jerks. These symptoms may progress to hyperthermia, hypertonicity, rhabdomyolysis, renal failure, convulsions, coma, and death. Thus, when switching to or from an SSRI and MAOI, a 2-week "washout period" should be implemented (5 weeks appropriate for fluoxetine given its longer half life). Hypertensive crisis may also be seen as a side effect of MAOIs. This generally occurs when MAOIs are taken with tyramine-rich foods (wine, cheese, etc.). Additional side effects include orthostatic hypertension, drowsiness, weight gain, sexual dysfunction, dry mouth, sleep dysfunction, numbness and parasthesias (if pyridoxine deficiency), seizures, and edema (if liver toxicity).

Atypical antipsychotic side effects include metabolic syndrome, weight gain, hyperlipidemia, and hyperglycemia. At times, atypical antipsychotic agents may be used in conjunction with an SSRI to treat mood symptoms.

Bibliography

American Psychiatric Association. *Diagnostic and statistical manual of mental disorders: DSM-5.* 5th ed. Washington, DC: American Psychiatric Association; 2013.

Beauregard M, Paquette V, Levesque J. Dysfunction in the neural circuitry of emotional self-regulation in major depressive disorder. *Neuroreport.* 2006;17(8):843–6.

Belmaker RH, Agam G. Major depressive disorder. *New Engl J Med.* 2008;358(1):55–68.

Cotter D, Mackay D, Landau S, Kerwin R, Everall I. Reduced glial cell density and neuronal size in the anterior cingulate cortex in major depressive disorder. *Arch Gen Psychiatry.* 2001;58(6):545–53.

Fava M, Kendler KS. Major depressive disorder. *Neuron,* 2000;28(2):335–41.

Holmes AJ, Pizzagalli DA. Spatiotemporal dynamics of error processing dysfunctions in major depressive disorder. *Arch Gen Psychiatry.* 2008;65(2):179–88.

Malaria

Epidemiology and Demographics: Malaria is a parasitic disease caused by sporozoites of the *Plasmodium* genus. Greater than 200 million infections were reported in 90+ countries in 2016 alone. There is no sex predominance, and it can afflict any age group. Children are disproportionately at risk for death, since children younger than 5 years of age constitute 70% of the 445,000 malaria deaths annually. Depending on the species, incubation after initial infection can range from a week to a month, wherein patients are often asymptomatic.

Plasmodium species are widespread globally. They are most commonly seen in Africa, but also can be found in Latin America, the Caribbean, Asia, Eastern Europe, and the South Pacific.

Disorder Description: Malaria is caused by the *Plasmodium* genus, most commonly by five major species (the first two being the most widespread and common): *P. vivax, P. falciparum, P. malariae, P. ovale,* and *P. knowlesi.* The parasites are transmitted primarily by mosquitos (mostly *Anopheles* species). *P. falciparum* causes the most severe symptoms and mortality, with more frequent systemic and cerebral involvement. Risks of infection are tied to exposure (e.g., living in or traveling to endemic areas), but risks of severe morbidity and mortality are linked to immunocompromise, age (mostly younger patients, as noted above), and pregnant women.

Once clinically suspected, rapidly performed diagnostic tests can detect antibodies, but are less specific for acute infections and only provide qualitative rather than quantitative results. PCR testing can provide confirmation, but blood smear microscopy is still the gold standard, as it can also help quantify infection burden.

Symptoms

Localization site	Comment
Cerebral hemispheres	Cerebral malaria (encephalopathy, seizures, delirium), microinfarctions, cerebral edema, elevated intracranial pressure
Mental status and psychiatric aspects/complications	Encephalopathy, autoimmune encephalitis
Ocular – retinal	Retinal hemorrhages
Outside CNS	Fever, headache, chills, hypovolemia Anemia, hepatic dysfunction

Secondary Complications: Secondary complications are largely related to the severity of systemic disease as the sporozoites parasitize red blood cells (RBC), resulting in RBC adherence to microvasculature. Hypoglycemia, anemia, and hemolysis are common initially, which can cascade into renal failure, hepatic dysfunction, coagulopathy (including possibly disseminated intravascular coagulation), circulatory collapse, and even respiratory distress (largely from acidosis). This can result in hepatomegaly, jaundice, splenomegaly (with potential splenic rupture), and thrombocytopenia. Cerebral malaria can result in residual deficits including hemiplegia, cortical blindness, deafness, chronic epilepsy, language deficits, and cognitive deficits. In fact, a post-malarial autoimmune encephalitis can rarely occur, within 2 months of resolution of the acute illness.

Treatment Complications: Depending on the severity of infection and patient risk factors for mortality, hospitalization may or may not be necessary. There are a variety of anti-malarial drugs used. In areas of chloroquine-sensitive *Plasmodium* species (reference to regularly updated CDC guidelines and maps is helpful), use of chloroquine, hydroxychloroquine, atovaquone-proguanil, mefloquine, quinine + tetracycline/doxycycline combination may be appropriate. However, in resistant areas, WHO guidelines include utilization of artemisinin-containing combination regimens.

Specific complications are related to adverse reactions based on the specific drug(s) chosen. These can range from general gastrointestinal symptoms and hematological symptoms (e.g., anemia, thrombocytopenia, leukopenia) to more severe neurological symptoms of myopathy and mild neuropathy.

Bibliography

Lee H, Halverson S, Ezinwa N. Mosquito-borne diseases. *Prim Care.* 2018;45(3):393–407.

Salvana EMT, Salata RA, King CH. Parasitic infections of the central nervous system. In Aminoff MJ, Josephson SA, eds. *Aminoff's neurology and general medicine.* 5th ed. London: Academic Press; 2014. pp. 947–51.

World Health Organization. World malaria report 2017. Geneva (Switzerland): World Health Organization; 2017.

Male Hypoactive Sexual Desire Disorder

Epidemiology and Demographics: The prevalence of male hypoactive sexual desire disorder varies widely based on age and geographic location. Approximately 6% of men aged 18–24 years and 41% of men aged 66–74 years have problems with sexual desire. However, a persistent lack of interest in sex for 6 months or longer affects only 1.8% of men (ages 16–44 years).

Disorder Description: As stated in the DSM-5, male hypoactive sexual desire disorder can be defined as:

A. Persistently or recurrently deficient (or absent) sexual/erotic thoughts or fantasies and desire for sexual activity. The judgment of deficiency is made by the clinician, taking into account factors that affect sexual functioning, such as age and general and sociocultural contexts of the individual's life.

B. The symptoms in Criterion A have persisted for a minimum duration of approximately 6 months.

C. The symptoms in Criterion A cause clinically significant distress in the individual.

D. The sexual dysfunction is not better explained by a nonsexual mental disorder or as a consequence of severe relationship distress or other significant stressors and is not attributable to the effects of a substance/medication or another medical condition.

Differential Diagnosis: Differential diagnosis should include nonsexual mental disorders, substance/ medication use, another medical condition, interpersonal factors, and other sexual dysfunctions.

In nonsexual mental disorders, there may also be a lack of interest. In major depressive disorder, for example, there may be lack of interest or pleasure in all or most activities. This may account for lack of sexual desire as well, and in such cases an additional diagnosis of hypoactive sexual desire disorder should not be given.

In substance/medication use, the use of some substance may account for hypoactive sexual desire, and hypoactive sexual desire disorder would not be the diagnosis. It is important to consider sexual side effects of psychotropic medications. The estimated incidence of selective serotonin reuptake inhibitor (SSRI)-induced sexual dysfunction ranges from approximately 15 to 80%. With the exception of buproprion, most of the other SSRIs and selective serotonin–norepinephrine reuptake inhibitors (SNRIs) as well as neuroleptics (both typical and atypical) are associated with sexual dysfunction. This is usually dose dependent and reversible when the drug is stopped. A 14-week prospective observational study (STAR*D) of 1473 patients treated with citalopram found that: decreased libido occurred in 54%, difficulty achieving orgasm occurred in 36%, and among 574 males, erectile dysfunction occurred in 37%. A cross-sectional survey of 704 patients who had started SSRIs or SNRIs estimated that sexual dysfunction occurred in approximately 50%. Women are treated with SSRI medications more frequently than men and are thus more likely to be affected by SSRI-related sexual dysfunction. On the other hand, several randomized trials have established that sexual dysfunction occurs less often with buproprion than with SSRIs. A network meta-analysis of 37 randomized trials ($n > 14,000$ depressed patients) found that the incidence of sexual dysfunction was less with bupropion than escitalopram, paroxetine, or sertraline. In addition, one prospective study ($n = 31$ patients with fluoxetine-induced sexual dysfunction) found that after switching from fluoxetine to buproprion, sexual functioning was much or very much improved in 81%.

In another medical condition, such as hypogonadism, diabetes mellitus, thyroid dysfunction, and central nervous system disease, there may be secondary hypoactive sexual desire, and thus a diagnosis of hypoactive sexual desire disorder should not be given.

In the context of interpersonal factors, such as severe relationship distress or other stressors, there may be an associated loss of sexual desire in a male, but in these cases a diagnosis of male hypoactive sexual desire disorder would not be accurate.

In up to one-half of men with hypoactive sexual desire disorder, there are comorbid erection problems. In a slightly lower proportion of these men, there are ejaculation problems. Thus, the presence of another sexual dysfunction does not rule out male hypoactive sexual desire disorder.

Finally, if a man's low sexual desire is explained by his self-identification as asexual, then the diagnosis of male hypoactive sexual desire disorder is not made.

Secondary Complications: Male hypoactive sexual desire disorder may negatively affect one's partner relationships. Furthermore, male hypoactive sexual desire disorder is often comorbid with major depressive disorder and other mental disorders, as well as endocrine abnormalities.

Treatment Complications: Treatment usually consists of counseling, but pharmacologic therapy may also be used. Testosterone supplementation has been shown to be effective for short-term treatment. Testosterone supplementation side effects include acne, increased risk of blood clots, worsening sleep apnea (and thus daytime sleepiness), decreased testicular size, aggression and mood swings, breast enlargement, and increased risk of heart attack and stroke.

Another treatment, albeit only modestly more effective than placebo, is Flibanserin. Its side effects include dizziness, sleepiness, and nausea.

Bibliography

American Psychiatric Association. *Diagnostic and statistical manual of mental disorders: DSM-5.* 5th ed. Washington, DC: American Psychiatric Association; 2013.

Meuleman EJ, Van Lankveld JJ. Hypoactive sexual desire disorder: An underestimated condition in men. *BJU Int.* 2005;95(3):291–6.

Segraves KB, Segraves RT. Hypoactive sexual desire disorder: Prevalence and comorbidity in 906 subjects. *J Sex Marital Ther.* 1991;17(1):55–8.

Stoléru S, Redouté J, Costes N, et al. Brain processing of visual sexual stimuli in men with hypoactive sexual desire disorder. *Psychiatry Res.* 2003;124(2):67–86.

Malignant Hyperthermia (MH)

Epidemiology and Demographics: Reported frequency of malignant hyperthermia (MH) is 1 in 100,000 in patients receiving anesthetics (frequency is probably underestimated due to atypical cases and mild reactions). Occurs in all ethnic groups, males more than females in a ratio of 2:1. Over 90% have no family history of MH and over 50% have previous uneventful exposure to general anesthetics. When inherited, it is an autosomal dominant trait, with a defect in the ryanodine receptor (RYR1), the primary channel for release of intrasarcoplasmic calcium.

Disorder Description: Manifests clinically as a hypermetabolic crisis when an MH-susceptible (MHS) individual is exposed to a volatile anesthetic (halothane, isoflurane, enflurane, sevoflurane, desflurane) or succinylcholine. Clinical signs are variable but tend to occur in a similar order: masseter spasm, hypercarbia, sinus tachycardia, generalized muscle rigidity, tachypnea, cyanosis, hyperthermia, sweating, cola colored urine, ventricular tachycardia/fibrillation, and excessive bleeding. Diagnosis is best accomplished by the caffeine halothane contracture test.

Symptoms

Localization site	Comment
Cerebral hemispheres	Hypercarbia can produce encephalopathy with confusion
Mental status and psychiatric aspects/complications	Patient may be restless and agitated, with alteration in mental status. Can have cardiac arrest as a complication from ventricular fibrillation with subsequent cerebral edema, herniation, and death
Muscle	Muscle rigidity may be limited to masseter spasm, most frequently observed after administration of succinylcholine
	Generalized muscle rigidity noted with inhalational anesthetics. Delayed complication of muscle weakness

Secondary Complications: Muscle breakdown can result in myoglobinuria and renal failure as well as hyperkalemia and increased body temperature. Hyperkalemia further worsens cardiac instability and ventricular arrhythmias. Eventually hemodynamic instability may cause multi-organ failure. Disseminated intravascular coagulation can occur.

Treatment Complications: Treatment involves aborting the anesthetic as soon as possible, hyperventilating the patient with 100% oxygen, placement of activated charcoal filters in the breathing circuit to rapidly reduce the concentration of potent inhalational anesthetic to less than 5 ppm, initiation of IV dantrolene, correction of electrolyte disturbances, and use of cooled IV fluids and cooling blankets. Because rapid correction and avoiding hypothermia are both important, devices used for targeted temperature management are particularly effective.

Bibliography

Rosenbaum HK. Malignant hyperthermia. *MedLink Neurology*. Updated Jun 8, 2015. San Diego: MedLink Corporation. Available from www.medlink.com/article/malignant_hyperthermia. Accessed Aug 24, 2018.

Malingering

Epidemiology: Malingering is a common occurrence in hospitalized patients. One study showed that 46–60% of cases of social security disability exams were judged as malingering. Malingering is more common in males than females. Malingering is a diagnosis of exclusion after medical tests have been performed, and found to be negative for pathology.

Description: Malingering is not a mental disorder. Malingering is the exaggeration or fabrication of signs or symptoms for the purpose of a secondary gain. Common secondary gains are room and board, drugs, exemption for work or service, reduction of criminal sentences, financial, and avoiding police. Elements from history that suggest malingering are legal involvement, significant discrepancy between objective findings and reported symptoms, failure to cooperate with the evaluation or treatment, and presence of anti-social personality disorder.

Malingering patients often present with vague and multiple physical complaints that are inconsistent with any one medical condition. Most often pick symptoms that are highly subjective and difficult to prove (or disprove). They often eagerly and dramatically describe symptoms, and have a marked inconsistency between history and mental status exam. They may also use technical medical terms and demand specific medications. They often have a history of many long hospital stays, and their symptoms often remit as soon as their secondary gain is acquired.

Malingerers may report anxiety or depression, and try to convince the examiner of how much their function is impaired and how much they are bothered by the symptoms. When malingering is suspected, objective tests are crucial. The Minnesota Multiphasic Personality Inventory-2 (MMPI-2) may pick up distortions in both physical and psychologic symptoms. Direct confrontation is not advised because this often results in the patient becoming angry and fleeing from treatment. Strategies that allow the patient to save face are generally more successful.

Differential Diagnosis: Malingering should be differentiated from factitious disorder imposed on self (Munchausen syndrome). In factitious disorder imposed on self, a patient may feign symptoms, but in the absence of any external goal or reward. In factitious disorder, the symptoms are feigned so that the individual may assume the "sick role."

Secondary Complications: Malingering may result in fines and/or incarceration.

Treatment Complications: Because malingering is a conscious deception and not a medical disorder, medical treatment is not appropriate.

Bibliography

American Psychiatric Association. *Diagnostic and statistical manual of mental disorders: DSM-5.* 5th ed. Washington, DC: American Psychiatric Association; 2013.

Mittenberg W, Patton C, Canyock EM, Condit DC. Base rates of malingering and symptom exaggeration. *J Clin Exp Neuropsychol.* 2002;24(8):1094–102.

Pankratz L, Erickson RC. Two views of malingering. *Clin Neuropsychol.* 1990;4(4):379–89.

Rogers R, ed. *Clinical assessment of malingering and deception.* New York: Guilford Press; 2008.

Stern T, et al. *Massachusetts General Hospital handbook of general hospital psychiatry.* Philadephia, PA: Saunders; 2010.

Manganese Toxicity

Epidemiology and Demographics: May be absorbed via inhalation or ingestion. Mostly occupational exposure in miners and industrial workers.

Disorder Description: Initially non-specific symptoms like asthenia, restlessness, apathy, and cramping. Miners seem to be more likely to develop "manganese madness" with compulsive acts, delusions, and hallucinations. A few months later, the extrapyramidal syndrome begins with all of the classic parkinsonian manifestations: bradykinesia, masked face, hypophonia, micrographia, tremor, stooped posture, and gait disturbance.

Symptoms

Localization site	Comment
Brainstem	Substantia nigra NOT affected
Basal ganglia	A classic cause of toxin-induced parkinsonism Manganese accumulates in the globus pallidus

Bibliography

Cersosimo MG, Koller WC. The diagnosis of manganese-induced parkinsonism. *Neurotoxicology.* 2006;27(3):340–6. PMID:16325915.

Chu N-S, Huang C-C, Calne DB. Manganese. In Spencer PS, Schaumburg HH, eds. *Experimental and clinical neurotoxicology.* 2nd edition. Oxford, UK: Oxford University Press; 2000. pp. 752–5.

Mania

Epidemiology and Demographics: In the United States, the 12-month prevalence of bipolar I disorder is approximately 0.6% and bipolar II disorder is approximately 0.8%.

Disorder Description: As stated in DSM-5, a manic episode can be defined as:

A. A distinct period of abnormally and persistently elevated, expansive, or irritable mood and abnormally and persistently increased goal-directed activity or energy, lasting **at least 1 week** and present most of the day, nearly every day (or any duration if hospitalization is necessary).

B. During the period of mood disturbance and increased energy or activity, three (or more) of the following symptoms (four if the mood is only irritable) represent to a significant degree

and represent a noticeable change from usual behavior:

i. Inflated self-esteem or grandiosity.

ii. Decreased need for sleep (e.g., feels rested after only 3 hours of sleep).

iii. More talkative than usual or pressure to keep talking.

iv. Flight of ideas or subjective experience that thoughts are racing.

v. Distractibility (i.e., attention too easily drawn to unimportant or irrelevant external stimuli), as reported or observed.

vi. Increase in goal-directed activity (either socially, at work or school, or sexually) or psychomotor agitation (e.g., purposeless non-goal-directed activity).

vii. Excessive involvement in activities that have a high potential for painful consequences (e.g., engaging in unrestrained buying sprees, sexual indiscretions, or foolish business investments).

C. The mood disturbance is sufficiently severe to cause marked impairment in social or occupational functioning or to necessitate hospitalization to prevent harm to self or others, or there are psychotic features.

D. The episode is not attributable to physiologic effects of a substance (e.g., a drug of abuse, a medication, or other treatment) or to another medical condition.

As stated in DSM-5, a hypomanic episode can be defined as:

A. A distinct period of abnormally and persistently elevated expansive or irritable mood and abnormally and persistently increased activity or energy, lasting **at least 4 consecutive days** and present most of the day, nearly every day.

B. During the period of mood disturbance and increased energy and activity, three (or more) of the following symptoms (four if the mood is only irritable) have persisted and represent a noticeable change from usual behavior, and have been present to a significant degree:

i. Inflated self-esteem or grandiosity.

ii. Decreased need for sleep (e.g., feels rested after only 3 hours of sleep).

iii. More talkative than usual or pressure to keep talking.

iv. Flight of ideas or subjective experience that thoughts are racing.

v. Distractibility (i.e., attention too easily drawn to unimportant or irrelevant external stimuli), as reported or observed.

vi. Increase in goal-directed activity (either socially, at work or school, or sexually) or psychomotor agitation (e.g., purposeless non-goal-directed activity).

vii. Excessive involvement in activities that have a high potential for adverse consequences (e.g., engaging in unrestrained buying sprees, sexual indiscretions, or foolish business investments).

C. The episode is associated with an unequivocal change in functioning that is uncharacteristic of the individual when not symptomatic.

D. The disturbance in mood and the change in functioning are observable by others.

E. The episode is not severe enough to cause marked impairment in social or occupational functioning or to necessitate hospitalization. If there are psychotic features, the episode is, by definition, manic.

F. The episode is not attributable to the physiologic effects of a substance (e.g., a drug of abuse, a medication, other treatment).

Differential Diagnosis: Neurologic or other medical causes of mania must be ruled out such as cerebrovascular accident (CVA), brain tumors, mild traumatic brain injury (TBI), HIV, hyperthyroidism, tertiary syphilis, neurodegenerative disorders, and MS. These may appear clinically like mania, but have other core features. Strokes in the right orbital frontal lobe, temporal lobe, basal ganglia, or thalamus have been associated with mania. Tertiary syphilis can present with mania. However, this will be accompanied with dysarthia, facial and limb hypotonia, intention tremors of the face, tongue, and hands; with reflex abnormalities. As for neurodegenerative disorders, frontotemporal dementias, Huntington's disease, and basal ganglia calcification are associated commonly with mania. A manic or hypomanic episode is not itself a diagnosis, but occurs in the context of bipolar I or bipolar II disorder, respectively.

Secondary Complications: As mentioned above, manic and hypomanic episodes occur in the context of mood disorders. Complications of the episodes themselves include interpersonal, societal, and financial problems, usually secondary to rash and adverse decisions during mania. See entries for *Bipolar I Disorder*, *Bipolar II Disorder*, and *Bipolar and Related Disorder due to Another Medical Condition*.

Treatment Complications: Treatments and associated side effects are discussed in the entries for *Bipolar I Disorder* and *Bipolar II Disorder*.

Selective serotonin reuptake inhibitors (SSRIs) used to treat major depressive disorder and other disorders may trigger mania. SSRI side effects include nausea, diarrhea, insomnia, headache, anorexia, weight loss, sexual dysfunction, restlessness (akathisia-like), serotonin syndrome (fever diaphoresis, tachycardia, hypertension, delirium, neuromuscular excitability), hyponatremia, and seizures (0.2%).

Mood stabilizers are the treatment of choice for bipolar patients. Most frequently used are valproic acid and lithium, specifically for bipolar I. For valproic acid, patients need to have labwork such as complete blood count (CBC) and liver function tests prior to initiation. For lithium, patients must have labwork such as metabolic panel, paying close attention in particular to renal function tests. Valproic acid side effects include headache, nausea, vomiting, somnolence, thrombocytopenia, dyspepsia, dizziness, diarrhea, tremor, weight changes, hepatotoxicity, pancreatitis, SIADH (syndrome of inappropriate antidiuretic hormone secretion), hyponatremia, pancytopenia, and hyperammonemia. Lithium side effects include hypothyroidism, tremor, polyuria, polydipsia, weight gain, diarrhea, vomiting, cognitive impairment, acne, edema, coma, seizures, arrhythmias, syncope, goiter, and diabetes insipidus.

Suggested Reading

American Psychiatric Association. *Diagnostic and statistical manual of mental disorders: DSM-5.* 5th ed. Washington, DC: American Psychiatric Association; 2013.

McDonald WM, Krishnan KR, Doraiswamy PM, et al. Occurrence of subcortical hyperintensities in elderly subjects with mania. *Psychiatry Res.* 1991;40(4):211–20.

Pares P. Mania following deep brain stimulation for Parkinson's disease. *Neurology.* 2002;59(9):1421–4.

Peet M. Induction of mania with selective serotonin re-uptake inhibitors and tricyclic antidepressants. *Br J Psychiatry.* 1994;164(4):549–50.

Starkstein SE, Mayberg HS, Berthier ML, et al. Mania after brain injury: neuroradiological and metabolic findings. *Ann Neurol.* 1990;27(6):652–9.

Young RC, Biggs JT, Ziegler VE, Meyer DA. A rating scale for mania: reliability, validity and sensitivity. *Br J Psychiatry.* 1978;133(5):429–35.

Maple Syrup Urine Disease

Epidemiology and Demographics: Autosomal recessive; consanguinity leads to higher rates in certain populations (e.g., Mennonites in the United States). Other rates are recorded as ~1/180,000.

Disorder Description: Maple syrup urine disease (MSUD) belongs to a group of conditions known as **amino-acidopathies** (including phenylketonuria, hereditary tyrosinemia, nonketotic hyperglycinemia, and homocystinuria), presenting with encephalopathy and vomiting, or liver failure in the first days to months of life. They are a heterogeneous group of disorders, with the severe form of nonketotic hyperglycinemia presenting as unremitting seizures with hypotonia and hiccoughs; tyrisonemia presenting in a neonate with bleeding diathesis due to liver disease, or later in infancy with a renal Fanconi syndrome. MSUD classically presents at the end of the first week of life with feeding difficulties, lethargy, coma, seizures, and urine with a characteristic odor of maple syrup.

MSUD is an amino-acidopathy associated with a defect in the metabolism of branched chain amino acids – leucine, isoleucine, and valine. Enzyme deficiency allows accumulation of these amino acids and leads to encephalopathy and progressive neurodegeneration.

MSUD is caused by a deficiency in the BCKD (branched chain alpha ketoacid dehydrogenase) complex (Chr 19), which catalyzes decarboxylation of branched chain amino acids to branched acyl-CoAs. Accumulation of leucine, which is rapidly transported across the blood–brain barrier, causes neurologic issues, whilst elevation of plasma isoleucine is associated with the maple syrup odor.

Various forms exist: classic (infantile onset), intermediate, or intermittent forms – based on residual BCKD enzyme activity. All children are at risk of metabolic decompensation during periods of stress and protein catabolism – illness, trauma, surgery. A partially thiamine-responsive form also exists.

Post birth, untreated neonates with **classic** (infantile form) MSUD have elevated plasma concentrations of branched-chain amino acids (BCAAs) (leucine, isoleucine, and valine) and allo-isoleucine by 12–24 hours. By age 2–3 days, ketonuria, irritability, and poor feeding are present; and the characteristic odor of maple syrup is usually present. The disease is usually not detected until age 4–5 days, when deepening encephalopathy ensues, manifesting as lethargy, intermittent apnea, opisthotonus, seizures, and stereotyped movements such as "fencing" and "bicycling." By 7–10 days, if left untreated, coma and respiratory failure may occur. Classic MSUD in neonates is a medical emergency.

Intermediate forms are characterized by acute crises of severe metabolic encephalopathy during sufficient catabolic stress.

Acute transient ataxia has also been reported in well-controlled patients with classic MSUD.

Diagnosis is made by assessing plasma amino acids and finding elevated branched-chain amino acids and the presence of alloisoleucine. Plasma leucine is greatly elevated, with a ratio of leucine: valine:isoleucine of approximately 4:2:1. Plasma allo-isoleucine >5 μmol/L is diagnostic. Genetic testing confirms the diagnosis. Differential diagnoses include other inborn errors of metabolism associated with predominant neurologic deterioration such as urea cycle defects and organic acidemias (i.e., propionic or isovaleric acidemias, methylmalonic acidemia with homocystinuria, multiple carboxylase deficiency).

Symptoms

Localization site	Comment
Cerebral hemispheres	Acute encephalopathy – lethargy, confusion, seizures, coma – usually in acute metabolic crises
	Central hypotonia, dystonia
Cerebellar	Intermittent ataxia even in well-controlled individuals with classic MSUD – etiology unknown

Treatment Complications: Treatment and prevention of acute metabolic decompensation via dietary restriction of branched chain amino acids. MSUD has been added to some newborn screening programs and early dietary intervention (preferably before symptom onset) leads to good outcomes. Dietary management aims to maintain stable plasma BCAA concentrations and ratios. Use of a "sick-day" formula recipe (devoid of leucine and enriched with calories, isoleucine, valine, and BCAA-free amino acids) combined with rapid and frequent amino acid monitoring allows many catabolic illnesses to be managed in the outpatient setting. Prognosis is good for those who are diagnosed early, treated promptly, and who follow a strict lifelong diet.

Bibliography

Frazier DM, et al. Nutrition management guideline for maple syrup urine disease: An evidence- and consensus-based approach. *Mol Genet Metab.* 2014;112(3):210–17.

NORD. Maple syprup urine disease. http://rarediseases.org/rare-diseases/maple-syrup-urine-disease/. Accessed Jun 20, 2016.

Strauss KA, Puffenberger EG, Morton DH. Maple syrup urine disease. Jan 30, 2006. Updated May 9, 2013. In Pagon RA, Adam MP, Ardinger HH, et al., eds. *Gene Reviews*®. Seattle (WA): University of Washington, Seattle; 1993–2016. Available from: www.ncbi.nlm.nih.gov/books/NBK1319/. Accessed Aug 25, 2018.

Marchiafava–Bignami Disease

Epidemiology and Demographics: Marchiafava–Bignami disease occurs predominantly in men and in chronic alcoholics.

Disorder Description: A rare neurologic disorder characterized by demyelination and necrosis of the corpus callosum. Clinical presentation varies as it is difficult to differentiate symptoms of alcohol abuse alone from those of this disorder. Presentation ranges from seizures, tremor, hallucinations, and delirium tremors to progressive dementia, dysarthria, slowing of movement, problems with balance and gait, hemiparesis, emotional disturbances, aphasia,

stupor, or coma. It can have an acute, chronic, or subacute course.

Symptoms

Localization site	Comment
Cerebral hemispheres	Seizures, unsteadiness, hemiparesis, aphasia, stupor, coma
Mental status and psychiatric aspects/complications	Dementia, hallucinations, emotional disturbances
Cerebellum	Ataxia, dysarthria
Peripheral neuropathy	Sensory, motor, autonomic nerve dysfunction, loss of reflexes, decreased vibratory and position sense

Secondary Complications: Alcoholism can lead to peripheral neuropathy, myopathy, nutrtitional deficiencies, cardiac problems, and eventual death.

Bibliography

Ropper AH, Samuels MA, Klein JP. Diseases of the nervous system caused by nutritional deficiency. In *Adams & Victor's principles of neurology*, 10th ed. New York, NY: McGraw-Hill; 2014. Chapter 41.

Rosa A, Demiati M, Cartz L, Mizon JP. Marchiafava-Bignami disease, syndrome of interhemispheric disconnection, and right-handed agraphia in a left-hander. *Arch Neurol.* 1991;48:986.

Mastoiditis

Epidemiology and Demographics: Mastoiditis is the second most common complication of acute otitis media (AOM) in children less than 2 years old with an annual incidence of 37/100,000 children in 2011. Rarely, mastoiditis can occur in adult populations, especially elderly. Intracranial complications of mastoiditis are rare at 0.1% in the era of antibiotic treatment.

Disorder Description: Mastoiditis is a suppurative mastoid air cell infection complicated by AOM. The most common pathogen is *Streptococcus pneumoniae*. Patients with mastoiditis usually present with ear pain, postauricular tenderness/erythema, and protrusion of the auricle. A clinical specimen from the middle ear is important for diagnosis. CT of the temporal bone is diagnostic with loss of trabeculae. Signs of intracranial involvement are severe earache, seizures, fever, constant and persistent headache, nausea and vomiting, or focal neurologic symptoms. Drainage of pus and empiric antibiotics such as vancomycin and cefepime are indicated. Mastoidectomy is performed for severe cases. Extension of the infection can lead to intracranial or extracranial complications.

Symptoms

Localization site	Comment
Cerebral hemispheres	Epidural/subdural abscess, otitis meningitis, otitic hydrocephalus
	Intracranial extension can result in cerebral (temporal lobe) abscess or cerebral venous thrombosis
Mental status	Altered mental status can occur with meningitis/abscess
Cerebellum	Cerebellar abscess
Vestibular system (and non-specific dizziness)	Labyrinthitis
Base of skull	Lateral sinus thrombosis (sigmoid sinus thrombosis) is a frequent complication of mastoiditis. Patients usually present with gradual, persistent earache followed by headache, signs of increased intracranial pressure, cranial neuropathies
Cranial nerves	Cranial neuropathies, especially facial nerve palsy (direct bony erosion and extension). Gradenigo syndrome (otorrhea, retroorbital pain, ipsilateral abducens palsy)
Ear	Hearing loss due to external auditory canal obstruction or middle ear effusion

Secondary Complications: Intracranial and extracranial spread can lead to permanent neurologic deficits including hearing loss.

Treatment complications: Antibiotics for the treatment of mastoiditis presenting as a complication of chronic otitis should include coverage for *Staphylococcus aureus*, *Pseudomonas*, and enteric Gram-negative rods, as well as *Streptococcus pneumoniae* and *Haemophilus influenzae*. If patients do not respond to conservative therapy with IV antibiotics, further intervention involves mastoidectomy for debridement of necrotic bone. Myringotomy is an adjunct to mastoidectomy for the treatment of acute mastoiditis. When cholesteatoma is present, a tympanomastoidectomy is performed to remove both the necrotic bone in the mastoid and cholesteatoma.

Bibliography

Marom T, et al. Trends in otitis media-related health care utilization in the United States, 2001–2011. *JAMA Pediatr*. 2014;168(1):68–75.

Wald ER. Acute mastoiditis in children: Clinical features and diagnosis. In Post TW, ed. *UpToDate*. Waltham, MA. Last updated Jan 3, 2017. www.uptodate.com/contents/acute-mastoiditis-in-children-clinical-features-and-diagnosis. Accessed Aug 25, 2018.

Measles (Rubeola)

Epidemiology and Demographics: Prior to vaccination in 1963, the incidence of measles in the United States was estimated at 3–4 million with 500 deaths annually. After introduction of vaccine, the incidence of measles dramatically decreased to fewer than 500 cases annually. In 2011, 220 measles cases were reported in America. Worldwide, measles remains a huge burden: 145,700 patients died from measles in 2013. Children under the age of 5 are at risk.

Disorder Description: Measles is caused by a virus from the Paramyxoviridae family. It is a highly contagious disease transmitted by airborne spread and direct person-to-person contact. It is characterized by flu-like symptoms, conjunctivitis, coryza, cough, and Koplik spots, followed by exanthema. Transient immunosuppression caused by measles virus can lead to secondary infection. Pneumonia is the most common cause of measles-associated mortality.

Symptoms

Localization site	Comment
Cerebral hemispheres	1. Encephalitis usually occurs within 5 days after rash starts. Patient presents with headache, fever, vomiting, stiff neck, convulsion, or even coma. CSF shows lymphocytic pleocytosis and elevated protein. It can be fatal or complicated by severe neurodevelopmental impairment
	2. Acute disseminated encephalomyelitis (ADEM) is thought to be caused by autoimmune process after the infection. It usually occurs within 14 days after rash starts. Symptoms are similar to encephalitis but can also develop ataxia, myoclonus, choreoathetosis paraplegia, or urinary incontinence. CSF findings are similar to encephalitis
	3. Subacute sclerosing panencephalitis (SSPE) is a post-infection progressive degenerative disease that typically occurs 7 to 10 years after the infection. The risk of developing SSPE increases with decreasing age at infection but decreases with vaccination
	4. Measles inclusion body encephalitis (MIBE) usually occurs 1–6 months after infection in immunocompromised patients. Symptoms include seizure, myoclonus, and altered mental status. Inclusion body in neurons is diagnostic
Cerebellum	Both ADEM and SSPE can present with ataxia
Spinal cord	Patients with acute disseminated encephalomyelitis can present with symptoms of paraplegia, quadriplegia, incontinence, back pain, and sensory loss

Secondary Complications: Immunosuppression caused by measles virus can lead to severe central nervous system infection including encephalitis. About one-fourth of the children with encephalitis have neurologic sequelae. Keratitis and corneal ulceration can lead to blindness. Vitamin A deficiency was reported to be associated with increased rate of post-measles complications.

Treatment Complications: The treatment for measles is mainly supportive. Vitamin A supplementation was recommended by WHO. No significant treatment complications have been reported.

Bibliography

Centers for Disease Control and Prevention. Measles. In Hamborsky J, et al., eds. *Epidemiology and prevention of vaccine-preventable diseases (The Pink Book)*. 13th ed. Washington DC: Public Health Foundation; 2015. Chapter 13.

Gans H, Maldonado YA. Measles: Epidemiology and transmission. Last updated May 25, 2017. In Post TW, ed. *UpToDate*. Waltham, MA. www .uptodate.com/contents/measles-epidemiology-and-transmission. Accessed Aug 25, 2018.

Moss WJ, et al. Measles. *The Lancet*. 2012;379(9811):153–64.

Measles, Mumps, and Rubella Vaccine

Epidemiology and Demographics: Measles, mumps, and rubella (MMR) vaccine is included as part of routine vaccination programs globally. The seroconversion rates from the vaccine of measles, mumps, and rubella are 96–99%, 84–100%, and 95%, respectively.

Disorder Description: The vaccine is composed of live virus vaccines against measles, mumps, and rubella.

Symptoms

Localization site	Comment
Cerebral hemispheres	Acute disseminated encephalomyelitis, seizures, subacute sclerosing panencephalitis, and aseptic meningitis
Mental status and psychiatric aspects/complications	Headache, irritability, and malaise
Cerebellum	Ataxia
Vestibular system (and non-specific dizziness)	Dizziness and syncope
Cranial nerves	Deafness and retrobulbar neuritis
Spinal cord	Transverse myelitis
Peripheral neuropathy	Guillain–Barré syndrome, paresthesia, and polyneuropathy

Localization site	Comment
Muscle	Arthropathy, arthralgia, arthritis, and myalgia

Secondary Complications: Adverse reactions to MMR include fever, rash, lymphadenopathy, joint complaints, hypersensitivity reactions, development of immune thrombocytopenia, and seizures.

Treatment Complications: Controversial possible post-vaccination encephalopathy with ataxia, seizures, and altered mental status has been reported. The Institute of Medicine has contended there is no causal connection between MMR vaccine and autism.

Bibliography

Demicheli V, Rivetti A, Debalini MG, Di Pietrantonj C. Vaccines for measles, mumps and rubella in children. *Cochrane Database Syst Rev.* 2012:CD004407.

Elliman D, Sengupta N, El Bashir H, Bedford H. Measles, mumps, and rubella: prevention. *BMJ Clin Evid.* 2007;2007:pii:0316.

Hendriksz T, Malouf P, Foy JE. Advisory Committee on Immunization Practices (ACIP) of the Centers for Disease Control and Prevention Vaccines for measles, mumps, rubella, varicella, and herpes zoster: immunization guidelines for adults. *J Am Osteopath Assoc.* 2011;111(10 Suppl 6):S10–2.

McLean HQ, Fiebelkorn AP, Temte JL, et al. Prevention of measles, rubella, congenital rubella syndrome, and mumps, 2013: summary recommendations of the Advisory Committee on Immunization Practices (ACIP). *MMWR Recomm Rep.* 2013;62:1.

White SJ, Boldt KL, Holditch SJ, Poland GA, Jacobson RM. Measles, mumps, and rubella. *Clin Obstet Gynecol.* 2012;55(2):550–9. DOI: 10.1097/GRF.0b013e31824df256.

Medication-Overuse Headache

Epidemiology and Demographics: This type of headache has been reported to have a worldwide prevalence of 1–2%. Other studies suggest a prevalence of 0.5–7.2%. One study carried out in a Norwegian cohort showed an incidence of 0.72 per 1000 person-years. Studies suggest a bias of women over men at a ratio of 3–4:1. The condition is most common in the age group above 40 years. The prevalence tends to decrease with increasing age, especially over 65 years. In children, the prevalence is 0.3–0.5%.

Disorder Description: This condition is described as having a headache for more than 15 days out of a month, regular overuse of medication for more than 3 months of at least one medication for headache, and the quality of headache worsened with medication use. In the case of simple analgesics, the time criteria is at least 15 days out of a month; in the instance of triptan, ergots, opioids, or combination analgesics, the time criteria is at least 10 days out of a month. The formal criteria for diagnosing this condition do not account for the dosage of medication or the characterization of headache.

Symptoms

Localization site	Comment
Head	There are no formal criteria in terms of location or other characteristic in the diagnosis of this condition

Secondary Complications: Overuse of medications used in the treatment of headache has established side effects. Simple analgesics have known gastrointestinal complications. Other reported medications used in this condition like opioids or combination analgesics have known side effects as well. However, there is no specific condition or complication to medication-overuse headache outside of established and reported side effects to medications.

Treatment Complications: Some studies suggest a relapse rate of 20–40% within the first year after withdrawal of medication overuse. Fewer patients relapse after 12 months.

Bibliography

Kristoffersen ES, Lundqvist C. Medication-overuse headache: a review. *J Pain Res.* 2014;7:367–78. DOI:10.2147/JPR.S46071.

Kudrow L. Paradoxical effects of frequent analgesic use. *Adv Neurol.* 1982;33:335–41.

Mathew NT, Kurman R, Perez F. Drug induced refractory headache: clinical features and management. *Headache.* 1990;30(10):634–8.

Mehuys E, Paemeleire K, Van Hees T, et al. Self-medication of regular headache: a community pharmacy-based survey. *Eur J Neurol.* 2012;19(8):1093–9.

Medulloblastoma

Epidemiology and Demographics: Medulloblastoma is the most common central nervous system malignancy in children (20% of all childhood brain tumors and 30% to 40% of all posterior fossa childhood brain tumors). It occurs slightly more commonly in males than in females (1.3 to 1). There is no racial difference. It is more common within the first 10 years with a bimodal distribution, peaking at 3 to 4 years of age and again later at 8 to 10 years of age.

Disorder Description: Medulloblastoma is composed of biologically different subsets of tumors arising from stem and/or progenitor cells of the cerebellum. WHO has described the variants of medulloblastoma as classic, nodular-desmoplastic, large cell/anaplastic, and medulloblastoma with extensive nodularity.

Symptoms

Localization site	Comment
Mental status and psychiatric aspects/complications	Infants: developmental delay, anorexia, and increased irritability
	Children: nonspecific fatigue, declining academic performance, and personality changes
Brainstem	Diplopia: sixth nerve paresis due to increased intracranial pressure or direct infiltration of the tumor into the brainstem
	Facial weakness, hearing loss, and associated unilateral cerebellar deficits (cerebellopontine angle extension more common in adults)
Cerebellum	Limb ataxia: present early and causes unsteadiness
Cranial nerves	Nystagmus and diplopia (IV or VI palsy)
	Setting-sun sign: paralysis of upgaze (in very young children)
Spinal cord	Paraplegia/monoplegia due to spinal cord compression is very rare
Specific spinal roots	Radicular pain due to leptomeningeal spread

Treatment Complications: Children can develop long-term neurocognitive deficits due to radiotherapy. Posterior fossa syndrome can occur following surgery, which is characterized by mutism, cerebellar dysfunction, supranuclear cranial nerve palsy, and hemiparesis. It occurs 12–48 hours after surgery.

Bibliography

De Bont JM, Packer RJ, Michiels EM, Den Boer ML, Pieters R. Biological background of pediatric medulloblastoma and ependymoma: a review from a translational research perspective. *Neuro-oncology.* 2008;10(6):1040–60.

Kieffer-Renaux V, Bulteau C, Grill J, et al. Patterns of neuropsychological deficits in children with medulloblastoma according to craniospatial irradiation doses. *Dev Med Child Neurol.* 2000;42(11):741–5.

Taran SJ, Taran R, Malipatil N, Haridas K. Paediatric medulloblastoma: an updated review. *West Indian Med J.* 2016;65(2):363–8.

Meige Syndrome (Oromandibular Dystonia + Blepharospasm)

Epidemiology and Demographics: Meige syndrome, or idiopathic cranial dystonia, has its peak onset at 60 years. Women are more affected than men with a preponderance ranging from 3:2 to 2:1. The prevalence rate is estimated at 5–10/100,000. The disorder is usually sporadic but a few reports describe a familial occurrence.

Disorder Description: Meige syndrome refers to blepharospasm associated with dystonic movements of other muscle groups in the face, neck, and limbs. There may be a variety of movements including abnormal eye closure, opening and closing of the mouth, tensing of the platysma, pursing of the lips, protrusion of the tongue, contractions of the soft palate, turning of the neck, etc. The earliest symptom is usually a specific action dystonia, which may then generalize. There are often sensory tricks (geste antagoniste), which may relieve symptoms. The etiology is unknown but may involve dysfunction in the basal ganglia-thalamo-cortical circuits.

Secondary Complications: Patients who are severely affected by blepharospasm may be rendered functionally blind. Sudden unexpected eye closure during activities may also result in injury such as when driving. Dystonia affecting the jaw, soft palate, and lower facial muscles may result in difficulty with speech and swallowing; there may also be unintended injury to the lips, gums, teeth, and recurrent jaw dislocation.

Treatment Complications: First line treatment is focused botulinum toxin injections. However, patients may experience unintended weakness in the muscles targeted. When this occurs for blepharospasm, patients may experience eye closure weakness, dry eyes, blurred vision, and diplopia. If this occurs in the lower facial muscles and neck, patients may experience dysarthria, dysphagia, and neck weakness. Oral medications such as anticholinergics and benzodiazepines may result in intolerable side effects, especially in the elderly.

Bibliography

Balasubramaniam R, Ram S. Orofacial movement disorders. *Oral Maxillofac Surg Clin North Am.* 2008:20(2):273–85.

Colosimo C, Suppa A, Fabbrini G, Bologna M, Berardelli A. Craniocervical dystonia: clinical and pathophysiological features. *Eur J Neurol.* 2010;17(s1):15–21.

Kraft SP, Lang AE. Cranial dystonia, blepharospasm and hemifacial spasm: clinical features and treatment, including the use of botulinum toxin. *CMAJ: Can Med Assoc J.* 1988;139(9):837.

Melanoma

Epidemiology and Demographics: Primary central nervous system (CNS) melanomas are rare and represent only 0.07% of all brain tumors. Secondary CNS melanomas are more common and occur as a metastasis.

Disorder Description: Melanoma is a tumor originating from the melanocytes. They arise from melanocytes present in the leptomeninges in the cerebral convexity, in the skull base, posterior fossa, and spinal cord.

Symptoms

Localization site	Comment
Mental status and psychiatric aspects/complications	Confusion and personality changes
Brainstem	Ocular motility defects due to CN III, VI and facial weakness due to CN VII; can mimic midbrain and pons cavernoma with recurrent hemorrhages

Localization site	Comment
Cerebellum	Ataxia
Spinal cord	Spastic paraplegia, brachialgia, or other signs of myelopathy depending upon the level affected. Cauda equina compression with acute retention of urine (epidural compression)
Dorsal root ganglia	Polyradicular pain (tumor infiltration of plexus)
Unclear localization	Subarachnoid hemorrhage or intracerebral hemorrhage (rupture of the tumor)

Secondary Complications: Retinopathy (paraneoplastic, Recoverin-Ab CV2-Ab, Rod-Bipolar-Cell-Ab).

Treatment Complications:

- Chemotherapy: dacarbazine, temozolomide, paclitaxel, cisplatin, carboplatin, vinblastine: Hair loss, oral ulcers, loss of appetite, nausea and vomiting, diarrhea, opportunistic infections, pancytopenia, fatigue.
- Pembrolizumab, ipilimumab, interferon: skin rash, arthralgias, colitis, hepatitis, neuropathy, unusual severe headaches, blurry vision, fatigue, cough, constipation, and cytopenia.
- Brain irradiation can cause leukoencephalopathy.

Suggested Reading

Choi KN, Withers HR, Rotman M. Intracranial metastases from melanoma. Clinical features and treatment by accelerated fractionation. *Cancer.* 1985;56(1):1–9.

Hayward RD. Malignant melanoma and the central nervous system. A guide for classification based on the clinical findings. *J Neurol Neurosurg Psychiatr.* 1976;39(6):526–30.

Raizer JJ, Hwu WJ, Panageas KS, et al. Brain and leptomeningeal metastases from cutaneous melanoma: survival outcomes based on clinical features. *Neuro-oncology.* 2008;10(2):199–207.

Meniere's Disease

Epidemiology and Demographics: Idiopathic condition of the inner ear, affecting adults, with a female predilection. The prevalence of Meniere's in the United States is approximately 15 in 100,000.

Disorder Description: Meniere's disease is characterized by episodic vertigo, and hearing loss, tinnitus, and fullness in the affected ear. The pathophysiology is endolymphatic hydrops or abnormal fluid retention within the membranous labyrinth of the inner ear. Episodic vertigo occurs unpredictably, can last for hours at a time, and can be incapacitating. Balance is usually completely normal between attacks. Most cases are unilateral, and the audiogram will show low- and high-frequency sensorineural hearing loss in the affected ear. The differential diagnosis of episodic vertigo is vestibular migraine, but the latter does not cause unilateral hearing loss.

Symptoms

Localization site	Comment
Inner ear	Endolymphatic hydrops, causing episodic vertigo, sensorineural hearing loss, and subjective tinnitus and fullness
Cranial nerves	The cochleovestibular nerve is not affected
Central nervous system	The central nervous system is not affected

Secondary Complications: Patients are at risk of injury from falling. A small percentage of patients with a pernicious form of Meniere's disease experience *drop attacks*, a sudden loss of vestibular tone without warning.

In bilateral cases, hearing loss can be disabling. In severe cases, a cochlear implant might be needed. Tinnitus may be troublesome and occasionally disabling.

Treatment Complications: Treatment consists of salt-restricted diet, diuretics, betahistine, dexamethasone injections. Refractory cases can be treated with intratympanic gentamicin ("chemical labyrinthectomy"), vestibular nerve section, or surgical labyrinthectomy.

Thiazide diuretics can cause dehydration and hypokalemia. Acetazolamide can cause paresthesias, anorexia, and metabolic acidosis. Chemical or surgical deafferentation can result in permanent sensorineural hearing loss and gait ataxia.

Bibliography

Harcourt J, Barraclough K, Bronstein AM. Meniere's disease. *BMJ.* 2014;349. PMID: 25391837.

Silverstein H, Smouha E, Jones R. Natural history vs. surgery for Meniere's disease. *Otolaryngol Head Neck Surg.* 1989;100:6–16.

Wright T. Menière's disease. *BMJ Clin Evid.* 2015;2015:pii:0505. PMID: 26545070.

Meningioma

Epidemiology and Demographics: Meningiomas are the most common primary central nervous system tumors and account for about one-third of all primary brain and spinal tumors. The estimated number of new cases per year in the United States is nearly 26,000 with median age at diagnosis of 65 years. Meningiomas are more common in women.

Disorder Description: Meningiomas are tumors arising from the meninges, the protective layers surrounding the central nervous system. They are typically slow growing, rarely producing symptoms, and sometimes discovered incidentally on brain imaging.

Symptoms

Localization site	Comment
Cerebral hemispheres	Monoparesis of the contralateral leg (parasagittal), contralateral hemianopia (occipital lobe) **Kennedy-Foster syndrome**: anosmia with possible ipsilateral optic atrophy and contralateral papilledema (olfactory groove) Seizures (cortical irritation) Headache (compression)
Mental status and psychiatric aspects/complications	Apathy, disinhibited behavior (subfrontal location)
Brainstem	Facial weakness and hemiparesis (pons)
Cerebellum	Unsteady gait
Vestibular system (and non-specific dizziness)	Dizziness (left cerebellomedullary cistern)

Localization site	Comment
Base of skull	Tongue atrophy associated with fasciculation (foramen magnum)
Cranial nerves	Monocular loss of vision (optic nerve)
	Visual field deficits (depending on location along the optic tract)
	Multiple cranial nerve deficits (II, III, IV, V, VI), leading to decreased vision and diplopia (cavernous sinus)
	Sensorineural hearing loss with facial weakness (cerebellopontine angle meningioma)
Pituitary gland	Pan hypopituitarism (sella turcica)
Spinal cord	Progressive paraparesis and numbness
Conus medullaris	Paraparesis (extremely rare)
Specific spinal roots	Paraplegia with sensory level (thoracic), foot drop (L5 with compression of surrounding roots)
Unclear localization	Obstructive hydrocephalus (intraventricular meningiomas)

Secondary Complications: Neurofibromatosis Type 2, delayed effect of radiation, Cowden syndrome, and familial meningiomas.

Treatment Complications: Surgery can result in seizures and damage to surrounding normal structures. Gamma knife surgery can produce peritumorous changes, causing headaches, seizures, and focal neurologic signs and transient cranial nerve dysfunction. Side effects of radiation include headache, leukoencephalopathy, cognitive impairment, and hypopituitarism.

Bibliography

Gerganov V, Bussarsky V, Romansky K, et al. Cerebellopontine angle meningiomas. Clinical features and surgical treatment. *J Neurosurg Sci.* 2003;47(3):129–35.

Jiang XB, Ke C, Han ZA, et al. Intraparenchymal papillary meningioma of brainstem: case report and literature review. *World J Surg Oncol.* 2012;10:10.

Wofford JL, Moran WP, Wilson TA, Velez R. Clinical presentation of meningioma in the elderly. *J Am Geriatr Soc.* 1993;41(2):122–6.

Menkes Disease

Epidemiology and Demographics: The incidence of Menkes disease is 1:100,000–1:250,000 live births. A third are de novo mutations. There is no racial or ethnic predilection. The disease presents around the age of 2 months, mainly in males, and children die by the age of 3. However, very early intramuscular copper–histidine treatment may correct some of the neurologic symptoms.

Disorder Description: Menkes is a multisystemic disorder of copper metabolism – also known as trichopoliodystrophy or kinky hair, kinky vessel disease. It is an X-linked disorder, with majority of patients being males, characterized by progressive neurodegeneration and connective tissue disturbances. Menkes is caused by mutations in the ATP7A gene (Xq13.3) coding for an energy-dependent transmembrane protein involved in the delivery of copper to secreted enzymes and in the export of surplus copper from cells. The biochemical phenotype is characterized by low levels of copper in plasma, liver, and brain, with secondary reduced activity of copper-dependent enzymes. There is paradoxical copper retention in some tissues such as duodenum, kidney, spleen, and skeletal muscle.

The scalp hair of affected infants has a pathognomonic twisted (*pili torti*), "kinky" appearance, reminiscent of steel wool. Distribution is typically more on vertex of the head, with sparse or absent hair on back and sides. Other abnormalities such as trichoclasis (transverse fracture) or trichoptilosis (longitudinal splitting) may also be present.

Lack of copper enzymes leads to loss of developmental milestones, onset of hypotonia and seizures, and failure to thrive – usually between the ages of 6 and 8 weeks.

Symptoms related to the neuraxis are thought to be related to deficiency of dopamine B-hydroxlase, a copper-requiring enzyme critical to the catecholamine biosynthetic pathway. This leads to a lack of norepinephrine and excess of dihydroxyphenylalanine (DOPA). Cytochrome c oxidase is another copper-dependent enzyme, involved in the mitochondrial respiratory chain, leading to a subacute necrotizing encephalomyopathy.

Symptoms

Localization site	Comment
Cerebral hemispheres	Hypotonia, developmental regression, seizures
	Subdural and epidural hemorrhages due to connective tissue abnormalities
	Imaging – progressive cerebellar and cerebral atrophy, elongated and tortuous intracranial vessels, as well as bilateral subdural collections or bleeds
Cranial nerves	Retinal hypopigmentation, eyelid ptosis, partial optic nerve atrophy
Autonomic nervous system	Temperature instability, hypoglycemia

Secondary Complications: Vascular hemorrhages may lead to encephalopathy.

Bibliography

Kaler SG. ATP7A-related copper transport disorders. In Pagon RA, Adam MP, Ardinger HH, et al., eds. *Gene Reviews*®. Updated Aug 18, 2016. Seattle, WA: University of Washington, Seattle; 1993–2017. Available from: www.ncbi.nlm.nih.gov/books/NBK1413/.

Tumer Z, Moller LB. Menkes disease. *Eur J Hum Genet.* 2010;18:511–18.

Mescaline

Epidemiology and Demographics: No age, gender, or race predilection.

Disorder Description: An active ingredient of the peyote cactus, which is a small, spineless cactus found in the southwestern United States and northern Mexico. It is a naturally occurring psychedelic alkaloid of the phenethylamine class, known for its hallucinogenic effects similar to those of LSD and psilocybin.

Symptoms

Localization site	Comment
Cerebral hemispheres	Cerebral atrophy (chronic)
Mental status and psychiatric aspects/complications	Hallucinations (acute) Anxiety (acute) Paranoia (acute) Emotional lability (acute)

Localization site	Comment
Cerebellum	Ataxia (acute)
Cranial nerves	Nystagmus (acute) Photophobia (acute)
Plexus	Hyperreflexia (acute)
Muscle	Tremors (acute)
Neuromuscular junction	Increased activation of 5HT2A receptors (chronic) Noradrenergic excitability (chronic) Dopaminergic excitability (chronic)

Bibliography

Delgado J. Intoxication from LSD and other common hallucinogens. *UpToDate.* Updated Sep 20, 2017. www.uptodate.com/contents/intoxication-from-lsd-and-other-common-hallucinogens?source=machineLearning&search=mescaline&selectedTitle=1~4&sectionRank=1&anchor=H15#H15. Accessed Aug 28, 2018.

Mesial Temporal Sclerosis (MTS)

Epidemiology and Demographics: Mesial temporal sclerosis (MTS) exists in up to two-thirds of cases of refractory temporal lobe epilepsy. Equally prevalent in both sexes.

Disorder Description: The most common pathologic finding in drug-resistant mesial temporal lobe epilepsy. Etiology unclear, but studies have shown increased incidence among family members and an association with precipitating insults, such as prolonged febrile seizures. There is also evidence demonstrating that MTS is both a result and a cause of seizures.

MTS is characterized histologically by neuronal loss and gliosis involving the hippocampus (CA1 > CA4 > CA2–3), the amygdala, entorhinal cortex, uncus, and para-hippocampal gyrus. MRI features include hippocampal atrophy and increased signal intensity on T2-weighted imaging. EEG correlates include interictal anterior temporal spike wave discharges and temporal intermittent rhythmic delta activity.

Resective surgery significantly improves seizure frequency in patients with MTS, with temporal lobectomy having a success rate near 75%.

Symptoms

Localization site	Comment
Cerebral hemispheres	Focal seizures, often described as bland, with staring, oro-manual automatisms
	Auras involve epigastric rising sensation, nonspecific cephalic sensation, déjà vu, and fear
Mental status and psychiatric aspects/ complications	Postictally, can have disturbances of mood, cognition, language, and memory
	Patients with MTS have significantly higher rates of depression than those with neocortical temporal lesions. Also, a greater frequency of cognitive side effects and mood problems with antiepileptic drugs. Issues with verbal memory decline are common with dominant temporal lobe involvement

Secondary Complications: Refractory epilepsy resulting from MTS can contribute to substantial cognitive, psychologic, and social consequences.

Treatment Complications: The risks of temporal lobectomy include verbal memory impairments and naming difficulties in cases involving the dominant temporal lobe, and superior quadrantanopsia. Memory decline may depend on preoperative baseline functioning and seizure freedom postoperatively.

Bibliography

Cendes F. Febrile seizures and mesial temporal sclerosis. *Curr Opin Neurol.* 2004;17(2):161–4.

Garcia CS. Depression in temporal lobe epilepsy: a review of prevalence, clinical features, and management considerations. *Epilepsy Res Treat.* 2012;2012:809843.

Lewis DV. Losing neurons: selective vulnerability and mesial temporal sclerosis. *Epilepsia.* 2005;46(Suppl 7): 39–44.

Spano VR, Mikulis DJ. Mesial temporal sclerosis in epilepsy. *CMAJ.* 2011;183(15):E1151.

Metachromatic Leukodystrophy

Epidemiology and Demographics: Prevalence ranges from 1/40,000 to 1/100,000 in North Americans and Northern Europeans. Age of onset varies from 6 months to adulthood. It is more common in Habbanite Jews in Israel, Arabs living in Israel, and Navajo Indians in the United States.

Disorder Description: Autosomal recessive lysosomal storage disease. It affects the gene for the enzyme arylsulfatase A. This prevents the conversion of sulfatide to cerebroside. Cerebroside is a key component in myelin. Metachromatic leukodystrophy results in degeneration of myelin in the cerebrum, cerebellum, spinal cord, and peripheral nerves. It presents as progressively worsening motor function including problems with gait and spasticity. It can also produce a reduction in speech output, brisk reflexes early on with later involvement of peripheral nerves producing areflexia, and hypotonia. It causes problems with vision, optic atrophy, dysarthria, and dysphagia. There is no curative treatment at this time.

Symptoms

Localization site	Comment
Cerebral hemispheres	Spasticity, problems with vision, dysarthria, dysphagia, decreased speech output
Mental status and psychiatric aspects/complications	Slowed mental processing/ mental regression
Cerebellum	Problems with gait
Spinal cord	Worsening motor function, problems with gait
Peripheral neuropathy	Areflexia, hypotonia

Secondary Complications: Physical injury and infection are a risk secondary to motor, gait, vision, and swallowing problems.

Bibliography

Gustavson KH, Hagberg B. The incidence and genetics of metachromatic leucodystrophy in northern Sweden. *Acta Paediatr Scand.* 1971;60:585.

Heinisch U, Zlotogora J, Kafert S, Gieselmann V. Multiple mutations are responsible for the high frequency of metachromatic leukodystrophy in a small geographic area. *Am J Hum Genet.* 1995;56:51.

Holve S, Hu D, McCandless SE. Metachromatic leukodystrophy in the Navajo: fallout of the American-Indian wars of the nineteenth century. *Am J Med Genet.* 2001;101:203.

Ropper AH, Samuels MA, Klein JP. Inherited metabolic diseases of the nervous system. In *Adams & Victor's principles of neurology*, 10th ed. New York, NY: McGraw-Hill; 2014. Chapter 37.

Von Figura K, Gieselmann V, Jacken J. Metachromatic leukodystrophy. In Scriver CR, Beaudet AL, Sly WS, et al., eds. *The metabolic and molecular bases of inherited diseases*. 8th ed. New York: McGraw-Hill; 2001. p. 3695.

Zlotogora J, Bach G, Barak Y, Elian E. Metachromatic leukodystrophy in the habbanite Jews: high frequency in a genetic isolate and screening for heterozygotes. *Am J Hum Genet*. 1980 32:663.

Methamphetamine Abuse

Epidemiology and Demographics: Common abusers are young adolescent males, with no race predilection.

Disorder Description: Strong central nervous system stimulant composed of two isomeric forms of methamphetamine, a dextro-isomer and a levo-isomer. The more heavily abused component is the dextro-isomer. Common locations of high use are Asia, Oceania, and the United States. Methamphetamine and related compounds are now the second most commonly used illicit substance worldwide, after cannabis.

Symptoms

Localization site	Comment
Cerebral hemispheres	Seizures (acute) Gray matter atrophy degeneration (chronic) White matter hypertrophy (chronic) Coma (acute) Globus pallidus and hippocampus injury in methamphetamine-induced encephalopathy (chronic) Cerebral ischemia (stroke) (acute) Cerebral hemorrhage (acute) Transient ischemic attack (acute)
Mental status and psychiatric aspects/ complications	Psychosis with mood swings (acute) Delusions and violent behavior Euphoria (acute) Cognitive impairment (acute) Visual and auditory hallucinations
Cerebellum	Cerebellar atrophy (chronic)
Cranial nerves	Optic nerve atrophy (chronic)

Localization site	Comment
Spinal cord	Spinal cord infarction (acute)
Specific spinal roots	Lumbosacral radiculopathy (acute)
Plexus	Plexopathy (acute)
Muscle	Tremors (acute) Choreoathetosis (chronic): variation of rapid and slow jerking movements of distal muscle that are incorporated in semi-purposeful act Dyskinesia (impaired voluntary movement) Rhabdomyolysis (acute)
Neuromuscular junction	Dopaminergic neurotoxicity (increase in Parkinson's disease risk) Serotonergic neurotoxicity (increase in serotonin risk)

Secondary Complications

- **Cardiovascular** effects: hypertension with associated arrhythmias; vasospasm; accelerated atherosclerosis leading to stroke.
- **Coagulation** dysfunction combined with hypertensive effect results in hemorrhagic strokes.
- **Hepatic** complications:
  - acute liver failure may result in brain edema, amplified by hypoglycemia, hypoxia, and seizures;
  - hepatic myelopathy with rapidly progressing spastic paraparesis;
  - severe fatigue, cognitive dysfunction, and mood disorder.

Bibliography

Ardakani RK, Nahangi H, Yadegari M, Hosseini-Sharifabad M. The effects of long-term administration of methamphetamine on the cerebellum of the male mice: a stereological study. The Neuroscience Journal of Shefaye Khatam. www.shefayekhatam.ir/browse.php?a_id=453&sid=1&slc_lang=en. Accessed Aug 28, 2018.

Foroughipour M, Farzadfard M, Aghaee M, Ghabeli-Juibary A, Rezaietalab F. Methamphetamine related radiculopathy: case series and review of literature. *Asia Pacific J Med Toxicol*. 2013;2(2):71–5. DOI: 10.22038/apjmt.2013.894.

Gonzalez-Usigli HA. Chorea, athetosis, and hemiballismus. MSD Manuals. Revised Feb 2017. Available from www.merckmanuals.com/professional/neurologic-disorders/movement-and-cerebellar-disorders/chorea,-athetosis,-and-hemiballismus. Accessed Aug 28, 2018.

NIDA. Methamphetamine. National Institute on Drug Abuse website. www.drugabuse.gov/publications/research-reports/methamphetamine. September 19, 2013. Accessed August 28, 2018.

Won S, Hong RA, Shohet RV, Seto TB, Parikh NI. Methamphetamine-associated cardiomyopathy. *Clin Cardiol*. 2013;36(12):737–42. DOI:10.1002/clc.22195.

Methotrexate Toxicity

Disorder Description: Methotrexate works by inhibiting dihydrofolate reductase in a competitive manner and has multiple indications for usage. Pathophysiology of neurotoxicity is poorly understood. Postulated theories are depletion of folate, endothelial injury, and inhibition of catecholamine synthesis. No effective treatment available. Leucovorin doesn't help.

Symptoms

Localization site	Comment
Cerebral hemispheres	Acute stroke-like symptoms with aphasia or hemiparesis Posterior reversible leukoencephalopathy (PRES) with vision loss, seizures **Mineralizing microangiopathy**: non-inflammatory fibrosis and calcification (visible on imaging) of capillaries and venules in basal ganglia
Mental status and psychiatric aspects/complications	Delayed leukoencephalopathy develops years after with personality changes and learning disability
Cerebellum	Ataxia
Cranial nerves	Central scotomas and reduced vision (methotrexate-induced optic atrophy)
Spinal cord	Transient aseptic meningitis and transverse myelitis (lumbar puncture directed intrathecal injection in acute phase)

Bibliography

Aminoff MJ, Josephson SA. *Aminoff's neurology and general medicine*. London, UK: Academic Press; 2014.

Jahnke K, Korfel A, Martus P, et al. High-dose methotrexate toxicity in elderly patients with primary central nervous system lymphoma. *Ann Oncol*. 2005;16(3):445–9.

Wernick R, Smith DL. Central nervous system toxicity associated with weekly low-dose methotrexate treatment. *Arthritis Rheum*. 1989;32(6):770–5.

Microphthalmos/Nanophthalmos

Epidemiology and Demographics: Microphthalmos occurs in about 2 to 17 per 100,000 births. Sex distribution is approximately equal.

Disorder Description: Microphthalmos is a congenital structural eye abnormality. It can be thought of as a spectrum of phenotypes with variable penetrance with anophthalmia being complete absence of an eye, and coloboma being a segmental ocular defect. Microphthalmos represents a non-specific growth failure of the eye in response to prenatal insults and/or genetic defects.

A microphthalmic eye is at least 2 standard deviations below the age-adjusted mean axial length. Simple microphthalmos (also known as nanophthalmos) is a small but structurally normal eye whereas complex microphthalmos is associated with other congenital ocular abnormalities. Microphthalmos can be isolated or part of a genetic syndrome and has been described as part of over 100 different syndromes.

Symptoms

Localization site	Comment
Cranial nerves	CHARGE syndrome (Coloboma, Heart abnormalities, Atresia of the choanae, Retardation of growth, Genitourinary abnormalities, and Ear abnormalities) is the most common form of syndromic microphthalmia. Patients may have cranial nerve abnormalities including facial palsy and difficulty swallowing
Pituitary gland	Bone Morphogenic Protein 4 gene expresses a signaling molecule that has a critical role in embryonic development. Mutations in this gene have been associated with a spectrum of abnormalities including anophthalmia/microphthalmia, hypopituitarism, other brain abnormalities, and digital abnormalities

Secondary Complications: Cataract is often found in association with microphthalmia. Ocular motility abnormalities are present in many microphthalmic patients (higher incidence of poor vision and subsequent sensory tropia). Anterior segment abnormalities, angle closure glaucoma, and retinal detachments are also associated complications.

Treatment Complications: In a newborn with anophthalmos or microphthalmos, the first step in management is to determine whether it is isolated or part of a syndromic phenotype. Further workup is determined by clinical exam. Molecular testing in the absence of systemic findings is low yield.

Management and treatment of ocular complications require regular ophthalmologic follow up to maximize visual potential. Management considerations include amblyopia treatment, or eye protections in eyes with little or no visual potential.

In anophthalmic or severely microphthalmic cases (when the eye is deemed to have no visual potential), there is often underdevelopment of the orbit, eyelids, and facial structure. There are reconstructive surgical options to improve the cosmetic appearance. These include lid surgery, orbital reconstruction with implants, and bone grafts. These have associated surgical complications.

Bibliography

Warburg M. Classification of microphthalmos and coloboma. *J Med Genet*. 1993;30:664–9.

Middle Cerebral Artery (MCA) Occlusion

Etiologies

The middle cerebral artery (MCA) can be occluded as a result of any major vascular disease category but the most common causes by far are atherosclerosis and cardioembolus.

Atherosclerosis is seen most frequently in patients with metabolic syndrome, prior coronary or peripheral vascular artery disease, a strong family history of atherosclerosis, and a history of cigarette smoking. The occlusion usually occurs at the origin of the MCA from the ICA or at the distal portion of the MCA trunk, often referred to as the "trifurcation."

Cardioembolic MCA strokes occur most frequently in patients with atrial fibrillation, valvular heart disease, an acute anterior wall myocardial infarction, or in patients with a patent foramen ovale associated with an atrial septal aneurysm and may result from occlusion of either the primary trunk of the MCA or its more distal branches.

Less common but important causes of MCA occlusion include vasculitis, coagulopathies, and dissection of the internal carotid artery.

Disorder Description

MCA syndromes result from ischemic injury to the cerebral hemispheres as a result of thromboembolic occlusion of the vessel. Because the MCA is the dominant vessel of the cerebral hemisphere, even occlusions of its secondary branches produce significant neurologic syndromes.

The MCA is a medium sized, muscular artery, which originates from the distal internal carotid artery after the cavernous sinus and travels in the subarachnoid space. The MCA trunk travels horizontally in the Sylvian fissure to the surface of the cerebral hemisphere and then splits into three major branches (the "trifurcation"). The MCA trunk gives rise to large penetrating arteries that serve the basal ganglia, internal capsule, and insular cortex, known as the "Deep Territory" of the hemispheres, before its trifurcation near the lateral surface of the cerebral hemisphere.

The important major branches are the:
- superior division, serving the frontal lobe;
- inferior division, serving the lateral temporal lobe (the medial temporal lobe is served by the posterior cerebral artery);
- anterior temporal branch, serving the anterior temporal lobe.

Note that the parietal lobe may be served by either the superior or inferior division. The branch serving the parietal lobe is referred to as the dominant branch for the particular individual.

As a leptomeningeal artery, the distal branches of the MCA anastomose freely with one another and with distal branches of the anterior and posterior cerebral arteries, forming important collaterals on the surface of the hemispheres since blood can flow either antegrade or retrograde in the distal territories.

Proximal MCA occlusion in the presence of excellent distal collaterals from anterior cerebral artery (ACA) and/or posterior cerebral artery (PCA) can result in the deep territory only being infarcted.

(This may resemble a lacunar syndrome, but the difference is that insular cortex is affected when MCA stem is involved.)

Clinical Syndromes

Symptoms:

1. Sensorimotor, hand = face > leg
2. Language – grammar/syntax vs rate/rhythm (prosody)
3. Gerstmann syndrome vs apraxia/neglect
4. Frontal eye fields
   With right hemisphere infarction with apraxia of eyelid opening (cerebral ptosis)
5. Insula – autonomic (EKG, arrhythmias)
6. Basal ganglia and internal capsule (pure motor)

The MCA delivers blood flow to the cerebral hemispheres, therefore all clinical syndromes reflect impairment of some portion of the cerebral hemispheres. Also, because the dominant and non-dominant hemispheres contribute differentially to aspects of human behavior, there are important differences in the resulting clinical syndromes.

The variable presence of PCA and ACA collaterals has important consequences for the variability of the MCA syndromes so that generalizations should be modified in any individual.

Deep territory MCA ischemia may involve the basal ganglia, the genu of the internal capsule, and the insular cortex.

- Involvement of the basal ganglia and genu of the internal capsule typically produces contralateral hemiplegia or hemiparesis. The typical pattern of face and arm involvement greater than leg that results from ischemia in the superior division of the MCA (see below) may not be apparent when the deep territory is involved. There is little or no right–left asymmetry.

- Insular cortex ischemia can create significant autonomic changes, including hyper- or hypotension, brady- or tachy-arrhythmias, and EKG changes suggestive of acute myocardial infarction. Recent observations suggest that insular involvement may result in altered consciousness. The combination of hemiparesis, dysautonomia, and lethargy may suggest the presence of intracerebral hemorrhage.

Right–left insula asymmetries may exist but there is substantial overlap.

Inferior division MCA ischemia affects the lateral surface of the posterior temporal lobe.

- Temporal lobe involvement frequently produces disturbances of memory and behavior, primarily manifested as anxiety and frustration not in keeping with the patient's personality. This subtle syndrome may become apparent when it is recognized that the patient also has visual hemianopia or superior quadrantanopia ("pie in the sky" due to involvement of Meyer's loop of the optic radiations). Involvement of either hemisphere can produce this syndrome.

- However, there are important asymmetries in accompanying cognitive disorders. In particular, involvement of the dominant hemisphere (left hemisphere in right handers) can result in classical Wernicke's aphasia and Gerstmann's syndrome. Wernicke's aphasia is a combination of fluent expressive (paraphasic) and receptive aphasias, which can occur independently to varying degrees in any individual. The complete Gerstmann's syndrome involves acalculia, right/left disorientation, finger agnosia, and alexia without agraphia. Partial Gerstmann's syndromes are more common than the complete syndrome.

- Ischemia in the inferior division of the non-dominant hemisphere also produces important cognitive disturbances including aprosodias, apraxias, and visuo-spatial neglect syndromes. These can be challenging to recognize and to treat.

Superior division MCA ischemia regularly alters function in the frontal lobe. For the sake of this discussion, it is assumed that the Superior Division is the dominant division, serving the parietal lobe as well as the frontal lobe. Ischemia produces a characteristic sensorimotor syndrome as well as more subtle behavioral disturbances.

- The classical sensorimotor syndrome of the superior division of the MCA is due to ischemia in the rolandic artery, which serves the pre- and post-central gyri. The result is weakness with congruent sensory disturbance that primarily involves the face and arm but largely spares the leg (which is on the interhemispheric surface in the ACA territory). Dysarthria and hand weakness with clumsiness are often prominent. Tone and deep tendon reflexes may be increased or decreased acutely but a Babinski sign is usually present. Both tone and reflexes usually increase within 2 or 3 days.

- The frontal eye fields (FEF) receive blood flow through the superior MCA division. FEF ischemia produces a gaze paresis to the same side as the hemiparesis but also produces important contralateral hemineglect and apraxia since the FEF are integral to attentional mechanisms. This may produce sensorimotor disturbances out of proportion to the degree of weakness or sensory loss.

- Broca's area is usually served by the superior division of the MCA and therefore non-fluent aphasia is often a prominent component of this arterial obstruction when the dominant hemisphere is involved. Similarly, however, the syndrome resulting from the non-dominant hemisphere produces an expressive aprosodia, essentially flat, monotonic speech devoid of expressive qualities.

- Posterior parietal lobe impairment produces apraxias that are as complex as they are subtle. Neglect syndromes, apraxias, dysphagia, cerebral ptosis, and transcortical sensory aphasias can accompany injury to the dominant MCA division. While they can appear acutely when either the non-dominant or dominant hemisphere is involved, they are more likely to persist when the non-dominant hemisphere is affected. The only exception to this is that transcortical aphasias are more likely to persist in the dominant hemisphere.

Anterior temporal branch ischemia is difficult to recognize as it may produce no observable neurologic deficits. By analogy with temporal lobe surgery for removal of gliomas or control of epilepsy, there may be no demonstrable deficits when the anterior temporal pole of the non-dominant hemisphere is affected. There is risk of language or memory disturbance when the dominant hemisphere is affected if the ischemic region extends posteriorly.

Secondary Complications

Common complications of an MCA stroke include falls, deep vein thrombosis, dysphagia with aspiration, and other physical injuries related to trauma that occur because of neglect syndromes.

While seizures are not common, neither are they rare and often occur with significant delays from the initial stroke, even years later. Seizures at onset may indicate a cardioembolic source.

The "malignant MCA syndrome" occurs when there is a life-threatening increase in intracranial pressure due to complete infarction of the MCA territory, usually in patients with little or no atrophy prior to the stroke, as is often the case in younger patients.

Treatment Complications

Intravenous thrombolysis with tissue plasminogen activator (tPA) or intra-arterial thrombolysis, either with mechanical devices or with tPA, are associated with a risk of intracerebral hemorrhage. Such hemorrhages vary from asymptomatic related to hemorrhagic transformation in the previously ischemic tissue all the way to catastrophic life-threatening deterioration due to massive bleeding.

Systemic bleeding or bleeding into large acute strokes can result from secondary prevention measures, including use of heparin, warfarin, direct thrombin, and Factor Xa inhibitors, or dual anti-platelet agents. Chronic anti-coagulation and anti-thrombotic measures increase the risk of subdural hematomas.

Craniectomy performed for malignant MCA syndrome requires a careful decision process due to poor quality of life that may be associated with increasing age and involvement of the dominant hemisphere.

Migraine with Aura

Epidemiology and Demographics: This condition has been reported with wide prevalence and incidence. The definition of migraine with aura encompasses a variety of headache types. The general consensus so far is that there is no preference for either sex in terms of prevalence and the overall prevalence is widespread.

Disorder Description: The presence of aura with migraine headaches can involve vision, motor symptoms, sensation, and language. There is controversy whether or not aura precipitates migraine headaches or migraine with aura is one entity. This type of headache is typically unilateral but there are reports of bilateral presentations. Some studies suggest that aura can exist alone without migraine headache. In these situations, careful consideration must be used to ensure that no vascular etiology is responsible for aura-like symptoms.

Symptoms

Localization site	Comment
Cerebral hemispheres	Involvement of either unilateral or bilateral hemispheres. Brainstem is also involved especially with aura presentations

Secondary Complications: Migraine headache with aura can persist for a long time leading to status migrainosus. In these situations, headache symptoms may be so severe that careful monitoring and strong abortive therapy are needed as in a hospital setting.

Treatment Complications: Abortive therapy like triptans can be used for severe migraine headaches. Side effects of this medication include vasoconstriction and can lead to strokes, especially in patients who have vascular risk factors. Excessive and prolonged use of nonsteroidal anti-inflammatory drugs can cause gastrointestinal complications.

Bibliography

Charles A. Migraine: a brain state. *Curr Opin Neurol.* 2013;26:235–9.

Charles A, Hansen JM. Migraine aura: new ideas about cause, classification and clinical significance. *Curr Opin Neurol.* 2015;28: 255–60.

Petrusic I, Zidverc-Trajkovic J. Cortical spreading depression; origins and paths as inferred from the sequence of events during migraine aura. *Funct Neurol.* 2014;29: 207–12.

Miosis (Small Pupil)

Epidemiology and Demographics: Miosis can affect all races/ethnicities of either sex at any age.

Disorder Description: Miosis is a small pupil due to poor dilation. Abnormally small pupil due to efferent dysfunction is addressed here. Unilateral abnormally small pupils are apparent on exam as anisocoria that is greater in dark compared with light environments. When the disorder is bilateral, findings can include small pupils that do not dilate in the dark. Horner syndrome consists of ipsilateral miosis and mild ptosis due to dysfunction of the sympathetic tract. First and second order Horner syndrome can sometimes be distinguished from third order Horner syndrome by the presence of ipsilateral anhidrosis.

Symptoms

Localization site	Comment
Brainstem	Lateral medullary injury (Wallenberg syndrome) can include Horner syndrome (1st order), ataxia, ipsilateral facial numbness, contralateral body numbness, vertigo, and dysphagia
	Hypothalamic, midbrain, or pontine injury can cause Horner syndrome (1st order), typically in association with other symptoms localizing to the brainstem
Base of skull	Cavernous sinus lesions can affect the 3rd order sympathetic neurons in association with ipsilateral ocular motility deficits (CN III, IV, VI) and facial numbness (V1, V2)
Cranial nerves	Trigeminal autonomic cephalgias such as cluster headache can include Horner syndrome both during and between attacks. During attacks there is associated pain, conjunctival redness, tearing, and rhinorrhea.
	Microvascular ischemia to the sympathetic neuron can cause isolated Horner syndrome (3rd order)
Spinal cord	Cervical and upper thoracic spinal cord or disc disease or manipulation can cause Horner syndrome through injury to the 2nd or 3rd order sympathetic neurons. This can be associated with other signs of spinal cord dysfunction

Localization site	Comment
Plexus	Injury to second order sympathetic neurons associated with brachial plexus injury is associated with peripheral motor and sensory deficits of the upper extremity that localize to the brachial plexus
Mononeuropathy or mononeuropathy multiplex	The second order sympathetic neurons can be affected by lesions in the lung apex or mediastinum (e.g., pancoast tumor, neuroblastoma), and neck intervention (e.g., surgery)
	The third order sympathetic neurons can be affected by carotid injury (e.g., dissection), which is typically painful and can be associated with ocular or brain ischemia. Oral trauma can also damage the 3rd order sympathetic neurons
Muscle	Topical application of pilocarpine causes pupillary constriction through cholinergic stimulation
	Prior inflammation of the iris can cause synechiae, which mechanically limit dilation of the pupil
Unclear localization	Systemic opiate administration is associated with miosis

Secondary Complications: The miotic pupil does not typically cause symptoms. The ptosis associated with Horner syndrome is also mild and typically neither occludes the visual axis nor disrupts eyelid function.

Treatment Complications: Surgical overcorrection of ptosis, which can be performed for psychosocial reasons, can cause eyelid retraction and ocular surface dryness.

Bibliography

Reede DL, Garcon E, Smoker WR, Kardon R. Horner's syndrome: clinical and radiographic evaluation. *Neuroimaging Clin N Am.* 2008;18(2):369–85.

Mitral Regurgitation

Epidemiology and Demographics: Mitral regurgitation (MR) in patients with rheumatic fever is more commonly seen in men than in women. Significant MR has been cited in approximately 2% of the US population.

Disorder Description: The primary causes of MR include mitral valve prolapse, rheumatic fever, cardiomyopathy, infective endocarditis, mitral annular calcification, and coronary artery disease. Less common causes include trauma and exposure to certain drugs. The different causes lead to varying mechanisms of dysfunction of the mitral valve, which ultimately leads to a flow of blood in two directions: the normal direction from the left atrium to the left ventricle then through the aortic valve, and the abnormal direction from the left ventricle back into the left atrium. The mitral leaflets that present with MR may have normal motion, increased motion (prolapse), restricted leaflet opening, or restricted leaflet closure.

Symptoms

Localization site	Comment
Cerebral hemispheres	Embolic complications that occur as a result of secondary atrial fibrillation with resultant left atrial thrombi may result in cortical/subcortical infarction/microemboli
Mental status and psychiatric aspects/complications	Light-headedness, dizziness, confusion, and infrequently syncope/presyncope may result from uncontrolled atrial fibrillation with a rapid ventricular response
Brainstem	Embolic events as a result of atrial fibrillation may affect function
Cerebellum	Embolic events as a result of atrial fibrillation may affect function
Vestibular system (and nonspecific dizziness)	Embolic events as a result of atrial fibrillation may affect function
Base of skull	Embolic events as a result of atrial fibrillation may affect function

Secondary Complications: Left ventricular dysfunction, pulmonary hypertension, and atrial fibrillation may all occur as a result of MR.

Treatment Complications: Many treatments, including ACE inhibitors and mitral valve repair or replacement for some. Complications of valve replacement include death, stroke, blood loss, myocardial infarction, atrial fibrillation, and atrial flutter. Complications of the prosthetic valve include thrombosis and infective endocarditis.

Bibliography

American Heart Association. Problem: mitral valve regurgitation. Feb 18, 2013. Available from www.heart.org/HEARTORG/Conditions/More/HeartValveProblemsandDisease/Problem-Mitral-Valve-Regurgitation_UCM_450612_Article.jsp. Accessed Jun 23, 2015.

Mayo Clinic Staff. Mitral valve regurgitation. Feb 18, 2015. Available from www.mayoclinic.org/diseases-conditions/mitral-valve-regurgitation/home/ovc-20121849. Accessed Jun 23, 2015.

Otto CM, Bonow RO. Valvular heart disease. In Mann DL, Zipes DP, Libby P, Bonow RO, Braunwald E, eds. *Braunwald's heart diseases: a textbook of cardiovascular medicine.* 10th ed. Philadelphia: Elsevier/Saunders; 2015. pp. 1479–94.

Mitral Stenosis

Epidemiology and Demographics: About 66% of patients with mitral stenosis are women. The most common cause of mitral stenosis is rheumatic fever, and symptoms of mitral stenosis manifest from a few years after infection up to more than 20 years after infection. Although symptoms may develop as early as childhood, symptoms are most often seen between 45 and 65 years of age in developed countries. Severe disease is much more prevalent and is more likely to manifest in the teenage years in undeveloped countries.

Disorder Description: The most common cause of mitral stenosis is rheumatic fever that leaves scarring on the mitral valve and hence leads to valve deformity. This deformity causes obstruction of blood flow into the left ventricle, which therefore increases blood volume in the left atrium causing resultant left atrial enlargement. Progression of mitral stenosis is much more rapid in tropical and subtropical areas than in the United States and Western Europe.

Symptoms

Localization site	Comment
Cerebral hemispheres	A fixed stenotic mitral valve may result in some degree of cerebral hypoperfusion although this is typically not as significant as aortic stenosis
Mental status and psychiatric aspects/complications	When significant hypoperfusion occurs, confusion, lightheadedness, dizziness (presyncope), and rarely even syncope may occur
Brainstem	Same as above
Cerebellum	Same as above
Vestibular system (and non-specific dizziness)	Same as above
Base of skull	Same as above

Secondary Complications: Pulmonary hypertension, atrial fibrillation (related to how severely obstructed the mitral valve is), a thromboembolic event, and a predisposition for infective endocarditis all may result from mitral stenosis.

Treatment Complications: Treatments include mitral valve replacement and rarely valvuloplasty. Complications of mitral valve replacement include death, stroke, blood loss, myocardial infarction, atrial fibrillation, and atrial flutter, and complications of the prosthetic valve include thrombosis and infective endocarditis.

Bibliography

American Heart Association. Problem: mitral valve stenosis. Aug 4, 2014. Available from www.heart.org/HEARTORG/Conditions/More/HeartValveProblemsandDisease/Problem-Mitral-Valve-Stenosis_UCM_450370_Article.jsp. Accessed Jun 23, 2015.

Mayo Clinic Staff. Mitral valve stenosis. Aug 22, 2014. Available from www.mayoclinic.org/diseases-conditions/mitral-valve-stenosis/basics/definition/con-20022582. Accessed Jun 23, 2015.

Otto CM, Bonow RO. Valvular heart disease. In Mann DL, Zipes DP, Libby P, Bonow RO, Braunwald E, eds. *Braunwald's heart diseases: a textbook of cardiovascular medicine.* 10th ed. Philadelphia: Elsevier/Saunders; 2015. pp. 1469–79.

Mitral Valve Prolapse

Epidemiology and Demographics: The incidence of mitral valve prolapse (MVP) is two times greater in women than in men, although more severe symptoms are seen more often in men over the age of 50 years than in women. Overall, the incidence of MVP in the population is about 2.4%.

Disorder Description: MVP has been linked to both genetic and non-genetic causes/predispositions. MVP is genetically transmitted via an autosomal trait that has been linked to loci on several chromosomes; many of these are associated with disorders of connective tissues. Women are more likely to be found with MVP syndrome while men are more likely to be found with myxomatous disease as the cause for MVP. The result of MVP is an improper closing of the mitral valve, which is defined by an upward bulging of the mitral leaflets back into the left atrium. The majority of patients with MVP remain asymptomatic for many years with few complications.

Symptoms

Localization site	Comment
Mental status and psychiatric aspects/ complications	Typically associated with anxiety and may result in mood-related problems possibly related to transient and unpredictable palpitations and their associated arrhythmias. Occasionally associated with accessory pathways/Wolff–Parkinson–White syndrome, and atrial arrhythmias when present may result in central nervous system hypoperfusion

Secondary Complications: Common result is mitral regurgitation (see entry for *Mitral Regurgitation*).

Treatment Complications: Patients with MVP in the past may have been thought to be more prone to infective endocarditis. More recently, the American Heart Association has not recommended antibiotic prophylaxis for patients with MVP. Most patients do not require treatment but treatments include beta blockers, heart rhythm medications, and if severe, mitral valve repair or replacement. Complications of valve replacement include death, stroke, blood loss, myocardial infarction, atrial fibrillation, and atrial flutter, and complications of the prosthetic valve include thrombosis and infective endocarditis.

Bibliography

American Heart Association. Problem: mitral valve prolapse. Apr 24, 2015. Available from www.heart.org/HEARTORG/Conditions/More/HeartValveProblemsandDisease/Problem-Mitral-Valve-Prolapse_UCM_450441_Article.jsp. Accessed Jun 23, 2015.

Mayo Clinic Staff. Mitral valve prolapse. Apr 5, 2014. Available from www.mayoclinic.org/diseases-conditions/mitral-valve-prolapse/basics/definition/con-20024748. Accessed Jun 23, 2015.

Otto CM, Bonow RO. Valvular heart disease. In Mann DL, Zipes DP, Libby P, Bonow RO, Braunwald E, eds. *Braunwald's heart diseases: a textbook of cardiovascular medicine.* 10th ed. Philadelphia: Elsevier/Saunders; 2015; pp. 1494–1497.

Mollaret Meningitis

Epidemiology and Demographics: True Mollaret meningitis is exceedingly rare, and since the advent of improved tests for viral detection, more cases can be attributed to viral causes. Only a handful of idiopathic, "genuine" cases have been reported in the literature. Women are at higher risk for this complication than men.

Disorder Description: Mollaret meningitis is an idiopathic aseptic recurrent meningitis first described by Mollaret in 1944. It is now recognized that most cases are likely secondary to herpes simplex type 2 (HSV-2) infection. Women often develop the initial episode during acquisition of genital HSV-2, with subsequent recurrent episodes.

Symptoms

Localization site	Comment
Unclear localization	Characterized by recurrent attacks of sudden onset meningitis – headaches, photophobia, and mild fever – that usually last for 2–7 days, with complete recovery but unpredictable recurrences. Focal neurologic symptoms and encephalopathy do not occur. Recurrent herpes simplex virus meningitis is clinically indistinguishable from cases of idiopathic Mollaret's meningitis

Secondary Complications: This is a benign condition with full recovery between episodes, though recurrence of meningitis can be regarded as a complication.

Treatment Complications: Antiviral treatment with acyclovir is curative. Acyclovir is generally well tolerated with rare side effects, but renal, hepatic, neurologic, and hemopoietic toxicity does occur.

Bibliography

Farazmand P, Woolley PD, Kinghorn GR. Mollaret's meningitis and HSV2 infections. *Int J STD AIDS.* 2011;22(6):306–7. DOI: 10.1258/ijsa.2010.010405.

Pearce JMS. Mollaret's meningitis. *Eur Neurol.* 2008;60:316–17.

Poulikakos PJ, Sergi EE, Margaritas AS, et al. A case of recurrent benign lymphocytic (Mollaret's) meningitis and review of the literature. *J Infect Public Health.* 2010;3(4):192–5. Copyright © 2010 King Saud Bin Abdulaziz University for Health Sciences.

Steel JG, Dix RD, Baringer JR. Isolation of herpes simplex type 1 in recurrent (Mollarets) meningitis. *Trans Am Neurol Assoc.* 1981;106:37–42.

Molybdenum Cofactor Deficiency and Isolated Sulfite Oxidase Deficiency

Epidemiology and Demographics: Estimated to occur in 1/100,000–1/200,000 newborns worldwide, although this may be an underestimate as many cases are thought to be underdiagnosed. No known racial or ethnic predilection.

Disorder Description: Molybdenum cofactor deficiency (MoCD) is a severe neonatal metabolic disorder of purine and pyrimidine metabolism, characterized by rapidly progressive neurologic damage. The genetic defects of MOCS1, MOCS2, or GPHN genes are autosomal recessive in nature. They are associated with the biosynthesis of the molybdenum cofactor, essential for the function of four enzymes – sulphite oxidase (SUOX), xanthine dehydrogenase (XDH), aldehyde oxidase, and mitochondrial amidoxime reducing component (mARC). These molybdenum-dependent enzymes are essential for xanthine and sulfite (from methionine and homocysteine) metabolism. Since isolated sulfite oxidase deficiency and MoCD have virtually identical phenotypes, the central nervous system (CNS) toxicity appears to be secondary to loss of function of sulfite oxidase.

The resultant loss of enzyme function leads to toxic accumulation of sulphite, S-sulfocysteine, xanthine, and hypoxanthine. Biochemical abnormalities include decreased serum uric acid and increased urine sulfite levels due to the combined enzymatic deficiency of XDH and SUOX. Deficiency of SUOX leads to the substitution of sulfite metabolites instead of cysteine in connective tissues, such as the lens, leading to lens dislocation. The pathogenesis of CNS effects is unknown, but may be related to sulfite accumulation or lack of sulfite in the CNS.

Pregnancy and delivery are typically normal, although there are some reports of depressed APGAR scores. Enzyme deficiency typically results in early onset in infancy of poor feeding, intractable seizures, and encephalopathy. Opisthotonus may be present. The condition is usually fatal by early childhood. In milder cases, onset is later (~15 months of age) and more likely to have mild or no developmental delays or in some cases present with tone or movement abnormalities. Physical examination may reveal narrow bifrontal diameter and deep-set eyes. Examination of eyes shows dislocated lens and lack of light response.

Diagnosis is made via quantitative plasma and urine amino acids, looking specifically for cysteine metabolite S-sulfocysteine. Plasma uric acid levels are decreased in MoCD but can be normal in isolated sulfite oxidase deficiency.

Symptoms

Localization site	Comment
Cerebral hemispheres	Epilepsy
	Feeding difficulties, hypotonia
	Imaging of sulfite oxidase deficiency – multiple cystic lesions in basal ganglia and cerebellum with ventriculomegaly, neuronal loss, and decreased white matter density
Cerebellar and basal ganglia	Movement disorder, opisthotonic posturing (similar picture to severe hypoxic ischemic encephalopathy)
Cranial nerves	Eyes – ectopia lentis

Secondary Complications: Nephrolithiasis.

Treatment: A number of case reports have described treatment with Precursor Z (cyclic pyranopterin monophosphate), which may lead to an improvement in psychomotor development and IQ, and improved seizure control. High-dose thiamine and betaine have also been trialled. Genetic therapy with a *MOCS1* expression cassette being carried by AAV vectors is now being studied as a future treatment.

Bibliography

Bindu PS. Encephalopathy due to sulfite oxidase deficiency. Orphanet rare diseases portal. Updated Jan 2012. Available from www.orpha.net/consor/cgi-bin/OC_Exp.php?Expert=833. Accessed Aug 28, 2018.

Veldman A, Santamaria-Araujo JA, Sollazzo S, et al. Successful treatment of molybdenum cofactor deficiency type A with cPMP. *Pediatrics.* 2010;125(5):e1249–54. DOI: 10.1542/peds.2009–2192. Epub Apr 12, 2010.

Monoclonal Gammopathy of Uncertain Significance (MGUS)

Epidemiology and Demographics: Monoclonal gammopathy of uncertain significance (MGUS) is a frequent finding in older adults, occurring in 3% of the population above 50 and in as many as 8% over age 80 years.

Disorder Description: Monoclonal gammopathy refers to an immunoglobulin present in serum produced by a clonal population of lymphoplasmacytic cells. In MGUS, the monoclonal immunoglobulin is detectable in serum at a concentration less than 3 g/dL but does not cause bone lesions, anemia, hypercalcemia, renal insufficiency, or hyperviscosity. The immunoglobulin can be IgG (most common), IgM, or light chain. Although technically asymptomatic ("unclear significance"), MGUS has been associated with peripheral neuropathies.

Symptoms

Localization site	Comment
Peripheral neuropathy	Patients with IgG MGUS (most common) can develop either a chronic demyelinating neuropathy indistinguishable from chronic inflammatory demyelinating polyneuropathy or a predominantly sensory axonal neuropathy.[1] Those with IgM MGUS typically have a chronic progressive, symmetric, demyelinating, distal sensorimotor neuropathy.[2] Some with IgM MGUS harbor anti-MAG IgM antibodies and have a characteristic clinical syndrome of distal predominantly sensory loss in legs, gait ataxia, and postural tremor in arms

Secondary Complications: MGUS can progress to overt multiple myeloma and should be monitored for routinely.

Treatment Complications: Immunomodulatory or antibody-depleting therapy (such as rituximab) is often used for progressive cases, which can significantly increase risk of infections in older adults with other comorbidities.

References

1. Di Troia A, Carpo M, Meucci N, et al. Clinical features and anti-neural reactivity in neuropathy associated with IgG monoclonal gammopathy of undetermined significance. *J Neurol Sci.* 1999;164:64–71.
2. Nobile-Orazio E, Manfredini E, Carpo M, et al. Frequency and clinical correlates of anti-neural IgM antibodies in neuropathy associated with IgM monoclonal gammopathy. *Ann Neurol.* 1994;36:416–24.

Movement Disorders and Pregnancy

Epidemiology and Demographics: Common movement disorders in pregnancy include restless leg syndrome (RLS), dystonia, tremor, ataxia, and chorea gravidarum.

The prevalence of RLS is 10–26% in pregnancy, significantly higher than in the general population (2.5–15%). More than half of pregnant women with existing RLS report worsening of symptoms.

Dystonia is not induced by pregnancy, but given its bimodal age of onset, many women are diagnosed in their reproductive years (mean age at diagnosis is 27) and undergo pregnancy with dystonia. Dystonia can either worsen or improve during pregnancy, but the majority remains unchanged.

With the decline in rheumatic fever, chorea gravidarum has become much rarer. In 1968 the incidence of chorea gravidarum was reported to be <0.001%. Lack of recent studies limits the accurate estimation of today's disease prevalence.

Pregnancy in patients with Parkinson's disease (PD) is rare; about 400 women under age 50 are diagnosed with PD each year. Huntington disease (HD) also occurs later in life, in the 5th to 6th decade, except for the Westphal variant or juvenile onset HD, which makes up about 10% of all HD patients.

Onset may be any time during pregnancy and even puerperium. RLS is more common in the third trimester.

Disorder Description: Movement disorders result from a misbalance of dopamine in the basal ganglia, which is comprised of the caudate, putamen, globus pallidus, subthalamic nucleus, thalamus, and substantia nigra. Loss of inhibition of the indirect circuitry, which helps prevent unwanted muscle contractions, results in hyperkinetic movements, such as in chorea; loss of inhibition of the direct pathway, on the other hand, causes bradykinesia and parkinsonian signs. The pathophysiology of RLS is poorly understood.

Several of the movement disorders are inheritable, including the autosomal dominant form of RLS and certain types of dystonia (DYT gene). Wilson disease should be considered in young persons who develop movement disorders due to copper deposition in the basal ganglia. Rheumatic fever and other rheumatologic diseases such as antiphospholipid syndrome and lupus predispose to chorea gravidarum. Hyperemesis gravidarum can lead to ataxia by B1 deficiency or dystonia by treatment with neuroleptics. In addition to neuroleptics, antiepileptics, sympathomimetics, and even antihistamines can induce dystonia, chorea, or tremor.

Symptoms

Localization site	Comment
Basal ganglia	Restless leg syndrome: • An irresistible urge to move the legs in order to relieve discomfort, particularly in the evenings and during inactivity. The discomfort is transiently relieved by movement • Periodic limb movements of sleep are commonly present Dystonia: • Characterized by involuntary muscle contractions that result in abnormal posturing and can be painful • Symptoms tend to fluctuate. For example, there is a diurnal nature to dopa-responsive dystonia. Other dystonias may be triggered by certain positions • Tremors, called dystonic tremors, may overlay the dystonia • A "sensory trick" is a touch maneuver that reduces or aborts the dystonia Chorea gravidarum: • Random, "dance-like" irregular movements of the limbs and face. The movements are constant and therefore patients are unable to hold still in a certain position • Movements can appear semi-purposeful as they are incorporated into goal-directed movements, such as combing one's hair or reaching for objects • Disappears during sleep

Secondary Complications: In Wilson disease and Huntington disease, psychiatric symptoms are quite prominent. Irritability, depression, and personality change are the most common psychiatric manifestations and may precede the onset of movement dysfunction by many years. Sometimes patients are incorrectly diagnosed with psychiatric disorders before the correct diagnosis is made.

Treatment Complications: Iron replacement therapy is effective in iron-deficient RLS patients, in addition to standard treatment with dopamine agonists like pramipexole and ropinirole. However, dopamine agonists have been associated with fetal malformations in animal models. Levodopa, on the other hand, while more prone to augmentation than dopamine agonists, is generally safer in pregnancy and is the drug of choice compared with dopamine agonists. Levodopa is also used with good response in dopa-responsive dystonia. Trihexyphenidyl, an anticholinergic drug, and tetrabenazine, with both monoaminergic and dopamine antagonistic properties, are alternative treatment options for generalized dystonia, while botulinum toxin B (FDA category C) has been reported to be efficacious and safe in focal dystonia. However, these medications have limited safety data during pregnancy, so they should be used with caution.

In all pregnancy-induced movement disorders, symptoms typically resolve after delivery. Therefore prolonged treatment is often unnecessary.

Many dopaminergic agents are FDA category C drugs and are not recommended during breastfeeding; despite some data reporting minimal adverse effects in humans, they should still be used with caution during pregnancy. Fetal complications like intrauterine growth retardation, digit malformation, and even death have been demonstrated in animals. Since treatment is purely symptomatic, discussion with the patient regarding risks and benefits is essential.

Bibliography

Grover A, Clark-Bilodeau C, D'Ambrosio CM. Restless leg syndrome in pregnancy. *Obstet Med.* 2015;8(3):121–5.

Kranick SM, Mowry EM, Colcher A, Horn S, Golbe LI. Movement disorders and pregnancy: a review of the literature. *Mov Disord.* 2010;25(6): 665–71.

Manconi M, Govoni V, De Vito A, et al. Pregnancy as a risk factor for restless legs syndrome. *Sleep Med.* 2004;5(3):305–8.

Pathania M, Upadhayaya S, Lali BS, Sharma A. Chorea gravidarum: a rarity in West still haunts pregnant women in the East. *BMJ Case Rep.* 2013; pii: bcr2012008096. DOI: 10.1136/bcr-2012-008096.

Robottom BJ, Reich SG. Exposure to high dosage trihexyphenidyl during pregnancy for treatment of generalized dystonia: case report and literature review. *Neurologist.* 2011;17(6):340–1.

Moyamoya

Epidemiology and Demographics: Most prevalent in Japan, Korea, China, Taiwan, India, and other Asian countries, moyamoya disease has been reported in various races and countries including the United States, Greece, and Turkey. It is the most common pediatric cerebrovascular disease in Japan, with a prevalence of approximately 3 in 100,000 and girls twice as commonly affected as boys. Incidence in Europe is about one-tenth that in Japan and the incidence in the United States is 0.086 in 100,000. A 10–15% familial occurrence in Japanese and other Asian populations indicates genetic susceptibility. Nearly 18% of patients can be asymptomatic, with an annual stroke risk of 3%.

Disorder Description: "Moyamoya disease" is an idiopathic nonatherosclerotic and noninflammatory condition with progressive stenosis of the bilateral (sometimes unilateral) terminal internal carotid artery and the proximal portions of the anterior cerebral and middle cerebral arteries with prominent collateral arterial circulation. Moyamoya means "puffy"; it describes the angiographic appearance of the collateral circulation.

"Moyamoya phenomenon" is used to describe the similar angiographic finding but in the presence of conditions such as hematologic abnormalities (sickle cell, lupus anticoagulant, factor V Leiden), atherosclerosis, vasoconstrictive drugs (cocaine), cranial irradiation, Grave's disease, infections (HIV, chronic meningitis, leptospirosis), tumors (craniopharyngioma, neurofibromatosis, optic glioma), and syndromes (Down, Alagille, Costello).

The clinical manifestations of moyamoya are variable and include transient ischemic attack (TIA), ischemic stroke (more common in children), hemorrhagic stroke (more common in adults), and epilepsy.

Symptoms

Localization site	Comment
Cerebral hemispheres	Transient ischemic attacks occur in approximately 40% and ischemic stroke in approximately 30%
	TIAs are usually motor related and usually remain unilateral, but may switch sides. Symptomatic episodes of ischemia may be triggered by exercise, crying, coughing, straining, fever, hyperventilation, or playing wind instruments
	Hemorrhagic symptoms (typically an altered level of consciousness) predominate in older patients, with a frequency of approximately 60%. Re-bleeds are common
	Seizures, either focal (motor, sensory) or generalized (secondary to stroke, ischemic or hemorrhagic) can occur. Seizures may be a manifestation of cerebral ischemia in 25% of pediatric cases
	Cerebral hypoperfusion rarely causes movement disorders such as hemidystonia, hemichoreoathetosis, paroxysmal exercise-induced dyskinesia, and "limb-shaking TIAs"
Mental status	Patients could present with intellectual dysfunction ranging from mental slowness to profound retardation from underlying strokes. In adults, executive functioning appears to be more impaired than memory and perception; however, their overall level of cognitive dysfunction is less severe than in children

Secondary Complications: Younger patients tend to have ischemic events while older patients can have hemorrhagic stroke. Re-bleeding is reported at a rate of 33 to 61%. It would be a challenge to medically manage a patient who has ischemic and hemorrhagic events (recurrent or concurrent). In addition to the collaterals, arterial aneurysms and pseudoaneurysms can occur.

Treatment Complications: For acute stroke, symptomatic treatment aims at reducing elevated intracranial pressure, improving cerebral blood flow, and controlling seizures. In cases with hemorrhagic stroke, ventricular drainage and/or hematoma, removal is often required. During hospitalization, it is important to control pain and avoid hypotension, hypocarbia, hyperthermia, and hypovolemia.

For secondary prevention of stroke, antiplatelet agents are preferred rather than warfarin unless there is coexisting hematologic disease. The risk of hemorrhage is higher with warfarin.

Surgical revascularization, either direct (superficial temporal or middle meningeal artery to middle cerebral artery) or indirect (multiple techniques), may be indicated in symptomatic or asymptomatic patients with poor vascular reserve or inadequate perfusion.

Bibliography

Singhal AB. *Moyamoya disease*. Medlink Neurology. Updated Dec 1, 2015. San Diego: MedLink Corporation. Available from www.medlink.com.

Mucormycosis, Cerebral

Epidemiology and Demographics: This is a rare disease with unclear epidemiology, owing to the need for biopsy or autopsy for a confirmation of the diagnosis.

Disorder Description: Invasive mucormycosis is an infection with *Mucorales* species and, based on location, can be rhinocerebral, pulmonary, cutaneous, gastrointestinal, disseminated, or unusual, such as endocarditis. In this entry, cerebral mucormycosis is discussed. As it usually spreads from nasal passages and involves the orbit, the term rhino-orbito-cerebral mucormycosis (ROCM) is also employed.

Cerebral mucormycosis has almost exclusively been described in diabetics and immunocompromised patients. Open head injury and intravenous drug use may predispose to direct cerebral infection.

Symptoms: ROCM develops after inhalation of fungal spores into the paranasal sinuses. The invading fungus spreads to invade the palate, paranasal and cavernous sinuses, orbit, and brain. The initial symptoms are of sinusitis and periorbital cellulitis. With the spread of infection, multiple cranial nerve palsies, orbital inflammation, eyelid edema, proptosis, headache, and acute vision loss may develop.

Localization site	Comment
Cerebral hemispheres	Abscess formation, watershed infarcts/ischemia from large vessel occlusion, venous infarcts from venous sinus thrombosis

Localization site	Comment
Mental status and psychiatric aspects/complications	Drowsiness from brainstem involvement and raised intracranial pressure, which can be secondary to mass effect of abscess or hydrocephalus
Brainstem	Diffuse involvement may occur with cranial nerve palsies and declining consciousness
Cerebellum	Abscess formation and direct infection may extend to cerebellum and cause ataxia, nystagmus, and secondary hydrocephalus. Tonsillar herniation can lead to death
Vestibular system (and nonspecific dizziness)	May be involved
Base of skull	May be involved
Cranial nerves	Involved by brainstem infection or cavernous sinus thrombosis
Pituitary gland	May be involved

Secondary Complications: The aggressive spread of infection necessitates early and aggressive surgical debridement. This is a key part of management but frequently involves disfiguring facial surgery.

Intracranial abscesses may need drainage, and secondary hydrocephalus will need shunting. Mucormycosis can spread to the lungs, and angioinvasion may also lead to disseminated infection, which has a fatality rate of 98%.

Treatment Complications: Repeated debridement and aggressive surgery are needed, leading to disfigurement. Antifungal treatment with IV amphotericin/micafungin/posaconazole is needed for several months, and is associated with hypersensitivity, electrolyte abnormalities, nephrotoxic potential, blood dyscrasias, and other side effects.

Bibliography

Centers for Disease Control and Prevention. Mucormycosis. Available from www.cdc.gov/fungal/diseases/mucormycosis/index.html. Accessed Aug 28, 2018.

Gonzalez CE, Rinaldi MG, Sugar AM. Mucormycosis. *Infect Dis Clin North Am*. 2002;16:895–914.

Petrikkos G, Skiadda A, Lortholary O, et al. Epidemiology and clinical manifestations of mucormycosis. *Clin Infect Dis.* 2012;4(suppl_1):S23–S34.

Spellberg B, Edwards J Jr, Ibrahim A. Novel perspectives on mucormycosis: pathophysiology, presentation, and management. *Clin Microbiol Rev.* 2005;18(3):556–69.

Multifocal Demyelinating Chronic Inflammatory Demyelinating Polyneuropathy (CIDP) (Multifocal Acquired Demyelinating Sensory and Motor Neuropathy, MADSAM), Lewis–Sumner Syndrome, Motor and Sensory Demyelinating Mononeuropathy Multiplex, Multifocal Motor and Sensory Demyelinating Neuropathy, Multifocal Inflammatory Demyelinating Neuropathy

Epidemiology and Demographics: Mean age in the early to mid-50s, but can range from 18 years to elderly.

Disorder Description: Asymmetric sensorimotor demyelinating polyneuropathy, usually in the distribution of discrete nerves, clinically resembles mononeuropathy multiplex. Arms are usually involved before legs. Patient may have relapsing or progressive course. As with chronic inflammatory demyelinating polyneuropathy (CIDP), the disorder is responsive to steroids or intravenous immunoglobulin (IVIG).

Symptoms

Localization site	Comment
Mononeuropathy or mononeuropathy multiplex	Asymmetric sensorimotor demyelinating polyneuropathy, usually in the distribution of discrete nerves, mostly in the upper extremities

Secondary Complications: Trouble with mobility and activities of daily living.

Treatment Complications: Although rare, IVIG can have risk of hypercoagulability causing stroke, pulmonary emboli, and deep vein thrombosis. Can have side effects from steroid.

Bibliography

Katirji B, Kaminski HJ, Ruff RL. *Neuromuscular disorders in clinical practice.* 2nd ed. New York: Springer-Verlag New York; 2014.

Multifocal Motor Neuropathy; Also Called Multifocal Motor Neuropathy with Conduction Block

Epidemiology and Demographics: The prevalence is about 0.6 to 2 per 100,000. Men are affected more than women (2.7:1). Onset is usually between 20 and 50 years old with mean onset between 30 and 40 years old.

Disorder Description: Slow progressive asymmetric multifocal weakness and atrophy without sensory abnormalities. Most classic presentation is a man with slowly progressive asymmetric hand weakness out of proportion to the degree of atrophy over several months to years. Wrist drop and hand weakness are common initial symptoms. May develop fasciculations or cramps. Muscle atrophy occurs late in the disease. Reflexes are variable. Anti-GM1 antibody is present in 30–80% of the patients.

Symptoms

Localization site	Comment
Mononeuropathy or mononeuropathy multiplex	Asymmetric. Multifocal motor mononeuropathy. Electrodiagnostic evidence shows persistent, multifocal, conduction blocks in motor nerves outside common entrapment sites

Secondary Complications: Trouble with mobility and activities of daily living.

Treatment Complications: Although rare, intravenous immunoglobulin has a risk of hypercoagulability causing stroke, pulmonary emboli, and deep vein thrombosis. Steroid and plasma exchange are ineffective.

Bibliography

Katirji B, Kaminski HJ, Ruff RL. *Neuromuscular disorders in clinical practice.* 2nd ed. New York: Springer-Verlag New York; 2014.

Multi-infarct Dementia

Epidemiology and Demographics: Multi-infarct dementia or vascular dementia (VaD) is the second most common form of dementia after Alzheimer's disease (AD) in most clinical series, and it makes up 10 to 20% of cases in North America and Europe. The relative preponderance of the two diseases may be reversed in countries such as Japan and China. Prevalence is estimated at 6 to 12 cases per 1000 person-years over the age of 70 years. The metabolic syndrome, a cluster of cardiovascular risk factors that include obesity, hypertension, insulin resistance, and dyslipidemia, is associated with incident vascular dementia to varying degrees.

Disorder Description: Multi-infarct dementia is best understood as a heterogeneous syndrome rather than a distinct disorder, in which the underlying cause is cerebrovascular disease in some form and its ultimate manifestation is dementia. Post stroke dementia can occur after multiple "silent" strokes, in association with cerebral amyloid angiopathy or cerebral autosomal dominant arteriopathy (CADASIL). Clinical features of multi-infarct dementia can be cortical (aphasia, agnosia, apathy, abulia, apraxia, executive dysfunction, or amnesia, etc.) or subcortical (slowed response times, focal motor signs, gait disturbance, bladder urgency, pseudobulbar palsy, memory deficits, etc.).

Symptoms

Localization site	Comment
Cerebral hemispheres	Cortical syndrome – this could occur secondary to an embolic phenomenon. In primarily cortical VaD, cognitive features are specific to the areas affected: - Medial frontal: executive dysfunction, abulia, or apathy. Bilateral medial frontal lobe infarction may cause akinetic mutism - Left parietal: aphasia, apraxia, or agnosia - Right parietal: hemineglect (anosognosia, asomatognosia), confusion, agitation, visuospatial and constructional difficulty - Medial temporal: anterograde amnesia Subcortical syndrome – in subcortical pathology, both lacunar infarcts and chronic ischemia affect the deep cerebral nuclei and white matter pathways. These often disrupt frontal lobe and other cortico-cortico circuits, producing deficits attributable to remote brain areas Characteristic features include focal motor signs, early presence of gait disturbance (marche à petit pas or magnetic, apraxic gait, or parkinsonian gait), history of unsteadiness and frequent, unprovoked falls, early urinary frequency, urgency, and other urinary symptoms not explained by urologic disease, pseudobulbar palsy, personality and mood changes, abulia, apathy, depression, emotional incontinence, cognitive disorder characterized by relatively mild memory deficit, psychomotor retardation, and abnormal executive function
Mental status and psychiatric aspects/complications	There may be coexistent depression. Also, frank psychosis, agitation, wandering behavior, mood issues may be seen during the course of dementia

Secondary Complications: Multi-infarct dementia shortens life expectancy to about 50% of normal at 4 years from initial evaluation, but females, those with higher education, and those who perform well on some neuropsychologic tests do better. Depression is common in multi-infarct dementia and can occur in 20% of the patients. Coexistent Alzheimer's dementia can give rise to a "mixed dementia" pattern.

Treatment Complications: Treatment of hypertension is important but hypotension may accelerate the dementia. Memantine, galantamine, and donepezil have modest benefits. Addition of an antiplatelet agent provides no further benefit. Measures of general application to dementia of all kinds are also appropriate, including referral to community services and local support groups, consideration of caregiver stress, and legal and ethical issues such as driving, competency, and advance directives.

Bibliography

Hachinski V. Optimizing the Hachinski Ischemic Scale. *Arch Neurol.* 2012;69:169–75.

Multiple Myeloma

Epidemiology and Demographics: Multiple myeloma is a relatively rare cancer with a lifetime risk of 0.7%. Median survival from diagnosis of central nervous system involvement is from 6 weeks to 5 months. It accounts for 0.9% of all cancer deaths.

Disorder Description: Multiple myeloma is a neoplasm in which there is proliferation of a single clone of plasma cells. Myeloma cells can affect the nervous system by direct infiltration, immunologic dysfunction, and due to metabolic derangements.

Symptoms

Localization site	Comment
Cerebral hemispheres	Hemiparesis, seizures (plasmacytoma), stroke (due to hyperviscosity syndrome)
Mental status and psychiatric aspects/complications	Confusion and coma (direct parenchymal involvement vs myelomatous meningitis)
Base of skull	Nonspecific pain with lytic bone lesions
Cranial nerves	Diplopia (III, VI), visual field deficits (II), and facial weakness (VII) due to leptomeningeal involvement or lytic lesions of foramina and sphenoid/petrous bones

Localization site	Comment
Pituitary gland	Hypopituitarism due to sella invasion
Spinal cord	Epidural spinal cord compression: pain; paraplegia/monoplegia and sensory disturbances depending on the level involved (most commonly thoracic level)
Peripheral neuropathy	Sensory loss of lower limbs (symmetric, mixed sensorimotor neuropathy) Osteosclerotic myeloma: gradual, motor, demyelinating neuropathy of upper limbs
Unclear localization	Numb chin syndrome: numbness of chin, lower lip, lower teeth, and buccal gingiva (can be seen in other head and neck cancers)

Secondary Complications

Uremic encephalopathy: delirium, myoclonus, and seizures.

Hypercalcemia: fatigue, confusion, muscle weakness, asterixis, and myalgia.

Amyloidosis: causes peripheral neuropathy, which is both an autonomic and distal axonal sensorimotor neuropathy.

Treatment Complications: Bortezomib can cause blood pressure fluctuations, rash, and peripheral neuropathy. Melphalan can cause bleeding diathesis, flu-like symptoms, rash, nausea, and vomiting.

Bibliography

Denier C, Lozeron P, Adams D, et al. Multifocal neuropathy due to plasma cell infiltration of peripheral nerves in multiple myeloma. *Neurology.* 2006;66(6):917–8.

Dispenzieri A, Kyle RA. Neurological aspects of multiple myeloma and related disorders. *Best Pract Res Clin Haematol.* 2005;18(4):673–88.

Schluterman KO, Fassas AB, Van Hemert RL, Harik SI. Multiple myeloma invasion of the central nervous system. *Arch Neurol.* 2004;61(9):1423–9.

Multiple Sclerosis (MS)

Epidemiology and Demographics: Incidence is 2–3 times higher in women. In children, incidence is only 0.3 to

0.4% of all cases. Risk of developing symptoms peaks at age 30 and drastically decreases by age 60. It is most prevalent (30–80 per 100,000) in Canada, northern United States, and northern Europe. It is least prevalent in areas near the equator (1 per 100,000). Fifteen percent to 20% of MS patients have an affected relative.

Disorder Description: An autoimmune demyelinating disease resulting in impairment of saltatory conduction. It is thought that a viral or an infectious process may activate the disease in patients who have a genetic predisposition. Demyelinated nerve fibers are highly sensitive to conduction and increased heat or exercise can bring about symptoms. Patients may have an insidious slow progressive course of disease (primary progressive multiple sclerosis) with occasional plateaus, or more commonly, relapsing and remitting with symptom onset occurring over hours or days (relapsing–remitting multiple sclerosis). Secondary progressive multiple sclerosis starts off as relapsing–remitting type, followed by progressive worsening of disease with or without relapses. MS commonly presents as tingling in one limb, band-like sensation in the trunk likely due to involvement of the posterior column of the spinal cord, weakness, diplopia, ataxia, optic neuritis, dysarthria, facial pain/numbness, or vertigo. Treatment is with disease-modifying agents such as natalizumab, cyclophosphamide, glucocorticoids, azathioprine, dalfampridine, or cladribine.

Symptoms

Localization site	Comment
Cerebral hemispheres	Numbness, weakness, hyperreflexia
Mental status and psychiatric aspects/complications	Fatigue, slowing of mental processing, lack of motivation
Brainstem	Diplopia, dysarthria, vertigo
Cerebellum	Ataxia
Cranial nerves	Optic neuritis, blurry vision, loss of vision, vertigo, diplopia, dysarthria, afferent pupillary defect
Spinal cord	Sensory disturbances, weakness, hyperreflexia, bladder dysfunction
Dorsal root ganglion	Sensory disturbances

Secondary Complications: Weakness, difficulty walking, and difficulty swallowing can lead to severe disability and recurrent infections.

Treatment Complications: Steroid therapy can lead to psychosis, confusion, weight gain, hyperglycemia, myopathy, glaucoma, cataracts, osteoporosis, or vertebral fractures.

Natalizumab infusion can lead to JC virus activation and subsequent progressive multifocal leukoencephalopathy.

Bibliography

Ropper AH, Samuels MA, Klein JP. Multiple sclerosis and other inflammatory demyelinating diseases. In *Adams & Victor's principles of neurology*, 10th ed. New York, NY: McGraw-Hill; 2014. Chapter 36.

Multiple Sclerosis in Pregnancy

Epidemiology and Demographics: Overall incidence rates of multiple sclerosis (MS) are 3.6 cases per 100,000 person-years (95% CI 3.0, 4.2) in women and 2.0 (95% CI 1.5, 2.4) in men, nearly twice as frequent in onset in women compared with men. The incidence of the disease increases as one travels further north or south from the equator. If exposure to a higher risk environment occurs during adolescence (before 15 years of age), migrating to a lower risk latitude does not mitigate the MS risk.

The age of onset peaks between 20 and 30 years. Almost 70% of patients manifest symptoms between ages 21 and 40 with rare onset prior to 10 or after 60 years of age.

Latitude at early life and genetic factors both play a role in the occurrence of MS. The incidence of MS in first-degree relatives is 20 times higher than in the general population. Monozygotic twin studies show a concordance rate of 30%, while dizygotic twins show a concordance rate of less than 5%.

Disorder Description: The most established effect of pregnancy on the course of MS is a reduction in relapse rates in the last trimester by 70–80%. This is likely due to the immunotolerant state of pregnancy in general. However, disease activity often reappears aggressively in the first few months after delivery, temporarily overshooting pre-pregnancy levels. The most helpful and accurate counseling is to inform patients that pregnancy has no negative effect on long-term MS prognosis.

Multiple sclerosis is a chronic autoimmune, inflammatory neurologic disease of the central nervous system (CNS). The inflammatory target is myelinated axons in the CNS; MS destroys the myelin and the axons, and therefore specifically is active in the white matter of the brain, and myelinated tracts in the brainstem, cerebellar connections, and spinal cord.

The course of MS is highly varied and unpredictable. In 85% of patients, the disease is characterized initially by episodes of reversible neurologic deficits, called relapsing–remitting MS. Secondary progressive MS may develop in some patients with relapsing–remitting disease. Treatment with disease-modifying agents helps delay progression to this form of MS in which the course continues to worsen with or without periods of remission or plateaus. Other more severe and treatment-resistant forms include primary progressive MS and progressive-relapsing MS.

The diagnosis is determined by evidence of: (1) at least two different lesions (plaques or scars) in the white matter of the CNS (the space dissemination criterion); (2) at least two different episodes in the disease course (the time dissemination criterion); and (3) chronic inflammation of the CNS, as determined by analysis of the CSF (the inflammatory criterion).

Symptoms

Localization site	Comment
Optic nerve	Partial loss of vision and pain in one eye
Medial longitudinal fasciculus injury (MLF), which connects the sixth cranial nerve (CN VI) nucleus on one side of the pons to the medial rectus subnucleus of the third cranial nerve (CN III) in the contralateral midbrain	Internuclear ophthalmoplegia
White matter of brain and/or spinal cord	Limb weakness Spasticity Sensory disturbance: numbness and paresthesias, pain Fatigue
Spinal cord	Difficulty with bladder and/or bowel control, sexual dysfunction

Localization site	Comment
Cervical spinal cord	Lhermitte sign, an electric shock-like pain that radiates down the spine or into the legs when the neck is flexed
Cerebellum	Ataxia, nystagmus, "scanning speech" (slow, hesitant speech)
Widespread white matter of brain	Cognitive difficulties

Secondary Complications: Secondary complications include urinary tract infections, pneumonias, osteoporosis pressure sores, and depression.

Treatment Complications: None of the oral disease-modifying therapies (DMTs) is recommended for use while pregnant or breast-feeding, and most women discontinue these medications prior to pregnancy. However, based on individualized decision-making, women with MS may continue glatiramer acetate (GA) or interferon beta when they feel this is their best option, with little evidence thus far of increased risk of major malformations. No DMTs are recommended during breast-feeding. For acute exacerbations of MS during pregnancy, methylprednisolone appears to have little effect on fetal development. Because methylprednisolone is metabolized before crossing the placenta it should be used instead of dexamethasone.

Bibliography

Alonso A, Hernán MA. Temporal trends in the incidence of multiple sclerosis: A systematic review. *Neurology.* 2008;71(2):129–35.

Alroughani A, Altintas A, Jumah MA, et al. Pregnancy and the use of disease-modifying therapies in patients with multiple sclerosis: benefits versus risks. *Mult Scler Int.* 2016;2016:1034912.

Coyle PK. Management of women with multiple sclerosis through pregnancy and after childbirth. *Ther Adv Neurol Disord.* 2016(3):198–210.

Multiple System Atrophy (MSA; Shy–Drager Syndrome)

Epidemiology and Demographics: The age-adjusted prevalence of all forms of multiple system atrophy (MSA) is estimated as up to 4.4 per 100,000. MSA is more common in men, with symptoms typically beginning in the 6th decade. Smoking tobacco is significantly less frequent in MSA. Farming is an independent risk factor for MSA. While 97% of patients with MSA develop autonomic dysfunction, the early diagnosis of MSA was previously unclear because diagnosis of clinically significant dysfunction of the autonomic nervous system without peripheral nerve lesions had not been fully characterized. More recent evaluation of how MSA is diagnosed revealed that formal autonomic testing was done in 38% of patients (cardiovascular function tests in 32%, urodynamics tests in 14%, respiratory tests in 9%, and sudomotor function tests in 8% of patients).[1]

Disorder Description: MSA was first identified in 1960 by Drs. Shy and Drager when they described the condition as having orthostatic syncope, impotence, and urinary dysfunction with later development of the parkinsonian symptoms of gait disturbance, dysarthria, constipation, and bowel and bladder incontinence. In contrast to the ganglionic and postganglionic autonomic nerve dysfunction found in Parkinson's disease (PD), the dysautonomia in MSA is central and/or preganglionic. The central dysautonomia may be responsible for MSA cases of supine hypertension, global anhidrosis, respiratory insufficiency, and the "cold hands" sign (cold, dusky, violacious appearance of the hands). Using more recent diagnostic criteria for dystonia, nearly half of patients with MSA will develop dystonia, particularly anterocollis, potentially leading to secondary fibrotic and myopathic changes, unrelated to dopaminergic therapy. In addition, patients with MSA frequently manifest cerebellar and pyramidal signs. Rarely, patients have fasciculations and iris atrophy. The most common patient presentations of MSA are impotence among males and urinary incontinence among females. Other common signs and symptoms of dysautonomia in early MSA include orthostatic hypotension, arrhythmias, constipation, dysphagia, gastroesophageal reflux, seborrheic dermatitis, blepharitis, hyperhidrosis, sialorrhea, and dyspnea. A Unified Multiple System Atrophy Rating Scale (UMSARS) has been developed and validated to assess the severity of illness.

Shy–Drager syndrome or multi-system atrophy (MSA) is a sporadic neurodegenerative disorder with oligodendroglial alpha-synuclein inclusion as its main neuropathologic feature. MSA has a prodromal premotor phase, with clinical manifestations including sexual dysfunction, urinary urge incontinence, urinary retention, orthostasis, respiratory difficulties including inspiratory stridor, and REM behavior abnormalities. The premotor symptoms may precede the main motor symptoms by years. MSA clinical manifestations include autonomic failure and either poorly levodopa-responsive parkinsonism (MSA-P) due to striatal degeneration or cerebellar ataxia (MSA-C) or both. It is important to note that up to 40% of the patients may respond to levodopa in the early phase of the disease. The cerebellar symptoms include wide-based gait, uncoordinated limb movement, action tremor, and positional nystagmus. The disease course is quite aggressive, leading to death within 8 years of onset.

Symptoms

Localization site	Comment
Caudate/putamen/globus pallidus/ substantia nigra pars compacta/ motor cortex	Striatal neurodegeneration and parkinsonism including bradykinisia and akinetic rigidity and tremor
Autonomic nervous system	Postural instability and orthostasis, erectile dysfunction in men, increased urinary frequency, urgency, and incontinence
Locus coeruleus & mesopontine neurons	REM sleep abnormality
Dentate gyrus of the hippocampus	Amnestic symptoms
Cerebellum	Mainly in the MSA-C type, leading to ataxia, dysarthria, limb ataxia, and cerebellar oculomotor dysfunction
Neurovascular involvement	Raynaud's phenomena

Secondary Complications: Secondary radiculopathy, high fall risk, urgent gastrointestinal conditions, muscle pain.

Respiratory difficulties including inspiratory stridor can develop in approximately 30% of the patients. Some of these patients might respond well to continuous positive airway pressure.

Treatment Complications: The management is mainly symptom based, and the parkinsonism symptoms are unfortunately poorly responsive to levodopa therapy. Physical therapy could potentially be useful for fall prevention. Measures such as adequate fluid intake, high-salt diet, and frequent smaller meals, as well as compression stockings could be used in treatment of orthostatic symptoms. Speech therapy for dysarthria and swallowing evaluation for dysphagia are often needed.

Erectile dysfunction medications can exacerbate hypotension. Oromandibular dystonia is associated with dopaminergic therapy. Side effects or adverse effects of intramuscular botulinum toxin injections into the vocal cord, sternocleidomastoid, or other muscles in the treatment of dystonia may occur.

Reference

1. Jankovic J, Rajput AH, McDermott MP, Perl DP. The evolution of diagnosis in early Parkinson disease. Parkinson Study Group. *Arch Neurol.* 2000;57(3):369–72.

Suggested Reading

Dąbrowska M, Schinwelski M, Sitek EJ, et al. The role of neuroimaging in the diagnosis of the atypical parkinsonian syndromes in clinical practice. *Neurol Neurochir Pol.* 2015;49(6): 421–31.

Fanciulli A, Wenning GK. Multiple-system atrophy. *NEJM.* 2015;372(3):249–63.

Iodice V, Lipp A, Ahlskog JE, et al. Autopsy confirmed multiple system atrophy cases: Mayo experience and role of autonomic function tests. *J Neurol Neurosurg Psychiatry.* 2012;83:453–9.

Köllensperger M, Geser F, Ndayisaba JP, et al. Presentation, diagnosis, and management of multiple system atrophy in Europe: final analysis of the European multiple system atrophy registry. *Mov Disord.* 2010;25(15): 2604–12.

Tada M, Onodera O, Tada M, et al. Early development of autonomic dysfunction may predict poor prognosis in patients with multiple system atrophy. *Arch Neurol.* 2007;64(2):256–60.

Wenning GK, Stefanova N. Recent developments in multiple system atrophy. *J Neurol.* 2009;256: 1791–808.

Multiple System Atrophy-Cerebellar Type (MSA-C)

Epidemiology and Demographics: The reported incidence of multiple system atrophy (MSA) is about 0.6 cases per 100,000 person-years. After the age of 50, the incidence increases to 3 cases per 100,000, with mean age of onset being 54 years. There are two main clinical subtypes, based on the motor features present. The first type is the poorly levodopa-responsive parkinsonism (MSA-P) type, and the second type is the cerebellar ataxia (MSA-C) type. The MSA-P type is more than twice as common as the MSA-C type in Europe and North America.

Disorder Description: MSA involves widespread neurodegeneration affecting the substantia nigra, the sensorimotor striatum, dopaminergic terminals in the putamen, the inferior olive, the pontine nuclei, the cerebellar vermis, as well as other brainstem nuclei, and the intermediolateral cell column within the spinal cord. Early diagnosis of MSA-C could be challenging, but it is one of the differential diagnoses in the case of adult onset cerebellar ataxia. Other differential diagnoses include idiopathic late-onset cerebellar ataxia, which is also known as sporadic adult-onset ataxia of unknown etiology. A detailed clinical history, family history, and comprehensive neurologic examination, as well as MRI brain neuroimaging can indeed aid with determining the final diagnosis.

Symptoms

Localization site	Comment
Prominent olivopontocerebellar atrophy	Ataxia
Autonomic dysfunction	Orthostatic hypotension, urinary frequency, urgency, and incontinence
Putamen, nigrostriatal pathway	Rigidity, akinisia, tremor, dysphagia
Neurovascular involvement	Raynaud's phenomena

Secondary Complications: Orthostatic hypotension could lead to increase in fall risk. The treatment of parkinsonism is quite challenging with no long-term robust treatment.

Treatment Complications: As stated in the entry for *Multiple System Atrophy (MSA; Shy–Drager Syndrome)*, MSA-C (as well as MSA-P) is poorly responsive to levodopa. There is a reported transient response to levodopa in 40% of cases, but 90% of patients become levodopa unresponsive. Treatment of orthostatic hypotension in MSA-C can include increased fluid intake and high salt diet and compression stockings, as well as pharmacologic agents pyridostigmine, fludrocortisone, and midodrine. The treatment of urinary incontinence could range from anticholinergic agents such as oxybutynin or toleterodine to intermittent self-catheterization or permanent indwelling catheter.

Bibliography

Fanciulli A, Wenning GK. Multiple-system atrophy. *New Engl J Med*. 2015;372:249–63.

Lin DJ, Hermann KL, Schmahmann JD. Multiple system atrophy of the cerebellar type: Clinical state of the art. *Mov Disord*. 2014;29(4):294–304.

Lin IS, Wu RM, Lee-Chen GJ, Shan DE, Gwinn-Hardy K. The SCA17 phenotype can include features of MSA-C, PSP and cognitive impairment. *Parkinsonism Relat Disord*. 2007;13(4):246–9.

Wenning GK, Stefanova N. Recent developments in multiple system atrophy. *J Neurol*. 2009;256:1791–808.

Mumps Meningoencephalitis

Epidemiology and Demographics: Since the pre-vaccine era, there has been a more than 99% decrease in mumps cases in the United States. However, clustered outbreaks are not uncommon. In 2015–16, outbreaks were reported from several university campuses.

Disorder Description: The mumps virus is an RNA virus and belongs to the genus *Rubulavirus* in the family Paramyxoviridae.

Aseptic meningitis is the most common neurologic complication of mumps virus infection; it occurs in up to 10% of patients. Mumps encephalitis is rare. Widespread vaccination has been associated with virtual disappearance of this complication.

Symptoms

Localization site	Comment
Cerebral hemispheres	Aseptic meningitis is the most common complication, occurring in 1 to 10% of mumps patients. It can occur before, during, or after mumps parotitis. In some series, up to 50% of patients with mumps meningitis did not have a preceding parotitis
	Clinical manifestations typically include headache, low-grade fever, and mild nuchal rigidity. Seizures and altered consciousness may occur with encephalitis Encephalitis was previously rare and has gone unreported for some decades; previous reports mention encephalopathy, recurrent seizures, hemiplegia, gait apraxia
Mental status and psychiatric aspects/complications	Headache and neck stiffness with meningitis, seizures, altered mentation, and cognitive impairment with encephalitis
Cerebellum	Cerebellitis and ataxia have been reported
Cranial nerves	Previously a leading cause of sensorineural deafness. Facial palsy has been reported
Spinal cord	Transverse myelitis, polyradiculitis, and Guillain–Barré syndrome mentioned in isolated case reports
Mononeuropathy or mononeuropathy multiplex	Facial nerve palsy reported

Secondary Complications: The neurologic course of mumps is usually benign, with fever and signs of meningeal irritation lasting less than 5 days. It is usually followed by full recovery. Systemic complications such as orchitis followed by infertility occur more frequently. Death is extremely rare.

Treatment: Supportive treatment.

Bibliography

Anderson LJ, Seward JF. Mumps epidemiology and immunity: the anatomy of a modern epidemic. *Pediatr Infect Dis J*. 2008;27:S75.

Bruyn HB, Sexton HM, Brainerd HD. Mumps meningoencephalitis: a clinical review of 119 cases with one death. *Calif Med*. 1957;86(3):153–60.

Centers for Disease Control and Prevention. Mumps cases and outbreaks. Updated June 27, 2018. www.cdc.gov/mumps/outbreaks.html. Accessed Apr 6, 2017.

Dourado I, Cunha S, Teixeira MG et al. Outbreak of aseptic meningitis associated with mass vaccination with a urabe-containing measles-mumps-rubella vaccine: implications for immunization programs. *Am J Epidemiol.* 2000;151(5):524–30.

Johnstone JA, Ross CAC, Dunn M. Meningitis and encephalitis associated with mumps infection: a 10-year survey. *Arch Dis Child.* 1972;47(254): 647–51.

Mclean DM, Bach RD, Larke RP, McNaughton GA. Mumps meningoencephalitis, Toronto, 1963. *Can Med Assoc J.* 1964;90:458.

World Health Organization. Mumps reported cases. Jul 15, 2018. http://apps.who.int/immunization_monitoring/globalsummary/timeseries/tsincidencemumps.html. Accessed Sep 6, 2018.

Muscle Cramps

Epidemiology and Demographics: Muscle cramps are normal, and highly common. Weekly, in a normal population, the prevalence per person is about 35%. There is no sex predominance. Pregnant females are at greater risk. It can occur at any age, but has a higher frequency among the elderly. There is no geographic distribution.

Disorder Description: Muscle cramps are exceedingly common and are defined as sudden, painful, sustained contractions with motor units firing at frequencies up to 200 Hz. Frequently, they are seen in motor neuron disease (i.e., amyotrophic lateral sclerosis, Kennedy's disease).

Cramps are frequently a result of increased motor axon excitability or unstable polarization from myriad biochemical changes. They can recur if the muscle is prematurely returned to its unstretched state. Lack of exercise and mobility is a risk factor for cramping. There are many substances, medications, and metabolic states that can predispose to cramping. Ethanol and sequelae of cirrhosis both do so, as do medications such as nifedipine, cimetidine, terbutaline, salbutamol, clofibrate, diuretics, and penicillamine. Metabolic derangements such as diarrhea, emesis, uremia, exercise, pregnancy, hypothyroidism, and hypoadrenalism can also contribute. Disorders of glycogen, lipid, or mitochondrial metabolism are more likely to cause cramping.

There are no specific tests used for diagnosis as this is mostly a clinical entity. However, cramps can be elicited during electromyography and seen as high-frequency discharge.

Symptoms

Localization site	Comment
Muscle	Sudden, involuntary, and painful contraction, localized, with visible, palpable muscle hardening and often associated abnormal posturing of joints

Secondary Complications: Generally cramps are benign, but if they sustain without ceasing, they can cause morbidity due to risk of turning into tetany.

Treatment Complications: Massaging and stretching help relieve the contraction. Other conservative measures include avoiding offending drugs, hydrating, electrolyte replacement, and prophylactic stretching. Reduction of nerve and muscle irritability can be achieved with quinine, procainamide, diphenhydramine, and warmth. Antiepileptic drugs, such as phenytoin (starting at 100–200 mg), carbamazepine (starting at 100–200 mg), and gabapentin (starting at 300 mg) that block sodium channels can theoretically also reduce spontaneous membrane discharges. Vitamin E starting at 1000 IU has also been used. Pharmacologic intervention is typically given at night to aid sleep. That being said, actual utility of pharmacologic intervention is debatable, as there is a 40–50% efficacy rate just for placebo.

Typically conservative measures are utilized, so the rate of complications from treatment is exceedingly low. Adverse effects are dictated by the drug that is chosen, if at all. As such, quinine is no longer used given potential fatal hypersensitivity reactions and thrombocytopenia, and that arrhythmias as well as permanent vision loss can also occur at higher dosages. Carbamazepine can cause hyponatremia. Phenytoin can cause alopecia, gingival hyperplasia, and nystagmus at toxic levels.

Bibliography

Amato AA, Russell JA. *Neuromuscular disorders.* New York: McGraw-Hill; 2008. pp. 143–56

Longo DL, Kasper DL, Fauci A, et al., eds. *Harrison's principles of internal medicine.* 17th ed. New York: McGraw-Hill Education/Medical; 2016. pp. 1292, 1412, 1462–4.

Myasthenia Gravis

Epidemiology and Demographics: Prevalence in the United States is 14–20/100,000. Most common age at onset is the second and third decades in women and seventh and eighth decades in men. Juvenile onset MG is rare.

Disorder Description: MG is an autoimmune post-synaptic neuromuscular junction disorder. Antibodies most commonly against acetylcholine receptors, and less commonly against muscle-specific kinase, are present in serum in 80–90% of patients. Seronegative MG refers to patients with MG with unidentified autoantibodies.

Symptoms

Localization site	Comment
Neuromuscular junction	Ocular myasthenia: Fluctuating ptosis, ophthalmoparesis
	Generalized MG: In addition to above, fluctuating proximal generalized weakness with improvement after rest, and worsening at the end of the day or in warm weather. Also with fluctuating dysphagia, dysarthria, and shortness of breath. Weakness of head extension and flexion

Secondary Complications: MG exacerbation and crisis are possible complications that lead to hospitalization, intensive care unit stays, respiratory failure with intubation, and hospital acquired complications.

Treatment Complications: Pyridostigmine treatment may lead to increased secretions, diarrhea, and muscle cramps. Immunosuppressive treatment may lead to increased chance of infections, leukopenia, and hepatotoxicity. Steroid complications may occur.

Bibliography

Amato AA, Russell JA. *Neuromuscular disorders.* 2nd ed. New York: McGraw-Hill Medical; 2016.

Katirji B, Kaminski HJ, Ruff RL. *Neuromuscular disorders in clinical practice.* 2nd ed. New York: Springer-Verlag New York; 2014.

Myasthenia Gravis and Pregnancy

Epidemiology and Demographics: Myasthenia gravis (MG) affects approximately 1 million persons worldwide and has a prevalence of 0.02%. MG is twice as common in women as men and has an onset in the second and third decades, which are reproductive years. There is little evidence that MG has a greater incidence of onset during pregnancy than during the nonpregnant state. The course of MG during pregnancy is variable, with exacerbation occurring in 40% of affected women while the remainder either improve (30%) or have no meaningful change (30%). HLA-B8 and DR3 serotype is associated with the onset of MG in this age group. Environmental factors that predispose to MG exacerbation include infection, general anesthesia, emotional stress, and some medications (aminoglycosides, ciprofloxacin, chloroquine, procaine, lithium, phenytoin, beta-blockers, procainamide, statins).

Disorder Description: MG is an autoimmune disease in which antibodies are developed against the acetylcholine receptor or muscle-specific kinase, leading to decreased transmission across the neuromuscular junction causing weakness. The presentation is classically fluctuating weakness or fatigability. Repetitive stimulation on nerve conduction study may show a small decrement in the compound muscle action potential. An extension of the physical exam to include the ice pack test for ptosis or tensilon test for muscle weakness can also be helpful in the diagnosis.

Symptoms

Localization site	Comment
Neuromuscular junction	Fatigability and fluctuating weakness in the following distributions: • Extraocular muscle weakness or ptosis is present initially in 50% • First complaint may be specific focal weakness, and should prompt an assessment of weakness at other sites, especially extraocular movements • Bulbar muscle weakness such as fatigue with mastication and swallowing • Limb weakness usually more severe proximally than distally • Weakness of head extension and flexion • Generalized weakness without ocular muscle weakness is rare

Secondary Complications: Transient neonatal myasthenia in newborn babies may occur irrespective of the mother's disease status. Expectant mothers should aim to deliver in hospitals. All newborns should undergo a neurologic examination with neonatal critical care available.

During labor and delivery, regional anesthesia may be used safely while neuromuscular blockade should be avoided. Likewise, magnesium should be used with caution for treatment of eclampsia in MG patients because it blocks calcium entry in the presynaptic nerve terminal and further decreases acetylcholine transmission. Fatigue may also be more pronounced in MG patients.

Treatment Complications: Pregnancy issues should be discussed with female MG patients prior to conception, given the above potential treatment complications. Specifically, thymectomy, if indicated, should be undertaken several months prior to pregnancy since the clinical benefit is realized several months after the surgery. Thymectomy is an important consideration since it may reduce the need for medication during pregnancy.

For symptomatic management, oral pyridostigmine is first-line.

Prednisone is the first-line immunosuppressive therapy and is not contraindicated for MG exacerbations during pregnancy. Cyclosporine and azathioprine (formerly FDA category C and D, respectively) may also be used. Mycophenilate (category D) and methotrexate (category X) are not recommended due to their teratogenic risk.

For myasthenic crisis, should it occur during pregnancy, PLEX and intravenous immunoglobulin (category C) may be used in pregnancy for a short-term response.

Prednisone may exacerbate gestational diabetes. Intravenous cholinesterase inhibitors may produce uterine contractions and therefore should be avoided. Teratogenic immunomodulating therapy should be avoided if possible due to teratogenic risk.

Bibliography

Chaudhry SA, Vignarajah B, Koren G. Myasthenia gravis during pregnancy. *Can Fam Physician*. 2012;58(12):1346–9.

Sanders DB, Wolfe GI, Benatar M, et al. International consensus guidance for management of myasthenia gravis: Executive summary. *Neurology*. 2016;87(4):419–25.

Wolfe GI, Kaminski HJ, Aban IB, et al.; MGTX Study Group. Randomized trial of thymectomy in myasthenia gravis. *N Engl J Med*. 2016;375(6):511–22.

Mycoplasma pneumoniae Encephalitis

Epidemiology and Demographics: *Mycoplasma pneumoniae* is transmitted by respiratory droplets. Overall, 1% of the population is infected annually in the United States. The cumulative attack rate in families approaches 90%, and immunity is not long lasting.

CNS manifestations occur in approximately 0.1% of all patients with *M. pneumoniae* infections, typically causing encephalitis. The prognosis is guarded with 20 to 60% suffering neurologic sequelae.

Disorder Description: *M. pneumoniae* is an atypical bacterium characterized by the absence of a peptidoglycan cell wall, resulting in resistance to several antibacterial agents.

Symptoms

Localization site	Comment
Cerebral hemispheres	Encephalitis is the most frequent manifestation
Mental status and psychiatric aspects/complications	Encephalitis reported with altered consciousness, subsequent alterations in behavior such as Kluver Bucy syndrome reported. Intracranial hypertension, coma, psychosis, hemiparesis, seizures, and acute disseminated encephalomyelitis also mentioned in literature
	Aseptic meningitis with headache and photophobia also reported
Brainstem	Intracranial hypertension can put pressure on the midbrain; direct brainstem involvement may occur
Cerebellum	Cerebellar ataxia described
Vestibular system (and non-specific dizziness)	Ataxia frequently reported
Cranial nerves	Cranial nerve palsies occur
Spinal cord	Transverse myelitis can occur
Anterior horn cells	Polyradiculitis
Dorsal root ganglia	Polyradiculitis
Peripheral neuropathy	Rarely present as peripheral neuropathy

Secondary Complications: With spinal cord involvement, permanent neurologic sequelae. Severe, even fatal, cases are known.

Treatment Complications: The pneumonia is usually treated with macrolide or fluoroquinolone antibiotics; however, CNS involvement is possibly auto-immune with cross-reactivity of *M. pneumoniae* antigens to galactocerebroside. Immunosuppressive treatment has not demonstrated clear benefit for adults, although steroids may have a role in the treatment of children with neurologic disease.

Bibliography

Bitnun A, Ford-Jones E, Blaser S, Richardson S. Mycoplasma pneumoniae encephalitis. *Semin Pediatr Infect Dis.* 2003;14:96.

Daxboeck F. Mycoplasma pneumoniae central nervous system infections. *Curr Opin Neurol.* 2006;19:374.

Foy HM, Kenny GE, Cooney MK, Allan ID. Long-term epidemiology of infections with Mycoplasma pneumoniae. *J Infect Dis.* 1979;139:681.

Gücüyener K, Simşek F, Yilmaz O, et al. Methyl-prednisolone in neurologic complications of Mycoplasma pneumonia. *Indian J Pediatr.* 2000;67(6):467–9.

Tsiodras S, Kelesidis T, Kelesidis I, et al. Mycoplasma pneumoniae-associated myelitis: a comprehensive review. *Eur J Neurol.* 2006;13:112.

Mycotic Aneurysm

Epidemiology and Demographics: In adults, 2 to 6% of intracranial aneurysms are stated to be of infective origin with a higher percentage in children. In persons with endocarditis, the frequency of infective aneurysms ranges from 4 to 15% depending on study design, with proven ruptured bacterial aneurysms accounting for 1 to 2%. About 20% are multiple. Men and women are equally affected. The mean age at presentation is approximately 30 years, and no age is exempt.

Disorder Description: Infective aneurysms develop when septic emboli lodge in the vasa vasorum causing necrosis of the arterial wall with resultant fusiform (usual) and saccular (uncommon) dilatation of the artery at more distal locations compared with intracranial noninfective aneurysms. Initially, a bland infarct may result. Secondary hemorrhage occurs in 40% with or without aneurysm formation distal to the occlusion due to the friability of the

vessel wall. Mycotic aneurysms can develop anywhere but are most commonly seen in the intracranial arteries, followed by visceral arteries and upper or lower extremity arteries, typically occurring at arterial bifurcations. Blood cultures are positive in 50 to 85% of cases. *Streptococcus* and *Staphylococcus* are the most common etiologies.

Infective aneurysms are suspected in persons with endocarditis or sepsis when neurologic symptoms are unexplained by systemic illness. Headache, transient focal neurologic signs, encephalopathy, cranial neuropathies, or aseptic meningitis may antedate aneurysm rupture. A careful history will often reveal congenital or valvular heart disease, pulmonary arteriovenous fistula, recent cardiovascular procedure, or the use of intravenous drugs. Examination may show signs of bacterial endocarditis including Roth spots, Janeway lesions, splinter hemorrhages, enlarged spleen, or changing heart murmur.

Symptoms

Localization site	Comment
Cerebral hemispheres	Bleeding due to rupture is the most common mode of presentation of infective aneurysms. Intracranial bleeding occurs in about one-half of cases, whereas septic embolism resulting in infarction is present in about a third of cases
	Sudden severe headache with associated stiff neck, focal signs such as hemiparesis with or without alteration of consciousness, seizures, and confusion are common initial symptoms indicating subarachnoid hemorrhage, intracerebral hemorrhage, or septic infarction
	Fever, intermittent headache, malaise, and lethargy due to systemic toxicity may precede other neurologic symptoms by a few days. Because these aneurysms frequently coexist with other neurologic complications of sepsis, such as meningitis or cerebral abscess, the initial symptoms of aneurysm rupture can be atypical
	Warning leaks, common in saccular aneurysms, and transient ischemic attacks infrequently precede the discovery of the aneurysm. Subdural and extradural hemorrhages are exceptional
	HIV-associated aneurysms tend to present with ischemic strokes involving the arterial territory supplied by the affected artery and with headaches
	The aneurysms themselves may cause focal neurologic signs by compression

Localization site	Comment
Mental status and psychiatric aspects/ complications	Lethargy progressing to coma could occur with complications such as hemorrhage, hydrocephalus, cerebral edema, herniation
Brainstem	Infarct and hemorrhages could result in brainstem syndromes
Cerebellum	Infarct and hemorrhages could result in cerebellar syndromes
Cranial nerves	Coexisting meningitis, sinus infection, cavernous thrombophlebitis may result in cranial neuropathy
Spinal cord	Osteomyelitis of the thoracic and lumbar spine from aortic aneurysms may result in paraplegia, bladder dysfunction, back pain Lumbar vertebral erosions may occur from the aneurysms resulting in lumbago
Peripheral neuropathy	Infected aneurysms can impinge on the nerves supplying the extremities, for example brachial artery aneurysm can cause wrist drop from radial nerve compression
Muscle	Psoas abscess – extension of infection from an aortic or iliac aneurysm to the psoas muscle may cause flank pain, inguinal pain, and limping
Unclear localization	Enlarging or ruptured carotid or subclavian artery aneurysm may compress the structures of the neck leading to stenosis or deviation of the trachea or impingement of the laryngeal nerves resulting in hoarseness of voice

Secondary Complications: Complications may include cerebral edema and infarction, hemorrhage, vasospasm, abscess formation, and hydrocephalus, the last usually being due to subarachnoid hemorrhage or basal meningitis. Persons harboring fungal aneurysms have mortality rates of over 90%, whereas those with bacterial aneurysms have a mortality rate of approximately 30% despite antibiotic treatment. Serial angiography has demonstrated that more than 50% of aneurysms will resolve with antibiotic treatment.

Treatment Complications: Antibiotic therapy is mandated for all cases of infective aneurysms and is begun as soon as the diagnosis (most often in association with infective endocarditis) is suspected, and continued for at least 6 weeks but may be prolonged in cases with myocardial abscess, prosthetic heart valve, and in immunosuppressed individuals.

Endovascular therapy (occlusion of parent artery with coil/balloon/glue/onyx vs stent placement) is indicated in case of ruptured mycotic aneurysms that do not have a hematoma producing mass effect or increased intracranial pressure and whose aneurysm does not involve an eloquent vascular territory. The need for antiplatelet therapy (combination aspirin and clopidogrel) before and after stent placement to prevent thromboembolic complications is an area of potential concern in a patient with a ruptured aneurysm.

Surgical candidates are those patients with aneurysmal rupture with an intraparenchymal hematoma producing mass effect or increased intracranial pressure, ruptured aneurysm, and in stable condition but who experience failure of endovascular therapy because of risks to eloquent parent arteries, and unruptured, enlarging aneurysms that involve an eloquent vascular territory.

Once a diagnosis of infective aneurysm is confirmed, anticoagulant therapy to prevent further embolization is contraindicated because these drugs are ineffective in preventing embolization from infected valves and increase the risk of catastrophic cerebral hemorrhage.

Bibliography

Chun JY, Smith W, Halbach VV, et al. Current multimodality management of infectious intracranial aneurysms. *Neurosurgery.* 2001;48(6):1203–13; discussion 1213–4.

Mandell G. Infective endarteritis and mycotic aneurysms. In Mandell G, Bennett J, Dolin R, eds. *Principles and practice of infectious disease.* Philadelphia: Churchill Livingstone; 2000. pp. 888–92.

Myocardial Infarction

Epidemiology and Demographics: Most commonly seen in men over the age of 45 years and women over the age of 55 years. According to the Centers for Disease Control and Prevention, each year, 735,000 Americans experience a myocardial infarction (MI).

Disorder Description: Coronary atherosclerosis is the cause of almost every myocardial infarction, and it is often seen with superimposed coronary thrombosis. The result is ischemia due to the lack of blood supply, which therefore results in necrosis (infarction) of heart tissues. Risk factors include age over 45 years in men and over 55 years in women, family history of coronary artery disease, hypertension, hypercholesterolemia, diabetes, obesity, and smoking history.

Symptoms

Localization site	Comment
Cerebral hemispheres	Particularly associated with atrial as well as ventricular arrhythmias, which may cause cerebral hypoperfusion and hypoxia. Associated with presyncope, syncope, and sudden death

Secondary Complications: Myocardial infarction may lead to arrhythmias, heart failure, heart rupture, and valvular problems.

Treatment Complications: May result in atrial and ventricular arrhythmias with resultant central nervous system hypoperfusion, presyncope, syncope, and/or sudden death. Atrial fibrillation may result in a higher risk of cerebrovascular events.

Bibliography

American Heart Association. About heart attacks. May 15, 2015. Available from www.heart .org/HEARTORG/Conditions/HeartAttack/ AboutHeartAttacks/About-Heart-Attacks_ UCM_002038_Article.jsp. Accessed Jun 23, 2015.

Mayo Clinic Staff. Heart attack. Nov 15, 2014. Available from www.mayoclinic.org/diseases-conditions/heart-attack/basics/definition/con-20019520. Accessed Jun 23, 2015.

Scirica BM, Morrow DA. ST-elevation myocardial infarction: pathology, pathophysiology, and clinical features. In Mann DL, Zipes D, Libby P, Bonow RO, Braunwald E, eds. *Braunwald's heart disease: A textbook of cardiovascular medicine.* 10th ed. Philadelphia, PA: Elsevier/Saunders; 2015; pp. 1071–85.

Myoclonic Epilepsy with Ragged Red Fibers (MERRF)

Epidemiology and Demographics: Myoclonic epilepsy with ragged red fibers (MERRF) is a very rare disease, with prevalence estimates at around 1/400,000. There is no sex predominance, but it is maternally inherited. Myoclonus, the first symptom, typically presents in late adolescence or young adulthood. It is more common in Northern Europe.

Disorder Description: MERRF is a multisystem disorder characterized by myoclonus, typically the first symptom (though not specific to MERRF), followed by generalized epilepsy, ataxia, weakness, and dementia.

It is a maternally inherited mitochondrial disorder, involving mutations in the mitochondrial MT-TK gene. Most commonly (nearly 80%), there is an A to G mutation at nucleotide 8344 (8344A>G) encoding tRNA(Lys); other mutations include m.8356T>C, m.8363G>A, and m.8361G>A.

The characteristic diagnostic finding is "ragged red fibers" on Gomori trichrome stain from clumps of diseased mitochondria that accumulate in muscle fiber subsarcolemma. Serum CK is normal or mildly elevated, but lactate and pyruvate are commonly elevated and increase further with physical activity. Nerve conduction studies may show axonal polyneuropathy; EMG frequently demonstrates myopathic potentials.

Symptoms

Localization site	Comment
Cerebral hemispheres	Epilepsy/seizures
Mental status and psychiatric aspects/complications	Dementia
Cranial nerves	Sensorineural hearing loss, optic atrophy, pigmentary retinopathy
Spinal cord	Pyramidal signs (corticospinal signs, positive Babinski, hyperreflexia)
Peripheral neuropathy	Sensorimotor polyneuropathy with pes cavus
Muscle	Weakness, atrophy, spasticity
Unclear localization	Short stature, multiple lipomatosis

Secondary Complications: There are multiple, though less common, systemic findings. Lactic acidosis is prevalent. Cardiac arrhythmias with conduction block are possible.

Treatment Complications: There is no treatment for the underlying disorder. Rather, management is symptomatic/supportive. Seizures are treated with antiepileptic drugs. Aerobic exercise can be helpful, while physical therapy can improve motor ability. Complications of treatment depend on the antiepileptic drug chosen.

Bibliography

Amato AA, Russell JA. *Neuromuscular disorders*. New York: McGraw-Hill; 2008. pp. 143–56.

DiMauro S, Hirano M. MERRF. GeneReviews®. Jun 3, 2003. Updated Jan 29, 2015. Seattle (WA): University of Washington, Seattle; 1993–2017.

Tobon A. Metabolic myopathies. *Continuum (Minneap Minn)*. 2013;19(6 Muscle Disease):1571–97.

Myoclonus Dystonia

Epidemiology and Demographics: Myoclonus dystonia presents in childhood or adolescence but can sometimes present in adulthood, especially if the diagnosis is initially missed. Described age range is from 6 months of age to 80+ years old. Males and females are equally affected. Frequency of the condition is unknown. It is found world-wide.

Disorder Description: Myoclonus dystonia is an autosomal dominant condition that is most commonly linked to chromosome 7 at the epsilon sarcoglycan (*SGCE*) gene. It is commonly referred to as DYT11 dystonia. It presents in childhood with myoclonus that usually affects the arms and the neck. More than 50% of the time, it is accompanied by focal or segmental dystonia that can affect the arms, neck, or trunk. Cervical dystonia and writer's cramp are frequently seen. The motor symptoms of the condition are typically alcohol responsive, but this can be variable. Other genes implicated in the myoclonus dystonia phenotype include *DRD2* and *TOR1A*, but these mutations have only been described in single families with the phenotype.

Symptoms

Localization site	Comment
Cerebral hemispheres	Epilepsy is rare
Mental status and psychiatric aspects/complications	Depression, anxiety, obsessive-compulsive disorder, attention deficit hyperactivity disorder, and panic attacks
Spinal cord	Myelopathy if the cervical dystonia is severe
Peripheral nerve	Peripheral neuropathy from alcoholism if present

Secondary Complications: Because of the alcohol responsive nature of the motor symptoms, alcohol dependence is commonly seen in patients with myoclonus dystonia.

Treatment Complications: Anticholinergics can impair cognition and should not be used in elderly patients. There is danger of potential benzodiazepine dependence with prolonged clonazepam and lorazepam use. Botulinum toxin for focal dystonia can cause reversible muscle weakness and/or dysphagia. Deep brain stimulation can worsen cognitive impairment or exacerbate underlying mood disorders.

Bibliography

Hess CW, Raymond D, Aguiar Pde C, Frucht S, et al. Myoclonus-dystonia, obsessive-compulsive disorder, and alcohol dependence in SGCE mutation carriers. *Neurology*. 2007;68:522–4.

Kinugawa K, Vidailhet M, Clot F, et al. Myoclonus-dystonia: An update. *Mov Disord*. 2009;24:479–89.

Raymond D, Ozelius L. Myoclonus-dystonia. May 21, 2003. Updated Jan 26, 2012. In Pagon RA, Adam MP, Ardinger HH, et al., eds. *GeneReviews* [Internet]. Seattle (WA): University of Washington, Seattle; 1993–2016.

Zimprich A, Grabowski M, Asmus F, et al. Mutations in the gene encoding epsilon-sarcoglycan cause myoclonus-dystonia syndrome. *Nat Genet*. 2001;29:66–9.

Myophosphorylase Deficiency (McArdle's Disease)

Epidemiology and Demographics: Autosomal recessive, 1:100,000. Some heterozygous individuals (1:160) can be symptomatic with enzyme activity of 20–40% of normal. Specific genetic mutations exist in varied ethnic groups.

Disorder Description: McArdle's disease is a glycogen storage disease (type V) caused by a defect in a skeletal muscle isoform of glycogen phosphorylase. The disease is caused by a mutation in the PYGM gene, which encodes the mycophosphorylase enzyme, leading to a pure myopathy. (Other glycogen storage diseases affect liver and heart isoforms as well, causing other organ involvement.)

Myophosphorylase initiates the breakdown of muscle glycogen by removing (1,4)-α-glucosyl units from the outer branches of glycogen, leading to liberation of glucose-1-phosphate. This in turn undergoes glycolysis, creating lactate and pyruvate in hypoxic conditions, which act as alternate energy sources for the Krebs cycle. In the absence of the enzyme, patients with McArdle's are unable to metabolise their muscle glycogen stores.

There is great clinical heterogeneity, with most patients presenting with exercise intolerance, or acute crises associated with rhabdomyolysis and myoglobinuria. Both isometric muscle contraction and dynamic muscle activity can induce rhabdomyolysis. Patients often demonstrate a "second wind" phenomenon – whereby resting allows them to return to exercise.

About a third of patients present with fixed weakness and wasting (proximal > distal). The marked decrease in skeletal muscle phosphorylation potential leads to the accumulation of phosphate and ADP leading to premature muscle atrophy and contractures.

Other muscle glycolytic defects (such as other glycogen storage diseases including phosphorylase kinase deficiency) can manifest similarly. General exercise intolerance and a high creatine phosphokinase (CPK) at rest (~ 1500–3000 U/L) and following exercise (10,000 U/L) may be the first clue. The second wind phenomenon is unique to McArdle's. The ischemic forearm test (where no change in lactic acid is measured, denoting the absence of anaerobic consumption of glycogen) is suggestive, but false negatives occur. Confirmation of the diagnosis is via molecular genetics or muscle biopsy.

Symptoms

Localization site	Comment
Muscular system	A pure myopathy: exercise intolerance or acute crises after static or dynamic intense exercise

Secondary Complications: Complications include marked muscle breakdown (rhabdomyolysis) and myoglobinuria causing renal failure

Treatment Complications: Management is comprised of:
Dietary advice – a complex carbohydrate-rich diet as well as pre-exercise ingestion of carbohydrates can markedly improve exercise tolerance.
Medically supervised aerobic training of low to moderate intensity.
Prevention of exercise overexertion – especially high loads on low muscle mass.

Bibliography

Goldstein J, Austin S, Kishnani P, et al. Phosphorylase kinase deficiency. May 31, 2011. In Pagon RA, Adam MP, Ardinger HH, et al., eds. *GeneReviews*® [Internet]. Seattle (WA): University of Washington, Seattle; 1993–2016.

Luica A, Nogales-Gadea G, Pérez M, et al. McArdle disease – what do neurologists need to know? *Nat Clin Pract Neurol.* 2008;4(10):568–77. DOI: 10.1038/ncpneuro0913

Martín MA, Lucía A, Arenas J, et al. Glycogen storage disease type V. Apr 19, 2006. Updated Jun 26, 2014. In Pagon RA, Adam MP, Ardinger HH, et al., eds. *GeneReviews*® [Internet]. Seattle (WA): University of Washington, Seattle; 1993–2016.

Myotonic Dystrophy Type 1

Epidemiology and Demographics: Myotonic dystrophy Type 1 (DM1) is an autosomal dominant disorder with an incidence of approximately 13.5/100,000 and a prevalence of 3–5/100,000. DM1 is the most common form of myotonic dystrophy diagnosed in children. There is no sex predominance, as males and females are affected approximately equally. It can present at any age. It presents in four subtypes: classic adult-onset, congenital, childhood-onset, and late-onset. There is no geographic predominance, but it is the most common muscular dystrophy among adults of European ancestry.

Disorder Description: It is important to think of DM1 as not only a muscular disease, but also a systemic disorder with effects on multiple organ systems. It predominantly affects facial, oropharyngeal, long finger flexor, and foot/toe dorsiflexor muscles. Proximal weakness is not present early. Myotonia (delayed muscular relaxation) is identified easier in the distal muscles.

DM1 is caused by a (CTG) trinucleotide repeat expansion of the gene DMPK on chromosome 19q13.3. In DM1, age of onset and disease severity correlate well with CTG repeat size.

Creatine kinase tends to be normal or mildly elevated. EMG will reveal myopathy signs and myotonic discharges. The definitive diagnosis is based on genetic analysis.

Symptoms

Localization site	Comment
Muscle	Predominantly affects facial, oropharyngeal, long finger flexor, and foot/toe dorsiflexor muscles. Presence of myotonia

Secondary Complications: Patients can develop early onset cataracts, cardiac arrhythmias and conduction blocks, endocrine dysfunction, and cognitive impairment.

Treatment Complications: There is no proven treatment for this disease. Management is supportive and requires a multidisciplinary approach.

Bibliography

Udd B. The myotonic dystrophies: molecular, clinical, and therapeutic challenges. *Lancet Neurol.* 2012;11(10):891–905.

Wicklund MP. The muscular dystrophies. *Continuum (Minneap Minn).* 2013;19(6):1535–70.

Myotonic Dystrophy Type 2

Epidemiology and Demographics: Myotonic dystrophy Type 2 (DM2) has a lower prevalence than DM1 in the United States, though some reports suggest similar prevalence to DM1 in Europe. Symptoms present later in life compared with DM1; DM2 most often presents in middle age or later. There is no

geographic predominance, but it is the most common muscular dystrophy among adults of European ancestry. Can affect males and females.

Disorder Description: DM2 is an autosomal dominant dystrophy. Muscle pain and stiffness often predominate and clinical and EMG myotonia may be absent. Weakness is predominant proximally. In most patients, the systemic manifestations in DM2 are less frequent and milder than in DM1.

DM2 is caused by a (CCTG) trinucleotide repeat expansion of the gene DMPK on chromosome 19q13.3. In DM2, age of onset and disease severity do not correlate well with CCTG repeat size.

Creatine kinase tends to be normal or mildly elevated. EMG will reveal myopathy signs and myotonic discharges. The definitive diagnosis is based on genetic analysis.

Symptoms

Localization site	Comment
Muscle	Predominantly affects proximal muscles. Presence of myotonia. Although often the deep finger flexors are also substantially affected

Secondary Complications: Patients can develop early onset cataracts, cardiac arrhythmias and conduction blocks, endocrine dysfunction, and cognitive impairment.

Treatment Complications: There is no proven treatment for this disease. Management is supportive and requires a multidisciplinary approach.

Bibliography

Udd B. The myotonic dystrophies: molecular, clinical, and therapeutic challenges. *Lancet Neurol.* 2012;11(10):891–905.

Wicklund MP. The muscular dystrophies. *Continuum (Minneap Minn).* 2013;19(6):1535–70.

NADH CoQ Reductase Deficiency

Epidemiology and Demographics: Prevalence of adult mitochondrial disease is 1/5000. A third are de novo mutations, with no racial or ethnic predilection. Like all mitochondrial disorders, its mode of inheritance can be maternal (mitochondrial DNA is coded by the mother), X-linked dominant, or autosomal recessive. Mutations in any of 38 nuclear-encoded (nuclear DNA) and 7 mitochondrial-encoded (MiDNA) subunits can cause the disorder. There are also a number of proteins that are involved in the correct processing and assembly of complex I, the total number of which as yet remains unknown.

Disorder Description: NADH-coenzyme Q reductase (complex I) deficiency is the most frequent mitochondrial disorder of childhood, comprising around a third of all mitochondrial disorders. The condition is caused by mutations in multiple genes, coding for various subunits of a complex that is part of the mitochondrial respiratory chain. Complex I plays critical roles in transferring electrons from reduced NADH to coenzyme Q10 (CoQ10, ubiquinone) and in pumping protons to maintain the electrochemical gradient across the inner mitochondrial membrane. This electrochemical gradient is subsequently harnessed by complex V (ATP synthase) to synthesize ATP and generate reactive oxygen species (ROS).

There is a poor correlation between genotype and phenotype, with clinical pictures (e.g., individuals with external ophthalmoplegia) having varying genetic causes, such as a large mtDNA deletion, a single nucleotide variant of mtDNA (e.g., m.3243A>G), or a heterozygous pathogenic variant in a nuclear gene causing a secondary mtDNA abnormality. Alternately, the same pathogenic variant may cause a range of very different clinical syndromes (e.g., the m.3243A>G single nucleotide variant may cause chronic progressive external ophthalmoplegia [CPEO], diabetes mellitus and deafness, or severe encephalopathy with recurrent strokes and epilepsy).

A number of clinical subtypes are recognized, including:

a. Leigh syndrome manifests as marked and often fatal lactic acidosis, seizures, and characteristic findings on MRI (see below).

b. MELAS – lactic acidosis with stroke-like episodes.

c. Other – single organ involvement such as hypertrophic cardiomyopathy (HCM), Leber's hereditary optic neuropathy (LHON), leukoencephalopathy, pure myopathy, and hepatopathy with tubulopathy. Fatal infantile lactic acidosis is also recognised.

The majority of affected individuals develop symptoms during the first year of life and have a rapidly progressive disease course, resulting in a fatal outcome in childhood.

Symptoms

Localization site	Comment
Cerebral hemispheres	Seizures – respond variably to traditional antiepileptic drugs. Sodium valproate is contraindicated given its effect on carnitine metabolism
	Migraine headaches – can be a herald of stroke
	Metabolic stroke – varying non-vascular distributions, often sparing white matter (MELAS)
	Imaging: MRS – often with high lactate peak particularly in basal ganglia
	MELAS – cortical and subcortical areas of destruction, involving parietal and basal ganglia. Not necessarily corresponding with vascular territories
	Leigh syndrome – T2 hyperintense bilateral brainstem & basal ganglia
Cranial nerves	Progressive extraocular ophthalmoplegia (PEO) and retinopathy
	Sensorineural hearing loss
	Eyelid ptosis
Autonomic nervous system	Cardiac manifestations – either hypertrophic cardiomyopathy or arrhythmia
	Other autonomic manifestations – orthostasis, syncope, temperature instability, GI dysmotility
Myopathy	Exercise intolerance and poor stamina due to energy failure

Secondary Complications: Hepatopathy can cause encephalopathy.

Treatment Complications: Few studies have shown clinical efficacy of any treatment, with many studies suggesting that coenzyme Q10 and carnitine supplementation should be tried. Coenzyme Q10 can cause liver function test changes and nausea.

Bibliography

Fassone E, Shamima R. REVIEW Complex I deficiency: clinical features, biochemistry and molecular genetics. *J Med Genet.* 2012;49:578–90.

Gorman GS, Schaefer AM, Ng Y, et al. Prevalence of nuclear and mitochondrial DNA mutations related to adult mitochondrial disease. *Ann Neurol.* 2015;77(5):753–9. DOI:10.1002/ana.24362.

Lightowlers RN, Taylor RW, Turnbull DM. Mutations causing mitochondrial disease: What is new and what challenges remain? *Science.* 2015;349(6255):1494–9. DOI: 10.1126/science.aac7516.

Narcolepsy

Epidemiology and Demographics: Prevalence of narcolepsy type 1 is 0.02 to 0.18% of the population in the United States and Western Europe. The prevalence of narcolepsy type 2 is uncertain as it is not as well studied; however, it has been estimated to be 0.02 to 0.03%. There is a slight male predominance. Bimodal distribution, peak in adolescence (15 years) and second peak at 35 years. Etiology unknown; however, increased incidence noted after 2009 H1N1 influenza outbreak and streptococcal infections. Close association with human leukocyte antigen (HLA) subtypes DR2/DRB1*1501 and DQB1*0602.

Disorder Description: Excessive daytime somnolence (irresistible urge to sleep during the day) for at least a period of 3 months. Some patients may have signs of REM-sleep dissociation such as cataplexy (narcolepsy type 1). Cataplexy, which is specific for narcolepsy, is defined as more than one episode of a brief symmetric loss of muscle tone with retained consciousness. Strong emotional reactions are typical precipitants of cataplexy. Nocturnal sleep is typically disrupted with an inability to maintain continuous sleep. Other associated symptoms include hypnagogic hallucinations (transition from wake to sleep) and hypnapompic hallucinations (transition from sleep to wake) as well as sleep paralysis (inability to move voluntarily during sleep to wake transitions).

Diagnosis is made based on clinical symptoms of daytime irrepressible need to sleep (as described above) and presence of a mean sleep onset latency of ≤8 minutes and two or more sleep-onset REM periods (SOREMPs) on a Multiple Sleep Latency Test (MSLT). A SOREMP on the previous night's nocturnal polysomnogram can replace one SOREMP on an MSLT.

Narcolepsy type 1 vs type 2: Narcolepsy type 1 is diagnosed if cataplexy is present or CSF hypocretin levels are low (<110 pg/mL or less than one-third of mean values from normal individuals) even in the absence of cataplexy. Narcolepsy type 2 is diagnosed if cataplexy is absent and CSF hypocretin-1 concentration is >110 pg/mL or less than one-third of mean values from normal individuals. Differential diagnosis includes insufficient sleep time, obstructive sleep apnea, idiopathic hypersomnolence, and hypersomnolence due to medication or other medical problems.

Symptoms

Localization site	Comment
Forebrain	Lateral hypothalamus. Loss of hypocretin-containing neurons, ?autoimmune basis
Mental status and psychiatric aspects/complications	Sleepiness, depression, social dysfunction

Secondary Complications: Weight gain, depression, and social and workplace dysfunction are very common among narcolepsy patients.

Treatment Complications: Evaluate for and treat any other coexisting sleep disorders such as obstructive sleep apnea. Behavioral techniques such as sleep hygiene, scheduled naps, and maintaining a regular sleep schedule. Sodium oxybate, a sodium salt of gamma hydroxybutyrate (GHB), improves sleep quality, reduces daytime sleepiness, and is the most effective and only FDA-approved treatment for cataplexy.

Stimulants, such as modafinil/armodafinil, methylphenidate, and amphetamines, may also be used to help maintain wakefulness during the day.

Other treatments for cataplexy include REM-suppressing agents such as venlafaxine and fluoxetine.

Modafinil and armodafinil are hepatically metabolized and inducers of the cytochrome P450 enzyme system, which may affect the metabolism of other drugs. Methylphenidate and amphetamines are both central nervous system stimulants and can cause systemic hypertension and psychiatric events such as psychosis, anorexia, and anxiety.

Sodium oxybate treatment can cause rapid sedation and has potential for abuse. It should not be used with alcohol or other sedating medications such as benzodiazepines or opioids due to potential for respiratory depression. Abrupt withdrawal of cataplexy-suppressing medications can lead to status cataplecticus.

Bibliography

American Academy of Sleep Medicine. *International classification of sleep disorders.* 3rd ed. Darien, IL: American Academy of Sleep Medicine; 2014.

Andlauer O, Moore IVH, Hong SC, et al. Predictors of hypocretin (orexin) deficiency in narcolepsy without cataplexy. *Sleep.* 2012;35:1247–55.

Dauvilliers Y, Arnulf I, Mignot E. Narcolepsy with cataplexy. *Lancet.* 2007;369:499–511.

Wang J, Greenberg H. Status cataplecticus precipitated by abrupt withdrawal of venlafaxine. *J Clin Sleep Med.* 2013;9(7):715–6.

Zeman A, Britton T, Douglas N, et al. Narcolepsy and excessive daytime sleepiness. *BMJ.* 2004;329:724.

Nasopharyngeal Cancer

Epidemiology and Demographics: Nasopharyngeal malignant tumors can produce metastasis to any part of the body. However, the central nervous system through its proximity to the nasopharynx is the site of most of the complications. The rate of neurologic involvement is about 30%. Incidence is less than 1/100,000 in the United States.

Disorder Description: Nasopharyngeal cancers can be difficult to recognize early because of their insidious manner of growth, their lack of specificity of initial symptoms, and the relative inaccessibility of the nasopharynx to routine examination. Neurologic manifestations may occur early or late during the disease, and may at times be the earliest recognizable abnormalities. Cranial nerves are the most commonly affected and the ones traversing the middle fossa (CN V and VI) are the most susceptible to injury.

Symptoms

Localization site	Comment
Cerebellum	Dysmetria, truncal ataxia, and intention tremor (paraneoplastic)
Cranial nerves	Hearing loss, tinnitus, or a feeling of fullness or pressure in the ear (due to collection of serous fluid in the ear)
	Diplopia, sensory loss of the face, and loss of vision
Spinal cord	Sensory loss of the lower limbs (metastatic invasion of the spinal cord)
Unclear localization	Opsoclonus and myoclonus (paraneoplastic)

Treatment Complications: Complications of radiotherapy include hearing impairment, trismus, dysphagia, xerostomia, and temporal lobe necrosis.

Bibliography

American Cancer Society. What are the key statistics about nasopharyngeal cancer? Updated Aug 8, 2016. Available from www.cancer.org/cancer/nasopharyngeal-cancer/about/key-statistics.html. Accessed Sep 9, 2018.

Rosenbaum HE, Seaman WB. Neurologic manifestations of nasopharyngeal tumors. *Neurology.* 1955;5(12):868–74.

Turgman J, Braham J, Modan B, Goldhammer Y. Neurological complications in patients with malignant tumors of the nasopharynx. *Eur Neurol.* 1978;17(3):149–54.

Neck Neoplasms

Epidemiology and Demographics: Neck neoplasms are more common in men after 40 years of age and represent about 3% of all cancers.

Disorder Description: Neck cancers originate from the mucosal surface in most instances and hence are squamous cell carcinomas or their variants. The most common risk factors are chronic tobacco and alcohol use. Neurologic complications can result from direct infiltration of the tumor or due to metastasis. They can also result from medication side effects and paraneoplastic syndromes.

Symptoms

Localization site	Comment
Cerebral hemispheres	Cerebral metastasis: extremely rare, can cause seizure and focal neurologic deficits
Mental status and psychiatric aspects/ complications	Headache and personality changes (frontal lobe syndrome) **Anti-HU encephalomyelitis**: laryngeal carcinoma (paraneoplastic)
Cranial nerves	Dysphonia due to invasion of vagus nerve or recurrent laryngeal nerve
	Dysphagia: invasion of tongue and pharyngeal musculature and X and XII nerves
	Glossopharyngeal neuralgia: invasion of IX nerve
	Multiple cranial nerve palsy from leptomeningeal spread
Plexus	Brachial plexopathy: pain
Peripheral neuropathy	Sensory neuropathy (paraneoplastic): pharynx small cell carcinoma
Neuromuscular junction	Eaton Lambert (paraneoplastic): small cell carcinoma of larynx

Secondary Complications: Nutritional deficiencies such as Wernicke's encephalopathy due to: (1) dysphagia and trismus; (2) anorexia due to malignancy and chemotherapeutic agents; (3) risk factors causing the tumors such as alcoholism and smoking.

Treatment Complications

Surgery:

Chronic pain, reduced range of motion of shoulder, voice changes.

Injury to the cranial nerves during neck dissection: spinal accessory nerve, hypoglossal nerve, vagus nerve and facial nerve.

Horner's syndrome: injury to the sympathetic fibers accompanying carotid artery results in ipsilateral ptosis, miosis, but with preserved facial sweating.

Carotid artery injury.

Radiotherapy:

Cervical cord myelopathy, cranial neuropathy, and brachial plexopathy.

Chemotherapy:

Cisplatin: peripheral sensory neuropathy, ototoxicity, and focal encephalopathy.
5-Fluorouracil: acute cerebellar syndrome.

Bibliography

Clouston PD, Sharpe DM, Corbett AJ, Kos S, Kennedy PJ. Perineural spread of cutaneous head and neck cancer. Its orbital and central neurologic complications. *Arch Neurol.* 1990;47(1):73–7.

Heroiu Cataloiu AD, Danciu CE, Popescu CR. Multiple cancers of the head and neck. *Maedica (Buchar).* 2013;8(1):80–5.

Ruzevick J, Olivi A, Westra WH. Metastatic squamous cell carcinoma to the brain: an unrecognized pattern of distant spread in patients with HPV-related head and neck cancer. *J Neurooncol.* 2013;112(3):449–54.

Neisseria meningitis

Epidemiology and Demographics: Rates of meningococcal disease have been declining in the United States since the late 1990s. In 2015, there were about 375 cases of meningococcal disease reported in total.

Rates of disease are highest in children younger than 1 year, followed by a second peak in those aged 16 through 23 years.

Meningococcal infection displays seasonal variation in attack rates, which are highest in February/ March and lowest in September. Crowding, poor sanitation, and malnutrition make developing countries more susceptible to the spread of infection to epidemic proportions. Nasopharyngeal carrier status, complement deficiency, use of eculuzimab, HIV, and other states of immunosuppression can predispose to infection. In developed countries, age less than 5 years, lower socioeconomic status, freshman year of college, college dormitories, military recruits, black race, and attendees at day care centers pose a higher risk.

Disorder Description: This gram-negative diplococcus is the leading cause of meningitis in children and young adults in the United States. It is also the second most common cause of meningitis in adults. As compared with the other common types of bacterial meningitis (*Streptococcus pneumoniae*, *Haemophilus influenzae*), meningococcal meningitis should be suspected when the course is more fulminant. Delirium and stupor may supervene in a matter of hours. Petechial rash is present in 50%; lividity of the lower extremities and circulatory collapse frequently accompany. Meningitis, however, can occur with or without meningococcal sepsis.

Symptoms

Localization site	Comment
Cerebral hemispheres	Focal cerebral signs are not as common as with the other bacterial meningitides. Collection of purulent material in cerebral fissures can lead to seizures, direct pressure-mediated neurologic deficits, or Todd's paralysis
	Infectious vasculitis with occlusion of surface cerebral veins and consequent cerebral infarction can occur
	Sympathetic sterile subdural effusions are not uncommon in infants; these are sterile but may cause neurologic signs by mass effect
Mental status and psychiatric aspects/ complications	Raised intracranial pressure, probably primarily as a consequence of toxin-mediated edema seems to be the main etiology of the declining level of consciousness
Brainstem	Raised ICP with pressure on brainstem, tonsillar herniation with pressure on the upper cervical cord are complications associated with mortality
Cerebellum	Pressure from herniated cerebellar tonsils on the upper cervical cord can lead to quadriparesis and respiratory failure
Cranial nerves	Cranial nerve palsies are more frequent with S. pneumoniae, where the nerve can be invaded by purulent exudate. Raised intracranial pressure can lead to papilledema with vision changes and lateral rectus palsy. In contrast to the other forms of meningitis, deafness and other enduring cranial nerve deficits are unusual
Pituitary gland	Hypothalamic–pituitary dysfunction is an uncommon complication after bacterial meningitis
Spinal cord	Spinal cord abscess, epidural abscess, polyradiculitis, and spinal cord infarction secondary to vasculitis of the spinal artery
Anterior horn cells	Polyradiculitis has been described
Dorsal root ganglia	Polyradiculitis has been described
Conus medullaris	Conus medullaris syndrome has been described

Localization site	Comment
Unclear localization	Raised intracranial pressure as a consequence of toxin-mediated edema seems to be the main etiology of the declining level of consciousness, and may also lead to papilledema with vision changes, lateral rectus palsy, tonsillar herniation, and death

Secondary Complications: Mortality can approach 5%. The case to fatality ratio for meningococcal disease is approximately 10%, and 11 to 26% of survivors have serious sequelae, including neurologic disability (e.g., focal neurologic deficits, seizures, etc.), limb loss, and deafness.

Acute fulminating cases of meningococcal septicemia (Waterhouse–Friderichsen syndrome) occur mainly in children younger than 10 years of age and are characterized by vomiting, diarrhea, extensive purpura, disseminated intravascular coagulation, cyanosis, convulsions, shock, coma, and often death within hours despite appropriate treatment; many of these cases have meningitis and adrenal insufficiency with hemorrhage into the adrenal glands or adrenal infarction.

Treatment Complications: The US Centers for Disease Control and Prevention recommends routine vaccination with quadrivalent meningococcal conjugate vaccine of adolescents 11 to 18 years of age and vaccination of persons 2 to 55 years of age who have an increased risk of invasive meningococcal disease.

Treatment is straightforward in early cases with antimicrobials; cefotaxime/ceftriaxone are agents of choice. With treatment delay, complications include circulatory shock, purpura fulminans, and disseminated intravascular coagulation (DIC). Intensive care and high mortality are expected in this setting. Fluids should not be restricted unless signs of SIADH (syndrome of inappropriate antidiuretic hormone secretion) or increased intracranial pressure are evident.

Long-term complication of hearing loss may require cochlear implants.

Bibliography

Brandtzaeg P, Ovstebøo R, Kierulf P. Compartmentalization of lipopolysaccharide production correlates with clinical presentation in meningococcal disease. *J Infect Dis.* 1992;166:650.

Centers for Disease Control and Prevention. Meningococcal disease. Updated Apr 9, 2018. www.cdc.gov/meningococcal/index.html. Accessed Sep 9, 2018.

Heckenberg SG, de Gans J, Brouwer MC, et al. Clinical features, outcome, and meningococcal genotype in 258 adults with meningococcal meningitis: a prospective cohort study. *Medicine (Baltimore)*. 2008;87:185.

Julayanont P, Ruthirago D, DeToledo JC. Bacterial meningitis and neurological complications in adults. *SWRCCC*. 2016;4(14):5–16.

Ropper A, Samuels M. Disease of the peripheral nervous system. In *Adams and Victor's principles of neurology*. 9th ed. New York: McGraw-Hill Education/Medical; 2009.

Nemaline Rod Myopathy

Epidemiology and Demographics: Nemaline rod myopathy is not common, with reported rates of 1 out of 50,000 births. There is no sex predominance. There is no specific age of onset. Clinical reports describe a wide spectrum, from severe congenital forms to mild adult-onset forms. There is no clear geographic predominance.

Disorder Description: Nemaline rod myopathy (NRM) is characterized by the presence of thread-like appearing, electron-dense nemaline bodies or rods within myofibers, also seen on modified Gomori-trichrome stain, where the rods would be seen as small, red-staining bodies in the subsarcolemma and perinuclear regions.

NRM is a genetic disorder, with at least 10 identified genes. There are dominant mutations of skeletal muscle α-actin 1 (ACTA1), recessive mutations of nebulin (NEB) genes, muscle specific cofilin 2 (CFL2), troponin T1 slow skeletal type (TNNT1), β-tropomyosin 2 (TPM2), α-tropomyosin 3 (TPM3), kelch-like family member 40 (KLHL40), kelch-like family member 41 (KLHL41), and muscle-specific ubiquitin ligase (KBTBD13) genes, as well as severe and often fatal recessive mutations of leiomodin 3 (LMOD3).

Genetic testing is the mainstay. Electromyography (EMG) can demonstrate early recruitment of small-amplitude, short-duration muscle unit action potentials (MUAPs) in affected muscles. Muscle biopsy is rarely done, but may show type 1 fiber predominance and hypotrophy, but only in congenital/early onset forms, not adult onset forms.

Symptoms

Localization site	Comment
Muscle	Patients present with initial prominent axial and limb-girdle weakness. This can progress to distal muscles. However, distal or predominately lower extremity weakness only has been documented

Secondary Complications: Congenital forms are more prone to scoliosis due to weakness, but can have reasonable mobility, albeit usually at a delayed time frame to normal peers. Some patients do progress to require continuous ambulatory assistance or wheelchairs. Respiratory issues can develop, due to axial weakness, resulting in at least nightly noninvasive respiratory assistance progressing up to ventilation via tracheostomy. Bulbar weakness makes nutrition and communication difficult.

Treatment Complications: Treatment is supportive, with focus on monitoring respiratory function and mobility improvement. There is no cure.

There are no common complications of treatment, save the known risk factors based on a case by case situation from supportive procedures of respiratory or nutrition assistance.

Bibliography

Amato AA, Russell JA. *Neuromuscular disorders*. New York: McGraw-Hill; 2008. pp. 578, 582–583.

Mah JK, Joseph JT. An overview of congenital myopathies. *Continuum (Minneap Minn)*. 2016;22(6):1932–53.

Neuroacanthocytosis

Epidemiology and Demographics: Very rare group of familial disorders. Even distribution between males and females in autosomal forms. McLeod syndrome is X-linked recessive.

Disorder Description: A group of basal ganglionic degenerative disorders with finding of acanthocytes on peripheral blood smear. Although the diseases are grouped together because of characteristic acanthocytes, blood smear is neither specific (acanthocytes can be seen with liver disease or following splenectomy) nor sensitive (often missed with routine smears; yield can be improved by incubation with 1:1 of heparinized normal saline prior to fixation).

The Levine–Critchley syndrome is caused by autosomal recessive mutation in the *VPS13A* gene presenting in early adulthood. The McLeod syndrome is caused by X-linked recessive mutation in *XK* presenting in middle age. Huntington's disease-like 2 (HDL2) is caused by an autosomal dominant mutation in *JPH3* presenting in early adulthood. Pantothenate kinase-associated neurodegeneration (PKAN) is caused by an autosomal recessive mutation in *PANK2* presenting in childhood.[1]

Symptoms

Localization site	Comment
Cerebral hemispheres	Levine–Critchley, McLeod, HDL2 associated with atrophy of caudate nucleus. PKAN has characteristic iron deposition in pallidum visualized as "eye of the tiger" on MRI. Levine–Critchley and McLeod develop as hyperkinetic disorder. Levine–Critchley associated with characteristic tongue protrusion dystonia in which the tongue pushes *out* the food bolus after first contacting it.[2] HDL2 generally presents with chorea, dystonia, and parkinsonism. PKAN occurs in children with dystonia, parkinsonism, and retinitis pigmentosa
Mental status and psychiatric aspects/ complications	Can present as impairment of memory and executive function progressing to psychosis or obsessive-compulsive disorder. Some will initially meet DSM criteria for schizophrenia with both positive and negative symptoms
Cerebellum	Gait instability and dysdiadochokinesia can be present though hard to separate clinically from other concurrent movement disorders
Peripheral neuropathy	Mild axonal neuropathy with clinical findings of areflexia and distal mild sensory-motor neuropathy in Levine–Critchley[3]
Muscle	Mild myopathy that can be hard to detect clinically. Creatine kinase (CK) levels are usually mildly elevated in Levine–Critchley

Secondary Complications: Cardiomyopathy suggests McLeod syndrome, which has characteristic weak expression of Kell antigen on erythrocytes.

Treatment Complications: No specific treatment. Supportive treatment with neuroleptics for psychosis can mask emerging movement disorders. Antiepileptic treatment can also cause cognitive slowing.

References

1. Jung HH, Danek A, Walker RH. Neuroacanthocytosis syndromes. *Orphanet J Rare Dis*. 2011;6:68.
2. Walker RH. Untangling the thorns: advances in the neuroacanthocytosis syndromes. *J Mov Disord*. 2015;8:41–54.
3. Walker RH, Jung HH, Danek A. Neuroacanthocytosis. *Handb Clin Neurol*. 2011;100:141–51.

Neuroacanthocytosis with Abetalipoproteinemia (Bassen–Kornzweig Syndrome)

Epidemiology and Demographics: Incidence less than 1 in a million (rare).

Disorder Description: Caused by autosomal recessive inheritance of mutation in gene encoding microsomal triglyceride transfer protein (MTP) and marked by severe hypocholesterolemia and malabsorption of lipid-soluble vitamins with consequent neurologic injury (particularly from vitamin E deficiency).

Symptoms

Localization site	Comment
Cerebellum	Ataxia and dysmetria usually beginning by second decade
Cranial nerves	Retinal degeneration starting often with loss of night vision progressing to blindness. Ptosis and ophthalmoplegia can also be seen
Syndromes with combined spinal cord and peripheral nerve lesions	Dorsal column dysfunction and peripheral neuropathy from central and peripheral demyelination resulting in loss of proprioception, vibratory sense, and deep tendon reflexes

Secondary Complications: Chronic diarrhea from steatorrhea starting from infancy. Hepatic steatosis and elevated serum transaminase levels can occur. Coagulopathy infrequently occurs.

Treatment Complications: Lifelong treatment with low-fat diet and high-dose oral fat-soluble vitamin supplementation can be difficult to comply with.

Bibliography

Lee J, Hegele RA. Abetalipoproteinemia and homozygous hypobetalipoproteinemia: a framework for diagnosis and management. *J Inherit Metab Dis.* 2014;37:333–9.

Neuroferritinopathy (Hereditary Ferritinopathy, Neurodegeneration with Brain Iron Accumulation)

Epidemiology and Demographics: Neuroferritinopathy is a very rare disease with fewer than 100 cases reported. The prevalence is unknown. The disorder presents in adulthood, usually by the 4th decade, but earlier and later presentations have been observed ranging from early teens to 6th decade.

Disorder Description: Neuroferritinopathy is a progressive neurologic disorder that presents with a movement disorder (chorea or dystonia) in one or two limbs, which progresses to involve other limbs within 5–10 years. The movement disorder then generalizes to include the face and voice, with abnormal speech and facial dyskinesias as well as dysarthria and dysphagia. Cognitive decline accompanies the movement disorder. Cerebellar symptoms can also be seen.

MRI imaging is distinctive among the NBIA (neurodegeneration with brain iron accumulation) disorders and reveals abnormal iron accumulation that progresses to increased signal on T2-weighted imaging followed by cystic change involving the putamina, globus pallidi, caudate nuclei, substantia nigra, and red nuclei.

Neuroferritinopathy is an autosomal dominant disorder caused by truncating mutations in exon 4 of the *FTL* gene, located on chromosome 19.

Symptoms

Localization site	Comment
Cerebral hemispheres	Basal ganglia: iron deposition and cystic change due to neuronal loss involving the putamina, globus pallidi, caudate nuclei, substantia nigra, red nuclei
Mental status and psychiatric aspects/ complications	Frontal/subcortical deficits Disinhibition Emotional lability
Cerebellum	Cerebellar ataxia

Secondary Complications: Poor caloric intake and malnutrition may occur due to difficulty with facial movements.

Contractures and decreased mobility occur due to the movement disorder.

Treatment Complications: The movement disorder can be treated with typical medications for dystonia or chorea, all of which have side effects (levodopa, tetrabenazine, diazepam, clonazepam, botulinum toxin injections).

Bibliography

Chinnery PF. Neuroferritinopathy. Apr 25, 2005. Updated Dec 23, 2010. In Pagon RA, Adam MP, Ardinger HH, et al., eds. *GeneReviews®* [Internet]. Seattle (WA): University of Washington, Seattle; 1993–2016. Available from: www.ncbi.nlm.nih.gov/books/NBK1141/. Accessed Aug 30, 2018.

Crompton DE, Chinnery PF, Bates D, et al. Spectrum of movement disorders in neuroferritinopathy. *Mov Disord.* 2005;20:95–9.

McNeill A, Birchall D, Hayflick SJ, et al. T2 and FSE MRI distinguishes four subtypes of neurodegeneration with brain iron accumulation. *Neurology.* 2008;70:1614–9.

OMIM. Neurodegeneration with brain iron accumulation 3; NBIA3 (606159). www.omim.org/entry/606159. Accessed Sep 9, 2018.

Wills AJ, Sawle GV, Guilbert PR, Curtis AR. Palatal tremor and cognitive decline in neuroferritinopathy. *J Neurol Neurosurg Psychiatry.* 2002;73:91–2.

Neurofibromatosis Type 1 (NF1)

Epidemiology and Demographics: Incidence of neurofibromatosis type 1 (NF1) is 1/2500–3500.

Disorder Description: Autosomal dominant disorder caused by defects in NF1 gene on chromosome 17q11.2, which is a tumor suppressor gene. It encodes for the protein Neurfibromin. NF1 is characterized by central nervous system (CNS) and peripheral nervous system (PNS) tumors and cutaneous manifestations.

Symptoms

Localization site	Comment
Cerebral hemispheres	Megalencephaly leading to macrocephaly
	Unidentified bright objects: basal ganglia and thalamus T2 hyperintensities on MRI; significance of these lesions not known
Mental status and psychiatric aspects/ complications	In children, attention deficit hyperactivity disorder (ADHD), autism spectrum disorders, behavioral abnormalities, and psychosocial issues
Brainstem	**Unidentified bright objects:** brainstem T2 hyperintensities on MRI; significance of these lesions not known
Cerebellum	**Unidentified bright objects:** cerebellum T2 hyperintensities on MRI; significance of these lesions not known
Cranial nerves	**Optic nerve glioma:** progressive deterioration of vision
Pituitary gland	Hypothalamus compression by optic chiasma glioma can cause precocious puberty
Spinal cord	**Dumb-bell tumor:** the intraspinal component may compress the spinal cord to produce bladder and bowel incontinence, sensory level, and paraplegia/monoplegia
Specific spinal roots	Neurofibromas may involve spinal nerve roots causing radicular pain
Peripheral neuropathy	Neurofibroma, plexiform neurofibroma, and malignant peripheral nerve sheath tumors cause pain and mononeuropathy of the involved nerves

Secondary Complications: Vasculopathy leading to hypertension, stenosis, aneurysms, and arteriovenous malformation of cerebral circulation resulting in intracranial hemorrhage and seizures.

Treatment Complications: Permanent residual deficits after excision of the CNS tumor and cosmetic disfigurement after excision of superficial cutaneous tumors. Complications of radiotherapy include transformation to malignant peripheral nerve sheath tumors, development of brain tumors, and moyamoya disease.

Bibliography

Batista PB, Bertollo EM, de Souza Costa D, et al. Neurofibromatosis: part 2 – clinical management. *Arq Neuropsiquiatr.* 2015;73(6):531–43.

Fox CJ, Tomajian S, Kaye AJ, et al. Perioperative management of neurofibromatosis type 1. *Ochsner J.* 2012;12(2):111–21.

Pastar Z, Lipozencić J, Budimcić D, Tomljanović-veselski M. Neurofibromatosis: review of the literature and case report. *Acta Dermatovenerol Croat.* 2006;14(3):167–71.

Neurofibromatosis Type 2 (NF2)

Epidemiology and Demographics: Autosomal dominant disorder occurring in 1/35,000–50,000. Most commonly presents between the ages of 20 and 30 years, but 30% of cases present in childhood.

Disorder Description: Neurofibromatosis type 2 (NF2) occurs due to mutation of the NF2 gene on chromosome 22q, which codes for the protein merlin or schwannomin. NF2 gene is a tumor suppressor gene and hence mutation results in multiple central nervous system tumors. Mutation can be inherited or occur de novo.

Symptoms

Localization site	Comment
Cerebral hemispheres	Meningiomas can cause seizure
Cerebellum	Ataxia secondary to schwannoma and meningioma in the cerebellopontine angle
Cranial nerves	Bilateral vestibular schwannoma (most characteristic) and schwannoma of other cranial nerves with hearing loss, tinnitus, and facial numbness
Spinal cord	Meningioma, schwannoma, and ependymoma occur and cause back pain, sensory loss, and quadriparesis/paraparesis or monoparesis according to the location
Peripheral neuropathy	Peripheral nerve schwannoma causing mononeuropathy
Unclear localization	Ocular manifestation: cataracts, epiretinal membranes, and retinal hamartomas

Treatment Complications: Bevacizumab can cause an increase in blood pressure and bleeding tendencies, and bowel perforation. Complications of stereotactic radiosurgery include facial neuropathy, trigeminal neuropathy, and vestibular dysfunction.

Bibliography

Asthagiri AR, Parry DM, Butman JA, et al. Neurofibromatosis type 2. *Lancet.* 2009;373(9679):1974–86.

Mathieu D, Kondziolka D, Flickinger JC, et al. Stereotactic radiosurgery for vestibular schwannomas in patients with neurofibromatosis type 2: an analysis of tumor control, complications, and hearing preservation rates. *Neurosurgery.* 2007;60(3):460–8.

Pastar Z, Lipozencić J, Budimcić D, Tomljanović-Veselski M. Neurofibromatosis: review of the literature and case report. *Acta Dermatovenerol Croat.* 2006;14(3):167–71.

Neurolathyrism

Epidemiology and Demographics: Neurolathyrism occurs in poor countries, where it is caused by excessive consumption of the grass pea legume (*Lathyrus sativus*). Since the grass pea is drought-resistant, this disease is more common in times of famine. Epidemics have followed famine in Ethiopia (last in 1996), Bangladesh, India, and China over the last century. It is more common in males.

Disorder Description: It is considered a nutritional disorder. The grass pea legume contains the neurotoxin β-N-oxalyl-L-α,β-diaminopropionic acid (L-β-ODAP). This chemical compound acts as a glutamate receptor agonist, eliciting sustained stimulation of AMPA receptors in the spinal cord. This sustained stimulation triggers a signaling cascade of reactions that results in cell death. Clinically, it presents as irreversible acute to subacute extremity weakness that eventually progresses into spastic paresis.

Onset of weakness is typically 3 to 6 months after heavy consumption of the seeds, and progression to spasticity is fast.

Symptoms

Localization site	Comment
Brain	Limited data given prevalence among low socioeconomic status in developing countries
	One study using imaging (n=2) suggests normal cortical motor mapping, corticospinal fibers, supplementary motor area (SMA), and cerebellum
Mental status and psychiatric aspects/ complications	Cognition is unaffected
Spinal cord	Unclear pathogenic mechanism since disease is prevalent only in areas where neuropathology is not possible. Likely due to axonal dysfunction at the spinal level, with relative preservation of the cortical cell bodies
	Affects the lower extremities mainly, and sometimes progressing to involve the upper extremities. Can be asymmetric. No sensory involvement. No sphincter, bowel or bladder involvement
Peripheral neuropathy	Rare, and occurs as distal sensory lower limb neuropathy

Treatment Complications: Supportive treatment with centrally acting muscle relaxants such as tolperisone can be uncommonly associated with exacerbation of muscle weakness or headache.

Bibliography

Bick A, Meiner Z, Gotkine M, Levin N. Using advanced methods to study neurolathyrism. *IMAJ.* 2016;18:341–5.

Ngudi D. Research on motor neuron diseases konzo and neurolathyrism: trends from 1990 to 2010. *PloS Negl Trop Dis.* 2012;6(7):11759.

Tan RY, Xing G-Y, Zhou G-M, et al. Toxin β-ODAP activates integrin β1 and focal adhesion: A critical pathway to cause neurolathyrism. *Sci Rep.* 2017;7:40677.

Neuromyelitis Optica (NMO)

Epidemiology and Demographics: The prevalence of neuromyelitis optica (NMO) ranges from 0.5 to 10 per 100,000. Recurrent NMO is more common in women than men with a ratio ranging from 5:1 to 10:1, respectively. It is more common among African, East Asian, and Latin American populations.

Disorder Description: An inflammatory disorder of the central nervous system caused by immune-mediated demyelination and axonal damage mainly of the optic nerves and spinal cord. Serum NMO-IgG Ab binds Aquaporin 4 antigen (AQP4), a water channel protein found in the spinal cord gray matter, and periaqueductal and periventricular areas as well as at the blood–brain barrier. NMO presents as optic neuritis and/or transverse myelitis. It has a relapsing course and may lead to vision loss. Transverse myelitis or demyelination of the spinal cord usually involves three or more spinal cord vertebrae in NMO. It can lead to bladder dysfunction, sensory loss below the segment of spinal cord affected, and limb weakness. The typical treatment is high-dose intravenous steroids for 3–5 days or plasma exchange followed by starting an immunosuppressive agent such as azathioprine, methotrexate, mycophenolate, or rituximab.

Symptoms

Localization site	Comment
Brainstem	Nausea, vomiting, hiccups
Cranial nerves	Vision disturbance or vision loss
Spinal cord	Sensory loss, bladder dysfunction, limb weakness

Treatment Complications: Steroid therapy can lead to psychosis, confusion, weight gain, hyperglycemia, myopathy, glaucoma, cataracts, osteoporosis, or vertebral fractures.

Plasma exchange complications include anaphylaxis, hypocalcemia, and depletion of immunoglobulins and coagulation factors.

Rituximab can lead to hepatitis B reactivation, JC virus infection, and subsequent progressive multifocal leukoencephalopathy, or death.

Bibliography

Asgari N, Lillevang ST, Skejoe HP, et al. A population-based study of neuromyelitis optica in Caucasians. *Neurology*. 2011;76:1589.

Cabrera-Gómez JA, Kurtzke JF, González-Quevedo A, Lara-Rodríguez R. An epidemiological study of neuromyelitis optica in Cuba. *J Neurol*. 2009;256:35.

Crout T, Parks LP, Majithia V. Neuromyelitis optica (Devic's syndrome): an appraisal. *Curr Rheumatol Rep*. 1999;18(8):54.

Flanagan EP, Cabre P, Weinshenker BG, et al. Epidemiology of aquaporin-4 autoimmunity and neuromyelitis optica spectrum. *Ann Neurol*. 2016; Feb 17. DOI: 10.1002/ana.24617. [Epub ahead of print]

Jung JS, Bhat RV, Preston GM, et al. Molecular characterization of an aquaporin cDNA from brain: candidate osmoreceptor and regulator of water balance. *Proc Natl Acad Sci USA*. 1994;91:13052.

Mealy MA, Wingerchuk DM, Greenberg BM, Levy M. Epidemiology of neuromyelitis optica in the United States: a multicenter analysis. *Arch Neurol*. 2012;69:1176.

Papais-Alvarenga RM, Carellos SC, Alvarenga MP, et al. Clinical course of optic neuritis in patients with relapsing neuromyelitis optica. *Arch Ophthalmol*. 2008;126:12.

Sellner J, Boggild M, Clanet M, et al. EFNS guidelines on diagnosis and management of neuromyelitis optica. *Eur J Neurol*. 2010;17:1019.

Uzawa A, Mori M, Kuwabara S. Neuromyelitis optica: concept, immunology and treatment. *J Clin Neurosci*. 2014;21:12.

Wingerchuk DM. Neuromyelitis optica: effect of gender. *J Neurol Sci*. 2009;286:18.

Neuromyotonia (Isaac Syndrome)

Epidemiology and Demographics: Exact prevalence is not known, but it is not a common disease. There is no sex predominance. Typically, patients are adolescents or adults; most are symptomatic before age 40 years. There is no geographic predominance.

Disorder Description: Neuromyotonia is primarily an acquired disorder, likely autoimmune (close to 80%). There are antibodies against voltage-gated calcium channels (VGKC) on motor nerves, resulting in continuous excitability or hyperexcitability. Neuromyotonia can also be monophasic (possibly post-infectious), relapsing–remitting, or chronic.

Neuromyotonia is sporadic, though reportedly there are some families with autosomal dominant inheritance. Thus, neuromyotonia has three etiologies: acquired (likely autoimmune), paraneoplastic, and hereditary.

Serum and cerebrospinal fluid (CSF) VGKC antibodies may be detected via radioimmunoassay. Autoimmune markers may also be present in CSF, such as increased protein, immunoglobulins, and oligoclonal bands. Nerve conduction studies are typically normal for motor and sensory modalities, though some patients may have a concomitant peripheral neuropathy. The classic finding is of high-pitched abrupt decrescendo neuromyotonic discharges on needle electromyography (though it is not specific, as these discharges have been found in other disorders, such as myasthenia, amyloidosis, etc.). Blocks and neuromuscular blockades will decrease these discharges. Myokymic discharges, otherwise known as grouped fasciculation potentials, as well as fasciculation potentials, doublets, triplets, multiplets, and complex repetitive discharges can also be found.

Symptoms

Localization site	Comment
Mental status and psychiatric aspects/ complications	Confusion, hallucinations, or insomnia
Peripheral neuropathy	Numbness and paresthesias may develop from a concomitant peripheral neuropathy
Muscle	Diffuse fasciculations and myokymia (muscle twitching), muscle stiffness, and cramps. This may result in a stiff posture, with slight trunk flexion, shoulder elevation and abduction, carpopedal spasm, plantarflexion, facial grimacing, as well as flexion of elbows, wrists, hips, and knees. This may be focal or diffuse, and affects more distal muscles rather than axial and proximal muscles. It is non-painful but worsens with voluntary activity, and persists into sleep

Secondary Complications: Due to continuous muscle involvement, there may be excessive sweating, as well as dyspnea, dysphagia, and voice changes. This can all result in weight loss.

Treatment Complications: Immunomodulatory therapy in the form of plasmapheresis, intravenous immunoglobulin, azathioprine, and corticosteroids have been effective for short-term benefit. Botulinum toxin has aided in the short term, blocking the neuromuscular transmission. Anticonvulsants, such as phenytoin, carbamazepine, and gabapentin, as well as antiarrhythmics such as mexiletine aid in decreasing excitability, and reduce or relieve the stiffness, muscle spasms, and pain. Baclofen and other muscle relaxants can aid patients as well with symptomatic therapy.

A common risk of immunomodulation is heightened risk of infections. Complications related to steroid therapy (hyperglycemia, osteoporosis, cataracts, infections, weight gain, steroid-induced myopathy) can develop. Botulinum toxin can cause respiratory dysfunction and toxicity. Phenytoin can cause nystagmus at toxic doses, gingival hyperplasia, agranulocytosis, and anemia, as well as GI side effects. Carbamazepine can cause hyponatremia, agranulocytosis, and anemia. Both antiepileptic drugs carry potential teratogenic risks.

Bibliography

Amato AA, Russell JA. *Neuromuscular disorders*. New York: McGraw-Hill; 2008. pp. 144–56.

Neuro-Ophthalmic Disorders in Pregnancy

Epidemiology and Demographics: Many conditions in pregnancy present with visual symptoms – visual aura in migraines, papilledema in venous sinus thrombosis and idiopathic intracranial hypertension, visual loss from pituitary tumor enlargement, occipital lobe visual changes from pre-eclampsia/eclampsia and posterior reversible encephalopathy syndrome, ophthalmoplegia from Wernicke encephalopathy, ptosis or diplopia in myasthenia gravis, and optic neuritis in multiple sclerosis. These topics are discussed in detail in dedicated sections.

Other neuro-ophthalmic disorders of vascular etiology include diabetic retinopathy, retinal artery occlusion, and pre-eclampsia/eclampsia-related vision changes. A minority of pregnant women (about 10%) experience progression of existing diabetic retinopathy. The risk of stroke is increased during pregnancy and even more so in the puerperium, and can present as retinal vascular occlusion.

No specific time frame associated with pregnancy-related neuro-ophthalmic disease has been identified. Stroke and MS exacerbations are more common postpartum.

Predisposing factors include migraine (visual aura), excessive weight gain (IIH), coagulopathy (venous thrombosis and retinal vascular occlusion), existing pituitary adenoma, hyperemesis gravidarum (B1 deficiency leading to Wernicke encephalopathy), myasthenia gravis, multiple sclerosis, and diabetes mellitus (diabetic retinopathy). The course of gestational diabetes is too short for diabetic retinopathy to develop; therefore, those who are at risk are pregnant women who have underlying long-standing diabetes.

Disorder Description: Pregnancy-associated edema of the lens and cornea can cause refractive errors resulting in myopic shift, and is considered a normal phenomenon. Accumulation of fluid under the retinal epithelium causes a focal retinal detachment that shows as a white subretinal exudate on funduscopic exam. Fluid retention under the retinal epithelium can cause central serous chorioretinopathy. It is a rare condition with an incidence of 0.008% but can be exacerbated by pregnancy.

Central or branch retinal artery occlusion results in ischemia of the retina. On fundoscopy, the retina appears pale. Venous occlusions are more prone to retinal hemorrhage.

Symptoms

Localization site	Comment
Cerebral hemispheres	Posterior reversible encephalopathy syndrome: • Edema of the occipital lobe causes unilateral or bilateral visual field disturbances • Migraine • Patients may experience visual aura such as blurry vision or scintillating scotoma prior to headache onset

Localization site	Comment
Cranial nerves	Idiopathic intracranial hypertension Venous sinus thrombosis: • Papilledema on exam, accompanied by headache, nausea, and vomiting • Multiple sclerosis • Optic neuritis, characterized by loss of color vision (especially red), decreased visual acuity, and pain with eye movement • Multiple sclerosis activity is usually decreased during pregnancy and increased postpartum. If a patient develops optic neuritis during pregnancy, the NMO (neuromyelitis optica) antibody should be checked
Globe	Retinal artery occlusion: • Acute monocular painless vision loss • An afferent pupillary defect may be present • Retinal pallor, and a clot in the retinal artery may be seen on dilated eye exam • Central serous chorioretinopathy • Decreased visual acuity and metamorphopsia

Secondary Complications: Depending on the etiology of the neuro-ophthalmic disorder, the visual disturbance may become permanent if left untreated, such as in retinal vascular occlusion and MS. Other causes like PRES and pre-eclampsia/eclampsia have more severe systemic consequences such as cerebral edema, seizures, and brain hemorrhage.

Treatment Complications: For edema in the cornea and lens and central serous chorioretinopathy, no treatment is necessary. The conditions almost always resolve spontaneously after delivery.

Diabetic retinopathy is best prevented with good glycemic control. Laser photocoagulation can treat proliferative diabetic retinopathy by controlling neovascularization.

For retinal artery occlusion, treatment is similar to that of ischemic stroke. Ocular massage, paracentesis, and carbogen treatment have been used but with little effect on the natural history of the disease. More recently, intra-arterial tissue plasminogen activator (tPA) has become more widely used and may have some benefit if employed within 6 hours of symptom onset. Intra-arterial tPA is associated with a higher rate of systemic and intracranial hemorrhage than intravenous tPA.

Magnesium treatment for the eclamptic angiopathy spectrum can result in magnesium toxicity, whose symptoms include urine retention, hypotension, muscle weakness, and respiratory distress. Calcium gluconate helps reverse the toxicity.

Bibliography

Cugati S, Varma DD, Chen CS, Lee AW. Treatment options for central retinal artery occlusion. *Curr Treat Options Neurol.* 2013;15(1):63–77.

Digre KB. Neuro-ophthalmology and pregnancy: what does a neuro-ophthalmologist need to know? *J Neuroophthalmol.* 2011;31(4):381–7.

Errera M, Kohly RP, da Cruz L. Pregnancy-associated retinal diseases and their management. *Surv Ophthalmol.* 2013;58(2):127–42.

Grant AD, Chung SM. The eye in pregnancy: ophthalmologic and neuro-ophthalmologic changes. *Clin Obstet Gynecol.* 2013;56(2):397–412.

Neuropathies Common to Pregnancy Including Delivery Syndromes and Compressive Neuropathies

Epidemiology and Demographics: The most common acquired neuropathies during pregnancy are Bell's palsy, carpal tunnel syndrome, and compressive neuropathies during labor and delivery.

The incidence of Bell's palsy is approximately 15 per 100,000 without gender predilection. It is estimated to be three times more common in pregnant women (45 per 100,000 births) than in nonpregnant women.

Carpal tunnel syndrome, or median nerve entrapment at the wrist, is more common in women overall and even more so during pregnancy. A wide range of incidence has been reported, but in prospective studies, it is estimated to be about 43%, compared with 1–5% in the general population.

Of peripartum compressive neuropathies, the common peroneal nerve is most commonly affected (81%), followed by the sciatic nerve (15%), and femoral nerve (4%). Ulnar and radial neuropathies, and lumbosacral radiculopathy are rare.

The above neuropathies an occur at any time during and after pregnancy, but particularly during the third trimester, delivery, and immediate postpartum period. Women over 30 years of age are at higher risk.

Excessive weight gain or edema during pregnancy may predispose women to carpal tunnel syndrome or compressive neuropathies. Epidural anesthesia, prolonged labor, lithotomy positions involving extreme hip flexion, external rotation, or abduction of the thigh have been associated with lumbosacral plexopathy and lower extremity peripheral neuropathy. Fetal macrosomia and malpositioning can also cause stretch injury to the plexus, and the use of forceps may inadvertently compress the femoral or obturator nerve against the pelvis.

Genetically, PMP22 deletion is a risk factor of compressive neuropathies, while SEPT9 mutation is associated with pregnancy-related Parsonage–Turner syndrome. Gestational diabetes has not been found to be a risk factor for carpal tunnel syndrome.

Disorder Description: Compression of a peripheral nerve results in neuropraxia, destruction of myelin surrounding the axon (which remains intact), and clinically manifests as focal sensory loss or weakness. This is due to slowed conduction across the site of compression. With time, the axon can degenerate causing denervation and subsequent muscle atrophy, known as axonotmesis.

Altered immunity during the pregnant state is likely related to Parsonage–Turner syndrome and Bell's palsy, but the exact pathophysiology is not well defined. Most cases are idiopathic.

Diagnosis is made clinically, but nerve conduction studies and needle electromyography (NCS/EMG) can be used to support the finding.

Symptoms

Localization site	Comment
Cranial nerve	Bell's palsy • Paralysis of both upper and lower facial muscles. Onset may be painful
Plexus	Lumbosacral plexopathy • L5 dermatome and muscles are usually most affected, which include knee flexion, ankle dorsiflexion, inversion, and eversion Parsonage–Turner syndrome • Also known as brachial neuritis, it is a painful neuropathy at the shoulder that frequently presents with scapular winging, but other nerves can be affected as well

Localization site	Comment
Peripheral neuropathy	Carpal tunnel syndrome • Numbness in the distribution of the median nerve distal to the wrist. Weakness is often detected in the abductor pollicis brevis Sciatic and common peroneal neuropathy • Both can present as postpartum foot drop. However, weakness in both ankle inversion (tibial nerve) and eversion localize the injury more proximally than the common peroneal nerve to the sciatic nerve Femoral and obturator neuropathy • In femoral neuropathy, there is weakness of knee extension (quadriceps muscles) and loss of sensation in the anterior thigh. If the compression is proximal to the inguinal ligament, hip flexion (iliopsoas) is also weak • Obturator neuropathy results in weakness in leg adduction and loss of sensation in the medial thigh Meralgia paresthetica • A purely sensory neuropathy caused by compression of the lateral femoral cutaneous nerve, which results in tingling and numbness of the lateral thigh

Secondary Complications: If the patient has additional symptoms such as pain, edema, and erythema in the vicinity of the suspected nerve compression site, it should raise concern for a hematoma and pelvic imaging (CT or MRI) should be obtained without delay.

Treatment Complications: Treatment is typically conservative as most peripheral and compressive neuropathies resolve postpartum. Rest and avoidance of aggravating positions promote recovery. Persistent symptoms may require splinting or bracing to maintain the nerve in neutral position. Physical therapy is also helpful.

Medical management should only be used for debilitating symptoms during pregnancy since these neuropathies will resolve postpartum. Most pharmacologic treatments have not been proven safe for pregnancy; however, if needed, corticosteroids are effective for Parsonage–Turner syndrome and Bell's palsy. Positive sensory symptoms such as tingling and burning sensation may be treated with anticonvulsants (carbamazepine, gabapentin, phenytoin) or tricyclic antidepressants, but note that many of these medications are FDA category C or D.

Surgical intervention such as carpal tunnel release is usually reserved for severe cases that result in denervation and muscle weakness, and can almost always be postponed until after delivery.

Compressive neuropathies are preventable. Frequent repositioning and prudent use of surgical support systems like stirrups and shoulder straps should be undertaken in every patient. Postpartum sensory loss or weakness warrants a thorough neurologic evaluation, with follow up nerve conduction study and EMG.

There is no risk associated with conservative treatments. Surgery should ideally be postponed until postpartum. Risk of surgery is generally low, the highest rate of complications being incomplete release of the compressed nerve (about 5%).

Bibliography

Bradshaw AD, Advincula AP. Postoperative neuropathy in gynecologic surgery. *Obstet Gynecol Clin North Am.* 2010;37(3):451–9.

Padua L, Aprile I, Caliandro P, et al.; Italian CTS Study Group. Carpal tunnel syndrome in pregnancy. *Neurology.* 2002;59(10):1643–6.

Sax TW, Rosenbaum RB. Neuromuscular disorders in pregnancy. *Muscle Nerve.* 2006;34:559–71.

Yoram C, Lavie O, Granovsky-Grisaru S, Aboulafia Y, Diamant YZ. Bell palsy complicating pregnancy. *Obs Gyn Survey.* 2000;55(3):184–8.

Neuropathy with IgM Binding to Myelin-Associated Glycoprotein (MAG)

Epidemiology and Demographics: The prevalence of IgM monoclonal gammopathy neuropathy is about 5–31% in patients with IgM monoclonal gammopathy. About 50% of patients with IgM monoclonal gammopathy neuropathy have antibodies that bind to myelin-associated glycoprotein (MAG).

Disease Description: IgM autoantibodies target myelin-associated glycoprotein, a cell surface glycoprotein in Schwann cells and uncompacted myelin. This causes a symmetric demyelinating sensorimotor neuropathy, affecting distal more than proximal nerves, which is slowly progressive, usually over years. Sensory symptoms are predominant (earlier than motor); gait disorder; sensory ataxia; difficulty with tandem gait is usually the early sign that is out of proportion to the degree of sensory loss. Weakness develops in 80% (legs and toes). Tremor in hands is also common.

Symptoms

Localization site	Comment
Peripheral neuropathy	• Demyelinating sensorimotor peripheral polyneuropathy with predilection for distal segments of nerves and no conduction blocks • Symmetric, sensory loss and ataxia more than motor • Predominantly distal (legs more than arms) • Neuropathic action tremor

Treatment Complications: Although rare, intravenous immunoglobulin may have risk of hypercoagulability causing stroke, pulmonary emboli, and deep vein thrombosis. Chemotherapeutic agents such as rituximab increase risk of decreased immunity, leukopenia, neutropenia, thrombocytopenia, cardiotoxicity, and pulmonary toxicity.

Bibliography

Katirji B, Kaminski HJ, Ruff RL. *Neuromuscular disorders in clinical practice.* 2nd ed. New York: Springer-Verlag New York; 2014.

Neuropathy with IgM Binding to Sulfatide

Epidemiology and Demographics: This is a relatively rare disease. There is no predilection for either sex. Usually affects individuals over age 50 years. Incidence is unknown.

Disorder Description: This disease is caused by IgM or IgG against sulfatide. Patients may present with numbness in the toes and it slowly progresses to the proximal lower extremities. By the time the numbness involves the knees, the fingertips begin to experience numbness. Other patients may present with walking difficulty and tremor. Still others may present with ataxia and burning pain.

Symptoms

Localization site	Comment
Dorsal root ganglia	Antibodies may bind to dorsal root ganglia
Peripheral neuropathy	Peripheral nerve myelin sheaths

Treatment Complications: Immunomodulators can be tried. Intravenous immunoglobulins may cause headaches, fatigue, or myalgias. Rituximab may cause headache, neuropathy, insomnia, and pain.

Bibliography

Campagnolo M, et al. Polyneuropathy with anti-sulfatide and anti-MAG antibodies: Clinical, neurophysiological, pathologic features and response to treatment. *J Neuroimmunol.* 2015;281:1–4.

Neuromuscular Disease Center. Anti-sulfatide antibodies in sensory-motor neuropathies. http://neuromuscular.wustl.edu/antibody/sulfatide.html. Accessed Aug 31, 2018.

Niacin (Vitamin B3) Deficiency: Pellagra

Epidemiology and Demographics: Niacin deficiency is mostly seen in people in developing countries where corn-based diets are eaten (China, Africa, and India). In the United States, niacin deficiency is found mainly in alcoholics, but it is also found in patients with congenital defects of intestinal and kidney absorption of tryptophan (Hartnup disease) or patients with carcinoid syndrome (in which there is increased conversion of tryptophan to serotonin).[1,2] Isoniazid, a medication used to treat tuberculosis, is a structural analog of niacin and can precipitate niacin deficiency. Other drugs causing niacin deficiency by inhibiting the conversion of tryptophan to niacin are 5-fluorouracil, pyrazinamide, 6-mercaptopurine, hydantoin, ethionamide, phenobarbital, azathioprine, and chloramphenicol.[3]

Disorder Description: Pellagra is characterized by dermatitis, diarrhea, and dementia. The early symptoms may be mistaken for psychiatric disorder due to nonspecific symptoms. Patients complain of insomnia, fatigue, irritability, anxiety, and depression. Initially poor concentration, apathy, and a mild impairment of memory are noticed. Sometimes an acute confusional psychosis can be seen with niacin deficiency.[1] If niacin deficiency is not treated, patients develop dementia. Rash appears initially as a scaly dermatitis in sun exposed skin, followed by hyperpigmentation. Inflammation of mucous membranes causes diarrhea and glossitis. Subacute combined degeneration (posterior and lateral columns) has been described with niacin deficiency. Sensory motor axonal peripheral neuropathy is less common and is difficult to distinguish from neuropathic beriberi.[1,4,5]

An acute cerebral syndrome is described by Jolliffe and coworkers in alcoholic patients consisting of clouding of consciousness, progressing to extrapyramidal symptoms, rigidity and tremors of the extremities, uncontrollable grasping and sucking reflexes, and coma. Most of these patients improved when treated with glucose, saline, and large doses of nicotinic acid.[1,6]

Symptoms

Localization site	Comment
Cerebral hemispheres **Motor cortex (Betz cells)**	Irritability, insomnia, anxiety, depression
	Seizures
	Apathy
	Dementia
	Sometimes acute psychosis
Cerebellum (dentate nucleus)	Gait disturbances
Basal ganglia	Extrapyramidal symptoms, tremors
Spinal cord (dorsal column and lateral column)	Subacute combined degeneration
Peripheral neuropathy	Sensory motor peripheral neuropathy

Treatment Complications: Niacin is used as an antihyperlipidemic agent. It reduces total and LDL cholesterol.[7] Common side effects of niacin are flushing, nausea, vomiting, pruritus, hives, elevation in serum aminotransferases, and constipation.[8] A niacin-induced myopathy has also been described.[9] Caution should be used in patients with a history of gout, since niacin is also known to elevate serum uric acid concentration. Higher doses of naicin can cause hepatotoxicity and gastrointestinal side effects.[10]

References

1. Ropper AH, Samuels MA, Klein JP. *Adams and Victor's principles of neurology*. 10th ed. New York: McGraw-Hill Education/Medical; 2014.
2. Kasper DL, Fauci AS, Hauser SL, et al., eds. *Harrison's principles of internal medicine*. 19th ed. New York: McGraw-Hill Education/Medical; 2015.
3. Wan P, Moat S, Anstey A. Pellagra: a review with emphasis on photosensitivity. *Br J Dermatol*. 2011;164:1188.
4. Bomb BS, Bedi HK, Bhatnagar LK. Post-ischaemic paresthesiae in pellagrins. *J Neurol Neurosurg Psychiatry*. 1977;40:265.
5. Ishii N, Nishihara Y. Pellagra among chronic alcoholics: Clinical and pathological study of 20 necropsy cases. *J Neurol Neurosurg Psychiatry*. 1981;44:209.
6. Jolliffe N, Bowman KM, Rosenblum LA, Fein HD. Nicotinic acid deficiency encephalopathy. *JAMA*. 1940;114:307.
7. Altschul R, Hoffer A, Stephen JD. Influence of nicotinic acid on serum cholesterol in man. *Arch Biochem Biophys*. 1955;54:558.
8. DiPalma JR, Thayer WS. Use of niacin as a drug. *Annu Rev Nutr*. 1991;11:169.
9. Gharavi AG, Diamond JA, Smith DA, Phillips RA. Niacin-induced myopathy. *Am J Cardiol*. 1994;74:841.
10. Vilter RW, Mueller JF, Bean WB. The therapeutic effect of tryptophane in human pellagra. *J Lab Clin Med*. 1949;34:409.

Nightmare Disorder

Epidemiology and Demographics: Prevalence is unknown, but it is more common in children, with an age of onset from 3 to 6 years. Sex predominance is unknown.

Specific personality types may predispose to this disorder. Pharmacologic agents affecting neurotransmitters norepinephrine, serotonin, and dopamine are associated with nightmares. These agents include antidepressants, antihypertensives, and dopamine-receptor agonists.

Disorder Description: Nightmare disorder is characterized by recurrent, highly dysphoric dreams causing significant distress, occurring during REM sleep and often resulting in awakening. Emotions are typically negative and involve intense fear, anxiety, or terror but can also include anger, rage, embarrassment, and disgust. Individuals are typically able to recall details of the nightmare upon awakening. Occasional nightmares are common in children, occurring in 60–75% of children starting as early as 2.5 years of age, but this does not constitute a nightmare disorder.

Few polysomnographies during nightmares are available but can show abrupt awakenings from REM sleep preceded by accelerated heart rate and respiratory rates.

Symptoms

Localization site	Comment
Unclear localization	Unclear but the activation-synthesis hypothesis states that during dreaming the activated brain generates its own information by a pontine brainstem neuronal mechanism

Treatment Complications: Psychotherapy aimed at resolving conflict has been the treatment of choice historically, but little evidence is available supporting its use. Other therapies are available including imagery rehearsal therapy (IRT), a form of cognitive behavioral therapy in which the individual rescripts the nightmare and rehearses the new scenarios using imagery. Exposure, relaxation, and rescripting therapy (ERRT) is another type of cognitive behavioral therapy that is designed for nightmares related to trauma, which combines IRT with exposure and relaxation therapy. Other treatments include lucid dreaming, eye movement desensitization and reprocessing, and hypnosis.

Prazosin, an alpha-1 adrenergic receptor antagonist that crosses the blood–brain barrier, has been used in treatment of nightmares and is thought to work by reducing noradrenergic tone during sleep. Other medications, though not as well studied, are available for use as potential therapy including clonidine, trazodone, and risperidone. Benzodiazepines, though often used, are ineffective in reducing nightmares.

Side effects of prazosin include decreases in blood pressure or dizziness.

Bibliography

American Academy of Sleep Medicine. *International classification of sleep disorders.* 3rd ed. Darien, IL: American Academy of Sleep Medicine; 2014.

Hobson JA, McCarley RW. The brain as a dream state generator: an activation-synthesis hypothesis of the dream process. *Am J Psychiatry.* 1977;134:1335–48.

Krakow B, Hollifield M, Johnston L, et al. Imagery rehearsal therapy for chronic nightmares in sexual assault survivors with posttraumatic stress disorder: a randomized controlled trial. *JAMA.* 2001;286: 537–45.

Nadorff MR, Lambdin KK, Germain A. Pharmacological and non-pharmacological treatments for nightmare disorder. *Int Rev Psychiatry.* 2014;26:225–36.

Nielsen T, Zadra A. Idiopathic nightmares and dream disturbances associated with sleep-wake transitions. In Kryger MH, Roth T, Dement WC, eds. *Principles and practice of sleep medicine.* 5th ed. Philadelphia: Saunders; 2010. pp. 1106–15.

Nitrous Oxide and the Inhalation Anesthetics

Epidemiology and Demographics: Common users are young males/adolescents. No race predilection.

Disorder Description: The inhalation agents are most deserving of the title general anesthetics. They are excellent hypnotics resulting in analgesia and skeletal muscle relaxation. Nitrous oxide, commonly known as "laughing gas," is an inorganic inhalation agent that is colorless, odorless to sweet-smelling, and non-irritating to the tissues.

Symptoms

Localization site	Comment
Cerebral hemispheres	Ischemic encephalopathy (acute), reduction of oxygen resulting in neurologic complications
Mental status and psychiatric aspects/ complications	Euphoria (acute) Amnesia (chronic) Derealization (chronic) Cataplexy (acute) Psychosis (chronic)
Brainstem	Dysregulation of sleep–wake cycle (acute)
Cerebellum	Ataxia (acute)
Pituitary gland	Disruption of the hypothalamus–pituitary–adrenal (HPA) axis (disruption of anterior pituitary hormones) (chronic)
Spinal cord	Paresthesias (acute)
Anterior horn cells	Decrease in muscle (acute)
Conus medullaris	Analgesic effect (acute)
Cauda equina	Analgesic effect (acute)
Specific spinal roots	Analgesic effect (acute)

Localization site	Comment
Plexus	Analgesic effect (acute)
Mononeuropathy or mononeuropathy multiplex	Paresthesias (acute)
Peripheral neuropathy	Peripheral neuropathy (chronic) Polyneuropathy (chronic)
Muscle	Hypotonia (acute)
Syndromes with combined spinal cord and peripheral nerve lesions	Subacute combined degeneration neuropathy secondary to nitrous oxide ("laughing gas") abuse that had affected vitamin B12 activation

Secondary Complications: Indirect effects on neurologic system. Inactivation of vitamin B12 by nitric oxide enzymes causes vitamin B12 dysfunction, resulting in peripheral neuropathy.

Bibliography

Becker DE, Rosenberg M. Nitrous oxide and the inhalation anesthetics. *Anesth Progr.* 2008;55(4):124–31. DOI:10.2344/0003-3006-55.4.124.

Drug Addiction Treatment. Health effects of nitric oxide abuse. www.drugaddictiontreatment.com/types-of-addiction/club-drugs/health-effects-of-nitrous-oxide-abuse/. Accessed Aug 31, 2018.

McCann SM, Kimura M, Karanth S, Yu WH, Rettori V. Nitric oxide controls the hypothalamic-pituitary response to cytokines. *Neuroimmunomodulation.* 1997;4:98–106. DOI:10.1159/000097327.

Shoults K. Case report: Neurologic complications of nitrous oxide abuse. *BCMJ.* 2016;58(4):192–4.

Nocardia

Epidemiology and Risk Factors: In the United States, it has been estimated that 500–1000 new cases of nocardiosis occur every year. The male-to-female ratio is 3:1.

Nocardia species are typically found in standing water, decaying plants, and soil. Infection can occur when soil containing *Nocardia* gets into open wounds or cuts. However, nocardiosis most commonly occurs in the lungs by inhalation of dust containing the bacteria. Central nervous system (CNS) disease is present in approximately 20% of nocardiosis cases and most commonly results from dissemination of infection from a pulmonary or cutaneous site.

Immunocompromised individuals are at risk, but about a third of reported cases are in otherwise healthy individuals.

Disorder Description: *Nocardia* is an aerobic, gram-positive actinomycetes-like bacterium that uncommonly affects humans. In the United States, nocardiosis most often shows up as a lung infection. From the lungs, it can spread to other parts of the body. The brain is the most common site of disseminated infection.

Symptoms

Localization site	Comment
Cerebral hemispheres	The hallmark is development of a brain abscess. In one review of 131 cases of nocardial brain abscess, focal deficits occurred in 42%, nonfocal findings in 27%, and seizures in 30%. The abscesses were multiple in 38%. Mortality is three times higher than that of other bacterial brain abscesses (30% vs 10%) Sagittal sinus thrombosis, hemorrhagic and ischemic infarcts have been described
Mental status and psychiatric aspects/ complications	Mental status changes are as per location of brain abscess and features of raised intracranial pressure. Any part of the brain may be affected, and multiple abscesses can occur. Brainstem involvement and seizures can lead to declining consciousness
Brainstem	Brainstem abscesses have been described
Cranial nerves	Endophthalmitis and subretinal abscess have been reported. Brainstem involvement may lead to other cranial nerve involvement
Spinal cord	Spinal cord abscess and cord compression have been described. Cervical spine abscess can lead to quadriplegia
Unclear localization	Meningitis can occur with or without an associated brain abscess

Secondary Complications: Long-term sequelae of lobar abscess includes functional deficit subserved by the focal region of the brain. Seizures and cognitive impairment may occur.

Treatment Complications: Surgical intervention/aspiration of brain abscess for diagnosis and treatment along with prolonged antibacterial courses are required, traditionally with trimethoprim/sulfamethoxazole and imipenem. If multiorgan failure occurs, amikacin is preferred. Given that subspecies of *Nocardia* exhibit differential susceptibilities, formal antimicrobial susceptibility testing is always necessary to ensure optimal antibiotic treatment. Treatment is protracted for up to a year in CNS nocardiosis. Treatment complications include morbidity of surgery and hypersensitivity to medication.

Bibliography

Anagnostou T, Arvanitis M, Kourkoumpetis TK, et al. Nocardiosis of the central nervous system: experience from a general hospital and review of 84 cases from the literature. *Medicine (Baltimore)*. 2014;93(1):19–32.

Brown-Elliott BA, Brown JM, Conville PS, Wallace RJ Jr. Clinical and laboratory features of the *Nocardia* spp. based on current molecular taxonomy. *Clin Microbiol Rev*. 2006;19:259.

Centers of Disease Control and Prevention. Nocardiosis. Updated Feb 24, 2017. www.cdc.gov/nocardiosis/. Accessed Aug 31, 2018.

Mamelak AN, Obana WG, Flaherty JF, Rosenblum ML. Nocardial brain abscess: treatment strategies and factors influencing outcome. *Neurosurgery*. 1994;35:622.

Non-arteritic Anterior Ischemic Optic Neuropathy (NAION)

Epidemiology and Demographics: The incidence of non-arteritic anterior ischemic optic neuropathy (NAION) increases with age and is estimated at 2.3–10.3/100,000 in the United States. The disease is most prevalent in the 50-year-old and above age group. Women have a slight predominance over men (1.2:1). Caucasians are more affected than all other populations. Comorbid vascular risk factors (hypertension, diabetes mellitus, and hyperlipidemia) are associated with this disease.

Disorder Description: The central retinal artery and the short and long posterior ciliary arteries are the major branches off the ophthalmic artery and are the predominant blood supply to the optic nerve. Anterior ischemic optic neuropathy is characterized by visual loss associated with optic disc swelling and eventual optic disc atrophy. It results from ischemia of the caudal segment of the globe, i.e., the vessels that supply the optic nerve as it exits the eye, resulting in optic disc swelling and subsequent atrophy. This distinguishes AION from posterior ischemic optic neuropathy, in which little to no swelling occurs as the ischemia affects a more posterior segment of the optic nerve. AION is further subdivided into an arteritic and a non-arteritic form. In both, the end result of the ischemia leads to visual loss.

Non-arteritic AION may result from venous insufficiency that occurs when the tributary venules receiving blood from the optic nerve capillaries drain into the central retinal vein posterior to the optic nerve head.

Symptoms

Localization site	Comment
Cranial nerves	Painless visual loss secondary to ischemia to optic nerve, usually first noticed upon awakening. The cup:disc ratio is usually small on funduscopic exam, and the disc is pale and edematous

Secondary Complications: Bilateral visual loss (20% of cases).

Treatment Complications: Treatment of non-arteritic AION is linked to treatment of vascular risk factors such as hypertension and diabetes mellitus. These treatments can lead to hypotension and hypoglycemia. Some advocate for the use of levodopa, though its efficacy in treatment of NAION is controversial. This treatment can be complicated by extrapyramidal side effects.

Bibliography

Johnson LN, Guy ME, Krohel GB, Madsen RW. Levodopa may improve vision loss in recent-onset, nonarteritic anterior ischemic optic neuropathy. *Ophthalmology*. 2000;107:521–6.

Levin LA, Danesh-Meyer HV. Hypothesis: a venous etiology for nonarteritic anterior ischemic optic neuropathy. *Arch Ophthalmol*. 2008;126:1582–5.

Miller NR, ed. Anterior ischemic optic neuropathy. In *Walsh and Hoyt's clinical neuro-ophthalmology*. Vol 1. Baltimore: Williams & Wilkins; 1982. pp. 212–26.

Nonconvulsive Status Epilepticus (NCSE)

Epidemiology and Demographics: Incidence of nonconvulsive status epilepticus (NCSE) varies by age and subtype, and is estimated at around 2–8/100,000. Incidence rate increases with age. In elderly patients (>60 years), rate of 55–86/100,000 reported. In the ICU setting the rate is estimated to be at least 10% of patients. Overall, it has been shown that NCSE accounts for 30–63% of all status epilepticus.

Disorder Description: NCSE is commonly defined epidemiologically as 30 minutes or more of continuous or intermittent electrographic seizures without prominent motor features. Approximately 15% of patients may have nonconvulsive seizures on EEG after clinical cessation of convulsive status epilepticus. May manifest as change in behavior or altered mental state, with bizarre behaviors, language disturbance, perceptual changes, or lethargy and obtundation. NCSE can occur in comatose patients or noncomatose patients. May be accompanied by subtle motor manifestations such as lip and lid twitching or gaze abnormalities.

Electrographically classified as generalized or focal in origin and further subdivided by clinical features or other specific EEG patterns. EEG is essential for diagnosis. Causes include pre-existing epilepsy, acute systemic infection, acute brain injury, inflammatory disorders, and hypoxic–anoxic encephalopathy. The underlying cause is the most relevant prognostic factor for recovery.

Treatments generally include intravenous benzodiazepines as first line, phenytoin and valproate as second line therapies, and levetiracetam, lacosamide, topiramate, barbituates, or other sedative agents such as propofol or midazolam as additional options.

Symptoms

Localization site	Comment
Cerebral hemispheres	Absence, myoclonic absence, or focal status epilepticus. Associated with palpebral myoclonia, limb and oro-alimentary automatisms, dystonic posturing, twitching of the face or limbs, rhythmic nystagmus or gaze deviation
Mental status and psychiatric aspects/complications	Alterations in awareness. Odd confusional behaviors. Amnesia. Psychosis less common

Secondary Complications: NCSE is associated with higher rates of mortality in critically ill patients and may be associated with poorer outcomes for recovery or other cognitive sequelae. Underlying etiology is usually the main indicator of prognosis. Patients with established epilepsy typically have a better prognosis then patients with acute CNS injury.

Treatment Complications: Benzodiazepines are sedating and can cause respiratory depression. Antiepileptic drugs may be associated with a number of idiosyncratic reactions. Phenytoin infusion may induce cardiovascular instability, ataxia, dizziness, frozen glove syndrome, and rash. Valproate side effects include weight gain, hyperactivity, transaminitis, thrombocytopenia, and pancreatitis. The combination of valproic acid and lamotrigine may increase the risk of Stevens–Johnson syndrome. Most common side effect of levetiracetam is change in behavior/agitation.

Bibliography

Fernandez-Torre JL, Kaplan PW, Hernandez-Hernandez MA. New understanding of nonconvulsive status epilepticus in adults: treatments and challenges. *Expert Rev Neurother.* 2015;15(12):1455–73.

Meierkord H, Holtkamp M. Non-convulsive status epilepticus in adults: clinical forms and treatment. *Lancet Neurol.* 2007;6(4):329–39.

Trinka E, Cock H, Hesdorffer D, et al. A definition and classification of status epilepticus: Report of the ILAE Task Force on Classification of Status Epilepticus. *Epilepsia.* 2015;56(10):1515–23.

NREM-Related Parasomnias

Disorders of arousal, which include confusion arousals, sleepwalking, and sleep terrors, are recurrent episodes of incomplete awakening from slow wave (N3) NREM sleep. They usually occur during the first third of sleep with absent or inappropriate responsiveness when others intervene during the episode. There is no or little recollection of the episode.

Obesity Hypoventilation Syndrome

Epidemiology: The prevalence of obesity hypoventilation syndrome (OHS) is unknown; however, it is correlated to obstructive sleep apnea (OSA). The current estimated prevalence of OSA is ~6% of the general population, and it is estimated that 20% of these patients will have OHS.

Disorder Description: OHS consists of obesity sleep-disordered breathing and chronic alveolar hypoventilation during the daytime. The cutoff levels for hypoventilation of these patients are >45 mmHg $PaCO_2$ and PaO_2 <70 mmHg. In most patients the breathing dysfunction during sleep is a form of OSA. In this context it is important to distinguish OHS from severe hypothyroidism, neuromuscular diseases, or Arnold–Chiari type II malformations. The resulting sleep disturbances can result in severe daytime sleepiness and somnolence and the effects of sleep deprivation are seen as well. Complications from increased PCO_2 can be seen also.

Symptoms

Localization site	Comment
Cerebral hemispheres	Hypoxia, increased cranial pressure, thickened speech, incorrect choice of words, CSF acidosis, increased cranial pressure
Mental status and psychiatric aspects/ complications	Fatigue, irritability, difficulty in concentration, sleepiness, memory impairment, cognitive dysfunction
Cranial nerves	Nystagmus, loss of accommodation
Muscles	Tremor of hands

Secondary Complications: Untreated OHS can lead to pulmonary arterial hypertension and worsening hypoxemia. Resulting sleep deprivation will impair cognitive function. Hypersomnolence, and mood and cognitive disturbances are common among these patients. Other consequences of chronic hypercapnia and hypoxemia include risk of respiratory failure and need for hospitalization particularly in association with simultaneous respiratory illness.

In addition, pulmonary hypertension with cor pulmonale, polycythemia vera, and neurocognitive dysfunction may be seen.

Treatment Complications: Treatment includes weight loss, continuous positive airway pressure, and the use of noninvasive ventilation in the form of bilevel positive airway pressure. Other modes of noninvasive ventilation such as average volume assured pressure support also have utility in management of this condition.

Noninvasive positive-pressure ventilation (NIPPV) has many risks including increased infection risk of the upper and lower respiratory tract, increased risks of epistaxis, and increased risk of GI tract perforation. Feeding intolerance is often seen using NIPPV. Pharmacotherapy using medroxyprogesterone can lead to increased risk of venous thromboembolism.

Bibliography

Alchanatis M, Zias N, Deligiorgis N, et al. Sleep apnea-related cognitive deficits and intelligence: an implication of cognitive reserve theory. *J Sleep Res.* 2005;14:69–75.

American Academy of Sleep Medicine. *International classification of sleep disorders.* 3rd ed. Darien, IL: American Academy of Sleep Medicine; 2014.

Engleman HM, Douglas NJ. Sleepiness, cognitive function, and quality of life in obstructive sleep apnoea/hypopnoea syndrome. *Thorax.* 2004;59:618–22.

Engleman HM, Ringshott RN, Martin SE, Douglas NJ. Cognitive function in the sleep apnea/hypopnea syndrome (SAHS). [Abstract]. *Sleep.* 2000;15(23):102–8.

Littleton SW, Mokhlesi B. The Pickwickian syndrome – obesity hypoventilation syndrome. *Clin Chest Med.* 2009;30(3):467–78. DOI: 10.1016/j.ccm.2009.05.004

Mokhlesi B. Obesity hypoventilation syndrome: a state-of-the-art review. *Respir Care.* 2010;55(10):1347–62.

Ropper AH, Samuels MA, Klein JP. The acquired metabolic disorders of the nervous system. In *Adams and Victor's principles of neurology.* 10th ed. New York: McGraw-Hill; 2014. p. 1132.

Obsessive-Compulsive Disorder

Epidemiology and Demographics: In the United States, the 12-month prevalence of obsessive-compulsive disorder (OCD) is 1.2%, and the international prevalence is 1.1–1.8%. Adult females are more frequently affected than adult males, but male children are more frequently affected than female children.

Disorder Description: As stated in the DSM-5, obsessive-compulsive disorder can be defined as:

A. Presence of obsessions, compulsions, or both:

Obsessions are defined as:

1. Recurrent and persistent thoughts, urges, or images that are experienced at some time during the disturbance as intrusive and unwanted, and that in most individuals cause marked anxiety or distress.

2. The individual attempts to ignore or suppress such thoughts, urges, or images, or to neutralize them with some other thought or action (i.e., by performing a compulsion).

Compulsions are defined as:

1. Repetitive behaviors (e.g., hand washing, ordering, checking) or mental acts (e.g., praying, counting, repeating words silently) that the individual feels driven to perform in response to an obsession or according to rules that must be applied rigidly.

2. The behaviors or mental acts are aimed at preventing or reducing anxiety or distress, or preventing some dreaded event or situation; however, these behaviors or mental acts are not connected in a realistic way with what they are designed to neutralize or prevent, or are clearly excessive.

B. The obsessions or compulsions are time-consuming (e.g., take more than 1 hour per day) or cause clinically significant distress or impairment in social, occupational, or other important areas of functioning.

C. The obsessive-compulsive symptoms are not attributable to the physiologic effects of a substance (drug of abuse, medication) or another medical condition.

D. The disturbance is not better explained by the symptoms of another mental disorder (e.g., excessive worries as in generalized anxiety disorder, preoccupation with appearance as in body dysmorphic disorder, hair pulling as in trichotillomania, skin picking as in excoriation disorder, stereotypies as in stereotypic movement disorder, ritualized eating behavior as in eating disorders, preoccupation with substances or gambling as in substance-related and addictive disorder, preoccupation with having an illness as in illness anxiety disorder, sexual urges or fantasies as in paraphilic disorders, impulses as in disruptive/impulse control/conduct disorder, guilty ruminations as in major depressive disorder, thought insertion or delusional preoccupations as in schizophrenia spectrum or other psychotic disorders, or repetitive patterns of behavior as in autism spectrum disorder).

Differential Diagnosis: Differential diagnosis should include anxiety disorders, other obsessive-compulsive and related disorders, eating disorders, tics and stereotyped movements, psychotic disorders, and other compulsive-like behaviors.

In anxiety disorders, the recurrent thoughts are generally regarding real-life concerns, whereas OCD obsessions usually include irrational, odd, or magical content, and compulsions are usually linked to the obsessions in OCD.

In major depressive disorder thoughts are usually mood-congruent (negative thinking) and not necessarily experienced as intrusive or distressing and ruminations are not linked to compulsions as in OCD.

In other obsessive-compulsive and related disorders, there may also be obsessions and/or compulsions. Such obsessions or compulsions are generally limited to a certain context. For example, in trichotillomania, the compulsive behavior is limited to hair pulling in the absence of obsessions. In hoarding disorder, symptoms focus exclusively on difficulty parting with objects.

In eating disorders, obsessions and compulsions are limited to concerns about weight and food.

In tics and stereotyped movements, the occurrences are typically less complex than compulsions and are not aimed at neutralizing obsessions. Whereas compulsions are usually preceded by obsessions, tics are generally preceded by premonitory sensory urges.

It is important to note that there are two neuropsychiatric conditions that frequently present with OCD symptoms as part of their manifestation: Tourette syndrome (TS) and pediatric autoimmune neuropsychiatric disorder associated with streptococcal infections (PANDAS). TS is a childhood-onset neuropsychiatric disorder characterized by multiple motor tics and one or more vocal tics that persist for at least 1 year. The diagnostic criteria for PANDAS include: prepubertal onset; OCD or chronic tic disorder; relapsing–remitting course of the disease; motor hyperactivity or reduced fine motor coordination; onset of the disease or symptoms exacerbation temporally related to streptococcal infections. It is interesting that streptococcal infections have also been suggested to relate to TS. These two disorders warrant the evaluation of all tic disorder patients for OCD and vice versa.

Another association to note is that of OCD and multiple sclerosis. In 2012, a cross-sectional study was done on 112 patients with MS. The frequency of OCD in patients with MS was 16.1%. The conclusion was that OCD might be considered in quantifying disability of MS and suggested that all MS patients be screened for OCD.

In the psychotic disorder delusional disorder, there are no obsessions followed by compulsions, and in schizophrenia and related disorders, there are hallucinations or problems in formal thought processes.

In other compulsive-like behaviors, such as paraphilias, gambling, and substance use, there may be compulsions, but they generally result in pleasure of the individual, distinguishing these occurrences from OCD.

In obsessive-compulsive personality disorder, there are not necessarily intrusive thoughts, images, or urges, or compulsions in response to such obsessions. Instead, obsessive-compulsive personality disorder is characterized by an enduring and pervasive maladaptive pattern of excessive perfectionism and rigid control. OCD and obsessive-compulsive personality disorder are not mutually exclusive diagnoses.

Secondary Complications: OCD can detrimentally impact various domains of life. Excessive time may be spent obsessing and performing compulsions, and may result in tardiness to obligations or missed deadlines. Obsessions about harm may make interpersonal relationships difficult as they may be perceived as dangerous. Obsessions about symmetry may make completion of school or work projects difficult or impossible. Contamination obsessions may result in non-adherence to medication regimens or avoidance of doctors' offices and/or hospitals. Excessive washing may result in dermatologic problems.

Treatment Complications: First line treatment for OCD is selective serotonin reuptake inhibitors (SSRIs).

Refractory cases may be treated with clomipramine (serotonin selective tricyclic antidepressants [TCAs]) or atypical antipsychotics.

SSRI side effects include nausea, diarrhea, insomnia, headache, anorexia, weight loss, sexual dysfunction, restlessness (akathisia-like), serotonin syndrome (fever diaphoresis, tachycardia, hypertension, delirium, neuromuscular excitability), hyponatremia, and seizures (0.2%).

TCAs are highly protein bound and lipid soluble and thus have many drug interactions. They have antihistaminic properties including sedation and weight gain; antiadrenergic properties including orthostatic hypotension, dizziness, reflex tachycardia, and arrhythmias; and antimuscarinic effects including dry mouth, constipation, urinary retention, blurry vision, tachycardia, and exacerbation of narrow angle glaucoma. TCAs are lethal in overdose and thus suicide risk should be carefully assessed. Symptoms of overdose include agitation, tremors, ataxia, arrhythmias, delirium, hypoventilation (secondary to central nervous system depression), myoclonus, hyperreflexia, seizures, and coma. Serotonergic effects are also seen in TCAs including erectile/ejaculatory dysfunction in males and anorgasmia in females.

Atypical antipsychotic side effects include metabolic syndrome, weight gain, hyperlipidemia, and hyperglycemia.

Bibliography

Abramowitz JS, Taylor S, McKay D. Obsessive-compulsive disorder. *Lancet.* 2009;374(9688):491–9.

American Psychiatric Association. *Diagnostic and statistical manual of mental disorders: DSM-5.* 5th ed. Washington, DC: American Psychiatric Association; 2013.

Baxter LR, Phelps ME, Mazziotta JC, et al. Local cerebral glucose metabolic rates in obsessive-compulsive disorder: a comparison with rates in unipolar depression and in normal controls. *Arch Gen Psychiatry.* 1987;44(3):211–18.

Baxter LR, Schwartz JM, Bergman KS, et al. Caudate glucose metabolic rate changes with both drug and behavior therapy for obsessive-compulsive disorder. *Arch Gen Psychiatry.* 1992;49(9):681–9.

Hirschtritt ME, Lee PC, Pauls DL, et al.; Tourette Syndrome Association International Consortium for Genetics. Lifetime prevalence, age of risk, and genetic relationships of comorbid psychiatric disorders in Tourette syndrome. *JAMA Psychiatry*. 2015;72(4):325–33.

Spinello C, Laviola G, Macrì S. Pediatric autoimmune disorders associated with streptococcal infections and Tourette's syndrome in preclinical studies. *Front Neurosci*. 2016;10:310.

Stein DJ. Obsessive-compulsive disorder. *Lancet*. 2002;360(9330):397–405.

Obstructive Sleep Apnea, Adult

Epidemiology and Demographics: In adults age 30–70 years, approximately 13% of men and 6% of women have moderate to severe sleep disordered breathing (Apnea Hypopnea Index [AHI] ≥15). In addition, it is estimated that 14% of men and 5% of women have an AHI ≥5 plus symptoms of daytime sleepiness. This disorder is more prevalent in men, with a ratio of 2:1. However, this difference declines in older age as the risk for obstructive sleep apnea (OSA) is higher in post-menopausal women. OSA is more prevalent in middle-aged men and post-menopausal women.

The major predisposing factors for OSA are excess body weight, morphology (soft tissue and craniofacial structure), and collapsibility of the airway. In addition abnormalities in ventilatory control play a role. Menopause also increases the risk of OSA among women.

Disorder Description: Obstructive sleep apnea is characterized by repetitive obstructions of the upper airway, each episode lasting for a minimum of 10 seconds. Complete obstructions (apneas) or partial obstructions (hypopneas) can result in sleep fragmentation from frequent arousals, intermittent hypoxia, and heart rate variability. Events tend to be longer and associated with more severe oxygen desaturations during REM sleep.

Excessive daytime sleepiness is a common complaint among patients with OSA. Women may also report symptoms of insomnia, mood disturbances, and poor sleep quality.

Diagnosis is made based on diagnostic polysomnography or home sleep apnea testing. Presence of OSA syndrome is defined based on an AHI ≥ 5/hour with symptoms of excessive daytime sleepiness. AHI ≥ 5/hour and < 15/hour constitutes mild disease, AHI ≥ 15/hour and < 30/hour constitutes moderate disease, and AHI ≥ 30/hour is severe disease.

Symptoms

Localization site	Comment
Mental status and psychiatric aspects/ complications	Mood disturbances, including depression, anxiety. Excessive daytime sleepiness and decreased ability to perform complex tasks

Secondary Complications: There is evidence that OSA is an independent risk factor for various comorbidities, including systemic hypertension and diabetes mellitus. OSA is also frequently observed in patients with atrial fibrillation, stroke, and coronary artery disease and may be an independent risk factor for these conditions. The excessive daytime sleepiness associated with OSA puts some patients at risk for motor vehicle accidents as well.

Treatment Complications: Standard therapy for obstructive sleep apnea includes continuous positive airway pressure therapy, which delivers positive airway pressure through a nasal or full face mask to prevent upper airway collapse. Other treatment options include mandibular advancement oral appliance, maxillofacial surgery, and uvulopalatalpharyngoplasty.

CPAP may be uncomfortable for some patients, leading to nonadherence. Some patients might develop central sleep apnea as a result of this.

Maxillomandibular advancement therapy carries the risks of occlusal changes and temporomandibular joint discomfort.

Bibliography

American Academy of Sleep Medicine. *International classification of sleep disorders*. 3rd ed. Darien, IL: American Academy of Sleep Medicine; 2014.

Peppard PE, Young T, Barnet JH, et al. Increased prevalence of sleep-disordered breathing in adults. *Am J Epidemiol*. 2013;177:1006–14.

White DP, Younes MK. Obstructive sleep apnea. *Compr Physiol*. 2012;2(4):2541–94.

Occipital Lobe Epilepsy (OLE)

Epidemiology and Demographics: Occipital lobe epilepsy (OLE) accounts for 2–13% of focal epilepsy syndromes. In benign occipital epilepsies of childhood, age of onset is between 3 and 15 years. Affects both sexes equally.

Disorder Description: Seizure originating from within the occipital lobe. A common feature in OLE is visual phenomena in the early part of seizures. This can include visual auras and/or elementary visual hallucinations, ictal blindness, contralateral eye and head deviation, eye movement sensations, blinking, and eyelid flutter.

Localization on EEG may be challenging due to deep occipital lobe foci, and rapid seizure propagation due to a high degree of functional connectivity. Studies have reported that occipital spike and wave discharges are detected in 17% of patients interictally and 30% ictally.

May occur secondary to cortical malformations, such as dysgenesis or occipital periventricular heterotopias; or due to toxic-metabolic conditions such as reversible posterior leukoencephalopathy. Can present as part of neurodegenerative disorders such as Lafora body disease, myoclonic epilepsy with ragged red fibers (MERRF), and with occipital calcifications associated with celiac disease. Childhood OLE may be genetic in origin, which includes: early onset childhood occipital epilepsy (Panayiotopoulos type), late-onset childhood occipital epilepsy (Gastaut type), and idiopathic photosensitive occipital epilepsy.

Management has improved with high-resolution MRI, careful video-EEG monitoring, and FDG-PET. Intracranial EEG should be performed to localize focus in patients with suspected lesional OLE and refractory seizures. Significant improvement in seizure control with resection of area has been reported in up to 80% of cases. In early childhood occipital epilepsy, seizures spontaneously remit by the end of adolescence and rarely recur.

Symptoms

Localization site	Comment
Cerebral hemispheres	Seizures with elementary visual hallucinations, illusions, blindness, eye movements, blinking, secondary generalization
	Headache in Gastaut type
	Absent visual symptoms, prolonged autonomic seizures (pallor, nausea, salivation) in Panayiotopoulos type
	EEG with occipital spikes

Localization site	Comment
Mental status and psychiatric aspects/ complications	Limited studies evaluating cognitive functions in children with benign occipital epilepsies, showing dysfunction relating to visuomotor coordination, memory, and attention
	Adults with OLE have been shown to have subtle difficulties in processing and mental manipulation of visual spatial data

Secondary Complications: Syncope, emesis in Panayiotopoulos syndrome. Migraines associated with Gastaut type.

Treatment Complications: Postoperative visual field deficits can occur if symptomatic lesions are removed surgically. Carbamazepine is recommended for the idiopathic childhood epilepsies, but may be associated with hyponatremia, leukopenia, transaminitis, and issues such as bone loss and decreased libido in adults.

Bibliography

Piazzini A, et al. Visuoperceptive impairment in adult patients with occipital lobe epilepsies. *Epilepsy Behav.* 2009;15(2):256–9.

Polat M, et al. Neurocognitive evaluation in children with occipital lobe epilepsy. *Seizure.* 2012;21(4):241–4.

Yang PF, et al. Intractable occipital lobe epilepsy: clinical characteristics, surgical treatment, and a systematic review of the literature. *Acta Neurochir (Wien).* 2015;157(1):63–75.

Occipital Neuralgia

Epidemiology and Demographics: There are no epidemiological studies that document the incidence or prevalence of occipital neuralgia. Case reports are limited and involve few patients.

Disorder Description: The hallmark presentation of occipital neuralgia involves paroxysmal lancinating pain that is described as stabbing, shooting, electric, or shock-like. The pain originates in the occiput and radiates to the vertex. A dull aching pain can persist between these exacerbations. Symptoms are associated with allodynia of the scalp in the distribution of the nerve (C2, C3 branches). The etiology of this condition is unknown and is considered to be idiopathic.

Symptoms

Localization site	Comment
Spinal cord	Involvement of dermatomes and nerves from the branches of cervical roots 2 and 3

Treatment Complications: Symptomatic management is standard of care (massage, physical therapy, warm or cold compresses). However, antiepileptic drugs have been used with success in reducing frequency and severity of attacks. These drugs have not been studied extensively. Occipital nerve block is also a consideration but small case reports show that the pain returns, with average length of relief of 31 days.

Bibliography

Afridi SK, Shields KG, Bhola R, Goadsby PJ. Greater occipital nerve injection in primary headache syndromes: prolonged effects from a single injection. *Pain*. 2006;122:126–9.

Dougherty C. Occipital neuralgia. *Curr Pain Headache Rep*. 2014;18:411.

Hammond SR, Danta G. Occipital neuralgia. *Clin Exp Neurol*. 1978;15:258–70.

Oculogyric Crisis

Epidemiology and Demographics: Oculogyric crisis makes up about 6% of all myo-dystonic reactions to medications. It is the most common of ocular dystonic reactions and is likely underreported.

Disorder Description: Oculogyric crisis is a dystonic reaction involving the upward deviation of the eyes, in response to medication or medical conditions. Drugs that may cause oculogyric crisis include antipsychotics, metoclopramide, carbamazepine, and lithium, the most common mechanism being D2-receptor antagonism. This is usually very uncomfortable and described as being painful.

Epilepsy may manifest as "oculogyric seizures" and should be considered in a case of oculogyric crisis.

Secondary Complications: Because oculogyric crisis is usually in response to medications, and in particular antipsychotic medications, a mood or psychotic disorder is often comorbid. Other dystonic reactions that often coexist with oculogyric crisis include torticollis and blepharospasm. Dystonic reactions can be life-threatening if they involve the airway (laryngospasm) or diaphragm. Additional extra-pyramidal side effects that can be seen with neuroleptic drugs include Parkinsonism (bradykinesia, cogwheel rigidity, pill-rolling tremor, and bradykinesia) and akathisia (an uncomfortable, subjective sense of restlessness that may manifest as fidgeting).

Treatment Complications: Treatments for acute dystonic reactions include benztropine and diphenhydramine (anticholinergics), anti-Parkinson's agents (L-dopa), and muscle relaxants (clonazepam).

Anticholinergic side effects include dry mouth, blurred vision, constipation, drowsiness, urinary retention, altered mental status, and hallucinations. L-dopa may cause dyskinesia, bradykinesia, syncope, depression, suicidal ideation, hallucinations, psychosis, dizziness, headache, anxiety, depression, mood changes, and compulsive behaviors. Clonazepam may cause respiratory depression, dependency/abuse, seizures, suicidality, syncope, central nervous system stimulation, impaired coordination, dizziness, depression, fatigue, dysarthria, amnesia, impaired concentration, disinhibition, libido changes, irritability, and diplopia.

Bibliography

American Psychiatric Association. *Diagnostic and statistical manual of mental disorders: DSM-5*. 5th ed. Washington, DC: American Psychiatric Association; 2013.

FitzGerald PM, Jankovic J. Tardive oculogyric crises. *Neurology*, 1989;39(11):1434.

Lee MS, Kim YD, Lyoo CH. Oculogyric crisis as an initial manifestation of Wilson's disease. *Neurology*. 1999;52(8):1714–5.

Leigh RJ, Foley JM, Remler BF, Civil RH. Oculogyric crisis: a syndrome of thought disorder and ocular deviation. *Ann Neurol*. 1987;22(1):13–17.

Ohtahara Syndrome (Early Infantile Epileptic Encephalopathy, EIEE)

Epidemiology and Demographics: Early infantile epileptic encephalopathy (EIEE) is one of the earliest presenting epileptic encephalopathies. Typically, the syndrome develops within the first few weeks to months of infancy.

Disorder Description: Presentation consists of the rapid development of tonic spasms lasting up to 10 seconds, up to hundreds of times per day. Many patients will die during infancy; those who survive typically have significant cognitive and motor impairment, often with difficult to control epilepsy.

The electroencephalogram consists of a pattern of bursts of high-amplitude spikes and polyspikes coincident with the tonic seizures, followed by periods of EEG suppression (burst suppression pattern).

There is a wide range of potential causes including associations with various gene mutations.

Antiepileptic drugs (AEDs) and adrenocorticotropic hormone (ACTH) are the primary treatments.

Symptoms

Localization site	Comment
Cerebral hemispheres	Tonic seizures at onset. Other types may occur, and syndrome may evolve into others as the patient ages. EEG shows burst suppression at onset. Associated with a wide range of brain structural abnormalities on MRI involving the cerebral cortices
Mental status and psychiatric aspects/ complications	Severe intellectual disability common

Treatment Complications: AEDs may be associated with cognitive impairment, ataxia, dizziness, and more rarely severe allergic reactions, liver failure, or pancreatitis. ACTH may be associated with changes in blood pressure and glycemic control, and an increased risk of infection.

Bibliography

Beal JC, Cherian K, Moshe SL. Early-onset epileptic encephalopathies: Ohtahara syndrome and early myoclonic encephalopathy. *Pediatr Neurol.* 2012;47(5):317–23.

Oligodendroglioma

Epidemiology and Demographics: Accounts for up to 25% of all diffuse gliomas, 2-4% of all the primary central nervous system (CNS) neoplasias, and 6% of the CNS tumors in children. Typically occurs from 40 to 65 years of age; more frequent in males compared with females (2:1). No difference among the races.

Disorder Description: An infiltrative neoplasm arising from the glial system, demonstrating features of the oligodendroglia, commonly located in the cerebral hemispheres, extremely rare in the brainstem, and less than 1.5% will localize in the spinal cord. It was initially defined and diagnosed by histology; however, with the 2016 update of the *World Health Organization (WHO) classification of CNS tumors*, the diagnosis currently requires the demonstration of the IDH (isocitrate dehydrogenase) gene family mutation and the 1p/19q co-deletion. In the setting of non-available molecular testing or inconclusive genetic results, a histologically typical oligodendroglioma should be diagnosed as "not otherwise specified" (NOS). The WHO classification includes: oligodendroglioma WHO grade II – anaplastic oligodendroglioma WHO III (IDH-mt, 1p19q co-deleted) and oligodendroglioma NOS – anaplastic oligodendroglioma NOS (IDH-mt, 1p19q co-deleted *indeterminate*).

Symptoms

Localization site	Comment
Cerebral hemispheres	Often superficial with extension to the cortex and subcortical white matter (corticomedullary junction), frontal lobes > parietal > temporal. The overall clinical presentation will be determined by the location of the tumor. Focal neurologic deficits, signs of increased intracranial pressure: severe headaches, vomiting, papilledema, more than 75% will present with seizure either generalized tonic–clonic or focal complex seizures
Mental status and psychiatric aspects/ complications	These conditions may be present prior to the oligodendroglioma, potentially causing delay in diagnosis, or the tumor may simulate these symptoms/conditions resulting in the etiology being overlooked or misdiagnosed: psychosis, mania, depression, anxiety, delirium, schizophrenia, anorexia nervosa, cognitive dysfunction
Brainstem, cerebellum	Although described as a clinical surprise, there is a handful of cases in the literature; more frequent in children, presenting with nausea, vomiting, dysphagia, dysarthria, diplopia, ataxia, altered mental status including coma
Spinal cord	Urinary retention, constipation, sensorimotor deficits (weakness, pain)

Secondary Complications: Permanent neurologic impairment associated with location of the mass, hydrocephalus, blindness, herniation, epilepsy, aphasia, apraxia, ataxia, genitourinary dysfunction, coma, death.

Treatment Complications

- Temozolomide: nausea, vomiting, diarrhea, transaminitis, pancytopenia, infertility.
- PCV:
  - *P*rocarabazine: hypertensive crises, irreversible peripheral neuropathy
  - Lomustine (also called *C*CNU): thrombocytopenia-bleeding diathesis, leukopenia, blindness, pulmonary toxicity, nephrotoxicity
  - *V*incristine: peripheral neuropathy, constipation, alopecia
- Radiation therapy: anorexia, pancytopenia, bleeding diathesis, infections, fatigue, weakness, weight loss.

Bibliography

Alvarez JA, Cohen ML, Hlavin ML. Primary intrinsic brainstem oligodendroglioma in an adult. *J Neurosurg.* 1996;85(6):1165–9. DOI:10.3171/jns.1996.85.6.1165.

Bunevicius A, Deltuva VP, Deltuviene D, Tamasauskas A, Bunevicius R. Brain lesions manifesting as psychiatric disorders: eight cases. *CNS Spectr.* 2008;13(11):950–8.

Hodges SD, Malafronte P, Gilhooly J, et al. Rare brainstem oligodendroglioma in an adult patient: Presentation, molecular characteristics and treatment response. *J Neurol Sci.* 2015;355 (1-2):209–10. DOI:10.1016/j.jns.2015.05.019.

Lachi PK, Irrakula M, Ahmed SF, et al. Clinical profile and outcomes in brainstem glioma: An institutional experience. *Asian J Neurosurg.* 2015;10(4):298–302. DOI:10.4103/1793-5482.162709.

Mohindra S, Savardekar A, Bal A. Pediatric brainstem oligodendroglioma. *J Neurosci Rural Pract.* 2012;3(1):52–4. DOI:10.4103/0976-3147.91940.

Onchocerciasis

Epidemiology and Demographics: Transmitted through repeated bites of the Simulium blackfly. The main burden is in sub-Saharan Africa, and in limited areas in the Americas and Yemen. The World Health Organization (WHO) estimates that at least 25 million people are infected with *Onchocerca volvulus* worldwide; of these people, 300,000 are blind and 800,000 have some sort of visual impairment.

Usually, many bites are needed before being infected, so people who travel for short periods of time (generally less than 3 months) to affected areas have a low chance of becoming infected with *O. volvulus.*

Disorder Description: Onchocerciasis, or river blindness, is a neglected tropical disease caused by the parasitic worm *Onchocerca volvulus.* Some people do not experience symptoms, but many do, which include itchy skin rashes, nodules under the skin, and vision changes. The inflammation caused by larvae that die in the eye results in blindness.

Symptoms

Localization site	Comment
Cerebral hemispheres	Nodding syndrome is an epileptic disorder of unknown etiology that occurs in children in East Africa in association with onchocerciasis. It causes progressive cognitive dysfunction, neurologic deterioration, stunted growth, and a characteristic nodding of the head
Mental status and psychiatric aspects/complications	The treatment of onchocerciasis with ivermectin can lead to encephalopathy, particularly when there is co-infection with *Loa loa* Probable *Loa loa* Encephalopathy Temporally Related to Mectizan Treatment (PLERM) is defined as: coma (without seizures, usually with fever) occurring in a previously healthy person with no other underlying cause for the coma – onset of progressive disturbances of the central nervous system within 5 days of treatment with ivermectin, without remission; and post-treatment blood smear showing >10,000 *L. loa* microfilariae per milliliter (mf/mL), and/or CSF testing positive for *L. loa* microfilariae
Cranial nerves	Leading cause of blindness in endemic areas
Dorsal root ganglia	Onchocercal itch and its neurologic basis is an area of investigation. The itching is caused by the presence of the parasites in subcutaneous tissues, but further potentiation and the disabling nature of the itch may have another basis as well, which is presently poorly understood

Treatment Complications: The treatment of onchocerciasis with ivermectin can lead to encephalopathy, particularly when there is co-infection with *Loa loa*. This clinical entity (PLERM) is described in the table above.

Bibliography

Centers for Disease Control and Prevention. Parasites – Onchocerciasis (also known as river blindness). Aug 10, 2015. www.cdc.gov/parasites/onchocerciasis/index.html. Accessed Sep 2, 2018.

Johnson T, Tyagi R, Lee P, et al. Nodding syndrome may be an autoimmune reaction to the parasitic worm Onchocerca volvulus. *Sci Transl Med.* 2017;9(377):eaaf6953.

Njamnshi A, Bisseck AZ, Etya'ale D. Onchocerciasis: neurological involvement. In Bentivoglio M, Cavalheiro E, Kristensson K, Patel N, eds. *Neglected tropical diseases and conditions of the nervous system.* New York, NY: Springer; 2014. pp. 147–64.

Twum-Danso NA, Meredith S. Variation in incidence of serious adverse events after onchocerciasis treatment with ivermectin in areas of Cameroon co-endemic for loiasis. *Trop Med Int Health.* 2003;8(9):820–31.

WHO. Signs, symptoms and treatment of onchocerciasis. www.who.int/onchocerciasis/symptoms/en/. Accessed Sep 2, 2018.

Ophthalmoplegic Migraine

Epidemiology and Demographics: A rare, episodic condition mostly seen in children, with average age of onset at 10 years. There are exceptionally rare cases of this condition occurring during infancy. Although this condition occurs in adults, the child and adult versions are largely considered to be the same.

Disorder Description: This condition is defined as at least two attacks of migraine headaches associated with cranial nerve III, IV, and/or VI neuropathy. Imaging studies should not reveal any parasellar orbital fissure or posterior fossa lesion.

Symptoms

Localization site	Comment
Cerebral hemispheres	Many studies reveal transient enhancement of cranial nerve III root on imaging. Other studies suggest breakdown of blood–brain barrier and associated vasospasm as etiology of symptoms
Cranial nerves	Other studies suggest involvement of trigeminal nerve as triggering migraine symptoms

Secondary Complications: There are usually no secondary complications. Most studies reveal that these headaches resolve spontaneously. The longest duration of headache symptoms on record is 84 days.

Treatment Complications: Symptoms resolve spontaneously; abortive treatment is rarely used.

Bibliography

Ambrosetto P, Nicolini F, Zoli M, et al. Ophthalmoplegic migraine: from questions to answers. *Cephalalgia.* 2014;34(11):914–19.

Daroff RB. Ophthalmoplegic migraine. *Cephalalgia.* 2001;21:81.

Friedman A, Harter D, Merritt H. Ophthalmoplegic migraine. *Arch Neurol.* 1962;7:320–7.

Lal V. Ophthalmoplegic migraine: Past, present and future. *Neurol India.* 2010;58:15–19.

Opioid Intoxication

Epidemiology and Demographics: Males 18 years of age and older are the biggest abusers of medication. No race predilection.

Disorder Description: Includes morphine, heroin, oxycodone, and synthetic (man-made) opioid narcotics. Common occurrence in the United States; 22 million worldwide. Opioids can be administered intravenously, subcutaneously, intranasally, orally, or by inhaling. The various effects on the human body are indicated below.

Symptoms

Localization site	Comment
Cerebral hemispheres	Cerebral ischemia (acute)
Mental status and psychiatric aspects/complications	Confusion (acute)
	Delirium (acute)
	Anxiety (acute)
	Irritability (acute)
	Euphoria (acute)
Brainstem	Insomnia (acute)
Cranial nerves	Miosis (acute)
Pituitary gland	Dysregulation of hypothalamus–pituitary–adrenal axis: growth hormone/prolactin

Localization site	Comment
Spinal cord	Spinal analgesia (acute)
Specific spinal roots	Spinal analgesia (acute)
Plexus	Spinal analgesia (acute)
Mononeuropathy or mononeuropathy multiplex	Analgesic effects (acute)
Peripheral neuropathy	Analgesic effects (acute)
Muscle	Tremors (acute)
	Myalgia (acute)
	Rhabdomyolysis (acute)
Neuromuscular junction	Dysregulation of the dopamine receptors (chronic)

Secondary Complications

Complications that indirectly affect the nervous system via:

Cardiovascular complications: dysrhythmias resulting in strokes.

Respiratory complications: acute respiratory distress syndrome results in cerebral hypoxia.

Hepatic complications: liver failure resulting in hepatic encephalopathy.

Gastric complications: gastric dysmotility from narcotic bowel syndrome can result in metabolic encephalopathy.

Renal complications: renal failure resulting from rhabdomyolysis can result in uremic encephalopathy.

Treatment Complications

Complications of detoxification are those of opiate withdrawal (see entry for *Opiate Withdrawal*). Methadone may acutely cause sedation, euphoria, a "drug high," or insomnia. Longer term use has been associated with impaired cognition.

Buprenorphine may cause sedation and other potential opiate-related symptoms. The opioid naltrexone may cause mood changes, hallucinations, insomnia, anxiety, and other opiate withdrawal symptoms.

Clonidine, which may be used to treat anxiety and agitation associated with heroin abuse, may cause sedation or rarely induce altered mentation and hallucinations.

Bibliography

Delta Medical Center. Opioid abuse signs, symptoms and effects. www.deltamedcenter.com/addiction/opiates/effects-symptoms-signs. Accessed Sept 2, 2018.

Hazelden Betty Ford Foundation. Signs of addiction. www.hazeldenbettyford.org/articles/addictive-substances-effects-and-withdrawal-symptoms. Accessed Sept 2, 2018.

Narconon. What parts of the body may be severely damaged by painkiller abuse? www.narconon.org/drug-abuse/prescription/painkillers/body-damage.html. Accessed Sept 2, 2018.

Symptoma. Opioid withdrawal. www.symptoma.com/en/info/opioid-withdrawal. Accessed Sept 2, 2018.

Opioid Withdrawal

Epidemiology and Demographics: Men aged 18 years and over are common users.

Disorder Description: Around 26.4 million and 36 million people around the globe abuse opioid drugs. Opioid drugs can cause physical dependence in humans. The list of drugs consists of codeine, morphine, heroin, meperidine, hydrocodone, methadone, and hydromorphone.

Opioid withdrawal symptoms can start from hours after last dose and last for months. Symptoms include:

- Nausea
- Muscle cramping
- Depression
- Agitation
- Anxiety
- Opiate cravings

Symptoms

Localization site	Comment
Cerebral hemispheres	Withdrawal-induced neuronal activation occurs in lateral and ventrolateral columns of neurons, and particularly the caudal ventrolateral periaqueductal gray matter
Mental status and psychiatric aspects/complications	Depression (acute) Anxiety (acute)

Localization site	Comment
Cranial nerves	Mydriasis (chronic)
Muscle	Muscle cramping
Neuromuscular junction	GABA receptor dysregulation

Treatment Complications: Methadone may acutely cause sedation, euphoria, a "drug high" or insomnia. Longer term use has been associated with impaired cognition.

Buprenorphine may cause sedation and other potential opiate-related symptoms. The opioid naltrexone may cause mood changes, hallucinations, insomnia, anxiety, and other opiate withdrawal symptoms.

Clonidine, which may be used to treat anxiety and agitation associated with opiate withdrawal, may cause sedation or rarely induce altered mentation and hallucinations.

Bibliography

American Addiction Centers. Opioid withdrawal timelines. http://americanaddictioncenters .org/withdrawal-timelines-treatments/opiate/. Accessed Sep 9, 2018.

Compton WM, Yolkow ND. Abuse of prescription drugs and the risk of addiction. *Drug Alcohol Depend.* 2006;83(Suppl 1): S4–S7.

NIH. Opiate and opioid withdrawal. Update Aug 14, 2018. https://medlineplus.gov/ency/ article/000949.htm. Accessed Sep 9, 2018.

Optic Atrophy

Epidemiology and Demographics: Optic atrophy can affect all races/ethnicities of either sex at any age.

Disorder Description: Optic atrophy is an examination finding (i.e., optic disc pallor). Occasionally it can be seen as decreased optic nerve caliber on orbital or neuro-imaging. Optic atrophy reflects chronic injury to the optic nerve and takes 2–3 months to develop following the initial injury. It does not indicate the cause of the injury. Pattern of vision loss, history of visual symptoms, and associated current or past symptoms guide the differential diagnosis.

Symptoms

Localization site	Comment
Vestibular system (and nonspecific dizziness)	Diabetes insipidus, diabetes mellitus, optic atrophy, and deafness (DIDMOAD) is a progressive inherited condition most often inherited in an autosomal recessive pattern
Base of skull	Lesions of the skull base or dura, such as meningiomas, metastatic disease, fibrous dysplasia, sinus mucoceles, and pachymeningitis can cause optic neuropathy and eventually optic atrophy through compression of the intracranial optic nerve. There can be associated cranial neuropathies, but the optic nerves can be affected in isolation. Vascular compression by aneurysm or ectatic carotid artery can cause optic nerve compression
Cranial nerves	Prior intrinsic optic nerve diseases with incomplete recovery often develop optic atrophy. These include non-arteritic ischemic optic neuropathy, ischemic optic neuropathy due to giant cell arteritis, optic neuritis, other inflammatory optic neuropathy, infectious optic neuropathy, vitamin/mineral deficiency (e.g., B12, copper), traumatic injury, and inherited optic neuropathies such as dominant optic atrophy and Leber hereditary optic neuropathy
	Inflammatory, infectious, or neoplastic processes affecting the subarachnoid space can cause compression of the optic nerve within the optic nerve sheath. If this is a distributed process there may be associated meningeal symptoms. However, focal processes can affect the optic nerves in isolation
Pituitary gland	Pituitary adenoma and other suprasellar masses can compress the optic chiasm and lead to optic atrophy. These can affect the neighboring cavernous sinuses, impacting CN III, IV, V1, and V2 within them to cause extraocular movement limitations, diplopia, and facial numbness
Spinal cord	Dorsal column symptoms associated with optic atrophy raise suspicion for a nutritional cause such as vitamin B12 or copper deficiency
Muscle	Enlarged extraocular muscles, for example from thyroid orbitopathy or orbital myositis, can compress the optic nerves. These can be associated with ocular motility limitations
Unclear localization	Mass lesions in the orbit can also cause compression of the optic nerve with or without orbital signs and symptoms

Secondary Complications: Visual hallucinations can occur in the setting of bilateral vision loss from any cause, including optic atrophy due to "release" of deafferented visual system. Patients typically have insight into these.

Bibliography

Lee AG, Chau FY, Golnik KC, Kardon RH, Wall M. The diagnostic yield of the evaluation for isolated unexplained optic atrophy. *Ophthalmology*. 2005;112(5):757–9.

Van Stavern GP, Newman NJ. Optic neuropathies. An overview. *Ophthalmol Clin North Am*. 2001;14(1):61–71.

Optic Glioma

Epidemiology and Demographics: These tumors can grow in various parts of the optic tract (one or both optic nerves, optic chiasm, etc.), and they have the potential to spread along these pathways. Most of these tumors occur in children under the age of 10 years.

Disorder Description: Grade I pilocytic astrocytoma and grade II fibrillary astrocytoma are the most common tumors affecting these structures. Higher-grade tumors may also arise in these locations. Although the cause is unknown, optic glioma has been linked to neurofibromatosis Type 1. Grade I pilocytic astrocytomas are the more common. They have also been known to grow along with hypothalamic gliomas.

Symptoms

Localization site	Comment
Mental status and psychiatric aspects/complications	Vary from mild to severe; memory deficit, daytime sleeping, loss of appetite, memory deficits, depression, anorexia with loss of appetite and body fat
Cranial nerves	Symptoms due to tumor growing and pressing on optic nerves and nearby structures: Involuntary eyeball movement, outward bulging of one or both eyes, squinting, vision loss in one or both eyes that starts with loss of peripheral vision and ultimately complete blindness. Strabismus
Cerebral hemispheres	Diencephalic syndrome
Base of skull	Hormonal disturbances: delayed growth, loss of appetite

Treatment Complications: Radiation therapy side effects such as localized brain edema. Chemotherapy systemic adverse events such as depressed immune status and risk of superimposed infections.

Bibliography

Parsa CF, Hoyt CS, Lesser RL, et al. Spontaneous regression of optic gliomas: thirteen cases documented by serial neuroimaging. *Arch Ophthalmol*. 2001;119(4):516–29.

Optic Neuritis (Demyelinating Optic Neuritis, Optic Nerve Inflammation)

Epidemiology and Demographics: Demyelinating optic neuritis newly affects 1–5/100,000 individuals annually. It affects females three times more often than males and most commonly occurs in the 4th decade of life. It is more common in the northern United States and Western Europe. Age of onset is typically between 20 and 40 years.

Disorder Description: Optic neuritis refers to inflammation of the optic nerve. In this entry we use the term to exclusively refer to demyelinating optic neuritis of the type associated with neuromyelitis optica or multiple sclerosis (MS). Classically this presents with unilateral vision loss associated with pain on eye movements. The natural history is nadir of vision loss within 7 days and gradual improvement starting within 30 days, with over 80% of patients recovering excellent vision in the affected eye.

Sometimes optic neuritis is used more broadly to refer to any inflammatory or infectious optic neuropathy. Inflammatory causes can include sarcoidosis, lupus, and sinusitis-associated. Infectious causes can include *Bartonella henselae*, Lyme disease, syphilis, toxoplasmosis, and tuberculosis.

Patients usually complain of pain on eye movement. It follows an acute to subacute course. More than half of patients will develop further demyelinating disease and MS within 5 years. For patients who do not develop MS, the cause may be postinfectious. Oral steroids may increase relapse of optic neuritis, so intravenous steroids are the treatment of choice as they may quicken recovery.

Symptoms

Localization site	Comment
Cerebral hemispheres	Concurrent or previous symptoms localizing to the cerebral hemispheres raise suspicion for MS
Mental status and psychiatric aspects/ complications	Concurrent or previous symptoms of mental status changes or psychiatric disturbance raise suspicion for MS
Brainstem	Concurrent or previous symptoms localizing to the brainstem raise suspicion for MS
Cerebellum	Concurrent or previous symptoms localizing to the cerebellum raise suspicion for MS
Vestibular system (and non-specific dizziness)	Concurrent or previous symptoms localizing to the vestibular system raise suspicion for MS
Cranial nerves	Optic neuritis affects the optic nerve, causing vision decrease, blurry vision, color vision decrease, and afferent pupillary defect. If the inflammation is in the orbital segment of the optic nerve there is associated pain on eye movements. If the inflammation involves the distal optic nerve there may be optic disc swelling
Spinal cord	Concurrent or previous symptoms localizing to the spinal cord raise suspicion for MS or neuromyelitis optica

Secondary Complications: Though recovery is typically excellent, it can be incomplete. When one eye is affected there can be poor depth perception and binocular inhibition, where the vision with the affected eye detracts from the good vision in the fellow eye.

Isolated optic neuritis is associated with future development of MS. Presence of lesions on MRI brain at the time of optic neuritis is associated with increased risk of MS development.

Treatment Complications: Acute optic neuritis is frequently treated with a short course of high-dose steroids, which are associated with insomnia, anxiety, appetite increase, and risk of gastric ulcers in the short term. Steroid therapy can also lead to psychosis, confusion, weight gain, hyperglycemia, myopathy, glaucoma, cataracts, osteoporosis, or vertebral fractures.

Severe cases are sometimes treated with plasmapheresis, which has risks associated with catheter placement and can lead to electrolyte imbalance and coagulopathy.

Bibliography

Balcer LJ. Optic neuritis. *N Engl J Med.* 2006;354: 1273–80.

Eggenberger ER. Inflammatory optic neuropathies. *Ophthalmol Clin North Am.* 2001;14(1):73–82.

Optic Neuritis Study Group. The clinical profile of optic neuritis. Experience of the Optic Neuritis Treatment Trial. *Arch Ophthalmol.* 1991;109(12):1673–8.

Percy AK, Nobrega FT, Kurland LT. Optic neuritis and multiple sclerosis. An epidemiologic study. *Arch Ophthalmol.* 1972;87:135.

Rodriguez M, Siva A, Cross SA, et al. Optic neuritis: a population-based study in Olmsted County, Minnesota. *Neurology.* 1995;45:244.

Ropper AH, Samuels MA, Klein JP. Disturbances of vision. In *Adams & Victor's principles of neurology.* 10th ed. New York, NY: McGraw-Hill; 2014. Chapter 13.

Optic Neuropathy, Compressive

Epidemiology and Demographics: Compressive optic neuropathy can affect any race/ethnicity of either sex at any age.

Disorder Description: Compression of the optic nerve causes dysfunction of the optic nerve and vision loss. Typically it initially affects the peripheral vision and progresses over time to affect central vision and visual acuity. Compression in the orbit can be associated with optic nerve head swelling. Both orbital and intracranial compression can initially present with a normal appearing optic nerve head. Optic nerve head atrophy can develop months after permanent injury to the optic nerve has occurred.

Symptoms

Localization site	Comment
Base of skull	Lesions of the skull base or dura, such as meningiomas, metastatic disease, fibrous dysplasia, sinus mucoceles, and pachymeningitis can cause optic neuropathy and eventually optic atrophy through compression of the intracranial optic nerve. There can be associated cranial neuropathies, but the optic nerves can be affected in isolation
	Vascular compression by aneurysm or ectatic carotid artery can cause optic nerve compression

Localization site	Comment
Cranial nerves	Inflammatory, infectious, or neoplastic processes affecting the subarachnoid space can cause compression of the optic nerve within the optic nerve sheath. If this is a distributed process there may be associated meningeal symptoms. However, focal processes can affect the optic nerves in isolation
Pituitary gland	Sellar and suprasellar masses can compress the optic nerves where they form the chiasm, classically causing bitemporal visual field loss. If these invade the neighboring cavernous sinuses there can be associated eye movement limitations, diplopia, and facial numbness from involvement of the cranial nerves that travel through it them
Muscle	Enlarged extraocular muscles, for example from thyroid orbitopathy or orbital myositis, can compress the optic nerves. These can be associated with ocular motility limitations and proptosis
Unclear localization	Mass lesions in the orbit can also cause compression of the optic nerve with or without orbital signs and symptoms

Treatment Complications: Surgical treatment of any lesion compressing the optic nerve can cause further injury to the optic nerve and progressive vision loss. Both acute and delayed radiation injury can occur to cause further vision loss in cases treated with radiation therapy.

Bibliography

Van Stavern GP, Newman NJ. Optic neuropathies. An overview. *Ophthalmol Clin North Am.* 2001;14(1):61–71.

Orbital Arteriovenous Fistula

Epidemiology and Demographics: Arteriovenous (AV) fistulas can affect any age group and any sex. Orbital AV fistulas are rare.

Disorder Description: AV fistulas are an acquired abnormal connection between an artery and vein without an intervening capillary bed. In the orbit, these lesions tend to be low flow, unlike carotid-cavernous fistulas that may be high or low flow, and may be spontaneous or related to trauma. In the orbit, AV fistulas develop from branches of the ophthalmic artery and anterior cerebral fossa veins as well as between the recurrent meningeal artery and superior or inferior ophthalmic veins. They can be isolated, but may also be associated with other facial or intracranial AV fistulas.

Symptoms: Patients will present with signs and symptoms similar to carotid–cavernous sinus fistulas: proptosis, chemosis, dilated conjunctival and retinal vessels, and dilated supraorbital vein.

Localization site	Comment
Cranial nerves	Carotid–cavernous fistula may present with similar ocular symptoms to orbital fistulas, but, in addition, may have numerous cranial nerve palsies, including CN III, IV, V, and VI as well as Horner syndrome from lesions that affect the sympathetics as they travel through the sinus
Unclear localization	AV fistulas of the orbit may be associated with other fistulas in the facial and intracranial vasculature

Secondary Complications: Complications of AV fistulas include exposure from proptosis and chemosis, which may both prevent normal eyelid closure. Optic nerve compression from large apical lesions is another complication that must be assessed.

Treatment Complications: Low flow AV fistulas may be observed as many will spontaneously close, but this may lead to corneal exposure or optic nerve compression if the lesions cause progressive symptoms. The definitive diagnosis of these lesions is by angiography, which carries a small but known risk of complications including bleeding, false aneurysm, ocular and cerebral ischemia from occlusion of the internal carotid artery, and death. When there are visual symptoms, surgical intervention with coiling or other embolization techniques may in themselves cause similar complications.

Bibliography

Frankefort N, Salu P, Van Tussenbfoek F. Orbital arteriovenous fistula with symptoms contralateral to the arterial supply. A case report. *Bull Soc Belge Ophthalmol.* 2005;296:63–7.

Ohtsuka K, Hashimoto M. Clinical findings in a patient with spontaneous arteriovenous fistulas of the orbit. *Am J Ophthalmol.* 1999;127(6):736–7.

Orbital Hemorrhages

Epidemiology and Demographics: Retrobulbar hemorrhage or hematoma may affect any age or sex, as they are usually related to trauma or may present as a complication after retrobulbar anesthetic injection or orbital surgery. Spontaneous rupture of arteriovenous anomalies has been reported, but is considered very rare compared with their intracranial counterparts.

Disorder Description: Retrobulbar hemorrhage most commonly results from damage to the infraorbital artery and may occur after an orbital floor fracture or its repair. Other vessels that can hemorrhage include the anterior and posterior ethmoidal arteries in the medial wall, and the zygomaticotemporal and zygomaticofacial arteries in the lateral wall as well as orbital veins. When performing surgery along the medial and lateral walls, care should be taken to identify and cauterize these vessels to mitigate postoperative hemorrhage. Resection of fat during blepharoplasty may also rupture small vessels supplying these anterior fat pads.

The posterior orbit is bound by bone for 360 degrees, while the orbital septum forms the anterior boundary of the orbit along with the eyelids and canthal tendons. These anterior structures limit anterior displacement of orbital contents, and together, these landmarks form an "orbital compartment" that has limited ability to expand. A hemorrhage in the orbit can create a compartment syndrome, leading to pressure on the optic nerve and other orbital structures and secondary vision loss if not addressed promptly.

Symptoms: Patients with orbital compartment syndrome present with rapid onset ocular pain, proptosis, periorbital ecchymosis, chemosis, limitation of eye movements, diplopia, and decreased vision.

Secondary Complications: Retrobulbar hemorrhage or hematoma may lead to compressive optic neuropathy, retinal ischemia, and irreversible vision loss in as little as 90 minutes. Ischemic changes to the extraocular muscles may also result in impaired ocular motility and secondary diplopia.

Treatment Complications: The treatment for retrobulbar hemorrhage is prompt surgical decompression by lateral canthotomy and inferior cantholysis. These incisions are usually left open and close by secondary intention, but may result in abnormalities of the eyelids including entropion, ectropion, and ptosis. More aggressive treatment may be needed in selected cases, including superior cantholysis and even surgical bony decompression of the orbit, usually by fracturing of the orbital floor. Surgical bony decompression may result in diplopia and enophthalmos.

Bibliography

Lima V, Burt B, Leibovitch I, et al. Orbital compartment syndrome: the ophthalmic surgical emergency. *Surv Ophthalmol.* 2009;54(4):441–9.

Moin M, Kersten RC, Bernardini F, et al. Spontaneous hemorrhage in an intraorbital arteriovenous malformation. *Ophthalmology.* 2000;107(12):2215–9.

Popat H, Doyle PT, Davies SJ. Blindness following retrobulbar haemorrhage: it can be prevented. *Br J Oral Maxillofac Surg.* 2007;45(2):163–4.

Orbital Inflammation (Orbital Pseudotumor)

Epidemiology and Demographics: Idiopathic orbital inflammation is uncommon, with prevalence of around 10% among patients with orbital disease. It can occur at any age and has no sex or racial predilection. It can affect any part of the orbit including the sclera (scleritis), eye muscles (myositis), and lacrimal gland (dacryoadenitis), or it may diffusely involve the entire orbit.

Disorder Description: Orbital inflammation is commonly idiopathic. In the other cases, specific systemic disorders may be identified, including sarcoidosis, IgG4-related disease, Wegener's granulomatosis, and histiocytic disorders. Patients may present with proptosis, restricted eye motility, and eye pain that make it difficult to distinguish clinically from orbital cellulitis or thyroid eye disease. Neuroimaging may show enhancement of the retro-orbital fat or of an extraocular muscle, involving the tendon. Orbital inflammatory disease is exquisitely sensitive to steroids, and a lack of prompt response should raise suspicion about the diagnosis.

Symptoms

Localization site	Comment
Unclear localization	Orbital myositis is usually an idiopathic inflammation of one or more ocular muscles. Symptoms include prominent and rapid onset double vision and pain with eye movements, ptosis, and eyelid edema. Signs include conjunctival injection over the affected muscle and chemosis. Any muscle may be affected, although the superior rectus/levator complex and medial rectus have been shown to be the most often affected

Localization site	Comment
	Dacryoadenitis is inflammation of the lacrimal gland. Patients present with superolateral eyelid swelling and redness that is tender to palpation. There can be inferonasal displacement of the globe, but diplopia is not a common finding. The etiology in these cases may be idiopathic, but viral, sarcoidosis, lymphoma are other etiologies for which biopsy is recommended
	Orbital cellulitis most commonly occurs secondary to spread of infection from a neighboring sinusitis. It may rapidly lead to vision loss and it may also spread outside the orbit, leading to meningitis, cavernous sinus thrombosis, or septicemia. These patients must be observed closely and treated aggressively
	Graves' disease is a systemic autoimmune disease that can affect many organs. In the orbit, it can cause inflammation of the orbital fat and eye muscles leading to proptosis, exposure keratopathy, eyelid retraction, and even compressive optic neuropathy

Secondary Complications: Vision loss from compressive optic neuropathy and exposure keratopathy from proptosis.

Treatment Complications: Orbital inflammatory conditions are usually treated initially with steroids. Steroid dependence and other complications from long-term steroid use including mental status changes and sleep disturbance. These complications may be mitigated by early transition to steroid-sparing medications.

Bibliography

Demirci H, Shields CL, Shields JA, et al. Orbital tumors in the older adult population. *Ophthalmology*. 2002;109(2):243–8.

Rootman J, Robertson W, Lapointe JS. Inflammatory diseases. In Rootman J, ed. *Diseases of the orbit: a multidisciplinary approach*. Philadelphia: J.B. Lippincott; 1988. pp. 143–204.

Orbital Tumors

Epidemiology and Demographics: The most common orbital tumor in children is the infantile hemangioma, while in adults it is the encapsulated venous malformation (cavernous hemangioma). The most common primary malignant orbital tumor in children is rhabdomyosarcoma, while the most common metastatic lesion is neuroblastoma. In adults, the most common primary malignant orbital tumor is lymphoma, and the risk increases with age, but without clear sex predilection. The most common metastatic tumor in adults is breast in women and lung in men.

Disorder Description: Many orbital tumors are isolated to the orbit. They most commonly cause proptosis, but may also cause hypoglobus or hyperglobus, depending on the location of the tumor. Tumors located in the orbital apex may also present with optic neuropathy from compression of the optic nerve. Those with secondary complications are listed below.

Symptoms

Localization site	Comment
Pineal gland	Retinoblastoma (RB) is considered an intraocular tumor rather than an orbital tumor, and is the most common malignant intraocular tumor of childhood. It often presents with leukocoria (white pupil) or strabismus (eyes misaligned). If treated early, a cure can usually be achieved. If untreated, retinoblastoma may extend intracranially along the optic nerve into the central nervous system with a poor prognosis. Rarely, patients with either unilateral or bilateral RB may also develop a neuroectodermal tumor of the pineal gland
Base of skull	Neurofibromatosis Type 1 (NF1) is an autosomal dominant condition that may result in sphenoid wing dysplasia with pulsatile proptosis and optic nerve gliomas, usually in childhood. Large hypothalamic lesions may cause headache and obstruction of the third ventricle. NF1 may also cause subcutaneous neurofibromas in the eyelid, giving it an "S" shaped deformity that is pathognomonic
	Sphenoid wing meningioma may cause ipsilateral proptosis, ophthalmoplegia, and optic nerve dysfunction if it involves the optic canal. These lesions often involve the anterior and middle cranial fossae as well as the zygomatic fossa, and have an increased incidence in patients with NF1
Cranial nerves	Neurofibromatosis Type 2 is associated with bilateral acoustic neuromas and optic nerve sheath meningiomas

Localization site	Comment
Unclear localization	Neuroblastoma may be primary in the neck or orbit or metastatic from the adrenal gland. In the neck, along the sympathetic chain, it may cause Horner syndrome. Neuroblastoma may be associated with paraneoplastic syndrome, which may cause opsoclonus (involuntary conjugate multidirectional saccades)
	Orbital lymphoma (OL) may be primary or it may be a manifestation of systemic lymphoma, although the clinical and radiographic findings are similar for both. OL is most likely to be mucosa-associated lymphoid tissue lymphoma. OL can be difficult to distinguish from orbital inflammatory syndrome (OIS), but it is less likely to have pain and more likely to have a mass lesion than is OIS. The classic subconjunctival "salmon patch" may be present in anterior lesions, but regardless of location, they tend to mold to surrounding structures, rather than indent or displace them. Usually, these lesions are easily biopsied, and a systemic oncologic workup should be initiated. Radiation is the treatment of choice for isolated OL, while systemic disease requires chemotherapy. A small percentage of localized OL may develop systemic lymphoma

Secondary Complications: Compressive optic neuropathy may result from an orbital tumor, especially if it is located near the apex of the orbit or in the optic nerve or its nerve sheath. Exposure keratopathy may result if an orbital tumor causes severe proptosis.

Treatment Complications: Vision loss may result from surgical treatment of optic nerve or nerve sheath tumors, or from radiation to treat them. Retrobulbar hemorrhage may result from surgical treatment of orbital tumors, as may diplopia if the extraocular muscles are manipulated during tumor resection.

Bibliography

Hatef E, Roberts D, McLaughlin P, Pro B, Esmaeli B. Prevalence and nature of systemic involvement and stage at initial examination in patients with orbital and ocular adnexal lymphoma. *Arch Ophthalmol.* 2007;125(12):1663–7.

Shields JA, Shields CL, Scartozzi R. Survey of 1264 patients with orbital tumors and simulating lesions. The 2002 Montgomery Lecture, Part 1. *Ophthalmology.* 2004;111:997–1008.

Orofacial Dyskinesia/Facial Chorea

Epidemiology and Demographics: Spontaneous orofacial dyskinesia typically affects the elderly. The prevalence ranges from 1% to 38% of the population. It seems to be more common in nursing home patients with dementia. There may be a 2–3 to 1 female-to-male predominance.

Disorder Description: Orofacial dyskinesia is defined as involuntary, repetitive, stereotypical movement of the face, jaw, and tongue. It may be seen in most inherited (Huntington's disease) and acquired causes of chorea (Sydenham's chorea, structural lesions, etc.). Dyskinesias may also be spontaneous or medication induced (tardive dyskinesia). Spontaneous orofacial dyskinesia in the elderly is strongly associated with ill-fitting dentures, oral pain, and the perception of inadequate oral hygiene. The clinical presentation is typically milder compared with tardive orofacial dyskinesia and improves with appropriately fitted dentures.

Symptoms

Localization site	Comment
Mental status and psychiatric aspects/complications	Spontaneous orofacial dyskinesia of the elderly is often associated with dementia
Muscle	Hypertrophy of tongue and jaw muscles Pain and muscle spasm

Secondary Complications: Tooth wear and fracture, prosthesis damage and displacement, orofacial pain, temporomandibular joint dislocation, dysphagia, and chewing difficulties with inadequate nutrition with weight loss.

Treatment Complications: Focused botulinum toxin injections may be attempted but may result in side effects of dysphagia. Pharmacotherapy is often poorly tolerated.

Bibliography

Balasubramaniam R, Ram S. Orofacial movement disorders. *Oral Maxillofac Surg Clin North Am.* 2008;20(2):273–85.

Evidente VGH, Adler CH. Hemifacial spasm and other craniofacial movement disorders. *Mayo Clin Proc.* 1998;73(1): 67–71.

Kraft SP, Lang AE. Cranial dystonia, blepharospasm and hemifacial spasm: clinical features and treatment, including the use of botulinum toxin. *CMAJ*. 1988;139(9):837–44.

Orthostatic Tremor (OT)

Epidemiology and Demographics: Orthostatic tremor (OT) is considered rare, but there are limited epidemiological data. Women may be affected slightly more frequently, as suggested by two reviews. Age of onset varies, although the mean onset of symptoms is in the sixth decade.

Disorder Description: OT is characterized by unsteadiness on standing accompanied by a rapid 13- to 18-Hz tremor of the legs. The high frequency of the tremor results in fusion of the muscle contractions and may appear like rippling of the muscles. The tremor can be heard with a stethoscope placed over the affected thigh or calf, sounding rather like a distant "helicopter." Symptoms characteristically improve on walking or sitting down. Patients tend to shift the weight on their leg or walk on the spot or tend to lean against a wall to minimize symptoms. There may be co-existing tremor of the trunk or outstretched arms.

The syndrome can be primary or secondary and associated with a variety of disorders, most commonly parkinsonism, but can occur with dementia with Lewy bodies or progressive supranuclear palsy, head trauma, thiamine deficiency, alcohol use, pontine/cerebellar infarcts, rarely with monoclonal gammopathy, Grave's disease, and small cell cancer.

Symptoms

Localization site	Comment
Mental status and psychiatric aspects/ complications	Dementia may precede or may occur years after the onset of OT if associated with Parkinson's disease or dementia with Lewy bodies
Cerebellum	Cerebellar lesions may be responsible in some secondary cases

Secondary Complications: OT can have a serious impact on quality of life and can cause depression. Falls can occur, but are rare.

Treatment Complications: Response to treatment is poor. Clonazepam, gabapentin, and primidone may help.

Levodopa may play a role in treatment if associated with Parkinson's disease. Deep brain stimulation (ventral intermediate nucleus of the thalamus) may be tried in refractory cases.

Bibliography

Gerschlager W, Brown P. Orthostatic tremor – a review. *Handb Clin Neurol*. 2011;100:457–62.

Osler–Weber–Rendu Syndrome (Hereditary Hemorrhagic Telangiectasia)

Epidemiology and Demographics: Epidemiologic studies suggest likely prevalence rates of hereditary hemorrhagic telangiectasia (HHT) of between 1/5000 and 1/8000 with much higher rates described in certain geographically isolated populations (e.g., 1/1330 in Afro-Caribbean residents of Curacao and Bonaire). It is inherited as an autosomal dominant condition with varying penetrance and expression.

Disorder Description: Combination of epistaxis, gastrointestinal bleeding, and iron deficiency anemia associated with characteristic telangiectasia on the lips, oral mucosa, and fingertips. Occurrence of arteriovenous malformations (AVMs) in characteristic locations helps make the diagnosis of HHT. The life-threatening complications result from arteriovenous malformations in the pulmonary (50%), hepatic (30%), and cerebral (10%) circulations.

Pulmonary AVMs (PAVMs) allow systemic venous blood to bypass the normal pulmonary circulation, resulting in paradoxical embolic stroke, brain abscess, and migraines. These symptoms are often the first manifestations of a pulmonary arteriovenous malformation and even of hereditary hemorrhagic telangiectasia itself. Cerebral AVMs can bleed and cause hemorrhagic stroke; hepatic AVMs can result in high output cardiac failure or other pathologies, and on occasion require liver transplantation.

Cerebrovascular malformations include classical nidal AVMs, micro AVMs (nidus <1 cm), high flow arteriovenous fistulae (AVFs; generally found in children), and telangiectasias. Cerebral arteriovenous shunts affect approximately 10% of HHT patients, are often multiple, and are usually silent. The latter may be less frequent than those seen in non-HHT cerebral AVMs, in part due to the lower frequency of associated aneurysms.

Symptoms

Localization site	Comment
Cerebral hemispheres	High flow shunts through AVFs in young infants can present with systemic circulatory overload or hydrovenous dysfunction (e.g., macrocephaly, hydrocephalus). Other presentations include seizures, ischemia of the surrounding tissue due to a steal effect, or hemorrhage
	Migraine occurs in HHT more commonly than in those without HHT. The migraines are clinically indistinguishable but tend to occur more in patients with pulmonary AVMs
Spinal cord	Spinal AVMs are less common but may present with para- or quadriplegia and back pain

Secondary Complications: Hemorrhage can be primary intracerebral or subarachnoid depending on the source of the bleed, AVM, or aneurysm, respectively. Pulmonary AVMs can cause right to left shunting and result in brain abscess. Polycythemia and hypoxemia with cyanosis, and clubbing can occur with pulmonary AVMs.

A rare syndrome combines HHT with juvenile polyposis of the intestine, and it may be pertinent to consider this, since the risk of cancer is high.

Treatment Complications: AVMs of the lung and brain are treated even when asymptomatic given the high rate of catastrophic complications. AVMs of the skin, oral mucosa, gastrointestinal system, and liver are treated when symptoms occur. This distinction determines routinely recommended screening for AVMs in patients with HHT.

If contrast ECHO shows pulmonary shunting, even if no pulmonary AVM is detected by chest CT, a lifetime recommendation for prophylactic antibiotic treatment protocol with dental cleaning and other procedures with risk for bacteremia is advised due to the high risk of paradoxical embolus or cerebral abscess.

Cerebral AVMs >1.0 cm in diameter are usually treated using neurovascular surgery, embolotherapy, and/or stereotactic radiosurgery. Management of spinal AVMs is challenging.

Anticoagulants such as warfarin and nonsteroidal anti-inflammatory agents such as aspirin and ibuprofen that interfere with platelet function should be avoided unless required for treatment of other medical conditions.

Bibliography

McDonald J, Bayrak-Toydemir P, Pyeritz RE. Hereditary hemorrhagic telangiectasia: An overview of diagnosis, management, and pathogenesis. *Genet Med.* 2011;13:607–16. DOI:10.1097/GIM.0b013e3182136d32.

Osteoarthritis

Epidemiology and Demographics: Prevalence is 3.6% of the population (27 million people in the United States). More common in patients over 60 years of age; 10% prevalence in males and 18% in females. In those younger than 45 years of age, the prevalence in men and women is equal.

Disorder Description: Osteoarthritis is a joint disease involving breakdown of joint cartilage and underlying bone. Risk factors include obesity and those that have jobs with daily positions resulting in high level of joint stress.

Localization site	Comment
Hands, feet, spine, large weight-bearing joints	Pain, joint stiffness more common in the morning, hard bony enlargements called Heberden's nodes on small joints
Knee	Pain, stiffness, and joint effusion

Secondary Complication: Osteophyte formation can cause complications including root compression and hypomineralization of the bone.

Complication of Treatment: Nonsteroidal anti-inflammatory drugs can cause gastrointestinal side effects. Oral opioids should not be used in osteoarthritic patients as first line treatment, which may cause lightheadedness, drowsiness, and addiction.

Bibliography

Arden N, Blanco F, Cooper C, et al. *Atlas of osteoarthritis.* New York: Springer Healthcare Communications. 2015; p. 21.

Mayo Clinic. Swollen knee. www.mayoclinic.org/diseases-conditions/swollen-knee/symptoms-causes/syc-20378129. Accessed Sep 3, 2018.

Osteoblastoma

Epidemiology and Demographics: Accounts for 1% of all primary bone tumors and 5% of spinal tumors, 80% presenting in the 3rd decade of life with a higher predominance of males over females (2–3:1).[1-4] No predominance by race. More commonly found in the posterior arch of the vertebral column, although in the cervical spine, the vertebral body is affected at a higher frequency.[1]

Disorder Description: Osteoblastoma is a benign bone-producing tumor that is histologically indistinguishable from osteoid osteoma. Some literature considers both as a subset of the same tumor, although osteoblastomas are larger in size, appear in an older population, have a more aggressive tendency, and are able to extend to adjacent tissue but do not metastasize. Two types of osteoblastoma have been described: conventional and aggressive. The frequency of presentation is slightly higher in the vertebral column compared with the large bones.[5] The diagnosis is confirmed with biopsy. In imaging studies there is evidence of a well-demarcated lesion, with noticeable edema surrounding it, potentially leading to misdiagnosis of a malignant tumor.

Symptoms

Localization site	Comment
Cerebral hemispheres	Described in the calvarial bone frontoparietal region,[5] occipital bone with compression of the posterior fossa causing obstructive hydrocephalus[6] and local deformities, and ethmoid bone causing eye proptosis and nasal obstruction. Reported in sphenoid and maxilla bone
Base of skull	Palpable mass in the retroauricular region, severe headaches, obstructive hydrocephalus
Cranial nerves	When the temporal bone is involved, rarely will cause 7th and 8th cranial nerve compression; if lower cranial nerves are involved, will cause dysarthria, dysphagia, dysphonia, hoarseness, syncope, near syncope, dysesthesia, facial palsy
Spinal cord	Resistant pain neck and spine, stiffness, pathologic compression fractures developing scoliosis
Specific spinal roots	Radicular pain

Localization site	Comment
Muscle	Paraspinal muscle contraction causing torticollis
Rare presentation	Increased intracranial pressure syndrome has been described secondary to dominant transverse-sigmoid sinus junction compression caused by a small temporal bone osteoblastoma[7,8]

Secondary Complications: Pathologic fractures, spinal deformities, aneurysmal bone cysts, scoliosis, torticollis, local deformities, restrictive lung disease from scoliosis, and chronic pain.

Treatment Complications

- Partial and wide end-block resection: blood loss, wound infection/dehiscence, implant failure, local regression, fractures, and prolonged hospital stay and healing time.
- Chemotherapy (including methotrexate, doxorubicin, cisplatin): nausea, vomiting, anorexia, alopecia, pancytopenia, bleeding diathesis, fatigue, weakness, reversible peripheral neuropathy (cisplatin), leukoencephalopathy (methotrexate), cardiomyopathy (doxorubicin), and infertility.
- Radiation therapy: the side effects will vary depending on the dose and area at which it is aimed, including sunburn-like changes, hair loss, nausea, diarrhea, dry mouth, headaches, developmental delay, peripheral neuropathy, and infertility.

References

1. Stavridis SI, Pingel A, Schnake KJ, Kandziora F. Diagnosis and treatment of a C2-osteoblastoma encompassing the vertebral artery. *Eur Spine J.* 2013;22(11):2504–12. DOI:10.1007/s00586-013-2875-5.

2. Kandziora F, Pingel A. Posterior-anterior resection of a cervical spine osteoblastoma. *Eur Spine J.* 2010;19(6):1041–3. DOI: 10.1007/s00586-010-1461-3.

3. Gutteck N, Mendel T, Held A, Wohlrab D. Cervical spine osteoblastoma in children: selective diagnostics as the basis for effective surgical management. *Orthopade.*

2010;39(1):92–6. DOI: 10.1007/s00132-009-1530-7.

4. Samdani A, Torre-Healy A, Chou D, Cahill AM, Storm PB. Treatment of osteoblastoma at C7: a multidisciplinary approach. A case report and review of the literature. *Eur Spine J.* 2009;18(Suppl 2):196–200. DOI: 10.1007/s00586-008-0806-7.

5. Miller C, Khan R, Lemole GM Jr, Jacob A. Osteoblastoma of the lateral skull base: work-up, surgical management, and a review of the literature. *J Neurol Surg Rep.* 2013;74(1):37–42. Epub 2013 Jun 13. DOI: 10.1055/s-0033-1346978.

6. Han X, Dong Y, Sun K, Lu Y. A huge occipital osteoblastoma accompanied with aneurysmal bone cyst in the posterior cranial fossa. *Clin Neurol Neurosurg.* 2008;110(3):282–5. Epub 2007 Dec 4.

7. Boaro A, Marton E, Mazzucco GM, Longatti P. Osteoblastoma mimicking an idiopathic intracranial hypertension syndrome. *J Pediatr Neurosci.* 2017;12(1):87–90. DOI:10.4103/jpn. JPN_167_16.

8. Miller C, Khan R, Lemole GM Jr, Jacob A. Osteoblastoma of the lateral skull base: Work-up, surgical management, and a review of the literature. *J Neurol Surg Rep.* 2013;74:37–42.

Osteochondroma

Epidemiology and Demographics: Osteochondroma is the most common benign bone tumor. Affects primarily children and adolescents, and after development will remain with the individual for the rest of their lives, accounting for 40% of all benign tumors of the bone, 9% of all bone tumors, and less than 0.5% of spinal tumors (cervical spine > thoracic). Seen slightly more frequently in men compared with women (1.5–2:1), and is more common in Caucasians. Prevalence is 2/100,000 individuals in the general population

Disorder Description: Exophytic tumor overlying the bone, also known as osteocartilaginous exostosis, growing from cartilaginous tissue in the secondary ossification centers. Classified as single and sporadic with lower malignant potential, or multiple and hereditary multiple exostoses (autosomal dominant). The underlying mechanism for solitary and multiple osteochondromas has been associated with a loss of function mutation in the EXT1 or EXT2 genes located on chromosomes 8 and 11, causing deficiency of glycosyltransferases and therefore deficiency of heparan sulphate, a key component of skeletal development. Will typically be found incidentally or will cause local compression of the surrounding structures hence the clinical presentations and subsequent complications.

Symptoms

Localization site	Comment
Cerebral hemispheres	Meningeal/clivus osteochondromas causing diplopia, obstructive hydrocephalus
Spinal cord	Intraspinal osteochondromas present with compressive myelopathy, quadriparesis, quadriplegia, hemiparesis, ambulatory dysfunction, transverse myelopathy
Mononeuropathy or mononeuritis multiplex	Pain; sciatica found in sacral osteochondroma; peroneal mononeuropathy seen in osteochondromas of the fibular head
Peripheral neuropathy	Associated with local compression depending on the location of the mass
Muscle	Torticollis, reactive myositis
Unclear localization	Vocal cord compression from ostechondroma arising from C4–C5 causing airway dislocation and acute onset of respiratory distress, dysphagia and paralysis of left vocal cord

Secondary Complications: Local deformities, aneurysms of the compressed vessels, and peripheral neuropathy.

Treatment Complications: Complications of partial and wide end-block resection include blood loss, wound infection/dehiscence, implant failure, local regression, fractures, and prolonged hospital stay and healing time.

References

Castro-Castro J, Rodiño-Padín J, Touceda-Bravo A, Castro-Bouzas D, Pinzón-Millán A. Cervical spine osteochondroma presenting with torticollis and hemiparesis. *Neurocirugia (Astur).* 2014;25(2):94–7. Epub 2013 Oct 16.

Certo F, Sciacca G, Caltabiano R, et al. Anterior, extracanalar, cervical spine osteochondroma associated with DISH: description of a very rare tumor causing bilateral vocal cord paralysis, laryngeal compression and dysphagia. Case report and review of the literature. *Eur Rev Med Pharmacol Sci.* 2014;18(1 Suppl):34–40.

Herget GW, Kontny U, Saueressig U, et al. Osteochondroma and multiple osteochondromas: recommendations on the diagnostics and follow-up with special consideration to the occurrence of secondary chondrosarcoma. *Radiologe.* 2013; 53(12):1125–36.

Huegel J, Sgariglia F, Enomoto-Iwamoto M, et al. Heparan sulfate in skeletal development, growth, and pathology: the case of hereditary multiple exostoses. *Dev Dyn.* 2013;242(9):1021–32. Epub 2013 Jul 29.

Mnif H, Koubaa M, Zrig M, Zammel N, Abid A. Peroneal nerve palsy resulting from fibular head osteochondroma. *Orthopedics.* 2009;32(7):528.

Sciubba DM, Macki M, Bydon M, et al. Long-term outcomes in primary spinal osteochondroma: a multicenter study of 27 patients. *J Neurosurg Spine.* 2015;22(6):582–8. DOI:10.3171/2014.10. SPINE14501.

Tian Y, Yuan W, Chen H, Shen X. Spinal cord compression secondary to a thoracic vertebral osteochondroma. *J Neurosurg Spine.* 2011;15(3):252–7. Epub 2011 May 20.

Osteoma

Epidemiology and Demographics: Usually found in children and adolescents between ages 10 and 35 years. More common in males. Responsible for 10% of all benign bone lesions.

Disorder Description: Osteoid osteoma is a benign skeletal neoplasm composed of osteoid and woven bone. It is of unknown etiology. X-rays, CT, or MRI are used for diagnosis.

Symptoms

Localization site	Comment
Bone involved	Focal bone pain at the site of the tumor worse at night. It increases with activity. It is exquisitely relieved by small doses of aspirin. It is rarely larger than 1.5 cm in diameter

Secondary Complications: Intra-articular tumors may show joint effusion associated with a premature loss of cartilage. Regional osteoporosis may appear.

Spinal involvement may cause alignment abnormalities, which may manifest as scoliosis, kyphosis, or hyperlordosis.

Bibliography

Davies AM, Wellings RM. Imaging of bone tumors. *Curr Opin Radiol.* 1992;4(6):32–8.

Osteomalacia

Epidemiology and Demographics: Osteomalacia is considered to be a rare disease by the office of the Rare Diseases of The National Institute of Health, which means that it affects fewer than 200 thousand people in the US population.

Disorder Description: Characterized by incomplete mineralization of normal osteoid tissue following closure of the growth plates. Renal osteodystrophy refers to osteomalacia seen in patients with chronic renal insufficiency, which in addition may cause fractures. The risk factors are vitamin D deficiency due to decreased sunlight exposure and insufficient intake of calcium and vitamin D as well as primary hypophosphatemia.

Symptoms

Localization site	Comment
Affected bone	Nonspecific bone pain and tenderness, rarely hypotonia, waddling gait. "Milkman's syndrome" refers to bone insufficiency-related fractures that are bilateral and symmetric
Vertebrae	Fracture
Arms and legs	Bowing deformities
Skull	Basilar invagination
Neonate	Posterior flattening and squaring of the skull
Other	Oncogenic osteomalacia. Rare paraneoplastic syndrome associated with neoplasms that produce fibroblast growth factor

Bibliography

Mankin HJ. Rickets, osteomalacia and renal osteodystrophy. An update. *Orthop Clin North Am.* 1990;21(1):81–96.

Osteomyelitis

Epidemiology and Demographics: Occurs in 1/5000 children. Vertebral osteomyelitis is seen in 2.4 cases/100,000 of population. One case per 1000 in neonates is reported. Seen more in males than in females. Foot puncture causes 30–40% of cases of osteomyelitis in diabetes mellitus.

Disorder Description: Osteomyelitis is an acute or chronic inflammatory process of the bone and its structure due to infection. It may be localized or it may spread through the periosteum, cortex, marrow, and cancellous tissue. Two primary categories of acute osteomyelitis are described:

Hematogenous osteomyelitis is seen in children, due to bacterial feeding from the blood. Common site is the rapidly growing and highly vascular metaphysis of growing bone. Vertebral osteomyelitis due to hematogenous seeding can be seen due to urinary tract infection or skin infection. Slow clinical development and insidious onset are reported.

Direct or contiguous inoculation osteomyelitis due to direct contact of the tissue and bacteria during trauma or surgery.

Chronic osteomyelitis and osteomyelitis secondary to peripheral vascular disease have also been described.

Symptoms

Localization site	Comment
General symptoms	Fever, fatigue, malaise, irritability, restriction of movements, local edema, erythema, and tenderness
Newborns (less than 4 months)	*Staphylococcus aureus*, *Enterobacter* species, group A and group B *Streptococcus*
Children aged 4 months to 4 years	*Staphylococcus aureus*, group A *Streptococcus*, *Haemophilus influenzae*, *Enterobacter* species
Adults	*Staphylococcus aureus*, *Enterobacter*, or *Streptococcus*, tuberculosis bacteria

Secondary Complications: Bone abscess, paravertebral epidural abscess, bacteremia, fracture, loosening of the prosthetic implant, draining of the tissue and sinus tracts.

Bibliography

Kaplan SL. Osteomyelitis in children. *Infect Dis Clin North Am.* 2005;19(4):787–97, vii.

Zimmerli W. Clinical practice. Vertebral osteomyelitis. *N Engl J Med.* 2010;362(11):1022–9.

Osteoporosis

Epidemiology and Demographics: In the United States, 9.9 million have osteoporosis. Caucasians and Asians are at increased risk.

Disorder Description: Osteoporosis is a chronic progressive disease. It is also the most common metabolic bone disease, characterized by low bone mass and microarchitectural deterioration of bone tissue resulting in fragile bone. Fractures can occur. Osteoporosis may be due to estrogen deficiency, aging, calcium deficiency, or vitamin D deficiency.

Symptoms

Localization site	Comment
Vertebral fractures	Back pain, respiratory compromise, increased risk of pneumonia, worsening posture, and kyphosis
Hip fracture	Pain, difficulty ambulating

Secondary Complications: Vertebral compression fractures often occur with minimal stress like coughing, lifting, or bending.

Hip fractures can occur due to falls. Secondary complications of hip fractures include nosocomial infections and pulmonary thromboembolism. Deep vein thrombosis also can occur.

Treatment Complications: Vertebroplasty and kyphoplasty may increase risk of adjacent level vertebral fractures after the procedures.

Bibliography

Lynn SG, Sinaki M, Westerlind KC. Balance characteristics of persons with osteoporosis. *Arch Phys Med Rehabil.* 1997;78(3):273–7.

Osteosarcoma

Epidemiology and Demographics: Most common primary malignancy of the bone. Overall rare, with an incidence of 3 cases per million-population-years. Occurs in a bimodal fashion, with the first peak in 1st to 2nd decade of life, coinciding with the pubertal growth spurt, defining the association between the osteosarcoma and adolescence. The second occurs in the 7th decade; this is a secondary malignancy related typically to Paget's. The incidence is higher in males compared with females (in spinal osteosarcoma the incidence seems to be slightly higher in females); higher incidence in young Blacks and Hispanics compared with elderly Whites. It primarily affects the long bones, but spinal involvement is seen in up to 14% of the cases. Highest incidence is in the sacrum (30%), followed by the thoracolumbar spine (25%) and the cervical spine (<25%). The head and neck have been described in about 6% of the cases, involving the base of the skull and the facial bones.

Disorder Description: Highly malignant tumor, characterized by the production of osteoid tissue. By the World Health Organization definition, a core biopsy is always required, dividing them into surface and central tumors. The classification includes: tumor grade I (low grade), II (high grade); tumor extension A (intraosseous involvement only), B (intra- and extraosseous extension); presence of distant metastases III. The etiology of this neoplasia is unknown, although there is evidence for a potential viral cause. The known environmental cause is ionizing radiation. Regarding risk factors for developing osteosarcoma, Paget's disease of the bone is present in 1% of patients with osteosarcoma, and in the pediatric population with retinoblastoma or genetic mutation of p53, the incidence of osteosarcoma is 500 times higher compared with the general population.

Symptoms

Localization site	Comment
Base of the skull, cranial nerves	Dysphagia, dysphonia, hoarseness, lateral tongue deviation, unilateral/bilateral soft palate palsy, diplopia
Spinal cord	Sacrum > thoracolumbar > cervical, main feature is pain, pathologic fractures, myelopathy-paraplegia/quadriplegia, paresthesias
Cauda equina	Fecal and urinary incontinence
Specific spinal roots	Intercostal root pain, non-mechanical radicular arm and leg pain

Secondary Complications: Pathologic fractures, spinal deformities, thoracic-respiratory restriction, quadriplegia, facial deformities, dysphagia, and dysarthria.

Treatment Complications

- Wide end-block resection includes: blood loss, wound infection/dehiscence, implant failure, local regression.
- Chemotherapy (including methotrexate, doxorubicin, cisplatin, carboplatin, ifosfamide, cyclophosphamide, etoposide, gemcitabine, topotecan): nausea, vomiting, anorexia, alopecia, pancytopenia, bleeding diathesis, fatigue, weakness, hemorrhagic cystitis (ifosfamide, cyclophosphamide, etoposide), reversible peripheral neuropathy (cisplatin, carboplatin), acute myeloid leukemia (etoposide), leukoencephalopathy (methotrexate), cardiomyopathy (doxorubicin), infertility.
- Radiation therapy: the side effects will vary depending on the dose and area at which it is aimed, including sunburn-like changes, hair loss, nausea, diarrhea, dry mouth, headaches, developmental delay, peripheral neuropathy, and infertility.

Bibliography

Fischgrund JS, ed. *Orthopaedic knowledge update 9.* Rosemont, IL: American Academy of Orthopaedic Surgeons; 2008.

Huvos AG. *Bone tumors: diagnosis treatment and prognosis.* Vol 2. Philadelphia: W.B. Saunders. Co; 1991.

Katonis P, et al. Spinal osteosarcoma. *Clin Med Insights Oncol.* 2013;7:199–208. PMC. Web. Jun 5, 2017.

McIntyre JF, Smith-Sorensen B, Friend SH, et al. Germline mutations of the p53 tumor suppressor gene in children with osteosarcoma. *J Clin Oncol.* 1994;12:925–30.

Mirabello L, Troisi RJ, Savage SA. Osteosarcoma incidence and survival rates from 1973 to 2004: data from the Surveillance, Epidemiology, and End Results Program. *Cancer.* 2009;115(7):1531–43.

Ozaki T, Flege S, Liljenqvist U, et al. Osteosarcoma of the spine: experience of the Cooperative Osteosarcoma Study Group. *Cancer.* 2002;94(4):1069–77.

Otosclerosis

Epidemiology and Demographics: Genetic disease of the inner ear; autosomal recessive with incomplete penetrance. Female predominance, and more common in Caucasian and Indian patients than in African Americans. Although the prevalence of otosclerosis in the general population approximates 0.3%, autopsy studies have found pathologic otosclerosis in as high as 10% of examined temporal bones. Otosclerosis becomes symptomatic in early adulthood.

Disorder Description: Otosclerosis is a genetic disorder of the inner ear. The pathophysiology is remodeling of the otic capsule bone, which ordinarily does not occur postnatally. The disease causes conductive hearing loss when the stapes footplate is affected. Sensorineural hearing loss may occur as well ("cochlear otosclerosis"). Vestibular symptoms occur infrequently, with an incidence perhaps no greater than in the general population. Endosteal involvement by otosclerosis can be associated with vestibular hair cell loss that may contribute to vestibular symptoms. Otosclerosis patients with vertigo may have abnormalities on VEMP testing (vestibular myogenic evoked potentials).

Symptoms

Localization site	Comment
Inner ear	Conductive or sensorineural hearing loss, +/– tinnitus; vestibular symptoms are uncommon
Cranial nerves	The cochleovestibular nerve is not affected
Central nervous system	The central nervous system is not affected

Secondary Complications: Diplacusis, an abnormal perception of pitch, in the affected ear.

Treatment Complications: Conductive hearing loss is treated by surgical stapedectomy. Vertigo is not uncommon after stapedectomy, but is usually self-limited. Other potential complications of stapedectomy are dysgeusia, sensorineural hearing loss, and a "dead ear" in 1–2% of cases.

Bibliography

Causse JB, Causse JR, Cezard R, et al. Vertigo in postoperative follow-up of otosclerosis. *Am J Otol.* 1988;9:246–55.

Grayeli AB, Sterkers O, Toupet M. Audiovestibular function in patients with otosclerosis and balance disorders. *Otol Neurotol.* 2009;30:1085–91.

Hlzll Ö, Kaya S, Schachern PA, et al. Quantitative assessment of vestibular otopathology in otosclerosis: A temporal bone study. *Laryngoscope.* 2016;126:E118–22.

Lin KY, Young YH. Role of ocular VEMP test in assessing the occurrence of vertigo in otosclerosis patients. *Clin Neurophysiol.* 2015;126:187–93.

Ovarian Cancer

Epidemiology and Demographics: Ovarian cancer is the 7th leading cause of death in the world, with an incidence of 50,000 new cases per year and a 5-year survival rate of 30–40% across the globe in the later stages. Highest mortality rate is in White females followed by Hispanics; lower in Blacks and Asians. In the United States, the overall mortality associated with ovarian cancer has declined compared with the 1990s. Risk factors include: nulliparity, hormonal replacement therapy, and genetic predisposition expressed by the presence of BRCA1-2 accounting for 15% of the hereditary cases.

Disorder Description: Ovarian cancer accounts for less than 6% of cases of central nervous system neoplastic involvement. Neurologic complications are associated with the location of the metastatic disease or regional or distant involvement, lumbosacral plexus, brain, spinal cord, and dural/leptomeningeal involvement; 20% of these metastases occur from hematogenous spreading. The majority of spinal cord metastases are extramedullary causing compression syndromes; only 1% will be associated with intramedullary location. Brain metastases from gynecologic tumors are rare and typically supratentorial, although there is an infratentorial predilection as well, with an estimated incidence of 1–3%. Thirty-five percent are accounted for by choriocarcinoma, which in fact has a bleeding tendency.

Paraneoplastic syndromes have been described with gynecologic disorders and include limbic encephalitis, opsoclonus, retinal degeneration, and cerebellar degeneration.

Symptoms

Localization site	Comment
Cerebral hemispheres	Headache, seizures, focal deficits depending on local mass effect, lethargy
Cerebellum	Cerebellar degeneration: axial and appendicular ataxia, dizziness, nausea, vomiting, dysarthria

Localization site	Comment
Cauda equina	Transverse myelitis, saddle anesthesia, bowel and bladder dysfunction
Plexus	Lumbosacral plexus involvement presenting with severe pain preceding weakness, sensory motor disturbances in general
Peripheral neuropathy	Involving peroneal nerve: no dorsiflexion or eversion of the ipsilateral foot, lateral femoral cutaneous causing meralgia paresthetica, ilioinguinal, iliohypogastric, genitofemoral, femoral, and obturator neuropathy, lower extremity weakness

Secondary Complications: Seizures, peripheral neuropathies, ambulatory dysfunction, endocrinopathies, and myelopathy.

Treatment Complications:

- Surgery: neuropathies (femoral most commonly described), neuromas.
- Local radiation: lumbosacral plexopathy, myokymia, Brown–Sequard syndrome.
- Whole brain radiation therapy: headache, cognitive deficits, memory loss, intellectual disability, personality changes, seizures, change in mental status, local edema, cerebral vasculopathies, primary hypothalamic dysfunction, meningiomas, sarcomas, gliomas
- Chemotherapy: reversible distal sensorimotor peripheral neuropathy typically seen with platinum-based chemotherapeutic agents, headache, confusion, ataxia, seizures, encephalopathy, myelopathy, hearing loss, cranial neuropathies.

Bibliography

Breast Cancer Linkage Consortium. Cancer risks in BRCA2 mutation carriers. *J Natl Cancer Inst.* 1999;91(15):1310–6.

Newton HB, Malkin MG. *Neurological complications of systemic cancer and antineoplastic therapy.* (Neurological Disease and Therapy series: Vol 96). Boca Raton, FL: CRC Press; 2016. p. 307.

Reid BM, Permuth JB, Sellers TA. Epidemiology of ovarian cancer: a review. *Cancer Biol Med.* 2017;14(1):9–32.

Wentzensen N, Poole EM, Trabert B, et al. Ovarian cancer risk factors by histologic subtype: an analysis from the Ovarian Cancer Cohort Consortium. *J Clin Oncol.* 2016;34(24):2888–98. Epub 2016 Jun 20.

Paget's Disease of the Bone

Epidemiology and Demographics: One to three million people in the United States suffer from this disease; male to female ratio is 1.2:1. Highest prevalence is noted in persons older than 65 years.

Disorder Description: Paget's disease of the bone is a localized disorder of bone remodeling, which typically begins with excessive bone resorption followed by an increase in bone formation. The affected bone is mechanically weak, larger, less compact, more vascular, and more susceptible to fracture.

Symptoms

Localization site	Comment
Axial skeleton, particularly lumbar spine and sacral spine	May be asymptomatic. Increased alkaline phosphatase may be noted. Bone pain is the most common symptom, which is worse at night. Fractures may occur
Femur	Hip pain worse with weightbearing, relieved with rest. Fractures may occur.
Skull	Enlarged or deformed, may lead to hydrocephalus, basilar invagination, cerebellum or brainstem compression syndrome
Cranial nerves	Hearing loss, deafness, tinnitus, vertigo, optic nerve and visual field affectation

Secondary Complications: Uncommon, but a potentially fatal complication is the development of osteosarcoma causing increased bone pain with an enlarging soft tissue mass and a lytic lesion, which can also lead to pathogenic fracture.

Bibliography

Dove J. Complete fracture of the femur in Paget's disease of the bone. *J Bone Joint Surg Br.* 1980;62–B(1):12–7.

Lyles KW, Siris ES, Singer FR, Meunier PJ. A clinical approach to diagnosis and management of Paget's disease of bone. *J. Bone Miner Res.* 2001;16(8):1379–87.

Palatal Myoclonus or Palatal Tremor

Epidemiology and Demographics: This is a rare movement disorder that is seen equally in females and males.[1] There have only been a limited number of case series and case reports. The two types that have been described are essential and symptomatic. Essential palatal myoclonus (EPM) does not have a clear causative lesion. The age range was 4–74 years, with average age of onset being 29.4 +/− 16.8 years.[2] In a case series with symptomatic palatal myoclonus (SPM), it has been seen as young as 18 months and as old as 91 years with average age of onset being 49.2 +/− 16.7 years. Overall, the onset of essential palatal myoclonus was concluded to have a younger age of onset than the symptomatic form.[1] The symptomatic form of palatal myoclonus is more common in males than in females.[1,2]

Disorder Description: This condition involves continuous jerks of the soft palate. EPM is a result of contractions of the tensor veli palatini muscle, and there is an audible ear click,[1-3] which is loud enough to be heard by people other than the patient. It has been demonstrated that the ear clicks heard secondary to closure of the eustachian tube in EPM are not a feature of SPM.[4] The movements can often be altered and transiently suppressed. It has been suggested that in many cases, essential palatal myoclonus may represent a psychogenic movement disorder[5,6]; in other cases, there may be a genetic link. The psychogenic palatal tremor is intermittent, under voluntary control, increases with attention toward the patient, and decreases with distractibility. SPM is the more common form of palatal myoclonus and occurs when there is a structural lesion in the brainstem or cerebellum. A distinguishing feature of this subtype is the absence of an audible ear click.[1,2] In SPM, the levator veli palatini muscle is responsible for the rhythmic movements of the soft palate, and nearly always SPM is associated with synchronous movements of the eyes, larynx, pharynx, face, diaphragm, and cervical muscles.[4] It is often associated with hypertrophy of the inferior olive. Causes may include cerebrovascular disease, degenerative disease, encephalitis, demyelinating disease, tumors, and brain trauma involving pathways between the dentate, red, and inferior olivary nuclei.[1,4] SPM has also been reported to occur with Hashimoto's encephalopathy (which improved when the underlying condition was treated). SPM is more likely to persist during sleep, while EPT may disappear during sleep.[1]

Symptoms

Localization site	Comment
Cerebral hemispheres	Some cases have been reported to occur as a sequela of cortical infarct
Mental status and psychiatric aspects/complications	Psychogenic causes are thought to be responsible for EPM in some cases. Speech has been reported to be dysarthric with ongoing palatal tremor. Psychiatric manifestations include suicide attempts due to bothersome ear clicks
Brainstem	Ipsilateral dentate nucleus, contralateral red nucleus, central tegmental tract, and inferior olivary nucleus are the causative regions thought to be responsible for SPM
Cerebellum	Superior cerebellar peduncle and olivocerebellar fibers are sites that may be involved in symptomatic palatal tremor
Vestibular system (and nonspecific dizziness)	Symptoms of ongoing ear clicks are representative of EPM
Cranial nerves	CN V (trigeminal nerve) innervates the tensor veli palatini, which is responsible for EPM CN IX and X innervate levator veli palatini, which is responsible for SPM
Muscle	Levator veli palatini is responsible for the rhythmic movements of SPM. Tensor veli palatini muscle is the likely cause of ear clicks in EPM

EPM and psychogenic disorder may either coexist or may be mistaken for one another.[1,5]

Secondary Complications: Besides the clicking that is associated with EPM, which may induce frustration for the patient, other complications have been associated with both EPM and SPM. Palatal myoclonus can be accompanied by pharyngeal and laryngeal myoclonic movements. When this occurs, severe respiratory difficulties may become apparent for the patient. Some cases of dysarthria and dysphagia have also been reported.

Treatment Complications: One of the treatment options for palatal myoclonus is botulinum toxin injections into the affected muscles. Palatal weakness has been reported as a complication of this treatment. Another treatment option is oral benzodiazepines, which may cause addiction or sedation.

References

1. Deuschl G, Mischke G, Schenck E, Schulte-Monting J, Lucking CH. Symptomatic and essential rhythmic palatal myoclonus. *Brain*. 1990;113:1645–72.
2. Zadikoff C, Lang AE, Klein C. The 'essentials' of essential palatal tremor: a reappraisal of the nosology. *Brain*. 2006;129:832–40.
3. Vieregge P, Klein C, Gehrking E, Kurtke D. The diagnosis of 'essential' palatal tremor. *Neurology*. 1997;49:248–9
4. Deuschl G, Toro C, Hallett M. Symptomatic and essential palatal tremor. 2. Differences of palatal movements. *Mov Disord*. 1994;9(6):676–8.
5. Kadakia S, McAbee G. Volitional control of palatal myoclonus. *Mov Disord*. 1990;5:182–3.
6. Williams DR. Psychogenic palatal tremor. *Mov Disord*. 2004;19:333–5.

Pancreatic Cancer

Epidemiology and Demographics: Gastrointestinal cancers are responsible for 24% of the deaths related to cancer. Among the gastrointestinal cancers is pancreatic cancer, which recently has been recognized as the 3rd leading cause of cancer-related death in the United States With an incidence of 45,000 cases/year, it is typically diagnosed during the 6th to 7th decade of life. It occurs more often in males. Although gastrointestinal cancers in general may be associated with brain metastases, leptomeningeal, bone, and spinal cord metastases are uncommon with pancreatic cancer. While pancreatic brain metastases occur in less than 0.2% of cases (>60% as a single lesion), more recent reports suggest the metastatic disease associations may be increasing.

Disorder Description: Pancreatic cancer is a fatal disease, and a true oncologic challenge, given its dismal prognosis with a 100% mortality. It is associated with several, albeit uncommon, paraneoplastic syndromes or additional neoplasms. These include neuroendocrine tumors, Zollinger–Ellison syndrome, insulinomas, glucagonomas, anti-GAD antibody encephalomyelitis, anti-Purkinje cell antibodies with opsoclonus-ataxia, Miller–Fisher syndrome, chronic inflammatory demyelinating polyneuropathy, and cerebellar degeneration.

Symptoms

Localization site	Comment
Cerebral hemispheres	Seizures, hydrocephalus, venous sinus thrombosis with subsequent cerebral hemorrhage, cerebral hemorrhage from disseminated intravascular coagulation, embolic or thrombotic cerebrovascular accident. Encephalomyelitis
Mental status and psychiatric aspects/complications	Encephalopathy, hepatic encephalopathy with liver metastasis, stupor, coma Depression, anxiety
Cerebellum	Opsoclonus, ataxia
Unclear localization	Asterixis
Cranial nerves	Cranial neuropathies
Spinal cord	Myelopathy
Cauda equina	Bladder and bowel symptoms
Specific spinal roots	Radiculopathy
Plexus	Severe pain, gastroparesis

Secondary Complications: Hydrocephalus, chronic pain, CIPD, ambulatory dysfunction, and focal neurologic deficits.

Treatment Complications:
- Surgery: hemorrhage, infection.
- Whole brain radiation therapy (WBRT): optic neuritis, brainstem necrosis with co-therapy with gemcitabine.
- Stereotactic radiosurgery for brain metastasis: hemorrhage.
- Chemotherapy: gemcitabine associated with paresthesias in 20% of the cases, autonomic neuropathy.

Bibliography

Lemke J, Scheele J, Kapapa T, et al. Brain metastasis in pancreatic cancer. *Int J Mol Sci.* 2013;14(2): 4163–73. DOI:10.3390/ijms14024163.

Makarova-Rusher OV, Ulahannan S, Greten TF, Duffy A. Pancreatic squamous cell carcinoma: a population-based study of epidemiology, clinicopathologic characteristics and outcomes. *Pancreas.* 2016;45(10):1432–7.

Newton HB, Malkin MG. *Neurological complications of systemic cancer and antineoplastic therapy.* (Neurological Disease and Therapy series: Vol 96). Boca Raton, FL: CRC Press; 2016. p. 330.

Patchell RA, Tibbs PA, Walsh JW, et al. A randomized trial of surgery in the treatment of single metastases to the brain. *N Engl J Med.* 1990;322:494–500.

Pancreatitis

Epidemiology and Demographics: Pancreatitis is a relatively uncommon disease that can occur in acute or chronic forms. The incidence of acute pancreatitis is estimated at 40 cases/100,000 adults per year. The incidence of chronic hepatitis has been reported to be 4/100,000. Acute pancreatitis tends to affect men more than women.

Disorder Description: Pancreatitis occurs as a result of inflammation in the pancreas cells. Chronic pancreatitis presents with abdominal pain that can be severe, nausea and vomiting, weight loss, and malabsorption. Acute pancreatitis presents with severe abdominal pain, nausea and vomiting, anorexia, and symptoms from its complications such as edema, fever due to infection and abscess formation, and jaundice. Pancreatic encephalopathy occurs in about 1–2% of patients with acute pancreatitis and ranges from mild problems with attention span to delirium or coma.

Symptoms

Localization site	Comment
Cerebral hemispheres	Seizure
Mental status and psychiatric aspects/complications	Anxiety, delirium, pancreatic encephalopathy

Secondary Complications: Excessive alcohol use is a common risk factor for chronic pancreatitis, which can also cause peripheral neuropathy or myopathy. Patients with chronic pancreatitis can develop diabetes mellitus, which can cause neuropathy among other neurologic complications. Chronic pancreatitis can lead to neurologic complications from nutritional deficiencies.

Bibliography

Majumder H, Chari ST. Chronic pancreatitis. *Lancet.* 2016;387:1957–66.

Rana-Guajardo AC, Cámara-Lemarroy CR, Rendón-Ramírez EJ, et al. Wernicke encephalopathy presenting in a patient with severe acute pancreatitis. *JOP.* 2012;13:104.

Ruggieri RM, Lupo I, Piccoli F. Pancreatic encephalopathy: a 7-year follow-up case report and review of the literature. *Neurol Sci.* 2002;23:203–5.

Tsai HH, Hsieh CH, Liou CW, et al. Encephalopathy and acute axonal sensorimotor polyneuropathy following acute pancreatitis: a case report and review of the literature. *Pancreas.* 2005;30(3): 285–7.

Panic Attack

Epidemiology and Demographics: In the United States, the 12-month prevalence of panic attacks is 11.2% in adults. Females are more frequently affected than males. Panic attacks may occur in children, but are rare until puberty. Prevalence decreases with increasing age after onset and does not appear to differ according to race.

Disorder Description: Panic attack is not itself a mental disorder and can occur in the context of any anxiety disorder or other mental disorder, and some medical conditions. Thus, "panic attack" is generally used as a specifier, as in "depressive disorder with panic attacks."

As stated in DSM-5, a panic attack is defined as: An abrupt surge of intense fear or intense discomfort reaching a peak within minutes, and during which time four (or more) of the following symptoms occur:

i. Palpatations, pounding heart, or accelerated heart rate
ii. Sweating
iii. Trembling or shaking
iv. Sensations of shortness of breath or smothering
v. Feelings of choking
vi. Chest pain or discomfort
vii. Nausea or abdominal distress
viii. Feeling dizzy, unsteady, light-headed, or faint
ix. Chills or heat sensations
x. Paresthesias (numbness or tingling sensations)
xi. Derealization (feelings of unreality) or depersonalization (being detached from oneself)
xii. Fear of losing control or "going crazy"
xiii. Fear of dying

Differential Diagnosis: Differential diagnosis should include other paroxysmal episodes, anxiety disorder due to another medical condition, substance/medication-induced anxiety disorder, and panic disorder.

In other paroxysmal disorders, there may be a current surge of an emotional state, but this state is not fear. Some examples of other paroxysmal disorders include "anger disorder" and "grief disorder."

In anxiety disorder due to another medical condition, a surge of fear is secondary to a medical condition. Examples of conditions that may cause anxiety include hyperthyroidism, hyperparathyroidism, pheochromocytoma, vestibular dysfunctions, seizure disorders, and cardiopulmonary conditions (e.g., arrhythmias, supraventricular tachycardia, asthma, chronic obstructive pulmonary disease). The history, physical examination, and laboratory testing should determine the etiology of the condition causing anxiety.

In substance/medication-induced anxiety disorder, intoxication with stimulants may induce a panic attack. Conversely, withdrawal from a depressant may induce the panic attack. It should be determined whether the individual had panic attacks prior to the onset of excessive drug use. In cases wherein there is onset of panic attacks after 45 years of age, or in those wherein atypical features (loss of consciousness, vertigo, incontinence) are seen, an underlying medical condition or substance use should be carefully considered.

Panic disorder is characterized by repeated, unexpected panic attacks. These are necessary, but not sufficient for the diagnosis of panic disorder. See entry for *Panic Disorder* for full criteria.

Secondary Complications: Panic attacks are associated with comorbid mental disorders including anxiety disorders, depressive and bipolar disorders, impulse control disorders, and substance use disorders. They are also associated with the increased likelihood of developing such disorders.

Treatment Complications: Because panic attack is a symptom and not a diagnosis, a panic attack in and of itself is often not treated. In the context of a medical condition or substance-induced panic attack, the underlying etiology should be treated. In a panic attack in the context of panic disorder, benzodiazepines can be used as abortive therapy and selective serotonin reuptake inhibitors (SSRIs) can be used as prophylaxis. See entry for *Panic Disorder*.

Side effects of benzodiazepines include drowsiness, impairment of intellectual function, motor coordination problems, and amnesia. Respiratory depression may occur in overdose, especially when combined with alcohol or other depressants. Withdrawal from benzodiazepines may cause seizures and can be life threatening.

SSRI side effects include nausea, diarrhea, insomnia, headache, anorexia, weight loss, sexual dysfunction, restlessness (akathisia-like), serotonin syndrome (fever diaphoresis, tachycardia, hypertension, delirium, neuromuscular excitability), hyponatremia, and seizures (0.2%).

Bibliography

American Psychiatric Association. *Diagnostic and statistical manual of mental disorders: DSM-5.* 5th ed. Washington, DC: American Psychiatric Association; 2013.

Breslau N, Schultz LR, Stewart WF, Lipton R, Welch KMA. Headache types and panic disorder: Directionality and specificity. *Neurology.* 2001;56(3):350–4.

Cox BJ, Swinson RP, Endler NS, Norton GR. The symptom structure of panic attacks. *Compr Psychiatry.* 1994;35(5):349–53.

Ley R. Agoraphobia, the panic attack and the hyperventilation syndrome. *Behav Res Ther.* 1985;23(1):79–81.

Reiman EM, Raichle ME, Butler FK, Herscovitch P, Robins E. A focal brain abnormality in panic disorder, a severe form of anxiety. *Nature.* 1984;310(5979):683–5.

Panic Disorder

Epidemiology and Demographics: Two million Americans are diagnosed with panic disorder every year with a 12-month prevalence of 2.7% and a lifetime prevalence of 4.7%. It occurs twice as commonly in females as compared with males. The average age of onset is 24 years; however, both younger and older individuals are affected.

Disorder Description: As stated in DSM-5, panic disorder can be defined as:

A. Recurrent unexpected panic attacks. The patient feels intense fear or discomfort that reaches a peak within minutes. During this period, four (or more) of the following symptoms occur:

[Note: The abrupt surge can occur from a calm state or an anxious state.]

1. Palpitations, pounding heart, or accelerated heart rate.
2. Sweating.
3. Trembling, shaking.
4. Sensations of shortness of breath or smothering.
5. Feelings of choking.
6. Chest pain or discomfort.
7. Nausea or abdominal distress.
8. Dizziness, unsteadiness, light-headedness or feeling faint.
9. Chills or heat intolerance.
10. Paresthesias (numbness or tingling sensations).
11. Derealization (feelings of unreality) or depersonalization (being detached from oneself).
12. Fear of losing control or "going crazy."
13. Fear of dying.

B. These symptoms are followed by at least 1-month duration of the following:

1. Persistent concern or worry about the reoccurrence of panic attacks or associated symptoms (e.g., losing control, having a heart attack, or "going crazy").
2. Significant maladaptive change in behavior related to these attacks (e.g., behaviors designed to avoid having panic attacks including avoidance of exercise or unfamiliar situations).

C. The disturbance is not attributable to the physiologic effects of a substance or another medical condition.

D. The disturbance is not better explained by another mental disorder.

[Note: Unlike panic disorder, panic attack, as a symptom, may occur in context of another mental or medical condition, and should have an identifiable trigger.]

Differential Diagnoses

Differential diagnosis	Similar symptoms	Distinguishing factors
Seizures	□ Abrupt onset □ Aura; i.e., fear □ Muscle tension □ Hypervigilance □ Fear of losing control	□ Detailed seizure history □ Peri-ictal memory impairment with or without LOC □ Abnormal EEG □ Motor symptoms
Vertigo	□ Anticipation of vertigo may lead to panic □ Hypersensitivity to visual stimuli □ Dizziness (vestibular dysfunction) □ Imbalance	□ History of dizziness and imbalance □ Nystagmus noted on physical exam
Headache/migraine	□ Aura □ Anticipation of headache may lead to panic □ Avoidance of triggers □ Nausea/vomiting	□ History of headache/migraine □ Sensitivity to smell, noise, and light □ Aura – blurred vision, and other visual disturbances
Parkinson's disease	□ Anxiety (during "off" period) □ Fear of embarrassment from Parkinson's symptoms: tremor or difficulty with gait □ Restlessness □ Autonomic instability	□ Detailed history □ Side effect of Parkinson's medication □ Rigidity/resting tremor □ Shuffling gait □ Flat facial affect
Transient ischemic attack	□ Paresthesia □ Episodic □ Resolution of symptoms	□ Older age □ Recovery time days to weeks. □ Neurologic symptoms or deficits
Multiple sclerosis	□ Tingling □ Numbness □ Loss of balance □ Dizziness □ Complete resolution of symptoms	□ Neurologic deficits □ Abnormal brain imaging

Treatment

- Selective serotonin reuptake inhibitors (SSRIs): e.g., fluoxetine, paroxetine, sertraline, citalopram, and escitalopram.
- Selective norepinephrine reuptake inhibitors: e.g., venlafaxine and duloxetine.
- Benzodiazepines: used for rapid onset of action while SSRI achieves full effect (usually 2–6 weeks), e.g., lorazepam, alprazolam, clonazepam, and diazepam. Clonazepam is preferred due to relatively longer half-life and less addiction risk.
- Cognitive behavioral therapy (CBT): targets the fear and behavioral patterns by exposure and restructuring therapy.
- Combination of CBT and SSRI/serotonin-norepinephrine reuptake inhibitors (SNRIs).

Bibliography

American Psychiatric Association. *Diagnostic and statistical manual of mental disorders.* 5th ed. Washington, DC: American Psychiatric Association; 2013.

Beletsky V, Mirsattari SM. Epilepsy, Mental health disorders, or both? *Epilepsy Res Treat.* 2012; Article ID 163731. http://dx.doi.org/10.1155/2012/163731.

Cassem NH, Stern TA, Rosenbaum JF, Jellinek MS, Fricchione GL. *Massachusetts General Hospital handbook of general hospital psychiatry.* 6th ed. St. Louis, MO: Mosby; 2004.

Kessler RC, Chiu WT, Jin R, et al. The epidemiology of panic attacks, panic disorder, and agoraphobia in the National Comorbidity Survery Replication. *Arch Gen Psychiatry.* 2006;63(4):415–24.

Lyketsos CG, Kozauer N, Rabins PV. Psychiatric manifestations of neurologic disease: Where are we headed? *Dialog Clin Neurosci.* 2007;9(2):111–24.

Nadarajan V, Perry RJ, Johnson J, Werring DJ. Transient ischemic attack: mimics and chameleons. *Pract Neurol.* 2013;14:23–31.

Rizzo M, Eslinger PJ. *Principles and practice of behavioral neurology and neuropsychology.* Philadelphia, PA: W.B. Saunders; 2004.

Pantothenate Kinase-Associated Neurodegeneration (PKAN)/ Hallevorden–Spatz

Epidemiology and Demographics: Pantothenate kinase-associated neurodegeneration (PKAN) is a rare disorder. It has been reported in select communities in which intra-familial marriages are common, such as the Agrawal community in the northern part of India.

Disorder Description: It is an autosomal recessive disorder, involving the PANK2 gene on chromosome 20, leading to iron deposition in the basal ganglia. PKAN is a major subtype of neurodegeneration with brain iron accumulation (NBIA). The symptoms usually present in infancy, involving motor and language development. Later on, the child's gait and motor skills are affected, and between the ages of 3 and 6, choreoathetosis and dystonia occur. As the disease progresses, further neurologic symptoms including dysarthria, spasticity, bilateral retinopathy, optic atrophy, and seizures, as well as learning disorders develop. The disease onset can also be in adulthood. In such cases, the disease presentation is more atypical, and symptoms can include slowly progressive chorea without dementia or can have clinical features of Tourette syndrome. Optic atrophy could be the initial sign and can present a few years prior to the other aforementioned symptoms.

Symptoms

Localization site	Comment
Optic atrophy	This could be the presenting sign and proceed other symptoms by several years
Cerebral cortex	Cortical atrophy with iron pigment deposits with secondary ventricular enlargement
Substantia nigra	Parkinsonism including gait abnormality, bradykinisia, rigidity, and tremor

Localization site	Comment
Cerebellum	Although this is more rare, it has been reported
Basal ganglia including globus pallidus and caudate	The basal ganglia involvement on MRI imaging is manifested as a low-intensity ring surrounding a high-signal-intensity region ("eye of the tiger" sign)
Muscle	Though less common, myopathic involvement with increase in creatine kinase level has been reported

Secondary Complications: Severe orobuccolingual dystonia may result in recurrent tongue biting and self-mutilation, and full-mouth dental extraction might be indicated. Soft resin bite guards can be used in such cases.

Treatment Complications: There is no specific treatment for this disorder, and the management is often symptom based. For example, in the context of parkinsonism, levodopa, anticholinergics, and oral or continuous intrathecal baclofen can prove efficacious. In treatment-resistant cases, stereotactic pallidotomy is a potential treatment option. In the case of dystonia, botulinum toxin might be considered.

Bibliography

Gordon N. Pantothenate kinase-associated neurodegeneration (Hallevorden-Spatz syndrome). *Eur Paediatr Neurol Soc.* 2002;(6):243–7.

Gregory A, Hayflick SJ. Neurodegeneration with brain iron accumulation. *Folia Neuropathol.* 2005;43(4):286–96.

Mikati MA, Yehya A, Darwish H, Karam P, Comair Y. Deep brain stimulation as a mode of treatment of early onset pantothenate kinase-associated neurodegeneration. *Eur J Pediatr Neurol.* 2008;13(1):61–4.

Schneider SA. *Movement disorder curricula.* New York, NY: Springer; 2017.

Shields DC, Sharma N, Gale JT, Eskandar EN. Pallidal stimulation for dystonia in pantothenate kinase-associated neurodegeneration. *Pediatr Neurol.* 2007;37(6):442–5.

Paracoccidioides brasiliensis

Epidemiology and Demographics: Infection endemic to Central and South America. Acute/subacute form in endemic areas only, and primarily affects children and young adults. Chronic form affecting male adults in their mid-40s presents many years after exposure in an endemic area. Nine percent to 25% of systemic cases have nervous system involvement.

Disorder Description: Myocotic infection that presents with granulomatous inflammation. There are two presentations, both more common in immunosuppressed individuals:

1. acute/subacute: disseminated lesions weeks or months after infection; and
2. chronic: oral mucosa, airways, lung, central nervous system (CNS) involvement years after infection.

Spinal fluid analysis is very unreliable for diagnosis.

When the nervous system is involved, symptoms depend on the location of involvement as indicated in the table below.

Symptoms

Localization site	Comment
Cerebral hemispheres	Chronic meningoencephalitis 17% Seizure 33%, hemiparesis 25%, headache 21%
Mental status	Confusion 13%
Brainstem/cranial nerves	Bulbar signs 8%
Cerebellum	Ataxia 25%
Spinal cord	Very rare

Secondary Complications: Hydrocephalus in 21% of CNS cases; both communicating and non-communicating forms are possible. Frequently residual hyperdense or calcified lesions on non-contrast head CT.

Treatment Complications: Side effects of antifungals only. Treatment is typically with trimethoprim–sulphamethoxazole or amphotericin B.

Bibliography

de Almeida SM. Central nervous system paracoccidioidomycosis: an overview. *Braz J Infect Dis.* 2005;9(2):126–33.

Martinez R. Epidemiology of paracoccidioidomycosis. *Rev Inst Med Trop Sao Paulo.* 2015:57(Suppl 19):11–20.

Paraganglioma

Epidemiology and Demographics: Rare neoplasia with unknown incidence. Classified as sporadic and hereditary, with sporadic predominance in adulthood up to 75% and 30–40% hereditary in childhood. Diagnosed predominantly between the 3rd and 5th decades of life, with female predominance in the sporadic cases. Known with malignant potential defined by the World Health Organization as the presence of metastatic disease, and up to 20% will have a malignant diagnosis.

Disorder Description: A rare subset of catecholamine-secreting or non-secreting neuroendocrine tumor. Originates from glomus cells, embryonically derived from neural crest, chromaffin negative (subtle difference from pheochromocytoma). These chemoreceptors are located adjacent to the vasculature.

Paragangliomas are part of the autonomic nervous system, symmetrically located along the neuroaxis, dichotomized as being either sympathetic secreting tumors of predominantly norepinephrine, located in lower mediastinum, abdomen, and pelvis, or parasympathetic non-secreting neoplasia, typically located in the skull base, neck, and upper mediastinum. Histologically similar to ependymomas, with similar cuboidal/polygonal small cells clustered in a way known as "zellballen." The immunophenotype of this tumor includes positive testing for chromogranin, synaptophysin, neuron-specific enolase, serotonin, neurofilament, glial fibrillary acidic protein, and neural cell adhesion molecule; negative testing for S-100 protein. The mutation associated with hereditary cases is in the mitochondrial succinate dehydrogenase enzyme complex (SDH-A, SDH-B, SDH-C), and the following syndromes have a particular susceptibility for the development of paragangliomas: multiple endocrine neoplasia 2A-2B, neurofibromatosis type 1, and von Hippel–Lindau.

Symptoms

Localization site	Comment
Cerebral hemispheres	Syncope
Mental status and psychiatric aspects/complications	Anxiety, apprehension
Vestibular system	Nausea, vomiting, dizziness, vertigo, tinnitus

Localization site	Comment
Cauda equina	Saddle anesthesia
Specific spinal roots	Radicular pain, local paresthesias

Secondary Complications: Hypertension, malignant arrhythmias, and sudden death.

Treatment Complications:

- Surgery: hemorrhage, malignant hypertension, arrhythmias, multiorgan failure.
- Embolization: hemorrhage, skin necrosis, cranial nerve deficits, stroke, hearing loss.
- Radiotherapy: mucositis, skin rash, hypoacusis, hypopituitarism, xerostomia, bone necrosis.

Bibliography

Abermil N, Guillaud-Bataille M, Burnichon N, et al. TMEM127 screening in a large cohort of patients with pheochromocytoma and/or paraganglioma. *J Clin Endocrinol Metab*. 2012;97:E805–9.

Anderson J, Gulant RW. Paraganglioma of the cauda equina: a case report. *J Neurol Neurosurg Psychiatry*. 1987;50:100–3.

Bayley JP, Kunst HP, Cascon A, et al. SDHAF2 mutations in familial and sporadic paraganglioma and phaeochromocytoma. *Lancet Oncol*. 2010;11:366–72.

Kirmani S, Young WF. Hereditary paraganglioma-pheochromocytoma syndromes. May 21, 2008. Updated Nov 6, 2014. In Pagon RA, Adam MP, Ardinger HH, et al., eds. *GeneReviews®* [Internet]. Seattle (WA): University of Washington, Seattle; 1993–2017.

Papathomas TG, de Krijger RR, Tischler AS. Paragangliomas: update on differential diagnostic considerations, composite tumors, and recent genetic developments. *Semin Diagn Pathol*. 2013;30(3):207–23. DOI: 10.1053/j.semdp.2013.06.006.

Paragonimus Infection (Paragonimiasis)

Epidemiology and Demographics: The main species causing infection is *Paragonimus westermani*, which occurs primarily in Asia, particularly China. Other species have been isolated from Africa and Central/South America. Although rare in the United States, several cases have been associated with ingestion of uncooked crawfish during river raft float trips in Missouri.

Disorder Description: Paragonimus is a lung fluke (flatworm) that infects the human lungs. Infection occurs through ingestion of undercooked crab, shellfish, or crayfish infected with metacercariae. Serious cases of paragonimiasis occur when the parasite travels from the lungs to the central nervous system.

After ingestion, the larvae travel through the duodenal wall and ultimately through the diaphragm to reach the lungs. Coughing up the flukes releases them back to the atmosphere, and they find their way to water and are ingested by snails, which get eaten by crabs and crayfish to complete the cycle.

Symptoms: Cough, fever, and symptoms like chronic bronchitis/tuberculosis, hemoptysis, abnormal CXR, eosinophilia, and sputum peppered with clumps of fluke eggs can occur. Central nervous system spread is an infrequent complication.

Localization site	Comment
Cerebral hemispheres	Meningitis tends to occur as an acute manifestation and is the initial presenting feature in one-third of cases. The parasite can penetrate the meninges and invade brain parenchyma, leading to meningitis, encephalitis, arachnoiditis, hemorrhage, or a space-occupying lesion. Temporal and occipital lobe involvement is most frequent
	Chronic manifestations include headache, vomiting, seizures, visual disturbances (particularly diplopia and homonymous hemianopsia), and motor or sensory disturbances related to a space-occupying lesion. Up to 10 cerebral cysts may be seen, predominantly in the temporal and occipital lobes
	On MRI, multiple cystic, ring-enhancing lesions with surrounding edema may be seen. Calcification of the lesions occurs in approximately 50%. The appearance has been described as being like "soap-bubble calcifications" on skull imaging or as having a "grape cluster" quality. Hydrocephalus and localized hemorrhages may be seen. The characteristic appearance of paragonimiasis is the "tunnel sign," which shows the track of the adult worm
Mental status and psychiatric aspects/ complications	Brainstem involvement, hydrocephalus, and seizures can lead to decreased consciousness

Localization site	Comment
Brainstem	Brainstem abscesses have been described
Spinal cord	Spinal cord involvement is rare, epidural involvement is more common than intradural
	MRI of the lumber spine may reveal multiple well-defined intradural masses and chronic arachnoiditis
	Although the route of infection to the spinal canal is not yet known, the theory of direct migration of larvae from the lung or direct dissemination via CSF is assumed

Treatment Complications: Complications include those related to surgery, epilepsy, and cerebral edema. Praziquantel/triclabendazole treatment is given along with surgical drainage of abscess/shunting for hydrocephalus, antiepileptics, steroids, and other supportive treatment. Anthelminthic treatment may lead to hypersensitivity and arrhythmias.

Bibliography

Centers for Disease Control and Prevention. Paragonimiasis. www.cdc.gov. Accessed Sep 4, 2018.

Johnson RJ, Jong EC, Dunning SB, et al. Paragonimiasis: diagnosis and the use of praziquantel in treatment. *Rev Infect Dis* 1985; 7:200.

Kim MK, Cho BM, Yoon DY. Imaging features of intradural spinal paragonimiasis: A case report *Br J Radiol*. 2011 Apr; 84(1000): e72–e74.

Oh SJ. Spinal paragonimiasis. *J Neurol Sci* 1968; 6:125–40

Xia Y, Ju Y, Chen J, You C. Cerebral paragonimiasis: a retrospective analysis of 27 cases. *J Neurosurg Pediatr* 2015; 15:101.

Parainfluenza

Epidemiology and Demographics: Caused by four viruses, HPIV1 to HPIV4. Ubiquitous virus; 90% of adults have antibodies that are incompletely protective. Each serotype has a different seasonality:
- PIV1: biannual fall epidemics
- PIV2: annual fall epidemics
- PIV3: spring but variable
- PIV4: unknown

Disorder Description: Presents as a typical upper and/or lower respiratory, flu-like illness. Communicated through droplets, and outbreaks are common. Immunocompromised individuals are at increased risk for severe disease. Neurologic involvement is uncommon. Diagnosed with nasal swab antigen or PCR test.

Mild encephalopathy with reversible splenial lesions (MERS) is more common in influenza A and B, but has been reported with parainfluenza. This condition may be associated with hyponatremia, CSF pleocytosis, and EEG changes, including generalized and occipital slowing and focal spikes.

Symptoms

Localization site	Comment
Cerebral hemispheres	Seizure. Reversible lesions in the splenium of the corpus callosum
Meninges	Case reports of meningoencephalitis
Mental status and psychiatric aspects/complications	Confusion/delirium in MERS
Vestibular system (and non-specific dizziness)	<1/1000

Secondary Complications: Communicating hydrocephalus. High risk of having co-infections, particularly in the immunocompromised, so workup should always exclude other bacterial or fungal infections.

Treatment Complications: Treatment is supportive.

Bibliography

Aminoff MJ, Josephson SA, eds. *Aminoff's neurology and general medicine*. 5th ed. London, UK: Elsevier; 2014.

Ka A, Britton P, Troedson C, et al. Mild encephalopathy with reversible splenial lesion: An important differential of encephalitis. *Eur J Paediatr Neurol*. 2015;19(3):377–82.

Fry AM, Curns AT, Harbour K, et al. Seasonal trends of human parainfluenza viral infections: United States, 1990–2004. *Clin Infect Dis*. 2006;43(8):1016–22. Epub 2006 Sep 13.

Paraneoplastic Autonomic Neuropathy

Epidemiology and Demographics: Uncommon syndrome, <1% with morbidity and mortality resulting from severe dysautonomia. No predilection by race, although there are discrepancies regarding gender.

Disorder Description: Autoimmune dysautonomia associated with a malignancy, with damage to the autonomic system. Has multiple clinical manifestations, with a typical enteric plexus lesion, leading to impaired motility and autonomic gastroparesis. Subacute global autonomic impairment, involving multiple limbs of the autonomic nervous system. Other paraneoplastic syndromes may coexist. Associated commonly with small cell lung cancer and thymoma. Classically associated with anti-Hu antibodies, voltage-gated potassium channel antibodies, or ganglionic nicotinic acetylcholine receptor antibodies; 30% of the patients seropositive for the nicotinic acetylcholine receptor antibodies were positive for a malignancy even though it is the most common nonparaneoplastic cause of ganglionopathy. All patients with rapid onset of severe autonomic failure warrant screening for occult malignancy.

Symptoms

Localization site	Comment
Plexus	Sympathetic impairment with prominent orthostatic hypotension, syncope, and impaired sweating
	Parasympathetic involvement: xerostomia, xerophthalmia, urinary retention, erectile dysfunction, difficulty with vision in bright light due to fixed pupils, hemodynamic instability, gastrointestinal dysmotility, severe constipation, nausea, early satiety due to lack of gastric emptying, abdominal distention, and weight loss

Secondary Complications: Syncope, falls, and weight loss.
Treatment Complications:
- Immunomodulation: neurotoxicity, cognitive impairment, myositis, headache, paresthesia, insomnia, tremor, severe encephalopathy, seizures or even status epilepticus, motor polyneuropathy, depression, anxiety, lethargy, leukoencephalopathy, and endocrinopathies.
- Surgical resolution of primary tumor.

Bibliography

Bataller L, Dalmau J. Paraneoplastic disorders of the nervous system. *Continuum (Minneap Minn)*. 2005;11(5, Neuro-Oncology):69–92. DOI: 10.1212/01.con.0000293680.24426.ae.

Honnorat J, Antoine J-C. Paraneoplastic neurological syndromes. *Orphanet J Rare Dis*. 2007;2:22. DOI:10.1186/1750-1172-2-22.

Lancaster E. Paraneoplastic disorders. *Continuum (Minneap Minn)*. 2015;21(2, Neuro-Oncology): 452–75. DOI: 10.1212/01.CON.0000464180.89580.88.

Muppidi S, Vernino S. Paraneoplastic neuropathies. *Continuum (Minneap Minn)*. 2014;20(5, Peripheral Nervous System Disorders):1359–72. DOI: 10.1212/01.CON.0000455876.53309.ec.

Paraneoplastic Encephalomyelitis

Epidemiology and Demographics: Uncommon rapidly progressive paraneoplastic syndrome, which may precede the diagnosis of the malignancy. Described more commonly in men up to 45–50 years of age. Associated with testicular tumors, gynecologic and lung neoplasias, manifesting usually as limbic/brainstem encephalitis and myelitis.

Disorder Description: Rapidly progressive autoimmune disorder that involves the central nervous system (hippocampus, cerebellum, brainstem, and spinal cord), dorsal root ganglia, and autonomic system, with a diagnosis based upon the dominant symptoms from involvement of two or more areas, typically presenting as a combination between limbic encephalitis and cerebellar degeneration.

The antibodies described in this paraneoplastic disease include anti-Hu antibody, CRMP5, Ma2, amphiphysin, and GlyR antibodies.

Symptoms

Localization site	Comment
Cerebral hemispheres	Epilepsia partialis continua, encephalopathy, seizures, mutism
	Depression, anxiety, confusion, lethargy, aphasia, hallucinations
Mental status and psychiatric aspects/ complications	Cognitive impairment
Cerebellum	Appendicular and truncal ataxia, dysarthria

Localization site	Comment
Vestibular system	Dizziness, nausea, vomiting
Spinal cord	Myelopathy, paraparesis, tetraparesis
Dorsal root ganglia	Dysesthesia to all modalities, more pronounced in proprioception, sensory ataxia

Secondary Complications: Dependence, frequent falls, depression, epilepsy, and tremor.

Treatment Complications:

- Immunomodulation: neurotoxicity, cognitive impairment, myositis, headache, paresthesia, insomnia, tremor, severe encephalopathy, seizures or even status epilepticus, motor polyneuropathy, depression, anxiety, lethargy, leukoencephalopathy, and endocrinopathies.
- Surgical resolution of primary tumor.

Bibliography

Bataller L, Dalmau J. Paraneoplastic disorders of the nervous system. *Continuum (Minneap Minn).* 2005;11(5, Neuro-Oncology):69–92. DOI: 10.1212/01.con.0000293680.24426.ae.

Honnorat J, Antoine J-C. Paraneoplastic neurological syndromes. *Orphanet J Rare Dis.* 2007;2:22. DOI:10.1186/1750-1172-2-22.

Lancaster E. Paraneoplastic disorders. *Continuum (Minneap Minn).* 2015;21(2, Neuro-Oncology):452–75. DOI: 10.1212/01.CON.0000464180.89580.88.

Muppidi S, Vernino S. Paraneoplastic neuropathies. *Continuum (Minneap Minn).* 2014;20(5, Peripheral Nervous System Disorders):1359–72. DOI: 10.1212/01.CON.0000455876.53309.ec.

Paraneoplastic Limbic Encephalitis

Epidemiology and Demographics: Limbic encephalitides are part of the paraneoplastic syndromes, described more commonly in women and young children, although seen in both sexes. The neoplasias associated with the presence of this entity will vary depending on the demographics of the patient and the antibodies present, and include thymomas, small cell lung cancer, neuroendocrine tumors, breast cancer, and ovarian teratomas. Neurologic recovery has been described with appropriate treatment, with a mean hospital stay length of up to 3 months. The mortality described is 5%, and the relapse is up to 25%, commonly with non-removed tumors or sub-optimally treated.

Disorder Description: Autoimmune encephalitis has been recently more recognized. The limbic encephalitis includes an array of antibodies: NMDA-receptor, anti-AMPA-receptor, anti-GABA B-receptor, anti-LGI1, anti-Ma2, anti-Hu or CV2/CRMP5 antibodies. Characterized by a viral-like prodrome, with subsequent development of psychiatric symptoms, decreased sensorium, abnormal movements and posturing, including seizures, and autonomic dysfunction.

Anti-NMDA receptor (NMDA-R) encephalitis is the most common, with up to 4% presence of NMDA receptor antibodies positive in this population; these antibodies will alter the synapse. More than half of the women over 18 years of age will have unilateral or bilateral ovarian teratomas, with an increased frequency in black women compared with white women, decreasing to a 10% probability with younger females. In men, testicular germ cell tumors have been described.

Anti-AMPA receptor (AMPA-R) encephalitis is described in middle-aged women; over 70% of cases have been associated with thymus, lung, or breast neoplasias.

Anti-GABA B receptor (GABAB-R) is described in the over 60 years age group; no sex preference, and associated with small cell lung cancer and neuroendocrine tumors.

Anti-LGI1 limbic encephalitis is associated with thymomas. These antibodies target voltage-gated potassium channels. It is also associated with autosomal dominant lateral temporal lobe epilepsy and partial epilepsy with auditory features.

Symptoms

Localization site	Comment
Cerebral hemispheres	Seizures, non-convulsive status epilepticus, myoclonus, oro-facial, limb, and trunk dyskinesias; dystonic postures Dysarthria, dysphagia
Mental status and psychiatric aspects/ complications	Short-term memory loss, confusion, irritability, depression, insomnia, behavioral changes, psychosis
Peripheral neuropathy	Autonomic dysfunction
Unclear localization	Viral prodrome, respiratory dysfunction

Secondary Complications: Intubation, cognitive dysfunction, infections, and intensive care neuropathy.

Treatment Complications

- Surgery: inherent to each particular tumor resection, hemorrhage, infection.
- Immunotherapy–immunosuppression: weight gain, hypertension, hyperglycemia, nausea, vomiting, abdominal distention, diarrhea, infections.

Bibliography

Bataller L, Dalmau J. Paraneoplastic disorders of the nervous system. *Continuum (Minneap Minn).* 2005;11(5, Neuro-Oncology):69–92. DOI: 10.1212/01.con.0000293680.24426.ae.

Honnorat J, Antoine J-C. Paraneoplastic neurological syndromes. *Orphanet J Rare Dis.* 2007;2:22. DOI:10.1186/1750-1172-2-22.

Lancaster E. Paraneoplastic disorders. *Continuum (Minneap Minn).* 2015;21(2, Neuro-Oncology):452–75. DOI: 10.1212/01. CON.0000464180.89580.88.

Muppidi S, Vernino S. Paraneoplastic neuropathies. *Continuum (Minneap Minn).* 2014;20(5, Peripheral Nervous System Disorders):1359–72. DOI: 10.1212/01. CON.0000455876.53309.ec.

Rosenfeld MR, Dalmau, JO. Paraneoplastic disorders of the CNS and autoimmune synaptic encephalitis. *Continuum (Minneap Minn).* 2012;18(2, Neuro-Oncology):366–83. DOI: 10.1212/01.CON.0000413664.42798.aa.

Paraneoplastic Motor Neuron Disease

Epidemiology and Demographics: The paraneoplastic motor neuron diseases include myasthenia gravis (MG) and Lambert–Eaton myasthenic syndrome. MG is typically seen in the 6th decade of life accompanied by a thymoma, although can be seen in the 3rd decade of life as well, with equal sex distribution. Lambert–Eaton myasthenic syndrome presents in 50% of the patients with lung cancer. It is described in patients older than 40 years with male predominance, and it is the most common paraneoplastic syndrome seen with small cell lung cancer.

Disorder Description: The most common motor neuron paraneoplastic disorders include MS and Lambert–Eaton myasthenic syndrome, characterized by the presence of autoantibodies to the neuromuscular junction and peripheral membrane protein. The expression of antigens by the tumor leads to the mechanism of action, stimulating the immune activity of T cells and/or antibodies, directed against not only the tumor, but also nerves and muscles.

MG is characterized by the presence of autoantibodies against acetylcholine receptor (AChR) and less frequently antibodies against muscle-specific tyrosine kinase (MuSK). Other antibodies described include those against membrane proteins titin, ryanodine, myosine, actin, and actinin. When AChR are positive, 15% are associated with thymoma, conversely at least 50% of the patients diagnosed with thymoma will develop MG. Thymoma is a rare tumor linked to autoimmunity. This is related to dysregulation of lymphocyte selection, as well as stimulation of the proliferation of autoreactive T lymphocytes and of B lymphocytes that give rise to autoantibodies. Electrodiagnostic studies will help to differentiate and confirm the diagnosis.

Symptoms

Localization site	Comment
Cerebral hemispheres	Fluctuating encephalopathy
Mental status and psychiatric aspects/ complications	Insomnia
Muscle	Myositis with associated myocarditis, arrhythmias, heart failure, sudden death, myokymia, fibrillations
Neuromuscular junction	Fatigable muscle weakness, respiratory muscle weakness, dyspnea, sexual dysfunction, constipation. Fatigable bulbar muscles causing diplopia, dysphagia, dysarthria, dry cough, nasal voice, neck weakness, ptosis
Unclear localization	Chest pain, superior vena cava syndrome

Secondary Complications: Dysarthria, hoarseness, overall weakness, and functional disability.

Treatment Complications:

- Thymectomy: recurrent laryngeal nerve damage (dysarthria, respiratory weakness), myasthenic crisis, hemorrhage, and infection.

- Immunotherapy–immunosuppression: Weight gain, hypertension, hyperglycemia, nausea, vomiting, abdominal distention, diarrhea, and infections.

Bibliography

Turk HM, et al. Paraneoplastic motor neuron disease resembling amyotrophic lateral sclerosis in a patient with renal cell carcinoma. *Med Princ Pract*. 2009;18(1):73–5.

Paraneoplastic Opsoclonus–Myoclonus

Epidemiology and Demographics: This paraneoplastic syndrome is described in 40% of small cell lung cancer (SCLC) patients, 20% of cases of breast cancer and ovarian cancer, and 2–3% of neuroblastomas in children. No predominance by gender, and the age of presentation is associated with the epidemiology of the primary tumor.

Disorder Description: Paraneoplastic-autoimmune, neurobehavioral, and movement disorder characterized by opsoclonus described as chaotic multidirectional saccades, truncal–appendicular myoclonus and ataxia. The clinical presentation in children is associated with hypotonia, irritability, behavioral changes, and psychomotor retardation. The etiologies are varied, including idiopathic, infectious, toxic-metabolic, and neoplasias. As part of the paraneoplastic spectrum, the tumors described include SCLC, gynecologic cancers, and neuroblastoma in children. Many autoantibodies have been described, although in most patients with the paraneoplastic presentation the antibodies will be non-detectable. The presence of antibody suggests the involvement of a humoral immune mechanism, including: anti-Hu antibody, most commonly seen in SCLC and 10% in neuroblastoma; anti-Ri Ab, typically seen in gynecologic cancers; and others mentioned are CRMP5, amphiphysin, Yo, and anti-Ma2, the latter associated with brainstem or cerebellar encephalitis. Although the exact pathophysiology of the opsoclonus is unclear, there have been some descriptions regarding the disinhibition of the fastigial nucleus of the cerebellum; for the rest of the neuropathologic abnormalities there are descriptions of loss of neurons in the medulla, Purkinje and granular cerebellar cell damage, and brainstem gliosis.

Symptoms

Localization site	Comment
Cerebral hemispheres	Encephalopathy, stupor, coma
Mental status and psychiatric aspects/ complications	Irritability, sleep disorder, cognitive decline
Cerebellum	Appendicular or truncal ataxia and myoclonus, truncal titubation, opsoclonus described as an intermittent, sometimes constant chaotic involuntary ocular multidirectional movement with vertical, horizontal, rotatory saccades with inter-saccadic events Vomiting. Dysarthria
Brainstem	Ophthalmoplegia
Unclear localization	Myoclonus

Secondary Complications: Cognitive and behavioral impairment, disability, and dependence.

Treatment Complications

- Immunotherapy: fatigue, rash, pruritus, infection, bleeding risk, depression, irritability.
- Plasma exchange therapy: infections, bleeding, myoclonus, pain.
- Surgery of primary tumor with intrinsic complications associated with the procedure itself.

Bibliography

Arroyo HA, Tringler N. Opsoclonus-myoclonus syndrome. *Medicina (B Aires)*. 2009;69(1 Pt 1): 64–70.

Bataller L, Dalmau J. Paraneoplastic disorders of the nervous system. *Continuum (Minneap Minn)*. 2005;11(5, Neuro-Oncology):69–92. DOI: 10.1212/01.con.0000293680.24426.ae.

Blumkin L, Lerman-Sagie T. Opsoclonus myoclonus ataxia syndrome in Israel. *Harefuah*. 2010;149(1):24–8, 63.

Catsman-Berrevoets CE, Aarsen FK, van Hemsbergen ML, et al. Improvement of neurological status and quality of life in children with opsoclonus myoclonus syndrome at long-term follow-up. *Pediatr Blood Cancer*. 2009;53(6):1048–53.

Honnorat J, Antoine J-C. Paraneoplastic neurological syndromes. *Orphanet J Rare Dis*. 2007;2:22. DOI:10.1186/1750-1172-2-22.

Matsumoto H, Ugawa Y. Paraneoplastic opsoclonus-myoclonus syndrome: a review. *Brain Nerve.* 2010;62(4):365–9.

Paraneoplastic Optic Neuropathy–Retinopathy

Epidemiology and Demographics: These paraneoplastic disorders are infrequent. The most common neoplasias associated with them are melanoma and small cell lung cancer (SCLC), gynecologic including ovarian, endometrial and cervical, followed by breast cancer; known high mortality associated with the presence of the malignancy. The melanoma-associated retinopathy is slightly more frequent than the cancer-associated retinopathy with male predominance compared with females (5:1), and typical age of diagnosis at 60 years.

Disorder Description: The paraneoplastic optic retinopathy is a classic, although rare, acquired autoimmune retinopathy characterized by the triad of photosensitivity, ring scotoma, and attenuation of retinal arterioles but overall normal fundoscopy, in the appropriate clinical setting; typically precedes the diagnosis of cancer. This paraneoplastic retinopathy is associated with the synthesis of antirecoverin (anti-retinal) antibodies against the rhodopsin membrane, described in SCLC. This syndrome is also known as cancer-associated retinopathy (CAR). The other neoplasia associated with this paraneoplastic syndrome is the metastatic melanoma (melanoma-associated retinopathy, MAR) with antibodies against the bipolar cells of the retina.

There is another paraneoplastic entity described that is an optic neuritis associated with several antibodies, mainly anti-CV2/CRMP5 (collapsin response-mediator protein-5) and anti-Hu. The majority of these patients have SCLC.

Symptoms

Localization site	Comment
Brainstem	Subacute painless bilateral visual loss, presence of flickering lights, with cone dysfunction expressed by: worsening visual acuity, color vision impairment, photosensitivity, central scotoma. Rod dysfunction expressed by: impaired dark adaptation, night blindness, peripheral field defects
Cerebellar	Ataxia

Secondary Complications: Blindness.

Treatment Complications:

- Immunotherapy: optic neuritis, infection, neuropathy, rash, and endocrinopathies.

Bibliography

Bataller L, Dalmau J. Paraneoplastic disorders of the nervous system. *Continuum (Minneap Minn).* 2005;11(5, Neuro-Oncology):69–92. DOI: 10.1212/01.con.0000293680.24426.ae.

Honnorat J, Antoine J-C. Paraneoplastic neurological syndromes. *Orphanet J Rare Dis.* 2007;2:22. DOI:10.1186/1750-1172-2-22.

Lancaster E. Paraneoplastic disorders. *Continuum (Minneap Minn).* 2015;21(2, Neuro-oncology):452–75. DOI: 10.1212/01. CON.0000464180.89580.88.

Nicolle MW. Myasthenia gravis and Lambert-Eaton myasthenic syndrome. *Continuum (Minneap Minn).* 2016;22(6, Muscle and Neuromuscular Junction Disorders):1978–2005. DOI: 10.1212/ CON.0000000000000415.

Paraneoplastic Sensory Neuronopathy – Ganglionopathy

Epidemiology and Demographics: This paraneoplastic syndrome is uncommon; predominantly seen in females (80%) and whites (98%), with mean age of onset at 60 years. About 20% of all cases of sensory neuronopathy are related to an underlying malignancy; the other described etiologies include Sjögren syndrome or a toxic metabolic syndrome in the setting of chemotherapy. Up to 16% of all paraneoplastic sensory neuronopathies are seronegative. The mean survival time is 28 months after diagnosis.

Disorder Description: Autoimmune disorder also known as sensory ganglionopathy, characterized by the destruction of the dorsal root ganglia; known entity associated with malignancy. Characterized by progressive asymmetric paresthesias, dysesthesias, and numbness in the limbs and trunk, with less frequently cranial nerve involvement. In electrophysiologic studies there are small-amplitude or absent sensory nerve action potentials with relative preservation of motor conduction velocities.

This syndrome is associated with small cell lung cancer, but has also been described in extrapulmonary conditions such as lymphoma, neuroblastoma, and thymoma. The described antibodies in this syndrome include antineuronal nuclear antibody type 1 (ANNA-1), commonly known as anti-Hu, which may be found in serum or CSF and is highly predictive of the presence of malignancy. Additional antibodies described include collapsin response mediator protein-5 (CRMP-5), also known as anti-CV2.

Symptoms

Localization site	Comment
Brainstem	Anosmia and/or dysgeusia, and hearing difficulties suggestive of proximal sensory involvement
Cerebellum	Cerebellar ataxia as well
Anterior horn cells	Preserved strength
Dorsal root ganglia	Progressive asymmetric painful or numbing dysesthesias. Impaired sensation to all modalities, particularly proprioception, causing sensory ataxia and pseudo-athetoid movements with closed eyes. Typically upper limbs are involved first
Peripheral neuropathy	Decreased or abolished reflexes
Unclear localization	Autonomic dysfunction

Secondary Complications: Frequent falls, disability, and dependence.
Treatment Complications: Complications are those associated with surgical treatment of primary tumor.

Bibliography

Bataller L, Dalmau J. Paraneoplastic disorders of the nervous system. *Continuum (Minneap Minn).* 2005;11(5, Neuro-Oncology):69–92. DOI: 10.1212/01.con.0000293680.24426.ae.

Honnorat J, Antoine J-C. Paraneoplastic neurological syndromes. *Orphanet J Rare Dis.* 2007;2:22. DOI:10.1186/1750-1172-2-22.

Lancaster E. Paraneoplastic disorders. *Continuum (Minneap Minn).* 2015;21(2, Neuro-oncology):452–75. DOI: 10.1212/01. CON.0000464180.89580.88.

Muppidi S, Vernino S. Paraneoplastic neuropathies. *Continuum (Minneap Minn).* 2014;20(5, Peripheral Nervous System Disorders):1359–72. DOI: 10.1212/01.CON.0000455876.53309.ec.

Nicolle MW. Myasthenia gravis and Lambert-Eaton myasthenic syndrome. *Continuum (Minneap Minn).* 2016;22(6, Muscle and Neuromuscular Junction Disorders):1978–2005. DOI: 10.1212/CON.0000000000000415.

Vernino S. Paraneoplastic disorders affecting the neuromuscular junction or anterior horn cell. *Continuum (Minneap Minn).* 2009;15(1, Myasthenic Disorders and ALS):132–46. DOI: 10.1212/01.CON.0000300011.79845.eb.

Parietal Lobe Epilepsy

Epidemiology and Demographics: Represents 4.4% to 6% of all epilepsies, can occur at any age, and affects males and females equally.

Disorder Description: Seizures originating from the parietal lobe. Most commonly involves primary sensory cortex presenting with subjective sensation complaints. Clinical manifestations become more apparent once seizures propagate.

Etiologies may include tumors, congenital anomalies, post-inflammatory brain scarring, and vascular lesions. More recent surgical series have a high incidence of cortical dysgenesis.

Antiepileptic drugs are considered first-line treatment. Patients refractory to medication should be evaluated for resective surgery. Surface EEG rarely localizes a seizure focus. Techniques such as combined EEG and functional magnetic resonance imaging (EEG–fMRI) may be useful to refine localization.

Symptoms

Localization site	Comment
Cerebral hemispheres	Somatosensory auras: burning sensation, tingling, or numbness sometimes spreading from the face to hand, arm, and leg. Visual hallucinations, kinesthetic illusions, sensations of ocular movement, distortions of body shape, or perceived absence of body parts. Disruptions of language and comprehension. Later clonus and secondary generalization

Treatment Complications: Transient Gerstmann syndrome and primary limb or hemisensory deficits may occur postoperatively with surgical interventions.

Bibliography

Kim DW, et al. Parietal lobe epilepsy: the semiology, yield of diagnostic workup, and surgical outcome. *Epilepsia*. 2004;45(6):641–9.

Salanova V. Parietal lobe epilepsy. *J Clin Neurophysiol*. 2012;29(5):392–6.

Parinaud Syndrome

Epidemiology and Demographics: Occurs sporadically in association with a structural abnormality of the dorsal midbrain. Classically, it has been associated with three major groups: (1) children with brain tumors in the pineal gland or midbrain (pinealoma/intracranial germinoma are the most common), (2) women in their 20s to 30s with multiple sclerosis, and (3) older adults following stroke of the upper brainstem. Obstructive hydrocephalus can occur in any age group independent of underlying etiology resulting in the syndrome.

Disorder Description: Parinaud syndrome is also called the Sylvian aqueduct syndrome, the pretectal syndrome, the dorsal midbrain syndrome, and the Koerber–Salus–Elschnig syndrome.

Parinaud syndrome is a supranuclear paralysis of vertical gaze resulting from impaired function of the mesencephalon (rostral interstitial nucleus of Cajal). The classic triad includes vertical gaze abnormalities (especially upgaze), convergence-retraction nystagmus, and pupillary abnormalities (large with light-near dissociation). The constellation is variable and could include some or many of the following: downward gaze preference or tonic downward deviation of the eyes ("setting-sun sign"), primary position upbeat or downbeat nystagmus, impaired convergence and divergence, excessive convergence tone, skew deviation (often with the higher eye on the side of the lesion), bilateral upper eyelid retraction (Collier "tucked-lid" sign), and bilateral ptosis.

It is commonly caused by tumors in the pineal region (e.g., dysgerminomas), tectal tumors, or intrinsic lesions of the dorsal midbrain (e.g., infarction, infection, and demyelination). Other etiologies include arteriovenous malformations, giant aneurysms of the posterior fossa, and obstructive hydrocephalus (with expansion of the aqueduct and pressure on the dorsal midbrain).

Symptoms

Localization site	Comment
Cerebral hemispheres	Hydrocephalus may cause increased intracranial pressure resulting in varying degrees of altered consciousness including coma
	"Setting sun" sign is one of the cardinal features in a child with developing obstructive hydrocephalus
Brainstem	Rarely horizontal eye movements may be involved

Secondary Complications: Tectal masses most commonly result in hydrocephalus with associated headaches, nausea, and vomiting. Bilateral papilledema may accompany the syndrome.

Treatment Complications: Most patients improve within a few months of treating the hydrocephalus. Significant upgaze palsy can be relieved with bilateral inferior rectus recessions. Retraction nystagmus and convergence movement are usually improved with this procedure as well.

Bibliography

Baloh RW, Furman JM, Yee RD. Dorsal midbrain syndrome: Clinical and oculographic findings. *Neurology*. 1985;35:54.

Lee AG, Brazis PW. *Clinical pathways in neuro-ophthalmology: an evidence-based approach*. New York: Thieme; 1998.

Parkinson's Disease (PD)

Epidemiology and Demographics: Parkinson's disease (PD) prevalence increases with age, from 41/100,000 for ages 40–49 years to 1900/100,000 for ages 80 years and above.[1] Predominant age at presentation is 60 years. The prevalence is approximately 7.5 million worldwide, about 1 million of whom are in the United States. Incidence of PD ranges from 8 to 18.6 per 100,000 person-years.[2] PD affects men and women of all races, occupations, and countries, but some studies have shown a slightly greater risk for men than women.

Disorder Description: PD is a neurodegenerative disorder characterized clinically by the cardinal symptoms of bradykinesia, rigidity, and tremor. According to the Braak theory, neurodegeneration begins in the medulla and olfactory nucleus and progresses towards the cortex in a caudal to rostral direction.[3] Two hallmark features are intra-cytoplasmic proteinaceous inclusions, called "Lewy" bodies, in the nervous system and degeneration of dopaminergic neurons in the substantia nigra. The non-dopaminergic pathology of inclusion body deposition is considered to occur first, resulting in the non-motor symptoms of PD such as constipation, anosmia, rapid eye movement (REM) sleep behavior disorder, and cardiac denervation. Traditionally these symptoms are not responsive to dopaminergic therapy. The classic motor symptoms include bradykinesia, resting tremor, rigidity, and gait disturbances. Specific symptoms that are a result of bradykinesia include micrographia, masked facies, reduced eye blinking, and a soft voice or hypophonia. Oropharyngeal dysphagia may occur.[4]

Factors that confer increased risk include pesticide exposure (agent orange, rotenone, paraquat, and maneb), rural living or farming, and drinking well water, while cigarette smoking and caffeine intake appear to reduce risk. Vascular insults and brain trauma in older patients result in a 44% increased risk of developing PD over the next 5–7 years.[5] Earlier concerns of welding and manganese toxicity causing parkinsonism remain controversial.

The cause of the more common, sporadic PD (85–90% of cases) is currently unknown, but environmental factors are suspected to contribute in patients older than 50 years, while genetic factors are of greater importance in those younger. Familial PD (10–15% of cases) has been identified with specific gene mutations with autosomal dominant inheritance, PARK 1,4 at the alpha-synuclein locus and PARK-8 at the LRRK2 locus. Parkin gene mutation is the more commonly responsible gene in PD patients less than 40 years of age.[6]

Symptoms

Localization site	Comment
Cerebral hemispheres	Spectrum of mild cognitive impairment to dementia
Basal ganglia	Inability to initiate movement, bradykinesia, rigidity
Mental status and psychiatric aspects/ complications	Mood disorders such as depression, anxiety, panic attacks, psychosis with visual hallucinations

Localization site	Comment
Brainstem	Dysfunction in sleep center results in REM sleep behavior disorder (RBD). Autonomic nervous system dysfunction includes orthostatic hypotension, constipation, and genitourinary disturbances
Cranial nerves	Dysphagia, anosmia, and cardiac denervation

Secondary Complications: Depression is very common in PD with more than half of the patients affected. Psychosis with visual hallucinations are generally formed and are non-threatening. Visual hallucinations may be indicative of impending dementia.

Most patients with PD die from complications resulting from aspiration pneumonia as a result of dysphagia, which can also cause dehydration and malnutrition. Additionally, they can become injured as a result of orthostasis.

Treatment Complications: Nausea and vomiting are known to occur if a peripheral decarboxylase inhibitor is not given along with levodopa. Peripherally converted dopamine can access the dopamine receptors within the area postrema of the brain, thereby triggering symptoms of nausea. Acute dopaminergic effects can also include orthostatic hypotension.

Dyskinesias may be experienced during levodopa therapy, which are generally choreiform in nature; however, they may present as dystonic movements, myoclonus, or other movement disorders.

An additional levodopa induced motor complication is fluctuation in response to therapy, which is termed the "on–off" effect. When treatment response is effective it is considered "on." It is described as "off" when medication effect wears off and parkinsonism features reappear. Other possible variations of this fluctuation are the "wearing off" effect in which the duration of drug benefit progressively decreases, and the "delayed-on" and "no-on" effects in which patients experience a delay in onset or no response to therapy.

Impulse control disorders that include gambling and acts of hypersexuality appear to occur more frequently with dopamine agonists. The drugs that are currently used in this class include ropinirole, pramipexole, rotigotine, and apomorphine. Some related side effects of these agents include nausea, vomiting, orthostatic hypotension, and lower extremity edema. Chronic use of dopaminergic agents can result in hallucinations, cognitive impairment, and sedation.

Patients who use catechol-O-methyl transferase (COMT) inhibitors can experience side effects that include diarrhea and orange urine (approximately 10% of patients using entacapone). Although virtually not used, fatal hepatotoxicity has been reported with tolcapone. Centrally acting anticholinergics may cause cognitive impairment, urinary dysfunction, and glaucoma, thereby limiting its use, particularly in the elderly.

References

1. Pringsheim T, Jette N, Frolkis A, Steeves TD. The prevalence of Parkinson's disease: a systematic review and meta-analysis. *Mov Disord.* 2014;29:1583.
2. de Lau LM, Breteler MM. Epidemiology of Parkinson's disease. *Lancet Neurol.* 2006;5:525.
3. Braak H, Del Tredici K, Rub U, de Vos RAI et al. Staging of brain pathology related to sporadic Parkinson's disease. *Neurobiol. Aging.* 2003;24:197–211.
4. Gelb DJ, Oliver E, Gilman S. Diagnostic criteria for Parkinson disease. *Arch Neurol.* 1999;56:33.
5. Gardner RC, Burke JF, Nettiksimmons J, et al. Traumatic brain injury in later life increases risk for Parkinson disease. *Ann Neurol.* 2015;77(6):987–95.
6. Klein C, Schneider SA, Lang AE. Hereditary parkinsonism: Parkinson disease look-alikes – an algorithm for clinicians to "PARK" genes and beyond. *Mov Disord.* 2009;24:2042.

Parotid Cancer

Epidemiology and Demographics: The parotid malignancies constitute 3–4% of all head and neck neoplasias. Incidence of 1–2/100,000 population, with mean age of presentation being 60 years of age; typically affects females more than males (4:1). Survival at 10 years is 69% with normal facial function vs 37% with partial and 13% with complete paralysis. Most common histologic subtype is mucoepidermoid (34%).

Disorder Description: Parotid malignancies will present with facial palsy in 5% of the cases; typically seen in tumors involving the medial lobe of the parotid, with perineural invasion in 86% of the patients with complete paralysis. The histologic types include mucoepidermoid carcinoma, adenoid cystic carcinoma, adenocarcinoma, carcinoma pleomorphic, acinic cell carcinoma, and squamous cell carcinoma.

Symptoms

Localization site	Comment
Cerebral hemispheres	Occipital headaches
Brainstem	Facial nerve palsy with progression over time, persistent ear pain, lack of recovery, persistent facial paresthesias
Cerebellum	Ataxia, dizziness, nausea, vomiting
Base of skull	Cavernous sinus syndrome ophthalmoplegia, loss of corneal reflex, sensory loss in V1, hypoacusis

Secondary Complications: Facial nerve palsy, auriculotemporal nerve damage with Frey's syndrome, characterized by re-innervation flushing, sweating in the ipsilateral cheek while eating.

Treatment Complications

- Surgery: hemorrhage, infection, necrosis, facial nerve damage, chronic pain, paresthesias, changes of speech, and swallowing.
- Radiation: Brainstem encephalopathy, myelopathy, baroreflex failure, radiation necrosis, and leukoencephalopathy.

Bibliography

Gaeta M, Frosina P, Loria G, Di Pietro A, De Renzis C. A case of perineural metastatic diffusion along the facial nerve: its computed tomographic demonstration and the radiotherapy considerations. *Radiol Med.* 1994;87(6):870–2.

Kumar PP, Patil AA, Ogren FP, Johansson SL, Reeves MA. Intracranial skip metastasis from parotid and facial skin tumors: mechanism, diagnosis, and treatment. *J Nat Med Assoc.* 1993;85(5)369–74.

Newton HB, Malkin MG. *Neurological complications of systemic cancer and antineoplastic therapy.* (Neurological Disease and Therapy series: Vol 96). Boca Raton, FL: CRC Press; 2016. p. 80.

Renehan AG, Gleave EN, Slevin NJ, McGurk M. Clinico-pathological and treatment-related factors influencing survival in parotid cancer. *Br J Cancer.* 1999;80(8):1296–300.

Tullio A, Marchetti C, Sesenna E, et al. Treatment of carcinoma of the parotid gland: The results of a multicenter study. *J Oral Maxillofac Surg.* 2001;59(3):263–70.

Paroxysmal Hemicrania and Chronic Paroxysmal Hemicrania

Epidemiology and Demographics: This condition is seen in the third or fourth decade of life. Seen in both men and women equally. The prevalence of this condition is unknown as there are no studies looking at this directly. However, given the similarity of this condition to cluster headache, some estimate that paroxysmal hemicrania has a prevalence of 1 in 50,000.

Disorder Description: This type of headache is characterized by strictly unilateral pain. The incidence of either left- or right-side headache is of equal frequency. A small percentage (3–15%) present with alternating side attacks. The pain can be orbital, supraorbital, temporal, or a combination of these sites. Further, the pain can spread to the occiput, neck, shoulder, maxilla, periauricular region, and oral cavity. Involvement of occiput is seen in 40% of cases. Most cases report severe headache pain. The diagnosis of paroxysmal hemicrania must include at least one cranial autonomic feature. Lacrimation is the most common reported associated symptom. Other side effects include conjunctival injection, rhinorrhea, nasal congestion, ptosis, facial flushing, eyelid edema, and facial sweating. Attacks can occur up to 50 times in a day. Some patients report triggers for this type of headache like exercise, neck movement, alcohol, bending downward, coughing, warm environment, cold weather, or a strong smell.

The chronic form of this condition accounts for almost 80% of all paroxysmal hemicrania cases. This condition must be continuous for more than 1 year or occur with a brief period of remission of less than 1 month to fit the diagnosis.

Symptoms

Localization site	Comment
Cerebral hemispheres	Some studies suggest a role for posterior hypothalamus, ventral midbrain, red nucleus, and substantia nigra. The hypothalamus is thought to be central to the cranial autonomic features

Secondary Complications: This type of headache can be refractory to treatment. Rarely, some cases have been reported of patients undergoing deep brain stimulation with varying degrees of success.

Treatment Complications: Excess use of indomethacin, the treatment for paroxysmal hemicrania, can lead to tachyphylaxis – a rare occurrence. In these patients, the effectiveness of the medication decreases substantially and relatively quickly, likely secondary to increased tolerance.

Bibliography

Antonaci F, Sjaastad O. Chronic paroxysmal hemicrania (CPH): a review of the clinical manifestations. *Headache.* 1989;29:648–56.

Boes CJ, Matharu MS, Goadsby PJ. The paroxysmal hemicraniatic syndrome. *Cephalalgia.* 2003;23:24–8.

Cittadini E, Matharu MS, Goadsby PJ. Paroxysmal hemicrania: a prospective clinical study of 31 cases. *Brain.* 2008;131(Pt4):1142–55.

Prakash S, Patell R. Paroxysmal hemicrania: an update. *Curr Pain Headache Rep.* 2014;18:407.

Paroxysmal Kinesigenic Dyskinesia (PKD)

Epidemiology and Demographics: Paroxysmal kinesigenic dyskinesia (PKD) is the most common type of the paroxysmal movement disorders, including non-kinesigenic (PKND), exercise-induced dyskinesia (PED), and paroxysmal hypnogenic dyskinesia (PHD), which has been further identified as autosomal dominant nocturnal frontal lobe epilepsy. Women present a better prognosis and a higher chance of complete remission than men, but the male-to-female ratio was higher in sporadic cases but not in familial cases.[1] Precise prevalence is currently unknown.

Disorder Description: PKD is a paroxysmal dyskinesia precipitated by sudden, voluntary movements. It is characterized by recurrent attacks of chorea and/or involuntary dystonia and tends to be autosomal dominant and familial in nature.[2,3] Consciousness is preserved, and patients respond to treatment with carbamezapine or phenytoin.[1] PKD is frequently preceded by infantile convulsions.[4] Migraine and hemiplegic migraine were the most common associated phenotypes.[4] Women also indicated improvement of attacks while pregnant, indicating the potential for hormonal influence in PKD, but further studies are needed for verification.[1]

The major PKD gene has been identified as *PRRT*, a small, proline-rich transmembrane protein present on chromosome 16pq11.2.[5] This disease-causing mutation that reduces the level of PRRT2, and therefore the gene's interaction with SNAP25, a protein that facilitates synaptic exocytosis, reduces the restriction of presynaptic exocytosis and thereby results in excessive neurotransmitter release.[4] This finding, as well as a potential increase in glutamine release, shows that the limited neurotransmitter release regulation could result in migraines.[4]

PNKD attacks are often triggered by alcohol, coffee, or strong emotions. They tend to last longer than PKD attacks, often 10 minutes to 1 hour, but can extend to 12 hours.[4] These attacks, however, are infrequent and occur only a few times a year.

PED is the rarest of the aforementioned paroxysmal movement disorders. Attacks of dystonia occur, which are induced by physical exertion after long periods of exercise. PED is also associated with migraine, hemiplegia, ataxia, and epilepsy.[2,4]

Symptoms

Localization site	Comment
Cerebellum	Among regions of highest expression levels of SNAP25 and PRRT2, indication of possible association of hyperexcitability and symptomatic dystonia/chorea[4]

Secondary Complications: Hur et al. conducted a case report on paroxysmal dyskinesia secondary to the 2009 H1N1 infection.[6] Neurologic complications including seizures and encephalopathy were more common, while secondary movement disorders such as chorea and dystonia were rarely reported. Aspiration pneumonia can result from dysphagia, and complications sustained from a fall are the usual causative factors that lead to mortality.

References

1. Bruno MK, Hallett M, Gwinn-Hardy K, et al. Critical evaluation of idiopathic paroxysmal kinesigenic dyskinesia: new diagnostic criteria. *Neurology*. 2004;63(12):2280–7.
2. Bhatia KP. Familial (idiopathic) paroxysmal dyskinesias: an update. *Semin Neurol*. 2001;21(1):69–74.
3. Van Rootselaar AF, van Westrum SS, Velis DN, Tijssen MA. The paroxysmal dyskinesias. *Pract Neurol*. 2009;9(2):102–9.
4. Gardiner AR, Jaffer F, Dale RC, et al. The clinical and genetic heterogeneity of paroxysmal dyskinesias. *Brain*. 2015;138(12):3567–80.
5. Wang JL, Cao L, Li XH, et al. Identification of Prrt2 as the causative gene of paroxysmal kinesigenic dyskinesias. *Brain*. 2011;134(12):3493–501.
6. Hur YJ, Hwang T. Secondary paroxysmal dyskinesia associated with 2009 H1N1 infection. *Korean J Pediatr*. 2013;56(1):42–4.

Paroxysmal Nocturnal Hemoglobinuria (PNH)

Epidemiology and Demographics: Paroxysmal nocturnal hemoglobinuria (PNH) is a rare disease that is present worldwide with estimated incidence less than 10 per million per year. Affects men and women equally.

Disorder Description: Caused by an acquired mutation in hematopoietic stem cells in the *PIGA* gene encoding a cell membrane glycolipid anchor, which is important for many pathways including inhibition of complement-mediated erythrocyte lysis. For unclear reasons, acquired aplastic anemia can often precede the diagnosis of PNH. Clinical symptoms can be from episodic hemolysis or thrombotic events.

Symptoms

Localization site	Comment
Cerebral hemispheres	Can cause cerebral venous thrombosis (most frequently in superior sagittal sinus, lateral sinuses, or cortical veins) affecting cerebral function diffusely by increased intracranial pressure or more focally in cases of cortical vein thrombosis[1]
Mental status and psychiatric aspects/ complications	Venous sinus thrombosis can initially present as headache and confusion
Unclear localization	Headache frequently accompanies PNH even without venous thrombosis[2]

Secondary Complications: Patients can have cytopenias from concurrent aplastic anemia or myelodysplastic syndrome. Thrombosis can affect other locations including pulmonary veins, hepatic veins, and mesenteric veins. Thromboembolism is a major cause of morbidity. Spontaneous intravascular hemolysis occurs with characteristic nocturnal hemoglobinuria.

Treatment Complications: Eculizumab, a humanized monoclonal antibody to complement component C5, is an approved therapy that reduces the risk of thrombosis and hemolysis but is associated with life-threatening *Neisseria* infections, including meningitis.

References

1. Meppiel E, Crassard I, Peffault de Latour R, et al. Cerebral venous thrombosis in paroxysmal nocturnal hemoglobinuria: a series of 15 cases and review of the literature. *Medicine (Baltimore)*. 2015;94:e362.
2. Schrezenmeier H, Muus P, Socié G, et al. Baseline characteristics and disease burden in patients in the International Paroxysmal Nocturnal Hemoglobinuria Registry. *Haematologica*. 2014;99:922–9.

Patent Ductus Arteriosus

Epidemiology and Demographics: Although symptoms may not manifest until later in life, patent ductus arteriosus (PDA) is a congenital heart defect, which is therefore present from birth. For children born at term, incidence is estimated in the 0.02%–0.06% range, with higher rates in preterm births.

Disorder Description: Shortly after birth (2 or 3 days), the ductus arteriosus, which is patent in the fetus and connects the pulmonary artery to the descending aorta, usually closes. There are several characterizations of severity of a ductus that remains open, which depends on the size of the duct and how the systemic and pulmonary vascular resistance differ. There is no certain cause of patent ductus arteriosus (PDA), but risk factors include premature birth, a family history of genetic heart problems, infection in the mother during pregnancy with rubella, and birth at altitudes greater than 10,000 feet.

Symptoms

Localization site	Comment
Cerebral hemispheres	Hypoperfusion with syncope/presyncope related to secondary arrhythmias as well as embolic complications
Mental status and psychiatric aspects/complications	Lightheadedness, fatigue, confusion, and potential focal central nervous system (CNS) problems that may affect the various CNS areas indicated below
Brainstem	Same as above
Cerebellum	Same as above
Vestibular system (and nonspecific dizziness)	Same as above
Base of skull	Same as above

Secondary Complications: A small PDA may not be problematic but a large PDA may lead to a number of problems. Atrial arrhythmias and dyspnea may present in a larger PDA, along with left ventricular volume overload and pulmonary hypertension (possibly Eisenmenger syndrome) resulting from increased pulmonary circulation. Heart failure may also occur and there is an increased risk for infective endocarditis.

Treatment Complications: Treatments include transcatheter occlusion and surgical closure via ductal ligation and/or division. All carry a relatively low risk of complications or death.

Bibliography

Mayo Clinic Staff. Patent ductus arteriosus (PDA). Dec 16, 2014. Available from www.mayoclinic.org/diseases-conditions/patent-ductus-arteriosus/basics/complications/con-20028530 Accessed Jul 6, 2015.

Webb GD, Smallhorn J, Therrien J, Redington AN. Congenital heart disease. In Mann DL, Zipes DP, Libby P, Bonow RO, Braunwald E, eds. *Braunwald's heart disease: A textbook of cardiovascular medicine.* 10th ed. Philadelphia, PA: Elsevier/Saunders; 2015. pp. 1413–14.

Patent Foramen Ovale

Epidemiology and Demographics: The foramen ovale does not close in approximately 25% of people.

Disorder Description: A fetus has a foramen ovale, which is a tunnel between the septum secundum and septum primum that allows blood to flow from the right atrium to the left atrium to help bypass pulmonary circulation. A patent foramen ovale results when this tunnel fails to close. The reasons for this failure are not clearly understood.

Symptoms

Localization site	Comment
Cerebral hemispheres	Embolic complications that typically present as focal areas of infarction
Mental status and psychiatric aspects/ complications	Depression following transient ischemic attack (TIA) and stroke are common with occasional central nervous system deficits depending on the areas affected
Brainstem	Embolic events may affect this area
Cerebellum	Same as above
Vestibular system (and nonspecific dizziness)	Same as above
Base of skull	Same as above

Secondary Complications: Patent foramen ovale may be cited as a potential cause of stroke or TIA. The open connection between the right and left heart provides an avenue for thrombus to travel from the right venous side to the left arterial side (paradoxical embolization to systemic circulation).

Treatment: Anticoagulants are used if cryptogenic stroke occurs, and transcatheter closure is also a viable treatment option.

Bibliography

Mayo Clinic Staff. Patent foramen ovale. Jul 16, 2015. Available from www.mayoclinic.org/diseases-conditions/patent-foramen-ovale/basics/causes/con-20028729. Accessed Jul 19, 2015.

Webb GD, Smallhorn J, Therrien J, Redington AN. Congenital heart disease. In Mann DL, Zipes DP, Libby P, Bonow RO, Braunwald E, eds. *Braunwald's heart disease: A textbook of cardiovascular medicine.* 10th ed. Philadelphia, PA: Elsevier/Saunders; 2015. pp. 1409–10.

Peduncular Hallucinosis

Epidemiology and Demographics: This is a rare disorder reported in the literature primarily as case reports.

Disorder Description: Patients complain of vivid colorful hallucinations in the setting of any lesion (e.g., stroke, hemorrhage, tumor) affecting the pons, thalamus, or midbrain. The hallucinations may be lilliputian at times. The patients are generally aware that the hallucinations are false.

Symptoms

Localization site	Comment
Mental status and psychiatric aspects/ complications	Cognitive and sleep disorders are commonly seen in association with this disorder
Brainstem	Visual hallucinations

Secondary Complications: This is associated with cognitive disturbances and abnormal sleep patterns.

Treatment Complications: There have been case reports of successful treatment with atypical antipsychotics. These medications are often sedating and may lead to parkinsonism and neuroleptic malignant syndrome.

Bibliography

Benke T. Peduncular hallucinosis: A syndrome of impaired reality monitoring. *J Neurol.* 2006;253:1561–71.

Penney L, Galameau D. Peduncular hallucinosis: A case report. *Oschner J.* 2014(Fall);14(3): 456–8.

Perilymphatic Fistula (PLF)

Epidemiology and Demographics: Perilymphatic fistula (PLF) affects the inner ear and can occur sporadically as a result of trauma or a chronic middle ear infection. Spontaneous PLF probably does not exist; superior semicircular canal dehiscence (SCD) should be suspected in these cases. The incidence of PLF is unknown but it is considered a rare disorder likely affecting fewer than 200,000 individuals.

Disorder Description: PLF is an abnormal communication between the membranous labyrinth and the middle ear. Common etiologies include erosion of the inner ear by cholesteatoma, traumatic fractures of the temporal bone, or otosyphilis. Patients with PLF complain of position or pressure-induced vertigo. The hallmark sign of PLF is vertigo and deviation of the eyes with external pressure on the tragus (positive fistula test). As in SCD, increasing middle ear pressures will elicit a response.

Symptoms

Localization site	Comment
Inner ear	Dehiscence of bone resulting in a third window phenomenon with vestibular symptoms +/− hearing loss and tinnitus
Cranial nerves	The cochleovestibular nerve is not affected
Central nervous system	The central nervous system is not affected

Secondary Complications: Imbalance and vertigo in these patients may result in increased risk for injuries or falls. Hearing loss may occur as result of sudden changes in middle ear pressures.

Treatment Complications: PLF resulting from cholesteatoma requires a tympanomastoidectomy with exteriorization of cholesteatoma sac and minimal dissection over the fistula to avoid sensorineural hearing loss. PLF resulting from blunt trauma may initially be managed with bed rest, head elevation, laxatives, and monitoring of hearing/vestibular function. Cases failing conservative management may undergo middle ear exploration with fat patching of the oval and round windows. When otosyphilis is suspected, serum should be sent for fluorescent treponemal antibodies; the treatment is benzathine penicillin and steroids.

Repair of a PLF via cholesteatoma resection or patching of the oval/round window carries the risk of profound sensorineural hearing loss.

Bibliography

Friedland DR, Wackym PA. Clinical forum: a critical appraisal of spontaneous perilymphatic fistulas of the inner ear. *Am J Otol.* 1999;20:261–76.

Minor LB. Labyrinthine fistulae: pathobiology and management. *Curr Opin Otolaryngol Head Neck Surg.* 2003;11:340–6.

Smouha EE, Bojrab DI. Lateral semicircular canal fistula. In *Cholesteatoma.* New York, NY: Thieme; 2011. p. 88.

Perineuritis

Epidemiology and Demographics: Most patients (90% or more) are 50 years of age or older. Gender predilection, frequency of condition, and geographic distribution vary based upon cause.

Disorder Description: Thickening of perineurium focally around some fascicles with associated degeneration or loss of perineural cells with or without inflammation.

Potential causes include:
a. Diabetes: most common cause of perineuritis
b. Chronic inflammatory demyelinating polyradiculoneuropathy
c. Cryoglobulinemia: monoclonal antibodies, hepatitis C, hepatitis A or B, HIV, Epstein–Barr virus, bacterial infections, immune disorders (lupus, scleroderma, Sjögren's, rheumatoid arthritis), lymphoproliferative disorders (myeloma, Hodgkin's lymphoma, non-Hodgkin's B cell lymphoma, macroglobulinemia, chronic lymphocytic leukemia, hairy cell leukemia, lymphoblastic lymphadenopathy)
d. Spanish toxic oil
e. Weight loss
f. Collagen vascular disorders
g. Sepsis
h. Wegener's granulomatosis: causes optic perineuritis
i. Giant cell arteritis: causes optic perineuritis
j. Sarcoidosis: causes optic perineuritis
k. Syphilis: causes optic perineuritis
Risk factors include:
a. Diabetes
b. Infection with hepatitis C, hepatitis A or B, HIV, or Epstein–Barr virus
c. Autoimmune disorders
d. Cancer: lymphoma or leukemia
e. Sepsis
f. Ingestion of adulterated Spanish rapeseed oil (Spanish toxic oil)

Symptoms

Localization site	Comment
Cranial nerves	Optic perineuritis – vision loss of the peripheral visual field progressing for longer than 2 weeks (arcuate scotoma). Central and color vision preserved, pain on eye movement, swollen or normal optic disc, diplopia, chemosis and/or subtle ptosis may be present. Patients are typically 45 years of age or older
Mononeuritis multiplex	Paresthesias, pain, and restless legs. More common with Type III cryoglobulinemia, acute or subacute onset, asymmetric symptoms involving distal more than proximal extremities, both sensory and motor nerves can be involved

Secondary Complications: Visual disturbances: blurred vision, double vision, and vision loss. Pain and weakness in lower extremities.

Treatment Complications: The steroid methylprednisolone is commonly used to treat this condition. Methylprednisolone causes an increased risk of infection, hyperglycemia, avascular necrosis of the hip, psychosis, Cushing's disease, and osteoporosis.

Bibliography

Hickman SJ. Optic perineuritis. *Curr Neurol Neurosci Rep.* 2016;16(2):16.

Sorenson EJ, Sima AA, Blaivas M, Sawchuk K, Wald JJ. Clinical features of perineuritis. *Muscle Nerve.* 1997;20(9):1153–7.

Periodic Limb Movement Disorder

Epidemiology and Demographics: Among US undergraduate college students aged 17–25 years between 2009 and 2010, the prevalence of periodic limb movement disorder or restless leg syndrome (PLMD/RLS) was 8%, and women were at a greater risk.[1] There were no significant differences in risk by ethnicity.[1] The prevalence of PLMD among University of Alabama students aged 17–25 years between 2010 and 2011 was 8.4% specifically for RLS and 7.8% (132/1684) for PLMD.[2] PLMD is thought to be rare as periodic limb movements (PLMs) are typically associated with RLS, REM sleep behavior disorder, or narcolepsy and represent a distinct diagnosis from PLMD. PLMs are associated with RLS in more than 80% of cases[3,4]; however, PLMD can occur without RLS.[3] The rate of diagnosis of PLMD by the Diagnostic Interview for Sleep Patterns and Disorders has substantial specificity for diagnosing PLMD (specificity = 0.88%, sensitivity = 0.67%), and the rate of diagnosis using this standardized tool was significantly higher than the clinician diagnosis.[5] The most objective diagnostic tool is a sleep-related parameter measured by polysomnography or actigraphy, particularly the Periodic Limb Movements in Sleep (PLMS), PLM index (PLMI), PLMs arousal index (PLMS-AI), and sleep efficiency.[4]

Disorder Description: PLMs are episodic, involuntary muscle contractions that occur during sleep typically leading to repetitive limb movements during sleep.[4] Higher frequency of PLMs ($\geq$15 PLMs/hour of sleep) is associated with genetic polymorphisms (BTBD9, TOX8/BCo34767, MEIS1, MAP2K5/SKOR1, PTPRD).[3] The disorder most often affects the lower extremities, including the toes, ankles, knees, and hips, and occasionally the upper extremities.[4]

Symptoms

Localization site	Comment
Mental status and psychiatric aspects/complications	Daytime sleepiness and fatigue Less commonly poor physical or mental health, decrements in academic performance, difficulty concentrating, poorer lifestyle factors including substance use, reduced physical activity, and less social engagement
Brainstem	Sleep rhythm disruption
Cranial nerves	Cardiac arrhythmias
Muscle	Congestive heart failure

Secondary Complications: Limb movements may be associated with an arousal or awakening, thereby disrupting the sleep rhythms.[4] PLMD is associated with other disorders, including depression, cardiovascular disease, REM sleep behavior disorder, narcolepsy, Parkinson's disease, and multiple system atrophy.[3] Daytime impairments found among people with sleep disorders may include sleepiness and fatigue, poor physical or mental health, decrements in academic performance, difficulty concentrating, poorer lifestyle factors including substance use, reduced physical activity, and less social engagement.[2] However, college students with PLMD were not found to have significant differences in working memory capacity span task or a higher incidence of a mental health disorder.[2] There is a significant association of PLMD with cardiovascular disorders, including congestive heart failure, and increased risk of atrial fibrillation and coronary artery disease.[3]

References

1. Gaultney JF. The prevalence of sleep disorders in college students: impact on academic performance. *J Am Coll Health*. 2010;59(2): 91–7.
2. Petrov ME, Lichstein KL, Baldwin CM. Prevalence of sleep disorders by sex and ethnicity among older adolescents and emerging adults: Relations to daytime functioning, working memory and mental health. *J Adolesc*. 37;2014:587–97.
3. Moore H, Winkelmann J, Lin L, et al. Periodic leg movements during sleep are associated with polymorphisms in BTBD9, TOX3/BC034767, MEIS1, MAP2K5/SKOR1, and PTPRD. *Sleep*. 2014;37(9):1535–42.
4. Aurora RN, Kristo DA, Bista SR, et al. The treatment of restless legs syndrome and periodic limb movement disorder in adults – an update for 2012: practice parameters with an evidence-based systematic review and meta-analyses. *Sleep*. 2012;35(8):1039–62.
5. Merikangas KR, Zhang J, Emsellem H, et al. The structured Diagnostic Interview for Sleep Patterns and Disorders: rationale and initial evaluation. *Sleep Med*. 2014;15:530–5.

Periodic Paralysis

A group of rare disorders that present as transient painless muscle weakness. This includes:

Hypokalemic periodic paralysis
Thyrotoxic periodic paralysis
Hyperkalemic periodic paralysis
Anderson syndrome
Paramyotonia congenita

Hypokalemic Periodic Paralysis (HypoPP). Further divided into three subtypes (depending on channel involvement):

(a) HypoPPtype 1 – mutation of CACNL1AS (involving L type of calcium channel)
(b) HypoPPtype 2 – mutation of SCN4A (involving sodium channel)
(c) HypoPPtype 3 – mutation of KCNE3 (involving potassium channel)

The most common type of periodic paralysis is hypokalemic periodic paralysis. The prevalence of HypoPP is about 1/100,000.[1] HypoPP has an autosomal dominant inheritance pattern. Men are more affected than women and penetrance is incomplete mainly in women.[2]

Attacks begin in teen years or young adulthood. Attacks are characterized by proximal muscle weakness (legs > arms) with hyporeflexia or areflexia. Consciousness is preserved. Attacks last for hours usually. Myotonia is absent. Diurnal variation (more weakness during night or early morning than midday) has been noticed. Frequency of attacks is about once or twice a week. Cranial and bulbar muscles are usually not involved. Involvement of respiratory muscles is rare but fatal.

Precipitating factors include heavy carbohydrate meals, heavy exercise followed by period of rest, and administration of insulin.

During attacks, serum potassium is low.[3] During attacks, motor nerve conduction studies reveal lower compound muscle action potentials and electromyography reveals electrical silence.[4] Inter-attack muscle biopsy reveals centrally placed vacuolar or tubular aggregates.[4] Provocative test by giving glucose load is considered dangerous. Genetic testing is preferred for diagnosis.

Life-threatening cardiac arrhythmias have been reported during attacks with low serum potassium level.[4,5] Later, patient also develops progressive proximal myopathy.[4,6]

Secondary causes of hypokalemic periodic paralysis should be excluded such as primary hyperaldosteronism, use of diuretics, renal potassium wasting, gastrointestinal potassium loss (diarrhea), and steroid use, etc.[4]

Treatment: Acute treatment should be provided with oral potassium.[4] Preventive treatments include: (1) nonpharmacologic measures such as a low-carbohydrate diet and avoiding vigorous exercise; and (2) pharmacologic measures – use of carbonic anhydrase inhibitors such as acetazolamide.[2,4,7] Sometimes triamterene or spironolactone is also added in refractory cases.[4,7]

Thyrotoxic Periodic Paralysis: A sporadic HypoPP usually seen in Asian populations.[4,5] It is associated with hyperthyroidism, and most common cause is Grave's disease.[4,8-13] Men are more commonly affected than women.[4]

Attacks usually begin around 3rd decade. Symptoms of thyrotoxicosis either precede or occur simultaneously with attack. Attacks are characterized by proximal weakness (legs > arms) with or without hyporeflexia. Patients also complain of muscle aches and pains.[14]

Degree of hypokalemia during attack is variable.[15] Labs may reveal high thyroxine and low thyroid-stimulating hormone during attack.[16]

Cardiac arrhythmias and electrocardiogram changes are noticed also with thyrotoxic HypoPP.

Treatment: Acute treatment is replacement of potassium and monitoring for rebound hyperkalemia, and intravenous propranolol.[17-18] Prophylactic treatment involves treatment of hyperthyroidism and use of propranolol.[19]

Hyperkalemic Periodic Paralysis (HyperPP): This is a rare autosomally inherited disorder. It results from mutation affecting sodium channels (SCN4A gene).

Prevalence of HyperPP is about 1/200,000.[20] Women and men appear to be equally affected.

Attacks usually begin in childhood and are characterized by proximal muscle weakness. Attacks are usually brief in duration lasting from minutes to hours. Bulbar and respiratory muscles are spared. Myotonia is present in between the attacks.[4,21]

Precipitating factors include fasting, pregnancy, emotional stress, rest following exercise, exposure to cold, and potassium ingestion.[4]

Cardiac arrhythmias have been reported in HyperPP.[22] Later in disease, patient develops progressive proximal myopathy.[23]

During attacks, serum potassium level may be high or normal. In between attacks, electromyography studies reveal myotonia. Sometimes an exercise test performed during electromyography helps to confirm the diagnosis.[24,25] Muscle biopsy eventually shows vacuolar changes that are more peripheral. Genetic testing is preferred.

Treatment: Acute treatment is usually not required as attacks are brief. Mild attacks can be aborted with exercise. Severe attacks are treated with thiazide diuretics, beta agonist agents, or intravenous calcium.[1,4,26] For prophylactic treatment, carbonic anhydrase inhibitors (acetazolamide),

beta agonists, and thiazide diuretics are useful.[27-29] Patients remain paralysed for hours when they recover from general anesthesia.[30] Mexiletine is used to treat myotonia.

Anderson's Syndrome: A rare syndrome characterized by periodic paralysis, cardiac arrhythmias, and periodic paralysis. It has autosomal dominant inheritance pattern and is caused by mutation affecting potassium channels. Attacks begin in childhood. Patient also develops long QT syndrome and permanent proximal muscle weakness. Dysmorphic features are short stature, scoliosis, clinodactyly, hypertelorism, small or prominent low-set ears, micrognathia, and broad forehead.[4]

Paramyotonia Congenita: A rare autosomal dominant inherited disease caused by mutation in sodium channels (SCN4A).

Clinical features include periodic paralysis and myotonia. Attacks of weakness are either spontaneous or precipitated by exposure to cold. Symptoms begin either during infancy or early childhood. Myotonia gets worse with exercise compared with other myotonic syndromes. Later in disease, patient develops progressive proximal myopathy.[4]

During attack, serum potassium level is normal or high. Creatinine kinase may be elevated. Routine nerve conduction studies are normal, but compound muscle action potentials reduce in amplitude with cooling of limb. Electromyography reveals myotonia that disappears with cooling as muscle becomes inexcitable.[4]

Treatment: Acute attacks rarely need treatment as weakness is mild. Avoidance of cold and vigorous exercise is advised. Prophylactic treatment with mexiletine or thiazide diuretics can be helpful.[4]

References

1. Fontaine B. Periodic paralysis. *Adv Genet.* 2008;63:3.
2. Ke Q, Luo B, Qi M, et al. Gender differences in penetrance and phenotype in hypokalemic periodic paralysis. *Muscle Nerve.* 2013;47:41.
3. Miller TM, Dias da Silva MR, Miller HA, et al. Correlating phenotype and genotype in the periodic paralyses. *Neurology.* 2004;63:1647.
4. Kasper DL, Fauci AS, Hauser SL, et al., eds. *Harrison's principles of internal medicine.* 19th ed. New York: McGraw-Hill Education/Medical; 2015.

5. Ober KP. Thyrotoxic periodic paralysis in the United States. Report of 7 cases and review of the literature. *Medicine (Baltimore)*. 1992;71:109.

6. Links TP, Zwarts MJ, Wilmink JT, et al. Permanent muscle weakness in familial hypokalaemic periodic paralysis: Clinical, radiological and pathological aspects. *Brain*. 1990;113(6):1873.

7. Venance SL, Cannon SC, Fialho D, et al. The primary periodic paralyses: diagnosis, pathogenesis and treatment. *Brain*. 2006;129:8.

8. Chen YC, Fang JT, Chang CT, Chou HH. Thyrotoxic periodic paralysis in a patient abusing thyroxine for weight reduction. *Ren Fail*. 2001;23:139.

9. Pompeo A, Nepa A, Maddestra M, et al. Thyrotoxic hypokalemic periodic paralysis: An overlooked pathology in western countries. *Eur J Intern Med*. 2007;18:380.

10. Hannon MJ, Behan LA, Agha A. Thyrotoxic periodic paralysis due to excessive L-thyroxine replacement in a Caucasian man. *Ann Clin Biochem*. 2009;46:423.

11. Chou HK, Tsao YT, Lin SH. An unusual cause of thyrotoxic periodic paralysis: triiodothyronine-containing weight reducing agents. *Am J Med Sci*. 2009;337:71.

12. Manoukian MA, Foote JA, Crapo LM. Clinical and metabolic features of thyrotoxic periodic paralysis in 24 episodes. *Arch Intern Med*. 1999;159:601.

13. Pothiwala P, Levine SN. Analytic review: thyrotoxic periodic paralysis: a review. *J Intens Care Med*. 2010;25:71.

14. Hsieh MJ, Lyu RK, Chang WN, et al. Hypokalemic thyrotoxic periodic paralysis: clinical characteristics and predictors of recurrent paralytic attacks. *Eur J Neurol*. 2008;15:559.

15. Shiang JC, Cheng CJ, Tsai MK, et al. Therapeutic analysis in Chinese patients with thyrotoxic periodic paralysis over 6 years. *Eur J Endocrinol*. 2009;161:911.

16. Griggs RC, Bender AN, Tawil R. A puzzling case of periodic paralysis. *Muscle Nerve*. 1996;19:362.

17. Lu KC, Hsu YJ, Chiu JS, et al. Effects of potassium supplementation on the recovery of thyrotoxic periodic paralysis. *Am J Emerg Med*. 2004;22:544.

18. Birkhahn RH, Gaeta TJ, Melniker L. Thyrotoxic periodic paralysis and intravenous propranolol in the emergency setting. *J Emerg Med*. 2000;18:199.

19. Conway MJ, Seibel JA, Eaton P. Thyrotoxicosis and periodic paralysis: improvement with beta blockade. *Ann Intern Med*. 1974;81:332.

20. Jurkat-Rott K, Lehmann-Horn F. Genotype-phenotype correlation and therapeutic rationale in hyperkalemic periodic paralysis. *Neurotherapeutics*. 2007;4:216.

21. Venance SL, Cannon SC, Fialho D, et al. The primary periodic paralyses: diagnosis, pathogenesis and treatment. *Brain*. 2006;129:8.

22. Gould RJ, Steeg CN, Eastwood AB, et al. Potentially fatal cardiac dysrhythmia and hyperkalemic periodic paralysis. *Neurology*. 1985;35:1208.

23. Bradley WG, Taylor R, Rice DR, et al. Progressive myopathy in hyperkalemic periodic paralysis. *Arch Neurol*. 1990;47:1013.

24. McManis PG, Lambert EH, Daube JR. The exercise test in periodic paralysis. *Muscle Nerve*. 1986;9:704.

25. Kuntzer T, Flocard F, Vial C, et al. Exercise test in muscle channelopathies and other muscle disorders. *Muscle Nerve*. 2000;23:1089.

26. Hanna MG, Stewart J, Schapira AH, et al. Salbutamol treatment in a patient with hyperkalaemic periodic paralysis due to a mutation in the skeletal muscle sodium channel gene (SCN4A). *J Neurol Neurosurg Psychiatry*. 1998;65:248.

27. Bendheim PE, Reale EO, Berg BO. beta-Adrenergic treatment of hyperkalemic periodic paralysis. *Neurology*. 1985;35:746.

28. Riggs JE, Griggs RC, Moxley RT 3rd, Lewis ED. Acute effects of acetazolamide in hyperkalemic periodic paralysis. *Neurology*. 1981;31:725.

29. Cannon SC, George AL. Pathophysiology of myotonia and periodic paralysis. In Asbury AK, McKhann GM, McDonald WI, et al., eds. *Diseases of the nervous system*. 3rd ed. Cambridge, UK: Cambridge University Press; 2002. p. 1183.

30. Klingler W, Lehmann-Horn F, Jurkat-Rott K. Complications of anaesthesia in neuromuscular disorders. *Neuromuscul Disord*. 2005;15:195.

Peroneal Neuropathy

Epidemiology and Demographics: This is a relatively common disease that can occur in all ages. There is no predilection for either sex.

Disorder Description: The condition causes weakness of the dorsiflexors and everters of the affected foot and toes. Numbness occurs in the outside of the calf and the upper surface of the foot. Surgery can be a potential risk factor along with people who frequently cross their legs. Compression from a local cyst may occur in the popliteal area.

Symptoms

Localization site	Comment
Peripheral neuropathy	Peroneal nerve at the fibular head

Secondary Complications: Trips and falls from foot drop.

Treatment Complications: Surgical intervention may rarely cause injury to other nerves.

Bibliography

Brazis PW, et al., eds. Peripheral nerves. In *Localization in clinical neurology*. 6th ed. Philadelphia, PA: Lippincott Williams and Wilkins; 2011. Chapter 2.

Stewart JD. Foot drop: where, why and what to do? *Pract Neurol.* 2008;8(3):158–69. DOI: 10.1136/jnnp.2008.149393.

Persistent Depressive Disorder (Dysthymia)

Epidemiology and Demographics: DSM-5 definition of persistent depressive disorder is a combination of the DSM-IV diagnoses of dysthymia and a major depressive episode. The 12-month prevalence in the United States of persistent depressive disorder is 0.5%, compared with 1.5% for major depressive disorder.

Disorder Description: According to DSM-5, this disorder represents a consolidation of DSM-IV-defined chronic major depressive disorder and dysthymic disorder.

A. Depressed mood for most of the day, for more days than not, as indicated by either subjective account or observation by others, for at least 2 years. (In children and adolescents, mood can be irritable, and duration must be at least 1 year.)

B. Presence, while depressed, of two (or more) of the following:
    i. Poor appetite or overeating
    ii. Insomnia or hypersomnia
    iii. Low energy or fatigue
    iv. Low self-esteem
    v. Poor concentration or difficulty making decisions
    vi. Feelings of hopelessness

C. During the 2-year period (1 year for children or adolescents) of the disturbance, the individual has never been without the symptoms in Criteria A and B for more than 2 months at a time.

D. Criteria for a major depressive disorder may be continuously present for 2 years.

E. There has never been a manic episode or a hypomanic episode, and criteria have never been met for cyclothymic disorder.

F. The disturbance is not better explained by a persistent schizoaffective disorder, schizophrenia, delusional disorder, or other specified or unspecified schizophrenia spectrum and other psychotic disorder.

G. The symptoms are not attributable to the physiologic effects of a substance (e.g., a drug of abuse, a medication) or another medical condition (e.g., hypothyroidism).

H. The symptoms cause clinically significant distress or impairment in social, occupational, or other important areas of functioning.

Differential Diagnosis: Differential diagnosis should include major depressive disorder, psychotic disorders, depressive or bipolar and related disorder due to another medical condition, substance/medication-induced depressive or bipolar disorder, and personality disorders.

The diagnosis of major depressive disorder is distinguished from persistent depressive disorder by how long the symptoms are present. A major depressive episode does not last 2 years and thus would not be considered persistent depressive disorder.

In psychotic disorders (schizoaffective, schizophreniform, schizophrenia), depressive symptoms are common; however, a separate diagnosis of persistent depressive disorder is not made if the symptoms are only present during the course of the psychotic disorder.

In depressive or bipolar and related disorder due to another medical condition, the mood disturbance is judged (by history, physical exam, and laboratory findings) to be attributable directly to another medical condition.

In substance/medication-induced depressive or bipolar disorder, there are depressive symptoms, but they are etiologically related to a substance (e.g., a drug of abuse, medication, or toxin).

In persistent depressive disorder, there is often co-occurring personality disturbance. When one's presentation meets the criteria for both persistent depressive disorder and a personality disorder, both diagnoses are given.

Secondary Complications: Persistent depressive disorder may significantly decrease one's quality of life. It may lead to, or occur with, substance abuse. Relationship and family difficulties, as well as problems with school or work may occur. Additional complications include chronic pain and illness, suicidal thoughts and behavior, and personality disorders.

Treatment Complications: Treatment for persistent depressive disorder should include both psychotherapy and pharmacotherapy (combination is more effective than either alone). Pharmacotherapy may include selective serotonin reuptake inhibitors (SSRIs), tricyclic antidepressants (TCAs), and monoamine oxidase inhibitors (MAOIs). SSRI side effects include nausea, diarrhea, insomnia, headache, anorexia, weight loss, sexual dysfunction, restlessness (akathisia-like), serotonin syndrome (fever diaphoresis, tachycardia, hypertension, delirium, neuromuscular excitability), hyponatremia, and seizures (0.2%).

TCAs are highly protein bound and lipid soluble and thus have many drug interactions. They have antihistaminic properties including sedation and weight gain; antiadrenergic properties including orthostatic hypotension, dizziness, reflex tachycardia, and arrhythmias; and antimuscarinic effects including dry mouth, constipation, urinary retention, blurry vision, tachycardia, and exacerbation of narrow angle glaucoma. TCAs are lethal in overdose and thus suicide risk should be carefully assessed. Symptoms of overdose include agitation, tremors, ataxia, arrhythmias, delirium, hypoventilation (secondary to central nervous system depression), myoclonus, hyperreflexia, seizures, and coma. Serotonergic effects are also seen in TCAs including erectile/ejaculatory dysfunction in males and anorgasmia in females.

MAOI side effects include serotonin syndrome (especially when taken together with SSRIs or other drugs that also raise serotonin levels). Serotonin syndrome is characterized by lethargy, restlessness, confusion, flushing, diaphoresis, tremor, and myoclonus. These symptoms may progress to hyperthermia, hypertonicity, rhabdomyolysis, renal failure, convulsions, coma, and death. To avoid serotonin syndrome, a "washout period" of 2 weeks should be used between the discontinuation of either an SSRI or MAOI and the start of another. A 5-week period is necessary for fluoxetine washout. When taken with tyramine-rich foods (aged cheeses, wines, chicken liver, fava beans, etc.), MAOIs may cause hypertensive crisis. In hypertensive crisis, markedly elevated blood pressure along with headache, sweating, nausea, vomiting, photophobia, autonomic instability, chest pain, arrhythmias, and death can be seen. Other MAOI side effects include orthostatic hypotension, drowsiness, sexual dysfunction, dry mouth, sleep problems, liver toxicity, edema, and seizures. Patients with pyridoxine deficiency can have numbness or paresthesias, so they should be supplemented with vitamin B6.

Bibliography

American Psychiatric Association. *Diagnostic and statistical manual of mental disorders: DSM-5.* 5th ed. Washington, DC: American Psychiatric Association; 2013.

Thase ME, Fava M, Halbreich U, et al. A placebo-controlled, randomized clinical trial comparing sertraline and imipramine for the treatment of dysthymia. *Arch Gen Psychiatry.* 1996;53(9):777–84.

van Elst LT, Woermann FG, Lemieux L, Trimble MR. Amygdala enlargement in dysthymia – a volumetric study of patients with temporal lobe epilepsy. *Biol Psychiatry.* 1999;46(12):1614–23.

Weissman MM, Leaf PJ, Bruce ML, Florio L. The epidemiology of dysthymia in five communities: rates, risks, comorbidity, and treatment. *Am J Psychiatry.* 1988;145(7):815–19.

Williams JW Jr, Barrett J, Oxman T, et al. Treatment of dysthymia and minor depression in primary care: a randomized controlled trial in older adults. *JAMA.* 2000;284(12):1519–26.

Persistent Vegetative State

Epidemiology and Demographics: According to estimates cited in a consensus statement by the Multi-Society Task Force on persistent vegetative state (PVS), there are 10,000 to 25,000 adults and 4000 to 10,000 children in a PVS in the United States.[1] Head trauma is the most common acute cause of PVS in adults, and hypoxic–ischemic encephalopathy is the most common acute cause in children. Non-acute causes of PVS include degenerative disorders such as Alzheimer's dementia and developmental disorders such as anencephaly.[1]

Disorder Description: Patients in a vegetative state are unaware of their surroundings and lack self-awareness, yet have intact sleep–wake cycles with intermittent periods of wakefulness, as well as partial or complete preservation of hypothalamic and brainstem autonomic functions. During periods of wakefulness, PVS patients may smile, cry, moan, or exhibit stereotyped reflexive movements, which are purposeless, rather than goal-directed. PVS describes a vegetative state that persists for at least 1 month in patients with degenerative, metabolic, or developmental disorders, or present at 1 month following traumatic brain injury (TBI) or non-TBI. PET scan during PVS shows decreased cerebral glucose metabolic rates, comparable to rates reported during deep general anesthesia of normal subjects. Despite the appearance of interactivity, PVS patients are in an unconscious state.[1]

Consciousness requires both wakefulness and awareness. Wakefulness is mediated by ascending stimuli from the pontine tegmentum, posterior hypothalamus, and thalamus. Awareness is mediated by cerebral cortical neurons and their connections to major subcortical nuclei. Comatose patients lack both wakefulness and awareness. PVS patients are intermittently awake, with intact though irregular sleep–wake cycles, but lack awareness. It is also important to distinguish PVS from locked-in syndrome, in which awareness is retained, but demonstration of awareness is limited by profound quadraparesis.[1]

Neuropathology of acute causes of PVS fall into two main patterns: diffuse laminar cortical necrosis (typically following global hypoxic–ischemic injury) and diffuse axonal injury (after trauma).[1] Disproportionately selective and severe thalamic injury was noted in one case study (of Karen Ann Quinlan), and Kinney et al. posit that the thalamus may play a critical role in the pathogenesis of PVS.[2] There is a lack of data regarding neuropathologic correlates of PVS resulting from degenerative, metabolic, or developmental disorders.[1]

Following an initial insult, a patient may be initially comatose, then subsequently recover to a PVS or better. Coma from TBI carries a better prognosis than non-traumatic coma. Recovery after prolonged coma from TBI has been described.[3] In a review of 434 patients in a vegetative state at 1 month post-TBI, 33% had recovered consciousness at 3 months post-TBI, 46% had recovered by 6 months, 52% by 12 months, and 7% after 12 months.[1] The AAN recommended in a 1995 summary statement that PVS can be judged to be permanent at 12 months post-TBI and at 3 months after non-TBI, with the caveat that special attention should be paid to signs of awareness in children during the first year post-TBI.[4]

Karen Ann Quinlan, a 21-year-old woman, suffered a cardiopulmonary arrest and hypoxic–ischemic brain injury in 1975, following accidental ingestion of sedatives with alcohol, and remained in a PVS for the next 10 years, eventually succumbing to a combination of pneumonia, endocarditis, and meningitis. Her case led to the establishment of medicolegal guidelines for the care of PVS patients.[2] Discussion with family regarding level of treatment is essential, including provision of medications, supplemental oxygen and use of antibiotics, sustaining measures such as dialysis, and artificial nutrition and hydration.[4] As per a position paper by the AAN in 1989, nutrition and hydration administered by artificial means (such as G-tube) is classified as a form of medical treatment, not a nursing procedure, and may be discontinued in accordance with practices governing withholding and withdrawing other forms of medical treatment in PVS patients.[5] Of note, end-of-life decision-making is largely governed by state law, and some states have more restrictive statutes that either exclude PVS from the clinical conditions for which life-sustaining treatment can be withdrawn or permit care to be withdrawn only if specifically authorized by an advance directive.[6]

PVS needs to be distinguished from minimally responsive state and from locked-in syndrome. Patients with locked-in syndrome are unable to speak and unable to move their limbs but retain intact consciousness and cognition. Communication with locked-in syndrome patients is challenging. Patients can usually communicate using blinking as a way to signal "yes/no" answers (e.g., "blink once if yes, blink twice if no"). Patients with retained eye movements can sometimes be trained to use eye movements to control a computer cursor.

The minimally conscious state describes patients whose level of behavior is slightly better than patients with PVS.[7] They may reach for objects such as a glass of water. They may follow visual input or auditory input for several seconds. They may respond inconsistently to commands such as "move your arm."

Symptoms

Localization site	Comment
Cerebral hemispheres	Irregular sleep–wake cycles, with periods of wakefulness during which eyes may be open, sustained visual pursuit is lacking, movements are purposeless, and there is no evidence of language comprehension or expression, self-awareness, or awareness of the environment[1]
Brainstem/ cranial nerves	Cardiopulmonary and autonomic functions mediated by the brainstem are intact Variably preserved cranial nerve reflexes, and some patients may demonstrate[1]: – unequal or irregular pupils – CN III palsy – internuclear ophthalmoplegia – impaired vestibulo-ocular reflex

Secondary Complications: Complications of PVS include muscle contractures and decubitus ulcers, as well as nutritional deficiencies, and patients often succumb to infection such as pneumonia or UTI. Preventive measures include daily physical therapy, skin care, frequent repositioning, feeding tube placement, and prompt antibiotic treatment when indicated. Mortality is 33% during the first year of PVS, often from pneumonia or UTI. If the PVS patient survives beyond the first year, the mortality rate decreases. Life expectancy for most PVS patients ranges from 2 to 5 years, though some survive longer, and the chance of surviving more than 15 years is approximately 1/15,000 to 1/75,000.[1]

Treatment Complications: Establishing level of treatment in PVS patients in consultation with family is critical, as is awareness of state laws governing provision of care, and involvement of ethics committees when necessary.

References

1. Multi-Society Task Force on PVS. Medical aspects of the persistent vegetative state. *N Engl J Med*. 1994;330:1499–579.

2. Kinney HC, Korein J, Panigrahy A, Dikkes P, Goode R. Neuropathological findings in the brain of Karen Ann Quinlan: the role of the thalamus in the persistent vegetative state. *N Engl J Med*. 1994;330:1469–75.

3. Posner JB, Saper CB. *Plum and Posner's diagnosis of stupor and coma*. 4th ed. Oxford: Oxford University Press; 2007.

4. Quality Standards Subcommittee of the American Academy of Neurology. Practice parameters: Assessment and management of patients in the persistent vegetative state (Summary statement). *Neurology*. 1995;45:1015–18.

5. No authors listed. Position of the American Academy of Neurology on certain aspects of the care and management of the persistent vegetative state patient. *Neurology*. 1989;39:125–6

6. Larriviere D, Bonnie RJ. Terminating artificial nutrition and hydration in persistent vegetative state patients: Current and proposed state laws. *Neurology*. 2006;66:1624–8.

7. Giacino JT, et al. The minimally conscious state: definition and diagnostic criteria. *Neurology*. 2002;58(3):349–53.

Pertussis

Epidemiology and Demographics: Available vaccine has drastically decreased the incidence of pertussis. Many cases are mild, so incidence data are unreliable. Booster vaccine is needed later in childhood. Predominantly affects children <6 years old, but all ages are susceptible.

Disorder Description: Also known as "whooping cough." Caused by *Bordetella pertussis* or *Bordetella parapertussis*. These are gram-negative, pleomorphic, and aerobic bacilli. Classically presents as paroxysms of severe coughing fits often causing vomiting. The infection does not directly affect the nervous system.

Diagnosis is through nasopharyngeal secretion swab.

Can be treated with erythromycin, azithromycin, and clarithromycin within 4 weeks of onset.

Symptoms

Localization site	Comment
Cerebral hemispheres	Encephalopathy

Secondary Complications: Seizures and encephalopathy can occur as complications of asphyxia. Seizures can occur as a complication of alkalosis related to vomiting.

Treatment Complications: Although early whole cell vaccines caused rare neurologic complications, newer acellular vaccines do not.

Bibliography

Cherry JD, Heininger U. Pertussis and other *Bordetella* infections. In Feigin RD, Cherry JD, Demmler-Harrison GJ, et al., eds. *Textbook of pediatric infectious diseases.* Vol. 1. Philadelphia, PA: Saunders/Elsevier; 2009. pp. 1683–706.

Sanghi V. Neurologic manifestations of diphtheria and pertussis. In Biller J, Ferro JM, eds. *Neurologic aspects of systemic disease Part III.* Handbook of Clinical Neurology. Vol 121. 3rd Series. Philadelphia, PA: Elsevier; 2014.

Phencyclidine (PCP)

Disorder Description: A hallucinogen that is a synthetic anesthetic also known as angel dust with variable routes of absorption via orally, smoked, insufflated, or injected.

Epidemiology and Demographics: The predominant users are males aged 25–34 years, with no race predilection.

Symptoms

Localization site	Comment
Cerebral hemispheres	Tonic–clonic seizures (acute)
	Intracranial hemorrhage (chronic)
Mental status and psychiatric aspects/ complications	Euphoria (acute)
	Hallucination (acute)
	Memory loss (chronic)
	Depression (chronic)
	Anxiety (chronic)
	Social withdrawal (chronic)
	Phobias (chronic)
	Violent manic behavior (chronic)
	Schizophrenic behavior (chronic)
	Cognitive difficulties (chronic)
	Speech difficulties (chronic)

Localization site	Comment
Brainstem	Autonomic instability (acute)
	Disruption of the sleep–wake cycle (acute)
	Decerebrate rigidity (acute) – patient lies in rigid extension with the arms internally rotated at the shoulders, elbows, knees, and hips extended, and fingers, ankles, and toes flexed
Vestibular system (and nonspecific dizziness)	Ataxia (acute)
Cranial nerves	Nystagmus (acute)
	Hyperacusis (acute)
	Diminished gag reflex (acute)
	Diminished corneal reflexes (acute)
Spinal cord	Paresthesias (acute)
Anterior horn cells	Paresthesias (acute)
Dorsal root ganglia	Paresthesias (acute)
Mononeuropathy or mononeuropathy multiplex	Paresthesias (acute)
Peripheral neuropathy	Decreased peripheral sensation (acute)
Muscle	Tremors (chronic)
	Catatonic rigidity muscle (acute)
Neuromuscular junction	Increases levels of dopamine (acute and chronic)
	Disrupts levels of glutamate (acute and chronic)

Secondary Complications: Indirectly affects nervous system

- Cardiovascular effects: can induce hypertensive crises resulting in cerebral hemorrhage.
- Respiratory effects: respiratory failure can lead to cerebral ischemia.
- Renal effects: acute renal failure leads to rhabdomyolysis and seizures.

Bibliography

Brenner S. PCP toxicity. Updated Feb 1, 2018. https://emedicine.medscape.com/article/1010821-overview. Accessed Sep 17, 2018.

Hallucinogens.com. PCP effects on the brain. http://hallucinogens.com/pcp/pcp-effects-on-the-brain/. Accessed Sep 6, 2018.

National Institute of Drug Abuse. What are the effects of common dissociative drugs on the brain and body? Feb 2015. www.drugabuse.gov/publications/research-reports/hallucinogens-dissociative-drugs/what-are-effects-common-dissociative-drugs-brain-body. Accessed Sep 6, 2018.

Phenylketonuria (PKU)

Epidemiology and Demographics: Incidence is 1/13,500 to 19,000 births in the United States. It is less common in the African American population.

Disorder Description: Phenylketonuria (PKU) is an inborn error of metabolism, characterized by deficiency of phenylalanine hydroxylase (PAH). PAH catalyzes the conversion of the amino acid phenylalanine to tyrosine. PAH deficiency leads to the acummulation of phenylalanine and its metabolites in the blood and in the brain. In developed countries, PKU is identified via testing at birth for inborn errors of metabolism.

There are different combinations of mutations that lead to different phenotypes, ranging from mild to moderate to severe. Classic PKU is of the severe phenotype.

High blood concentrations of phenylalanine result in brain toxicity due to its inhibitory effect on the transport of free L-amino acids that are needed for synthesis of neurotransmitters (DA and serotonin) across the brain–blood barrier.

If untreated, it can lead to microcephaly, severe intellectual disability, epilepsy, a musty odor, eczema, decreased hair and skin pigmentation, and structural brain changes. Main treatment consists of maintaining a phenylalanine-free diet. Prognosis depends both on the time of diagnosis and the severity of the disease.

Symptoms

Localization site	Comment
Cerebral hemispheres	Diffuse white matter injury is apparent on MRI
	A common finding is a symmetric increase in T2-weighted signal in the periventricular white matter. The severity of the changes seems to be proportional to dietary status
Mental status and psychiatric aspects/ complications	Cognitive outcome is correlated to the extent of control of blood phenylalanine concentration. However, their IQ scores, even when treated, are slightly lower than those of other family members
	Several studies have suggested that individuals with PKU show more internalizing behaviors and have higher rates of anxiety, depression, and avoidant personality

Treatment Complications: Treatment involves dietary restriction of foods with phenylalanine and aspartame. Administration of sapropterin may be considered and may be associated with headache, dizziness, or uncommonly hyperactivity or feeling of agitation.

Bibliography

Leuzzi V, et al. Biochemical, clinical and neuroradiological (MRI) correlations in late-detected PKU patients. *J Inherit Metab Dis.* 1995;18(5):624–34.

Leuzzi V, et al. The pathogenesis of the white matter abnormalities in phenylketonuria. A multimodal 3.0 Tesla MRI and magnetic resonance spectroscopy (1H MRS) study. *J Inherit Metab Dis.* 2007;30(2):209–16.

Rahja R, et al. Mental health and social functioning in early treated phenylketonuria: the PKU-COBESO study. *Mol Genet Metab.* (2013);110(Suppl): S57–S61.

Smith I, Knowles J. Behavior in early treated PKU: a systematic review. *Eur J Pediatr.* 2000;159(2):S89–93.

Pheochromocytoma

Epidemiology and Demographics: Rare subset of neuroendocrine neoplasia, with an incidence of 0.8 per 100,000 population-years; total value is likely an underestimate given that at least 50% are asymptomatic and are diagnosed postmortem. Diagnosed predominantly between the 4th and 5th decade of life, without gender predominance. Pheochromocytomas have a hereditary and a sporadic presentation, with familial favoring childhood presentation; the mutation associated with the hereditary cases is in the mitochondrial succinate dehydrogenase enzyme complex (SDH-A, SDH-B, SDH-C). The following syndromes are associated with the appearance of this catecholamine-secreting tumor: 50% in multiple endocrine neoplasia 2A–2B, 5% in neurofibromatosis type 1, and 20% in von Hippel–Lindau and Sturge–Weber. These neoplasia have malignant potential defined by the World Health Organization by the presence of metastatic disease; 10% will develop tumor, spread occurring up to 20 years post treatment.

Disorder Description: Sympathetic catecholamine-secreting neuroendocrine tumor, also known as adrenal paraganglioma, originating from glomus cells, derived from neural crest.

Since it is an adrenal paraganglioma, it will have the same histology as an adrenal neoplasm, i.e., cuboidal/polygonal small cells clustered in a fashion known as "zellballen." Positive staining: chromogranin, synaptophysin, S100 (sustentacular cells), PAS+ diastase-resistant hyaline globules and tenascin (strong in clinically malignant tumors), neuron-specific enolase, neurofilament, variable vimentin, bcl2, and focal HMB45. Negative staining: MelanA/Mart1, inhibin, and calretinin.

Symptoms

Localization site	Comment
Cerebral hemispheres	Episodic headache, blurry vision, syncope
Mental status and psychiatric aspects/ complications	Anxiety, panic attack-like symptoms: tremor, diaphoresis, nonexertional palpitations, pallor, feeling of imminent death, apprehension
Vestibular system	Nausea, vomiting

Secondary Complications: Episodic malignant hypertension, episodic hypotension, malignant arrhythmias, hyperglycemia, weight loss, polyuria, Takotsubo cardiomyopathy, myocardial infarct, pulmonary edema, sudden death.

Treatment Complications:
- Surgery: hemorrhage, malignant hypertension, myocardial infarct, arrhythmias, multiorgan failure, death.
- Embolization: hemorrhage, skin necrosis.
- Radiotherapy: mucositis, skin rash, hypoacusis, hypopituitarism, xerostomia, bone necrosis.

Bibliography

Abermil N, Guillaud-Bataille M, Burnichon N, et al. TMEM127 screening in a large cohort of patients with pheochromocytoma and/or paraganglioma. *J Clin Endocrinol Metab*. 2012;97: E805–9.

Anderson J, Gulant RW. Paraganglioma of the cauda equina: a case report. *J Neurol Neurosurg Psychiatry*. 1987;50:100–3.

Bayley JP, Kunst HP, Cascon A, et al. SDHAF2 mutations in familial and sporadic paraganglioma

and phaeochromocytoma. *Lancet Oncol.* 2010;11:366–72.

Fishbein L. Pheochromocytoma and paraganglioma: genetics, diagnosis, and treatment. *Hematol Oncol Clin North Am*. 2016;30(1):135–50. DOI: 10.1016/j.hoc.2015.09.006. Epub 2015 Oct 23. DOI:10.1016/j.hoc.2015.09.006

Hrabovsky EE, McLellan D, Horton JA, Klingberg WG. Catheter embolization: preparation of patient with pheochromocytoma. *J Pediatr Surg*. 1982;17(6):849–50.

Kirmani S, Young WF. Hereditary paraganglioma-pheochromocytoma syndromes. May 21, 2008. Updated Nov 6, 2014. In Pagon RA, Adam MP, Ardinger HH, et al., eds. *GeneReviews*® [Internet]. Seattle (WA): University of Washington, Seattle; 1993–2017.

Naguib M, Caceres M, Thomas CR Jr, Herman TS, Eng TY. Radiation treatment of recurrent pheochromocytoma of the bladder: case report and review of literature. *Am J Clin Oncol*. 2002;25(1):42–4.

Papathomas TG, de Krijger RR, Tischler AS. Paragangliomas: update on differential diagnostic considerations, composite tumors, and recent genetic developments. *Semin Diagn Pathol*. 2013;30(3):207–23. DOI: 10.1053/j.semdp.2013.06.006.

You D, Ren R, Chen E, et al. Radiotherapy for urinary bladder pheochromocytoma with invasion of the prostate: A case report and literature review. *Mol Clin Oncol*. 2016;4(6): 1060–2. Epub 2016 Mar 17.

Phospholipase A-Associated Neurodegeneration (Neuroaxonal Dystrophy)

Epidemiology and Demographics: This is a relatively rare condition. The list of references below contains reports of patients from as young as 14 months to young adults. There is no predilection for either sex.

Disorder Description: The PLA2G6 gene produces an enzyme that causes the chemical breakdown of glycerophospholipids. Patients may present with gradual weakness and cognitive dysfunction. Over time, the weakness may change into increased tone.

485

Symptoms

Localization site	Comment
Cerebellum	Progressive cerebellar atrophy
Peripheral neuropathy	Spheroid bodies in peripheral nerve biopsy

Secondary Complications: The decline in mental status and weakness may progress to affect the patient's ability for self care.

Treatment Complications: No disease-modifying treatments exist.

Bibliography

Beck G, Shinzawa K, Hayakawa H, et al. Deficiency of calcium-independent phospholipase A2 beta induces brain iron accumulation through upregulation of divalent metal transporter 1. *PLoS One*. 2015;10(10):e0141629. DOI:10.1371/journal.pone.0141629.

Bernardi B. MRI findings in patients with clinical onset consistent with infantile neuroaxonal dystrophy (INAD), literature review, clinical and MRI follow-up. *Neuroradiol J*. 2011;24(2):202–14. Epub 2011 May 11.

Illingworth MA, Meyer E, Chong WK, et al. PLA2G6-associated neurodegeneration (PLAN): Further expansion of the clinical, radiological and mutation spectrum associated with infantile and atypical childhood-onset disease. *Mol Genet Metab*. 2014;112(2):183–9. DOI:10.1016/j.ymgme.2014.03.008.

Pica

Epidemiology and Demographics: The prevalence of pica is unclear. Among those with an intellectual disability, the incidence of pica appears to be correlated with the severity of disability. Nutritional deficiencies are common causes of pica and need to be looked out for prior to considering psychiatric causes.

Disorder Description: As stated in DSM-5, pica can be defined as:

A. Persistent eating of non-nutritive, non-food substances over a period of at least 1 month.

B. The eating of non-nutritive, non-food substances is inappropriate to the developmental level of the individual.

C. The behavior is not part of a culturally supported or socially normative practice.

D. If the eating behavior occurs in the context of another mental disorder or medical condition, it is sufficiently severe to warrant additional clinical attention.

Differential Diagnosis: Differential diagnosis should include anorexia nervosa, factitious disorder, and non-suicidal self-injurious behavior as part of personality disorders.

In some presentations of anorexia nervosa, individuals may eat non-nutritive substances (e.g., paper) in an effort to control appetite. When the consumption of non-nutritive substances is primarily a method for weight control, the diagnosis of anorexia nervosa should be given.

In factitious disorder, individuals may consume non-nutritive substances in an effort to falsify physical symptoms. In these cases, there is an element of deception that is consistent with deliberate induction of injury or disease.

In non-suicidal self-injury or non-suicidal self-injurious behaviors in personality disorders, an individual may swallow potentially harmful objects (e.g., pins, needles, knives) in the context of maladaptive behavior patterns associated with personality disorders or non-suicidal self-injury.

Secondary Complications: Pica can significantly impair physical functioning, but is rarely the sole or primary cause of impairment of social functioning. Pica is often comorbid with other disorders in which social functioning impairment is characteristic. Certain items such as paint chips may contain lead or other toxic substances. Consumption of such materials may lead to intellectual disability and/or brain damage. Eating non-nutritive substances may also interfere with normal dietary habits and may thus lead to malnourishment. Eating some solid objects may lead to obstruction and cause constipation or tears in the esophageal and/or intestinal lining. This is particularly common in the case of hair-eating. Patients suffering from trichotillomania may rarely consume their pulled hair. The consumed hair can then cause a bezoar, usually in the stomach, and may lead to gastrointestinal obstruction. Pica may also be the cause of infection and fistula formation.

Treatment Complications: Treatment first should address dietary deficiencies and potential toxicities such as lead poisoning. Treatment includes psychosocial and family-guidance approaches, and behavior-modification therapy.

In cases of pica of psychogenic etiology that is refractory to psychosocial therapies, selective serotonin reuptake inhibitors (SSRIs) have been shown to have efficacy. SSRI side effects include nausea, diarrhea, insomnia, headache, anorexia, weight loss, sexual dysfunction, restlessness (akathisia-like), serotonin syndrome (fever diaphoresis, tachycardia, hypertension, delirium, neuromuscular excitability), hyponatremia, seizures (0.2%).

Bibliography

American Psychiatric Association. *Diagnostic and statistical manual of mental disorders: DSM-5.* 5th ed. Washington, DC: American Psychiatric Association; 2013.

Bhatia MS, Gupta R. Pica responding to SSRI: An OCD spectrum disorder? *World J Biol Psychiatry.* 2009;10(4–3):936–8.

Feldman MD. Pica: current perspectives. *Psychosomatics.* 1986;27(7):519–23.

Ruddock JC. Lead poisoning in children: with special reference to pica. *J Am Med Assoc.* 1924;82(21):1682–4.

Singhi S, Singhi P, Adwani GB. Role of psychosocial stress in the cause of pica. *Clin Pediatr.* 1981;20(12):783–5.

Pineoblastoma

Epidemiology and Demographics: Pineal region tumors represent less than 1% of all primary brain tumors in adults and between 2 and 5% of all childhood central nervous system neoplasias. These tumors tend to occur in children and young adults between the ages of 10 and 20 years (mean at 13 years of age), with adults presenting at 30 years of age. About 10 to 20% of the tumors, particularly pineoblastoma, have the potential to spread through the cerebrospinal fluid; rarely spreads elsewhere in the body. This usually occurs late in the disease.

Disorder Description: Results from the malignant transformation of pineal parenchymal cells show it has similar histologic and imaging features to the embryonal tumors (medulloblastoma, neuroectodermal tumors); however, it is molecularly distinct. It is a highly cellular tumor, composed of small, round blue cells that correspond to the appearance in imaging studies; lobulated, poorly defined, necrotic

with the tendency to involve adjacent brain structures. This neoplasm has a poor prognosis and is the most aggressive pineal parenchymal tumor, classified as a grade IV by the World Health Organization, with the potential to metastasize to the rest of the neuroaxis and recur despite treatment.

Symptoms

Localization site	Comment
Cerebral hemispheres	Obstructive hydrocephalus secondary to cerebral aqueduct occlusion causing altered mentation including lethargy, stupor, obtundation, coma, death. Diabetes insipidus
Brainstem	Compression of the tectum of the brainstem presenting as Parinaud syndrome, including absent vertical gaze, mydriasis with pupillary reflex to accommodation but diminished to light, anisocoria, convergence, and retraction nystagmus
Cerebellum	Ataxia, dysmetria from involvement of the superior cerebellar peduncle
Vestibular system (and nonspecific dizziness)	Nausea, vomiting, headache, diplopia
Pituitary gland	Parinaud syndrome due to the compression of the tectum of the brainstem

Secondary Complications: Diabetes insipidus, obstructive hydrocephalus, circadian rhythm disorders, vertical gaze palsy.

Treatment Complications:

- Intrinsic complications from ventriculoperitoneal (VP) shunting for obstructive hydrocephalus: infection, bleeding, obstruction, over-shunting, intracranial hypotension.
- Maximal surgical resection: pineal apoplexy, infections, progression of the deficits.
- Radiation: Severe headache migraine-like, severe vomiting, asthenia, fatigue. Vascular damage including stenosis-occlusion subsequently developing moyamoya-like pattern, aneurysms, microangiopathy; typically children are more prone to develop these events. Leukoencephalopathy. Pineal apoplexy.
- Chemotherapy: asthenia, weakness, nausea, vomiting, poor oral intake, dizziness, light-headedness, ataxia, weight loss.

Bibliography

Amato-Watkins AC, Lammie A, Hayhurst C, Leach P. Pineal parenchymal tumours of intermediate differentiation: An evidence-based review of a new pathological entity. *Br J Neurosurg.* 2016;30(1):11–5. DOI: 10.3109/02688697.2015.1096912.

Ito T, Kanno H, Sato K, et al. Clinicopathologic study of pineal parenchymal tumors of intermediate differentiation. *World Neurosurg.* 2014;81(5–6):783–9. DOI: 10.1016/j.wneu.2013.02.007.

Kwak J, Shim JK, Kim DS, et al. Isolation and characterization of tumorspheres from a recurrent pineoblastoma patient: Feasibility of a patient-derived xenograft. *Int J Oncol.* 2016;49(2):569–78. DOI: 10.3892/ijo.2016.3554.

Raleigh DR, Solomon DA, Lloyd SA, et al. Histopathologic review of pineal parenchymal tumors identifies novel morphologic subtypes and prognostic factors for outcome. *Neuro Oncol.* 2017;19(1):78–88. DOI: 10.1093/neuonc/now105.

Schild SE, Scheithauer BW, Schomberg PJ, et al. Pineal parenchymal tumors. Clinical, pathologic, and therapeutic aspects. *Cancer.* 1993; 72(3):870–80.

Pineocytoma

Epidemiology and Demographics: Pineocytomas are the second most common type of pineal parenchymal neoplasia after germinal cell. Benign mass that accounts for 14–27% of all pineal tumors and less than 1% of all central nervous system neoplasias. Typically found between 20 and 60 years of age, with slightly higher predilection for women compared with men (1:0.6).

Disorder Description: Pineocytoma is the most differentiated pineal neoplasia, arising from the pinealocytes. Relatively well-marginated, non-invasive, well-localized tumor; harbors large cysts and/or areas of calcification. Cells are arranged in clusters named pineocytomatous rosettes. Immunophenotype for diagnosis includes synaptophysin, neurofilament, and neuron-specific enolase, with variable chromogranin and 5-hydroxytryptamine (5-HT). Considered a low-grade tumor, pineocytoma is usually treated with either total surgical resection or partial resection, followed by local radiation therapy, with overall good prognosis and 5-year survival >80%; classified as a grade I by the World Health Organization.

Symptoms

Localization site	Comment
Cerebral hemispheres	Obstructive hydrocephalus secondary to cerebral aqueduct occlusion causing altered mentation including lethargy, stupor, obtundation, coma, death. Diabetes insipidus. Seizures
Mental status and psychiatric aspects/ complications	Obsessive-compulsive behavior, psychosis, impaired memory
Brainstem	Compression of the tectum of the brainstem presenting as Parinaud syndrome including absent vertical gaze, mydriasis with pupillary reflex to accommodation but diminished to light, anisocoria, convergence, and retraction nystagmus
Cerebellum	Ataxia, dysmetria from involvement of the superior cerebellar peduncle
Vestibular system (and nonspecific dizziness)	Nausea, vomiting, headache, diplopia, tinnitus, nystagmus, dizziness
Pituitary gland	Parinaud syndrome due to compression of the tectum of the brainstem
Other	Papilledema

Secondary Complications: Insomnia, irritability, personality changes, ataxia, diabetes insipidus, obstructive hydrocephalus, circadian rhythm disorders, vertical gaze palsy, muscle spasms.

Treatment Complications:
- Intrinsic complications from ventriculoperitoneal (VP) shunting for obstructive hydrocephalus: infection, bleeding, obstruction, over-shunting, intracranial hypotension.
- Maximal surgical resection: pineal apoplexy, infections, progression of the deficits.
- Radiation: Severe headache migraine-like, severe vomiting, asthenia, fatigue. Vascular damage including stenosis-occlusion subsequently developing moyamoya-like pattern, aneurysms, microangiopathy; typically children are more prone to develop these events. Leukoencephalopathy. Pineal apoplexy.
- Chemotherapy: asthenia, weakness, nausea, vomiting, poor oral intake, dizziness, lightheadedness, ataxia, weight loss, peripheral neuropathy, leukoencephalopathy.

Bibliography

Al-Hussaini M, Sultan I, Gajjar AJ, Abuirmileh N, Qaddoumi I. Pineal gland tumors: experience from the Seer database. *J Neurooncol.* 2009;94(3):351–8. DOI:10.1007/s11060-009-9881-9.

Ito T, Kanno H, Sato K, et al. Clinicopathologic study of pineal parenchymal tumors of intermediate differentiation. *World Neurosurg.* 2014;81(5–6):783–9. DOI: 10.1016/j.wneu.2013.02.007.

Kwak J, Shim JK, Kim DS, et al. Isolation and characterization of tumorspheres from a recurrent pineoblastoma patient: Feasibility of a patient-derived xenograft. *Int J Oncol.* 2016;49(2):569–78. DOI: 10.3892/ijo.2016.3554.

Mottolese C, Szathmari A, Beuriat PA. Incidence of pineal tumours. A review of the literature. *Neurochirurgie.* 2015;61(2–3):65–9. DOI: 10.1016/j.neuchi.2014.01.005.

Raleigh DR, Solomon DA, Lloyd SA, et al. Histopathologic review of pineal parenchymal tumors identifies novel morphologic subtypes and prognostic factors for outcome. *Neuro Oncol.* 2017;19(1):78–88. DOI: 10.1093/neuonc/now105.

Schild SE, Scheithauer BW, Schomberg PJ, et al. Pineal parenchymal tumors. Clinical, pathologic, and therapeutic aspects. *Cancer.* 1993; 72(3):870–80.

Piriformis Syndrome

Epidemiology and Demographics: This condition is relatively rare and is reported in women in their 30s and 40s.

Disorder Description: The piriformis muscle is right above the sciatic nerve. The muscle itself or scar tissue from previous surgery may contract and grow larger over time, eventually pressing on the sciatic nerve. External pressure/trauma may also cause the symptoms. When the sciatic nerve is compressed, patients may experience pain that starts in the gluteal muscles and radiates down the back of the leg. Some patients may walk into the office with the foot turned inward.

Symptoms

Localization site	Comment
Peripheral neuropathy	Sciatic nerve distribution

Secondary Complications: Anxiety from chronic pain and limitation of movement.

Treatment Complications: Nonsteroidal anti-inflammatory drugs (NSAIDs) may rarely cause cerebrovascular complications. Muscle relaxants and gabapentin may cause sedation. Injections may inadvertently injure the sciatic nerve.

Bibliography

Cass S. Piriformis syndrome: a cause of nondiscogenic sciatica. *Curr Sports Med Rep.* 2015;14(1):41–4. DOI: 10.1249/JSR.0000000000000110. Review.

Smoll NR. Variations of the piriformis and sciatic nerve with clinical consequence: a review. *Clin Anat.* 2010;23(1):8–17.

Pituitary Apoplexy

Epidemiology and Demographics: Pituitary apoplexy most often occurs in patients harboring large somatotroph or corticotroph macroadenomas. Pregnancy is another important risk factor for pituitary apoplexy. Incidence of pituitary apoplexy in patients with known pituitary adenomas ranges from 0.6% to 10%. Majority of patients are between 38 and 57 years old, and male-to-female ratio is 2:1.

Disorder Description: Acute pituitary apoplexy typically begins with sudden severe headache, often a "thunderclap" headache, often centered immediately between the eyes above the bridge of the nose. The presentation could involve other neurologic symptoms including visual disturbances, vomiting, meningeal irritation, fever, clouding of consciousness, or coma.

Upward extension of the pituitary hematoma involves the optic chiasm (producing early bitemporal hemianopsia), the olfactory pathways, and hypothalamus (altered electrolyte balance, vital signs, and thermoregulation). Downward extension into the sphenoid sinus leads to epistaxis and CSF rhinorrhea. Lateral extension into the cavernous sinus results in varying degree of involvement of cranial nerve III, IV, V, or VI.

Bleeding into the subarachnoid space could cause signs of meningeal irritation. Raised intracranial pressure could cause the altered vision, nausea, vomiting, and altered consciousness. Hemiparesis or seizures could rarely occur.

Symptoms

Localization site	Comment
Cerebral hemispheres	Involvement of the internal carotid artery in the lateral wall of the cavernous sinus could result in stroke
	Subarachnoid hemorrhage could result in signs of meningeal irritation and raised intracranial pressure
Mental status and psychiatric aspects/complications	Varying degree of altered mental status from lethargy, confusion to coma secondary to raised intracranial pressure
Base of skull	Extension into the sphenoid sinus could cause epistaxis or CSF rhinorrhea
Cranial nerves	A unilateral third nerve palsy is the most common cranial nerve abnormality (with impaired medial and downward gaze, diplopia, ptosis, and mydriasis), followed by nerve palsy of the sixth and fourth cranial nerves. Unilateral fifth cranial nerve involvement may occur with ipsilateral facial sensory loss
Pituitary gland	Rarely, cortisol-induced hyperglycemia and acute delirium can be the initial presentation of a pituitary adenoma hemorrhage with stormy release of the adrenocorticotrophic hormone
	Hypothalamic involvement may result in the syndrome of inappropriate antidiuretic hormone secretion, diabetes insipidus, or sympathetic dysregulation resulting in hypotension

Secondary Complications: Occasionally, the presentation is fulminant and can result in death. Raised intracranial pressure is a reliable predictor of potential mortality and mandates urgent neurosurgical intervention. Endocrine deficiency is variable but common (growth hormone deficiency in 90%, adrenocorticotrophic hormone and gonadotrophin deficiency in 66%, and thyroid-stimulating hormone deficiency in 40%). Prolactin deficiency is characteristic in apoplexy. Visual acuity and ophthalmoplegia improve with surgical decompression.

Treatment Complications: In the acute phase, it is imperative that fluid and electrolytes be managed adequately especially with diabetes insipidus. Corticosteroids must be administered to patients with adrenal insufficiency and thyroid function should be assessed. Urgent neurosurgical evaluation is essential if mental status deteriorates or hemodynamic status worsens. Long-term management includes careful evaluation and replacement of hormones. Neuroendocrine surveillance is indicated for recurrence of adenoma.

Bibliography

Nawar RN, AbdelMannan D, Selman WR, Arafah BM. Pituitary tumor apoplexy: a review. *J Intens Care Med.* 2008;23(2):75–90.

Vaphiades MS. Pituitary apoplexy. Medscape. Updated Sep 20, 2017. Available from https://emedicine .medscape.com/article/1198279-overview. Available from https://emedicine.medscape.com/ article/1198279-overview. Accessed Sep 25, 2018.

Pituitary Tumors: Non-prolactinoma

Epidemiology and Demographics: Pituitary adenomas are the most common intracranial neoplasm, with prevalence in the general population of about 10–20%. Pituitary adenomas account for 6–10% of all symptomatic intracranial tumors. Fifty to 60% of pituitary adenomas are non-prolactinomas.

Non-prolactinoma adenomas:

Growth hormone (GH)-secreting tumors – 20%.

Gonadotroph adenomas – 10–15%.

Null cell adenomas (non-functional) – 5–10%.

Corticotropin-secreting – 10–12% (F:M ratio 8:1, peak incidence 3rd–4th decade).

Thyroid-stimulating hormone (TSH)-secreting adenomas – 1% pituitary adenomas (F:M ratio 1.7:1).

Other pituitary tumors:

Craniopharyngiomas – the next most common neoplastic tumor after adenoma, account for about 1% of all intracranial tumors in adults and 10% of intracranial tumors in children.

Germinomas – 65% intracranial germ cell neoplasms, higher incidence in China and Japan compared with western countries, male predominance.

Chordomas are very rare and represent less than 0.5% of primary intracranial tumors.

Rathke cleft cysts are the most common type of cyst in sellar and suprasellar regions. Commonly found at the junction between anterior and posterior pituitary lobes. More common in adult females than males.

Arachnoid cysts develop from a duplication of the arachnoid and can develop anywhere in the brain. Less than 1% of all space-occupying lesions in the brain and occur mostly in children.

Additional rarer tumor types affecting the pituitary/sella include meningioma, metastasis, chondrosarcoma, glioma, sarcoma, carcinoma, ectopic pinealoma, plasmocytoma, subependymal giant cell astrocytoma, pituicytoma, non-germinomatous germ cell tumors such as teratomas, embryonal carcinomas, and chorioncarcinomas, epidermoid or dermoid cysts.

Disorder Description: Pituitary adenomas are sporadic collections of cells, particularly hormone-secreting cells, with different effects depending on the hormone secreted. In addition to complications associated with local mass effect such as visual loss and headache, presentation is dependent on which hormone is secreted. **Prolactinomas** are the most common type of secreting adenoma, but are discussed in more detail in the entry for *Prolactinoma*. **Growth hormone**-secreting adenomas present with acromegaly in adults and gigantism in children. Galactorrhea can be seen. **Corticotroph**-secreting adenomas are the most common cause of endogenous hypercortisolism, accounting for approximately 65–70% of all cases of Cushing syndrome. These particular adenomas are usually more invasive than other types of pituitary tumors and will occasionally first present with pituitary apoplexy. **Gonadotropin**-secreting adenomas (follicle-stimulating hormone [FSH], luteinizing hormone [LH]) account for 10–15% of all pituitary adenomas. Hypersecretion of FSH and LH will often present with hypopituitarism.

Craniopharyngiomas are benign epithelial tumors located along the craniopharyngeal duct, which extends from sella to suprasellar region. **Meningiomas** produce symptoms from local mass effect. **Metastases** to the sellar region are most commonly lung and breast carcinoma. Major complications with these lesions are diabetes insipidus and cranial nerve palsies.

Chorioncarcinomas account for 3–5% of intracranial germ cell neoplasms. Higher incidence in Japan and China compared with western countries. Occur in children, more often seen in pineal gland. **Rathke cleft cysts** are congenital deformities and are often incidentally found on MRIs performed for other reasons.

Symptoms

Localization site	Comment
Cerebral hemispheres	Located in sella turcica
	Pituitary stalk connects pituitary to hypothalamus
	Lesions that extend into the temporal lobes can induce seizure activity
Mental status and psychiatric aspects/ complications	Headache is a common feature of all pituitary tumors, particularly when they are large. Often associated with acromegaly, Rathke and arachnoid cysts
	Effects of hormones secreted in pituitary adenomas responsible for other psychiatric manifestations such as anxiety in thyrotropin-secreting adenoma and Cushing disease, depression and insomnia in Cushing disease, fatigue in acromegaly
Base of skull	If tumor mass extends into sinuses, possibility of CSF leak exists
Cranial nerves	– Field defects due to local mass effect on optic chiasm classically bitemporal hemianopsia
	– Cranial neuropathies or ophthalmoplegia with metastases, large expanding sellar masses, Sheehan syndrome/pituitary apoplexy, craniopharyngioma
	– Upward extension from an expanding sellar mass can cause distortion and compression of the pituitary stalk and/or hypothalamus, which in turn compromises the release of dopaminergic prolactin inhibition
	– Distortion and invasion of the pituitary stalk may also compromise the portal blood supply to the anterior pituitary gland, resulting in infarction or hemorrhage, which can manifest clinically as pituitary apoplexy with sudden visual loss, acute severe headache, meningismus, and ophthalmoplegia
	– Chordoma can present with palsies of 6th, 9th, 10th, 11th nerves
Pituitary gland	– Large masses within pituitary sella can compress normal pituitary, leading to hypopituitarism (hypogonadism, GH deficiency, central hypothyroidism, adrenal insufficiency)
	– Diabetes insipidus: primarily metastasis to sella, pituitary stalk lesion, hypophysitis, craniopharyngioma
	– Pituitary failure with large cystic masses
	– Endocrine deficits are frequently present, and affect GH secretion 75%, gonadotropins 40%, TSH 25%

Localization site	Comment
Peripheral neuropathy	Carpal tunnel in acromegaly, long-term effects of diabetes mellitus (DM) with Cushing disease
Muscle	Proximal muscle weakness in Cushing disease
Unclear localization	Hypertension, DM, sleep apnea, arthropathies and heart failure, precocious puberty with germ cell tumors in younger patients

Secondary Complications:

Cushing disease: Central obesity, dorsocervical and supraclavicular fat pads, DM, hypokalemia, kidney stones, polyuria, facial plethora, hirsutism, wide violaceous striae, ecchymoses, edema, acne, fungal infections, hyperpigmentation, hypertension, venous thrombosis, osteopenia/osteoporosis, proximal weakness/wasting, oligo-/amenorrhea, impotence/decreased libido, depression/anxiety, insomnia, headache.

Acromegaly: Hypertension, DM, sleep apnea, arthropathies, heart failure, edema, acne/oily skin, sweating, skin tags, prognathism, frontal bossing, acral enlargement, widened teeth spacing, arthropathy, colon polyps, thyroid nodules.

Diabetes insipidus: Excretion of excessive volumes of inappropriately dilute urine accompanied by increased fluid intake due to deficiency of antidiuretic hormone. Symptoms include urinary frequency, incontinence, nocturia, and enuresis.

Treatment Complications: For smaller tumors, medical management is often first-line. GH-secreting tumors are treated with octreotide, which has minimal side effects that include abdominal pain and diarrhea. Chronic therapy is associated with increased prevalence of cholelithiasis, particularly in patients with prior gallbladder disease. Discontinuing therapy is associated with recurrence of excess GH and insulin-like growth factor-1 (IGF-I) concentrations.

Surgical resection with transsphenoidal approach is a mainstay of therapy with rare complications; however, in 5–15% of cases, can develop diabetes insipidus (often transient). More rare complications include infection and CSF leak. Radiation therapy is rarely the first choice approach, but can be used as adjunctive therapy. Further complications include worsening of visual symptoms secondary to edema, tumor hemorrhage, and optic nerve necrosis in addition to developing malignant brain tumors, brain necrosis, and dementia. With radiation therapy, there is also danger of loss of pituitary function. At 10-year follow-up, more than 90% of patients have at least two or more deficient hormones, which can occur 2–25 years later.

Bibliography

Arafah BM, Nasrallah MP. Pituitary tumors: pathophysiology, clinical manifestations and management. *Endocr Relat Cancer.* 2001;8(4):287–305.

Chaudhary V, Bano S. Imaging of the pituitary: Recent advances. *Ind J Endocrinol Metab.* 2011;15(Suppl 3):S216–23. DOI:10.4103/2230-8210.84871.

Ironside JW. Best practice No 172: Pituitary gland pathology. *J Clin Pathol.* 2003;56:561–8.

Huguet I, Clayton R. Pituitary-hypothalamic tumor syndromes: Adults. Endotext [Internet]. South Dartmouth, MA: MDText.com, Inc.; 2000. Available from www.ncbi.nlm.nih.gov/books/NBK278946/. Accessed Jul 3, 2015.

Robertson GL. Diabetes insipidus: differential diagnosis and management. *Best Pract Res Clin Endocrinol Metab.* 2016;30(2):205–18.

Utz AL, Klibanski A. Pituitary disorders. *Continuum (Minneap Minn).* 2009;15(2, Neurology):17–36.

Plasma Cell Dyscrasias

Epidemiology and Demographics: Excluding monoclonal gammopathy of unclear significance (MGUS), symptomatic plasma cell dyscrasia is a disease of older adults affecting about 5/100,000 per year with increased incidence in those of African descent.

Disorder Description: Plasma cell dyscrasias are a group of disorders marked by clonal proliferation of plasma cells. In contrast to MGUS, there is usually evidence of end organ injury (such as bony lesions, hypercalcemia, renal insufficiency, and anemia). Typically the concentration of serum monoclonal protein is greater than 3 g/dL, and plasma cells form greater than 10% of cells in bone marrow biopsy. Plasma cell disorder can affect the nervous system by direct invasion (uncommon but significant) or by affecting the peripheral nervous system in diverse ways (more common).

Symptoms

Localization site	Comment
Cerebral hemispheres	Rarely, plasma cells can infiltrate brain parenchyma and present as focal or multi-focal mass-like lesions in the cerebral hemispheres[1]
Mental status and psychiatric aspects/ complications	Altered cognition, mood, or speech can occur either with rare parenchmymal or leptomeningeal infiltration. Hyperviscosity syndrome associated with markedly elevated immunoglobulin levels can also cause confusion. Hypercalcemia can cause cognitive decline[2]
Cerebellum	Vertigo and ataxia with hyperviscosity syndrome
Cranial nerves	Rare leptomeningeal infiltration causes multiple cranial neuropathies
Spinal cord	Plasmacytoma causing spinal cord compression. Pathologic fracture can also mechanically compress the spinal cord
Specific spinal roots	Leptomeningeal spread causing spinal root neuropathy

Peripheral neuropathy	Can cause multiple types of neuropathy[3]:
	1. Predominant sensory demyelinating neuropathy:
	   a. anti-MAG IgM causes syndrome of gait ataxia, distal sensory loss, and upper extremity tremor
	   b. chronic, symmetric progressive neuropathy clinically appearing like chronic inflammatory demyelinating polyneuropathy (CIDP) associated with IgG or IgA gammopathy
	2. Predominant sensory over motor axonal neuropathy:
	   a. symmetric distal painful neuropathy associated with cryoglobulinemia. Can have accompanying multiple mononeuropathies
	3. Predominant motor demyelinating neuropathy:
	   a. motor predominant clinical CIDP syndrome
	   b. POEMS – polyneuropathy, organomegaly, endocrinopathy, monocolonal gammopathy, and skin changes. Polyneuropathy is usually sensorimotor
	4. Sensorimotor neuropathy with autonomic dysfunction:
	   a. associated with amyloidosis with progressive distal sensorimotor neuropathy in combination with orthostasis and bowel/bladder/sexual dysfunction

Secondary Complications: Progressive plasma cell dyscrasia often has accompanying renal dysfunction, bony pain, and refractory anemia limiting treatment choices for neurologic diseases.

Treatment Complications: Treatment particularly with chemotherapeutic agents can cause treatment-related distal axonal painful neuropathy. Proteasome inhibitors such as bortezomib have been associated with central toxicity such as posterior reversible encephalopathy syndrome.

References

1. Malkani RG, Tallman M, Gottardi-Littell N, et al. Bing-Neel syndrome: an illustrative case and a comprehensive review of the published literature. *J Neurooncol.* 2010;96:301–12.
2. Sobol U, Stiff P. Neurologic aspects of plasma cell disorders. *Handb Clin Neurol.* 2014;120:1083–99.
3. Nobile-Orazio E. Neuropathy and monoclonal gammopathy. *Handb Clin Neurol.* 2013;115:443–59.

Platybasia

Disorder Description: Platybasia is an abnormality of the base of the skull resulting in flattening of the skull base. It may be developmental in origin or due to softening of the skull base bone allowing it to be pushed upwards. It may be associated with fusion of the first cervical vertebra to the skull.

Symptoms

Localization site	Comment
Base of skull	Pain at the back of the skull and upper part of the neck, cough-induced headache can be noted
Lower cranial nerve palsies	Dysphagia, dysphonia, and dysarthria

Treatment Complications: If asymptomatic, no treatment is indicated. If neural compression is present, decompression with conjunction with fusion of the skull to the upper cervical spine is suggested. Neurologic deficits due to surgical complications could occur.

Bibliography

Pearce JMS. Platybasia and basilar invagination. *Eur Neurol.* 2007;58:62–4.

POEMS Syndrome Neuropathy

Epidemiology and Demographics: Incidence unknown as this is a rare disorder. Age of onset is 50s to 60s. It is more common in males.

Disorder Description: Polyneuropathy, organomegaly, endocrinopathy, M protein, and skin changes (POEMS) is a neuropathy associated with multiple myeloma. Patients present with monoclonal plasma disorder and peripheral neuropathy. Presenting features include osteosclerotic lesions, weight loss, fatigue, papilledema, and Castleman's disease. Peripheral neuropathy begins with tingling in feet, paresthesias, followed by motor symptoms. Symptoms are progressive, symmetric, and proximal. Weakness is consistent with a motor chronic inflammatory demyelinating polyneuropathy.

Symptoms

Localization site	Comment
Cerebral hemispheres	Papilledema
Mental status and psychiatric aspects/complications	Fatigue
Peripheral neuropathy	Sensory disturbance, symmetric limb weakness proximal > distal, areflexia

Secondary Complications: Five-year risk of stroke in patients with POEMs syndrome is 13.4%.

Treatment Complications: There is no standardized treatment.

Bibliography

Dispenzieri A, Kyle RA, Lacy MQ, et al. POEMS syndrome: definitions and long-term outcome. *Blood.* 2003;101:2496.

Dupont SA, Dispenzieri A, Mauermann ML, et al. Cerebral infarction in POEMS syndrome:

incidence, risk factors, and imaging characteristics. *Neurology.* 2009;73:1308.

Poliovirus (Subtype Enterovirus)

Epidemiology and Demographics: Vaccines have eliminated wild infection in the United States, but occurs in other countries with lower vaccination rates.

Disorder Description: Spreads through fecal–oral route. One in 1000 infections lead to involvement of the motor neurons. Weakness starts 2–5 days after onset of headache, fever, and neck stiffness. Atrophy occurs 5 days later.

CSF can show elevated white blood cells (WBCs) and protein.

Symptoms

Localization site	Comment
Cranial nerves	10–15% with pharyngeal, laryngeal, or facial diplegia
Anterior horn cells	Legs more frequently involved than arms
Peripheral neuropathy	Legs more frequently involved than arms

Secondary Complications: Respiratory failure. Bone resorption causing hypercalcemia and renal calculi.

Post-polio syndrome occurs >10 years later with progressive weakness and pain, even in previously apparently uninvolved areas. Etiology is not known, but leading hypotheses are that a secondary injury or increased metabolic demand on the lower motor neurons causes failure of neurons that had previously compensated for loss during the primary disease.

Treatment Complications: Oral vaccine extremely rarely causes infection. With high immunization rates, the only infections reported were from oral vaccines, so they were switched to injection.

Bibliography

Aminoff MJ, Josephson SA, eds. *Aminoff's neurology and general medicine.* 5th ed. London, UK: Elsevier; 2014.

Poliovirus Vaccine

Epidemiology and Demographics: Most of the world is free of the poliovirus thanks to a world-wide vaccination program, except for some locations in Asia and Africa. The last outbreak of poliomyelitis in the United States was in 1979.

Disorder Description: Two vaccines are currently available: the live attenuated oral poliovirus vaccine (OPV) used mainly in the developing world; and the inactivated poliovirus vaccine (IPV) used in the developed world including the United States.

Symptoms of Polio

Localization site	Comment
Cerebral hemispheres	Encephalitis
Mental status and psychiatric aspects/ complications	Headache, altered mental status, confusion
Brainstem	Bulbar poliomyelitis: dysphagia, dysarthria, respiratory insufficiency, hemodynamic instability
Cerebellum	Ataxia (rare)
Cranial nerves	Cranial nerve palsy: VII, IX and X, and XI
Spinal cord	Spinal poliomyelitis
Anterior horn cells	Destruction of anterior horn cells leading to flaccid paralysis
Peripheral neuropathy	Destruction of the post-synaptic motor neurons: decreased reflexes and tone
Muscle	Proximal asymmetric weakness, legs more common than arms, can progress to flaccid paralysis

Secondary Complications: The OPV has been associated with vaccine-associated paralytic poliomyelitis and vaccine-derived poliomyelitis in very rare cases.

Treatment Complications: Treatment of poliomyelitis is mainly supportive: pain control, physical therapy, and mechanical ventilation if associated respiratory failure.

Bibliography

Aylward RB, Linkins J. Polio eradication: mobilizing and managing the human resources. *Bull World Health Org.* 2005;83(4):268–73.

Grist NR, Bell EJ. Paralytic poliomyelitis and nonpolio enteroviruses: studies in Scotland. *Rev Infect Dis.* 1984;6(Suppl 2):S385–6.

Howard RS. Poliomyelitis and the postpolio syndrome. *BMJ.* 2005;330(7503):1314–18.

Robbins FC, Nightingale EO. Selective primary health care: Strategies for control of disease in the developing world. IX. Poliomyelitis. *Rev Infect Dis.* 1983;5(5):957–68.

Webster P. A polio-free world? *The Lancet.* 2005;366(9483):359–60.

Polyarteritis Nodosa

Epidemiology and Demographics: Periarteritis or polyarteritis nodosa (PAN) is a relatively rare disorder with incidence of biopsy-proven cases of 0.7/100,000 and a prevalence of 6.3/100,000. The marked reduction in hepatitis B virus infection in many parts of the world has been associated with a parallel reduction in prevalence of PAN. It presents in older individuals, more often in males, with a male-to-female ratio of 1.5:1. It can occur in childhood but the disorder differs clinically from that in adults.

Disorder Description: PAN is a systemic necrotizing vasculitis that typically affects medium-sized muscular arteries, with occasional involvement of small muscular arteries. Most cases of PAN are idiopathic, although hepatitis B virus (HBV) infection, hepatitis C virus (HCV) infection, and hairy cell leukemia are important in the pathogenesis of some cases. The neurologic symptoms present early in the course of the disease and involve both the peripheral and the central nervous system. Peripheral nerve injury is related to damage of the vasa nervorum. Central nervous system injury due to vasculitis often reveals classic beading patterns in the vasculature on angiography.

The typical patient presents with constitutional symptoms of malaise, fever, and weight loss. Neurologic manifestations include peripheral nervous system symptoms or signs, especially mononeuritis multiplex in 38% to 70% of the patients. Asymmetric sensory and motor dysfunction affecting limbs in the distribution of different nerves are characteristic. Distal symmetric polyneuropathy or cranial neuropathy may occur (facial diplegia, oculomotor dysfunction, tonic pupils).

Central nervous system manifestations are less common (10%) and include diffuse encephalopathy, stroke, seizures, and intracerebral or subarachnoid hemorrhage. Spinal cord involvement is rare and may result from vasculitis of the spinal arteries or compression due to a subdural hematoma.

The other commonly involved organs outside of the nervous system include kidney (70%), skin (50%), joints with arthralgia (50%) and arthritis (20%), muscles with myalgias (50%), and the gastrointestinal system (30%). Hypertension is a common presentation (40%) due to renal involvement. It has a striking tendency to spare the lungs.

Symptoms

Localization site	Comment
Cerebral hemispheres	Manifestations of ischemic stroke largely depend on the location. Lacunar infarcts, cortical infarcts, or hemorrhages (deep or lobar or subarachnoid) can occur Seizures can occur secondary to the stroke
Mental status and psychiatric aspects/complications	Encephalopathy secondary to hypertension can present with varying degree of confusion, altered mentation and coma
Brainstem	Pontine lacunar infarcts are known to occur
Cranial nerves	Rarely, facial diplegia or oculomotor involvement may occur
Spinal cord	Vasculitis of the spinal arteries or compression due to a subdural hematoma can result in spinal cord syndromes with classic sensorimotor levels
Mononeuropathy or mononeuropathy multiplex	The classical presentation is an asymmetric polyneuropathy affecting named nerves (e.g., radial, ulnar, peroneal), typically with both motor and sensory deficits
Peripheral neuropathy	Distal symmetric progressive (sensorimotor, axonal)
Muscle	Myalgia, muscle pain, claudication

Secondary Complications: Prognosis and mortality are determined by severity of organ involvement, specifically the kidney, gastrointestinal system, coronary system, and central nervous system. Presence of aneurysms on visceral angiography portends poorer prognosis. Central nervous system complications can include hypertensive encephalopathy, intracranial hemorrhage, or stroke.

Treatment Complications: Diagnosis involves a combination of renal biopsy and visceral angiography. Long-term glucocorticoids are the mainstay of treatment for mild polyarteritis nodosa. Immunosuppressive medications such as azathioprine, methotrexate, or mycophenolate may be used to treat moderate or severe polyarteritis. All of these immunomodulators increase the risk of opportunistic infection. Use of angiotensin-converting enzyme (ACE) inhibitors is indicated to treat polyarteritis-associated hypertension but may be challenging in patients with elevated creatinine so that alternatives such as calcium channel blockers may be preferred.

Bibliography

Ramachandran TS, Roos RP. Periarteritis nodosa. Medlink Neurology. Updated Nov 14, 2017. San Diego: Medlink Corporation. Available from https://emedicine.medscape.com/article/330717-overview. Accessed Nov 25, 2018.

Younger DS. Vasculitis of the nervous system. *Curr Opin Neurol.* 2004;17:317–36.

Polycythemia Vera (PV)

Epidemiology and Demographics: Infrequent disorder with estimated incidence of about 2/100,000 per year with higher predominance in men. Primarily affects older adults but can be found in all age groups.

Disorder Description: A myeloproliferative disorder of elevated red blood cell mass (typically hemoglobin greater than 18.5 g/dL in men and 16.5 g/dL in women) strongly associated (>95%) with mutations in the *JAK2* gene.[1] Secondary cause for polycythemia such as chronic hypoxemia should be excluded. Symptoms are typically from vasomotor complications or from thrombosis.

Symptoms

Localization site	Comment
Cerebral hemispheres	Increased risk of arterial and venous thrombosis causing strokes. May also cause transient ischemic symptoms[2]
Cranial nerves	Visual blurring and transient blindness associated with delayed retinal blood flow

Secondary Complications: Characteristically associated with pruritus during a warm shower (aquagenic pruritus). Like thrombocythemia, can cause erythromelalgia (dysesthesias in hands and feet with associated color change). May also cause thrombosis in other venous locations such as the hepatic vein.

Treatment Complications: High-dose aspirin therapy also increases risk of hemorrhage in patients with PV. Treatment with chemotherapeutic agents may influence risk of later leukemia.

References

1. Cao M, Olsen RJ, Zu Y. Polycythemia vera: new clinicopathologic perspectives. *Arch Pathol Lab Med*. 2006;130: 1126–32.
2. Stuart BJ, Viera AJ. Polycythemia vera. *Am Fam Physician*. 2004;69:2139–44.

Polymyalgia Rheumatica

Epidemiology and Demographics: Predominant age at presentation is 50 years or older; median age at diagnosis is 72. Females affected more than males (2:1 ratio), and Caucasians are affected more than any other ethnic group. Polymyalgia rheumatica (PR) has been reported rarely in the black population. In the United States, 52.5 cases/100,000 persons aged 50 years or older. Prevalence is 0.5–0.7%.

Disorder Description: PR is a chronic inflammatory condition characterized by myalgias affecting the hip and shoulder girdles. The myalgias are associated with morning stiffness that lasts for more than an hour. This condition is associated with giant cell arteritis (GCA). Patients noted to have elevated erythrocyte sedimentation rate (ESR) and C-reactive protein (CRP). Patients respond rapidly to prednisone within 2–3 days.

Potential causes include:

Autoimmune process: Monocyte/macrophage activation. PR is associated with HLA-DR4 haplotype, high level of IL-6 associated with increased disease activity. Cell-mediated autoimmune injury to the elastic lamina of blood vessels.

Genetic predisposition: IL-6 and RANTES polymorphism seen in Spanish population.

Environmental factors: Exposure to viral infections (adenovirus, parvovirus B19, human parainfluenza virus).

Risk factors include:

Females older than 50 years of age.

Northern European descent – particularly Scandinavians.

Exposure to adenovirus, parvovirus B19, and human parainfluenza virus.

Genetic susceptibility based on the presence of IL-6 and/or RANTES polymorphisms.

PR is more common in northern Europe, with the highest incidence in Scandinavia and lower incidence in Mediterranean countries.

Symptoms

Localization site	Comment
Blood vessels supplying the synovium and bursae of shoulder and hip girdles	Pain and stiffness of neck, shoulders, thighs, and hips, especially after sleeping. Muscles are not affected directly. EMG studies and muscle biopsies are normal
Temporal artery	50% of people with temporal arteritis have polymyalgia rheumatica. Symptoms include headache, scalp tenderness, jaw stiffness, distorted vision
Unclear localization	Constant fatigue and lack of appetite, flu-like symptoms, low-grade fever, anemia

Secondary Complications:

Temporal arteritis

Chronic pain of the joints

Chronic fatigue

Vision changes

Persistent flu-like symptoms

Treatment Complications:

Steroids: Prednisone is commonly used to treat this condition. The use of prednisone causes an increased risk of infection, hyperglycemia, avascular necrosis of the hip, psychosis, Cushing disease, and osteoporosis.

Immunosuppressants: Methotrexate is the second-line choice of treatment when steroids are not effective. Methotrexate can cause patients to develop ulcerative stomatitis, aplastic anemia, agranulocytosis, leukoencephalopathy, seizures, Stevens–Johnson syndrome among other complications.

Bibliography

Buttgereit F, Dejaco C, Matteson EL, Dasgupta B. Polymyalgia rheumatica and giant cell arteritis: a systematic review. *JAMA*. 2016;315(22):2442–58.

Caylor TL, Perkins A. Recognition and management of polymyalgia rheumatica and giant cell arteritis. *Am Fam Physician*. 2013;88(10):676–84.

Polymyositis

Epidemiology and Demographics: Polymyositis is frequently found as an overlap disease or misdiagnosed; isolated polymyositis is uncommon. Incidence of polymyositis and closely linked dermatomyositis is 2/100,000 per year, while prevalence is estimated at 5–22/100,000. Females are more likely than males to develop polymyositis (2:1). Primarily affects patients over the age of 20 years. There is no specific geographic distribution.

Disorder Description: Polymyositis is an idiopathic inflammatory myopathy. Muscle weakness can develop alone, and frequently presents as neck flexor weakness and symmetric proximal arm and leg weakness over several weeks to months.

It is an acquired autoimmune disorder; the exact disease mechanism and cause are unclear. However, due to frequent comorbidity with cancer, it is thought that paraneoplastic processes contribute to polymyositis and the underlying autoimmune processes.

In diagnostic tests, serum CK is elevated, usually 5 to 50 times the normal value; it can also be used to monitor response to treatment. ESR and CRP can be normal. ANA (antinuclear antibody) is positive in 16–40% of patients. Electromyography studies will show increased insertional and spontaneous activity, small polyphasic motor unit action potentials, and early recruitment. Muscle biopsy will show significant evidence of inflammation and some necrosis, but unlike dermatomyositis, there is no evidence of immune deposits on microvasculature.

Symptoms

Localization site	Comment
Muscle	Symmetric and proximal muscle weakness (>90% of patients). Typically, deltoids and hip flexors, though neck flexor involvement is common. Distal muscle weakness is rare, if it occurs at all, and is usually mild without much impairment

Secondary Complications: There is an increased risk of cancer in polymyositis, though it is lower than in dermatomyositis. As with dermatomyositis, polymyositis is associated with interstitial lung disease and cardiac disease (conduction defects and arrhythmias, pericarditis, myocarditis, and eventual congestive heart failure). Polyarthritis can occur in up to 45% of patients. There is also an association with connective tissue diseases.

Treatment Complications: While there is no Class I evidence for treatment, currently, treatment is based on lifelong immunosuppression. Largely, corticosteroid therapy is first-line therapy. Other drugs such as methotrexate, azathioprine, or mycophenolate mofetil are frequently also added. If no improvement is found, intravenous immunoglobulins (IVIG) or rituximab may be added. In general, methotrexate tends to be avoided, due to risk of pulmonary toxicity.

Similar to dermatomyositis, complications related to steroid therapy (hyperglycemia, osteoporosis, cataracts, infections, weight gain, steroid-induced myopathy) can develop. Regarding methotrexate, pulmonary toxicity can occur. In general, opportunistic infections such as *Pneumocystis jirovecii* pneumonia are possible if no prophylaxis is in place.

Bibliography

Amato AA, Greenberg SA. Inflammatory myopathies. *Continuum (Minneap Minn)*. 2013;19(6):1615–33.

Mammen AL. Autoimmune myopathies. *Continuum (Minneap Minn)*. 2016;22(6):1852–70.

Polymyositis/Dermatomyositis versus Inclusion Body Myositis

Epidemiology and Demographics: From 0.5 to 8.4 cases per million population in the United States. Presents in adults older than 20 years of age (45–60 years of age most commonly). Dermatomyositis also noted in children (commonly 5–14 years of age). Inclusion body myositis (IBM) noted more frequently in adults older than 50 years of age. More common in women (2:1 ratio). Black population more commonly affected than Caucasians within the United States (5:1 ratio for polymyositis and 3:1 ratio for dermatomyositis). Men more commonly affected by IBM. Japanese population less affected than average by polymyositis.

Disorder Description: Polymyositis is an idiopathic inflammatory myopathy that causes symmetric, proximal muscle weakness. Dermatomyositis is an inflammatory myopathy similar to polymyositis that is associated with skin manifestations. Both present with similar clinical manifestations over weeks to months that are responsive to steroids. The two are best differentiated based on characteristic skin findings that are seen in dermatomyositis and muscle biopsy findings. IBM is classified as an inflammatory myopathy but contrary to its name, IBM shows minimal evidence of inflammation. It more commonly presents as an asymmetric distal weakness in older men. It is also diagnosed based on characteristic muscle biopsy findings.

Potential causes include:
T-cell (CD-8)-mediated cytotoxic processes
    directed against unidentified muscle antigen
    caused by:
      Autoimmune diseases
      Viral infections (see below)
      Malignancies: nasopharyngeal cancer, lung
        cancer, non-Hodgkin lymphoma, and
        bladder cancer
      Connective tissue disorders
      Medications (see below)
Anti Jo-1 antibodies (specific to polymyositis)
Anti-Mi-2 antibodies (specific to dermatomyositis)
Anti-SRP antibodies (specific to acute polymyositis
    with cardiac involvement)
    Risk factors include:
Human leukocyte antigen (HLA) – haplotypes A1,
    B8, and DR3
Infection:
    Coxsackievirus B1
    Human immunodeficiency virus (HIV)
    Human T-cell lymphotropic virus-1 (HTLV-1)
    Hepatitis B
    Influenza
    Echovirus
    Adenovirus
Medications:
    D-penicillamine
    Hydralazine
    Phenytoin
    Angiotensin-converting enzyme inhibitors
      (ACE-inhibitors)
    Statins

There is no specific higher proclivity to any specific region; however, individuals of Japanese descent have lower likelihood of developing polymyositis.

Symptoms

Localization site	Comment
Muscle	Polymyositis/dermatomyositis: weakness and/or loss of muscle mass in the proximal musculature as well as neck and torso flexors. Hip extensors severely affected. Dysphagia and other problems with esophageal motility. These conditions can also lead to interstitial lung disease and cardiac disease (cardiac failure and conduction abnormalities). Foot drop involving one or both feet has been noted
	Inclusion body myositis: Weakness affecting the quadriceps and finger flexors. Most common complaints including frequent tripping, difficulty climbing stairs, and trouble opening doors or gripping objects. There have been patient reports of severe thigh pain. Dysphagia has been noted in 40% to 85% of patients. Decline in aerobic capacity causing increased fatigue has also been noted

Secondary Complications:
    Weakness of the lower extremities.
    Finger flexor weakness.
    GI disturbances secondary to esophageal
      dysmotility.
Treatment Complications:
    Steroids: Prednisone is commonly used to treat
      this condition. The use of prednisone causes
      an increased risk of infection, hyperglycemia,
      avascular necrosis of the hip, psychosis,
      Cushing disease, and osteoporosis.
    Immunosuppressants: Methotrexate is the second-
      line choice of treatment when steroids are not
      effective. Methotrexate can cause patients to
      develop ulcerative stomatitis, aplastic anemia,
      agranulocytosis, leukoencephalopathy,
      seizures, Stevens–Johnson syndrome among
      other complications.

Bibliography

Dalakas MC, Hohlfeld R. Polymyositis and dermatomyositis. *Lancet.* 2003;362:971.

Dimachkie MM, Barohn RJ. Inclusion body myositis. *Neurol Clin.* 2014;32:629.

Polyneuropathy (Axonal)

Epidemiology and Demographics: As summarized by Hanewinckel et al., the prevalence is 1% and increases to 7% in the older population.

Disorder Description: Patients may present with paresthesias or pain and motor dysfunction in the feet first, followed by more proximal spread. In developing countries infectious causes such as leprosy are the most common cause. In industrialized nations, the common causes include diabetes, alcohol use, vitamin deficiencies, and drug side effects. Classified by cause, presentation, or axonal vs demyelinating.

Symptoms

Localization site	Comment
Mental status and psychiatric aspects/complications	Reduced quality of life
Peripheral neuropathy	Pain, numbness, tingling
Muscle	Weakness
Other	Gait difficulty and increased fall risk Can affect autonomic nervous system

Secondary Complications: In severe cases, sensory symptoms can also involve the thoracic and cervical nerves.

Treatment Complications: Medications such as gabapentin can cause sedation and renal impairment at high doses. Trial with tricyclic antidepressant medications can cause altered mental status. Opioids may cause sedation and respiratory suppression.

Bibliography

Brazis PW, et al., eds. Peripheral nerves. In *Localization in clinical neurology*. 6th ed. Philadelphia, PA: Lippincott Williams and Wilkins; 2011. Chapter 2.

Hanewinckel R, van Oijen M, Ikram MA, van Doorn PA. The epidemiology and risk factors of chronic polyneuropathy. *Eur J Epidemiol*. 2016;31:5–20. DOI:10.1007/s10654-015-0094-6.

Visser N. Chronic idiopathic axonal polyneuropathy is associated with the metabolic syndrome. *Diabetes Care*. 2013;36(4):817–22.

Posterior Cerebral Artery (PCA), Left Territory Infarction

Epidemiology and Demographics: Comprise approximately 5–15% of ischemic strokes. The frequency increases with age and is higher in males. All strokes are more likely to afflict those of African, Asian, Native American, and Hispanic descent than those of Caucasian descent.

Disorder Description: Blockage of one or more branches of the left posterior cerebral artery (PCA) leading to infarction of the supplied brain tissue. The blockage is most commonly caused by a cardioembolism but other possible causes include: vertebral artery dissection or atherosclerotic plaque leading to artery-to-artery embolism, and intrinsic PCA atherosclerosis. Rare causes include vasculitis, coagulopathies, and migrainous infarction. Standard vascular risk factors, including smoking, hypertension, hyperlipidemia, and diabetes, apply. In cardioembolic cases, atrial fibrillation, aortic plaque, and severe left ventricular dysfunction are more common causes. In the presence of a patent foramen ovale, systemic venous thrombosis could also be causative (paradoxical embolus).

Symptoms

Localization site	Comment
Cerebral hemispheres	Right homonymous hemianopia. Right hemisensory loss. Thalamic aphasia. Alexia without agraphia
Mental status and psychiatric aspects/ complications	Memory loss may occur. In bilateral infarction, transient alteration of consciousness may also be seen

Secondary Complications: Thalamic pain syndrome can lead to chronic neuropathic pain on the right side.

Treatment Complications: Hemorrhagic transformation of the infarct may be seen after thrombolysis or mechanical thrombectomy.

Bibliography

Arboix A, Arbe C, Garcia-Eroles L, et al. Infarctions in the vascular territory of the posterior cerebral artery: clinical features in 232 patients. *BMC Res Notes*. 2011;4:329–35.

Cereda C, Carrera E. Posterior cerebral artery territory infarctions. *Front Neurol Neurosci*. 2012;30:128–31.

Posterior Cerebral Artery (PCA), Right Territory Infarction

Epidemiology and Demographics: Comprise approximately 5–15% of ischemic strokes. The frequency increases with age and is higher in males. All strokes are more likely to afflict those of African, Asian, Native American, and Hispanic descent than those of Caucasian descent.

Disorder Description: Blockage of one or more branches of the left posterior cerebral artery (PCA) leading to infarction of the supplied brain tissue. The blockage is most commonly caused by a cardioembolism but other possible causes include: vertebral artery dissection or atherosclerotic plaque leading to artery-to-artery embolism and intrinsic PCA atherosclerosis. Rare causes include vasculitis, coagulopathies, and migrainous infarction. Standard vascular risk factors, including smoking, hypertension, hyperlipidemia, and diabetes, apply. In cardioembolic cases, atrial fibrillation, aortic plaque, and severe left ventricular dysfunction are more common causes. In the presence of a patent foramen ovale, systemic venous thrombosis could also be causative (paradoxical embolus).

Symptoms

Localization site	Comment
Cerebral hemispheres	Left homonymous hemianopia. Left hemisensory loss. Visual neglect. Prosopagnosia
Mental status and psychiatric aspects/ complications	Memory loss rarely occurs. In bilateral infarction, transient alteration of consciousness may also be seen

Secondary Complications: Thalamic pain syndrome can lead to chronic neuropathic pain on the left side.

Treatment Complications: Hemorrhagic transformation of the infarct may be seen after thrombolysis or mechanical thrombectomy.

Bibliography

Arboix A, Arbe C, Garcia-Eroles L, et al. Infarctions in the vascular territory of the posterior cerebral artery: clinical features in 232 patients. *BMC Res Notes*. 2011;4:329–35.

Cereda C, Carrera E. Posterior cerebral artery territory infarctions. *Front Neurol Neurosci*. 2012;30:128–31.

Posterior Ciliary Artery Thrombosis

Epidemiology and Demographics: This condition can be arteritic or nonarteritic and both forms are more common in Caucasians. The nonarteritic form (NAION – nonarteritic anterior ischemic optic neuropathy) is far more common, accounting for ~95% of cases. This has an incidence of 2–10/100,000 and has a mean age of onset of 60–70 years, although it can be seen at all ages. The arteritic form accounts for ~5% of cases with an incidence of 2/100,000 people. It is more common in females and has a mean age of onset of 70 years, with cases rare before age 60.

Disorder Description: The posterior ciliary artery supplies the choroid of the retina and the head of the optic nerve. Occlusion leads to anterior ischemic optic retinopathy. NAION is atherosclerotic in etiology. Risk factors include smoking, hypertension, and hyperlipidemia. AION is the most common cause of vision loss in giant cell (temporal) arteritis.

Symptoms

Localization site	Comment
Cranial nerves	Both forms cause painless vision loss over hours to days with the arteritic form being more rapid and severe

Secondary Complications: The vision loss is generally permanent. NAION is usually seen in conjunction with small vessel arteriosclerotic disease in other end organs. AION is an autoimmune disorder and often other such disorders are present.

Treatment Complications: Treatment of AION is with high-dose steroids and can lead to weight gain, infections, osteoporosis, diabetes, and avascular necrosis of the hip, among others.

Bibliography

Rodriguez Frontal M, Kerrison JB, Garcia R, Oria V. Ischemic optic neuropathy. *Semin Neurol*. 2007;27(3):221–32

Posterior Reversible Encephalopathy Syndrome (PRES)

Epidemiology and Demographics: Reported in individuals from 4 to 90 years of age, with mean age range of 39–47 years. Female predominance. Global incidence of posterior reversible encephalopathy syndrome (PRES) is unknown.

Disorder Description: PRES is a neurotoxic state that occurs as a result of cerebral blood perfusion abnormalities resulting in blood–brain barrier dysfunction with cerebral vasogenic edema. The vasogenic edema is most commonly in the parieto-occipital regions of the brain. Contrary to its name, regions beyond the posterior cerebrum have also been known to be affected in this condition. This condition is also known as *hypertensive encephalopathy* and *reversible posterior leukoencephalopathy*.

Potential causes include:

Severe hypertension:

    postpartum

    eclampsia/pre-eclampsia

    acute glomerulonephritis

Hemolytic uremic syndrome (HUS)

Thrombotic thrombocytopenic purpura (TTP)

Systemic lupus erythematosus (SLE)

Medication related:

    cisplatin

    interferons

    erythropoietin

    tacrolimus

    cyclosporine

    azathioprine

    L-asparginase

Bone marrow or stem cell transplantation

Sepsis

Hyperammonemia

    Risk factors include:

Hypertensive urgency or emergency

Post-partum female

Female with eclampsia or pre-eclampsia

Lupus

Sepsis

Immunosuppressive medications (as noted before)

No specific regions of the world have higher proclivity.

Symptoms

Localization site	Comment
Cerebral hemispheres	Symmetric vasogenic edema is most commonly seen in parieto-occipital regions sparing the calcarine and paramedian parts of the occipital lobe. Both cortical and subcortical regions may be affected. Watershed regions involving the frontal and inferior temporal areas have also been reported. Less commonly, edema can also be purely unilateral or not involve the cortical/subcortical matter at all. Infarction is noted in PRES in 10–15% of the cases, and hemorrhages are noted in 15% of the cases. Patients most commonly report visual abnormalities including: blurred vision, visual neglect, homonymous hemianopsia, visual hallucinations, and cortical blindness. In addition to this, headache and nausea/vomiting are common symptoms. Epileptic seizures have also been reported in patients with PRES. Patients with severe PRES can suffer from status epilepticus and can enter a comatose state
Mental status and psychiatric aspects/ complications	Altered mental status/encephalopathy is very common symptom in patients with PRES
Brainstem	Watershed regions affecting various areas of the brainstem have been reported. Less commonly, cases of PRES involving only the basal ganglia and brainstem have been reported
Cerebellum	Vasogenic edema in the cerebellum has also been reported. Vasogenic edema located in the brainstem and cerebellar regions can lead to transtentorial cerebellar herniation

Secondary Complications

1. Persistent visual changes including blindness.
2. Mental status changes including difficulty concentrating or focusing.
3. Inability to function independently because of persistent encephalopathy.
4. Death secondary to transtentorial herniation.

Treatment Complications: Antihypertensives are the mainstay of treatment for this condition. As such, overly aggressive use of antihypertensives can result in cerebral ischemia with resulting stroke/transient ischemic attack.

Bibliography

Fischer M, Schmutzhard E. Posterior reversible encephalopathy syndrome. *J Neurol.* 2017;264(8):1608–16.

Hinchey J, Chaves C, Appignani B, et al. A reversible posterior leukoencephalopathy syndrome. *N Engl J Med.* 1996;334:494.

Post-herpetic Neuralgia

Epidemiology and Demographics: This is a relatively common disease. As summarized by Christo et al., the incidence is 3/1000 per year and by 80 years of age, it increases to 10/1000 per year.

Disorder Description: Most people have dormant varicella zoster virus. When the virus is reactivated, patients can present with pain in the locations where the dormant virus tends to reside. Those areas include the thoracic, cervical, and trigeminal nerves. Burning pain develops after shingles rash resolves.

Symptoms

Localization site	Comment
Cranial nerves	Trigeminal nerves
Spinal cord	Cervical and thoracic (T4–6) levels

Secondary Complications: Visual disturbances if V1 division of trigeminal nerve is involved.

Treatment Complications: Potential diverse adverse central nervous system effects such as mood changes due to use of antiepileptic agents or antidepressants (used for analgesic effect). Sedation from opiates. Skin irritation from topical ointments.

Bibliography

Christo, PJ, et al. Post-herpetic neuralgia in older adults: evidence-based approaches to clinical management. *Drugs Aging.* 2007;24(1):1–19.

Denny-Brown D, et al. Pathologic features of herpes zoster: A note on 'geniculate herpes'. *Arch Neurol Psychiatr.* 1944;51:216.

Glynn C, et al. Epidemiology of shingles. *J R Soc Med.* 1990;83(10):617–9.

Johnson R. Herpes zoster and postherpetic neuralgia. *Expert Rev Vaccines.* 2010;9(Suppl 3):21–6.

Post-immunization Encephalomyelitis

Epidemiology and Demographics: Age of presentation varies based on vaccine. Most cases are in children (0–18 years of age), but individuals older than 18 years have also been affected after taking the influenza H1N1 and HPV vaccines. Slight male predominance (1.3:1 ratio) in the pediatric population, but not in adults. Frequency of condition is 0.1 to 0.2/100,000 persons vaccinated.

Disorder Description: Post-immunization encephalomyelitis is a form of acute disseminated encephalomyelitis (ADEM) that occurs after vaccination. Historically referred to as "neuroparalytic accident," post-immunization encephalomyelitis first became prominent after the introduction of Jenner's small pox (cow pox) vaccine in 1853 and Pasteur's rabies vaccine in 1885. Post-vaccination encephalomyelitis currently accounts for less than 5% of the present cases of ADEM. It should be noted that ADEM or any other adverse event that follows the administration of an inactivated component or live vaccination may be temporally associated with, but not necessarily the result of, the administration of the vaccine. Post-immunization encephalomyelitis is currently thought to be caused by *in vivo* infected neural tissue utilized in the preparation of the vaccine. This theory has been further supported by the fact that there has been a significant reduction in post-vaccination ADEM events after the development of vaccines utilizing recombinant proteins.

Potential causes include:

Rabies vaccine – sample preparation (extracted from rabbit brain and used particularly in developing countries)

Diphtheria–tetanus–pertussis (DTaP) vaccine

Smallpox vaccine

Measles–mumps–rubella (MMR) vaccine – most common cause of ADEM is non-neural MMR vaccine, though the ADEM rate is much higher with a live measles infection (1–2 per million vaccinated vs 1 in 1000 with live measles infection)

Japanese B encephalitis vaccine

Hog vaccine

Influenza vaccine (both intramuscular and intranasal preparations)

H1N1 (swine flu) vaccine

Human papilloma virus (HPV) vaccine (bivalent
and quadrivalent)

Hepatitis B vaccine

Polio vaccine

Pneumococcal pneumonia vaccine

Meningococcal vaccine

Hexavalent vaccine (combination vaccine
against diphtheria, tetanus, pertussis, polio,
Hemophilus influenzae B, and hepatitis B)

Risk factors include:

Genetic predisposition: mutation of the
SCN1A gene has been linked to an
increased susceptibility to post-vaccination
encephalomyelitis.

Recent neurotropic viral or bacterial infection:

Neurotropic viruses	Neurotropic bacteria
Measles	*Mycoplasma*
Mumps	*Leptospira*
Rubella	*Chlamydia*
Varicella	*Legionella*
Influenza A or B	*Borrelia*
Rocky Mountain spotted fever	*Campylobacter*
Human immunodeficiency virus (HIV)	*Streptococcus*
Human T-cell lymphotropic virus-1 (HTLV-1)	
Hepatitis A or B	
Herpes simplex virus	
Human herpes virus 6	
Epstein–Barr virus	
Cytomegalovirus (CMV)	
Vaccinia	
Coxsackie	

No particular geographic proclivity is known.

Symptoms

Localization site	Comment
Cerebral hemispheres	Patient may have focal cortical signs of aphasia, alexia, agraphia, and/or cortical blindness. In advanced cases, frontal release signs such as glabellar reflex, snout/sucking reflexes, and grasp may be present. Meningeal signs have also been reported. Although less common than in post-infection encephalomyelitis, seizures can occur in post-vaccination encephalomyelitis. MRI imaging may demonstrate demyelination in both gray and white matter, particularly the thalamus. This may not be apparent in hyperacute lesions but may develop later in a pathognomonic "sleeve-like" fashion. There is minimal axonal damage
Mental status and psychiatric aspects/ complications	Patient may demonstrate daytime somnolence with fluctuating alertness and orientation consistent with delirium. Adolescents and young adults can present with psychosis
Cerebellum	Patient may have symptoms of ataxia, dysmetria, and nystagmus
Brainstem/cranial nerves	Bilateral optic neuritis has been commonly observed in patients with post-immunization encephalitis. Patients with diminished visual acuity and afferent pupillary defect. Funduscopic exam has revealed bilateral optic disc pallor. Visual evoked potentials will be abnormal. Patients may have visual field deficits
Spinal cord	Patient can present commonly with focal motor weakness with some reports of diffuse motor weakness. Patient can have sensory abnormalities (can be paresthesias or numbness). Sensory levels have also been reported. Asymmetric reflex abnormalities may be present (hypo-/hyperreflexia). Babinski sign is noted. Imaging can demonstrate evidence of transverse myelitis
Unclear localization	Fever, malaise, and fatigue are commonly reported in patients with post-immunization encephalomyelitis. This is something that differentiates it from other demyelinating processes such as multiple sclerosis and neuromyelitis optica

Secondary Complications

Visual changes including blindness.
Persistent weakness and sensory changes.
Seizures.

Residual mental status changes and psychiatric disturbances.

Diminished executive functioning skills secondary to residual frontal lobe abnormalities.

Treatment Complications

Steroids: Methyprednisolone is commonly used to treat this condition. The use of methylprednisolone causes an increased risk of infection, hyperglycemia, avascular necrosis of the hip, psychosis, Cushing disease, and osteoporosis.

Intravenous immunoglobulin (IVIG): IVIG can induce reactions in patients with IgA deficiency. This occurs in 1/500–1000 patients. Serious anaphylactoid reactions occur soon after the administration of IVIG. Anaphylaxis associated with sensitization to IgA in patients with IgA deficiency can be prevented by using IgA-depleted immunoglobulin. The presence of IgG anti-IgA antibodies is not always associated with severe adverse reactions to IVIG. As IVIG can lead to thrombosis, it has also been known to cause stroke and acute myocardial infarction. Nephrotoxicity has also been linked to the use of IVIG. IVIG therapy can result in post-infusion hyperproteinemia, increased serum viscosity, and pseudohyponatremia. Aseptic meningitis is also a rare but well-recognized complication of IVIG therapy.

Plasmapheresis (for hyperviscosity syndrome): Hypocalcemia/hypomagnesemia before or after treatment, hypothermia during treatment, and transfusion-related reactions are also likely; hypotension may occur in patients taking angiotensin-converting enzyme (ACE) inhibitors, in particular while undergoing column-based plasmapheresis. Thrombocytopenia and hypofibrinogenemia may occur after plasmapheresis (especially if albumin is being used as a replacement product) and patients should be monitored for signs of bleeding.

Bibliography

Alper G. Acute disseminated encephalomyelitis. *J Child Neurol.* 2012;27(11):1408–25.

Huynh W, Cordato DJ, Kehdi E, Masters LT, Dedousis C. Post-vaccination encephalomyelitis: literature review and illustrative case. *J Clin Neurosci.* 2008;15(12):1315–22.

Post-infectious Encephalomyelitis

Epidemiology and Demographics: More than 80% of childhood cases occur in patients younger than 10 years, with a mean age range of 5 to 8 years. Somewhat less than 20% of cases occur in the second decade of life. Incidence in adulthood is unclear, accounting for less than 3% of the reported cases. Slight male predominance in the pediatric population (1.3:1 ratio), but not in adults. Varies based on infection. However, in the United States there is a decline in frequency of post-infectious encephalomyelitis (PIEM) as a result of vaccinations against infections. In other countries where immunizations are not so common, the rates of PIEM continue to be high. Before introduction of immunization, the incidence of PIEM after measles was 1/1000 cases. The incidence of PIEM was 1/10,000 cases for varicella-zoster, and 1/20,000 for rubella.

Disorder Description: PIEM is a form of acute disseminated encephalomyelitis (ADEM). It is a monophasic, primarily inflammatory demyelinating condition that occurs antecedent to or concomitant with an exanthematous or non-specific viral infection, though bacterial infections can also cause this condition. Research involving animal models indicates an infectious mechanism and a subsequent autoimmune response that ultimately causes central nervous system demyelination. The autoimmune response is mediated by T-cells that react to myelin antigens such as myelin basic protein, myelin oligodendrocyte glycoprotein, and proteolipid protein. B-cells and ganglioside antibodies have also been implicated in the mechanism of ADEM. The mean time to onset of neurologic disturbances after infection is 12 days with a range of 2 to 30 days. Most common symptoms at presentation include: unilateral or bilateral long tract signs, acute hemiparesis, change in mental status, and ataxia, either alone or in combination. Seizures were also present and were mainly of partial motor type.

Potential causes include:

Viral infection:

Measles

Mumps

Rubella

Varicella-zoster

Influenza A or B

Rocky Mountain spotted fever

HIV

HTLV-1

Hepatitis A or B

Herpes simplex virus
Human herpes virus 6
Epstein–Barr virus
Cytomegalovirus
Vaccinia
Coxsackie
Bacterial infection:
Mycoplasma
Leptospira
Chlamydia
Legionella cincinnatiensis
Borrelia
Campylobacter
Group A β-hemolytic streptococcus

Risk factors include a genetic predisposition. Mutation of the SCN1A gene has been linked to an increased susceptibility to post-vaccination encephalomyelitis.

A higher incidence of PIEM is seen primarily in underdeveloped regions of the world where preventative childhood immunization is not available. This includes areas of Asia, Africa, and South America.

Symptoms

Localization site	Comment
Cerebral hemispheres	Patient may have focal cortical signs of aphasia, alexia, agraphia, and/or cortical blindness. In advanced cases, frontal release signs such as glabellar reflex, snout/sucking reflexes, and grasp may be present. Meningeal signs have also been reported. Although less common than post-infection encephalomyelitis, seizures can occur in post-vaccination encephalomyelitis. MRI imaging may demonstrate demyelination in both gray and white matter, particularly the thalamus. This may not be apparent in hyperacute lesions but may develop later in a pathognomonic "sleeve-like" fashion. There is minimal axonal damage. Extrapyramidal (parkinsonian) sign and symptoms are commonly noted after Group A β-hemolytic streptococcus infection
Mental status and psychiatric aspects/ complications	Patient may demonstrate daytime somnolence with fluctuating alertness and orientation consistent with delirium. Adolescents and young adults can present with psychosis

Localization site	Comment
Cerebellum	Patient may have symptoms of ataxia, dysmetria, and nystagmus. Cerebellar syndrome is typically seen after varicella-zoster infection and typically carries a good prognosis
Brainstem/cranial nerves	Bilateral optic neuritis has been commonly observed in patients with post-immunization encephalitis. Patients with diminished visual acuity and afferent pupillary defect. Funduscopic exam has revealed bilateral optic disc pallor. Visual evoked potentials will be abnormal. Patients may have visual field deficits
Spinal cord	Patient can present commonly with focal motor weakness with some reports of diffuse motor weakness. Patient can have sensory abnormalities (can be paresthesias or numbness). Sensory levels have also been reported. Asymmetric reflex abnormalities may be present (hypo-/hyperreflexia). Babinski sign is noted. Imaging can demonstrate evidence of transverse myelitis
Unclear localization	Fever, malaise, and fatigue are commonly reported in patients with post-immunization encephalomyelitis. This is something that differentiates it from other demyelinating processes such as multiple sclerosis and neuromyelitis optica

Secondary Complications:
Visual changes including blindness.
Persistent weakness and sensory changes.
Seizures.
Residual mental status changes and psychiatric disturbances.
Diminished executive functioning skills secondary to residual frontal lobe abnormalities.

Treatment Complications:
Steroids: Methyprednisolone is commonly used to treat this condition. The use of methylprednisolone causes an increased risk of infection, hyperglycemia, avascular necrosis of the hip, psychosis, Cushing disease, and osteoporosis.

Intravenous immunoglobulin (IVIG): IVIG can induce reactions in patients with IgA deficiency. This occurs in 1/500–1000 patients. Serious anaphylactoid reactions occur soon after the administration of IVIG. Anaphylaxis associated with sensitization to IgA in patients with IgA deficiency can be prevented by using IgA-depleted immunoglobulin. The presence of IgG anti-IgA antibodies is not always associated with severe adverse reactions to IVIG. As IVIG can lead to thrombosis, it has also been known to cause stroke and acute myocardial infarction. Nephrotoxicity has also been linked to the use of IVIG. IVIG therapy can result in post-infusion hyperproteinemia, increased serum viscosity, and pseudohyponatremia. Aseptic meningitis is also a rare but well-recognized complication of IVIG therapy.

Plasmapheresis (for hyperviscosity syndrome): Hypocalcemia/hypomagnesemia before or after treatment, hypothermia during treatment, and transfusion-related reactions are also likely; hypotension may occur in patients taking angiotensin-converting enzyme (ACE) inhibitors, in particular while undergoing column-based plasmapheresis. Thrombocytopenia and hypofibrinogenemia may occur after plasmapheresis (especially if albumin is being used as a replacement product) and patients should be monitored for signs of bleeding.

Bibliography

Alper G. Acute disseminated encephalomyelitis. *J Child Neurol.* 2012;27(11):1408–25.

Wingerchuk DM. Postinfectious encephalomyelitis. *Curr Neurol Neurosci Rep.* 2003;3(3):256–64.

Post-Lumbar Puncture Headache

Epidemiology and Demographics: Thirty-two percent of patients who undergo a lumbar puncture (LP) develop a headache; however, this finding may be underreported as minor symptoms are not reported. Post-LP headache is more common in young adults (18–30 years). Young women with a lower body mass index and those who are pregnant are at higher risk of developing headaches after lumbar puncture. The incidence is less in the elderly for unclear reasons.

Disorder Description: Bilateral headaches that occur within 7 days of lumbar puncture. A common characteristic of this type of headache is worsening of symptoms within 15 minutes of sitting or standing upright, which resolves within 30 minutes of establishing recumbent position. Onset of headache is usually within 24–48 hours after dural puncture and can be delayed up to 12 days. Symptoms are often self-limited but can be severe enough to immobilize patient. Headache has been described as dull or throbbing in nature and can start in the frontal or occipital region then can later generalize. Sometimes, the headache pain can radiate down the neck and be associated with neck stiffness. Factors that can worsen symptoms include coughing, sneezing, straining, or ocular compression. Other associated symptoms include lower back pain, nausea, vomiting, vertigo, tinnitus, and rarely diplopia and cortical blindness.

Symptoms

Localization site	Comment
Cerebral hemispheres	Bilateral in nature; can start in frontal or occipital territory and then generalize
Cranial nerves	Rarely associated with cranial neuropathy

Secondary Complications: Local infection at site of lumbar puncture and inflammation; for persistent post-lumbar puncture headache for more than 72 hours, can undergo blood patch.

Treatment Complications: Use of oral or intravenous caffeine for resolution of headache symptoms puts patient at risk for recurrent headache. Blood patch has a 70–98% success rate; if blood patch is not successful, the procedure can be repeated to help seal dural hole caused by lumbar puncture.

Bibliography

Ahmed SV, Jayawarna C, Jude E. Post lumbar puncture headache: diagnosis and management. *Postgrad Med J.* 2006;82:713–16

Kuntz KM, Kokmen E, Stevens JC, et al. Post-lumbar puncture headaches: experience in 501 consecutive procedures. *Neurology.* 1992;42:1884–7.

Niall CT, Globerson JA, de Rosayro MA. Epidural blood patch for postdural puncture headache: it's never too late. *Anesth Anal.* 1986;65:895–6.

Olsen J, Bousser M-G, Diener H-C, et al. The international classification of headache disorders: 2nd edition. *Cephalalgia.* 2004;24:9–160.

Thomas S-R, Jamieson D-R, Muir K-W. Randomised controlled trial of atraumatic versus standard needles for diagnostic lumbar puncture. *BMJ* (*Clin Res Ed*). 2000;3210:986–90.

Turnbull DK, Shepherd DB. Post-dural puncture headache: pathogenesis, prevention and treatment. *Br J Anaesth*. 2003;91:718–29.

Post-transplant Encephalopathy and Other Complications

Epidemiology and Demographics: Post-transplantation encephalopathy (PTE) is a common complication following transplant procedures. Approximately 30% to 60% of patients may experience some type of neurologic complication following a transplant.[1,2]

Disorder Description: PTE is characterized by an alteration of consciousness, ranging from fluctuating delirium to coma. This alteration of consciousness can be accompanied by a variety of motor signs such as tremors, asterixis, and myoclonus.[2]

PTE can occur from a host of underlying disorders such as metabolic derangement, central nervous system or systemic opportunistic infections, and hypoxia–ischemia. PTE can also be seen as a direct result (or indirect result) of transplant medications. PTE is commonly known to occur in the setting of graft-versus-host disease.

Transplanted organ-specific complications have been cited in the medical literature.[2] Heart and pulmonary transplants have been associated with cerebral hypoxia and ischemia while bone marrow transplantation has been associated with prolonged thrombocytopenia and cerebral hemorrhage.[3] Cranial irradiation, also used in bone marrow recipients, has been associated with cerebral edema, which can cause an encephalopathy.[2] Different types of encephalopathies may coexist in a specific clinical setting, which poses a unique diagnostic challenge.[4]

Generally speaking, certain encephalopathies occur earlier in the post-transplantation period, while others occur later.[2] Hypoxic–ischemic encephalopathy is known to occur within the first 30 days post-transplant. Within the first 3 months, acute systemic rejection of the transplanted organ and resulting rejection encephalopathy is of concern. After 3 months, neurotoxicity from anti-rejection medications may develop as well as metabolic derangements which may lead to an encephalopathy.[2]

The diagnostic workup of post-transplant encephalopathy mirrors that of other encephalopathies. Imaging studies of the brain, such as MRI or CT, can be helpful to delineate ring-enhancing lesions that may be suggestive of an opportunistic infection. Note that non-specific atrophy and white matter lesions are typically seen in the MRI of brain of patients with graft-versus-host disease.[2] Routine blood work including a complete metabolic panel and therapeutic levels of anti-rejection medication can be helpful in diagnosing a uremic encephalopathy associated with renal transplant versus neurotoxicity from supra-therapeutic dosages of anti-rejection medications. Cerebrospinal fluid evaluation can further aid in the evaluation of any concomitant opportunistic infection that may have developed. EEG (electroencephalogram) is typically necessary to rule out convulsive versus non-convulsive status epilepticus, which can further complicate management of these patients.

Symptoms

Localization site	Comment
Cerebral hemispheres	Posterior reversible encephalopathy syndrome (PRES) with headache, altered mentation, seizures, and elevated blood pressure may occur with several transplant types. Uremic encephalopathy can be seen in patients following renal transplant during either acute or chronic rejection
	Effects of persistent uremia in renal transplant or encephalopathy from acute renal graft rejection. Neoplastic meningitis and central nervous system (CNS) deposits in patients with recurrent leukemia in context of undergoing bone marrow grafts. Cerebrovascular disease, coagulopathies, and endocarditis may occur in several conditions leading to transplants such as bone marrow transplants. Cerebral hypoxia in cardiac transplantation. Seizures associated with underlying conditions, coexisting metabolic aberrations, or hypoxia associated with assorted transplant procedures[4–6]
Brainstem	Central pontine myelinolysis (with altered mentation, quadriplegia, and pseudobulbar palsy) after hepatic, and less commonly hepatic or cardiac transplants, and associated with attempts to rapidly lower sodium concentrations

Localization site	Comment
Spinal cord	Due to an anatomic variation, the caudal spinal cord may be supplied by branches of the internal iliac arteries rather than by intercostal arteries. If the internal iliac artery is used to supply blood to the transplanted organ, this can lead to ischemia of the spinal cord[5]
Plexus	Brachial plexus injury and phrenic nerve injury can occur during the course of cardiac/lung transplant from stretch injuries[5]
Mononeuropathy or mononeuropathy multiplex	Chronic graft-versus-host disease can lead to systemic versus primary CNS vasculitis. This may present with focal entrapment neuropathies such as radial nerve palsy or peroneal nerve palsy (dropped wrist versus foot drop)
Peripheral neuropathy	Injuries to the femoral and lateral cutaneous nerves can occur during renal transplant. This is largely due to compression of the nerves during surgery.[5] Small-fiber and autonomic neuropathies are associated with uncontrolled diabetes most often seen in pancreatic transplant recipients
Muscle	Polymyositis in chronic graft-versus-host disease in bone marrow transplants
Neuromuscular junction	Myasthenic syndrome in chronic graft-versus-host disease in bone marrow transplants

Secondary Complications: Coagulopathy and its associated risks (e.g., cerebral hemorrhage) are common in patients with advanced hepatic disease that are candidates for liver transplantation.

Treatment Complications: Immunosuppressive agents such as cyclosporine or tacrolimus may cause an encephalopathy that resembles hypertensive encephalopathy with manifestations like altered mentation, mood changes, tremor, seizures, visual alterations, headaches, and other cortical deficits. PRES is one of the known complications of calcineurin inhibitors (cyclosporine and tacrolimus).[2] Sensory alterations such as paresthesias may occur. Direct epileptogenic effects of cyclosporine and monoclonal antibody therapies have been described.

Steroids notorious for risk of psychosis or less severe alterations in mood, myopathy, and steroid withdrawal problems if tapered too rapidly. Rare steroid-related epidural lipomatosis described. Monoclonal antibody treatment may cause an aseptic meningitis.

Immunosuppressive agents, such as cyclosporine and tacrolimus, in conjunction with corticosteroids, may predispose transplant patients to opportunistic systemic and CNS infections, thereby resulting in sepsis and a septic encephalopathy.[2] Immunosuppression may make patients vulnerable to incurring meningitis associated with agents like *Aspergillus*, *Listeria*, or *Cryptococcus*, brain abscess (e.g., *Toxoplasma*), or progressive multifocal leukoencephalopathy associated with JC virus. Post-transplant lymphoproliferative disorder may have CNS involvement.

Some antiepileptic agents may induce hepatic metabolism and result in lower levels of concomitant immunosuppressive therapies.

Assorted perioperative peripheral nerve injury syndromes may occur, such as brachial plexus insult from cardiac surgery and femoral nerve with renal transplants.

Meningitis may be a facet of the immune reconstitution inflammatory syndrome associated with rapid reduction in immunosuppressive therapy.

Several chemotherapeutic agents used in oncology may lead to the depletion of thiamine reserves and therefore predispose patients to Wernicke encephalopathy.[2]

References

1. Padovan CS, Sostak P, Straube A. [Neurological complications after organ transplantation]. *Der Nervenarzt*. 2000;71(4):249–58.
2. Živković SA. Neurologic complications after liver transplantation. *World J Hepatol*. 2013;5(8):409–16. DOI:10.4254/wjh.v5.i8.409.
3. Bashir. Neurologic complications of organ transplantation. *Curr Treat Options Neurol*. 2001;3(6):543–54.
4. Mathew RM, Rosenfeld MR. Neurologic complications of bone marrow and stem-cell transplantation in patients with cancer. *Curr Treat Options Neurol*. 2007;9(4):308–31.
5. Patchell RA. Neurological complications of organ transplantation and immunosuppressive agents. In Aminoff M, ed. *Neurology and general*

medicine. 4th ed. London: Churchill Livingstone; 2007. pp. 873–85.

6. Pruitt AA, Grus F, Rosenfeld MR. Neurological complications of solid organ transplantation. *The Neurohospitalist.* 2012;3(3):152–66.

Posttraumatic Stress Disorder (PTSD)

Epidemiology and Demographics: In the United States, the projected lifetime risk of posttraumatic stress disorder (PTSD) at age 75 is 8.7%. The 12-month prevalence in US adults is about 3.5%. PTSD rates are higher among veterans, police officers, firefighters, and emergency medical personnel than in those whose occupations do not increase the risk of exposure to trauma. The highest rates (a third to half of those exposed) are present in survivors of rape, military combat, internment, and genocide.

There is a higher prevalence of PTSD in some chronic migraine patients compared with those with another chronic headache condition (tension headaches) and healthy subjects, which should be considered when treating chronic migraine patients.

Disorder Description: As stated in DSM-5, posttraumatic stress disorder in adults can be defined as:

A. Exposure to actual or threatened death, serious injury, or sexual violence in one (or more) of the following ways:
   i. Directly experiencing the traumatic event(s)
   ii. Witnessing the event as it occurred to others
   iii. Learning that the event occurred to a close family member or friend
   iv. Experiencing repeated or extreme exposure to aversive details of the traumatic event (e.g., first responders collecting human remains, police officers repeatedly exposed to details of child abuse)

B. Presence of one or more of the following intrusive symptoms associated with the traumatic event, and beginning when the event occurred:
   i. Recurrent, involuntary, and intrusive distressing memories of the traumatic event
   ii. Recurrent distressing dreams wherein the content of the dream is related to the traumatic event
   iii. Dissociative reactions (e.g., flashbacks) wherein the individual feels or acts as if the traumatic event is recurring

   iv. Intense or prolonged psychologic distress at exposure to internal or external cues that symbolize or resemble an aspect of the traumatic event
   v. Marked psychologic reactions to internal or external cues that symbolize or resemble an aspect of the traumatic event

C. Persistent avoidance of stimuli associated with the traumatic event, beginning or worsening after the traumatic event occurred, as evidenced by one or both of the following:
   i. Avoidance of or efforts to avoid distressing memories, thoughts, or feelings about or closely associated with the traumatic events
   ii. Avoidance of or efforts to avoid external reminders that arouse distressing memories, thoughts, or feelings about or closely associated with the traumatic event

D. Negative alterations in thoughts and mood associated with the traumatic event, beginning or worsening after the traumatic event occurred, as evidenced by two or more of the following:
   i. Inability to remember an important aspect of the traumatic event (usually due to dissociative amnesia and not due to other factors such as head trauma or substance use)
   ii. Persistent and exaggerated negative beliefs or expectations about oneself, others, or the world
   iii. Persistent, distorted thoughts about the cause or consequences of the traumatic event that lead the individual to blame him/herself or others
   iv. Persistent negative emotional state
   v. Markedly diminished interest or participation in significant activities
   vi. Feeling of detachment or estrangement from others
   vii. Persistent inability to experience positive emotions (e.g., inability to experience happiness, satisfaction, or loving feelings)

E. Marked alterations in arousal and reactivity associated with the traumatic event that began or worsened after the event occurred, as evidenced by two or more of the following:
   i. Irritable behavior and angry outbursts (with little or no provocation) typically expressed as verbal or physical aggression toward people or objects
   ii. Reckless or self-destructive behavior

iii. Hypervigilance

iv. Exaggerated startle response

v. Problems with concentration

vi. Sleep disturbance (e.g., difficulty falling or staying asleep or restless sleep)

F. Duration of the disturbance is more than 1 month

G. The disturbance causes clinically significant distress or impairment in social, occupational, or other areas of functioning

H. The disturbance is not attributable to the physiologic effects of a substance (e.g., medication, alcohol) or another medical condition.

Differential Diagnosis: Differential diagnosis should include adjustment disorders, acute stress disorder, anxiety disorder/obsessive-compulsive disorder, major depressive disorder, personality disorders, dissociative disorders, conversion disorder, psychotic disorders, and traumatic brain injury.

In adjustment disorder, the stressful event can be of any severity, and need not satisfy criterion A of PTSD. This diagnosis is also made when criterion A of PTSD is satisfied but other criteria are absent.

In acute stress disorder, symptoms are present from 3 days to 1 month.

In obsessive-compulsive disorder, there are also recurrent intrusive thoughts, but these meet the criteria for obsession. Here the thoughts are not related to a traumatic event. In panic disorder and generalized anxiety disorder, the dissociative symptoms and depersonalization are not related to a traumatic event.

In major depressive disorder, the depression may or may not have been preceded by a traumatic event, and should be diagnosed if other PTSD symptoms are absent.

In personality disorders, the fixed and unhealthy thinking pattern occurs independent of traumatic exposure.

In dissociative disorders including dissociative amnesia, dissociative identity disorder, and depersonalization–derealization disorder, there may or may not be an association with other PTSD symptoms. There also may or may not be an association with a traumatic event. When all of the criteria for PTSD are fulfilled in addition to dissociative symptoms, the diagnosis "PTSD with dissociative symptoms" should be given.

In conversion disorder, there is a new onset of somatic symptoms. When criteria for PTSD are also fulfilled, the diagnosis of PTSD should be given instead of conversion disorder.

In psychotic disorders, illusions, hallucinations, and other perceptual disturbances are present. These symptoms may be seen in schizophrenia, depressive and bipolar disorders with psychotic features, in delirium and substance/medication-induced disorders, and psychotic disorders due to another medical condition. Flashbacks associated with PTSD must carefully be distinguished from these perceptual disturbances.

In traumatic brain injury, the injury may occur in the context of a traumatic event, and symptoms of PTSD may appear in conjunction with traumatic brain injury symptoms. Traumatic brain injury symptoms and PTSD are not mutually exclusive, and may occur in tandem and in response to the same event. Symptoms of the two may overlap, and thus the presence of symptoms that are specific to one diagnosis but not the other should be carefully assessed. For instance, in PTSD, re-experiencing and avoidance are characteristic symptoms, whereas in traumatic brain injury persistent disorientation and confusion are characteristic.

Secondary Complications: PTSD may lead to severe social, occupational, and physical disability, as well as high economic costs and high medical utilization. In veterans, PTSD has been associated with poor social and family relationships, absenteeism, lower income, and less education. PTSD has also been linked to an increase in suicidal ideation and attempts, and may be predictive of suicide attempts and/or completion. Reported rates of PTSD occur in over a third of patients hospitalized after traumatic injury such as motor vehicle accident, assaults, or fires. In a hospital setting, an event such as a traumatic amputation may trigger PTSD where the patient relives the surgery that was performed. These patients may go to a neurologist first in order to treat the phantom pain and neuralgia; therefore, it is important to be aware of this.

Another syndrome related to PTSD is PICS (post intensive care syndrome). Advances in critical care medicine have resulted in a growing population of survivors of critical illness. PICS constitutes new or worsening function in one or more of the following domains: cognitive, psychiatric, or physical function. Although the exact prevalence of PICS is unknown, it is estimated that one half or more will suffer from some component of PICS. The severity of cognitive impairment varies from mild to severe – from subtle difficulties in doing complex tasks to a profound inability to conduct one's ADL (activities of daily living). Areas that are commonly affected are: attention/concentration, memory, mental processing speed, and executive function. An observational study reported an incidence of PTSD of 10% in ICU survivors at both 3 and 12 months post hospitalization. Symptoms suggestive of PTSD include affective and behavioral responses to stimuli that promote flashbacks, hyperarousal, and severe anxiety, as well as intrusive recollection and avoidance of experiences that cause symptoms. Sexual dysfunction is common particularly in those with PTSD symptoms. One prospective observational study of 127 patients who spent more than 3 days in ICU reported sexual dysfunction in 44% of patients. Glucocorticoids are associated with a reduced risk for PTSD. Reduced levels of cortisol are thought to play a role in development of PTSD and it has been hypothesized that administration of glucocorticoids during critical illness may replenish cortisol levels thereby reducing risk of developing PTSD.

Treatment Complications: Selective serotonin reuptake inhibitors (SSRIs) are the first-line treatment for PTSD. SSRI side effects include nausea, diarrhea, insomnia, headache, anorexia, weight loss, sexual dysfunction, restlessness (akathisia-like), serotonin syndrome (fever, diaphoresis, tachycardia, hypertension, delirium, neuromuscular excitability), hyponatremia, seizures (0.2%).

Serotonin–norepinephrine reuptake inhibitors (SNRIs) are also effective for PTSD treatment. The side effect profile for SNRIs is very similar to that of SSRIs, but SNRIs tend to cause hypertension at higher doses. SNRIs also may cause dry mouth, constipation, and hepatotoxicity.

Prazosin, an alpha-1-receptor antagonist, is used to target nightmares and hypervigilance. It has been shown to reduce PTSD nightmares by lowering the hyperarousal component. Side effects include hypotension, headache, drowsiness, lethargy, weakness, blurred vision, nausea, vomiting, diarrhea, and constipation.

Augmentation with atypical antipsychotics may also be implemented in refractory cases. Atypical antipsychotic side effects include metabolic syndrome, weight gain, hyperlipidemia, and hyperglycemia.

Bibliography

American Psychiatric Association. *Diagnostic and statistical manual of mental disorders: DSM-5.* 5th ed. Washington, DC: American Psychiatric Association; 2013.

Rauch SL, van der Kolk BA, Fisler RE, et al. A symptom provocation study of posttraumatic stress disorder using positron emission tomography and script-driven imagery. *Arch Gen Psychiatry.* 1996;53(5):380–7.

Shin LM, Wright CI, Cannistraro PA, et al. A functional magnetic resonance imaging study of amygdala and medial prefrontal cortex responses to overtly presented fearful faces in posttraumatic stress disorder. *Arch Gen Psychiatry.* 2005;62(3):273–81.

Taylor HR. Prazosin for treatment of nightmares related to post traumatic stress disorder. *Am J Health Syst Pharm.* 2008;65(8):716–22.

Yehuda R. Post-traumatic stress disorder. *New Engl J Med.* 2002;346(2):108–14.

Yule W. Posttraumatic stress disorder. In Ollendick, King NJ, Yule W, eds. *International handbook of phobic and anxiety disorders in children and adolescents.* New York: Springer US; 1994. pp. 223–40.

Zarei MR, Shabani M, Chamani G, et al. Migraine patients have higher prevalence of PTSD symptoms in comparison to chronic tension type headache and healthy subjects: a case control study. *Acta Odontol Scand.* 2016;74(8):633–5.

Postural Orthostatic Tachycardia Syndrome (POTS)

Epidemiology and Demographics: Affects Caucasians more than other races, about 500,000 people in the United States (estimates of 11 million in the world). Young age (14–45 years) of presentation; females more than males (5:1).

Disorder Description: A disorder of autonomic instability with development of orthostatic symptoms (upright position) associated with a heart rate increment ≥30 (usually to ≥120 bpm) without orthostatic hypotension in the absence of medications that impair autonomic regulation or deconditioning. Patients present with lightheadedness, diminished concentration, tremulousness, nausea, and recurrent syncope commonly exacerbated by heat, illness, dehydration, and exercise. They may be incorrectly labeled as having panic disorder or chronic anxiety.

It is actually a syndrome with numerous causes involving abnormalities of sympathetic innervation. There is either a decrease of sympathetic innervation in the peripheral nervous system or increased central sympathetic drive.

Symptoms

Localization site	Comment
Cerebral hemispheres	Impaired cerebral perfusion causes lightheadedness, tremulousness, syncope, mental clouding (brain fog), and blurred or tunnel vision
	Orthostatic headache may occur (holocephalic/bifrontal) from reduced CSF orthostatic pressure
Mental status and psychiatric aspects/ complications	Sleep disturbances are known to occur. Anxiety is reported but this is usually a misinterpretation of the palpitations
Brainstem	Brainstem dysregulation may contribute to symptoms
Peripheral neuropathy	Length-dependent peripheral neuropathy in the neuropathic variant
	Impaired sweating in the lower limbs from dysautonomia of the peripheral nerves
	Dependent acrocyanosis
Other	Tachycardia, diaphoresis, palpitations

Secondary Complications: Relatively favorable prognosis. However, patients may experience insomnia, chronic fatigue, nausea, abdominal pain, bloating, and diarrhea.

Treatment Complications: Non-pharmacologic treatments including increased fluid intake (3 liters/day) and salt intake (1 g oral three times a day) are well tolerated. Compression stockings and abdominal binders may be uncomfortable (compliance may be a problem).

Pharmacologic treatment such as beta blockers and central sympathetic alpha 2 agonist clonidine can cause orthostatic hypotension; the alpha sympathomimetic midodrine can cause supine hypertension. If fludrocortisone is used in hypovolemic cases, it can cause supine hypertension, steroid myopathy, peripheral edema, and hyperglycemia.

Bibliography

Benarroch EE. Postural tachycardia syndrome. *Mayo Clin Proc*. 2012;87(12):1214–25.

Jacob G, Costa F, Shannon JR, et al. The neuropathic postural tachycardia syndrome. *N Engl J Med*. 2000;343:1008–14.

Raj SR. Postural orthostatic tachycardia syndrome (POTS). *Circulation*. 2013;127(23):2336–42.

Thieben MJ, Sandroni P, Sletten DM, et al. Postural orthostatic tachycardia syndrome: the Mayo Clinic experience. *Mayo Clin Proc*. 2007;82:308–13.

Potassium-Aggravated Myotonia

Myotonia Fluctuans: Rare autosomal dominant condition characterized by myotonia. Associated with a mutation in skeletal muscle sodium channel gene located on chromosome 17.[1] Myotonia fluctuans usually presents during first decade of life. Patients experience painless muscle stiffness at rest that improves with exercise. Myotonia is noticed in face, tongue, and extremities. Symptoms fluctuate in severity during day.[2] Symptoms are precipitated by potassium, cold, or fasting. Electromyography reveals myotonic discharges. Myotonia can be treated with sodium channel blocking agents such as mexiletine or tocainamide.

Myotonia Permanans: Rare autosomal dominant condition characterized by myotonia. Associated with a mutation in skeletal muscle sodium channel gene located on chromosome 17. Myotonia permanans usually presents during first decade of life. Patients experience painless muscle stiffness at rest that improves with exercise. Severe myotonia is noticed in face, extremities, and respiratory muscles leading to hypoxia. Neck and shoulder muscle hypertrophy is also noticed.[1,2] Symptoms are precipitated by potassium, cold, or fasting. Electromyography reveals myotonic discharges. Myotonia can be treated with sodium channel blocking agents such as mexiletine or tocainamide.

Acetazolamide-Responsive Sodium Channel Myotonia: Rare autosomal dominant condition characterized by myotonia. Associated with a mutation in skeletal muscle sodium channel gene located on chromosome 17.[3] Acetazolamide-responsive sodium channel myotonia usually presents during first decade of life. The characteristic feature of the disease is periodic worsening of myotonia mainly in face and hands. Symptoms are precipitated by cold or by ingestion of potassium. Severe stiffness and palpable rigidity are noticed after 15 minutes of potassium ingestion.[2,4,5] Electromyography reveals myotonia. Muscle biopsy reveals normal ratio of Type 1 and Type 2 fibers. Treatment with carbonic anhydrase inhibitor (acetazolamide) results in symptom resolution in 24 hours.

References

1. Tena Rosser AP. *Pediatric neurology: a case based review*. Lippincott Williams & Wilkins; 2007.
2. Ropper AH, Samuels MA, Klein JP. The myotonias, periodic paralyses, cramps, spasms, and states of persistent muscle fiber activity. In *Adams & Victor's principles of neurology*. 10th ed. New York, NY: McGraw-Hill; 2014. Chapter 50.
3. Patcek LJ, Tawil R, Griggs RC, Storvick D, Leppert M. Linkage of atypical myotonia congenita to a sodium channel locus. *Neurology*. 1992;42(2):431.
4. Science Direct. Potassium-aggravated myotonia. Available from www.sciencedirect.com/topics/neuroscience/potassium-aggravated-myotonia. Accessed Sep 25, 2018.
5. Trudell RG, Kaiser KK, Griggs R. Acetazolamide-responsive myotonia congenita. *Neurology*. 1987;37(3):488.

Prader–Willi Syndrome (Willi–Prader Syndrome; Prader–Labhart–Willi Syndrome)

Epidemiology and Demographics: Symptoms of Prader–Willi syndrome (PWS) are very age-specific, and begin in early infancy to age 2 years with hypotonia and feeding difficulties with poor suck, in many cases requiring a feeding tube. Between 2 and 6 years of age, symptoms include hypotonia with a history of poor suck in infancy and global developmental delay. Between ages 6 and 12 years, symptoms include a history of hypotonia in early childhood, a history of poor suck in infancy, global developmental delays, and excessive eating and central obesity. Over age 13 years to adulthood, symptoms include intellectual disability, delayed puberty, and behavioral problems.

The estimated prevalence of PWS is 1/10,000 to 1/30,000 in a number of populations.

Disorder Description: PWS is a neurodevelopmental disorder with numerous distinctive features, including:

1. Hypotonia: Can start perinatally and lead to decreased fetal movements in utero. At birth these babies have significant hypotonia with poor suck, poor cry, decreased reflexes, and lethargy. Over time, low tone improves, as does eating ability.
2. Global developmental delays: Motor and language milestones are significantly delayed. By school age, intellectual disability and learning disabilities are evident.
3. Delayed puberty due to hypogonadism, with small genitalia, infertility.
4. Hyperphagia and obesity: The eating behavior in PWS is hypothesized to be due to hypothalamic dysregulation of satiety. Children with PWS will hoard food and parents typically have to keep food locked up to prevent over-eating.
5. Endocrinopathies, including increased risk of diabetes mellitus type 2, hypothyroidism, and adrenal insufficiency.
6. Abnormal sleep with central and obstructive sleep apnea, oxygen desaturation, abnormal sleep architecture, also hypothesized to be due to hypothalamic dysfunction.
7. Neurobehavioral disturbances including autistic features, attention deficit/hyperactivity disorder, obsessive-compulsive disorder, and even psychosis.
8. Short stature, with and without documented growth hormone deficiency, small hands and feet.
9. Facial dysmorphology with almond-shaped eyes, thin upper lip, narrow forehead, hypopigmentation of skin, hair and eyes (as the *OCA2* gene for oculocutaneous albinism is located in this area).
10. Strabismus.
11. Bone issues include increased risk for hip dysplasia, osteopenia/osteoporosis leading to increased risk of fractures, scoliosis.

PWS is caused by mutations within the Prader–Willi critical region (PWCR) on chromosome 15 (15q11.2–q13). In PWS, this region is maternally inherited only due to either paternal deletion (70%), maternal uniparental disomy (UPD), or an imprinting defect.

Symptoms

Localization site	Comment
Cerebral hemispheres	Ventriculomegaly; decreased volume of brain tissue in the parietal-occipital lobe; Sylvian fissure polymicrogyria; incomplete insular closure; white matter lesions[1]
	Hypothalamic dysfunction
Mental status and psychiatric aspects/ complications	Temper tantrums; stubbornness; controlling and manipulative behavior compulsivity; difficulty with change in routine[2]; autism[3]; attention deficit/hyperactivity symptoms; insistence on sameness[4]
Pituitary gland	Reduced pituitary height[5]

Secondary Complications: Feeding issues/failure to thrive/malnutrition, hypotonia and weakness, sleep disturbances including sleep apnea.

Treatment Complications: Growth hormone replacement therapy has had concerns of worsening sleep apnea and increased morbidity and mortality.

References

1. Driscoll DJ, Miller JL, Schwartz S, et al. Prader–Willi syndrome. Oct 6, 1998. Updated Feb 4, 2016. In Pagon RA, Adam MP, Ardinger HH, et al., eds. *GeneReviews®* [Internet]. Seattle (WA): University of Washington, Seattle; 1993–2016. Available from: www.ncbi.nlm.nih.gov/books/NBK1330/. Accessed Sep 11, 2018.
2. Miller J, Kranzler J, Liu Y, et al. Neurocognitive findings in Prader-Willi syndrome and early-onset morbid obesity. *J Pediatr*. 2006;149:192–8.
3. Descheemaeker MJ, Govers V, Vermeulen P, Fryns JP. Pervasive developmental disorders in Prader-Willi syndrome: the Leuven experience in 59 subjects and controls. *Am J Med Genet A*. 2006;140:1136–42.
4. Wigren M, Hansen S. ADHD symptoms and insistence on sameness in Prader-Willi syndrome. *J Intellect Disabil Res*. 2005;49:449–56.
5. Iughetti L, Bosio L, Corrias A, et al. Pituitary height and neuroradiological alterations in patients with Prader-Labhart-Willi syndrome. *Eur J Pediatr*. 2008;167:701–2.

Pre-eclampsia

Epidemiology and Demographics: Pre-eclampsia affects 3 to 7% of pregnant women. Pre-eclampsia and eclampsia develop after 20 weeks' gestation; up to 25% of cases develop postpartum, most often within the first 4 days but up to 6 weeks postpartum. It is a leading cause of direct maternal mortality, accounting for 10–15% of deaths. The risk is greater for women older than 35 years or younger than 17 years.

Predisposing Factors: The strongest risk factors are pre-existing vascular disease. Antiphospholipid antibody syndrome carries the highest risk with 17% of affected women developing pre-eclampsia during pregnancy. Other strong risk factors in order of impact include pre-eclampsia in previous pregnancies, which increases the risk 7-fold from expected, preexisting chronic hypertension, obesity, vascular disorders (such as renal disease) or gestational diabetes, multifetal pregnancy, older age at pregnancy, family history of pre-eclampsia, and nulliparity.

Disorder Description: Pre-eclampsia is characterized by new-onset hypertension and new unexplained proteinuria after 20 weeks' gestation. Proteinuria is defined as >300 mg in a 24-hour urine collection. Alternatively, proteinuria is diagnosed based on a dipstick reading of 1+. Proteinuria, while typically present and highly supportive of the diagnosis, is not an absolute requirement for the diagnosis.

In the absence of proteinuria, pre-eclampsia is also diagnosed if pregnant women have new-onset hypertension accompanied by the new onset of thrombocytopenia (platelets <100,000/μL), renal insufficiency (serum creatinine >1.1 mg/dL or doubling of serum creatinine in women without renal disease), impaired liver function (aminotransferases > 2 times normal), pulmonary edema, cerebral or visual symptoms.

While the pathophysiology is poorly understood, placental factors initiate the illness. Pre-eclampsia begins with a pathologic placenta that releases anti-angiogenic vascular endothelial growth factors. These factors produce maternal disease by antagonizing the effects of maternal proangiogenic factors necessary for maintaining the vascular endothelium. Maternal hypertension and systemic vascular pathology is the end result. The cause of the initial placental disease is unknown. However, the effect of pre-eclampsia extends beyond delivery in that it predicts future cardiovascular disease in affected women.

Symptoms

Localization site	Comment
Cerebral hemispheres	Hyperreflexia
	Headaches, blurred vision, confused or altered mental status

Secondary Complications: Complications affecting the fetus include fetal growth restriction, abruptio placentae, and fetal death. Maternal complications include progression to eclampsia, which is among the most dire (discussed separately). Diffuse or multifocal vasospasm can result in hepatic infarction, hepatic rupture, intra-abdominal bleeding, pulmonary edema, and acute renal failure, any of which are potentially fatal.

Ten to 20% of women with severe pre-eclampsia or eclampsia develop the HELLP syndrome (hemolysis, elevated liver function tests, and low platelet count). Further, approximately 20% of women with HELLP syndrome develop disseminated intravascular coagulation, which carries a poor prognosis for both mother and fetus.

Treatment Complications: Prevention of pre-eclampsia should be undertaken in women with strong risk factors as outlined above. This consists of low-dose aspirin at 75–81 mg taken daily prior to 20 weeks' of pregnancy. One to 2 grams of calcium is recommended for the prevention of pre-eclampsia in all women, but especially those at high risk of developing pre-eclampsia.

The National Institute for Health and Care Excellence (NICE) guidance now recommends tight blood pressure control. Labetolol should be first-line treatment for hypertension over 150 mmHg systolic and 80–100 mmHg diastolic.

Magnesium sulfate is recommended in severe pre-eclampsia to prevent eclamptic seizures This is established in clinical practice for women with severe hypertension or proteinuria or with mild to moderate hypertension or proteinuria with the addition of clinical or laboratory abnormalities. A review by the Cochrane Collaboration from 2009 found that magnesium sulfate is also neuroprotective for the preterm infant (<37 weeks) and reduces risk of cerebral palsy by 15–50%.

NICE recommendations suggest conservative management below 34 weeks' gestation and that elective delivery before 34 weeks not be undertaken, unless the symptomatology is severe.

Adverse effects of magnesium sulfate include nausea, diarrhea, or vomiting, low blood pressure, irregular heartbeat, headache, and muscle aches. Magnesium exposure in utero is associated with low muscle tone and relatively lower than expected Apgar scores in newborns; however, there is no evident effect on longer term outcomes.

Bibliography

Bartsch E, Medcalf KE, Park AL, Ray JG. High Risk of Pre-eclampsia Identification Group. Clinical risk factors for pre-eclampsia determined in early pregnancy: systematic review and meta-analysis of large cohort studies. *BMJ*. 2016;353:i1753. DOI: 10.1136/bmj.i1753.

Duhig KE, Shennan AH. Recent advances in the diagnosis and management of pre-eclampsia. *F1000Prime Rep*. 2015;7:24. DOI: 10.12703/P7-24.

Powe CE, Levine RJ, Karumanchi SA. Preeclampsia, a disease of the maternal endothelium: the role of antiangiogenic factors and implications for later cardiovascular disease. *Circulation*. 2011;123(24):2856–69. DOI: 10.1161/CIRCULATIONAHA.109.853127.

WHO. *Recommendations for prevention and treatment of pre-eclampsia and eclampsia*. Geneva: World Health Organization; 2011.

Premature Ejaculation

Epidemiology and Demographics: Estimates of the annual prevalence of premature ejaculation vary widely. Internationally, more than 20–30% of men aged 18–70 complain of how rapidly they ejaculate. The new stricter definition of premature ejaculation in which ejaculation occurs within 1 minute upon vaginal penetration would only apply to 1–3% of men. Prevalence may increase with age.

Disorder Description: As stated in DSM-5, premature ejaculation can be defined as:

A. A persistent or recurrent pattern of ejaculation that occurs during partnered sexual activity within approximately 1 minute following vaginal penetration and before the individual wishes. (Note that although premature ejaculation may also be applied to those who engage in nonvaginal sexual activities, a specific duration criterion has not yet been established.)

B. The occurrence must have been present for at least 6 months and must occur on all or almost all occasions of sexual activity (in identified or all situational contexts).

C. The occurrence causes clinically significant distress in the individual.

D. The sexual dysfunction is not better explained by a nonsexual mental disorder, severe relationship distress, stressors, substance, medication, or another medical condition.

Differential Diagnosis: Differential diagnosis should include substance/medication-induced sexual dysfunction and ejaculatory concerns that do not meet diagnostic criteria.

In substance/medication-induced sexual dysfunction, ejaculation problems are due exclusively to substance use, intoxication, or withdrawal.

In ejaculatory concerns that do not meet diagnostic criteria, the patient may complain of early ejaculation and this may cause him distress, but the diagnosis of premature ejaculation would not be warranted.

Secondary Complications: Premature ejaculation may lead to a decrease in self-esteem, a sense of lack of control, and problems with sexual and partner relationships. It may also cause personal distress and/or decreased sexual satisfaction in the sexual partner. If ejaculation occurs prior to penetration, there may be difficulties with conception.

Treatment Complications: Selective serotonin reuptake inhibitors (SSRIs) are the first-line treatment for premature ejaculation. SSRI side effects include nausea, diarrhea, insomnia, headache, anorexia, weight loss, sexual dysfunction, restlessness (akathisia-like), serotonin syndrome (fever diaphoresis, tachycardia, hypertension, delirium, neuromuscular excitability), hyponatremia, seizures (0.2%).

If SSRIs fail or are not tolerated, clomipramine, a tricyclic antidepressant, may be used as second-line treatment. Its most common side effects include blurred vision, nausea, dry mouth, constipation, fatigue, weight gain, increased appetite, dizziness, tremor, headache, myoclonus, drowsiness, lethargy, restlessness, erectile dysfunction, and loss of libido.

Bibliography

American Psychiatric Association. *Diagnostic and statistical manual of mental disorders: DSM-5.* 5th ed. Washington, DC: American Psychiatric Association; 2013.

Hatzimouratidis K, Amar E, Eardley I, et al. Guidelines on male sexual dysfunction: erectile dysfunction and premature ejaculation. *Eur Urol.* 2010;57(5):804–14.

Waldinger MD. The neurobiological approach to premature ejaculation. *J Urol.* 2002;168(6):2359–67.

Waldinger MD, Hengeveld MW, Zwinderman AH. Paroxetine treatment of premature ejaculation: a double-blind, randomized, placebo-controlled study. *Am J Psychiatry.* 1994;151(9):1377–9.

Premenstrual Dysphoric Disorder

Epidemiology and Demographics: The annual prevalence of premenstrual dysphoric disorder (PMDD) in menstruating women is 1.8% to 5.8%, although it is believed that these estimates may be largely inflated because these epidemiological studies have generally been retrospective in design.

Disorder Description: PMDD is a marked change in mood and behavior that develops in the last week of the menstrual cycle before the onset of menses, which resolves in the first week post menses. According to DSM-5, PMDD is diagnosed if:

A. In the majority of menstrual cycles, five or more symptoms must be present in the last week before the onset of menses, begin to *improve* within a few days after the onset of menses, and become *minimal* or absent in the week postmenses.

B. One or more of the following symptoms must be present:
   i. Marked affective lability
   ii. Marked irritability or anger or increased interpersonal conflicts
   iii. Marked depressed mood, feelings of hopelessness, or self-deprecating thoughts
   iv. Marked anxiety, tension, or feelings of being keyed up or on edge

C. One or more of the following symptoms must additionally be present, to reach a total of five symptoms when combined with the above criterion B:
   i. Decreased interest in usual activities
   ii. Subjective difficulty in concentration
   iii. Lethargy, easy fatigability, or marked lack of energy
   iv. Marked change of appetite, overeating, or specific food cravings
   v. Hypersomnia or insomnia
   vi. A sense of being overwhelmed or out of control

vii. Physical symptoms such as breast tenderness or swelling, joint or muscle pain, a sense of "bloating," or weight gain

Differential Diagnosis: Differential diagnosis should include premenstrual syndrome (PMS), dysmenorrhea, bipolar disorder, major depressive disorder, and persistent depressive disorder (dysthymia).

Symptoms of PMS include breast tenderness, fatigue, cramping, bloating, irritability, aggressiveness, depression, inability to concentrate, food cravings, lethargy, and libido change. It is estimated that up to 40% of women of reproductive age are affected by PMS. Although PMS, like PMDD, has an onset of symptoms during the premenstrual phase of the menstrual cycle, symptoms are generally less severe. In PMS vs. PMDD, a minimum of five symptoms is not required, and there is no stipulation of affective symptoms.

Dysmenorrhea is characterized by painful menses, but does not come with affective changes.

In bipolar disorder, major depressive disorder, and persistent depressive disorder, symptoms may be similar to premenstrual dysphoric disorder, but when carefully charted, the symptoms do not follow the premenstrual pattern.

In some cases, women who have premenstrual symptoms may be using hormonal treatments such as contraceptives. If symptoms occur after the implementation of the medication, they may be due to the medication and not an underlying medical condition. If upon stopping hormonal treatment, the symptoms disappear, this would be consistent with the diagnosis of substance/medication-induced depressive disorder.

Secondary Complications: Symptoms may lead to distress and/or impairment in ability to function socially in the week preceding menses. This may manifest as marital problems or problems with children, colleagues, or friends. Chronic social issues should not be confused with those that occur only in association with PMDD.

Treatment Complications: Antidepressants such as selective serotonin reuptake inhibitors (SSRIs) have been shown to be effective in the treatment of premenstrual dysphoric disorder. SSRI side effects include nausea, diarrhea, insomnia, headache, anorexia, weight loss, sexual dysfunction, restlessness (akathisia-like), serotonin syndrome (fever diaphoresis, tachycardia, hypertension, delirium, neuromuscular excitability), hyponatremia, seizures (0.2%).

Oral contraceptives also are effective. The most common side effects of oral contraceptives include bloating, nausea, breast tenderness, and abnormal bleeding. Rarer and more serious side effects include cardiovascular disease, thromboembolic disease, and an increased incidence of certain cancers.

Bibliography

American Psychiatric Association. *Diagnostic and statistical manual of mental disorders: DSM-5.* 5th ed. Washington, DC: American Psychiatric Association; 2013.

Epperson CN, Haga K, Mason GF, et al. Cortical γ-aminobutyric acid levels across the menstrual cycle in healthy women and those with premenstrual dysphoric disorder: A proton magnetic resonance spectroscopy study. *Arch Gen Psychiatry.* 2002;59(9):851–8.

Grady-Weliky T. Premenstrual dysphoric disorder. *New Engl J Med.* 2003;348(5):433–8.

Yonkers KA, Halbreich U, Freeman E, et al. Symptomatic improvement of premenstrual dysphoric disorder with sertraline treatment: a randomized controlled trial. *JAMA.* 1997;278(12):983–8.

Yonkers KA, Brown C, Pearlstein TB, et al. Efficacy of a new low-dose oral contraceptive with drospirenone in premenstrual dysphoric disorder. *Obstet Gynecol.* 2005;106(3):492–501.

Primary Carnitine Deficiency

Epidemiology and Demographics: Incidence is ~1/20,000 to 1/70,000 live births, with ethnic variability. (Higher incidence in Faroe Islands: 1/1,300.) It is inherited in an autosomal recessive manner.

Disorder Description: Primary carnitine deficiency (PCD) is a metabolic disorder characterized by early childhood cardiomyopathy, often associated with weakness and hypotonia, failure to thrive, and recurrent hypoglycemia, hypoketotic seizures, and/or coma.

PCD is caused by a deficiency of the plasma membrane carnitine transporter, caused by mutations in the SLC22A5 gene on Chr 5q23.3. The transporter is essential for L-carnitine transport across the plasma membrane, and its deficiency leads to urinary carnitine wasting and carnitine deficiency. Intracellular carnitine is necessary for the transport of long chain fatty acids into the mitochondria for fatty acid oxidation. When fat is unavailable for energy production, glucose stores are consumed, resulting in hypoglycemia; and fat released from adipose tissue cannot be metabolized and accumulates in the liver, heart, and skeletal muscle leading to hepatic steatosis and lipid myopathy. The production of ketone bodies (used by the brain) is also impaired. Regulation of intra-mitochondrial free coenzyme A (CoA) is also affected, with accumulation of acyl-CoA esters causing inhibition of other pathways of metabolism, such as the Krebs cycle, and pyruvate and amino acid metabolism.

Three main organ systems are involved: cardiac – progressive cardiomyopathy; central nervous system – encephalopathy caused by hypoketotic hypoglycemia; and skeletal muscle – affected by myopathy. Young infants with primary carnitine deficiency usually present with hypoglycemic, hypoketotic encephalopathy, irritability, or seizures at the age of 2–6 months. Often periods of fasting involved with an intercurrent viral illness trigger acute episodes of decompensation. Developmental delay, lethargy, or hypotonia may also be a feature, as well as hepatomegaly, elevated liver transaminases, and secondary hyperammonemia.

Some children may present later, between the ages of 2 and 4 years, with cardiomyopathy or rapidly progressive heart failure. There have also been some descriptions of mild developmental delay as the only manifestation in rare cases. The adult presentation of PCD is rare and can present with fatigability, dilated cardiomyopathy, or arrhythmia. Secondary carnitine deficiency may be present in other metabolic disorders, particularly the organic acidemias.

Diagnosis is based on finding very low free and total carnitine concentrations (<5–10 µmol/L); and confirmed by skin fibroblast testing or genetic confirmation of SLC22A5 mutation. New-born screening is available in some European countries.

Symptoms

Localization site	Comment
Cerebral hemispheres	Hypotonia, developmental regression
	Episodes of metabolic decompensation – irritability, encephalopathy, coma; hypoglycemic seziures
Autonomic nervous system	Hyperammonemia may lead to respiratory depression
	Cardiac arrhythmia due to steatosis and arrhythmogenic effects of acylcarnitines

Secondary Complications: Cardiac arrhythmias and sudden death.

Treatment Complications: The mainstay of treatment is L-carnitine supplementation (100–400 mg/kg/day) and the prevention of hypoglycemia, which is very effective if commenced before organ damage occurs. Hypoglycemic episodes are treated with intravenous dextrose with the goal of return to an anabolic state. The prognosis is very good as long as oral carnitine supplementation is maintained.

L-carnitine can cause dizziness, vertigo, myasthenia, parasthesias.

Bibliography

El-Hattab AW. Systemic primary carnitine deficiency. Mar 15, 2012. Updated Jun 26, 2014. In Pagon RA, Adam MP, Ardinger HH, et al., eds. *GeneReviews*® [Internet]. Seattle (WA): University of Washington, Seattle; 1993–2015. Available from: www.ncbi.nlm.nih.gov/books/NBK84551/. Accessed Sep 12, 2018.

Magoulas PL, El-Hattab AW. Systemic primary carnitine deficiency: an overview of clinical manifestations, diagnosis, and management. *Orphanet J Rare Dis*. 2012;7:68. DOI: 10.1186/1750-1172-7-68.

Online Mendelian Inheritance in Man (OMIM). Carnitine deficiency, systemic primary; CDSP. McKusick VA, ed. Johns Hopkins University. Updated Jul 7, 2014. Entry Number 212140. Available at http://omim.org/entry/212140. Accessed Sep 12, 2018.

Primary Central Sleep Apnea

Epidemiology and Demographics: Prevalence is unknown; however, is estimated to be a rare disease. Some studies suggest a male predominance. Most common in the middle-aged to the elderly.

Predisposing Factors: The pathophysiology of primary central sleep apnea (CSA) is thought to be related to episodes of nocturnal hyperpnea that drive the $PaCO_2$ below the hypocapnic apnea threshold (HAT), which is the $PaCO_2$ below which respiratory motor output ceases and CSA occurs. Factors that increase ventilation such as high ventilatory chemosensitivity to CO_2 or those that raise the HAT (i.e., metabolic alkalosis) increase the propensity for the $PaCO_2$ to be driven below the HAT (low CO_2 reserve).

Disorder Description: Primary CSA has an unknown etiology and is caused by instability of the respiratory control system. It most often occurs in the transition from wakefulness to sleep (during stages N1 and N2 sleep) and is rare during N3 and REM sleep. Central apneas are apneas in which there is a cessation of airflow during sleep that is associated with the complete absence of respiratory effort. Central sleep apnea is associated with symptoms including frequent nocturnal awakenings and awakening with a gasping sensation as well as excessive daytime sleepiness and insomnia.

The diagnosis of primary CSA requires the following criteria: (1) one or more of the following – (a) sleepiness, (b) difficulty initiating or maintaining sleep, frequent awakenings, or nonrestorative sleep, (c) awakening short of breath, (d) snoring, (e) witnessed apneas; (2) (a) polysomnogram with ≥ 5 central apneas and/or central hypopneas per hour of sleep; (b) the number of central apneas and/or central hypopneas is >50% of the total number of apneas and hypopneas; (3) there is no evidence of daytime or nocturnal hypoventilation; (4) the disorder is not better explained by another sleep disorder, medical or neurologic disorder, medication use, or substance use disorder.

Symptoms

Localization site	Comment
Ventral medulla	CO_2-sensitive regions of the ventral medulla (retrotrapezoid nucleus) as well as other ventilatory control nuclei
Mental status and psychiatric aspects/ complications	Sleepiness, depression, social dysfunction

Secondary Complications: Daytime somnolence, depression, social and workplace dysfunction may occur in the setting of sleep fragmentation.

Treatment Complications: Treatment includes positive airway pressure (PAP), bilevel in the spontaneous times mode, or adaptive seroventilation. Acetazolamide may also be used as it lowers the CO_2 apneic threshold and decreases the propensity for hypocapnea-induced CSA.

Difficulty tolerating and compliance with PAP modalities is not uncommon and requires close clinical follow-up. Tachyphylaxis and paresthesias with acetazolamide may occur.

Bibliography

Dempsey JA, Smith CA, Przybylowski T, et al. The ventilator responsiveness to CO2 below eupnoea as a determinant of ventilator stability in sleep. *J Physiol.* 2004;560:1–11.

Eckert DJ, Jordan AS, Merchia P, et al. Central sleep apnea: Pathophysiology and treatment. *Chest.* 2007;131:595–607.

Jahaveri S, Dempsey JA. Central sleep apnea. *Compr Physiol.* 2013;3:141–63.

Sateia M, Berry RB, Bornemann MC, et al. *International classification of sleep disorders.* 3rd ed. Darien, IL: American Academy of Sleep Medicine; 2014.

Primary Coenzyme Q10 Deficiency

Epidemiology and Demographics: Unknown given rarity of the disease.

Disorder Description: Ubiquinone is a lipid-soluble component of virtually all cell membranes and has multiple metabolic functions. Coenzyme Q_{10} (CoQ_{10}) is the predominant human form of endogenous ubiquinone. It is synthesized in the mitochondrial inner membrane.

In addition to its role in the mitochondrial respiratory chain as an electron carrier from complex I and II to complex III, CoQ_{10} is now thought to be involved in a number of cellular functions.

Primary CoQ_{10} deficiency is an autosomal recessive condition with at least five major phenotypes:

1. Encephalomyopathy: recurrent myoglobinuria, brain involvement, and ragged red fibers. Generalized weakness, exercise intolerance, and recurrent myoglobinuria are symptoms of encephalomyopathic form. All patients have proximal muscle weakness. Brain involvement is variable and causes seizures, cognitive impairment, and cerebellar symptoms.

2. Severe infantile multisystemic disease: presents with infantile encephalopathy with renal involvement.

3. Cerebellar ataxia: most common phenotype. Cerebellar atrophy in all patients. Epilepsy (most common), pyramidal signs, intellectual disabilities, myopathic weakness, and delayed motor milestones are other symptoms. Muscle does not show ragged-red fibers.

4. Leigh syndrome: presents with growth retardation, ataxia, and deafness.

5. Isolated myopathy: presents with subacute onset of exercise intolerance and proximal limb weakness at variable ages. Muscle shows ragged-red fibers, and serum lactate and creatine kinase (CK) levels are elevated.

Treatment: Patients with all forms of coenzyme Q_{10} deficiency have shown clinical improvement with oral CoQ_{10} supplementation.

Bibliography

Quinzii CM, Dimauro S, Hirano M. Human coenzyme Q10 deficiency. *Neurochem Res.* 2007;32:723–7.

Primary CNS Angiitis (Vasculitis)

Epidemiology and Demographics: This disorder is quite rare with an unclear incidence but is estimated at 2/100,000. There is a male predominance (7:3). The mean age of presentation is around 50 years, although it can occur at any age and has been described in children.

Disorder Description: Disorder involving inflammation of blood vessels limited to the central nervous system. By definition, this occurs in the absence of any systemic vasculitis or other autoimmune disease. This leads to significant cerebral ischemia and multiple stroke, both ischemic and hemorrhagic.

Symptoms

Localization site	Comment
Cerebral hemispheres	Any manifestation of stroke is possible. There are usually multiple such events with stepwise progression. More common symptoms include hemiparesis, aphasia, ataxia, hemisensory loss, homonymous hemianopia. Seizures and headaches are frequent and often precede strokes
Mental status and psychiatric aspects/complications	Altered mental status. Memory loss. Personality change
Brainstem	Any brainstem stroke syndrome may occur but dysarthria
Cerebellum	Ataxia
Vestibular system	Vertigo
Cranial nerves	Diplopia. Monocular vision loss
Spinal cord	Paraparesis and urinary incontinence

Secondary Complications: Weight loss may be seen but is uncommon compared with systemic vasculitis.

Treatment Complications: Treatment involves long-term steroids or other anti-immune agents. Side effects of the former include weight gain, diabetes, osteoporosis, mania, and infection. Steroid sparing agents may lead to infection.

Bibliography

John S, Hajj RA. CNS vasculitis. *Semin Neurol.* 2014;34(4):405–12.

Rodriguez-Pla A, Monoch DA. Primary angiitis of the central nervous system in adults and children. *Rheum Dis Clin North Am.* 2015;41(1):47–62.

Primary CNS Lymphoma

Epidemiology and Demographics: Despite a recent increase in cases over the past 2 decades, primary CNS lymphoma (PCNSL) is relatively rare, representing less than 3% of all primary CNS tumors. There is an incidence of approximately 0.47 cases per 100,000 annually. PCNSL typically occurs in persons 65 years of age or older, who are immunocompetent. Prior to the institution of anti-retroviral therapy, PCNSL was common in patients with HIV and AIDS. EBV positive CNS lymphoma can occur in other immunocompromised patients, particularly those on immunosuppressive therapy, such as transplant patients.

Male-to-female ratio is 2:1 in immunocompromised patients, but in HIV-infected patients with PCNSL, nearly 95% are male.

PCNSL should be distinguished from systemic Hodgkin's and non-Hodgkin's lymphoma, which can have CNS involvement.

Disorder Description: PCNSL is a non-Hodgkin's lymphoma occurring within the CNS.

Contrast imaging of the brain typically reveals a single enhancing lesion, though in about one-third of cases multiple lesions are seen. Full spinal imaging may be indicated if there appears to be spinal cord involvement on exam.

Once a lesion is identified, diagnosis can be achieved by brain biopsy, CSF analysis with flow cytometry (particularly in cases of leptomeningeal enhancement), or vitrectomy or chorioretinal biopsy (in cases of ocular involvement). Pretreatment with steroids is not recommended as this can decrease the yield of biopsy. Pathology usually reveals diffuse large B-cell lymphoma.

Symptoms

Localization site	Comment
Cerebral hemispheres	Occurs in cerebral hemispheres, usually supratentorially in the frontal lobes, with predilection for periventricular location. Typical locations include the corpus callosum, basal ganglia, thalamus, but PCNSL can be found in any part of the brain. Signs and symptoms depend on part of cerebrum affected. Seizures may occur
Mental status	Cognitive, behavioral, and personality changes, particularly in the elderly. There may be evidence of psychomotor slowing and disorientation on exam. These symptoms are typically secondary to lesion burden and location in the cerebrum
Brainstem	Less typical location
Cerebellum	Less typical location, though usually involved when infratentorial compartment is affected. Presents with ataxia, dizziness, and other cerebellar symptoms. There are case reports of PCNLS affecting the cerebellopontine angle
Cranial nerves	Ocular involvement is not uncommon, particularly involving the posterior parts of the eye (vitreous body, choroidea, retina, and optic nerves). When occurring in isolation from CNS, it is referred to as primary intraocular lymphoma. Presenting symptoms include blurred vision, floaters, or vision loss
Pituitary gland	Case reports involving suprasellar region, presenting with hypopituitarism. Selective pituitary dysfunction may include syndrome of inappropriate antidiuretic hormone secretion (SIADH)
Spinal cord	Rarely can occur as a primary intramedullary spinal cord process, presenting with myelopathy and back pain, or even as a lower motor neuron process with areflexia and flaccid paralysis. Owing to the rarity of this entity, diagnosis is often delayed
Dorsal root ganglia	Extremely rare (case report)
Conus medullaris	Rare, can be involved in primary intramedullary spinal cord lymphoma
Cauda equina	Rare, can be involved in primary intramedullary spinal cord lymphoma. Cauda equina syndrome has been reported as the presenting feature of PCNSL with back pain, numbness, weakness, paresthesias, and bladder dysfunction

Localization site	Comment
Specific spinal roots	Very rarely involved
Plexus	Very rarely involved
Peripheral neuropathy	Rare, there are case reports of isolated peripheral nerve involvement (known as neurolymphomatosis)
Other	Symptoms of raised intracranial pressure (headache, vision changes, nausea/vomiting) Seizures (rare) Does not commonly present with constitutional symptoms, but sometimes reported. Leptomeningeal disease can occur and cause meningismus

Secondary Complications: Systemic metastases and/or relapses outside of the central nervous system are rare, affecting various organs such as the kidney, lymph nodes, testicles, GI tract, lung, and bone, among others. There are case reports of subcutaneous and cutaneous metastases. There is also a case report of PCNSL seeding along a ventriculoperitoneal shunt. There are case reports of PCNSL occurring with intracerebral hemorrhage or inducing paraneoplastic myasthenia gravis.

Treatment Complications: Treatment almost universally entails high-dose intravenous methotrexate-based induction (to induce remission). Often combination induction chemotherapy with another agent, such as rituximab or cytarabine, is used, although there is no clear consensus on what agent should be combined with methotrexate.

While a complete radiographic response is often observed, the high risk of recurrence necessitates a consolidation phase – typically with whole brain radiation or chemotherapy. Whole brain radiation is associated with neurotoxicity, and is sometimes avoided, especially in elderly patients who are particularly vulnerable to its neurotoxic effects.

Some protocols call for intraventricular or intrathecal chemotherapy. While this may result in improved survival rates, there is also a high rate of intra-Ommaya (portal through which to administer medication into the CSF) infection. Delayed neurotoxicity, particularly from whole brain radiation, manifests with various cognitive impairments, such as memory and attention deficits, and even dementia. Finally, methotrexate can cause nephropathy.

Bibliography

Al Bahrani B, Henderson C, Delaney G. Primary central nervous system lymphoma and subcutaneous metastases. *J Neurooncol.* 2000;47(2):141–4.

Carnevale J, Rubenstein JL. The challenge of primary central nervous system lymphoma. *Hematol Oncol Clin North Am.* 2016;30(6):1293–316.

Fitzsimmons A, Upchurch K, Batchelor T. Clinical features and diagnosis of primary central nervous system lymphoma. *Hematol Oncol Clin North Am.* 2005;19(4):689–703, vii.

Herrlinger U, Schabet M, Bitzer M, Petersen D, Krauseneck P. Primary central nervous system lymphoma: from clinical presentation to diagnosis. *J Neurooncol.* 1999;43(3):219–26.

Ko JH, Lu PH, Tang TC, Hsu YH. Metastasis of primary CNS lymphoma along a ventriculoperitoneal shunt. *J Clin Oncol.* 2011;29(34):e823–4

Korfel A, Schlegel U. Diagnosis and treatment of primary CNS lymphoma. *Nat Rev Neurol.* 2013;9(6):317–27.

Masroujeh R, Otrock ZK, Yamout B, Jabbour MN, Bazarbachi A. Myasthenia gravis developing in a patient with CNS lymphoma. *Int J Hematol.* 2010;91(3):522–4

Matsuyama J, Ichikawa M, Oikawa T, et al. Primary CNS lymphoma arising in the region of the optic nerve presenting as loss of vision: 2 case reports, including a patient with a massive intracerebral hemorrhage. *Brain Tumor Pathol.* 2014;31(3):222–8

Nayak L, Pentsova E, Batchelor TT. Primary CNS lymphoma and neurologic complications of hematologic malignancies. *Continuum (Minneap Minn).* 2015;21(2):355–72.

Rees J, Wen P, eds. *Blue books of neurology: Neuro-oncology.* Vol 36. Elsevier Inc. 2010; pp. 201–17.

Primary Cough Headache

Epidemiology and Demographics: This condition is mostly reported in patients older than 40 years.

Disorder Description: This condition is defined as sudden onset, lasting from 1 second to 30 minutes and brought on by and only in association with coughing, straining, or Valsalva's maneuver. A diagnosis of primary cough headache is one of exclusion. The clinician should always search for alternative explanation for etiology of this type of headache. The presentation of symptoms is usually bilateral. Some reports reveal an association with a recent respiratory infection with cough. In addition to sneezing, bending, stooping, or straining, an association with weightlifting has been reported. Subarachnoid hemorrhage should always be considered in this condition before arriving at primary cough headache.

Symptoms

Localization site	Comment
Cerebral hemispheres	Presentation can be unilateral or bilateral; some reports suggest overcrowding of posterior cranial fossa secondary to intracranial mass
Head and neck muscles and ligaments	Association with stretching of cervical ligaments and tendons in causing headache

Secondary Complications: Consideration of alternative etiologies before primary cough headache is important in the evaluation of a patient with complaints of cough-associated headache. There can be serious complications from a primary etiology if missed on clinical evaluation.

Treatment Complications: Published reports suggest a role for indomethacin (25–50 mg three times a day), therapeutic and diagnostic lumbar puncture, methysergide, acetazolamide (500–2000 mg daily), topiramate in treating this type of headache. There have been no reported treatment complications other than the known side effects of medications and known complications of lumbar puncture.

Bibliography

Cutrer FM, Boes CJ. Cough, exertional, and sex headaches. *Neurol Clin North Am.* 2004;22:133–49.

Headache Classification Subcommittee of the International Headache Society. The international classification of headache disorders. 2nd ed. *Cephalalgia.* 2004;24(Suppl 1):1–160.

Maheshwari PK, Pandey A. Unusual headaches. *Ann Neurosci.* 2012;19(4):172–6.

Primary Exertional Headache

Epidemiology and Demographics: Studies show there is a lifetime prevalence of 1%. There is no bias for either sex in the presentation of this type of headache.

Disorder Description: The exact cause of this condition is still unclear. An association exists with cardiac chest pain, specifically angina and unstable angina. In situations involving chest pain, the headache may be bilateral or unilateral. The headache has been described as throbbing in nature and not attributable to any other cause. Activities that can influence or cause this headache include running, rowing, tennis, and swimming. When evaluating patients with this differential diagnosis, always consider alternative factors like subarachnoid hemorrhage, pheochromocytoma, cardiac etiology, artery dissection, paranasal sinusitis, intracranial neoplasm, colloid cyst of third ventricle, hypoplasia of aortic arch after repair of coarctation.

Symptoms

Localization site	Comment
Cerebral hemispheres	One study suggests a link with craniovascular afferent nerves. Another study suggests a role of serotonin, bradykinin, histamine, and substance P that stimulate nociceptive intracranial receptors during headache, especially with decreased venous return to the heart

Secondary Complications: If secondary etiologies are not considered seriously, the primary etiology of this headache can go unnoticed and have serious complications.

Treatment Complications: There are no established treatments for this type of headache. Some suggest a "warm up" period before exercise or avoiding the specific activity outright. Indomethacin at doses of 25–150 mg daily has been reported to be helpful in these conditions, especially when taken 1 hour before exertional activity. Prophylaxis medications like beta blockers have also been used as suggested in some published reports.

Bibliography

Cutrer FM, Boes CJ. Cough, exertional, and sex headaches. *Neurol Clin North Am.* 2004;22:133–49.

Grace A, Horgan J, Breathnach K, et al. Anginal headache and its basis. *Cephalalgia.* 1997;17:195–6.

Maheshwari PK, Pandey A. Unusual headaches. *Ann Neurosci.* 2012;19(4):172–6.

Rasmussen BK, Olesen J. Symptomatic and nonsymptomatic headaches in a general population. *Neurology.* 1992;42:1225–31.

Primary Headache Associated with Sexual Activity

Epidemiology and Demographics: There are no large population studies that have studied primary headache associated with sexual activity. Reports in literature suggest that the pre-orgasmic type accounts for less than a third of all sexual activity-associated headache.

Disorder Description: There are two forms of this headache: pre-orgasmic and orgasmic. The pre-orgasmic form is characterized by a dull, bi-occipital, pressure-like or aching pain that appears during sexual activity and increases with mounting sexual excitement. The patient is often aware of increased contraction in neck and jaw muscles. These headaches often start mildly and intensify slowly and gradually with increasing sexual excitement. The median duration of this condition has been reported to be about 1 hour. The orgasmic form of this headache has a sudden and explosive onset followed by severe throbbing head pain that occurs just prior to or at the moment of orgasm. These types of headaches rapidly generalize to involve the entire head. Some reports suggest that the "active partner" is more likely to have sexual headache than the "passive partner."

Symptoms

Localization site	Comment
Cerebral hemispheres	Presentation is unilateral or bilateral. Pre-orgasmic type starts in the bi-occipital territory. Orgasmic type can be unilateral or bilateral and generalize rapidly to entire head

Secondary Complications: There are no specific complications from this headache. In the case of sudden onset headache symptoms, concern should be given to address and evaluate for alternative etiologies.

Treatment Complications: Indomethacin at a dose of 50–75 mg or naproxen 1–2 hours before sexual activity has been reported to be helpful. Propanolol at a dose of 40 mg 1–2 hours before sexual activity has also been reported to be helpful. Environmental concerns like anxiety associated with sexual activity can also be addressed with counseling. There have been no reported complications from these treatments.

Bibliography

Johns DR. Benign sexual headache within a family. *Arch Neurol.* 1986;43:1158.

Lance JW. Headaches related to sexual activity. *J Neurol Neurosurg Psychiatry.* 1976;39:1226.

Maheshwari PK, Pandey A. Unusual headaches. *Ann Neurosci.* 2012;19(4):172–6.

Primary Lateral Sclerosis

Epidemiology and Demographics: Listed under the rare diseases. Exact prevalence unknown. Presents normally in the 4th decade of life. Males and females are affected equally.

Disorder Description: Primary lateral scerosis (PLS) is a rare, progressive neuromuscular disorder that affects the upper motor neurons (UMNs) resulting in stiffness of the muscles of the lower extremities. It may progress to affect the upper extremities or the bulbar muscles.

Presents during midlife as progressive weakness and spasticity of the muscles of the lower extremities. It appears asymmetrically – tends to affect one leg, and then progresses to the other leg. Over time (mean 8 years), it may start affecting the lower motor neurons (LMNs) as well. Thus, it has been proposed by some that PLS may be a slowly progressive form of amyotrophic lateral sclerosis (ALS) that has a more benign prognosis. Rate of progression is variable from one patient to another. As it affects the bulbar muscles, it can cause dysphagia and dysarthria.

Though no one genetic mutation has been found, one paper identifies a Spanish family with autosomal dominant disease manifesting in the 5th or 6th decade of life with either dementia or PLS. A mutation of Arg573Gly was identified in this particular family. Alsin mutations cause ALS as well as juvenile forms of PLS. Other genetic causes of ALS and PLS are phenotypically overlapping.

Symptoms

Localization site	Comment
Cerebral hemispheres	30% have hyperintense lesions in T2 sequences of MRI (post-ischemic vs post-inflammatory) and 9% have subcortical vascular encephalopathy
Mental status and psychiatric aspects/ complications	One genetic cluster identified one family with a mutation with autosomal dominant inheritance. In this case, affected members had either PLS or dementia. Other study with a cohort of 76 patients failed to see a relationship but found that 20% of patients had pathologic crying or laughing
Spinal cord	UMNs affected first (asymmetric spasticity), and LMNs involved as disease progresses (weakness and tongue fasciculations)

Treatment Complications: Potential complications of antispasmodic agents include sedation, headache, or seizures.

Bibliography

Gomez-Tortosa E, et al. Familial primary lateral sclerosis or dementia associated with ARG573Gly TBK1 mutation. *J Neurol Neurosurg Psychiatry.* 2017;88(11):996–7. Post Script letter.

Wais V, et al. The concept and diagnostic criteria of primary lateral sclerosis. *Acta Neurol Scand.* 2017;136(3):204–11.

Primary Progressive Aphasia (PPA)

Epidemiology and Demographics: Age of onset in the majority of patients is before age 65 years, but the overall epidemiology of primary progressive aphasia (PPA) is unclear.

Disorder Description: PPA is a clinical syndrome characterized by an early, prominent isolated impairment of language, insidious in onset, progressive over time, and impairing activities of daily living. If a secondary cause of aphasia is present, such as a strategic stroke or tumor, a diagnosis of PPA cannot be made. Prominent early impairment in memory or prominent visuospatial disturbances also exclude a diagnosis of PPA.

Mesulum first coined the term PPA in 1982, in describing six patients without dementia who presented with a slowly progressive aphasia. A classification scheme for PPA was later proposed by Gorno-Tempini et al. in 2011, to standardize diagnostic criteria used by researchers. Specifically, three variants of PPA can be distinguished based exclusively on clinical criteria, or with additional support by available imaging (imaging-supported diagnosis) or pathology (diagnosis with definite pathology).

Agrammatic variant PPA (agPPA) is characterized by effortful speech in short phrases, with omissions of words without semantic meaning such as 'the' or 'not' (grammatical morphemes.) An apraxia of speech can be seen, with articulation errors. Prosody is impaired. Patients may have difficulty understanding complicated syntax, such as "The car that the truck hit was green." A written language production test, such as asking the patient to write a description of a picture, may reveal subtle grammatical errors. Of note, single-word comprehension and object knowledge are typically preserved in agPPA patients. Left posterior frontal and insular lobe atrophy may be seen on MRI, and hypoperfusion or hypometabolism may be seen on SPECT or PET. Notably, patients with corticobasal syndrome or progressive supranuclear palsy (PSP) can initially present with agPPA.

Semantic variant PPA (svPPA) is characterized by prominent severe deficits in naming and single-word comprehension, with relative preservation of other language domains. Patients may also have difficulty reading and writing words with irregular spellings (surface dyslexia/dysgraphia). Bilateral anterior temporal lobe atrophy (left worse than right) may be seen on MRI, and hypoperfusion or hypometabolism may be seen on SPECT or PET.

Logopenic variant PPA (lvPPA) is characterized by effortful speech with word-finding difficulties, without frank grammatical errors. Patients may occasionally make phonologic paraphasic errors. Prosody is normal. A deficit in phonologic short-term memory is a proposed underlying mechanism for lvPPA. In keeping with this hypothesis, lvPPA patients typically have difficulty repeating sentences, but are able to repeat single words. Left posterior perisylvian or parietal atrophy may be seen on MRI, and hypoperfusion or hypometabolism may be seen on SPECT or PET.

PPA has heterogeneous pathologic features, with most demonstrating tau-positive, ubiquitin/ TDP43-positive frontotemporal lobar degeneration pathology, and some demonstrating Alzheimer's disease (AD) pathology. Specifically, agPPA is linked to tau-positive pathology, svPPA is linked to ubiquitin-positive, TDP43-positive pathology, and lvPPA is linked to AD pathology. Progranulin (GRN) gene mutation has been observed in autosomal dominant cases of PPA. Interestingly, the same mutation can present as PPA in one patient, and behavioral variant frontotemporal dementia (bvFTD) in a family member. Mesulam et al. suggest that the varying presentation may be due to selective vulnerability of certain neural networks in different individuals, which may be either genetic or acquired.

Distinguishing PPA from AD is important clinically. Different aspects of ADLs (activities of daily living) are affected in the two disease processes, and different intervention strategies are used in PPA and AD. Specifically, some PPA patients may benefit from learning sign language, using voice synthesizers, or laptops with stored words or phrases.

Primary Torsion Dystonia

Epidemiology and Demographics: The frequency of DYT1 dystonia is estimated at 1/9000 in the Ashkenazi Jewish population.

Disorder Description: The term primary torsion dystonia (PTD) is based on an older classification system of dystonia in which disorders were classified based on age of onset, location, and etiology. PTD was defined as a monogenic dystonia classified by age of onset. Since then, significant discoveries have been made in the genes responsible for primary torsion dystonia, and the temporal profile of symptoms. What was previously thought of as PTD is now actually classified as several distinct diseases including DYT1 and DYT6 dystonia. DYT1 dystonia is the most commonly inherited dystonia. There is an autosomal dominant mode of inheritance with incomplete penetrance although some degree of anticipation has been reported. Mutations in the TOR1A gene cause abnormalities in the torsinA protein. It is more common in Ashkenazi Jews. Symptom onset may be as early as 9 years of age, and cases starting in adulthood have been reported. Symptoms usually begin with a focal action induced dystonia such as abnormal posturing of a foot when walking. DYT6 mutations occur in the Amish Mennonites.

It is caused by mutations in the THAP1 gene. DYT6 is inherited in an autosomal dominant fashion and is characterized by focal, predominantly cranio-cervical dystonia and dysphagia.

Symptoms

Localization site	
Cerebral hemispheres	Cortical involvement including the parietal and cingulate cortices
	Subcortical circuits involving sensorimotor basal ganglia and thalamus
Brainstem	Pontine lesions outside of the cerebello-cerebral-thalamo circuits
Cerebellum	Involved in network model with cerebral-thalamo circuits

Secondary Complications: Untreated sustained dystonic posturing may lead to orthopedic deformities including scoliosis and joint contractures.

Treatment Complications: Oral medications may cause anticholinergic effects and sedation. Botulinum toxin injections may cause transient unintended weakness and spread of toxin beyond the injected area.

Bibliography

Albanese A, Bhatia K, Bressman S, et al. Phenomenology and classification of dystonia: a consensus update. *Mov Disord*. 2013;28:863–73.

Bressman SB. Dystonia genotypes, phenotypes, and classification. *Adv Neurol*. 2004;94:101–7.

Fernandez H, Machado A, Pandya M. *Practical approach to movement disorders: diagnosis and management*. 2nd ed. New York, US: Demos Medical; 2014.

Fuchs T, Gavarini S, Saunders-Pullman R, et al. Mutations in the THAP1 gene are responsible for DYT6 primary torsion dystonia. *Nat Genet*. 2009;41(3):286–8.

Phibbs FT, Hedera P. Update on the genetics of movement disorders. *Continuum (Minneap Minn)*. 2010;16(1, Neurology):77–95.

Saunders-Pullman R. Genetics of dystonia. *Continuum (Minneap Minn)*. 2008;14(2, Neurology):65–89.

Progressive Multifocal Leukoencephalopathy (PML)

Epidemiology and Demographics: Occurs in immunosuppressed individuals. Classically known as an AIDS-defining illness in more recent years, it has occurred as a complication of monoclonal antibody therapies in multiple sclerosis and Crohn's disease.

Disorder Description: Caused by the ubiquitous JC virus. Leads to multifocal cerebral lesions resulting in abnormal neurologic symptoms based on location of those lesions. Progresses between 6 months and many years.

Diagnosed with clinical history in combination with positive CSF JC virus PCR.

Treatment is immune reconstitution.

Symptoms

Localization site	Comment
Cerebral hemispheres	Focal neurologic signs, seizures
Mental status and psychiatric aspects/complications	Encephalopathy, delirium
Brainstem	Dysphagia, dysarthria, diplopia
Cerebellum	Ataxia

Secondary Complications: Aspiration pneumonia, decubitus ulcers.

Treatment Complications: Immune reconstitution inflammatory syndrome (IRIS) is worsening of lesions due to increased vasogenic edema and potential tissue damage due to immune response to the virus. Can be managed with steroids if worsening is severe.

Bibliography

Aminoff MJ, Josephson SA, eds. *Aminoff's neurology and general medicine*. 5th ed. London, UK: Elsevier; 2014.

Bauer J, Gold R, Adams O, Lassmann H. Progressive multifocal leukoencephalopathy and immune reconstitution inflammatory syndrome (IRIS). *Acta Neuropathologica* [Online]. 2015;130(6):751–64.

Progressive Myoclonic Epilepsy

Epidemiology and Demographics: Rare. Onset typically in children and adolescents.

Disorder Description: A group of neurodegenerative diseases with similar clinical features characterized by disabling stimulus-induced or action myoclonus, generalized tonic–clonic seizures (GTCS), motor or gait abnormalities, and neuropsychiatric decline. Other seizure types such as tonic or absence may occur.

- Unverricht–Lundborg disease (EMP1): The most common. Autosomal recessive (AR) inheritance associated with cystatin B (CSTB) gene mutations. Onset ages 6–16 years. Symptoms may be relatively mild.
- Lafora body disease (EMP2): AR inheritance associated with laforin (EPM2A) or malin (EPM2B/NHLRC1) gene mutations. Typically of adolescent onset. Intracytoplasmic Lafora bodies seen on axillary skin biopsy. Seizures highly refractory, with rapid cognitive, visual, and motor deterioration.
- Myoclonic epilepsy with ragged red fibers (MERRF): Maternal inheritance. Several mutations in mitochondrial DNA have been described. Ragged red fibers on muscle biopsy. Generalized seizures more prominent in some forms, ataxia more so in others. Associated with short stature, hearing loss, optic atrophy, and cardiomyopathy.
- Neuronal ceroid lipofuscinoses (NCL): Usually AR inheritance, some AD. Lysosomal storage disease with at least 14 genetic subtypes and varying ages of onset from infancy to adulthood. Granular osmophilic deposits on skin biopsy, leukocyte enzyme and genetic testing diagnostic. Myoclonus less prominent in some forms or seen in late stages. Associated retinal abnormalities with visual loss, cognitive and motor deterioration, early death.
- Sialidosis: Autosomal recessive (AR) inheritance. Lysosomal storage disease associated with mutations in the α-N-acetyl neuraminidase-1 (NEU1) gene. Sialo-oligosaccharides may be found in urine, neuraminidase deficiency may be seen with leukocyte enzyme analysis. Age of onset variable, from infancy to adulthood. Macular cherry red spot, visual loss, hyperreflexia, and later onset myoclonus. Cognitive impairments with earlier onset disease.
- Dentatorubral-pallidoluysian atrophy (DRPLA): Autosomal dominant (AD) inheritance, with CAG trinucleotide repeat expansion of the DRPLA gene on chromosome 12. Larger repeat size associated with earlier onset and more severe symptoms. Myoclonus, seizures, choreathetosis, ataxia, dementia usually before 2nd decade.
- Gaucher disease (Type 3, Neuronopathic): AR inheritance. Lysosomal storage disease associated with gene mutations resulting in glucocerebrosidase deficiency. Gaze abnormalities, dementia, ataxia, spasticity, generalized seizures, in addition to myoclonus.
- Action myoclonus–renal failure syndrome (EPM4): AR inheritance, due to SCARB2 gene mutations. Myoclonus and renal dysfunction due to proteinuria with onset in the second or third decade. Relative sparing of cognitive function.
- Progressive myoclonus epilepsy–ataxia syndrome (EPM5): Onset between ages 5 and 10 years, with myoclonus, epilepsy, and ataxia secondary to the PRICKLE gene mutation. Relative sparing of cognitive function.
- "North Sea" progressive myoclonus epilepsy (EPM6): Due to mutations in the GOSR2 gene. Ataxia from age 2 years, myoclonus and epilepsy by age 6–7 years, and skeletal abnormalities such as scoliosis by adolescence. Relative sparing of cognitive function. Elevated creatine phosphokinase (CPK) levels.

Correct diagnosis of the underlying etiology is determined by inheritance pattern, age of onset, associated symptoms, genetic screening, skin or muscle biopsy, and enzyme testing. Prognosis is variable depending on the etiology of the syndrome. Intellectual disability ranges from mild cognitive impairment to a more rapidly progressive dementia. Lafora body disease, NCL, and Gaucher disease are eventually fatal, while later onset EMP1 may occur with a more indolent course with milder intellectual decline.

The treatment of myoclonus and seizures involves the broad-spectrum antiepileptic drugs (AEDs) such as valproate, levetiracetam, topiramate, and zonisamide. Clonazepam may also be useful.

Symptoms

Localization site	Comment
Cerebral hemispheres	Action or stimulus-induced myoclonus, GTCS, tonic, absence seizures. Dystonia, rigidity, spasticity, tremor. EEG associated with generalized spike or polyspike and wave discharges and a photoparoxysmal response. MRIs may show cortical and thalamic atrophy
Mental status and psychiatric aspects/ complications	Mild to severe cognitive impairments depending on etiology. Mood lability and depression common. Behavioral issues may occur. Excessive stimulation and stress may exacerbate myoclonus
Cerebellum	Ataxia may be observed
Cranial nerves	Retinal abnormalities and visual loss may be observed

Secondary Complications: Depression, anxiety, and increased suicidality are common, requiring long-term psychosocial support. Patients often have significant neurorehabilitation needs. Genetic counseling is important for family if a definite genetic cause has been determined. MERFF associated with short stature, hearing loss, optic atrophy, and cardiomyopathy with conduction abnormalities.

Treatment Complications: Valproate, and to a lesser extent topiramate and zonisamide, may be avoided in patients with known mitochondrial dysfunction. Valproate side effects include hyperactivity, weight gain, transaminitis, thrombocytopenia, pancreatitis, and known teratogenic effects. Levetiracetam may exacerbate mood disorders. Topiramate and zonisamide are associated with neuropsychiatric complaints, nephrolithiasis, metabolic acidosis, anhidrosis, and closed angle glaucoma. Benzodiazepines are sedating and can cause respiratory depression. An inappropriate selection of AEDs such as phenytoin, carbamazepine, oxcarbazepine, lamotrigine, gabapentin, or viagbatrin may exacerbate myoclonus and other seizure types.

Bibliography

Kalviainen R. Progressive myoclonus epilepsies. *Semin Neurol.* 2015;35(3):293–9.

Malek N, Stewart W, Greene J. The progressive myoclonic epilepsies. *Pract Neurol.* 2015;15(3):164–71.

Progressive Supranuclear Palsy (PSP)

Epidemiology and Demographics: Age of onset is typically in the 60s with an estimated prevalence of 5/100,000 persons.[1]

Disorder Description: Progressive supranuclear palsy (PSP) is a neurodegenerative condition characterized by vertical gaze palsy, early postural instability with falls, and progressive dementia. The distinguishing feature of PSP is vertical gaze palsy. Limitation of upgaze is frequently described for PSP, but is actually non-specific and can be seen with normal aging. Loss of voluntary downgaze can be key finding pointing to PSP in mildly demented patients with gait impairment and/or falls. Supranuclear paralyses of upgaze and lateral gaze may manifest one or more years after downward gaze impairment. Slow voluntary saccadic movement is another early finding. In contrast to voluntary eye movements, oculocephalics are preserved until late in the course of illness.[1] MRI reveals distinct midbrain atrophy. In sagittal section, the midbrain takes on a beaked appearance ("hummingbird sign").

Falls occur early in the disease course. The cause of falls is likely multifactorial, due to prominent postural instability, axial rigidity, bradykinesia, visual impairment, and cognitive impairment. Patients may suddenly "rocket" up out of a seated position in an impulsive attempt to stand, and fall backwards. This is known as the "rocket sign," and one manifestation of the frontal lobe dysfunction observed in PSP.[1]

Classically grouped with the Parkinson-plus syndromes, PSP is now also recognized as a frontotemporal dementia (FTD)-related disorder. About 20% of PSP patients initially present with behavioral changes, and up to 30% will meet criteria for behavioral variant frontotemporal dementia (bvFTD).[2] Common behavioral symptoms include executive dysfunction, apathy, and perseverative behaviors.[3] Cognitive impairment in PSP is classically described as subcortical in nature, with prominent cognitive slowing, prolonged thinking time on problem-solving tasks, and poor performance on timed verbal fluency tasks.[3] More recently, a cortical pattern of impairment has also been described, presenting with speech apraxia or non-fluent aphasia.[4]

The classic presentation of PSP described above is also known as Richardson syndrome. Other phenotypic variants of PSP include PSP-parkinsonism, PSP-pure akinesia with gait freezing, PSP-corticobasal syndrome, PSP-bvFTD, PSP-primary lateral sclerosis, and PSP-cerebellar. PSP is a tauopathy, and these different phenotypes can be attributed to tau deposition in different cortical and subcortical regions. Though the initial presentation differs for each variant, the clinical picture converges, and patients eventually develop vertical gaze palsy, postural instability, and falls.[1]

Symptoms

Localization site	Comment
Cerebral hemispheres	Cortex (in a portion of patients) – apraxia or aphasia[4]
	Subcortical structures – subcortical pattern of cognitive impairment
	Basal ganglia – parkinsonism
Brainstem	Midbrain – vertical gaze palsy, progressive to gaze paralysis
Cerebellum	Deep cerebellar nuclei (in PSP-cerebellar type) – ataxia[1]

Secondary Complications: Falls can cause significant injury. Dysphagia can lead to aspiration, and is a major cause of morbidity and mortality in PSP.[1]

Treatment Complications: Levodopa may have limited benefits for improving gait and tone for patients with the PSP-parkinsonism variant.[1] In general, however, PSP along with other Parkinson-plus syndromes shows a poor response to levodopa. Management of PSP is largely symptomatic. A multi-disciplinary approach is crucial. Early evaluation by physiotherapists to assess gait can help prevent falls and maximize mobility. Occupational therapists can assist patients to maintain independence with ADLs (activities of daily living). Speech pathologists can help with speech apraxia. Later in the disease course, regular swallow evaluations are essential for assessing dysphagia and making dietary adjustments as needed.

References

1. McFarland NR. Diagnostic approach to atypical parkinsonian syndromes. *Continuum (Minneap Minn)*. 2016;22:1117–42.
2. Finger EC. Frontotemporal dementias. *Continuum (Minneap Minn)*. 2016;22:464–89.
3. Kobylecki C, et al. Cognitive-behavioural features of progressive supranuclear palsy syndrome overlap with frontotemporal dementia. *J Neurol*. 2015;262:916–22.
4. Josephs KA, et al. Atypical progressive supranuclear palsy underlying progressive apraxia of speech and nonfluent aphasia. *Neurocase*. 2005;11:283–96.

Progressive Systemic Sclerosis (Scleroderma)

Epidemiology and Demographics: Systemic sclerosis is uncommon, with incidence at 9–19 cases per million per year, resulting in an estimated 100,000 cases in the United States. There is a female predominance, mostly at child-bearing ages, but declining after menopause. The most common age of onset is 30–50 years. Higher rates of scleroderma spectrum disorders are seen in the United States and Australia (United States more so than Australia) than in Japan or Europe. It is also more prevalent in African American populations than white populations, and often with more pulmonary involvement with worse outcomes.

Disorder Description: Progressive systemic sclerosis is also known as scleroderma (most commonly) or systemic sclerosis. It is a heterogeneous and multi-organ system connective tissue autoimmune disorder largely characterized by fibrosis and vasculopathy. Most commonly, cutaneous disease resulting in skin thickening, scarring, and joint calcification is seen. However, it frequently affects the lungs through fibrosis, and even pulmonary hypertension. GI tract can also be affected, mostly through inflammation and impaired motility. Renal involvement can result in failure, and worsens prognosis. Central nervous system involvement is rare. Most of its neuromuscular involvement is due to other organ failure or secondary to systemic processes. There can be entrapment, mostly located in carpal tunnel, but also sensory as well as sensorimotor neuropathies. Rarely there will be vascular ischemia causing mononeuritis multiplex. See below for further manifestations.

Scleroderma is an acquired sporadic autoimmune disorder. Etiology is precisely unclear, but there is consideration of environmental exposure and molecular mimicry (namely human cytomegalovirus, parvovirus B19, though without significant amounts of evidence). Anti-Scl-70 (anti-topoisomerase-I) and anti-U1-RNP positivity increases the risk of nervous system involvement.

Largely a clinical diagnosis. Antinuclear autoantibodies (ANA) are positive; anti-Scl-70 and anti-centromere positive (both are highly specific for systemic sclerosis). Anti-Scl-70 positivity is associated with decreased life span. Commonly anemia is present. Erythrocyte sedimentation rate is usually normal. Full-thickness skin biopsy may be needed. If there is myopathy related to systemic sclerosis, creatine kinase (CK) is rarely more than insignificantly elevated. Electromyography (EMG) will demonstrate decreased duration of motor unit potentials and increased frequency of polyphasic motor units. Muscle biopsy is rarely done, and at most would show mild abnormalities, including increased connective tissue, proliferation of intima in endomysial and perimysial blood vessels, and occasional perivascular infiltrates. However, if myositis develops, CK may exceed twice the normal level, EMG will be similar to polymyositis, and MRI can help delineate affected muscles.

Symptoms

Localization site	Comment
Cerebral hemispheres	Headache, seizures
Cranial nerves	Many cranial neuropathies have been reported. Most commonly, trigeminal nerve (CN V) is involved (5–15%). However, CN II–X (optic, oculomotor, trochlear, abducens, facial, auditory, and glossopharyngeal) have also been described
Spinal cord	Radiculopathy from compression (connective tissue disorder) Myelopathy: impaired vibratory sense, band-like paresthesias, hyperreflexia, impotence, and quadriparesis. Possibly due to compression and calcinosis
Plexus	Brachial plexopathy
Peripheral neuropathy	Entrapment: carpal tunnel syndrome (can be presenting sign) Symmetric sensory polyneuropathy Mixed sensory and motor polyneuropathy (may precede official diagnosis) Mononeuritis multiplex (mostly due to vasculitis and subsequent nerve infarction, which is rare) Cutaneous neuropathy Autonomic neuropathy

Localization site	Comment
Muscle	Mild, indolent type of proximal myopathy Myositis Weakness, possibly due to secondary atrophy from deconditioning, disuse atrophy. Chronic noninflammatory myopathy characterized (atrophy and fibrosis without elevated muscle enzyme levels). Inflammatory myositis (rare)

Secondary Complications: Scleroderma has diffuse systemic, though mostly non-neurologic, manifestations. Cutaneous and musculoskeletal manifestation includes thickened/scarred skin and joint calcinosis. Vascular presentations include Raynaud's phenomenon, and progress to frank vasculopathy including necrosis and digital ulcers. However, most concerning is pulmonary fibrosis and renal involvement, the latter of which portends poorly with respect to prognosis. Pulmonary and renal involvement can lead to pulmonary hypertension, as well as generalized uncontrolled hypertension, with associated hypertensive sequelae (stroke, vision changes, end organ damage, etc.), and even heart failure.

Treatment Complications: There is no single treatment for systemic sclerosis. Usually it is tailored to specific sequelae, such as ACE inhibitors for renal failure, PDE-5 inhibitors for pulmonary hypertension, diuresis for heart failure, etc. Prednisone and immunosuppressants such as mycophenolate mofetil are used, but more as therapy for pulmonary fibrosis and cutaneous manifestations. Treatment for trigeminal involvement is difficult as steroids may or may not help, and clinicians may need to resort to pain control through analgesics, antidepressants, anticonvulsants (i.e., carbamazepine, etc.), and other methods akin to chronic neuropathic pain. Treatment for entrapment neuropathies is largely conservative if not serious, and surgical if it is.

Complications of treatment depend on the clinical manifestations, resulting in specific therapies. Steroids and immunomodulators increase risk of illness or infection, or commonly cause gastrointestinal symptoms.

Bibliography

Averbuch-Heller L, Steiner I, Abramsky O. Neurologic manifestations of progressive systemic sclerosis. *Arch Neurol.* 1992;49:1292.

Denton CP, Khanna D. Systemic sclerosis. *Lancet.* 2017;390(10103):1685–99. DOI: 10.1016/S0140-6736(17)30933-9.

Hietaharju A, Jääskeläinen S, Kalimo H, Hietarinta M. Peripheral neuromuscular manifestations in systemic sclerosis (scleroderma). *Muscle Nerve.* 1993;16:1204.

Longo DL, Kasper DL, Fauci A, et al., eds. *Harrison's principles of internal medicine.* 17th ed. New York: McGraw-Hill; 2016. pp. 2906–106.

Prolactinoma

Epidemiology and Demographics: Prolactinomas are the most common type of secreting pituitary tumor, accounting for approximately 40% of all pituitary adenomas. They occur with an estimated incidence of 6–10 cases per million per year, which translates into a prevalence of approximately 60–100 cases per million. The majority of these prolactinomas are small, slow-growing, intrasellar microadenomas, which present more commonly in young women likely as a function of greater symptom burden caused by hyperprolactinemia. The larger macroadenomas tend to present more commonly in males and at a later age. It remains unclear if the difference between sexes is due to delayed diagnosis or whether gender-specific differences in tumor behavior exist. In the pediatric–adolescent age group, prolactinomas are rare and typically present in females as macroadenomas with symptoms of mass effect.

Disorder Description: Prolactinoma, or lactotroph adenoma, is a type of pituitary adenoma (a benign tumor of the anterior pituitary). Lesions smaller than 1 cm are classified as microadenomas, and lesions larger than 1 cm are macroadenomas. Prolactinomas are made of cells that produce the hormone prolactin, thereby usually causing hyperprolactinemia. There are no established risk factors for sporadic prolactinomas. Prolactinomas are rarely hereditary though can be seen in the setting of multiple endocrine neoplasia type 1 syndrome in association with parathyroid gland hyperplasia and pancreatic islet cell tumors. MEN-1 is inherited in an autosomal dominant fashion, affecting both sexes equally with no geographic or ethnic preference.

Symptoms

Localization site	Comment
Pituitary gland	Hypersecretion of prolactin causes oligoamenorrhea, infertility, and galactorrhea in women, hypogonadism, decreased libido, erectile dysfunction, infertility, gynecomastia (rare), and galactorrhea (rare) in men, and pubertal delay in children
	Hypopituitarism may result from compression of the pituitary stalk and resulting adrenal insufficiency, hypothyroidism, hypogonadism, or growth retardation
	Pituitary apoplexy results from local disruption of the arterial blood supply to the pituitary gland and may present acutely as headache, visual loss, diplopia, and altered mentation (rare)
Base of skull	Headaches may result from expansion of the sella turcica due to growth of the tumor
	CSF rhinorrhea may occur from downward extension of the tumor through the sphenoid sinus (rare)
Cranial nerves	Bitemporal hemianopia and diminished visual acuity may result from upward extension and compression of the optic chiasm and optic nerves
	Diplopia may result from lateral extension and compression of the oculomotor nerve
Mental status	Pituitary apoplexy may present as an acute alteration in alertness that may be confused for other medical or psychiatric disorders

Secondary Complications: Untreated prolactinomas causing amenorrhea in females will result in chronic estrogen deficiency leading to low bone mass and increased risk of fracture. Similarly in males, lower levels of testosterone from high prolactin levels can result in decreased bone mass as well as anemia.

Treatment Complications: Primary therapy for all prolactinomas regardless of size are dopamine agonists of which common side effects include headaches, nausea, postural hypotension, fatigue, anxiety, depression, and rarely psychosis. For large tumors in which medical therapy fails or is contraindicated, transphenoidal surgery or radiation therapy may be warranted. Complications include CSF leak, damage to internal carotid artery or optic nerves/chasm, and hypopituitarism.

Bibliography

Ciccarelli A, Daly AF, Beckers A. The epidemiology of prolactinomas. *Pituitary.* 2005;8(1):3–6.

Klibanski A. Clinical practice. Prolactinomas. *N Engl J Med.* 2010;362:1219–26.

Schlechte JA. Clinical practice. Prolactinoma. *N Engl J Med* 2003;349:2035–41.

Wong A, Eloy JA, Couldwell WT, Liu JK. Update on prolactinomas. Part 1: clinical manifestations and diagnostic challenges. *J Clin Neurosci.* 2015;22:1562–67.

Wong A, Eloy JA, Couldwell WT, Liu JK. Update on prolactinomas. Part 2: treatment and management strategies. *J Clin Neurosci.* 2015;22:1568–74.

Prolonged QT Syndrome

Epidemiology and Demographics: Can be inherited or acquired, both of which are more common in women. The inherited form has a prevalence of 1/7000 people and is responsible for 2000–3000 deaths annually in the United States. It usually becomes symptomatic in childhood. The acquired form is generally drug induced.

Disorder Description: Abnormalities of cardiac repolarization lead to prolongation of the QT interval. This can lead to torsade de pointe and ventricular tachycardia or fibrillation.

Symptoms

Localization site	Comment
Cerebral hemispheres	Syncope without premonitory symptoms, especially with physical activity or emotion. Seizure

Secondary Complications: Sudden cardiac death.

Treatment Complications: Beta blockers may cause fatigue, impotence, orthostasis, and exercise intolerance.

Bibliography

Kramer DB, Zimetbaum PJ. Long-QT syndrome. *Cardiol Rev.* 2011;19(5):217–25.

Vincent GM. The long QT syndrome. *Indian Pacing Electrophysiol J.* 2002;2(4):127–42.

Pronator Syndrome (also see Anterior Interosseous Nerve Syndrome)

Epidemiology and Demographics: As summarized by Rodner et al., the disease is rare in the United States, and the incidence and prevalence are not known.

Disorder Description: The pronator syndrome may present with the same symptoms as carpal tunnel syndrome of numbness in the first three fingers. It can also mimic some of the weakness found in the anterior interosseous nerve syndrome. Please see the table below for differentiating points among the differential diagnoses.

Symptoms

Carpal tunnel syndrome	Pronator syndrome	Anterior interosseous nerve syndrome
Reproduction of symptoms with percussion over the anterior aspect of the wrist or with prolonged flexion of the wrist	Patchy anterior forearm pain	
Awaken at night with pain and numbness	Mild weakness	Weakness in first, second, and third finger flexion, weak pronation with the elbow flexed. This is known as the Kiloh–Nevin sign, in other words, the "OK" sign
Sparing of the area over the thenar eminence	Numbness over the thenar eminence	No sensory symptoms

Localization site	Comment
Peripheral neuropathy	Median nerve

Secondary Complications: Pain limiting range of motion of the arm and over time may result in contractures in that extremity.

Treatment Complications: Local injection of anesthesia can be tried. Injections may rarely cause infection, blood loss, tissue or nerve injury. Nonsteroidal anti-inflammatory medications rarely can cause cerebrovascular complications.

Bibliography

Brazis PW, et al., eds. Peripheral nerves. In *Localization in clinical neurology*. 6th ed. Philadelphia, PA: Lippincott Williams and Wilkins; 2011. Chapter 2.

Rodner CM, Tinsley BA, O'Malley MP. Pronator syndrome and anterior interosseous nerve syndrome. *J Am Acad Orthop Surg*. 2013;21(5):268–75.

Propriospinal Myoclonus

Epidemiology and Demographics: Propriospinal myoclonus (PSM) is a very uncommon type of myoclonus originating from the spinal cord.[1] PSM has been reported more commonly in middle-aged individuals, but can affect all ages. Overall, due to its rarity, large-scale epidemiological research is lacking for this disorder. Case studies have been helpful in identifying that middle-aged persons are mainly affected; men may be more likely to have PSM than women.[1] Several studies have characterized various etiological agents that may affect all ages, such as diseases of the spinal cord (spinal lesions, trauma, post-operative complications, syringomyelia, arteriovenous [AV] fistula),[1] drugs, toxins, malignancy, and psychogenic or functional.[1]

Disorder Description: PSM is a myoclonic disorder of the axial musculature. It is characterized by a slow progression of electromyographic bursts, either rhythmic or arrhythmic, usually beginning in the mid-thoracic spinal cord region, propagating rostrally and caudally along the propriospinal pathways.[2–4] PSM is one of two forms of spinal myoclonus, the other being spinal segmental myoclonus. Contrary to PSM, spinal segmental myoclonus is usually secondary to a clear etiology and is confined to a specific myotome. The movements occur in flexion or extension, may or may not involve the limbs, and are usually stimulus sensitive. It is exaggerated when the patient is in the supine position. One study identified that the jerks in PSM spare the cranially innervated muscles.[5] The classical PSM jerks cannot be voluntarily suppressed.[1]

The disorder may be idiopathic, psychogenic, or secondary to an underlying factor. Idiopathic PSM includes the axial jerking movements without functional clinical clues in the patient's medical history, a normal spinal axis on imaging, a consistent EMG pattern characteristic of PSM, as well as absent "readiness potential" or Bereitschafts potential (BP) on EEG–EMG. The BP is usually associated with the preparation preceding a voluntary movement. Secondary causes share these characteristics, except for the presence of abnormal findings on spinal imaging or a positive history of exposure to a risk factor.[6] Psychogenic movements are not aggravated in the presence of other individuals and can be reduced by distracting the patient. Emotional and psychiatric disturbances can also be present. BP units may or may not be present in psychogenic PSM, but are certainly absent in idiopathic or secondary PSM.

An MRI is recommended to exclude a structural cause for myelopathy. Previously described in some cases, PSM was diagnosed without EMG or BP and with symptoms of optic neuritis, saddle anesthesia, or urinary incontinence. However, PSM does not classically present with those symptoms.

Polymyography is a highly recommended test that all patients with suspected PSM should undergo. A localized spinal generator with a characteristic propagation of slow conduction velocity signals will be present.

Symptoms

Localization site	Comment
Spinal cord	Mid-thoracic region of spinal cord site of initiation of propriospinal myoclonus, leading to abdominal wall, trunk, and cervical musculature myoclonic jerks. May include the upper and lower limbs

Secondary Complications: The reflex-sensitive nature of the myoclonic jerks of PSM can lead to some difficulties for the patient. The jerks can worsen in the supine position. Attempts to go to sleep can be very bothersome, and lead to insomnia. Some cases have also described symptoms related to tic disorders. If facial grimacing and tonic contractions of the eyes are present, this is not true PSM. This may then warrant functional or psychogenic workup.

Treatment Complications: Due to the heterogeneity of PSM, it can be very difficult to manage and treat the patient. Studies to exclude spinal cord pathology and proper myographic studies should be used to identify the pattern of PSM.

References

1. Roze E, Bounolleau P, Ducreux D, et al. Propriospinal myoclonus revisited: Clinical, neurophysiologic, and neuroradiologic findings. *Neurology.* 2009;72(15):1301–9.
2. Brown P. Propriospinal myoclonus: where do we go from here? *Mov Disord.* 2014;29(9):1092–3.
3. Brown P, Rothwell JC, Thompson PD, Marsden CD. Propriospinal myoclonus: evidence for spinal "pattern" generators in humans. *Mov Disord.* 1994;9(5):571–6.
4. Chokroverty S, Walters A, Zimmerman T, Picone M. Propriospinal myoclonus: a neurophysiologic analysis. *Neurology.* 1992;42(8):1591–5.
5. Chokroverty S. Propriospinal myoclonus. *Clin Neurosci.* 1995;3(4):219–22.
6. Antelmi E, Provini F. Propriospinal myoclonus: The spectrum of clinical and neurophysiological phenotypes. *Sleep Med Rev.* 2015;22:54–63.

Prostate Cancer

Epidemiology and Demographics: The most common malignancy in men; the number of new cases is approximately 130/1,000,000 men per year, and it causes 1–2% of deaths per year. In 2013, there was an estimated 2,850,139 men living with prostate cancer in the United States. Prostate cancer is commonly diagnosed in the 7th decade of life and has a greater prevalence in the West. In the United States, black men have a much greater incidence (58%) and mortality rates are twice as high as in white men, and Hispanics have lower incidence (14%) and mortality (17%) as compared with white men.

Disorder Description: Prostate cancer is a cancer of the prostate, which is often slow growing. It is initially confined to the prostate and if left untreated, can metastasize to lymph nodes and bones, most commonly the lumbar spine. Most common risk factors include family history, older age, smoking, radiation, and chronic urinary tract infections. BRCA2 and HOXB13 are some implicated genes.

Symptoms

Localization site	Comment
Cerebral hemispheres	Metastasis (via hematogenous spread; very rare, 1–2% incidence), limbic encephalitis as a paraneoplastic syndrome (rare), seizures
Mental status and psychiatric aspects/complications	Altered mental status secondary to cerebral metastasis/increased intracranial pressure (ICP)
Cerebellum	Metastasis (rare), paraneoplastic cerebellar degeneration
Pituitary gland	SIADH (syndrome of inappropriate antidiuretic hormone secretion), Cushing syndrome
Spinal cord	Spinal cord compression from vertebral metastases (lumbar most common); direct metastasis from spine
Specific spinal roots	Radiculopathy (vertebral metastasis causing nerve root compression)
Plexus	Sacral/pudendal plexus leading to autonomic dysfunction (urinary retention)
Peripheral neuropathy	Rarely as a paraneoplastic syndrome
Muscle	Dermatomyositis (rare; more commonly associated with other cancers)
Neuromuscular junction	Lambert–Eaton myasthenic syndrome (LEMS) (rare)
Meninges	Leptomeningeal carcinomatosis; epidural metastasis

Secondary Complications: Disseminated intravascular coagulation (DIC), thrombotic thrombocytopenic purpura (TTP), and hypercoagulable state of malignancy can lead to microthrombolism, embolic events, and bleeding diathesis causing infarcts and intracranial parenchymal hemorrhage, respectively. Liver dysfunction leading to hepatic encephalopathy.

Treatment Complications: The standard local treatments for prostate cancer (e.g., radical prostatectomy [RP], external beam radiation therapy [EBRT], brachytherapy, high-intensity focused ultrasound [HIFU], cryotherapy) are all associated with erectile dysfunction and impotence, to various degrees.

Rarely, RP is also associated with femoral nerve palsy and surgical orchiectomy can lead to sensory loss in the ipsilateral groin and lateral hemiscrotum secondary to ilioinguinal nerve injury.

Enzalutamide (an androgen antagonist) has been associated with seizures and PRES (posterior reversible encephalopathy syndrome).

Extramustine (an antineoplastic agent) causes increased risk of thromboembolism and stroke.

Gonadotropin-releasing hormone agonists have been associated with pituitary apoplexy in patients with pituitary adenoma and also spinal cord compression.

Bibliography

Attard G, Parker C, Eeles RA, et al. Prostate cancer. *Lancet*. 2016;387(10013):70–82.

Benjamin R. Neurologic complications of prostate cancer. *Am Fam Physician*. 2002;65(9):1834–40. Review.

Cuzick J, Thorat MA, Andriole G, et al. Prevention and early detection of prostate cancer. *Lancet Oncol*. 2014;15(11):e484–92.

Hong MK, Kong J, Namdarian B, et al. Paraneoplastic syndromes in prostate cancer. *Nat Rev Urol*. 2010;7(12):681–92.

Prosthetic Heart Valve

Epidemiology and Demographics: In the United States it is estimated that 60,000 to 95,000 patients undergo prosthetic heart valve procedures yearly.

Disorder Description: Heart valve disorders may lead to valve replacement with a prosthetic valve.

Symptoms

Localization site	Comment
Cerebral hemispheres	Can become stenotic with outflow tract obstruction leading to syncope and presyncope. Thrombus formation and the development of endocarditis, both of which may cause embolic and focal events of the central nervous system
Mental status and psychiatric aspects/ complications	Same as above

Localization site	Comment
Brainstem	Same as above
Cerebellum	Same as above
Vestibular system (and nonspecific dizziness)	Same as above
Base of skull	Same as above

Secondary Complications: Two major types of prosthetics: mechanical prostheses, which have a greater risk of thromboembolism, and bioprostheses, which have a greater risk of weakening of the valve.

Treatment Complications: Depending on the type of prosthesis and its location, anticoagulation may be needed. This in turn may be associated with risk of hemorrhage including intracerebral localizations.

Bibliography

Karden EM. Prosthetic heart valves. Feb 18, 2015. Available from http://emedicine.medscape.com/article/780702-overview#a4. Retrieved Jul 27, 2017.

Otto CM, Bonow RO. Valvular heart disease. In Mann DL, Zipes DP, Libby P, Bonow RO, Braunwald E, eds. *Braunwald's heart diseases: a textbook of cardiovascular medicine.* 10th ed. Philadelphia: Elsevier/Saunders; 2015; p. 1505.

Protein–Calorie Malnutrition

Epidemiology and Demographics: In developing countries, primary protein–energy malnutrition remains the most significant health problem that causes kwashiorkor and marasmus. In developed contries, protein-energy malnutrition is mostly secondary to other diseases and causes kwashiorkor- and marasmus-like syndromes.

Disorder Description: Protein–energy malnutrition occurs as a result of a relative or absolute deficiency of energy and protein. It may be primary, due to inadequate food intake, or secondary, as a result of other illness.

There are two distinct syndromes. Kwashiorkor, caused by a deficiency of protein in the presence of adequate energy, is typically seen in weaning infants at the birth of a sibling in areas where foods containing protein are insufficient. Marasmus, caused by combined protein and energy deficiency, is seen where adequate quantities of food are not available.

Kwashiorkor-like secondary protein–energy malnutrition occurs primarily in association with hypermetabolic acute illnesses such as trauma, burns, and sepsis. Marasmus-like secondary protein–energy malnutrition typically results from chronic diseases such as chronic obstructive pulmonary disease (COPD), heart failure, cancer, or AIDS. These two syndromes are estimated to be present in at least 20% of hospitalized patients.

Secondary Complications: *Wernicke disease* is characterized by nystagmus, abducens and conjugate gaze palsies, ataxia of gait, and mental confusion. These symptoms develop acutely or subacutely and may occur singly or in combination. Wernicke disease is caused by deficiency of thiamine and is observed mainly in alcoholics.

Korsakoff amnesic state: Korsakoff psychosis is a mental disorder in which retentive memory is impaired out of proportion to all other cognitive functions in an otherwise alert and responsive patient. This amnesic disorder, like Wernicke disease, is most often associated with the thiamine deficiency of alcoholism and malnutrition.

Beriberi is a disease of the heart and of the peripheral nerves, which may be affected separately. The symptoms of nutritional polyneuropathy are diverse. Many patients are asymptomatic and evidence of peripheral nerve disease is found only by clinical or electromyographic examination. The mildest neuropathic signs are thinness and tenderness of the leg muscles, loss or depression of the Achilles reflexes and patellar reflexes, and, at times, a patchy blunting of pain and touch sensation over the feet and shins. Most patients, however, are symptomatic and have weakness, paresthesias, and pain. The feet are always affected earlier and more severely than the hands. Beriberi is likely secondary to deficiency of the B vitamins.

Pellagra affects the skin, alimentary tract, and nervous systems. The early symptoms may be mistaken for those of a psychiatric disorder. Insomnia, fatigue, nervousness, irritability, and feelings of depression are common complaints; taken together they have the character of neurasthenia. It is known that pellagra may result from a deficiency of either nicotinic acid or tryptophan, the amino acid precursor of nicotinic acid. Nicotinic acid is formed from tryptophan, a process for which pyridoxine is essential.

Despite the frequency of folic acid deficiency and its hematologic effects, its role in the pathogenesis of nervous system disease has not been established. However, folate antagonists such as methotrexate are known to cause a neuropathy that is probably predicated on the vitamin deficiency. The polyneuropathy that occasionally complicates the chronic administration of phenytoin has also been attributed to folate deficiency. The folate deficiency of pregnancy is known to increase the incidence of neural tube defects.

The spinal cord, brain, optic nerves, and peripheral nerves are all affected by vitamin B12 deficiency, giving rise to a classic neurologic syndrome. The spinal cord is usually affected first and often exclusively. The term *subacute combined degeneration* is reserved for the spinal cord lesion of vitamin B12 deficiency and serves to distinguish it from other types of spinal cord diseases that happen to involve the posterior and lateral columns.

Bibliography

Papadakis MA, McPhee SJ. *Current medical diagnosis and treatment.* 58th ed. New York: McGraw-Hill Education; in press.

Ropper AH, Samuels MA, Klein JP. *Adams & Victor's principles of neurology.* 10th ed. New York, NY: McGraw-Hill; 2014.

Protein C Deficiency

Epidemiology and Demographics: Rare deficiency present in 1 in 20,000 without gender or ethnic predilection.

Disorder Description: When activated, Protein C cleaves procoagulant factors V and VIII. Inherited Protein C deficiency is an autosomal *heterozygous* disorder. Homozygosity can rarely cause a very severe thrombotic disorder presenting in infancy. Deficiency may also be caused by consumption (such as disseminated infection) or from decreased synthesis (such as from hepatic dysfunction).[1]

Symptoms

Localization site	Comment
Cerebral hemispheres	Primarily associated with increased risk of cerebral venous sinus thrombosis in the larger sinuses or cortical veins. Can also cause arterial ischemic stroke from paradoxical venous thromboembolism

Secondary Complications: Increased risk of venous thromboembolism particularly after paralysis from neurologic injury.

Treatment Complications: With Protein C deficiency, there is risk of warfarin-induced thrombosis including skin necrosis with initiation of warfarin therapy.

Reference

1. Goldenberg NA, Manco-Johnson MJ. Protein C deficiency. *Haemoph Off J World Fed Hemoph.* 2008;14:1214–21.

Protein S Deficiency

Epidemiology and Demographics: Protein S deficiency is present on testing in 0.1% or fewer of the population. Present in 2–8% of patients with venous thromboembolism.

Disorder Description: Protein S is a cofactor for activated Protein C, which inactivates thrombogenic factors Factor V and VIII. Deficiency can be inherited autosomally resulting in either deficient quantity or reduced activity. Acquired Protein S deficiency can occur in multiple states including pregnancy, oral contraceptive use, nephrotic syndrome, liver disease, or autoantibody against Protein S.[1]

Symptoms

Localization site	Comment
Cerebral hemispheres	Primarily associated with cerebral venous sinus thrombosis or paradoxical arterial ischemic stroke from venous thromboembolism. No clear increased risk of arterial thrombosis

Secondary Complications: Other venous thromboembolic complications.

Treatment Complications: Risk of warfarin-induced thrombosis with initiation of warfarin therapy in the setting of pre-existing Protein S deficiency.

Reference

1. D'Angelo A, Viganò D'Angelo S. Protein S deficiency. *Haematologica.* 2008;93:498–501.

Pseudallescheria boydii

Epidemiology and Demographics: Fungus found in stagnant and polluted water. Occurs in immunosuppressed and near drowning victims. Common in those with cystic fibrosis.

Disorder Description: Infection with *Pseudallescheria boydii* has two presentations:

1. mycetoma (99% of infections), a chronic, subcutaneous disease; and
2. pseudallescheriasis, involving the central nervous system, lungs, joints, and bone.

Transmitted via inhalation or skin breaks. Diagnosed with culture, cytology, or histology.

High mortality in central nervous system infection, up to 75%. No optimal treatment, although antifungals are used. Craniotomy and shunts can be used to manage complications related to mass effect.

Symptoms

Localization site	Comment
Cerebral hemispheres	Multiple brain abscesses can lead to focal neurologic signs, hydrocephalus, or herniation syndromes Can present as neutrophilic meningitis as well
Mental status and psychiatric aspects/complications	Encephalopathy possible depending on location of involvement
Brainstem/cranial nerves/cerebellum	Meningeal irritation involvement

Secondary Complications: Endocarditis can lead to stroke.

Treatment Complications: Often resistant to most antifungals.

Bibliography

Kershaw P, Freeman R, Templeton D, et al. Pseudallescheria boydii infection of the central nervous system. *Arch Neurol.* 1990;47(4):468–72.

Long S, Pickering LK, Prober CG, eds. *Principles and practice of pediatric infectious disease.* 4th ed. Edinburgh: Elsevier/Saunders; 2012.

Pseudomonas aeruginosa

Epidemiology and Demographics: Ubiquitous non-fermenting gram-negative bacillus. Risk factors are diabetes, chronic illness, old age, and immunosuppression. However, 10% of cases have no risk factors.

Disorder Description: Primary infection is the most common cause of malignant otitis externa (MOE), which presents with severe headache, ear pain tenderness, and mastoid pain. Otoscopic examination shows granulation tissue in the external auditory canal. Infection may then spread directly through the bone and into the meninges and/or brain. Bone scan and biopsy are useful for diagnosis.

Symptoms

Localization site	Comment
Cerebral hemispheres	Abscess causing mass effect and focal neurologic signs
Meninges	Frequently presents as chronic meningitis
Mental status and psychiatric aspects/complications	Encephalopathy
Cranial nerves	Seventh nerve palsy most common

Secondary Complications: Co-infection with *Staphylococcus aureus*. Hydrocephalus. Sepsis.

Treatment Complications: Frequent resistance to ciprofloxacin, so typically treated with pipercillin–tazobactam. Surgery may be indicated to remove bone or drain abscesses.

Bibliography

Aminoff MJ, Josephson SA, eds. *Aminoff's neurology and general medicine*. 5th ed. London, UK: Elsevier; 2014.

Roberts J, Larson-Williams L, Ibrahim F, Hassoun A. Malignant otitis externa (MOE) causing cerebral abscess and facial nerve palsy. *J Hosp Med*. 2010;5(7):E6–8.

Psilocybin

Epidemiology and Demographics: No gender or race predilection.

Disorder Description: Psilocybin is a psychedelic compound derived from a species of psilocybin mushrooms. When individuals ingest the compound, it gets converted to psilocin, which produces mind-altering effects on individuals lasting 2 to 6 hours.

Symptoms

Localization site	
Cerebral hemispheres	Seizures (acute)
Mental status and psychiatric aspects/complications	Euphoria (acute)
	Hallucinations (acute)
	Panic attack (acute)
	Distortion in time perceptions (acute)
	Hallucinogen-persisting perception disorder (chronic)
	Schizophrenia-like psychosis (chronic)
	Violent behavior (acute)
Cerebellum	Ataxia (acute)
Anterior horn cells	Tremors (acute)
Muscle	Tremors (acute)
Neuromuscular junction	Serotonin receptors dysregulation (chronic)

Bibliography

Longo LP, Johnson B. Addiction: Part I. Benzodiazepines – side effects, abuse risk and alternatives. *Am Fam Physician*. 2000;61(7):2121–8.

Wiegand TJ, Burns MM, Wiley JF. Clinical manifestations and evaluation of mushroom poisoning. Updated Dec 9, 2016. *UpToDate*. Waltham, MA. www.uptodate.com/contents/clinical-manifestations-and-evaluation-of-mushroom-poisoning?source=search_result&search=psilocybin&selectedTitle=2~8. Accessed Aug 8, 2018.

Psoas Abscess

Epidemiology and Demographics: Rare condition. Most common in men between the ages of 44 and 55 years. Risk factors are diabetes, human immunodeficiency virus (HIV) infection, renal failure, intravenous drug use, and immunosuppression. Additionally, trauma and hematoma formation can predispose to development of psoas abscess. Risk factors for secondary abscess include trauma and instrumentation in the inguinal region, lumbar spine, or hip region.

Disorder Description: Spread from either adjacent structures or by hematogenous spread. Infection can spread directly from the vertebral bodies, the abdominal aorta, the sigmoid colon, the appendix, the hip joint, and iliac lymph nodes.

In the case of hematogenous spread, *Staphylococcus aureus* and *Mycobacterium tuberculosis* are common pathogens.

Indirect spread of infection is often polymicrobial. Multiple pathogens are possible.

Symptoms

Localization site	Comment
Plexus	Mass effect from abscess formation can cause plexus dysfunction and injury
Muscle	Weakness of psoas and iliacus muscles impairs strength of hip flexion

Secondary Complications: Complications include destruction of adjacent structures, septic shock, deep vein thrombosis, hydronephrosis, bowel ileus, septic hip arthritis.

Treatment Complications: Plexus injury if surgical intervention needed.

Bibliography

Mallick IH, Thoufeeq MH, Rajendran TP. Iliopsoas abscesses. *Postgrad Med J.* 2004;80(946):459.

Mückley T, Schütz T, Kirschner M, et al. Psoas abscess: the spine as a primary source of infection. *Spine (Phila Pa 1976).* 2003;28(6):E106.

Psoas Hemorrhage

Epidemiology and Demographics: This occurs in 1.3–6.6% of patients treated with anticoagulants and 5.5–10.4% of hemophiliacs. It can also rarely be traumatic.

Disorder Description: Hemorrhage into the psoas muscle compresses the femoral nerve as it pierces the muscle.

Symptoms

Localization site	Comments
Mononeuropathy or mononeuropathy multiplex	Femoral neuropathy leads to weakness of the quadriceps muscles

Secondary Complications: If the hematoma involves the entire retroperitoneal area, anemia may result.

Treatment Complications: Reversal of anticoagulation may precipitate the clotting complication the mediations were being given to avoid.

Bibliography

Lefevre N, Bohu Y, Klouche S, Chewla N, Herman S. Complete paralysis of the quadriceps secondary to post-traumatic iliopsoas hematoma: A systematic review. *Eur J Orthopaed Surg Traumatol.* 2015; 25(1):39–43.

Parner SS, Carpenter JP, Fairman RM, Velazquez OC, Mitchell ME. Femoral neuropathy following retroperitoneal hemorrhage: case series and review of the literature. *Ann Vasc Surg.* 2006;20(4):536–40.

Psychogenic Dysphagia (Phagophobia)

Epidemiology and Demographics: The incidence and prevalence of psychogenic dysphagia are unknown. One study found that psychogenic dysphagic patients made up 3% of a large patient cohort seen at a swallowing center.

Disorder Description: Psychogenic dysphagia is the subjective difficulty with swallowing in the absence of radiologic and clinical findings. This is often accompanied with a "globus" sensation where the patient describes feeling like there is "something stuck in the throat."

Differential Diagnosis: Psychogenic dysphagia should be carefully differentiated from dysphagia caused by an identifiable underlying disturbance. Examples include esophageal atresia, achalasia, esophageal spasm, esophageal cancer, eosinophilic esophagitis, hiatal hernia, and gastroesophageal reflux, and these should be ruled out.

Eating disorders such as avoidant restrictive food intake disorder (ARFID) or anorexia nervosa may present with difficulty swallowing but can be differentiated if there is presence of food restriction due to fear of food or with intent of weight loss.

Secondary Complications: Psychogenic dysphagia may lead to aspiration and resultant pneumonia, dehydration, malnutrition, and weight loss.

Treatment Complications: Treatments generally include swallowing therapy, cognitive behavioral therapy, and video feedback modalities. There may be complications of treatments for obsessive-compulsive disorder, specific phobia, social phobia, or generalized anxiety disorder if any of these disorders underlie the psychogenic dysphagia.

Bibliography

American Psychiatric Association. *Diagnostic and statistical manual of mental disorders: DSM-5.* 5th ed. Washington, DC: American Psychiatric Association; 2013.

Barofsky I, Buchholz D, Edwin D, Jones B, Ravich W. Characteristics of patients who have difficulties initiating swallowing. Annual Meeting of the Dysphagia Research Society, Lake Geneva, WI, September, 1993.

Leopold NA. Dysphagia in drug-induced parkinsonism: a case report. *Dysphagia.* 1996;11(2):151–3.

Ravich WJ, Wilson RS, Jones B, Donner MW. Psychogenic dysphagia and globus: reevaluation of 23 patients. *Dysphagia.* 1989;4(1):35–8.

Tanidir C, Hergüner S. Mirtazapine for choking phobia: report of a pediatric case. *J Child Adolesc Psychopharmacol.* 2015;25(8):659–60.

Psychogenic Non-epileptic Seizures (PNES)

Epidemiology and Demographics: The incidence of psychogenic non-epileptic seizures (PNES) in the general population is unclear but is estimated to be 2–33/100,000. Approximately 5–25% of patients in outpatient epilepsy clinics are found to have PNES, and 25–40% of those in inpatient monitoring facilities are estimated to have PNES. There is a female predominance, and onset is commonly in the third decade of life. Samples with PNES had high rates of psychiatric comorbidity overall (53–100%), notably including posttraumatic stress disorder (PTSD), depression, personality and anxiety disorders.

Disorder Description: PNES are events that resemble epileptic seizures, but without the characteristic electrical discharges associated with epilepsy on EEG study.

Differential Diagnosis: Most importantly, PNES must be distinguished from epileptic seizures. Approximately 20% of true seizure patients also have psychogenic seizures making it even more important to investigate thoroughly. There are several clinical features that are useful for distinguishing one from the other. PNES usually last longer than 2 minutes (epileptic seizures often last less than 1–2 minutes) and eyes are generally closed (epileptic seizures characteristically have open eyes during the event). PNES often have vocalizations during the episode, and often no postictal symptoms and no incontinence. Epileptic seizures generally have early or no vocalizations during the episode, and frequently occur with incontinence, and a postictal state characterized by confusion, drowsiness, and headache. Video-EEG monitoring is the gold-standard for diagnosing PNES and for distinguishing it from epilepsy.

Secondary Complications: Only a minority (about a quarter to a third) of PNES patients achieve complete remission of their symptoms. Studies have found that PNES significantly decreases occupational status, even if episodes remit. Some studies suggest that it is not the PNES itself, but rather comorbid depression and psychologic issues that pose barriers to employment. PNES are also associated with an increased risk of suicide, which persists even if episodes remit. Patients also may develop new somatic complaints when their PNES remit. Such complaints include moderate to severe pain syndromes, with one study noting headaches in 77% of that population.

Treatment Complications: PNES treatment is often individualized based on provider preference and patient. Psychiatric interventions are commonplace, including cognitive behavioral therapy, traditional psychotherapy, and psychodynamic therapy. Since PTSD is very common in these patients, it is important to explore a history of abuse and offer therapeutic services for the management of symptoms.

Bibliography

Benbadis SR, Agrawal V, Tatum WO. How many patients with psychogenic nonepileptic seizures also have epilepsy? *Neurology.* 2001;57(5):915–17.

Benbadis SR, Hauser WA. An estimate of the prevalence of psychogenic non-epileptic seizures. *Seizure.* 2000;9(4):280–1.

Diprose W, Sundram F, Menkes DB. Psychiatric comorbidity in psychogenic nonepileptic seizures compared with epilepsy. *Epilepsy Behav.* 2016;56:123–30.

Ettinger AB, Devinsky O, Weisbrot DM, et al. Headaches and other pain symptoms among patients with psychogenic non-epileptic seizures. *Seizure.* 1999;8:424.

Ettinger AB, Devinsky O, Weisbrot DM, Ramakrishna RK, Goyal A. A comprehensive profile of clinical, psychiatric, and psychosocial characteristics of patients with psychogenic nonepileptic seizures. *Epilepsia*. 1999;40(9):1292–8.

Ettinger AB, Dhoon A, Weisbrot DM, Devinsky O. Predictive factors for outcome of nonepileptic seizures after diagnosis. *J Neuropsychiatry Clin Neurosci*. 1999;11:458.

Meierkord H, Shorvon S. The clinical features and prognosis of pseudoseizures diagnosed using video-EEG telemetry. *Neurology*. 1991;41(10):1643–3.

Psychogenic Pain (Psychalgia)

Epidemiology and Demographics: Psychogenic pain is estimated to have a prevalence of 40% in populations with chronic pain. It appears to be more common in females, and those with a family history of depression, alcohol, and pain.

Disorder Description: Psychogenic pain is not a diagnosable condition. Instead it is the description of pain that is associated with a psychologic, behavioral, or emotional stimulus given that medical or neurologic causes have been ruled out.

In the current nomenclature, the closest diagnosable condition to psychalgia is **somatic symptom disorder with predominant pain**. This is characterized by disproportionate and persistent thoughts about being in pain, persistently high levels of anxiety about being in pain, or devoting excessive time and energy to the symptom of pain. This must cause significant disruption of daily life typically for more than 6 months.

Secondary Complications: Psychogenic pain has been linked to an increase in the risk of suicide. It is hypothesized that a patient's burden of having a pain condition with an ambiguous etiology may be particularly difficult for patients, and may lead to hopelessness, frustration, and an increased suicide risk. Furthermore, when etiology of pain is not established, pain relief may be delayed or not given, further contributing to the suicide risk.

Treatment Complications: Psychogenic pain may be treated with psychotherapy, antidepressants such as selective serotonin reuptake inhibitors (SSRIs), serotonin–norepinephrine reuptake inhibitors (SNRIs), and analgesics used for general pain relief.

SSRI side effects include nausea, diarrhea, insomnia, headache, anorexia, weight loss, sexual dysfunction, restlessness (akathisia-like), serotonin syndrome (fever diaphoresis, tachycardia, hypertension, delirium, neuromuscular excitability), hyponatremia, seizures (0.2%).

Pain is frequently treated with opioid medications, which, in addition to their own side effects (nausea, vomiting, sedation, dizziness, constipation, respiratory depression), may lead to dependence.

Bibliography

American Psychiatric Association. *Diagnostic and Statistical Manual of Mental Disorders (DSM-5)*. 5th ed. American Psychiatric Pub; 2013.

Engel GL. "Psychogenic" pain and the pain-prone patient. *Am J Med*. 1959;26(6):899–918.

Ilgen MA, Kleinberg F, Ignacio RV, et al. Noncancer pain conditions and risk of suicide. *JAMA Psychiatry*. 2013;70(7):692–7.

Merskey HE. Classification of chronic pain: Descriptions of chronic pain syndromes and definitions of pain terms. *Pain*. 1986;Suppl 3:226.

Sriram T.G, Chaturvedi SK, Gopinath PS, Shanmugam V. Controlled study of alexithymic characteristics in patients with psychogenic pain disorder. *Psychother Psychosomat*. 1987;47(1):11–17.

Psychogenic Polydipsia

Epidemiology and Demographics: According to hospital surveys, psychogenic polydipsia (PP) is present in 6–17% of patients in inpatient psychiatric units. Women represent 60–80% of affected patients. While it is present in 10–20% of patients with schizophrenia, only 2–5% of those present with symptomatic hyponatremia. An association between affective disorders, anorexia nervosa, personality disorders, developmental disabilities, and PP has also been described.

Disorder Description: PP is water-seeking and excessive drinking often resulting in water intoxication and hyponatremia, not caused by a known physiologic condition. This is mediated, in part, by a reduced osmoregulation of thirst that is frequently seen in schizophrenic patients. PP may also be seen in the context of hypothalamic lesions affecting the thirst center located in the median preoptic nucleus.

Hypothalamic–pituitary sarcoidosis can also cause a discrepancy between osmotic thresholds for thirst and antidiuretic hormone (ADH) release resulting in polydipsia. PP may result in severe hyponatremia causing a wide range of central nervous system dysfunction, including seizures, coma, and death. Other complications of PP may include enuresis, hydronephrosis, renal failure, congestive heart failure, and osteoporosis.

Differential Diagnosis and Diagnostic Testing: PP is a diagnosis of exclusion, which can be achieved through the initial investigation of serum and urine sodium, as well as serum and urine osmolality. A complete metabolic panel, urinalysis, and BUN (blood urea nitrogen) should be ordered to exclude other etiologies, such as diabetes mellitus and osmotic diuresis. PP most commonly presents with a hypotonic and euvolemic hyponatremia.

Hyponatremia seen with PP or the syndrome of inappropriate ADH secretion (SIADH) is described when levels descend below 136 mEq/L. Both conditions are typically associated with serum osmolality below 280 mOsm/kg. However, the former (due to a dilutional effect) is associated with low urine osmolality (<100 mOsm/kg), whereas urine osmolality is greater than or equal to 100 mOsm/kg in SIADH (normal is 300–800 mOsm/kg). Similarly, urine sodium is less than 20 mEq/L in PP but greater than 30 mEq/L in SIADH.[1]

Further investigation is often warranted, especially to differentiate from diabetes insipidus. This can be done with a fluid deprivation test. The body's normal physiologic response to fluid deprivation is to conserve water through urine concentration (as is seen in a psychogenic polydipsia patient when deprived of fluid). The patient's urine would be very dilute before the water is restricted, <100 mOsm/kg H_2O, and achieves an osmolality of >600 mOsm/kg H_2O after restricting water and giving vasopressin. In contrast, when deprived of fluid, the diabetes insipidus patient continues to urinate large volumes of dilute urine. These results are diagnostic in a majority of cases; however, if results still remain equivocal, plasma arginine vasopressin (AVP), also known as ADH, can be measured both before and after water restriction. The plasma ADH is low before restriction in patients with PP and rises following the deprivation test.

Polydipsia and hyponatremia can be induced by a number of psychotropic drugs. While some stimulate thirst through their anticholinergic properties, others cause inappropriate ADH levels. Phenothiazines such as thioridazine, antiepileptic agents with psychotropic properties such as carbamazepine and oxcarbazepine, atypical neuroleptics (e.g., clozapine and aripiprazole), and selective and nonselective serotonin reuptake inhibitors (e.g., fluoxetine) may cause SIADH.[2]

Treatment Complications: Management of primary polydipsia includes fluid restriction to 1–1.5 L/day, as well as behavioral and pharmacologic therapy. Careful sodium monitoring and correction should take place to avoid the potentially fatal syndrome of central pontine myelinolysis (CPM). Once the patient is medically stable, cognitive and behavioral treatment should be initiated. Clozapine has been used in treatment of PP, but its efficacy is not confirmed in large trials, and it may further increase the risk of seizure characteristic to hyponatremia.[3]

References

1. Siegel AJ. Hyponatremia in psychiatric patients: update on evaluation and management. *Harv Rev Psychiatry*. 2008;16(1):13–24. DOI:10.1080/10673220801924308.
2. Bremner AJ Regan A. Intoxicated by water. Polydipsia and water intoxication in a mental handicap hospital. *Br J Psychiatry*. 1991;158: 244–50.
3. Whitchurch FT, Alexander J. Psychogenic polydipsia: Hidden or underdiagnosed? *Aust N Z J Psychiatry*. 2011;45(9):789–90. DOI:10.3109/00 048674.2011.585457.

Suggested Reading

Dundas B, Harris M, Narasimhan M. Psychogenic polydipsia review: Etiology, differential, and treatment. *Curr Psychiatry Rep*. 2007;9(3):236–41. DOI:10.1007/s11920-007-0025-7.

Hawken ER, Crookall JM, Reddick D, et al. Mortality over a 20-year period in patients with primary polydipsia associated with schizophrenia: A retrospective study. *Schizophr Res*. 2009;107 (2–3):128–33. DOI:10.1016/j.schres.2008.09.029.

Stuart CA, Neelon FA, Lebovitz HE. Disordered control of thirst in hypothalamic-pituitary sarcoidosis. *N Engl J Med*. 1980;303(19):1078.

Psychogenic Vertigo (Psychogenic Dizziness, Psychiatric Dizziness/Vertigo, Psychosomatic/Somatoform Vertigo)

Epidemiology and Demographics: Psychogenic vertigo is more common in females than males and was shown to make up 10.6% of patients with vertigo in a vertigo outpatient clinic.

Disorder Description: Psychogenic vertigo is not included as a diagnosis in the DSM-5. However, most studies cite the following definition: persistent (>3 months) dizziness with subjective imbalance, associated with hypersensitivity to movement. Symptoms may be exacerbated by visual stimuli of complexity, and there must not be an underlying physical neurotologic illness or medical condition causing dizziness. Further, imaging and balance function tests must yield non-diagnostic findings.

Differential Diagnosis: Psychogenic vertigo must be distinguished from vertigo of organic etiology including but not limited to Meniere's syndrome, benign positional vertigo, migraine-associated dizziness, and eighth nerve tumors.

Secondary Complications: There are several conditions that are commonly comorbid with psychogenic vertigo. In one study, 11.6% of patients also had a fear of heights or motion sickness before the current episode of vertigo; 20.7% of cases had a history of organic vestibular disease, including benign paroxysmal positional vertigo; 79.3% of patients had poor balance on balance assessment. There is also correlation with obsessive-compulsive personality disorder, narcissistic personality disorder, and avoidant personality disorder, as well as with panic disorder and other anxiety disorders.

Treatment Complications: Psychogenic vertigo patients are often treated successfully with psychotherapy to assess and decrease the underlying trigger(s), which may often be a cause of anxiety. Resistant cases may undergo cognitive-behavioral therapy, desensitization therapy, or potentially pharmacotherapy such as selective serotonin reuptake inhibitors (SSRIs).

SSRI side effects include nausea, diarrhea, insomnia, headache, anorexia, weight loss, sexual dysfunction, restlessness (akathisia-like), serotonin syndrome (fever diaphoresis, tachycardia, hypertension, delirium, neuromuscular excitability), and hyponatremia.

Bibliography

Furman JM, Jacob RG. Psychiatric dizziness. *Neurology.* 1997;48(5):1161–6.

Ödman M, Maire R. Chronic subjective dizziness. *Acta Oto-laryngologica.* 2008;128(10):1085–8.

Staab JP. Chronic dizziness: the interface between psychiatry and neuro-otology. *Curr Opin Neurol.* 2006;19(1):41–8.

Strupp M, Brandt T. Diagnosis and treatment of vertigo and dizziness. *Dtsch Arztebl Int.* 2008;105(10):173–80. http://doi.org/10.3238/arztebl.2008.0173.

Psychosis in Parkinson's Disease

Epidemiology and Demographics: Hospital-based studies have revealed psychosis in 20–30% of Parkinson's disease (PD) patients, with increasing prevalence as the disease progresses. Prior to the introduction of dopaminergic treatments, psychosis was found in 5–10% of PD patients. Up to 70% of patients with visual hallucinations were also found to have dementia. On average, psychotic symptoms are reported 10 or more years after initial diagnosis.

Disorder Description: Psychosis in PD embraces a specific collection of clinical features that differ from other psychotic disorders, including clear sensorium, retained insight, delusions, visual hallucinations, and sensory disturbances that worsen over time. In early stages, hallucinations are often mild, containing vivid, colorful figures of familiar persons or animals that the patient may try and interact with. Content of hallucinations often converts to frightening insects, rats, and serpents, inducing anxiety and panic attacks. Delusions are classically of paranoid nature involving persecution, spousal infidelity, or jealousy.

Psychosis in PD is usually characterized by hallucinations of a paranoid nature, but may also contain illusions, false sense of presence, and/or delusions. The psychotic features occur after the diagnosis of Parkinson's, must be continuous for 1 month, and are not better accounted for by another medical condition (schizophrenia and related disorders, delusional disorder, mood disorder with psychotic features) or another pathology associated with parkinsonism such as Lewy body dementia.

Differential Diagnosis: Psychosis in PD patients can be caused by a multitude of etiologies, both intrinsic and extrinsic, and a combination of both.

Intrinsic factors are most notably PD-induced progressive degeneration of the cholinergic pedunculopontine nucleus resulting in cognitive impairment and circadian rhythm disturbances, both of which serve as major psychogenic factors. This is evident in patients with REM sleep intrusion or rebound and subsequent psychotic behavior. As the majority of hallucinations are reported as visual, those with impaired performance on contrast and color discrimination tasks, impaired visual acuity, and ocular pathology are found to hallucinate more often. Increased age, disease duration and severity of disease, and depression put patients at higher risk.

Extrinsic factors are drug induced with anticholinergics inducing a toxic delirium and dopaminomimetics provoking a subacute dopaminomimetic psychosis. This is related to a functional alteration in the mesocorticolimbic area and dopamine receptor hypersensitivity, caused by long-term pulsatile dopaminergic treatment. There is no direct correlation between dose and duration of dopaminomimetic treatment nor levodopa plasma levels with the induction or severity of psychotic symptoms.

Psychosis in PD should be distinguished from psychosis due to other medical conditions (schizophrenia and related disorders, mood disorders with psychotic features, delusional disorders), or other causes associated with parkinsonism such as Lewy body dementia. In Lewy body dementia, cognitive deficits precede parkinsonism and psychosis. In turn, Parkinson's dementia begins with motor abnormalities and much later cognitive decline.

Treatment Complications: If a patient with PD presents with new onset confusion or psychosis, the first step is to rule out any identifiable cause unrelated to the disease itself such as infection, dehydration, electrolyte imbalance, or subdural hemorrhage. Non-parkinsonian medications should then be reduced if appropriate. If there is no resolution, a gradual withdrawal of antiparkinsonian therapies should be considered, removing those with a higher cognitive adverse effect to motor benefit ratio first: anticholinergics, amantadine, selegiline and dopamine receptor agonists, catechol-O-methyl transferase (COMT) inhibitors, and levodopa. Initiation of a relatively low D2 receptor blocker, clozapine and quetiapine, both atypical antipsychotic medications, has been shown to be efficacious in treatment of psychosis in PD patients with minimal worsening of parkinsonian symptoms. However, their metabolic and orthostatic hypotension side effects should be considered. In addition, clozaril requires ongoing systematic monitoring of blood cell count to prevent onset of agranulocytosis.

Psychosis associated with PD may be associated with the Parkinson drug regimens in some patients. However, stopping the offending agents may not be an option in PD patients. PD drugs should be decreased in dosage or discontinued in reverse order of the potency and efficacy: first anticholinergics, then MAO-B inhibitors, then COMT inhibitors, and dopamine agonists last. Electroconvulsive therapy has been very effective in treatment of depression and psychosis in PD patients. Maintenance electroconvulsive therapy should be considered in patients with recurrent psychopathology in patients with PD.

Bibliography

Fernandez HH, Friedman JH, Jacques C, Rosenfeld M. Quetiapine for the treatment of drug-induced psychosis in Parkinson's disease. *Mov Disord.* 1999;14:484.

Friedman JH. Parkinson disease psychosis: update. *Behav Neurol.* 2013;27(4):469–77.

Popeo D, Kellner CH. ECT for Parkinson's disease. *Med Hypotheses.* 2009;73(4):468–9. DOI: 10.1016/j.mehy.2009.06.053. PubMed PMID: 19660875.

Rabey JM, Treves TA, Neufeld MY, et al. Low-dose clozapine in the treatment of levodopa-induced mental disturbances in Parkinson's disease. *Neurology.* 1995;45:432.

Ravina B, Marder K, Fernandez HH, et al. Diagnostic criteria for psychosis in Parkinson's disease: report of an NINDS, NIMH work group. *Mov Disord.* 2007;22(8):1061–8.

Williams-Gray CH, Foltynie T, Lewis SJG, Barker RA. Cognitive deficits and psychosis in Parkinson's disease: a review of pathophysiology and therapeutic options. *CNS Drugs.* 2006;20(6):477–505. DOI:10.2165/00023210-200620060-00004.

Wolters E. Intrinsic and extrinsic psychosis in Parkinson's disease. *J Neurol.* 2001;248 (Suppl 3):22–8.

Zahodne LB, Fernandez HH. Pathophysiology and treatment of psychosis in Parkinson's disease: a review. *Drugs Aging.* 2008;25(8):665–82. DOI:10.2165/00002512-200825080-00004.

Psychotic Depression (Major Depressive Disorder with Psychotic Features)

Epidemiology and Demographics: In the United States, the 12-month prevalence of major depressive disorder is about 7%. Prevalence differs according to age with that in 18- to 19-year-olds being threefold higher than that in 60 years or older. Females have a 1.5 to 3-fold increased incidence of major depressive disorder relative to males.

In a large European survey, the point and lifetime prevalence of psychotic depression was 0.4%, and the mean age of onset was 29. It is more common in females, those who are unemployed, and those with a family history of bipolar disorder.

Disorder Description: Psychotic depression is the diagnosis of major depressive disorder with the specifier "with psychotic features." Patients must meet the same criteria as for major depressive disorder (below), and display psychotic features (hallucinations and/or delusions).

As stated in DSM-5, major depressive disorder can be defined as:

A. Five or more of the following symptoms have been present during the same 2-week period and represent a change from previous functioning; at least one of the symptoms is either (1) depressed mood or (2) loss of interest or pleasure.

   i. Depressed mood most of the day, nearly every day, as indicated by either subjective report (e.g., feels sad, empty, hopeless) or observation made by others (e.g., appears tearful). (In children and adolescents, this can manifest as irritability.)

   ii. Markedly diminished interest or pleasure in all, or almost all, activities most of the day, nearly every day (as indicated by either subjective account or observation).

   iii. Significant weight loss when not dieting or weight gain, or decrease or increase in appetite nearly every day.

   iv. Insomnia or hypersomnia nearly every day.

   v. Psychomotor agitation or retardation nearly every day (observed by others).

   vi. Fatigue or loss of energy nearly every day.

   vii. Feelings of worthlessness or excessive or inappropriate guilt (which may be delusional) nearly every day.

   viii. Diminished ability to think or concentrate, or indecisiveness, nearly every day

   ix. Recurrent thoughts of death, recurrent suicidal ideation without a specific plan, or a suicide attempt or a specific plan for committing suicide.

B. The symptoms cause clinically significant distress or impairment in social, occupational, or other important areas of functioning.

C. The episode is not attributable to the physiologic effects of a substance or to another medical condition.

D. The occurrence of the major depressive episode is not better explained by schizoaffective disorder, schizophrenia, schizophreniform disorder, delusional disorder, or other specified and unspecified schizophrenia spectrum and other psychotic disorders.

E. There has never been a manic episode or hypomanic episode.

Psychotic features specifier: Delusions and/or hallucinations are present:

Mood-congruent psychotic features: The content of all delusions and hallucinations is consistent with the typical depressive themes of personal inadequacy, guilt, disease, death, nihilism, or deserved punishment.

Mood-incongruent psychotic features: The content of the delusions or hallucinations does not involve typical depressive themes of personal inadequacy, guilt, disease, death, nihilism, or deserved punishment, or the content is a mixture of mood-incongruent and mood-congruent themes.

Differential Diagnosis: Differential diagnosis should include manic episodes with irritable mood or mixed episodes, mood disorder due to another medical condition, substance/medication-induced depressive or bipolar disorder, attention-deficit/hyperactivity disorder, adjustment disorder with depressed mood, and sadness.

In manic disorders with irritable mood or mixed episodes, there is the presence of manic symptoms, thus patients with depressive symptoms should be carefully examined for past manic episodes.

In a mood disorder due to another medical condition, there is a direct pathophysiologic link between the medical condition and the mood occurrence.

Substance/medication-induced depressive or bipolar disorder is characterized by depression or mania caused by intoxication or withdrawal of a substance.

In attention-deficit/hyperactivity disorder, there may also be distractibility and low frustration tolerance (as in major depressive disorder). The two disorders are not mutually exclusive; if criteria are met for each, both disorders should be diagnosed.

In adjustment disorder with depressed mood, the full criteria for major depressive disorder are not met (5 of 9 symptoms, most of the day, nearly every day for at least 2 weeks).

Episodes of sadness are fundamental aspects of the human experience. These episodes should not be diagnosed as major depressive disorder, unless they meet the full criteria (5 of 9 symptoms, most of the day, nearly every day for at least 2 weeks, causing clinically significant distress or impairment).

Secondary Complications: Impairment secondary to major depressive disorder can be severe. In some cases, the individual may exhibit complete incapacity to care for him- or herself, or is mute or catatonic. These individuals may also have more pain and physical illness and greater decreases in physical, social, and role functioning. The possibility of suicide exists throughout major depressive episodes. The most frequently described risk factor is a past history of suicide attempts or threats. However, most completed suicides are not preceded by previous attempts. Additional risk factors include male sex, being single or living alone, and having prominent feelings of hopelessness. Additionally, about 36% of those with psychotic depression were found to have a comorbid anxiety disorder. Five to 20% of those diagnosed with psychotic depression have their diagnosis eventually changed to bipolar disorder, and 10% are eventually diagnosed with schizoaffective disorder.

Treatment Complications: First-line treatment for major depressive disorder usually consists of selective serotonin reuptake inhibitors (SSRIs). This can be followed by tricyclic antidepressants (TCAs) and monoamine oxidase inhibitors (MAOIs), and possibly an atypical antipsychotic adjuvant (especially if there are psychotic features).

SSRI side effects include nausea, diarrhea, insomnia, headache, anorexia, weight loss, sexual dysfunction, restlessness (akathisia-like), serotonin syndrome (fever diaphoresis, tachycardia, hypertension, delirium, neuromuscular excitability), hyponatremia, seizures (0.2%).

TCAs are highly protein bound and lipid soluble and thus have many drug interactions. They have antihistaminic properties including sedation and weight gain; antiadrenergic properties including orthostatic hypotension, dizziness, reflex tachycardia, arrhythmias; and antimuscarinic effects including dry mouth, constipation, urinary retention, blurry vision, tachycardia, and exacerbation of narrow angle glaucoma. TCAs are lethal in overdose and thus suicide risk should be carefully assessed. Symptoms of overdose include agitation, tremors, ataxia, arrhythmias, delirium, hypoventilation (secondary to central nervous system depression), myoclonus, hyperreflexia, seizures, and coma. Serotonergic effects are also seen in TCAs including erectile/ejaculatory dysfunction in males and anorgasmia in females.

MAOI side effects include serotonin syndrome (usually when taken in combination with SSRIs). Serotonin syndrome first consists of lethargy, restlessness, confusion, flushing, diaphoresis, tremor, and myoclonic jerks. These may progress to hyperthermia, hypertonicity, rhabdomyolysis, renal failure, convulsions, coma, and death. Thus, when switching to or from an SSRI and MAOI, a 2-week "washout period" should be implemented (5 weeks if switching from fluoxetine [longer half life]). Hypertensive crisis may also be seen as a side effect of MAOIs. This generally occurs when MAOIs are taken with tyramine-rich foods (wine, cheese, etc.). Additional side effects include orthostatic hypertension, drowsiness, weight gain, sexual dysfunction, dry mouth, sleep dysfunction, numbness and parasthesias (if pyridoxine deficiency), seizures, and edema (if liver toxicity).

Atypical antipsychotic side effects include metabolic syndrome, weight gain, hyperlipidemia, and hyperglycemia.

Electroconvulsive therapy treatment, in which a small electrical current is administered to induce a seizure under general anesthesia, may also provide a clinical benefit. This seizure has mood boosting effects, and may help with the neurovegetative symptoms of depression. This treatment is effective and safe (even during pregnancy). Side effects include cognitive problems (short-term memory loss that is temporary).

Bibliography

American Psychiatric Association. *Diagnostic and statistical manual of mental disorders: DSM-5.* 5th ed. Washington, DC: American Psychiatric Association; 2013.

Greene KA, Dickman CA, Smith KA, Kinder EJ, Zabramski JM. Self-inflicted orbital and intracranial injury with a retained foreign body, associated with psychotic depression: case report and review. *Surg Neurol.* 1993;40(6):499–503.

Johnson J, Horwath E, Weissman MM. The validity of major depression with psychotic features based on a community study. *Arch Gen Psychiatry.* 1991;48:1075.

Ohayon MM, Schatzberg AF. Prevalence of depressive episodes with psychotic features in the general population. *Am J Psychiatry.* 2002;159:1855.

Shagass C, Naiman J, Mihalik J. An objective test which differentiates between neurotic and psychotic depression. *AMA Archiv Neurol Psychiatry.* 1993;75(5):461–71.

Psychotic Disorder Due to Another Medical Condition

Epidemiology and Demographics: The lifetime prevalence of psychotic disorder due to another medical condition is difficult to estimate given the wide variety of clinical presentations and medical etiologies. The lifetime prevalence is estimated to range from 0.21% to 0.54%. Individuals over 65 years old have a significantly higher prevalence compared with those in other age groups.[1]

Disorder Description: Psychosis broadly characterized by a combination of key features such as delusions, hallucinations, disorganized thinking, disorganized or abnormal motor behavior, and negative symptoms. We categorize psychiatric disorders as secondary when symptoms are due to a known medical illness or substance use, or as primary, or idiopathic, if the symptoms cannot be explained by another cause. Subcortical and limbic system lesions, as well as dopamine dysregulations, are thought to be implicated in the development of secondary psychosis.

As stated in DSM-5, psychotic disorder due to another medical condition can be defined as:

A. Prominent hallucinations or delusions.

B. Evidence from history, physical examination, and/or laboratory findings that the disturbance is a direct pathophysiologic consequence of another medical condition.

C. The disturbance is not better explained by another mental disorder.

D. The disturbance does not occur exclusively in the context of delirium.

E. The disturbance causes clinically significant distress or impairment in social, occupational, or other important areas of functioning.[1]

Differential Diagnosis: Differential diagnosis should include delirium, substance intoxication/withdrawal, and medication-induced psychosis.

In delirium, hallucinations and delusions commonly occur. However, a separate diagnosis of psychosis due to another medical condition is not given if such disturbances only occur in the context of delirium. If delusions are seen in the context of a neurocognitive disorder, this would be diagnosed as major or minor neurocognitive disorder with behavioral disturbances.

In substance/medication-induced psychotic disorder, there is evidence of prolonged substance use, withdrawal from a substance, or exposure to a toxin. Symptoms usually occur during or shortly after (<4 weeks) exposure or withdrawal. This is particularly prevalent in the context of medications used in neurologic diagnoses.

Below is the list of disorders that should be considered as underlying etiology of psychosis:

- Epilepsy
- History of head trauma
- Dementias:
  - Alzheimer's disease
  - Pick's disease
  - Lewy body disease
- Stroke
- Space-occupying lesions and structural abnormalities:
  - Primary brain tumors
  - Secondary brain metastases
  - Brain abscess/cysts
  - Tuberous sclerosis
  - Midline abnormalities
  - Cerebrovascular malformations
- Hydrocephalus
- Demyelinating diseases:
  - Multiple sclerosis
  - Leukodystrophies
  - Schilder's disease
- Neuropsychiatric disorders:
  - Huntington's disease
  - Wilson's disease

- Parkinson's disease
- Friedreich's ataxia
- Infections:
  - Viral encephalitis
  - Neurosyphilis
  - Lyme disease
  - HIV
  - Central nervous system (CNS) invasive parasites
  - Tuberculosis
  - Sarcoidosis
  - *Cryptococcus* infection
  - Prion disease
  - Autoimmune encephalitis
- Neurology medications:
  - Steroids
  - Anticonvulsants:
    - levetiracetam
    - lamotrigine
    - phenytoin
    - carbamazepine
    - vigabatrin
    - ethosuximide
    - phenacemide
    - barbiturates
  - Muscle relaxants:
    - baclofen
    - cyclobenzaprine
  - Parkinson's disease medications:
    - levodopa
    - COMT inhibitors
    - other dopaminergic agents
    - amantadine
    - anticholinergics
    - MAO-B inhibitors

Every patient that presents with psychotic symptoms warrants a workup for an organic cause. While often it is difficult to distinguish psychosis as primary or secondary, certain characteristics of symptoms may suggest a medical nature. An atypical presentation, for example, old age onset, specific predominating features, symptoms disproportionate to those expected from a typical psychotic disorder, may point toward a secondary cause. Development of psychosis following the onset of a medical condition tends to correlate with the course of the medical condition. Of course, one should consider the possibility of decompensation of underlying psychiatric illness by the ongoing medical condition and stressors associated with it. After completing a thorough anamnesis and exam, routine laboratory tests should be ordered including: a complete and differential blood count, erythrocyte sedimentation rate, glucose, electrolytes, thyroid function tests, liver function test, and a urine drug screen. If suspicion still persists or first line tests require further investigation, the following labs should be ordered: rapid plasma reagin, HIV testing, serum heavy metals, copper and ceruloplasmin levels, serum calcium, autoantibody titers, vitamin B12, folate levels, urine culture, and toxicology. Neuroimaging may be appropriate at this time and MRI, CT, PET, and SPECT scans should be considered. EEG, polysomnography, CSF testing, and karyotyping may also reveal potential secondary cause.

Treatment Complications: Treatment is generally symptomatic and should be aimed at resolving the underlying condition. In irreversible cases, such as a structural neurologic alternation, neuroleptics should be used with caution considering the higher risk of extrapyramidal symptoms in patients with underlying CNS pathology.

Bibliography

1. American Psychiatric Association. *Diagnostic and statistical manual of mental disorders: DSM-5.* 5th ed. Washington, DC: American Psychiatric Association; 2013.
2. Cummings J. Organic psychoses. Delusion disorders and secondary mania. *Psychiatr Clin North Am.* 1996;9(2):293–311.
3. Keshavan MS, Kaneko Y. Secondary psychoses: An update. *World Psychiatry.* 2013;12(1):4–15. DOI:10.1002/wps.20001.
4. Stern TA, Fricchione GL, Cassem NH, Jellinek M, Rosenbaum JF. *Massachusetts General Hospital handbook of general hospital psychiatry.* Philadephia, PA: Saunders; 2010.
5. Weisholtz DS, Dworetzky BA. Epilepsy and psychosis. *J Neurol Disord Stroke.* 2014;2(3):1069.

Ptosis

Epidemiology and Demographics: Can affect any age without sex predilection.

Disorder Description: Upper eyelid movement is controlled by three main muscles: the levator muscle, innervated by cranial nerve III, opens the eyelid along with the sympathetically innervated Muller muscle, which provides about 2 mm of eyelid elevation; the orbicularis oculi muscle, innervated by cranial nerve VII, closes the eyelid.

The most common form of ptosis is involutional, related to dehiscence of the levator aponeurosis from the upper eyelid tarsus, usually from age, but it is also seen in patients after ocular surgery or trauma, or in those who wear rigid gas permeable contact lenses. Congenital ptosis is related to abnormal levator muscle development and presents at birth. Neither of these conditions has neurologic consequences, although congenital ptosis may result in amblyopia, or decreased vision from occlusion of the eye and inadequate developmental stimulation of the visual system.

Ptosis may be caused by neurologic conditions, including third nerve palsy, Horner syndrome, myasthenia gravis, and myotonic dystrophy.

Symptoms

Localization site	Comment
Cerebral hemispheres	**Acute unilateral, usually right-sided hemispheric stroke** may cause complete bilateral cerebral ptosis. This is an important sign, as studies have shown that it may indicate imminent herniation (rare)
	Apraxia of eyelid opening (AEO) is disorder of execution of learned movement that cannot be accounted for by paralysis, weakness, incoordination, or sensory loss. It may be isolated, but more often seen in patients with Parkinson's disease or progressive supranuclear palsy. Patients with AEO cannot open their eyes, and they often elevate their brows in an attempt to get them open. They may also have blepharospasm
Cranial nerves	**Third nerve palsy** in adults is most commonly ischemic, related to vasculopathic risk factors. Other causes include trauma, tumor, and stroke, but the most feared cause is compression from a posterior communicating artery aneurysm. Ischemic third nerve palsies typically cause ptosis and motility abnormalities, but spare the pupil, while compressive third nerve palsies are more likely to be "complete," causing ptosis, motility abnormalities, and a dilated pupil. Pupil-sparing third nerve palsies may be observed, since they are usually ischemic and will resolve spontaneously, but complete third nerve palsies are a neuro-ophthalmic emergency, and immediate imaging is indicated to rule out an enlarging aneurysm
Muscle	**Myotonic dystrophy** is an autosomal dominant condition, characterized by progressive muscle wasting and weakness, associated with bilateral ptosis, lack of facial expression, and rarely diplopia
	Chronic progressive external ophthalmoplegia (CPEO) is a mitochondrial disorder that is mostly sporadic, but may be familial. Patients present with symmetric ophthalmoparesis and ptosis with poor levator function. Diplopia is rare due to symmetric ophthalmoparesis. A rare form of CPEO is Kearns–Sayre syndrome, which includes pigmentary retinopathy, ataxia, and heart block, which may be fatal
	Oculopharyngeal dystrophy may be autosomal dominant, and presents in middle age with progressive bilateral ptosis, dysphagia, facial weakness, and proximal limb weakness. Ophthalmoplegia may be another feature
Neuromuscular junction	**Myasthenia gravis (MG)** is caused by autoantibodies to the neuromuscular junction post-synaptic acetylcholine receptors that prevent normal neuromuscular communication. Patients present with fatigable ptosis and diplopia that may be unilateral or bilateral. MG may be purely ocular or systemic, in which case bulbar symptoms, involving speaking, chewing, and breathing, may be life-threatening
	Lambert–Eaton syndrome (LES) is a presynaptic transmission disorder, and may be caused by a primary autoimmune condition similar to MG, or it may be paraneoplastic. The autoantibodies in LES are directed against presynaptic voltage-gated calcium channels. Unlike MG, LES is associated with autonomic symptoms, and less with ophthalmoplegia and ptosis, although these may be present. It is important in patients with LES to rule out malignancy, most commonly small cell carcinoma of the lung
	Botulism is caused by *Clostridium botulinum* and blocks release of acetylcholine from the presynaptic nerve terminal. It mostly affects infants less than a year of age in endemic areas, but may also be caused by ingestion of honey or home-canned goods that have been inadequately sterilized. Patients present commonly with ophthalmoplegia, ptosis diplopia, bifacial weakness, and poorly reactive pupils. Infants usually present with hypotonia and poor suckling, and adults may also present with pharyngeal and limb weakness, respiratory difficulty, and constipation
Unclear localization/ sympathetic chain	**Horner syndrome** is caused by interruption of the sympathetic chain to the eye. This interruption may be caused by a lesion in the brainstem, a Pancoast tumor in the lung, carotid dissection in the neck, or other lesions along the sympathetic chain. It causes the classic triad of ptosis, miosis (small pupil), and anhidrosis on the affected side. The ptosis is typically about 2 mm, which is the amount of lift provided by the sympathetically innervated Muller muscle. Horner syndrome may also be congenital, where it is also associated with iris heterochromia, with the ipsilateral iris lighter in color than the contralateral side

Secondary Complications: Amblyopia may develop in children under the age of 7 years with significant uncorrected ptosis, and these patients should be treated without delay to prevent irreversible vision loss. Peripheral visual field loss may result in adults, which is reversible with manual eyelid elevation or surgical eyelid elevation.

Treatment Complications: The main complications of surgical treatment of ptosis are undercorrection, overcorrection, and infection. Overcorrection may result in painful corneal exposure, infection, and even perforation of the cornea if not addressed promptly. If frontalis suspension technique is used, extrusion and exposure of the sling material is a risk, as is donor site morbidity if autologous fascia lata is used.

Bibliography

Bever C, Aquino AV, Penn AS, et al. Prognosis of ocular myasthenia gravis. *Ann Neurol.* 1998;14: 516–9.

Defazio G, Livrea P, Lamberi P, et al. Isolated so-called paraxis of eyelid opening: Report of 10 cases and a review of the literature. *Eur Neurol.* 1998;39(4):204–10.

Pure Autonomic Failure (Bradbury–Eggleston Syndrome)

Epidemiology and Demographics: The presence of orthostatic hypotension increases with age and disease comorbidities. Most cases, as listed in the references below, occur in middle age or later. There has been no predilection for either sex.

Disorder Description: The central nervous system fails to sense the change in cardiovascular demands. Normally, blood pressure increases slightly when a person sits up from a supine position. When a person's blood pressure does not respond to the change in position, he or she experiences symptoms of lightheadedness.

Symptoms

Localization site	Comment
Cerebral hemispheres	Hypothalamic dysfunction, orthostatic hypotension
Spinal cord	Bladder and sexual dysfunction, intermediolateral spinal cord
Peripheral neuropathy	Failure of sympathetic nerve ending release of norepinephrine (sudomotor dysfunction)

Secondary Complications: Some patients progress to developing signs of Parkinson's disease or multiple system atrophy.

Treatment Complications: Compressive devices are a good option for patients with many contraindications for supine hypertension. However, the devices can cause overheating, especially in warm climates. Fludocortisone mainly works via constricting the blood vessels. This may worsen symptoms in patients with congestive heart failure. Midodrine may cause numbness or tingling in some patients. Droxidopa may cause headaches.

Bibliography

Ferguson-Myrthil N. Droxidopa for symptomatic neurogenic hypotension. *Cardiol Rev.* 2017;25(5):241–6. DOI: 10.1097/CRD.0000000000000151.

Idiaquez J. Pure autonomic failure. Bradbury Eggleston syndrome: Case report. *Rev Med Chil.* 2005;133(2):215–8. Epub Apr 7, 2005.

Kuritzky L, Espay AJ, Gelblum J, Payne R, Dietrich E. Diagnosing and treating neurogenic orthostatic hypotension in primary care. *Postgrad Med.* 2015;127(7):702–15, DOI: 10.1080/00325481.2015.1050340.

Pure Pallidal Degeneration

Epidemiology and Demographics: Lesions to the globus pallidus (GP) occur due to neuronal degeneration (rare),[1] carbon monoxide poisoning,[2] opiate addiction (5–10% of cases), and in vascular diseases.[3] Other causes of pallidal necrosis include 3,4-methylenedioxy-methamphetamine (MDMA), cocaine, and cyanide poisoning. Pallidal degeneration may also present within a syndrome that includes hypoprebetalipoproteinemia, acanthocytosis, and retinitis pigmentosa (HARP syndrome). Pure pallidal degeneration (PPD) is extremely rare; since 1995, cases have been scarce.[4] It is a disorder that occurs from age 5 to 14 years, but it has been reported in adults as well.[5,6]

Disorder Description: Pure lesions within the globus pallidus (GP) interna (GPi) result in the loss of inhibitor neurotransmitter pallidal projections to the thalamus, leading to hyperkinetic movements. Lesions within the globus pallidus externa (GPe) result in increased thalamic inhibition, which may explain the hypokinetic movements or dystonic symptoms seen in some cases.[4] Furthermore, as described by Aizawa et al., PPD can present with symptoms which include torsion dystonia, choreoathetosis, progressive rigidity, akinesia, abnormal postures, speech disturbances, and gait disturbances.[5,6] Bilateral lesions may be more common than unifocal lesions, and may present with symptoms of parkinsonism. In chronic presentations, patients may also experience personality changes. A case report by Galati and Stadler describe a schizophrenic patient who experienced a sustained remission after an occasional "selective" bilateral pallidal lesion induced by carbon monoxide intoxication.[2] Unilateral lesions can present with unilateral dystonic features.

Localization is to the globus pallidus interna or externa, bilaterally or unilaterally, inducing torsion dystonia, choreoathetosis, progressive rigidity, akinesia, abnormal postures, speech disturbances, and gait disturbances.[5,6]

Secondary Complications: Patients with pure pallidal degeneration predominantly experience movement disorders, which may affect gait and cause parkinsonism. Children presenting with PPD usually have normal mental development[4] but adults with PPD may present with mild cognitive abnormalities.

Treatment Complications: Most patients have a discouraging response to medication, with only limited cases responding to levodopa.

Bibliography

1. Feve AP, Fenelon G, Wallays C, Remy P, Guillard A. Axial motor disturbances after hypoxic lesions of the globus pallidus. *Mov Disord.* 1993;8(3):321–6.
2. Galati S, Stadler C. Schizophrenia symptoms relieved by CO-induced pallidal lesion: a case report. *J Neuropsychiatry Clin Neurosci.* 2013;25(2):E52–3.
3. Alquist CR, McGoey R, Bastian F, Newman W, 3rd. Bilateral globus pallidus lesions. *J La State Med Soc.* 2012;164(3):145–6.
4. Bucher SF, Seelos KC, Dodel RC, et al. Pallidal lesions: structural and functional magnetic resonance imaging. *Arch Neurol.* 1996;53:682–6.
5. Aizawa H, Kwak S, Shimizu T, et al. A case of adult onset pure pallidal degeneration. I. Clinical manifestations and neuropathological observations. *J Neurol Sci.* 1991;102(1):76–82.
6. Aizawa H, Kwak S, Shimizu T, Mannen T, Shibasaki H. A case of adult onset pure pallidal degeneration. II. Analysis of neurotransmitter markers, with special reference to the termination of pallidothalamic tract in human brain. *J Neurol Sci.* 1991;102(1):83–91.

Pyomyositis

Epidemiology and Demographics: Pyomyositis is a common disease, especially in tropical climates. Males are more commonly affected than females. It can occur at any age, but there is a bimodal distribution, with peaks in children 2–5 years of age and adults 20–45 years of age. Classically it has been found in tropical climes. However, it is increasingly being seen in temperate climates, typically in immunocompromised adults.

Disorder Description: Pyomyositis is defined as a purulent infection of skeletal muscle; frequently it is due to hematogenous spread, usually with abscess formation. There are three clinical stages. Stage 1 is characterized by mild infection (low-grade fever, mild leukocytosis, local crampy pain, erythema). Stage 2, at which patients commonly present, occurs 10–21 days after onset, and is characterized by worsening symptoms (namely frank fever, marked leukocytosis, severe muscle tenderness, edema, and likely an evident abscess with pus on aspiration). Stage 3 is progression to sepsis. Patients will be febrile and may meet systemic inflammatory response syndrome (SIRS)/sepsis criteria.

It is caused by local muscle infection, usually hematogenously spread from another site. Risk factors include immunodeficiency, trauma, intravenous drug use, concurrent infection, and malnutrition.

There is no specific test for pyomyositis, but signs of infection are indicative. There will be likely leukocytosis (likely left shift, though eosinophilia suggests concomitant parasitic infection), positive blood cultures, and positive wound culture/aspiration culture. ESR and CRP, acute phase inflammatory markers, are likely to be elevated. MRI of affected tissue is the optimal and most useful technique for specifically diagnosing pyomyositis. CT can be done if MRI is not available, and ultrasound can be helpful in localizing potential site of aspiration.

Symptoms

Localization site	Comment
Muscle	Myalgia/pain localized to single muscle group, commonly in lower extremities, though deeper proximal muscles, such as iliopsoas, truncal, paraspinal, and upper extremities can be affected
Outside central nervous system	Fever

Secondary Complications: Pyomyositis itself is frequently a secondary complication and does not directly cause many secondary complications.

Treatment Complications: Treating the underlying infection with appropriate antibiotics from culture data is paramount. In addition, percutaneous draining can not only help diagnosis, but improve resolution.

There are no specific complications of treatment, other than the known antibiotic adverse effects based on choice of antibiotic.

Bibliography

Bickels J, Ben-Sira L, Kessler A, Wientroub S. Primary pyomyositis. *J Bone Joint Surg Am.* 2002;84–A:2277.

Crum NF. Bacterial pyomyositis in the United States. *Am J Med.* 2004;117:420.

Pyridoxine Deficiency

Epidemiology and Demographics: More common in alcoholics and the elderly.

Disorder Description: Pyridoxine is essential for metabolism of hemoglobin, neurotransmitter production, gene expression, gluconeogenesis, and histamine synthesis. Deficiency may lead to failure of several processes.

Symptoms

Localization site	Comments
Cerebral hemispheres	Seizures
Mental status and psychiatric aspects/complications	Somnolence. Confusion
Peripheral neuropathy	Painful sensory neuropathy in stocking–glove distribution. Rare muscle weakness

Secondary Complications: Complications include seborrheic dermatitis, atrophic glossitis with ulcers, angular cheilitis, conjunctivitis, intertrigo, sideroblastic anemia, glucose intolerance.

Treatment Complications: Overcorrection can lead to pyridoxine toxicity (see entry for *Pyridoxine Toxicity*).

Bibliography

Combs GF. *The vitamins: fundamental aspects in nutrition and health.* San Diego: Elsevier; 2008. pp. 313–29.

Pyridoxine-Dependent Seizures

Epidemiology and Demographics: Rare, under-recognized, autosomal recessive genetic disorder. Prevalence between 1/20,000 and 1/600,000, affecting both males and females. Early onset, typically occurring in infancy.

Disorder Description: Neonatal encephalopathy and seizures, difficult to control with conventional antiepileptic drugs, but responding to pyridoxine (vitamin B6) supplementation. Most commonly due to mutations in the antiquitin (ALDH7A1) gene encoding the enzyme α-aminoadipic semialdehyde (AASA) dehydrogenase, resulting in abnormal lysine catabolism and accumulation of toxic substrates.

Intravenous pyridoxine or pyridoxal phosphate (PLP) should be administered early in infants presenting with refractory seizures until confirmatory testing is completed, as appropriate intervention may have a dramatic impact. Seizures may even occur prenatally, and vitamin B6 may be administered in pregnancy for those known to be at risk.

Diagnosis made in infants by measuring levels of AASA and Δ-1-piperidine-6-carboxylate (P6C) and testing for mutations in ALDH7A1. Pyridox(am)ine 50-phosphate oxidase (PNPO) deficiency may present in an identical manner, but may respond only to PLP. Lysine restriction, arginine supplementation, and folinic acid along with pyridoxine therapy may improve long-term outcome.

Symptoms

Localization site	Comment
Cerebral hemispheres	Focal or generalized seizures including infantile spasms, atonic and myoclonic types. Status epilepticus and epileptic encephalopathy are common
	EEG abnormalities relatively nonspecific, and may normalize after initiation of vitamin B6
	MRI may show white matter changes, callosal abnormalities, and atrophy
Mental status and psychiatric aspects/ complications	High risk for neurodevelopmental disability, with motor and speech delays or other long-term cognitive impairments of varying severity, even despite pyridoxine supplementation
	Mood disturbances, anxiety, attentional deficits, sleep disorders and tics also described

Secondary Complications: Epileptic encephalopathy in the neonate may present with emesis, abdominal distention, apnea, irritability, sleeplessness, and abnormal eye movements. Hypoglycemia and lactic acidosis have been described.

Treatment Complications: Pyridoxine infusion may be associated with apnea, and should only be done in a monitored setting. Oral supplementation associated with gastrointestinal symptoms and peripheral sensory neuropathy at high doses. PLP may be associated with liver enzyme abnormalities. Lysine restriction and arginine supplementation require monitoring of diet, caloric intake, and amino acid levels. High doses of pyridoxine, PLP, and folinic acid have been associated with increased seizures in patients where later testing showed these not to be indicated.

Bibliography

Basura GJ, et al. Clinical features and the management of pyridoxine-dependent and pyridoxine-responsive seizures: review of 63 North American cases submitted to a patient registry. *Eur J Pediatr.* 2009;168(6):697–704.

Bok LA, et al. Long-term outcome in pyridoxine-dependent epilepsy. *Dev Med Child Neurol.* 2012;54(9):849–54.

van Karnebeek CD, Jaggumantri S. Current treatment and management of pyridoxine-dependent epilepsy. *Curr Treat Options Neurol.* 2015;17(2):335.

Pyridoxine Toxicity

Epidemiology and Demographics: Seen with overdose of supplements but not described with food sources.

Disorder Description: Pyridoxine overdose is toxic to the dorsal root ganglia.

Symptoms

Localization site	Comments
Dorsal root ganglia	Painful sensory neuropathy in all extremities beginning both proximally and distally
Polyneuropathy	Distal weakness and atrophy may be seen in severe cases

Bibliography

Combs GF. *The vitamins: fundamental aspects in nutrition and health.* San Diego: Elsevier; 2008. pp. 313–29.

Perry TA, Weerasuriya A, Mouton PR, Holloway HW, Greig NH. Pyridoxine-induced toxicity in rats: a stereological quantification of the sensory neuropathy. *Exp Neurol.* 2004;190(1):133–44.

Rabbit Syndrome

Epidemiology and Demographics: Any patient taking antipsychotics may acquire rabbit syndrome (RS). This is characterized by rapid, rhythmic movements of the mouth. Middle-aged and elderly patients may be more susceptible.[1] Although not well studied, the syndrome may be more likely in women than men.[2] The prevalence of the syndrome ranges from 2.3% to 4.4% of patients treated with antipsychotics.[3] The syndrome occurs more commonly with typical rather than atypical antipsychotic use. This is most likely due to their greater dopaminergic receptor affinity. Haloperidol,[4] followed by other typical antipsychotics, such as the phenothiazines (fluphenazine, thioridazine, trifluoperazine), are the drugs that classically cause RS, followed by some atypical antipsychotics.[5] Of that class, risperidone has been found to have the most extrapyramidal symptoms, including RS. There is no timetable for initiation of the antipsychotic to onset of symptomatology; however, most cases occur with chronic exposure to the drugs.

Disorder Description: RS is a rapid, rhythmic, vertical motion of the mouth and lips induced by antipsychotics that resembles the chewing movements made by a rabbit. The movements occur at a frequency of approximately 5 Hz, and may produce a popping sound due to the rapid separation of the lips.[6] The movements can be brought on by an increased amount of anxiety and stress. They may also be seen during stage 1 non-REM sleep. The movements cannot be voluntarily controlled by the patient, which is commonly misdiagnosed as oral tardive dyskinesia (TD).[4] It is important to note that RS does not include the tongue movements nor the oral rotatory movements associated with TD.[4] RS may be present in conjunction with TD and drug-induced parkinsonism (DIP), thus making the diagnosis more challenging.

Although the mechanism behind RS remains unclear, it is likely that the dopaminergic antagonism of the typical antipsychotics is the underlying cause, similar to DIP and TD. Evidence suggests that discontinuation of the drug and supplementation with an atypical antipsychotic may improve symptoms. Atypical antipsychotics have less dopamine receptor antagonism. Furthermore, studies have described a potential hypercholinergic etiology. Anticholinergic agents trihexyphenidyl or biperiden have been successful treatments. This may represent a cholinergic and dopaminergic imbalance within the basal ganglia.[4]

Antipsychotic medications have been used for the treatment of schizophrenia, psychosis, mania, and Tourrette's syndrome. Studies have described that regardless of the underlying disease, a patient may be susceptible to developing RS.

Symptoms

Localization site	Comment
Basal ganglia	Facial movement abnormalities as described above
Mental status and psychiatric aspects/ complications	The rapid involuntary movements may lead to interference with interpersonal relationships

Secondary Complications: RS characteristically produces mild discomfort due to the involuntary control of the buccal musculature, but does not directly cause further complications. The popping sound that can be produced by the movements may negatively impact the individual's social interactions.

Treatment Complications: The majority of patients that are treated with typical antipsychotics have significant mental illness, such as schizophrenia and/or psychosis. Abrupt discontinuation would lead to further complications of the patient's underlying disability.

References

1. Schwartz M, Hocherman S. Antipsychotic-induced rabbit syndrome: epidemiology, management and pathophysiology. *CNS Drugs*. 2004;18(4):213–20.
2. Fornazzari L, Ichise M, Remington G, Smith I. Rabbit syndrome, antidepressant use, and cerebral perfusion SPECT scan findings. *J Psychiatry Neurosci*. 1991;16(4):227–9.
3. Wada Y, Yamaguchi N. The rabbit syndrome and antiparkinsonian medication in schizophrenic patients. *Neuropsychobiology*. 1992;25(3):149–52.
4. Catena Dell'osso M, Fagiolini A, Ducci F, et al. Newer antipsychotics and the rabbit syndrome. *Clin Pract Epidemiol Ment Health*. 2007;3:6.

5. Deshmukh DK, Joshi VS, Agarwal MR. Rabbit syndrome: a rare complication of long-term neuroleptic medication. *Br J Psychiatry*. 1990;157:293.
6. Villeneuve A. The rabbit syndrome. A peculiar extrapyramidal reaction. *Can Psychiatr Assoc J*. 1972;17(2, Suppl 2):SS69.

Rabies Virus

Epidemiology and Demographics: Transmitted through the saliva of an infected animal bite. In the United States most commonly transmitted from bats, raccoons, skunks, and foxes. Rare cases of transmission from organ transplants.

Rabies has not been identified in Antarctica, New Zealand, Japan, Sweden, Norway, Spain, some Caribbean Islands, or Hawaii.

Disorder Description: Symptoms can manifest from days to years after an exposure.

Two types are encephalitic and paralytic:

1. Encephalitic: Prodrome for about 1 week. Symptoms can include low-grade fever, chills, malaise, myalgias, weakness, fatigue, anorexia, sore throat, nausea, vomiting, headache, and occasionally photophobia. During the active infection phase there are pharyngeal spasms causing hydrophobia. This progresses to hyperactive encephalopathy then obtundation and coma.
2. Paralytic: flaccid paralysis worst in the bitten limb. Can mimic Guillain–Barré syndrome.

Symptoms

Localization site	Comment
Cerebral hemispheres	Encephalitis
Mental status and psychiatric aspects/complications	Alternating hyper- and hypoactivity
Brainstem	Early involvement including with autonomic instability
Multiple spinal roots	Paralytic form
Muscle	Spasms of head and neck muscles

Secondary Complications: Complications include aspiration pneumonia, asphyxiation, respiratory arrest, cardiac arrhythmia, stroke from cerebral vasospasm.

Treatment: Treatment is supportive for active infection, with some reports of survival. Prophylaxis after exposure is available with vaccination if there is no skin break or rabies immunoglobulin if there is a skin break. Most domestic animals are vaccinated.

Bibliography

Hankins DG, Rosekrans JA. Overview, prevention, and treatment of rabies. *Mayo Clin Proc*. 2004;79(5):671–6.
World Health Organization. WHO expert consultation on rabies. *WHO Tech Rep Ser* 2005;Abstract 931:88.

Radial Neuropathy

Epidemiology and Demographics: This is a relatively rare disease in the United States.

Disorder Description: The condition is due to impingement of the radial nerve.

Posterior cord: weakness of arm abduction and adduction, medial rotation and extension of the arm.

Axilla: weakness in wrist and finger extension with mild weakness in supination and flexion at the elbow. Additional weakness in extension at the elbow and numbness in the posterior forearm and arm.

Spiral groove: weakness in wrist and finger extension with mild weakness in supination and flexion at the elbow. There is numbness over the back of the hand.

Posterior interosseous neuropathy: Weakness in wrist and finger extension with mild weakness in supination and flexion at the elbow. Normal strength when one is flexing the elbow with the thumb pointed to the ceiling (when, e.g., hammering), extension at the elbow and extending at the wrist. No sensory symptoms.

Surgical intervention can be a risk factor.

Potential radial neuropathy sites

Posterior cord	Axilla	Spiral groove	PIN (posterior interosseous nerve)
Deltoid and latissimus dorsi are weak	Normal deltoid and latissimus dorsi	Normal tricep and no sensory loss to posterior forearm and arm	Normal brachioradialis, long head of extensor carpi radialis, triceps No cutaneous sensory loss
	Weak tricep and sensory loss to posterior forearm and arm		

Secondary Complications: Complications include muscle atrophy, numbness, contracture of upper extremity joint, and weakness.

Treatment Complications: Toxic metabolic encephalopathy from sedation used during surgery or post surgical infections.

Bibliography

Brazis PW, et al., eds. Peripheral nerves. In *Localization in clinical neurology*. 6th ed. Philadelphia, PA: Lippincott Williams and Wilkins; 2011. Chapter 2.

Gouse M. Incidence and predictors of radial nerve palsy with the anterolateral brachialis splitting approach to the humeral shaft. *Chin J Traumatol.* 2016;19(4):217–20.

Radiation to Brain and Spinal Cord

Epidemiology and Demographics: No specific age group affected. In children, girls have been reported to be more affected by post-radiation myelopathy. No specific incidence/prevalence rates are known.

Disorder Description: The most sensitive structures to radiation within the nervous system are thought to be oligodendroglia and Schwann cells, with neurons being less affected due to their post-mitotic state. Radiation toxicity is classified into three categories:

1. Acute reactions, which occur during the course of treatment and are caused by radiation-induced edema.
2. Early delayed reactions, occurring weeks to months after finishing radiation therapy. This reaction is caused by temporary inhibition of myelin synthesis.
3. Late delayed reactions, occurring months to years after radiation therapy. A very common type of late delayed reaction is radiation necrosis. This type of reaction is caused by damage to small and medium arterioles or by directly affecting glial cells.

Radiation myelopathy has been reported to occur in the cervical and thoracic region.

Potential causes include:
- Radiation for Hodgkin's lymphoma
- Radiation for nasopharyngeal and oropharyngeal cancers
- Radiation for medulloblastoma
- Radiation for breast cancer
- Radiation for pelvic malignancies
- Radiation for germ cell tumors
  Risk factors include:
- Age of the patient – infants and children have higher likelihood of complications
- Re-irradiation
- Exceeding the generally accepted tolerance doses of radiation
- Receiving concurrent chemotherapy that is known to cause peripheral neuropathy:
  - methotrexate (high-dose systemic and intrathecal)
  - platinum drugs (cisplatin, carboplatin, oxaliplatin)
  - taxanes (paclitaxel, docetaxel, cabazitaxel)
  - epothilones
  - plant alkaloids (vincristine, vinblastine, etoposide, vinorelbine)
  - thalidomide, lenalinomide, pomalidomide
  - bortezomib, carfilzomib
  - eribulin

No specific areas of the world have higher proclivity.

Symptoms

Localization site	Comment
Brain	Acute effects of radiation are caused by edema secondary to increased intracranial pressure. Most common symptom is headache. Acute effects are self-limited and do not require intervention. In rare cases, steroids may be required
	Early delayed toxicity occurs because of transient demyelination that occurs between 4 weeks and 4 months. Common symptoms include somnolence and worsening of neurologic deficits that are already present. Caution is advised in differentiating between recurrence of disease vs. early/late effects of radiation toxicity. Early/late effects are typically self-limited
	Effects of late delayed toxicity can be seen in several manifestations. These include: necrosis, atrophy, encephalopathy, infarction, hemorrhage, and neoplastic transformation. Necrosis, atrophy, and encephalopathy are the most common. Brain necrosis is noted typically 1–2 years after therapy is completed. Diagnosis is via biopsy, and treatment requires surgical removal of necrotic tissues. Steroids and anticoagulation have shown some benefit. Brain atrophy is typically seen 1 year after whole brain radiation. Imaging demonstrates large ventricle and periventricular white matter changes. Symptoms include dementia, memory problems, gait apraxia (similar to normal pressure hydrocephalus). There is no effective treatment for brain atrophy
Cervical spinal cord	Early delayed radiation myelopathy is known to cause Lhermitte's sign. This suggests demyelination of the posterior columns. In the cervical spinal cord the risk of delayed radiation myelopathy increases with increasing length of spinal cord irradiated.
Thoracic spinal cord	Late effects to the spinal cord are less common and generally more severe. Myelopathic syndrome typically develops involving a portion of the cord then progressing to involve the entire cord. The thoracic spinal cord is generally less sensitive to radiation injury than the cervical cord. For the thoracic spinal cord, published analyses do not indicate a definite relationship between irradiated rostral–caudal spinal cord volume and the risk of delayed myelopathy. Delayed radiation myelopathy usually presents with numbness or dysesthesias in the legs, followed by weakness and sphincter dysfunction, with an upper level of cord dysfunction ascending to lie within the irradiated area. Pain is usually not a prominent complaint. A *Brown–Sequard hemicord pattern* is fairly common early in the course. In most patients, the neurologic deficits progress over several weeks to months and often plateau, but rarely improve spontaneously

Localization site	Comment
Lumbar spinal cord	A rare syndrome of selective damage to lower motor neurons occurs following spinal irradiation for medulloblastoma, lymphoma, or germ cell tumors (particularly testicular cancer). This condition is called **radiation-induced motor neuron syndrome**. Patients develop roughly symmetric bilateral leg weakness beginning 4 to 14 months after completion of radiation. Examination shows muscle atrophy, fasciculations, normal or decreased muscle stretch reflexes, flexor plantar responses, and no sensory or sphincter involvement. Weakness is confined to the legs, even in patients who received irradiation to the entire spine. The syndrome usually progresses slowly over several months, and then stabilizes, but does not improve. Motor and sensory nerve conduction velocities are normal. Electromyographic evidence of diffuse denervation, including lumbar paraspinal muscles, is noted. Spine MR scans are typically normal. Lumbosacral anterior horn cells are believed to be the primary site of damage in these patients, but no published neuropathologic proof for this exists, and it is possible that the syndrome represents selective damage to proximal motor axons or to motor roots

Secondary Complications

1. Spinal cord hemorrhage
2. Cerebral hemorrhage
3. Radiation-induced cavernomas
4. Residual weakness and numbness of the upper and lower extremities
5. Persistent loss of bowel/bladder control
6. Chronic headache and neuropathic pain
7. Residual mental status deficits resulting in diminished executive functioning
8. Seizure disorder

Treatment Complications: Antiseizure medications use to treat seizure disorder can lead patients to develop metabolic disturbances, worsening of underlying psychiatric conditions, worsening somnolence/fatigue.

Narcotic pain medications used to treat chronic pain carry risk of addiction and tolerance. They also cause and worsen somnolence and fatigue.

Bibliography

Dropcho EJ. Neurotoxicity of radiation therapy. *Neurol Clin*. 2010;28(1):217–34.

Posner JB. Side effects of radiation therapy. In DeAngelis LM, Posner JB, eds. *Neurologic complications of cancer*. Philadelphia, PA: FA Davis; 1995. pp. 311–37.

Radiation to Peripheral Nerves/Plexuses

Epidemiology and Demographics: Age of presentation varies depending on age when radiation therapy received. However, the younger the age at the time of radiation, the higher the likelihood of neurologic complications secondary to radiation. No gender preference known. No specific prevalence or incidence known. However, peripheral nerve damage after radiation is uncommon as peripheral nerves are generally resistant to radiation. Peripheral nerve sheath tumors secondary to radiation are extremely rare.

Disorder Description: The peripheral nervous system consists of cranial nerves and spinal nerves. The brachial plexus is of particular concern during irradiation of the upper chest wall as it is located in the supraclavicular area and beneath the clavicles. The roots of the brachial plexus are formed by the anterior rami of spinal nerves C5–T1. The lumbosacral plexus plays a similar role in the innervation of the lower extremities. Damage to the plexus can produce a variety of sensory and motor deficits including pain, neuropathy, motor deficits, and functional disability. The peripheral nervous system is considered to be relatively resistant to damage by ionizing radiation. Complications secondary to radiation do not appear immediately, but can take years (a range of 5 years to 31 years) to develop to any level of clinical significance. Radiation to peripheral nerves can result in perineural fibrosis. Radiation has also been known to rarely cause benign tumors (neurofibromas) and malignant peripheral nerve sheath tumors (sarcomas). The nature and extent of radiation-induced tumors depends on: (1) total dose of radiation provided, (2) volume of the irradiated tissue, (3) the size of the daily dose, and (4) the time between doses of radiation. It is important to note that radiation-induced peripheral nerve tumors are hard to distinguish clinically from naturally forming peripheral nerve tumors as they demonstrate the same imaging features. Clinical evidence has revealed that 20 to 40 Gy of radiation delivered in a hypofractionated manner during intra-operative radiation therapy is sufficient to cause peripheral nerve neurofibromas.

Potential causes include:
a. Radiation for Hodgkin's lymphoma
b. Radiation for nasopharyngeal and oropharyngeal cancers
c. Radiation for medulloblastoma
d. Radiation for breast cancer
e. Radiation for pelvic malignancies
   Risk factors include:
a. Age of the patient – infants and children have higher likelihood for complications
b. Re-irradiation
c. Exceeding the generally accepted tolerance doses of radiation
d. Receiving concurrent chemotherapy that is known to cause peripheral neuropathy:
   i.   methotrexate (high-dose systemic and intrathecal)
   ii.   platinum drugs (cisplatin, carboplatin, oxaliplatin)
   iii. taxanes (paclitaxel, docetaxel, cabazitaxel)
   iv.   epothilones
   v.   plant alkaloids (vincristine, vinblastine, etoposide, vinorelbine)
   vi.   thalidomide, lenalinomide, pomalidomide
   vii. bortezomib, carfilzomib
   viii. eribulin

No specific areas of the world have higher proclivity.

Symptoms

Localization site	Comment
Cranial nerves	Olfactory, optic, facial, glossopharyngeal, hypoglossal, and vagus nerves most commonly affected following radiation after nasopharyngeal carcinoma. Symptoms include anosmia, visual loss, loss of tongue movement, loss of facial sensation, ageusia, loss of gag reflex, parasympathetic dysfunction
Brachial plexus/ peripheral nerves	Brachial plexus involvement commonly seen during radiation for Hodgkin's lymphoma and weeks to months after radiation for breast cancer. Post-radiation brachial plexopathy for most conditions appears typically weeks to months after radiation. Symptoms include sensory loss +/− weakness. Pain is usually absent. Other symptoms include myokymia and lymphedema. Presence of pain suggests recurrence of tumor. Radiation-induced plexopathy is not reversible

Localization site	Comment
Lumbar plexus/ peripheral nerves	Post-radiation lumbar plexopathy appears typically in less than 1 year (commonly 4–6 months) after radiation. The foot is affected initially with proximal muscle involvement occurring subsequently. Very rarely, spontaneous resolution has been reported. Radiation-induced lumbar plexopathy is typically not reversible

Secondary Complications

1. Residual sensory abnormalities involving taste, smell, vision, facial sensation.
2. Loss of gag reflex.
3. Residual weakness and sensory changes of the upper and lower extremities.
4. Cellulitis/lymphangitis.

Treatment Complications

1. Anticonvulsants: Gabapentin and pregabalin are commonly used for the treatment of this condition. Both of these medications are known to cause lower extremity edema. Additionally these medications are also known to cause Stevens–Johnson syndrome, increased risk of suicidality, depression, anaphylaxis. Abrupt withdrawal can cause seizure activity.
2. Tricyclic antidepressants: In cases where anticonvulsants are not effective, tricyclic antidepressants such as nortriptyline and amitriptyline are utilized. These medications are known to cause orthostatic hypotension and QT prolongation, and increase somnolence. They are also known to cause weight gain.
3. Selective serotonin/norepinephrine reuptake inhibitors: These medications are known to cause serotonin syndrome and SIADH (syndrome of inappropriate antidiuretic hormone secretion), and increase risk of suicidality and depression as well as mania/hypomania.

Bibliography

Dropcho EJ. Neurotoxicity of radiation therapy. *Neurol Clin.* 2010;28(1):217–34.

Posner JB. Side effects of radiation therapy. In *Neurologic complications of cancer*. Philadelphia, PA: FA Davis; 1995. pp. 311–37.

Radiculopathy

Epidemiology and Demographics: As summarized by Warren et al., the incidence of radiculopathy is 85 persons per 100,000. The incidence of lumbar radiculopathy is variable as different studies give different numbers.

Disorder Description: Back or neck pain with radiation down the limb is the usual presentation. Lumbar radiculopathy can be caused by anything that may invade the space of the spinal cord or nerve roots. For cervical radiculopathy in the younger patients, the cause is usually trauma. With increasing age, disc degeneration becomes the predominant cause.

Symptoms

Localization site	Comment
Spinal cord	Disc herniation
Cauda equina	Bowel or bladder dysfunction
Specific spinal roots	Narrowing of the neuroforamen

Secondary Complications: Weakness in muscles and decreased range of motion of the neck, back, or lower extremities due to pain.

Treatment Complications: Anti-inflammatory medications may rarely cause cerebrovascular complications. Acetaminophen may cause hepatic encephalopathy. Opiates can cause delirium, sedation, and other complications described throughout this text.

Bibliography

Alexander C. *Lumbosacral radiculopathy*. StatPearls. Treasure Island, FL: StatPearls Publishing; Jun 29, 2017.

Brazis PW, et al., eds. Peripheral nerves. In *Localization in clinical neurology*. 6th ed. Philadelphia, PA: Lippincott Williams and Wilkins; 2011. Chapter 2.

Warren M. *Cervical radiculopathy*. StatPearls. Treasure Island, FL: StatPearls Publishing; Jun 25, 2017.

Raeder's Paratrigeminal Neuralgia

Epidemiology and Demographics: This is a rare disease. As per the listed references, the disease has been reported only in males.

Disorder Description: Any external injury, pressure, inflammation of the ophthalmic division of the trigeminal nerve can cause this disease. Vasoactive intestinal polypeptide, calcitonin gene-related peptide, substance P, and neurokinin A have been found in certain animal studies.

Patients may complain of pain around their eyes. There may be a droopy eyelid or a small pupil when compared with the asymptomatic side.

Symptoms

Localization site	Comment
Cerebral hemispheres	Thalamus, hypothalamus
Brainstem	Spinal trigeminal nucleus, inferior olivary nucleus, preganglionic neurons of the parasympathetic system. Edinger–Westphal nucleus, superior and inferior salivary nucleus
Cranial nerves	Ophthalmic division of the trigeminal nerve, facial nerve
Spinal cord	Segments S2 to S4 of the spinal cord contain cell bodies of the parasympathetic system
Unclear localization	Cerebral arteries

Secondary Complications: Anxiety from chronic pain and vision changes may occur.

Treatment Complications: Nonsteroidal anti-inflammatory medications can rarely cause a cerebrovascular event.

Bibliography

Goadsby PJ. Raeder's syndrome: paratrigeminal paralysis of the oculopupillary sympathetic system. *J Neurol Neurosurg Psychiatry*. 2002;72(3):297.

Mokri B. Raeder's paratrigeminal syndrome. Original concept and subsequent deviations. *Arch Neurol*. 1982;39(7):395.

Tatsui C. Raeder's syndrome after embolization of a giant intracavernous carotid artery aneurysm: pathophysiological considerations. *Arq Neuropsiquiatr*. 2005;63(3A):676–80.

Rapid-Onset Dystonia–Parkinsonism Syndrome (RDP)

Epidemiology and Demographics: Rapid-onset dystonia–parkinsonism (RDP) is a rare dystonia-plus syndrome that develops in late adolescence to early adulthood, usually in one's 20s, though age of symptom onset ranges from 4 to 58 years.[1,2]

Disorder Description: RDP onset occurs over minutes to days, usually during a specific physical or psychologic stressor such as a febrile illness. The dystonia is more severe in the head and neck than in the lower body, and the parkinsonism is not levodopa-responsive and non-progressive.[3] Symptoms include dysarthria and dysphagia accompanied by bradykinesia, slow gait, and postural instability. Generally, the symptoms remain unchanged with only improvement in gait.[1,2]

At onset, patients have vague symptoms of dystonia involving the hand and arms. In nearly all patients, this was subtle and localized to the distal extremity. Generalized or truncal dystonia was never seen to precede symptoms. Clear progression face > arm > leg is a cardinal feature of mutation positive RDP, associated with sudden onset and bulbar symptoms.[4] RDP typically follows an autosomal dominant inheritance with variable expressivity and penetrance.[5,6]

Apart from the specific constellation of symptoms characterizing the disease, some important features help distinguish RDP from other acute dystonia syndromes. RDP is associated with only three parkinsonian features: bradykinesia, postural instability, and hypophonia. Absence of pain and tremors is a key feature distinguishing RDP from other acute dystonia syndromes.[4] RDP symptoms may be provoked by the presence of triggers such as physical or emotional stress, childbirth, and alcoholic binges. Clinical improvement (albeit minimal) helps to distinguish RDP from other dystonic syndromes.[5]

Symptoms

Localization site	Comment
Mental status and psychiatric aspects/ complications	Depression, social phobia, anxiety, schizoid tendencies such as psychosis
	Impairment was seen in attention, verbal fluency, coding tasks, visual memory, and verbal learning tasks compared with controls
Basal ganglia	Dystonia, bradykinesia, postural instability, hypophonia
Cranial nerves	Prominent bulbar findings: dysarthria, dysphonia, dysphagia; paroxysmal oculomotor abnormalities including oculogyric crisis[1]

RDP may have depressive and psychotic symptoms associated with the dystonia, which may lead to diagnostic dilemmas. Other dystonia phenotypes or inborn errors of metabolism such as Wilson disease may also present with these symptoms.[4]

Secondary Complications: No secondary complications have been observed to occur. Moreover, symptoms stabilize within a month of onset.

Treatment: High-dose benzodiazepine therapy has been beneficial in some patients, although treatment options are limited for RDP.[4]

References

1. Dobyns WB, Ozelius LJ, Kramer PL, et al. Rapid-onset dystonia-Parkinsonism. *Neurology*. 1993;43:2596–602.

2. Pittock SJ, Joyce C, O'Keane V, et al. Rapid-onset dystonia parkinsonism: a clinical and genetic analysis of a new kindred. *Neurology*. 2000;55:991–5.

3. Charlesworth G, Bhatia KP, Wood NW. The genetics of dystonia: New twists in an old tale. *Brain*. 2013;136(7):2017–37.

4. Sweney MT, Newcomb TM, Swoboda KJ. The expanding spectrum of neurological phenotypes in children with ATP1A3 mutations, alternating hemiplegia of childhood, rapid onset dystonia parkinsonism, CAPOS and beyond. *Pediatr Neurol*. 2015;52(1):56–64.

5. de Carvalho Aguiar P, Sweadner KJ, Penniston J, et al. Mutations in the Na+/K+-ATPase α3 gene ATP1A3 are associated with rapid onset dystonia parkinsonism. *Neuron*. 2004;43:169–75.

6. Brashear A, Dobyns WB, de Carvalho Aguiar P, et al. The phenotypic spectrum of rapid onset dystonia-parkinsonism (RDP) and mutations in the ATPIA3 gene. *Brain*. 2007;130(3):828–35.

Rasmussen Encephalitis

Epidemiology and Demographics: Seizures commonly start between 1 and 14 years of age, median age 6 years, but may occur in adults. Incidence between 1.7 and 2.4 per 100,000 per year in those below 18 years. Gender, geographical, and ethnic predominance have not been reported.

Disorder Description: Suspected immune-mediated inflammatory disorder that may preferentially affect one cerebral hemisphere. Often presents with medically intractable focal seizures and secondarily generalized tonic–clonic seizures (GTCS). Epilepsia partialis continua (EPC) in 50% of cases. Progressive inflammation and atrophy of the hemisphere occurs causing worsening hemiparesis or dysfunction of associated eloquent cortex. Earlier EEGs show unihemispheric slowing with or without epileptiform activity and unilateral seizure onset. Within months of acute stage, MRI brain shows unilateral enlargement of ventricular system, and T2/flair hyperintense lesions in gray and white matter. Serial MRIs will show worsening atrophy and progression of disease. Disease may become bihemispheric, as evident on pathology.

Cause believed to be secondary to a T-cell response to one or more antigenic epitopes with involvement of autoantibodies. Treatments include antiepileptic drugs, epilepsy surgery (hemispherectomy), and immunomodulatory therapies, such as steroids, intravenous immunoglobulin (IVIG), plasma exchange, T-cell inactivating chemotherapeutic agents (i.e., tacrolimus, aziathioprine), and the monoclonal antibody drugs (i.e., rituximab).

There are three disease stages:

prodromal – mild hemiparesis, low seizure frequency

acute – progressive hemiparesis, increase in seizure frequency (EPC), cognitive decline

residual – stable/permanent neurologic deficits, continued seizures

Symptoms

Localization site	Comment
Cerebral hemispheres	Focal seizures, EPC, secondarily GTCS
	Progressive paresis
	Unilateral cerebral hemispheric progressive atrophy on serial MRI
	EEG with focal slowing, and unilateral epileptiform discharges
Mental status and psychiatric aspects/ complications	Intermittent alterations of consciousness
	Progressive language deficits, cognitive decline

Secondary Complications: Progressive disability due to intellectual decline, progressive hemiparesis, dysphagia.

Treatment Complications: Surgery (hemispherectomy) curative for seizures, though may result in homonymous hemianopsia and hemiplegia. Prognosis for neurologic recovery of function better in patients operated on before late childhood. Steroids are associated with an increased risk for mood lability, psychosis, peptic ulceration, avascular necrosis, and infection. IVIG may be associated with flu-like symptoms during infusion and rarely anaphylaxis. Depending on the agent, other immunosuppressive drugs are associated with increased risk for infection, blood dyscrasias, renal or liver toxicity, among other side effects.

Bibliography

Daroff RB, Bradley WG, eds. *Bradley's neurology in clinical practice.* 6th ed. Philadelphia, PA: Saunders; 2012.

Varadkar S, et al. Rasmussen's encephalitis: clinical features, pathobiology, and treatment advances. *Lancet Neurol.* 2014;13(2):195–205.

Reactive Arthritis (Reiter's Syndrome)

Epidemiology and Demographics: Most common in young men (20 to 40 years of age); rarely occurs in children from enteric infections (symptoms after age 9 years). Enteric form has no gender predominance; venereal form has a male-to-female ratio of 5:1 to 10:1. More common in Caucasian than blacks. The frequency is estimated to be 3.5–5 cases per 100,000. Frequency related to prevalence of HLA-B27 in population.

Disorder Description: Reactive arthritis is an autoimmune process that occurs in response to a previous gastrointestinal or genitourinary infection. In some rare cases there have been reports of chlamydial infection of the respiratory system leading to this condition. The classic triad of symptoms includes: (1) non-infectious urethritis in men and cervicitis in women; (2) arthritis; and (3) conjunctivitis (iridocyclitis). When there is mucocutaneous involvement (pustular psoriasis), the condition is referred to as Feissenger–Leroy–Reiter syndrome. The clinical triad is present only in 30% of patients. In patients who develop the syndrome after an enteric infection, the symptoms of the triad tend to occur within 1 to 4 weeks after the infection. Reactive arthritis is associated with HLA-B27 haplotype on chromosome 6. HLA-B27 is an MHC Class I molecule involved in T-cell antigen presentation. It is thought that reactive arthritis develops with a cross-reactivity with specific types of microbial antigens that are disseminated into joints. Studies have reported that reactive arthritis and ankylosing spondylitis appear to be identical based on similar findings in long-term outcomes of the two conditions. Central and peripheral nervous system involvement in reactive arthritis is well recognized. In rare cases, there have also been reports of progressive myelopathy.

Potential causes include:

a. Genitourinary infection:
   i. *Chlamydia trachomatis*
   ii. *Neisseria* gonorrhea
   iii. *Ureaplasma urealyticum*
b. Gastrointestinal/respiratory infection:
   i. *Shigella flexneri*
   ii. *Salmonella enterica*
   iii. *Mycoplasma pneumoniae*
   iv. *Mycobacterium tuberculosis*
   v. *Cyclospora*
   vi. *Yersinia enterocolitica*
   vii. *Campylobacter jejuni*
   viii. *Clostridium difficile*
   ix. Beta hemolytic Group A *Streptococcus*
   x. *Streptococcus viridans*
c. Medications/iatrogenic:
   i. adalimumab
   ii. leflunomide
   iii. bacillus Calmette–Guerin (BCG) instillation for treatment of bladder cancer
   iv. tetanus and rabies vaccine

Risk factors include:

a. Caucasian males with HLA-B27 haplotype (HLA-B51 and HLA-DRB1 alleles also risk factors)
b. HIV infection or AIDS

There is higher proclivity to reactive arthritis in North America and Europe, particularly Finland and Norway. Higher proclivity is secondary to higher risk of infections. that lead to the development of reactive arthritis.

Symptoms

Localization site	Comment:
Brain	Cerebral vasculitis may result in patient developing seizure activity, headache, double vision, stroke, and encephalopathy
Cranial nerves	Glossopharyngeal neuralgia may present with patients complaining of sharp throat pain typically lasting seconds to minutes

Localization site	Comment:
Spinal cord	In cases of progressive myelopathy, sensory level, hyperactive knee and ankle jerks and Babinski sign may be present
Peripheral neuropathy	Axonal polyneuropathy may present with patient complaining of vague symptoms of paresthesias and numbness of the extremities in fashion similar to what is seen in diabetic neuropathy

Secondary Complications: Complications include stroke, neuropathy (cranial and peripheral), and myelopathy.

Treatment Complications: Reactive arthritis is a self-limited process. All treatments utilized for this condition are symptomatic or treat the underlying cause. Physical therapy, non-steroidal anti-inflammatory drugs, and corticosteroids are the medications most commonly utilized. Antibiotics may be given to treat underlying infection, and disease-modifying antirheumatic drugs such as sulfasalazine and methotrexate may be used safely and are often beneficial.

Bibliography

Carter JD, Hudson AP. Reactive arthritis: clinical aspects and medical management. *Rheum Dis Clin North Am*. 2009;35(1):21–44.

Kaarela K, Jäntti JK, Kotaniemi KM. Similarity between chronic reactive arthritis and ankylosing spondylitis. A 32–35-year follow-up study. *Clin Exp Rheumatol*. 2009;27(2):325–8.

Recurrent Isolated Sleep Paralysis

Epidemiology and Demographics: The prevalence of recurrent isolated sleep paralysis is unknown with no sex predominance. Age at onset is typically 14–17 years.

Predisposing factors include sleep deprivation, irregular sleep–wake schedules, stress. More common in supine position. Associations with bipolar disorder, anxiolytic medications, and sleep-related leg cramps have been reported.

Disorder Description: Recurrent isolated sleep paralysis is characterized by an inability to perform movements at sleep onset (hypnagogic) or on waking from sleep (hypnopompic) without a diagnosis of narcolepsy. There is preservation of atonia after an arousal from REM sleep with inability to speak or move the limbs, trunk, and head but respiration is not usually affected. There is preserved consciousness and individuals are able to fully recollect events surrounding the episode, which can last seconds to minutes. Episodes typically resolve spontaneously but can be aborted by external auditory or tactile stimulation or by intense efforts to move by the individual.

Symptoms

Localization site	Comment
Unclear localization	Sleep paralysis is a disassociated state with elements of REM sleep persisting into wakefulness

Recurrent isolated sleep paralysis is associated with psychiatric disorders including dissociative phenomena, anxiety disorders, panic disorder, and posttraumatic stress disorder.

Treatment Complications: Management includes reassurance, avoidance of sleep deprivation, and maintenance of regular sleep–wake schedules. In cases of frequent occurrence, substantial sleep disruption, or excessive distress, REM suppressive agents such as imipramine or fluoxetine may be used at bedtime.

Patients on imipramine should be monitored for QT prolongation. Anticholinergic effects should be monitored such as urinary retention, constipation, xerostomia, mental status changes.

Bibliography

American Academy of Sleep Medicine. *International classification of sleep disorders*. 3rd ed. Darien, IL: American Academy of Sleep Medicine; 2014

Schenck C, Mahowald M. REM sleep parasomnias in adults. In Barkoukis TJ, et al., eds. *Therapy in sleep medicine*. Philadelphia, PA: Elsevier; 2012. pp. 540–58.

Sharpless BA, Barber JP. Lifetime prevalence rates of sleep paralysis: a systematic review. *Sleep Med Rev*. 2011;15:311–5.

Recurrent Menstrual Psychosis

Epidemiology and Demographics: Menstrual psychosis is rare, and often goes unrecognized. In asylum studies performed in the late 19th century, 1–29/1000 female admissions were found to have menstrual psychosis. There are only about 80 confirmed cases in the literature. Most importantly, it is distinguished from other forms of psychosis by its perimenstrual association.

Disorder Description: A diagnosis of menstrual psychosis requires:

Acute onset against an otherwise normal functional background.

Short duration with complete recovery.

Psychotic features: hallucinations, delusions, mania, stupor, mutism, and delirium.

Periodicity in rhythm with the menstrual cycle.

The existence of recurrent menstrual psychosis is controversial and reports suggest that new-onset psychosis in a female in close proximity to menses is an early sign of bipolar disorder.

Differential Diagnosis: Differential diagnosis should include schizoaffective disorder, schizophreniform and brief psychotic disorder, delusional disorder, and schizotypal personality disorder, postpartum psychosis.

The key to distinguishing recurrent menstrual psychosis from these disorders is the periodicity of menstrual psychosis in synchronicity with the menstrual cycle. None of the schizophrenia-related disorders exhibits this timing. This requires careful record keeping of both the onset of menses and the onset of symptoms of menstrual psychosis. It can be differentiated from postpartum psychosis because menstrual psychosis is not associated with only the post-partum time period.

Secondary Complications: Recurrent menstrual psychosis may be associated with social, academic, and occupational dysfunction, due to the lack of functionality during the occurrence of the psychotic episode.

Treatment Complications: Typical and atypical antipsychotics may be used as treatment for recurrent menstrual psychosis. Side effects of typical antipsychotics include the extrapyramidal side effects such as parkinsonism (mask-like facies, bradykinesia, cogwheel rigidity, pill-rolling tremor), akathisia, and dystonia. Other side effects include hyperprolactinemia, sedation, weight gain, orthostatic hypotension, cardiac abnormalities, sexual dysfunction, anticholinergic side effects (dry mouth, tachycardia, urinary retention, blurry vision, constipation, worsening of narrow-angle glaucoma), tardive dyskinesia, and neuroleptic malignant syndrome. Atypical antipsychotic side effects are similar, but more frequently and to a larger extent include

metabolic syndrome, weight gain, hyperlipidemia, and hyperglycemia.

In addition to psychotropic medications, other approaches have been shown to be viable options. Thyroid hormones, for example, have been shown to be curative. Levothyroxine side effects include arrhythmias, congestive heart failure, hypertension, angina, pseudotumor cerebri (in pediatric population), craniosynostosis (in infants), and seizures. Less severe side effects include palpitations, increased appetite, tachycardia, nervousness, tremor, weight loss, diaphoresis, GI distress, insomnia, fever, headache, heat intolerance, and anxiety.

Progesterone has also been shown to be an effective treatment. Potential side effects of progesterone include thromboembolism, retinal thrombosis, optic neuritis, hypertension, stroke, myocardial infarction, breast or ovarian cancer, jaundice, depression, anxiety, anaphylaxis. Less serious side effects include headache, breast tenderness, depression, dizziness, fatigue, irritability, cough, chest pain, dysmenorrhea, constipation, and fluid retention.

Bibliography

Brockington I. Menstrual psychosis. *World Psychiatry*. 2005;4(1):9.

Brockington IF. Menstrual psychosis: a bipolar disorder with a link to the hypothalamus. *Curr Psychiatry Rep*. 2011;13(3):193.

Dennerstein L, Judd F, Davies B. Psychosis and the menstrual cycle. *Med J Aust*. 1983;1(11):524–6.

Felthous AR, Robinson DB, Conroy RW. Prevention of recurrent menstrual psychosis by an oral contraceptive. *Am J Psychiatry*. 1980;137(2):245–6.

Kramer MS. Menstrual epileptoid psychosis in an adolescent girl. *Am J Dis Child*. 1977;131(3):316–17.

Relapsing Polychondritis

Epidemiology and Demographics: Presents most commonly between 40 and 50 years of age, but can occur at any age. No gender preference. No race predominance. Frequency of condition is 3.5 cases per million.

Disorder Description: Relapsing polychondritis is characterized by inflammation and deterioration of cartilage. It is a condition that affects multiple systems in the body. It is a painful condition and can become life threatening if it affects the respiratory system, heart valves, or blood vessels. The involvement of the peripheral or central nervous system is relatively rare and only occurs in 3% of persons affected with this condition. It is sometimes seen in relation with concomitant vasculitis. The most common neurologic manifestations are palsies of the cranial nerves V and VII. Additionally hemiplegia, ataxia, myelitis, and polyneuropathy have been reported in the scientific literature. Very rare neurologic manifestations include aseptic meningitis, meningoencephalitis, stroke, focal or generalized seizures, and intracranial aneurysm. Magnetic resonance imaging of the brain shows multifocal areas of enhancement consistent with cerebral vasculitis in some cases.

The exact cause is unknown but is thought to be secondary to immune-mediated attack on proteins within the cartilage. There is a possible genetic cause as there is a higher familial predominance of the condition. However the exact genetic linkage is not known.

There are no known geographic areas with higher proclivity.

Symptoms

Localization site	Comment
Brain	Aseptic meningitis, cerebral vasculitis may result in patients developing stroke and/or focal or generalized seizures. Intracranial aneurysm may also occur
Cranial nerves	Palsies of trigeminal (CN V) and/or facial nerve (CN VII)
Spinal cord	Myelitis causing hemiplegia or paraplegia
Peripheral neuropathy	Compression of peripheral nerves secondary to cartilage inflammation may cause symptoms of numbness and/or paresthesias

Secondary Complications: Complications include stroke, neuropathy, intracranial aneurysm, peripheral neuropathy.

Treatment Complications: Patients treated with non-steroidal anti-inflammatory drugs for an extended period of time are likely to face complications associated with this class of medications.

Corticosteroids are also often used to treat this condition. Azathioprine and methotrexate are often used to reduce the side effects associated with corticosteroids. Prolonged steroid use can cause avascular necrosis of the hip, hyperglycemia, altered mentation/mania, and increased risk of infection secondary to immunosuppression. Methotrexate can cause patients to develop ulcerative stomatitis, aplastic anemia, agranulocytosis, leukoencephalopathy, seizures, Stevens–Johnson syndrome, among other complications. Azathioprine can cause patients to develop progressive multifocal leukoencephalopathy, lymphoma, and possibly other malignancies.

Cyclophosphamide is also used in severe manifestations of this disease. Cyclophosphamide can cause myelosuppression, bone marrow failure, hemorrhagic cystitis, pulmonary fibrosis, urinary bladder fibrosis, renal failure, congestive heart failure, SIADH (syndrome of inappropriate antidiuretic hormone secretion), sterility, among other complications.

Bibliography

Chopra R, Chaudhary N, Kay J. Relapsing polychondritis. *Rheum Dis Clin N Am*. 2013;39(2):263–76.

Langford CA. Relapsing polychondritis. In Kasper DL, Fauci AS, Hauser SL, et al., eds. *Harrison's principles of internal medicine*. 19th ed. New York: McGraw-Hill Education/Medical; 2015. p. 389.

REM Behavior Disorder

Epidemiology and Demographics: Overall prevalence is 0.38 to 0.5% with a male sex predominance. Age at onset is typically after age 50. Predisposing factors include male sex, age over 50, underlying neurologic disorders (Parkinson's disease, multiple system atrophy, Lewy body dementia, narcolepsy, cerebrovascular disease), smoking, head injury, pesticide exposure. Antidepressants (venlafaxine, serotonin reuptake inhibitors, but not buproprion), beta-blockers (bisoprolol, atenolol), anticholinesterase inhibitors, and selegiline have been implicated in iatrogenic REM behavior disorder (RBD).

Disorder Description: RBD is characterized by abnormal behaviors during REM sleep. In RBD, normal REM atonia is lost, and often patients present with dream enacting behavior usually of unpleasant, action-filled, violent dreams. The behaviors include both violent and non-violent behaviors and range from talking to kicking and punching. However, walking is uncommon. The individual typically awakens at the end of an episode and is alert and can coherently report a dream. RBD can emerge in children but is associated with narcolepsy, brainstem tumors, antidepressants, neurodevelopmental disorders. RBD may be the first symptom of a neurodegenerative process such as Parkinson's disease and may predate the onset of other symptoms by more than a decade, and one study showed RBD preceded the onset of a neurodegenerative process in about 51% of patients. In another study, patients with RBD were evaluated with (18)F-fluorodeoxyglucose PET imaging and Parkinson disease-related covariance pattern (PDRP) expression was seen in RBD patients and used as a marker for predicting future development of Parkinson disease or dementia with Lewy bodies.

Management of RBD should initially focus on patient and bed partner safety. Medications associated with RBD should be eliminated whenever possible and steps should be taken to identify and treat comorbid sleep disorders. Once offending medications are discontinued, many cases of RBD remit. Dream-enacting behaviors often resolve if underlying REM-related obstructive sleep apnea is treated. If violent behaviors persist, pharmacotherapy with clonazepam and/or melatonin can be initiated. Ninety percent of patients initially respond well to low doses of clonazepam (0.5 to 1.0 mg) at bedtime. Clonazepam reduces phasic EMG activity during REM with minimal effect on tonic muscle activity. High-dose melatonin (5 to 15 mg) suppresses both phasic and tonic REM motor activity and has been reported to be effective both as monotherapy or in combination with clonazepam. Other agents such as imipramine, carbamazepine, levodopa, pramipexole, donepezil, sodium oxybate, triazolam, zopiclone, quetiapine, and clozapine have been used with limited success.

Symptoms

Localization site	Comment
Brainstem	Interruption of the REM atonia pathway and/or disinhibition of multiple brainstem motor pattern generators are implicated, including pontine REM-on (precoeruleus and sublateral dorsal) and REM-off (ventral lateral portion of the peri-aqueductal gray matter and lateral tegmentum) nuclei

RBD is strongly linked with narcolepsy, type 1. Other associations include cerebrovascular disease, multiple sclerosis, progressive supranuclear palsy, Guillain–Barré syndrome, brainstem neoplasms, Machado–Joseph disease, mitochondrial encephalomyopathy, normal pressure hydrocephalus, Tourette syndrome, group A xeroderma, and autism.

Secondary Complications: Injuries including subdural hematoma, shoulder dislocation, cervical fracture, and lacerations severing arteries, tendons, and nerves.

Treatment Complications: Side effects due to clonazepam such as morning sedation, memory dysfunction, depression and personality changes, and aggravation of obstructive sleep apnea may occur. Melatonin can cause morning sedation and headaches.

Bibliography

American Academy of Sleep Medicine. International classification of sleep disorders, 3rd ed. Darien, IL: *American Academy of Sleep Medicine*; 2014.

Boeve BF, Silber MH, Ferman TJ, et al. Clinicopathologic correlations in 172 cases of rapid eye movement sleep behavior disorder with or without a coexisting neurologic disorder. *Sleep Med.* 2013;14: 754–62.

Devnani P, Fernandes R. Management of REM sleep behavior disorder: An evidence based review. *Ann Indian Acad Neurol.* 2015;18:1–5.

Holtbernd F, Gagnon JF, Postuma RB, et al. Abnormal metabolic network activity in REM sleep behavior disorder. *Neurology.* 2014;82:620–7.

Renal Cancer

Epidemiology and Demographics: Kidney cancer accounts for 3% of all US cancer cases. Renal cell carcinomas (RCC) originate in the renal cortex and account for 85% of all primary kidney cancer. Transitional cell carcinomas of the renal pelvis account for about 8%. Other parenchymal tumors of the kidney are far rarer. In the United States there are approximately 64,000 new cases and almost 14,000 deaths from RCC each year. The median age at diagnosis is 65. Men have a 2- to 3-fold higher risk than women. About 75% of patients present with localized disease, half of whom later develop metastatic disease. About 20–30% of patients have metastatic disease at presentation.

Disorder Description: Renal cancer is any primary malignancy of the kidney, renal cell carcinoma affecting the renal cortex being the most common. Flank and back pain, fatigue, anemia, hematuria, and weight loss are the most common presenting symptoms of kidney cancer. Common risk factors include von Hippel–Lindau disease, chronic dialysis, obesity, smoking, first-degree relative family history, and hypertension. Renal cell carcinoma metastasizes via the lymphatic system to local, regional, and mediastinal lymph nodes. It also metastasizes hematogenously to lung, bone, liver, and brain.

There are both central and peripheral nervous system complications of renal cancer, both more commonly associated with advanced stages of the cancer, therefore more complications arise as novel treatments prolong survival of renal cancer patients.

Symptoms

Localization site	Comment
Cerebral hemispheres	Brain metastases typically at gray/white matter junction. Patients present with headaches, motor deficits, ataxia, mental status changes, seizures
	Intra-tumoral hemorrhage is common, often with resultant stroke
	Leptomeningeal carcinomatosis is extremely rare
Mental status	Mental status changes secondary to brain metastases
Spinal cord	Rare metastases to intramedullary spinal cord. More commonly, metastases to thoracic, lumbar osseous spine with resultant local or radicular pain and sensorimotor deficits due to epidural spinal cord compression

Secondary Complications: Paraneoplastic complications: Rarely, paraneoplastic motor neuron disease presenting with symptoms mimicking amyotrophic lateral sclerosis. Paraneoplastic polymyositis presenting as weakness. Rarely, myasthenia gravis.

Hypercalcemia secondary to a paraneoplastic syndrome may present as lethargy, nausea, fatigue, confusion, weakness, and constipation.

Treatment Complications: Most common neurologic complication of treatment of metastatic renal cell carcinoma is sensory neuropathy (secondary to agents inhibiting tumor angiogenesis like sorafenib). Neuropsychiatric complications

secondary to immunotherapy (interferon-alpha, interleukin-2 [IL-2], etc.) occur in up to 30–50% of patients, including cognitive changes, delusions, hallucinations, depression. Less commonly, transient focal neurologic deficits, acute leukoencephalopathy, carpal tunnel syndrome, myositis, myasthenia gravis, brachial neuritis have been reported with IL-2.

Bibliography

Giglio P, Gilbert MR. Neurologic complications of cancer and its treatment. *Curr Oncol Rep.* 2010;12(1):50–9.

Palapattu GS, Kristo B, Rajfer J. Paraneoplastic syndromes in urologic malignancy: the many faces of renal cell carcinoma. *Rev Urol.* 2002;4(4):163–70.

Traul DE, Schiff D. Neurologic complications of genitourinary cancer. *Current Clinical Oncology: Cancer Neurology in Clinical Cancer.* Totowa, NJ: Humana Press; 2008.

Vogelzang NJ, Stadler WM. Kidney cancer. *Lancet.* 1998;352:1691–96.

Renal Failure, Acute

Epidemiology and Demographics: Acute renal failure complicates approximately 5% of hospital admissions and up to 30% of admissions to intensive care units. The incidence of acute kidney injury (AKI) has grown by more than fourfold in the United States since 1988 and is estimated to have a yearly incidence of 500/100,000 population, higher than the yearly incidence of stroke.

Disorder Description: Acute renal failure is a syndrome characterized by rapid decline in glomerular filtration rate (hours to days), retention of nitrogenous waste products, and perturbation of extracellular fluid volume and electrolyte and acid–base homeostasis.

Symptoms (Also See Entry for *Renal Failure, Chronic*)

Localization site	Comment
Mental status and psychiatric aspects/ complications	Altered mental status or seizures associated with electrolyte alterations such as hyponatremia or hypocalcemia

Secondary Complications

Uremia: Build up of nitrogenous waste products cause elevated BUN (blood urea nitrogen) concentration, which is a hallmark of AKI. BUN itself poses little direct toxicity at levels below 100 mg/dL. At higher concentrations, mental status changes can arise. Patient may exhibit asterixis and encephalopathy.

Hyponatremia: If severe can cause seizures.

Hyperkalemia: Potassium affects the cell membrane potential of cardiac, neural, and muscular tissues. Muscle weakness may be a symptom of hyperkalemia.

Hyperphosphatemia and hypocalcemia: Hypocalcemia is often asymptomatic but may cause perioral paresthesias, muscle cramps, seizures, carpopedal spasms, and prolongation of the QT interval on EKG.

Treatment Complications: Please see discussion of dialysis complications under entry for *Renal Failure, Chronic.*

Bibliography

Kasper DL, Fauci AS, Hauser SL, et al., eds. *Harrison's principles of internal medicine.* 19th ed. New York: McGraw-Hill Education/ Medical; 2015.

Renal Failure, Chronic

Epidemiology and Demographics: The most common cause of chronic kidney disease (CKD) in the United States and Europe is diabetic nephropathy, most often secondary to type 2 diabetes mellitus. Kidney disease, including mild to the most severe forms, occurs in up to one out of every ten individuals living in the United States.

Disorder Description: Also known as chronic kidney disease, the term chronic renal failure envelops the diverse potential etiologies and severities of renal dysfunction. It is more common in the elderly although it may be more severe and more progressive when it afflicts younger individuals.

Symptoms

Localization site	Comment
Cerebral hemispheres	Myoclonus
Mental status and psychiatric aspects/ complications	As the renal failure progresses it causes wide range of clinical manifestations, from subtle neuromuscular disease to mild memory, concentration, and sleep disturbance to hiccups, cramps, and twitching due to asterixis, myoclonus, seizures, and coma
Peripheral neuropathy	Peripheral neuropathy: usually becomes clinically evident after the patient reaches stage 4 CKD, although electrophysiologic and histologic evidence occurs at earlier stages. Initially, sensory nerves are involved more than motor, lower extremities more than upper, and distal parts of the extremities more than proximal. If dialysis is not initiated soon after onset of sensory neuropathy, motor involvement follows, including muscle weakness. Evidence of peripheral neuropathy without another cause (e.g., diabetes mellitus) is an indication for starting renal replacement therapy. Many of the complications described above will improve with dialysis, although subtle nonspecific abnormalities may persist Uremic polyneuropathy occurs in approximately 60% of patients with chronic renal failure and can affect motor, sensory, autonomic, and cranial nerves. Electrophysiologically, axonal loss and secondary demyelination is found
Muscle	Muscle cramps. Uremic myopathy usually appears in patients with a glomerular filtration rate (GFR) <25 mL/min and progression parallels the decline of renal function. It causes proximal limb weakness, muscle wasting, limited endurance, exercise limitation, and rapid fatigability. In general, physical exam, EMG, and muscle enzymes are normal

Secondary Complications: Uremia leads to disturbances in the function of virtually every organ system. After dialysis, neurologic symptoms improve, but level of azotemia correlates poorly with the degree of neurologic dysfunction.

Treatment Complications

Encephalopathy: Hemodialysis patients are at risk of Wernicke's encephalopathy because of not only low thiamine intake but probably also accelerated loss of thiamine.

Dialysis encephalopathy or dialysis dementia: Errors in dialysis water purification or the use of aluminum-containing dialysate and aluminum-containing phosphate binders to treat hyperphosphatemia cause accumulation of this element in many organs leading to microcytic anemia, osteomalacia, and dialysis encephalopathy.

Rejection encephalopathy: 80% of cases occur within 3 months of transplantation. Cytokine production secondary to the rejection may cause this.

Hypertensive encephalopathy: Patients display the encephalopathic symptom complex in combination with severe hypertension. Recombinant human erythropoietin for the correction of renal anemia causes hypertension in 35% of patients. Hypertensive encephalopathy occurs in 5%. MRI often demonstrates posterior reversible encephalopathy syndrome.

Dysequilibrium syndrome: Dialysis treatment may cause disequilibrium syndrome, which presents clinically with headache, nausea, muscle cramps and twitching, delirium, and seizures. It is self limited and subsides over hours to days.

Immunosuppressant-associated encephalopathy: Described with calcineurin inhibitors cyclosporine and tacrolimus. Common symptoms are tremor, headache, cerebellar or extrapyramidal signs. Neurotoxicity is more common when toxic levels accumulate in the body but may even be apparent at levels within therapeutic range.

Dementia: The incidence of multi-infarct dementia in this group is estimated at 3.7%, which is 7.4 times more frequent than the general elderly population.

Cerebrovascular disease: Ischemic stroke in renal failure mainly results from atherosclerosis, thromboembolic disease, or intradialytic hypotension. Hemodialysis is associated with a higher incidence of intracerebral hemorrhage and subarachnoid hemorrhage. Systemic anticoagulation in hemodialysis can be complicated by acute and chronic subdural hematoma.

Osmotic myelinolysis: Central pontine myelinolysis is clinically characterized by acute progressive quadriplegia, dysarthria, dysphagia, alteration of consciousness, horizontal and vertical gaze paralysis. Osmotic myelinolysis after rapid correction of prolonged

hyponatremia or less frequently hypernatremia by dialysis is a known problem. On the other hand, rapid serum sodium correction by hemodialysis occurs often, but only a few patients develop demyelination.

Opportunistic infections: Immunosuppression is the main cause of opportunistic infections. Uremic state itself can cause phagocytic dysfunction of polymorphonuclear leukocytes, leading to immunodeficiency especially against bacterial infection. This problem is even more prominent in patients with dialysis or renal transplants. Neurologic infections in patients with renal failure mainly present as acute, subacute or chronic meningitis, encephalitis, myelitis or brain abscess. Opportunistic pathogens include bacteria, fungi, viruses, and parasites.

Peripheral nervous system: Mononeuropathy of ulnar, median, and femoral nerves occurs because of ischemia, uremic tumoral calcinosis, and dialysis-associated amyloidosis. Acute femoral neuropathy is a known complication of renal transplantation due to preoperative compression of the nerve by retractors causing nerve ischemia. The incidence is estimated at about 2% with excellent chance of recovery.

Bibliography

Brouns R, De Deyn PP. Neurological complications in renal failure: a review. *Clin Neurol Neurosurg.* 2004;107:1–16.

Burn DJ, Bates B. Neurology and the kidney. *J Neurol Neurosurg Psychiatry.* 1998;65:810–21.

Kasper DL, Fauci AS, Hauser SL, et al., eds. *Harrison's principles of internal medicine.* 19th ed. New York: McGraw-Hill Education/Medical; 2015.

Lacerda G, Krummel T, Hirsch E. Neurologic presentations of renal diseases. *Neurol Clin.* 2010;28:45–59.

Repetitive Hand Use

Epidemiology and Demographics: As summarized by Ioannou et al., prevalence of focal dystonia is 29.5/100,000 people in the United States. This condition is seen more in musicians and writers.

Disorder Description: Just as the name of the disorder indicates, the disease is caused by overworked muscles. This may be due to occupations such as musicians and carpenters, or due to diseases such as Rett syndrome. A patient may complain of muscle spasms when trying to perform certain motions with his or her hand. There might be motor dysfunction, hand rigidity, paresthesias.

Symptoms

Localization site	Comment
Cerebral hemispheres	Basal ganglia
Mental status and psychiatric aspects/ complications	Anxiety and frustration
Muscle	Muscle and tendons

Secondary Complications: Limitation of movement, muscle atrophy, decrease in quality of life, detrimental to professional careers.

Treatment Complications: Botulinum toxin injections may be tried. They can occasionally cause extreme motor impairment.

Bibliography

Byl N. Treatment effectiveness for patients with a history of repetitive hand use and focal hand dystonia: a planned, prospective follow-up study. *J Hand Ther*. 2000;13(4):289–301.

Ioannou C. Objective evaluation of performance stress in musicians with focal hand dystonia: a case series. *J Mot Behav*. 2016;48(6):562–72.

Retinal Detachment

Epidemiology and Demographics: Retinal detachment (RD) is rare in the general population with estimated incidence of 5–18/100,000 people and varies widely across geographic location and ethnic groups. The most common form of RD (rhegmatogenous) appears to have higher incidence in the 60–70 age group, men, and young myopic patients.

Disorder Description: Retinal detachment describes the separation of the neurosensory retina from the underlying retinal pigment epithelium. There are three general mechanisms by which this occurs (in order of decreasing frequency): rhegmatogenous (detachment secondary to a hole or tear in the retina), tractional (abnormal adhesions at vitreoretinal interface pull on the retina), or exudative (fluid build up under the retina such as from inflammatory or neoplastic processes).

Symptoms

Localization site	Comment
Cerebral hemispheres	**Tuberous sclerosis** is a rare multi-system genetic disease associated with astrocytic tumors of the central nervous system (CNS), cutaneous lesions, intellectual disabilities, and seizures. Children with tuberous sclerosis often have seizures referred to as infantile spasms characterized by repetitive myoclonic spasms of the head, neck, and limbs. Astrocytic hamartomas of the retina are the principal ophthalmic manifestation of tuberous sclerosis. These can be seen in otherwise healthy individuals but in tuberous sclerosis these can be multifocal or bilateral. Generally these are benign tumors but can show progressive enlargement leading to retinal detachments
	Sturge–Weber syndrome (SWS) is a sporadic neurocutaneous disorder. Seizures are the most common neurologic abnormality. The main retinal abnormality is diffuse choroidal hemangioma, which can lead to total retinal detachment
	von Hippel–Lindau is an autosomal dominant neoplastic disorder associated with tumors of the central nervous system, retina, and visceral organs. In the eye, patients develop vascular tumors known as retinal capillary hemangioblastomas. These tumors tend to enlarge progressively without treatment and as these tumors grow, they can displace normal retinal structures. Intraretinal and subretinal exudates can accumulate ultimately leading to exudative retinal detachment. Fibrosis and hemorrhage associated with these tumors can also lead to tractional retinal detachments
Mental status and psychiatric aspects/ complications	**Norrie's disease** is a rare X-linked disorder characterized by congenital blindness, sensorineural hearing loss, and cognitive impairment. The ocular phenotype has been well described and is characterized by fibrous and vascular changes, and peripheral retinal ischemia presenting at birth that can progress to tractional retinal detachment. Other neurologic associations have been reported including seizure disorder and behavioral disturbances
	See **tuberous sclerosis** above. This is associated with intellectual disabilities
Vestibular system (and non-specific dizziness)	See **Norrie's disease** above. This is associated with sensorineural hearing loss

Localization site	Comment
Peripheral neuropathy	Diabetes mellitus is associated with a number of ocular manifestations particularly in the retina. Advanced diabetic retinopathy from ongoing ischemic insult to the retinal vasculature drives neovascularization or proliferative diabetic retinopathy. This neovascularization is associated with abnormal connective tissue formation particularly along the vitreo-retinal interface. This can create tractional forces on the retina resulting in tractional retinal detachments. These forces can also result in tears in the retina so combined tractional/rhegmatogenous detachments often occur in diabetic patients. Peripheral neuropathies are among the most common complications of diabetes, which are thought to occur due to damage to peripheral nerves secondary to prolonged exposure to elevated blood glucose levels
Unclear localization	Toxoplasmosis is a significant cause of infectious retinal disease and posterior uveitis in the immunocompetent host. Immunocompetent individuals generally are otherwise asymptomatic, but toxoplasmosis is the most common CNS infection in AIDS patients not receiving prophylaxis. In the eye, patients can develop retinal necrosis, retinal neovascularization, and secondarily tractional and retinal detachments

Secondary Complications: In a retinal detachment, the photoreceptors in the retina are separated from their blood supply. The macula, which is responsible for high resolution central visual acuity, is particularly susceptible to damage from retinal detachment. Central visual acuity may range from normal if the retinal detachment is peripheral, to hand motions if the detachment involves the central macula. Timing of retinal detachment repair and extent of macula involvement are important factors in visual outcome. Surgical advances now allow up to 95% of retinal detachments to be repaired by returning the retina to its proper anatomic position. However, not all patients return to their baseline visual acuity after successful surgical repair due to the factors described above.

Treatment Complications: The treatment of retinal detachments, particularly rhegmatogenous and tractional RDs, is surgical. As with any intraocular surgery, postoperative complications can include pressure elevation, cataracts, infection, and bleeding, all potentially negatively impacting vision. There are a number of complications unique to retinal detachment surgery. Proliferative vitreoretinopathy in which cells proliferate in the vitreous and on the retinal surface is the most common cause of failure after retinal detachment surgery. Phototoxicity to the retina from lighting used during surgery and damage to the retina and other ocular structures from substances such as air, nitric oxide, and silicone oil, which are used to tamponade the retina, have been reported. Diplopia can occur due to scleral buckles altering ocular alignment.

Bibliography

Edwards AO. Clinical features of congenital vitreoretinopathies. *Eye*. 2008;22:1233–42.

Retinal Migraine

Epidemiology and Demographics: A review of publications on retinal migraine reveals that this condition is rare. There are no epidemiological studies that evaluate prevalence or incidence. One journal article that reviewed retinal migraine suggests that this condition is seen mostly in women of childbearing age with history of migraine headaches with aura.

Disorder Description: The criteria for diagnosis involve at least two attacks of fully reversible monocular visual defects that last less than 60 minutes and must occur before, during, or after the headache. This condition is a diagnosis of exclusion as other causes must be ruled out. Many patients report a history of migraine headache with aura during these attacks. The headache is usually on the side of the vision loss. There are reported cases of permanent visual loss with these migraine headaches.

Symptoms

Localization site	Comment
Cerebral hemispheres	Involvement of retinal artery and optic nerves should always be evaluated in this condition before diagnosis of retinal migraine
Cranial nerves	Optic nerve involvement should be evaluated in this condition

Treatment Complications: There are no clear guidelines for management of retinal migraines. Outside of maintaining a healthy lifestyle, some suggest prophylactic medication to prevent further attacks. There are no established guidelines for prophylaxis. Some reports suggest a daily aspirin, calcium channel blocker, and other migraine headache prophylaxis medications. Triptans and ergots should be avoided due to increased risk of vasoconstriction.

Bibliography

Corbett JJ. Neuro-ophthalmic complications of migraine and cluster headaches. *Neurol Clin.* 1983;1:973–95.

Grosbert BM, Solomon S, Lipton RB. Retinal migraine.*Curr Pain and Headache Rep.* 2005;9:268–71.

Rothrock J, Walicke P, Swenson MR, et al. Migrainous stroke. *Arch Neurol.* 1988;45:63–7.

Retinitis Pigmentosa (Retinal Dystrophies)

Epidemiology and Demographics: Typical retinitis pigmentosa (RP) has an incidence of 1 in 5000 worldwide. It is a heterogeneous group of disorders but typically patients have presented for clinical diagnosis by age 30 years. The sex ratio depends on the inheritance pattern. Men may be more symptomatic with X-linked forms.

Disorder Description: RP encompasses a broad range of hereditary disorders affecting the photoreceptors and retinal pigment epithelium. The majority have a genetic basis and with current molecular capabilities, the responsible gene can be determined in about 40–50% of cases. There are autosomal dominant, autosomal recessive, and X-linked forms. Typically these are slowly progressive conditions leading to vision loss. Retinitis is a misnomer as inflammation is not a hallmark of these disorders. Classic funduscopic findings are pigment deposits in the mid-peripheral retina, attenuation of retinal vessels, and "waxy" optic nerve pallor.

Symptoms: Most forms of retinitis pigmentosa initially affect the rod photoreceptors, which impairs night vision and peripheral vision. Progressive constriction of peripheral vision is a hallmark of the disease. In most cases, central vision is spared until the late stages of disease. Patients can also complain of photopsias (flashing lights) in more advanced forms of the disease.

Localization site	Comment
Mental status and psychiatric aspects/ complications	**Bardet–Biedl syndrome** is a genetic disorder characterized by obesity, polydactyly, hypogonadism, and RP-like retinal degeneration. Intellectual disabilities, developmental delay, and behavioral abnormalities are commonly described
Spinal cord	**Abetalipoproteinemia** is a rare autosomal recessive lipid metabolism disorder. Fat malabsorption, diarrhea, and failure to thrive develop early in childhood. Spinocerebellar degeneration from vitamin E deficiency progresses to ataxia and lower extremity spasticity. Retinitis pigmentosa, either focal or diffuse, is the main ocular manifestation of this condition
Peripheral neuropathy	**Refsum disease** is an autosomal recessive disorder of lipid metabolism leading to the accumulation of the fatty acid phytanic acid in blood and tissues. This accumulation causes peripheral neuropathy, ataxia, hearing loss, retinitis pigmentosa, and dry, rough skin (ichthyosis)
Unclear localization	**Neuronal ceroid lipofuscinosis** (Batten's disease) is the general name for a group of neurodegenerative disorders characterized by accumulation of materials in lysosomes. Patients experience severe psychomotor retardation, leading to a vegetative state, seizures, and premature death. Retinal degeneration often leads to complete blindness in classic childhood forms of this disease

Secondary Complications: Secondary ocular complications of retinitis pigmentosa can occur, and thus these patients require routine ophthalmic monitoring. Cystoid macular edema in which cyst-like pockets of fluid can develop in the macula results in decreased vision. This is thought to be secondary to either leakage from the retinal vasculature or due to dysfunction in the retina's ability to pump out fluid. Vitreous abnormalities can often be seen clinically even in childhood and can prematurely detach. Retinal tears or detachments, however, are infrequent.

RP patients are also at risk of developing glaucoma, particularly primary angle closure glaucoma, and cataracts.

Treatment Complications: There are currently no FDA-approved treatments for retinal degenerations but treatment trials are ongoing. Vitamin A supplementation has been shown to have a mild effect in slowing the progression of vision loss in some studies. Hepatotoxicity and teratogenicity are the two major side effects with vitamin A use. Patients who develop cystoid macula edema may benefit from treatment with oral acetazolamide. Common side effects include paresthesias, fatigue, and drowsiness, and serious side effects include kidney damage and lactic acidosis.

Gene therapy and retinal prosthesis are two additional areas of research that are under way for retinitis pigmentosa.

Bibliography

Massof RW, Fishman GA. How strong is the evidence that nutritional supplements slow the progression of retinitis pigmentosa? *Arch Ophthalmol.* 2010;128(4):493–95. DOI:10.1001/archophthalmol.2010.46.

Pruett RC. Retinitis pigmentosa: clinical observations and correlations. *Trans Am Ophthalmol Soc.* 1983;81:693–735.

Rett Syndrome

Epidemiology and Demographics: Classic Rett syndrome is seen primarily in girls. After a period of neurotypical development, at 6–18 months of age there is a plateau in further development, followed by a regression of attained milestones. Later in childhood, there is a plateau of regression, followed by a static course complicated by acquired dystonia, and foot and hand deformities. Scoliosis and osteopenia can be seen in young adulthood. The prevalence of Rett syndrome in females is estimated to be 1:8500.[1]

Disorder Description: Rett syndrome is a neurodevelopmental disorder, seen mainly in girls, who after typical neurodevelopment up to 6–18 months have a plateau, followed by regression in motor and language skills as well as fits of inconsolable crying. Purposeful hand movement is lost, replaced by a characteristic hand-wringing stereotypy. Girls develop autistic features, anxiety, breathing irregularities, epilepsy, acquired microcephaly, impaired gait, and gastrointestinal dysmotility. Failure to thrive, scoliosis, vasomotor disturbance, and insensitivity to pain are common. Girls with Rett are also at risk for prolonged QT syndrome.

Rett syndrome is caused by mutations or deletions in the *MECP2* gene, an X-linked disorder thought to be lethal in affected males. Most mutations are not inherited, but *de novo*.

Symptoms

Localization site	Comment
Cerebral hemispheres	Microcephaly with closely packed neurons and with decreased dendritic spines and arbors[2]
Mental status and psychiatric aspects/ complications	Agitation, sleep disturbances
Brainstem	Abnormal breathing, heart rate, swallowing, peripheral vasomotor disturbances, sleep, bowel motility, salivation, and pain discrimination

Secondary Complications: Epilepsy, GI motility issues such as reflux and constipation, scoliosis, prolonged QT interval, and spasticity/dystonia are secondary complications that require medical interventions.

References

1. Laurvick CL, de Klerk N, Bower C, et al. Rett syndrome in Australia: a review of the epidemiology. *J Pediatr.* 2006;148:347–52.
2. Armstrong DD. Neuropathology of Rett syndrome. *J Child Neurol.* 2005;20:747–53.

Suggested Reading

Christodoulou J, Ho G. MECP2-related disorders. Oct 3, 2001. Updated Jun 28, 2012. In Pagon RA, Adam MP, Ardinger HH, et al., eds. *GeneReviews®* [Internet]. Seattle (WA): University of Washington, Seattle; 1993–2018. Available from www.ncbi.nlm.nih.gov/books/NBK1497/. Accessed Sep 15, 2018.

Reversible Cerebral Vasoconstriction Syndrome

Epidemiology and Demographics: Reversible cerebral vasoconstriction syndrome (RCVS) occurs between the ages of 20 and 50 years, and it affects women more than men. The mean age of onset is 42 years. Approximately 60% of the cases are secondary to a known precipitant, predominantly occurring during the early (1 week) postpartum period or after exposure to vasoactive substances.

Disorder Description: The classic clinical manifestation is recurrent sudden-onset and severe (thunderclap) headaches over 1–3 weeks, usually accompanied by nausea, vomiting, photophobia, confusion, and blurred vision. A prospective study of 67 patients with RCVS observed over 3 years reported that the main pattern of presentation (94%) was recurrent thunderclap headaches, occurring over a mean period of 1 week. Seizures and focal neurologic deficits have been infrequently reported, usually after onset of the headaches. The main neurologic entity in the differential is primary CNS arteritis (PCNSA) for which the clinical and radiologic findings may be identical.

Symptoms

Localization site	Comment
Brain	Affects cerebral vasculature

Secondary Complications: Early complications within the first week of onset of the syndrome include localized convexity non-aneurysmal subarachnoid hemorrhage (22%), intracerebral hemorrhage (6%), seizures (3%), and posterior reversible leukoencephalopathy (9%). Ischemic events, including transient ischemic attacks (16%) and cerebral infarction (4%), tend to occur later than hemorrhagic events, mostly during the second week. Transient ischemic attack symptoms most commonly include visual loss, followed by unilateral sensory symptoms, aphasia, and hemiparesis.

Diagnosis of RCVS is made by transfemoral cerebral angiography or through imaging with CT or magnetic resonance cerebral angiography. The direct transfemoral angiography is more sensitive than imaging angiography, with up to 30% of cases missed with imaging compared with direct angiography. Findings supporting the diagnosis are segmental narrowing and dilatation (string of beads) of cerebral vessels, which are bilateral and diffuse. The basilar artery, carotid siphon, or external carotid artery can be affected. The narrowing of arteries is a dynamic process; a repeat angiogram after a few days might show resolution of some vessels, with new constrictions often affecting more proximal vessels.

The first angiogram if performed within a week of clinical onset may be normal. Maximum vasoconstriction of the branches of the middle cerebral arteries (shown by magnetic resonance angiography) is reached a mean of 16 days after clinical onset.

Treatment Complications: There are no systematic treatment trials and the mainstay of treatment in the absence of cerebrovascular complications is rest, analgesia, and stopping any vasoactive medications. For prevention of vasospasm, nimodipine at a rate of 1–2 mg/hour, followed by an oral regimen (30–60 mg every 4 hours) tapered over the course of several weeks is a common treatment approach. Treatment is typically given for 4–8 weeks, although the optimal duration is unclear. The dose should be titrated and supportive measures taken to avoid systemic hypotension, to avoid precipitating cerebral infarction in the border zone arterial territories. Transcranial ultrasound measurement of systolic velocities in intracranial arteries has been used to assess treatment efficacy. The efficacy of treatment varies considerably between reports, ranging from 40 to 80%.

Bibliography

Calabrese LH, Dodick DW, Schwedt TJ, Singhal AB. Narrative review: reversible cerebral vasoconstriction syndromes. *Ann Intern Med.* 2007;146(1):34–44.

Chen SP, Fuh JL, Chang FC, et al. Transcranial color Doppler study for reversible cerebral vasoconstriction syndromes. *Ann Neurol.* 2008;63(6):751–7.

Ducros A. [Reversible cerebral vasoconstriction syndrome]. *Presse Med.* 2010;39(3):312–22.

Ducros A. Reversible cerebral vasoconstriction syndrome. *Lancet Neurol.* 2012;10:906–17.

Ducros A, Boukobza M, Porcher R, et al. The clinical and radiological spectrum of reversible cerebral vasoconstriction syndrome. A prospective series of 67 patients. *Brain.* 2007;130(Pt 12):3091–101.

Reversible Posterior Leukoencephalopathy (RPLS) and Posterior Reversible (Leuko-) Encephalopathy (PRES)

Epidemiology and Demographics: The true incidence is unknown as it has been described fairly recently. It can occur at any age but seems to be more common in women, even if one excludes cases caused by pregnancy.

Disorder Description: A disorder of diffuse or multifocal cerebral edema believed to be caused by acute hypertension (or at least an abrupt rise in blood pressure regardless of actual pressure) leading to endothelial dysfunction and extravasation of fluid. There are numerous etiologies, including hypertensive crisis, autoimmune diseases, immune-modulating/cytotoxic therapies (especially anti-rejection ones), eclampsia, and renal failure. It was initially seen in the posterior white matter, thus explaining the name, but was later found to affect any part of the brain including the gray matter. Coincident cerebral infarction is seen, due either to vasospasm or to constriction of small blood vessels adjacent to the edema field. Intracerebral hemorrhages may also be seen due to rupture of the dysfunctional vessels.

Symptoms

Localization site	Comment
Cerebral hemispheres	Seizures, including status epilepticus. Headache. Focal deficits, including hemiparesis, aphasia, hemianopia, hemisensory loss, etc.
Mental status and psychiatric aspects/complications	Encephalopathy
Brainstem	Focal deficits, including crossed motor and sensory signs and corticobulbar dysfunction
Cerebellum	Ataxia

Secondary Complications: Although the edema is reversible, there is commonly permanent damage, either microscopically or due to concomitant stroke or intracerebral hemorrhage. This may lead to development of epilepsy and persistent focal deficits. These patients frequently are also in the middle of a hypertensive crisis and may experience renal failure, myocardial dysfunction, hepatic failure, and retinal damage.

Treatment Complications: If the blood pressure is lowered too rapidly, ischemia may result.

Bibliography

Fugate JE, Rabinstein AA. Posterior reversible encephalopathy syndrome: clinical and radiological manifestations, pathophysiology, and outstanding questions. *Lancet Neurol.* 2015;14(9):914–25.

Larry C, Oppenheim C, Mas JL. Posterior reversible encephalopathy syndrome. *Handb Clin Neurol.* 2014;121:1687–701.

Rykken B, McKinney AM. Posterior reversible encephalopathy syndrome. *Semin Ultrasound CT MR.* 2014;35(2):118–35.

Rhabdomyolysis

Epidemiology and Demographics: Rhabdomyolysis is fairly common, particularly as there are many etiologies. It is most commonly seen after trauma, and large numbers of cases are seen in disaster situations. There is no predisposition to rhabdomyolysis based on sex. Any age is affected/at risk. There is no specific geographic distribution.

Disorder Description: Rhabdomyolysis is defined as muscle breakdown (i.e., rupture and necrosis), primarily of striated (skeletal) muscle, with release of cell degradation products and intracellular elements into bloodstream and extracellular space. The most common released substance is myoglobin, and at significantly high levels can cause renal dysfunction. Another substance released is creatinine kinase, an enzyme nonspecific to muscle, and present in brain and cardiac tissue; it is a common marker used in monitoring.

There are myriad causes. Any illness or injury to muscle will by definition result in rhabdomyolysis to some degree. Most commonly, notable rhabdomyolysis results from physical etiologies, such as trauma or crush injuries, but also compartment syndrome and even high-voltage electrical injuries can be responsible. Severe exercise and status epilepticus/status asthmaticus are also causes. Similarly, there are many metabolic etiologies, including hyperthermia (e.g., neuroleptic malignant syndrome), metabolic myopathies (McArdle's disease, phosphofructokinase deficiency, carnitine palmitoyl transferase deficiency, etc.), electrolyte abnormalities (through myotoxicity/myonecrosis), and endocrine disorders. Notably, metabolic myopathies are frequently inherited diseases that overall result in failure of energy delivery to the muscles due to myriad defects in metabolism (glucose, glycogen, lipid, or nucleosides). Toxic substances, such as toxins/venoms, alcohol (mostly through electrolyte abnormalities), and illegal drugs (heroin, cocaine, ecstasy, amphetamines, etc.) are known to result in myotoxicity and rhabdomyolysis. Prescribed drugs, such as colchicine, fibrates, statins, corticosteroids, selective serotonin reuptake inhibitors (SSRIs), narcotics, antiretrovirals (e.g., zidovudine), and even licorice toxicity can result in rhabdomyolysis. Infections, in particular pyomyositis or sepsis, can result in myotoxicity and myonecrosis. Ischemia, whether by compression or thromboembolism, also results in myotoxicity, and ultimately rhabdomyolysis, though mostly from reperfusion injury. Autoimmune, inflammatory, and neoplastic disorders can also cause rhabdomyolysis.

In diagnostic tests, urine and serum myoglobin may be increased, but are not reliably sensitive due to rapid hepatic metabolism. Creatine kinase (CK) levels are typically markedly elevated, though this occurs after serum myoglobin increases. Creatinine is frequently elevated due to creatine release and conversion, but as it is cleared faster than CK, it is less commonly seen.

Symptoms

There is limited central nervous system involvement.

Localization site	Comment
Muscle	Myalgia/muscle tenderness (diffuse vs localized, based on etiology), weakness
Outside nervous system	Dark urine (common), fever (less common)

Secondary Complications: Rhabdomyolysis is particularly dangerous with respect to secondary complications, namely renal failure from toxic levels of myoglobin release.

Treatment Complications: Treatment is largely comprised of aggressive early intravenous fluid hydration in efforts to increase renal clearance and decrease risk of renal failure. In disaster zones or crush injuries, due to volume loss or accumulation in injured limbs, as high as 10 L of intravenous fluids may need to be administered (supervised) to avoid renal failure. Forced diuresis (i.e., furosemide and other loop diuretics) may also be employed. Mannitol and bicarbonate (urine alkalinization) have been used as well after initial hydration, but evidence is sparse to inconclusive with respect to effectiveness. Should renal failure be severe enough, dialysis may be needed.

Complications of treatment are rare, and mostly related to patients with known comorbidities, namely fluid overload in heart failure patients.

Bibliography

Huerta-Alardín AL, Varon J, Marik PE. Bench-to-bedside review: Rhabdomyolysis – an overview for clinicians. *Crit Care.* 2005;9:158.

Vanholder R, Sever MS, Erek E, Lameire N. Rhabdomyolysis. *J Am Soc Nephrol.* 2000;11(8):1553–61.

Warren JD, Blumbergs PC, Thompson PD. Rhabdomyolysis: a review. *Muscle Nerve.* 2002;25:332.

Rheumatic Fever and Rheumatic Heart Disease

Epidemiology and Demographics: Incidence of acute rheumatic fever and rheumatic heart disease depends on treatment of initial streptococcal infection and therefore is much higher in low-income countries and communities. Worldwide incidence of acute rheumatic fever is 19 per 100,000 school-aged children. Incidence and prevalence of worldwide rheumatic heart disease is difficult to estimate but in studies about two-thirds of patients with acute rheumatic fever developed chronic cardiac conditions.

Disorder Description: Caused by group A streptococcus. Acute rheumatic fever is a non-supportive condition that occurs 2–3 weeks after a pharyngeal streptococcal infection manifested by arthritis or arthralgia, chorea, subcutaneous nodules, and erythema marginatum. Rheumatic heart disease refers to cardiac manifestations of acute rheumatic fever, including pericarditis, myocarditis, endocarditis, and valvulitis. Direct neurologic sequelae of acute rheumatic fever include Sydenham's chorea, which is caused by molecular mimicry with antibodies to streptococcus cross-reacting with neurons.

Symptoms

Localization site	Comment
Cerebral hemispheres	Stroke
	Sydenham's chorea
Mental status and psychiatric aspects/ complications	Confusion
Brainstem	Stroke
Cerebellum	Stroke

Secondary Complications: Embolic stroke due to atrial fibrillation and left ventricular thrombus, valvular regurgitation, cardiomyopathy, arrhythmia, heart block in rheumatic heart disease. These conditions have a clinically latent period and can progress over decades.

Treatment Complications: Antibiotics are used in secondary prevention after acute rheumatic fever to lower the incidence of the complications noted above and side effects of antibiotics. Surgical complications related to valve repair and replacement.

Bibliography

Bland EF, Duckett Jones T. Rheumatic fever and rheumatic heart disease; a twenty year report on 1000 patients followed since childhood. *Circulation*. 1951;4(6):836.

GBD 2013 Mortality and Causes of Death Collaborators. Global, regional, and national age-sex specific all-cause and cause-specific mortality for 240 causes of death, 1990–2013: a systematic analysis for the Global Burden of Disease Study 2013. *Lancet*. 2015;385(9963):117.

Meira ZM, Goulart EM, Colosimo EA, Mota CC. Long term follow up of rheumatic fever and predictors of severe rheumatic valvar disease in Brazilian children and adolescents. *Heart*. 2005;91(8):1019.

Tibazarwa KB, Volmink JA, Mayosi BM. Incidence of acute rheumatic fever in the world: a systematic review of population-based studies. *Heart*. 2008;94(12):1534.

Rheumatoid Arthritis

Epidemiology and Demographics: Uncommon before the age of 15. Incidence rises with age until 80 years. Most commonly starts in women at 40–50 years of age, later in men. Women are affected 3–5 times more often than men. No race predominance is known. Affects 0.5 to 1% of the world population. Incidence is 5 to 50 cases/100,000 population each year.

Disorder Description: Rheumatoid arthritis is an autoimmune condition that primarily affects the joints. It leads to patients developing red, swollen, and painful joints. In addition to this patients may also have low red blood cell count, pleuritis, and pericarditis. Patients can also have fever and fatigue. Symptoms have an insidious onset over weeks to months. Neurologic manifestations of the disease include peripheral neuropathy and mononeuritis multiplex. The most common peripheral neuropathy is carpal tunnel syndrome secondary to swelling around the wrist. Vertebral erosion is also seen and can lead to spinal cord compression. More specifically, patients are known to develop atlanto-axial dislocation secondary to erosion of the odontoid process and transverse ligaments.

Potential causes include:
- Genetic causes: HLA-DRB1*0401/0402, PTPN22, and PADI4 genes.
- Hormonal abnormalities.
- Environmental: smoking is the main environmental cause.
- Autoimmune: Exposure to a virus that may have led to an autoimmune response resulting in non-specific inflammation, followed by T-cell activation and finally chronic inflammation resulting in tissue injury from release of cytokines such as interleukin-1 (IL-1), tumor necrosis factor (TNF)-alpha, and IL-6.

Risk factors include:
- Smoking.
- Epstein–Barr virus (EBV) infection.
- Human herpes virus 6 (HHV-6) infection.
- Vitamin D deficiency: unclear if this a cause or a consequence of the rheumatoid arthritis.

There are no known geographic areas with higher proclivity.

Symptoms

Localization site	Comment
Spinal cord	C2 level cord compression secondary to atlanto-axial dislocation. Patient may develop quadriparesis or quadriplegia in severe cases
Peripheral neuropathy	Mononeuritis multiplex. Patient may complain of paresthesias or numbness of the hands, arms, legs, and/or feet

Secondary Complications: Cord compression can result in quadriplegia or quadriparesis. Peripheral neuropathy.

Treatment Complications

Disease modifying antirheumatic drugs (DMARDS): these are immunosuppressant medications and as such can cause patients to develop progressive multifocal leukoencephalopathy as well as other serious infections. This category of medications includes:
- methotrexate: can cause leukoencephalopathy
- hydroxycholoroquine
- sulfasalazine
- leflunomide
- TNF-alpha inhibitors (infliximab, certolizumab, and etanercept): can cause reactivation of latent tuberculosis
- abetacept
- anakinra
- rituximab
- toclizumab

Anti-inflammatory drugs:
1. NSAIDs: higher risk of GI complications and kidney complications
2. COX-2 inhibitors: higher risk of myocardial infarction
3. glucocorticoids

Bibliography

Majithia V, Geraci SA. Rheumatoid arthritis: diagnosis and management. *Am J Med*. 2007;120(11):936–9.

Scott DL, Wolfe F, Huizinga TW. Rheumatoid arthritis. *Lancet*. 2010;376(9746):1094–108.

Turesson C. Extra-articular rheumatoid arthritis. *Curr Opin Rheumatol*. 2013;25(3):360–6.

Turesson C, O'Fallon WM, Crowson CS, Gabriel SE, Matteson EL. Extra-articular disease manifestations in rheumatoid arthritis: incidence trends and risk factors over 46 years. *Ann Rheum Dis*. 2003;62(8):722–7.

Rickettsia rickettsii (Rocky Mountain Spotted Fever)

Epidemiology and Demographics: Present in North America, Central America, and parts of South America. Risk determined by exposure to ticks, which carry the disease. Higher risk of ticks in wooded areas and high grass. Increased risk with exposure to dogs living in the same areas. Transmission of bacteria occurs as early as 6 hours after bite. Different types of ticks carry the bacteria in different parts of the United States.

Disorder Description: Arthropod-transmitted bacteria, gram-negative rods. Typically, there is a persistent skin lesion at the site of the causative bite. Acute syndrome is characterized by fever, headache, arthralgia, myalgia, maculopapular and purpuric rash. Small percentage of infections occur without development of rash and are more severe due to delayed treatment. Neurologic involvement is rare, but can be severe.

Symptoms

Localization site	Comment
Cerebral hemispheres	Spontaneous hemorrhage. Seizure. Meningovasculitis and encephalitis. Risk of coma
Mental status and psychiatric aspects/complications	Delirium
Brainstem	With meningitis
Cerebellum	With meningitis
Cranial nerves	With meningitis

Secondary Complications: Hydrocephalus due to intracranial hemorrhage. Myocarditis, endocarditis, pneumonia. Chronic alcohol abuse and glucose-6-phosphate deficiency increase risk for more severe disease.

Treatment Complications: Difficult to confirm diagnosis; skin biopsy has highest yield. Doxycycline and azithromycin are typical treatments.

Bibliography

Biller J, Ferro JM, ed. *Neurologic aspects of systemic disease, Part III*. Handbook of Clinical Neurology, Vol 121 (3rd Series). San Diego: Elsevier; 2014.

Centers for Disease Control and Prevention. Rocky mountain spotted fever. Updated Aug 6, 2018. www.cdc.gov/rmsf/index.html. Accessed Sep 15, 2018.

Ring Chromosome 20 Syndrome

Epidemiology and Demographics: Rare disease of unknown prevalence, with approximately 60 patients reported. Symptoms often occur in childhood. Most cases lack family history of the disorder although familial cases have been reported.

Disorder Description: Rare disorder characterized by epilepsy, mild to severe mental impairment with behavioral difficulties, and malformations (microcephaly, facial dysmorphism, and cardiovascular anomalies) with an absence of a consistent pattern of dysmorphology.

Epileptic syndromes that have been described consist of:

1. Normal or nearly normal background EEG activity with trains of theta waves in fronto-central areas not significantly influenced by eye opening or level of vigilance.

2. Episodes of nonconvulsive status epilepticus (NCSE) consisting of a prolonged confusional state and long-lasting high-voltage slow waves with occasional spikes, usually frontal, sometimes unilateral on EEG.

3. Focal seizures and associated ictal terror with loss of consciousness, oroalimentary automatisms, and hypertonia, with frontal onset discharges of short duration. These events are refractory to pharmacologic treatment and patients also acquire psychomotor delay and major behavioral disturbances.

The mechanism underlying the development of epilepsy in ring chromosome 20 syndrome remains unknown but studies suggest a relationship between the mosaicism ratio and age at seizure onset, IQ, and malformation; but not with the response of epilepsy to drug treatment.

Symptoms

Localization site	Comment
Cerebral hemispheres	NCSE consisting of a prolonged confusional state
Mental status and psychiatric aspects/ complications	Intermittent alterations of consciousness. Bizarre behavior and amnesic symptoms. Mild to severe intellectual disability

Treatment Complications: Antiepileptic drugs (AEDs) may be associated with a number of idiosyncratic reactions, including multi-organ issues, and possible cognitive or psychiatric effects. Common side effects of AEDs include dizziness, fatigue, blurred vision, and gastrointestinal symptoms. Other reactions include rash, blood count abnormalities, liver toxicity, cognitive or mood complaints. There may be an increased risk of suicidality associated with AED use. Drug interactions are common.

Bibliography

Atkins L, Miller WL, Salam M. A ring-20 chromosome. *J Med Genet*. 1972;9(3):377–80.

Inoue Y, et al. Ring chromosome 20 and nonconvulsive status epilepticus. A new epileptic syndrome. *Brain*. 1997;120(Pt 6):939–53.

Nishiwaki T, et al. Mosaicism and phenotype in ring chromosome 20 syndrome. *Acta Neurol Scand*. 2005;111(3):205–8.

Porfirio B, et al. Ring 20 chromosome phenotype. *J Med Genet*. 1987;24(6):375–7.

Root Avulsion

Epidemiology and Demographics: Relatively rare.

Disorder Description: May be due to forceful hyperextension injuries sustained from a motor vehicle accident or birth trauma. Patients may complain of acute onset of pain, sensory changes, and weakness.

Symptoms

Localization site	Comment
Plexus	Brachial or lumbar plexopathy

Secondary Complications: Pain, muscle atrophy, other sensory disturbance.

Treatment Complications: Post-surgical pain.

Bibliography

Ferrante M. Brachial plexopathies: classification, causes and consequences. *Muscle Nerve.* 2004;30(5):547–68.

Zhong L. Microanatomy of the brachial plexus roots and its clinical significance *Surg Radiol Anat.* 2017;39(6):601–10.

Rosai-Dorfman Disease (Sinus Histiocytosis)

Epidemiology and Demographics: This disorder is extremely rare with cases only in the hundreds reported in the literature and an estimated incidence of 100 cases per year in the United States. There are no large-scale studies. It generally presents in the second and third decades of life with a mean age of 20.6 years. There is a 1.4:1 male-to-female predominance. Cases affecting the central nervous system tend to have a later age of onset (5th decade) and a stronger male predominance; however, only ~5% of cases involve the central nervous system (CNS) (fewer than 300 cases have been reported in the literature). It is less common in Asians than in other ethnic groups.

Disorder Description: This is an extremely rare disorder of abnormal but nonmalignant proliferation of non-Langerhans histiocytes. The histiocytes exhibit nondestructive phagocytosis of lymphocytes and erythrocytes, infiltrating lymph nodes or extra-nodal tissue. The etiology is unknown but is believed to be reactive. Some authors have suggested human herpesvirus 6 and Epstein–Barr virus as possible inciting infections but this is not yet proven. It most commonly presents as a massive enlargement of cervical (and less commonly other) lymph nodes with systemic signs of inflammation (e.g., fever) but can also affect extranodal areas. Such areas include skin, nose, paranasal sinuses, soft tissue, orbit, bone, salivary glands, and central nervous system.

Symptoms

Localization site	Comments
Cerebral hemispheres	Rarely affects the brain tissue itself. It generally is dural based and presents as would a meningioma with headaches and seizures. Focal deficits are uncommon
Spinal cord	Rarely affects spinal cord tissue but rather is dural based and presents as would a meningioma with myelopathy from external compression

Secondary Complications: Most cases are benign with spontaneous remission and few permanent symptoms. In the case of CNS involvement, symptoms are more severe and may require treatment.

Treatment Complications: Treatment is general surgical, particularly in the setting of a single large lesion causing symptoms. The risks of brain and/or spinal surgery include infection and damage to underlying neural tissue leading to permanent focal deficits. In systemic cases, steroids or chemotherapeutic agents may be used with complications including a weakened immune system and multiple or bizarre infections, nausea, pancytopenia. Steroids may also cause psychosis, diabetes, and avascular necrosis of the hip, among others.

Bibliography

Adeleye AO, Amir G, Fraifeld S, et al. Diagnosis and management of Rosai-Dorfman disease involving the central nervous system. *Neurol Res.* 2010;32(6):572–8.

Dalia S, Sagatys E, Sokol L, Kubal T. Rosai-Dorfman disease: tumor biology, clinical features, pathology, and treatment. *Cancer Control.* 2014;21(4):322–7.

Kroft S. Rosai-Dorfman disease: Familiar yet enigmatic. *Semin Diagn Pathol.* 2016;33(5):244–53.

Sandoval-Sus JD, Sandoval-Leon AC, Chapron JR, et al. Rosai-Dorfman disease of the central nervous system: report of six cases and review of the literature. *Medicine (Baltimore).* 2014;93(3):165–75.

Tian Y, Wang J, Ge Jz, Ma Z, Ge M. Intracranial Rosai-Dorfman disease mimicking multiple meningiomas in a child: a case report and review of the literature. *Childs Nerv Syst.* 2015;31(2):317–23.

Rt-PA

Description: A recombinant form of a natural fibrinolytic approved for use within the first 3–4.5 hours after onset of symptoms due to a cerebral infarct.

Treatment Complications: The most feared complication is hemorrhagic conversion of the infarct, which can in many cases cause symptoms worse than those of the initial stroke. Hemorrhages at other sites may occur. Angioedema is also possible, particularly if the patient is taking angiotensin-converting enzyme (ACE) inhibitors.

Bibliography

Jauch EC, Saver JL, Adams HP Jr, et al. American Heart Association Stroke Council; Council on Cardiovascular Nursing; Council on Peripheral Vascular Disease; Council on Clinical Cardiology. Guidelines for the early management of patients with acute ischemic stroke: a guideline for healthcare professionals from the American Heart Association/American Stroke Association. *Stroke*. 2013;44:870–947.

Rubella Virus (German Measles)

Epidemiology and Demographics: Incidence greatly reduced by vaccine; declared eliminated from the Americas in 2015, but depends on ongoing vaccination.

Disorder Description: Droplet transmission. Two- to 3-week measles-like illness, but milder, often with prominent arthralgia, lymphadenopathy, erythematous maculopapular rash that begins on the face and spreads caudally. One per 5000–6000 cases can develop encephalitis, which is usually self-limited and does not lead to long-term complications.

Symptoms

Localization site	Comment
Cerebral hemispheres	Fetal complications: cerebrovascular involvement, prominent white matter involvement, hydrocephalus Rare adult encephalitis
Brainstem	Risk of infarction in fetus. Demyelinating damage
Cerebellum	Risk of infarction in fetus. Demyelinating damage
Cranial nerves	Sensorineural hearing loss in fetus if exposed in first 16 weeks

Secondary Complications: Severe effect on the developing fetus, causing congenital rubella syndrome. Risk is higher earlier in pregnancy. Neurologically can lead to vascular and demyelinating pathology presenting with static encephalopathy, microcephaly, sensorineural hearing loss, cataracts, intrauterine growth restriction, and cardiac abnormalities. Also can have thrombocytopenia and purpura, hepatomegaly, and splenomegaly.

Treatment Complications: Treatment is symptomatic. Immunoglobulin may be given in pregnancy, but is incompletely effective.

Bibliography

Biller J, Ferro JM, ed. *Neurologic aspects of systemic disease, Part III*. Handbook of Clinical Neurology, Vol 121 (3rd Series). San Diego: Elsevier; 2014.

Pan American Health Organization. Americas region is declared the world's first to eliminate rubella. April 29, 2015. www.paho.org.ezproxy .med.nyu.edu/hq/index.php?option=com_con tent&view=article&id=10798%3Aamericas- free-of-rubella&catid=740%3Anews-press- releases&Itemid=1926&lang=en. Accessed Feb 1, 2017.

Rubenstein–Taybi Syndrome

Epidemiology and Demographics: Rubenstein–Taybi syndrome (RTS) is a rare genetic syndrome occurring in 1/125,000 births. Although an autosomal dominant disorder, the syndrome is usually a result of a de novo mutation, with parents most likely being unaffected. Thus, the occurrence in siblings is usually <1%, and affected individuals rarely reproduce, even though puberty/sexual development is normal. There is no clear sex predominance. It is present at birth, with a broad spectrum of presentations depending on the expressed phenotype. RTS is predominantly seen in those of European descent, though occasional cases of Black and Asian patients have been documented.

Disorder Description: RTS is a syndrome due to genetic mutations (deletions or pathogenic variants). It is caused by known mutations in two genes: CREBBP (40–60%) and EP300 (3–8%). About 30% have an unknown genetic basis.

Diagnosis is primarily based on clinical features, but is confirmed through cytogenetic testing to find the aforementioned genetic deficits. Monitoring of development, feeding, growth, hearing, and vision, as well as for cardiac, renal, and dental anomalies, especially in the first year of life, is most helpful since prenatal growth can be normal.

Symptoms

Localization site	Comment
Mental status and psychiatric aspects/ complications	Moderate to severe intellectual disability, as well as attention span deficits, noise sensitivity, impulsivity, and moodiness
Outside CNS	Variable, but distinctive facial features: arched brows, down-slanted palpebral fissures, low hanging columella, high palate, grimacing smile, and talon cusps. Also, coloboma and cataracts are possible
	Broad and often angulated thumbs and great toes, short stature, and weight gain
	Congenital heart defects, urinary and renal abnormalities, as well as cryptorchidism

Secondary Complications: Secondary complications are primarily related to the aforementioned extra-CNS symptoms. However, RTS patients are prone to laryngeal wall collapsibility, increasing difficulty of intubation, and risk of general anesthesia.

Treatment Complications: Treatment is largely symptomatic and supportive. Cognitive/developmental deficits are best treated with early intervention programs, special education, and vocational training as well as behavioral management. Treatment for other physical deficits (e.g., orthopedic surgeries for deformities, cardiac surgery for defects, ophthalmic surgery) may be warranted. Ancillary support groups and resources can help families; genetic counseling can assist patients and families.

Complications of treatment are largely limited to surgical procedures required on a case-by-case basis.

Bibliography

Spena S, Gervasini C, Milani D. Ultra-rare syndromes: the example of Rubinstein–Taybi syndrome. *J Pediatr Genet*. 2015;4(3):177–86.

Stevens CA. Rubinstein-Taybi syndrome. Aug 30, 2002. Updated Aug 7, 2014. In Pagon RA, Adam MP, Ardinger HH, et al., eds. *GeneReviews®* [Internet]. Seattle (WA): University of Washington, Seattle; 1993–2018. www .ncbi.nlm.nih.gov/books/NBK1526/. Accessed Sep 17, 2018.

Sanfilippo Syndrome

Epidemiology and Demographics: Sanfilippo syndrome is also known as mucopolysaccharidosis type III (MPS-III), constituting one of the five autosomal recessive, neurodegenerative lysosomal storage disorders relating to heparan sulfate, a structural protein. It is a genetic disorder, but can present heterogeneously with respect to severity and age of onset, though usually begins between the ages of 1 and 3 years with cognitive and behavioral issues. After 5–10 years, regression occurs, eventually resulting in vegetative state and death during teenage years. There is no clear sex predominance but incidence varies according to geographic region. For example, rates of 1/50,000 individuals born in the Netherlands, and and 1/66,000 in Australia have been noted.

Disorder Description: MPS-III is an autosomal recessive lysosomal storage disease, and although known to be related to heparan sulfate degradation, the exact mechanism of disease etiology is not entirely clear. Subtypes of this disease are defined by deficiencies in different enzymes within this process of heparan sulfate degradation.

MPS-III symptoms are related to deficiencies in enzymatic degradation of the structural glycosaminoglycan heparan sulfate, with resultant accumulation of breakdown products. However, the exact mechanism by which this results in the neurodegenerative symptoms is unknown.

Diagnosis begins with identification of clinical features, but is confirmed through assay of enzyme levels in tissue samples and gene sequencing, which can also be done prenatally.

Symptoms

Localization site	Comment
Mental status and psychiatric aspects/ complications	Hyperactivity, cognitive impairment, regression, neurodegeneration, and ultimately vegetative state and death
Outside CNS	Coarse facial features with broad eyebrows, dark eyelashes, dry and rough hair, and skeletal pathology that affects growth and causes degenerative joint disease, stiff joints, hirsutism, hepatosplenomegaly, macrocrania, hearing loss, diarrhea, dental caries

Secondary Complications: Secondary complications are primarily related to progressive degeneration, resulting ultimately in dysphagia, as well as cardiorespiratory issues, ultimately resulting in a vegetative state or death.

Treatment Complications: Treatment is largely symptomatic and supportive. Although enzymatic deficiencies can be supplemented, it does not cross the blood–brain barrier, resulting in no effective treatment of the critical neurodegenerative symptoms. Complications of treatment are largely limited to associated risks for the required supportive care.

Bibliography

Fedele AO. Sanfilippo syndrome: causes, consequences, and treatments. *Appl Clin Genet.* 2015;8:269–81. DOI:10.2147/TACG.S57672.

Sarcoid Myopathy

Epidemiology and Demographics: Incidence is highest for individuals younger than 40 years and peaks in the age-group from 20 to 29 years. A second peak is observed for women over 50. Affects both sexes with a slightly greater predominance among females. Occurs throughout the world in all races with an average incidence of 16.5/100,000 in men and 19/100,000 in women. Several studies suggest the presentation in people of African origin may be more severe and disseminated than for Caucasians, who are more likely to have asymptomatic disease. Occurs in 75% of those affected by sarcoidosis.

Disorder Description: Sarcoid myopathy may manifest as nodular myopathy, chronic myopathy, or acute myositis. Nodular myopathy is rare and manifests as multiple, tumor-like, palpable nodules in the muscles. Chronic myopathy occurs when myopathy is present in multiple muscle groups. The least common type of sarcoid myopathy is acute myositis. It usually occurs in the setting of acute arthritis. However since this form has a low prevalence, its normal characteristics, prognosis, and preferred treatment approaches are not well defined. It tends to occur early in the course of sarcoidosis and in patients younger than 40 years old. Patients with acute myositis typically have muscle swelling and experience diffuse pain emanating from the calf or thigh. Sometimes, sarcoid myositis may lead to contracture of the muscle and hypertrophy. Nonspecific associated symptoms include fatigue and fever.

Generalized muscle weakness occurs infrequently. It is important to note that since acute myopathy can mimic polymyositis, muscle biopsy may be needed to distinguish between the two conditions. Helpful imaging techniques include MRI, computed tomographic (CT) scan, or positron emission tomography (PET) where myopathy appears as star-shaped lesions within the muscle. Methotrexate has been shown to be effective in the treatment of acute sarcoid myositis. The use of intravenous immunoglobulins, mycophenolate, and anti-tumor necrosis factor (TNF)-α therapy in muscle sarcoidosis has not been established.

Potential causes include:

a. Genetics: presence of BTNL2 gene, HLA-DR alleles (HLA-B7-DR15 and HLA DR3-DQ2).
b. Infectious agents: mycobacteria, fungi, *Borrelia*, and *Rickettsia*.
c. Autoimmune: high prevalence of Th1 lymphokine.

Risk factors include:

a. Occupations with a high risk of exposure to chemicals and pesticides: firefighters, educators, military personnel, persons who work in industries where pesticides are used, law enforcement, and healthcare personnel.
b. History of treatment with TNF inhibitors (e.g., etanercept).
c. History of organ transplant.

The disease is most common in Northern European countries and the highest annual incidence of 60/100,000 is found in Sweden and Iceland. In the United Kingdom the prevalence is 16/100,000. In the United States, sarcoidosis is more common in people of African descent than Caucasians, with annual incidence reported as 35.5 and 10.9 per 100,000, respectively.

Symptoms

Localization site	Comment
Muscle	Muscle involvement is asymptomatic in less than 50% of sarcoid patients. Symmetric proximal muscle weakness, focal weakness may occur from presence of granulomas
	Non-specific symptoms: fever and fatigue
	Infrequent generalized muscle weakness

Localization site	Comment
	Presentation most commonly depends on the type of sarcoid myopathy:
	1. Nodular myopathy: multiple tumor-like palpable nodules in muscle, muscle biopsy reveals the presence of non-caseating granulomas in muscles
	2. Chronic myopathy: multiple muscle involvement, patients are commonly severely disabled. Unresponsive to steroid therapy
	3. Acute myositis: occurs commonly in those with acute arthritis, tends to occur early in the course of sarcoidosis, most of the individuals affected are younger than 40 years old. Patients have muscle swelling and complain of calf and/or thigh pain. Responds to methotrexate
	Muscle biopsy reveals the presence of non-caseating granulomas in muscles

Secondary Complications: Complications include peripheral neuropathy, central nervous system sarcoidosis, restrictive lung disease, heart failure.

Treatment Complications: Treatment complications related to methotrexate use are commonly seen and include thrombocytopenia, aplastic anemia, and agranulocytosis.

Bibliography

Chatham W. Rheumatic manifestations of systemic disease: sarcoidosis. *Curr Opin Rheumatol.* 2010;22:85–90.

Fayad F, Lioté F, Berenbaum F, Orcel P, Bardin T. Muscle involvement in sarcoidosis: a retrospective and follow-up studies. *J Rheumatol.* 2006;33:98–103.

Le Roux K, Streichenberger N, Vial C, et al. Granulomatous myositis: a clinical study of thirteen cases. *Muscle Nerve.* 2007;35:171–77.

Nemoto I, Shimizu T, Fujita Y, et al. Tumour-like muscular sarcoidosis. *Clin Exp Dermatol.* 2007;32:298–300.

Sarcoma

Epidemiology and Demographics: Rare, making up less than 1% of all new cancer diagnoses; combined soft tissue sarcomas and sarcomas of the bone. Incidence of 3–5/100,000 people annually. Slight male predominance of 1.4:1, median age at diagnosis is 59, bimodal distribution that peaks in 5th and

8th decades. Pediatric sarcomas make up 20% childhood cancers, most often bone sarcomas.

Disorder Description: Sarcomas are rare, malignant connective tissue tumors; there are over 50 subtypes. Most sarcomas are sporadic and idiopathic; however, some genetic defects and environmental factors have been implicated including carcinogens, viruses, and ionizing radiation. Genetic abnormalities usually fall into categories of abnormal gene and protein function, or predisposition to genetic instability. Approximately 3% of soft tissue sarcomas have been linked to a genetic syndrome including Li–Fraumeni syndrome, retinoblastoma, neurofibromatosis type 1 (NF-1), Gardener's and Werner's syndromes, familial adenomatous polyposis. Tumors are most commonly in the extremities, but also include gastrointestinal stromal tumors and head and neck tumors (5–15%). Sarcomas make up about 1% of malignant head and neck tumors in adults. Overall, survival in those with head and neck soft tissue sarcomas is poorer than other locations; thought to be at least in part due to incomplete resection. Alkylating agents increase risk of secondary sarcomas; vinyl chloride, arsenic, and anabolic steroids are chemicals found to increase risk. Kaposi sarcoma is the most common virus-related sarcoma. Ionizing radiation is known to increase risk of subsequent sarcoma development, even following unrelated malignancies such as carcinoma or lymphoma.

Symptoms

Localization site	Comment
Cerebral hemispheres	Brain tumors associated with Li–Fraumeni syndrome (genetic disorder that greatly increases one's risk of developing cancer during lifetime)
	Meningiomas, gliomas in NF2
	Aortic sarcoma as cause of embolic stroke
	Intracranial metastases
Mental status	Diplopia and headache with expanding skull base tumors such as chondrosarcoma
	Seizures secondary to intracranial metastases or complications of therapy
Brainstem	Astrocytoma in patients with Maffucci's syndrome (sporadic disease characterized by multiple enchondromas and hemangiomas) and Ollier's disease (similar to Maffucci's syndrome but no hemangiomas) as malignant transformation of enchondromas

Localization site	Comment
Cerebellum	Cerebellar degeneration as manifestation of paraneoplastic disease, endometrial sarcoma, for example
Vestibular system (and nonspecific dizziness)	Bilateral vestibular schwannomas in NF2
Base of skull	Chondrosarcoma accounts for 6% of skull base neoplasms
Cranial nerves	Optic pathway gliomas in NF1
	Optic neuropathies in sellar enchondromas, chondrosarcomas (particularly CN VI)
Pituitary gland	Pituitary adenoma in patients with Maffucci's syndrome and Ollier's disease (transformation of chondrosarcomas)
Spinal cord	Spinal cord compression from metastatic sarcoma, particularly rhabdomyosarcoma and Ewing's sarcoma but also myeloid sarcoma
Cauda equina	Spinal cord compression from metastatic sarcoma, particularly rhabdomyosarcoma and Ewing's sarcoma but also myeloid sarcoma
Plexus	Neurofibromas in neurofibromatosis
Peripheral neuropathy	Neurofibromas in NF1 and NF2. Neurofibromas in NF1 are prone to malignant degeneration with 1/10 lifetime chance of developing malignant peripheral nerve sheath tumors, which is greater rate than malignant transformation in NF2
	Peripheral neuropathy in patients treated with chemotherapy
Muscle	Rhabdomyosarcoma
Neuromuscular junction	Myasthenia gravis in rare inflammatory pseudotumor like follicular dendritic cell sarcoma (in setting of paraneoplastic pemphigus)

Secondary Complications: Because sarcomas are such a diverse group of tumors, secondary complications are variable. Most commonly related to local mass effect in whatever region of the body is affected. For example, secondary complications of gastrointestinal stromal tumor (GIST; the most common sarcoma of the gastrointestinal tract) are gastrointestinal bleeding and abdominal pain, whereas chondrosarcomas can present with dysarthria. Lungs are the most common site of metastasis and could in theory lead to SIADH (syndrome of inappropriate antidiuretic hormone secretion).

Treatment Complications: Peripheral neuropathies can be the sequelae of chemotherapy. Recurrent tumors or secondary tumors can occur from radiation therapy.

Incomplete surgical resection for head and neck tumors can predispose to more frequent recurrence.

Bibliography

Balcer LJ, Galetta SL, Cornblath WT, Liu GT. Neuro-ophthalmologic manifestations of Maffucci's syndrome and Ollier's disease. *J Neuroophthalmol.* 1999;19(1):62–6.

Bloch OG, Jian BJ, Yang I, et al. A systematic review of intracranial chondrosarcoma and survival. *J Clin Neurosci.* 2009;16(12):1547–51.

Galy-Bernadoy C, Garrel R. Head and neck soft-tissue sarcoma in adults. *Eur Ann Otorhinolaryngol Head Neck Dis.* 2016;133(1):37–42.

Gliem M, Panayotopoulos D, Feindt P, et al. Cerebellar degeneration as presenting symptom of recurrent endometrial stromal sarcoma with sex-cord elements. *Case Rep Neurol.* 2011;3(1):54–61.

Hui JY. Epidemiology and etiology of sarcomas. *Surg Clin North Am.* 2016;96(5):901–14.

Joseph JR, Wilkinson DA, Bailey NG, et al. Aggressive myeloid sarcoma causing recurrent spinal cord compression. *World Neurosurg.* 2015;84(3):866. e7–10.

Kramer ED, Lewis D, Raney B, Womer R, Packer RJ. Neurologic complications in children with soft tissue and osseous sarcoma. *Cancer.* 1989;64(12):2600–3.

Thomas DM, Ballinger ML. Etiologic, environmental and inherited risk factors in sarcomas. *J Surg Oncol.* 2015;111(5):490–5.

Wang L, Deng H, Mao M. Paraneoplastic pemphigus and myasthenia gravis, associated with inflammatory pseudotumor-like follicular dendritic cell sarcoma: response to rituximab. *Clin Case Rep.* 2016;4(8):797–9.

Yamashiro K, Funabe S, Tanaka, R, et al. Primary aortic sarcoma: A rare but critical cause of stroke. *Neurology.* 2015;84;755–6.

Sarcosporidiosis

Epidemiology and Demographics: Rare condition. Exists worldwide, but predominantly in Southeast Asia.

Disorder Description: Protozoan infection with *Sarcocystis.* Humans can be infected as accidental hosts and cysts may be deposited in skeletal and cardiac muscle through accidental ingestion of animal feces. Eventually cyst deterioration in the muscle leads to myositis and myocarditis characterized by vasculitis and fibrosis.

Infection of definitive host through ingestion of undercooked pork or beef usually does not cause systemic effects, but the stool of the host can cause accidental host-type infections. If there are systemic effects, they can include abdominal pain, diarrhea, and myalgia.

Symptoms

Localization site	Comment
Muscle	Cysts deposit in muscle and break down, causing pain and weakness

Secondary Complications: Death is very rare.

Treatment: Treatment not well established, only case reports of various anti-protozoal medications. Trimethoprim–sulfamethoxazole may be beneficial and steroids can be considered for myositis.

Bibliography

Fayer R, Esposito DH, Dubey JP. Human infections with Sarcocystis species. *Clin Microbiol Rev.* 2015;28(2):295–311.

Saturday Night Palsy

Epidemiology and Demographics: This is a relatively common condition. It is seen in anyone who has altered sensorium that may be caused by medications, toxins as alcohol, surgical procedure, or loss of consciousness.

Disorder Description: The level of radial nerve compression is usually against the humerus near the spiral groove. The patients may have difficulty extending the wrist and fingers backwards. There may also be numbness at the back of the forearm and hand. The following table shows differentiating characteristics between Saturday night palsy and other differential diagnoses.

Symptoms

C7 radiculopathy	Posterior cord	Above the spiral groove	At the spiral groove (Saturday night palsy)	Superficial radial nerve	Posterior interosseous nerve
Weak triceps and neck pain	Weak deltoid and sensory loss in the shoulder	Weak elbow, wrist, finger extension	Weakness of elbow, wrist, finger extension with paresthesia on the back of the hand	Paresthesia on the back of the hand	Weakness of finger extension and partial weakness of wrist extension

Secondary Complications: Axonal nerve injury, pain syndrome, and muscle atrophy.

Treatment Complications: Nonsteroidal anti-inflammatory medications can rarely cause cerebrovascular complications. Steroids can occasionally cause altered mental status or psychosis.

Bibliography

Brazis PW, et al., eds. Peripheral nerves. In *Localization in clinical neurology*. 6th ed. Philadelphia, PA: Lippincott Williams and Wilkins; 2011. Chapter 2.

Han BR, et al. Clinical features of wrist drop caused by compressive radial neuropathy and its anatomical considerations. *J Korean Neurosurg Soc.* 2014;55(3):148–51. DOI:10.3340/jkns.2014.55.3.148.

Kimbrough D, et al. Case of the season: saturday night palsy. *Semin Roentgenol.* 2013;48(2):108–10.

Schistosomiasis

Epidemiology and Demographics: The prevalence of schistosomiasis is highest in sub-Saharan Africa. Worldwide, it has been estimated that more than 200 million people are infected, and it may cause up to 200,000 deaths annually. Prevention based on mass treatment and water sanitation is important.

Disorder Description: Multiple types of parasitic blood flukes that vary based on geographic location. Most infections are asymptomatic. Symptomatic infection tends to affect the young. Symptoms are due to the host's immune response to the worm, which evades the immune system well.

Swimmer's itch is an immune reaction due to cutaneous entry of larvae of water-borne species that do not cause further infection.

Within 3–8 weeks of infection, acute schistosomiasis syndrome may develop, characterized by some combination of fever, urticaria, chills, myalgia, arthralgia, cough, diarrhea, and abdominal pain, usually associated with eosinophilia.

Chronic infection with repeated exposure over years is due to trapped eggs migrating to different organs, excluding the heart.

Symptoms

Localization site	Comment
Cerebral hemispheres/brainstem/cerebellum	Direct infection of cerebral vessels less common but can cause seizures, focal neurologic signs/symptoms
Spinal cord	Direct infection of blood vessels causes rapidly progressive transverse myelitis
Conus medullaris/cauda equina	Most common site involved

Secondary Complications: Secondary infections including bacteremia. Often co-infection with malaria. Bowel inflammation and ulceration. In liver, periportal fibrosis. In bladder, ulcerations, pseudopolyps, and chronic inflammation leading to bladder cancer.

Treatment Complications: Treatment is with corticosteroids followed by praziquantel. Symptoms can worsen with initiation of praziquantel. Early treatment before 4 weeks can be ineffective as treatment only affects mature worms. Treatment with corticosteroids can be for 2 weeks to 6 months and cause typical side effects associated with corticosteroid use.

Bibliography

Nascimento-Carvalho CM, Moreno-Carvalho OA. Neuroschistosomiasis due to Schistosoma mansoni: a review of pathogenesis, clinical syndromes and diagnostic approaches. *Rev Inst Med Trop Sao Paulo.* 2005;47(4):179.

Silva LC, Maciel PE, Ribas JG, et al. Treatment of schistosomal myeloradiculopathy with praziquantel and corticosteroids and evaluation by magnetic resonance imaging: a longitudinal study. *Clin Infect Dis.* 2004;39(11):1618–24. Epub Nov 8, 2004.

Schizoaffective Disorder

Epidemiology and Demographics: Schizoaffective disorder is less common than schizophrenia, with a lifetime prevalence of schizoaffective disorder of about 0.3%. Females are more commonly afflicted than males.

Disorder Description: As stated in DSM-5, schizoaffective disorder can be defined as:

A. An uninterrupted period of illness during which there is a major mood episode (major depressive or manic) concurrent with criterion A for schizophrenia (must include depressed mood).

B. In the absence of a mood episode, there must be delusions or hallucination for at least 2 weeks.

C. Symptoms that meet the criteria for a major mood episode are present for the majority of the total duration of the active and residual portions of the illness.

D. The disturbance is not attributable to the effects of a substance or another medical condition.

Differential Diagnosis: Differential diagnosis should include schizophrenia, schizophreniform, brief psychotic disorder, delusional disorder, schizotypal personality disorder, obsessive-compulsive disorder and body dysmorphic disorder, posttraumatic stress disorder, and autism spectrum disorder or communication disorders.

In major depressive disorder or bipolar disorder with psychotic features, delusions occur exclusively during a major depressive or manic episode, as opposed to schizoaffective disorder in which there are mood symptom-free periods that consist of delusions and/or hallucinations.

In schizophreniform disorder and brief psychotic disorder, the symptoms are of shorter duration than in schizophrenia: 1 day to 1 month for brief psychotic episode, and 1 month to 6 months for schizophreniform. In schizoaffective disorder,

like schizophrenia, symptoms are present for at least 6 months.

In delusional disorder, there are no hallucinations, disorganized thinking or behavior, or negative symptoms.

In schizotypal personality disorder, subthreshold symptoms are seen and are associated with persistent-personality features.

In obsessive-compulsive disorder and body dysmorphic disorder, there are prominent obsessions, compulsions, preoccupations with appearance and/or body odor, and/or repetitive features.

In posttraumatic stress disorder, flashbacks may have a hallucinatory quality and hypervigilance may be paranoid in nature, but these symptoms are associated with relating to and/or reliving a traumatic event.

Autism spectrum disorder and communication disorders have deficits in social interactions with repetitive and restrictive behaviors, in addition to other cognitive deficits.

Secondary Complications: Schizophrenia and schizoaffective disorders have a 5% suicide risk, with the presence of depressive symptoms increasing the risk. Schizoaffective disorder is associated with often severe social, academic, and occupational dysfunction (although dysfunction is not a criterion). There is substantial functional variability among individuals diagnosed with schizoaffective disorder.

Treatment Complications: Typical and atypical antipsychotics, in conjunction with supportive psychotherapy or cognitive behavioral therapy, are the conventional treatments for schizoaffective disorder. Side effects of typical antipsychotics include the extrapyramidal side effects including parkinsonism (mask-like facies, bradykinesia, cogwheel rigidity, pill-rolling tremor), akathisia, and dystonia. Other side effects include hyperprolactinemia, sedation, weight gain, orthostatic hypotension, cardiac abnormalities, sexual dysfunction, anticholinergic side effects (dry mouth, tachycardia, urinary retention, blurry vision, constipation, worsening of narrow-angle glaucoma), tardive dyskinesia (TD), and neuroleptic malignant syndrome. TD is characterized by choreoathetoid movements of the mouth, face, tongue, extremities, or trunk. This may include tongue writhing or thrusting, jaw movements, facial grimacing, and trunk writhing. TD risk increases with age, time of exposure to medications, and prior development of extrapyramidal symptoms. TD has been reported with all typical antipsychotics at a cumulative rate of 5% per year with higher risk in older populations. The typical antipsychotics are more likely to cause TD at all ages than the atypical ones, which is the major reason newer drugs have been prescribed more for maintenance use. Patients on these medications should be assessed for TD every 3 to 6 months throughout their treatment course (i.e., AIMs, or Abnormal Involuntary Movement Scale). Atypical antipsychotic side effects are similar, but more frequently and to a larger extent include metabolic syndrome, weight gain, hyperlipidemia, and hyperglycemia. Patients with related factors, including preexisting metabolic issues, obesity, diabetes or prediabetes, or high-risk lipid profiles, are more likely to have problems with these medications. Also, prescribers should be aware of neuroleptic malignant syndrome (NMS). The hallmark features are fever, muscle rigidity, mental status changes, autonomic instability, rhabdomyolysis, and creatine kinase elevation. The differential diagnosis is serotonin syndrome (hallmark is myoclonus), malignant hyperthermia (after exposure to halogenated inhalational anesthetic agents and succinylcholine), and malignant catatonia. (In malignant catatonia there is usually a behavioral prodome of some weeks characterized by psychosis, agitation, and catatonic excitement.)The condition is rare but potentially fatal. It should be treated as a medical emergency. The single strongest predictive factor is a prior episode of NMS. Other factors include recently initiated treatment, aggressive dosing, parenteral administration, acute medical illness, and dehydration. Also, some medical illnesses may mask NMS such as central nervous system (CNS) infection, systemic infections, seizures, acute hydrocephalus, acute spinal cord injury, heat stroke, acute dystonia, tetanus, CNS vasculitis, thyrotoxicosis, pheochromocytoma, and substance intoxication (PCP, ecstasy, cocaine, amphetamines).

Treatment of mood symptoms may include mood stabilizers such as lithium (for manic symptoms) or antidepressants such as selective serotonin reuptake inhibitors (SSRIs) (for depressive symptoms). Because of lithium's narrow therapeutic index, blood levels should be monitored. Symptoms of lithium toxicity include altered mental status, coarse tremors, convulsions, delirium, coma, and death. Lithium side effects include fine tremor, nephrogenic diabetes insipidus, GI disturbances,

weight gain, sedation, thyroid enlargement, hypothyroidism, arrhythmias, benign leukocytosis, and it may cause Ebstein's anomaly in the fetus if taken during the first trimester of pregnancy.

SSRI side effects include nausea, diarrhea, insomnia, headache, anorexia, weight loss, sexual dysfunction, restlessness (akathisia-like), serotonin syndrome (fever diaphoresis, tachycardia, hypertension, delirium, neuromuscular excitability), hyponatremia, seizures (0.2%).

Bibliography

American Psychiatric Association. *Diagnostic and statistical manual of mental disorders: DSM-5.* 5th ed. Washington, DC: American Psychiatric Association; 2013.

Beatty WW, Jocic Z, Monson N, Staton RD. Memory and frontal lobe dysfunction in schizophrenia and schizoaffective disorder. *J Nerv Ment Dis.* 1993;181(7):448–53.

Bilder RM, Goldman, RS, Volavka J, et al. Neurocognitive effects of clozapine, olanzapine, risperidone, and haloperidol in patients with chronic schizophrenia or schizoaffective disorder. *Am J Psychiatry.* 2002;159(6):1018–28.

Kane JM, Carson WH, Saha AR, et al. Efficacy and safety of aripiprazole and haloperidol versus placebo in patients with schizophrenia and schizoaffective disorder. *J Clin Psychiatry.* 2002;63(9):763–71.

Stoll AL, Banov M, Kolbrener M, et al. Neurologic factors predict a favorable valproate response in bipolar and schizoaffective disorders. *J Clin Psychopharmacol.* 1994;14(5):311–13.

Schizophrenia

Epidemiology and Demographics: The lifetime prevalence of schizophrenia is approximately 0.3–0.7%. The sex ratio differs across samples and populations. A disorder with more negative symptoms and longer duration has a higher incidence in males, whereas schizophrenia with more mood symptoms and brief presentations has an equal prevalence in males and females. In females, the disease may have a later onset.

Disorder Description: As stated in DSM-5, schizophrenia can be defined as:

A. At least two of the following, each present for a significant portion of time during a 1-month period (or less if treated successfully). At least one of these must be i, ii, or iii:

i. delusions
ii. hallucinations
iii. disorganized speech
iv. grossly disorganized or catatonic behavior
v. negative symptoms (i.e., diminished emotional expression or avolition)

B. For a significant portion of the time since the onset of the disturbance, level of functioning in one or more major areas including work, interpersonal relations, or self-care was markedly below the level achieved prior to the onset.

C. Signs of the disturbance are continuously present for at least 6 months. This period must include at least 1 month of symptoms (or less if successfully treated) that meet criterion A and may include periods of prodromal or residual symptoms.

D. Schizoaffective disorder and depressive or bipolar disorder with psychotic features have been ruled out because either: (1) no major depressive or manic episodes have occurred during active-phase symptoms or they have been present for a minority of the total duration of the active and residual periods of the illness; or (2) if mood episodes have occurred during active-phase symptoms, they have been present for a minority of the total duration of the active and residual periods of the illness.

E. The disturbance is not attributable to the physiologic effects of a substance or another medical condition.

F. If there is history of autism spectrum disorder or a communication disorder of childhood onset, the diagnosis of schizophrenia is made only if prominent delusions or hallucinations are present, in addition to other required symptoms of schizophrenia, for at least 1 month (or less if successfully treated).

Differential Diagnosis: Differential diagnosis should include schizoaffective disorder, schizophreniform and brief psychotic disorder, delusional disorder, schizotypal personality disorder, obsessive-compulsive disorder and body dysmorphic disorder, posttraumatic stress disorder, and autism spectrum disorder or communication disorders.

In major depressive disorder or bipolar disorder with psychotic features, delusions occur exclusively during a major depressive or manic episode.

In schizoaffective disorder, a major depressive or manic episode occurs concurrently with the active-phase symptoms and mood symptoms are present for the majority of the total duration of the active periods.

In schizophreniform disorder and brief psychotic disorder, the symptoms are of shorter duration than in schizophrenia: 1 day to 1 month for brief psychotic episode, and 1 month to 6 months for schizophreniform.

In delusional disorder, there are no hallucinations, disorganized thinking or behavior, or negative symptoms.

In schizotypal personality disorder, subthreshold symptoms are seen and are associated with persistent-personality features.

In obsessive-compulsive disorder and body dysmorphic disorder, there are prominent obsessions, compulsions, preoccupations with appearance and/or body odor, and/or repetitive features.

In posttraumatic stress disorder, flashbacks may have a hallucinatory quality and hypervigilance may appear paranoid in nature, but these symptoms are associated with relating to and/or reliving a traumatic event.

Autism spectrum disorder and communication disorders have deficits in social interactions with repetitive and restrictive behaviors, in addition to other cognitive deficits.

Secondary Complications: Schizophrenia is associated with often severe social, academic, and occupational dysfunction. Most individuals with schizophrenia are employed at lower level than their parents and most, especially men, do not marry and have limited social contacts outside of their family.

Treatment Complications: Typical and atypical antipsychotics are the conventional treatments for schizophrenia. Side effects of typical antipsychotics include the extrapyramidal side effects including parkinsonism (mask-like facies, bradykinesia, cogwheel rigidity, pill-rolling tremor), akathisia, and dystonia. For dystonia, prophylaxis with an anticholinergic agent, such as benztropine (1 to 2 mg twice daily), substantially reduces the likelihood of a dystonic reaction even in a high-risk patient. In an emergency such as laryngeal dystonia, intramuscular versions of benztropine and diphenhydramine can be given immediately. Dystonia is less common with the use of second-generation antipsychotics than with first-generation high-potency ones. For akathisia, dose reduction may improve symptoms or if relief is not obtained, then propranolol (10 to 20 mg two to four times a day) is often helpful. Other side effects include hyperprolactinemia, sedation, weight gain, orthostatic hypotension, cardiac abnormalities, sexual dysfunction, anticholinergic side effects (dry mouth, tachycardia, urinary retention, blurry vision, constipation, worsening of narrow-angle glaucoma), tardive dyskinesia, and neuroleptic malignant syndrome. Atypical antipsychotic side effects are similar, but more frequently and to a larger extent include metabolic syndrome, weight gain, hyperlipidemia, and hyperglycemia. Lastly, clozapine can be prescribed for treatment-resistant schizophrenia/psychosis. It is well known not to exacerbate extrapyramidal side effects. Its common side effects are seizures, neutropenia, agranulocytosis, myocarditis, QT prolongation, arrhythmias, torsades de pointes, stroke, syncope, hypotension, neuroleptic malignant syndrome (NMS), paralytic ileus, and pulmonary embolus. Due to the side effect profile, clozapine is not considered first-line treatment. Often, a long-acting injectable version of antipsychotics can be given to increase compliance (i.e., haloperidol decanoate, prolixin decanoate).

Bibliography

American Psychiatric Association. *Diagnostic and statistical manual of mental disorders: DSM-5*. 5th ed. Washington, DC: American Psychiatric Association; 2013.

Crow TJ, Ball J, Bloom SR, et al. Schizophrenia as an anomaly of development of cerebral asymmetry: a postmortem study and a proposal concerning the genetic basis of the disease. *Arch Gen Psychiatry*. 1989;46(12):1145–50.

Endicott J, Spitzer RL. A diagnostic interview: the schedule for affective disorders and schizophrenia. *Arch Gen Psychiatry*. 1978;35(7):837–44.

Friston KJ, Liddle PF, Frith CD, Hirsch SR, Frackowiak RSJ. The left medial temporal region and schizophrenia: a PET study. *Brain*. 1992;115(2):367–82.

Kapur S, Zipursky R, Jones C, Remington G, Houle S. Relationship between dopamine D2 occupancy, clinical response, and side effects: a double-blind PET study of first-episode schizophrenia. *Am J Psychiatry*. 2000;157(4):514–20.

Kay SR, Flszbein A, Opfer LA. The positive and negative syndrome scale (PANSS) for schizophrenia. *Schizophr Bull*. 1987;13(2):261.

Maurer K, Maurer K, Löffler W, Riecher-Rössler A. The influence of age and sex on the onset and early course of schizophrenia. *Br J Psychiatry*. 1993;162(1):80–6.

Weinberger DR, Berman KF, Zec RF. Physiologic dysfunction of dorsolateral prefrontal cortex in schizophrenia: I. Regional cerebral blood flow evidence. *Arch Gen Psychiatry*. 1986;43(2): 114–24.

Schizophreniform Disorder

Epidemiology and Demographics: It is estimated that the incidence of schizophreniform disorder is about fivefold lower than that of schizophrenia in the United States population and other developed countries. However, in developing countries the incidence may be higher, in some cases approaching the incidence of schizophrenia.

Disorder Description: As stated in DSM-5, schizophreniform disorder can be defined as:

A. At least two of the following, each present for a significant portion of time during a 1-month period (or less if treated successfully). At least one of these must be i, ii, or iii:
   i. delusions
   ii. hallucinations
   iii. disorganized speech
   iv. grossly disorganized or catatonic behavior
   v. negative symptoms (i.e., diminished emotional expression or avolition)

B. An episode of the disorder lasts for at least 1 month, but no more than 6 months. When a diagnosis must be made prior to the 6-month mark, it should be noted as "provisional".

C. Schizoaffective disorder and depressive or bipolar disorder with psychotic features have been ruled out because either: (1) no major depressive or manic episodes have occurred during active-phase symptoms, or (2) they have been present for a minority of the total duration of the active and residual periods of the illness.

D. The disturbance is not attributable to the physiologic effects of a substance or another medical condition.

Differential Diagnosis: Differential diagnosis should include schizoaffective disorder, schizophrenia and brief psychotic disorder, delusional disorder, schizotypal personality disorder, obsessive-compulsive disorder and body dysmorphic disorder, posttraumatic stress disorder, and autism spectrum disorder or communication disorders.

In major depressive disorder or bipolar disorder with psychotic features, delusions occur exclusively during a major depressive or manic episode.

In schizoaffective disorder, a major depressive or manic episode occurs concurrently with the active-phase symptoms and mood symptoms are present for the majority of the total duration of the active periods.

In brief psychotic disorder, the symptoms are of shorter duration (1 day to 1 month) than in schizophreniform disorder.

In schizophrenia, the same symptoms as in schizophreniform disorder are seen, but the duration is greater than 6 months.

In delusional disorder, there are no hallucinations, disorganized thinking or behavior, or negative symptoms.

In schizotypal personality disorder, sub-threshold symptoms are seen and are associated with persistent-personality features.

In obsessive-compulsive disorder and body dysmorphic disorder, there are prominent obsessions, compulsions, preoccupations with appearance and/or body odor, and/or repetitive features.

In posttraumatic stress disorder, flashbacks may have a hallucinatory quality and hypervigilance may be paranoid in nature, but these symptoms are associated with relating to and/or reliving a traumatic event.

Autism spectrum disorder and communication disorders have deficits in social interactions with repetitive and restrictive behaviors, in addition to other cognitive deficits.

Secondary Complications: The majority (two-thirds) of individuals diagnosed with schizophreniform disorder will progress to schizophrenia or schizoaffective disorder. These disorders are associated with often severe social, academic, and occupational dysfunction. Most with schizophrenia are employed at lower level than their parents and most, especially men, do not marry and have limited social contacts outside of their family. One-third of those with schizophreniform disorder will recover within 6 months, and these people have much better functional outcomes.

Treatment Complications: Typical and atypical antipsychotics are the conventional treatments for schizophreniform disorder. Side effects of typical antipsychotics include the extrapyramidal side effects including parkinsonism (mask-like facies, bradykinesia, cogwheel rigidity, pill-rolling tremor), akathisia, and dystonia. Other side effects include hyperprolactinemia, sedation, weight gain, orthostatic hypotension, cardiac abnormalities, sexual dysfunction, anticholinergic side effects (dry mouth, tachycardia, urinary retention, blurry vision, constipation, worsening of narrow-angle glaucoma), tardive dyskinesia, and neuroleptic malignant syndrome. Atypical antipsychotic side effects are similar, but more frequently and to a larger extent include metabolic syndrome, weight gain, hyperlipidemia, and hyperglycemia.

Bibliography

American Psychiatric Association. *Diagnostic and statistical manual of mental disorders: DSM-5.* 5th ed. Washington, DC: American Psychiatric Association; 2013.

Dazzan P, Murray RM. Neurological soft signs in first-episode psychosis: a systematic review. *Br J Psychiatry.* 2002;181(43):s50–s57.

Rubin P, Holm S, Friberg L, et al. Altered modulation of prefrontal and subcortical brain activity in newly diagnosed schizophrenia and schizophreniform disorder: A regional cerebral blood flow study. *Arch Gen Psychiatry.* 1991;48(11):987–95.

Weinberger DR, DeLisi LE, Perman GP, Targum S, Wyatt RJ. Computed tomography in schizophreniform disorder and other acute psychiatric disorders. *Arch Gen Psychiatry.* 1982;39(7):778–83.

Schizotypal Personality Disorder

Epidemiology and Demographics: Reported rates of schizotypal personality disorder in community samples range from 0.6% in a Norwegian sample to 4.6% in a US community sample. The prevalence in the clinical population appears to be low (0%–1.9%).

Disorder Description: According to DSM-5, schizotypal personality disorder can be defined as:

A. A pervasive pattern of social and interpersonal deficits marked by acute discomfort with, and reduced capacity for, close relationships as well as by cognitive or perceptual distortions and eccentricities of behavior, beginning by early adulthood and present in a variety of contexts, as indicated by five or more of the following:

i. Ideas of reference (excluding delusions of reference)

ii. Odd beliefs or magical thinking that influences behavior and is inconsistent with societal norms. In children and adolescents, it may manifest as bizarre fantasies and/or preoccupations

iii. Unusual perceptual experiences, including bodily illusions

iv. Odd thinking and speech (e.g., vague, circumstantial, metaphorical, overelaborate, or stereotyped)

v. Suspiciousness or paranoid ideation

vi. Inappropriate or constricted affect

vii. Odd, eccentric, or peculiar behavior or appearance

viii. Lack of close friends other than first-degree relatives

ix. Excessive social anxiety that does not diminish with familiarity and is often associated with paranoid fears rather than negative judgments about self.

B. Does not occur exclusively in the context of schizophrenia, a bipolar disorder, or depressive disorder with psychotic features, another psychotic disorder, or autism spectrum disorder.

Differential Diagnosis: Differential diagnosis should include other mental disorders with psychotic symptoms, neurodevelopmental disorders, personality change due to another medical condition, substance use disorders, and other personality disorders and personality traits.

In delusional disorder, schizophrenia, and bipolar or unipolar depression with psychotic features, there is a period of persistent psychotic symptoms. In the context of these disorders, the additional diagnosis of schizotypal personality disorder would only be warranted if the personality disorder was present before the psychotic symptoms and persisted in the absence of psychotic symptoms.

Neurodevelopmental disorders including communication disorders and autism spectrum disorder should also be considered in the differential. These disorders may be differentiated by the primacy and severity of impairment of language (not seen to same extent in schizotypal personality disorder).

In personality change due to another medical condition, one's difference in traits can be attributed to the effect of another medical condition on the central nervous system.

In substance use disorders, symptoms arise due to persistent substance use, and should be distinguished from symptoms associated with a personality disorder.

Schizotypal personality disorder can be distinguished from other personality disorders by its marked cognitive or perceptual distortions and marked eccentricity or oddness.

Secondary Complications: Individuals with schizotypal personality disorder often present to their physicians with concerns regarding comorbid anxiety or depression. In response to stress, those with schizotypal personality disorder may experience transient psychotic episodes (generally not of intensity or duration to warrant an additional diagnosis of brief psychotic episode or schizophreniform disorder). Thirty to 50% of those with schizotypal personality disorder also have a diagnosis of major depressive disorder. Also, there is common co-occurrence with schizoid, paranoid, avoidant, and borderline personality disorders.

Treatment Complications: Psychotherapy is generally considered the first-line treatment for schizotypal personality disorder. Typical and atypical antipsychotics have also been shown to be effective in small studies. Side effects of typical antipsychotics include the extrapyramidal side effects including parkinsonism (mask-like facies, bradykinesia, cogwheel rigidity, pill-rolling tremor), akathisia, and dystonia. Other side effects include hyperprolactinemia, sedation, weight gain, orthostatic hypotension, cardiac abnormalities, sexual dysfunction, anticholinergic side effects (dry mouth, tachycardia, urinary retention, blurry vision, constipation, worsening of narrow-angle glaucoma), tardive dyskinesia, and neuroleptic malignant syndrome. Atypical antipsychotic side effects are similar, but more frequently and to a larger extent include metabolic syndrome, weight gain, hyperlipidemia, and hyperglycemia.

Bibliography

American Psychiatric Association. *Diagnostic and statistical manual of mental disorders: DSM-5.*

5th ed. Washington, DC: American Psychiatric Association; 2013.

Chemerinski E, Triebwasser J, Roussos P, Siever LJ. Schizotypal personality disorder. *J Pers Disord.* 2013;27(5):652.

Ettinger U, Williams SC, Meisenzahl EM, et al. Association between brain structure and psychometric schizotypy in healthy individuals. *World J Biol Psychiatry.* 2012;13(7):544–9.

Goldberg SC, Schulz SC, Schulz PM, et al. Borderline and schizotypal personality disorders treated with low-dose thiothixene vs placebo. *Arch Gen Psychiatry.* 1986;43(7):680–6.

Gruzelier JH. Syndromes of schizophrenia and schizotypy, hemispheric imbalance and sex differences: implications for developmental psychopathology. *Int J Psychophysiol.* 1994;18(3):167–78.

Herpertz SC, Zanarini M, Schulz, CS, et al.; WFSBP Task Force on Personality Disorders. World Federation of Societies of Biological Psychiatry (WFSBP) guidelines for biological treatment of personality disorders. *World J Biol Psychiatry.* 2007;8(4):212–44.

Koenigsberg HW, Reynolds D, Goodman M, et al. Risperidone in the treatment of schizotypal personality disorder. *J Clin Psychiatry.* 2003;64(6):628–34.

Larrison AL, Ferrante CF, Briand KA, Sereno AB. Schizotypal traits, attention and eye movements. *Progr Neuropsychopharmacol Biol Psychiatry.* 2000;24(3):357–72.

Raine A, Benishay D. The SPQ-B: A brief screening instrument for schizotypal personality disorder. *J Pers Disord.* 1995;9(4):346–55.

Schwannoma, Vestibular

Epidemiology and Demographics: As summarized by Park et al., the median age is 50 years and the incidence is 1/100,000.

Disorder Description: The disease is caused by an overgrowth of the perineural elements of the Schwann cell. The patient may present with ringing in the ears and hearing impairment. There may be balance problems along with numbness in the face. There may also be facial muscle weakness. Sometimes there is a diagnosis or family history of neurofibromatosis Type 2.

Symptoms

Localization site	Comment
Brainstem	Tumor near vestibular nucleus

Secondary Complications: Very large tumors can compress the surrounding brain structures such as the cerebellum or brainstem and result in ataxia, altered sensorium, and hearing loss.

Treatment Complications: Surgical removal may result in CSF leak, infection, blood loss, hearing loss.

Bibliography

Lloyd SKW, King AT, Rutherford SA, et al. Hearing optimisation in neurofibromatosis type 2: A systematic review. *Clin Otolaryngol.* 2017;42(6):1329–37.

Park JK, Vernick DM, Ramakrishna N. Vestibular schwannoma. UpToDate. Available at www.uptodate.com/contents/vestibular-schwannoma-acoustic-neuroma. Accessed Sep 18, 2018.

Scleritis

Epidemiology and Demographics: Scleritis is most common in the 4th to 6th decades of life, and the peak incidence is in the 5th. Women are more likely to have scleritis than men (1.6:1). No report of any race predilection. The prevalence is estimated to be 6 cases/10,000 population.

Disorder Description: Scleritis is a chronic, painful, and potentially blinding inflammatory disease that affects the white of the eye, commonly known as the sclera. There are three major types of scleritis: diffuse scleritis (the most common), nodular scleritis, and necrotizing scleritis (the most severe). Scleritis may be the first sign of a connective tissue disorder. Scleritis can be classified as anterior scleritis and posterior scleritis. Anterior scleritis is the most common and accounts for about 98% of the cases. Anterior scleritis is subdivided into two types: non-necrotizing and necrotizing. Non-necrotizing scleritis is the most common, and is further divided into diffuse and nodular type based on morphology. Necrotizing scleritis accounts for 13% of the cases and is known to occur with or without inflammation. Posterior scleritis is characterized by flattening of the posterior aspect of the globe, thickening of the posterior coats of the eye (choroid and sclera), and retrobulbar edema.

Scleritis is usually caused by an autoimmune disease: immune complex-related vascular damage (type III hypersensitivity) and subsequent chronic granulomatous response (type IV hypersensitivity).

Risk factors include:
History of rheumatoid arthritis
History of systemic lupus erythematosus
History of relapsing polychondritis
History of spondyloarthropathies
History of Wegener's granulomatosis
History of polyartertis nodosa
History of giant cell arteritis
Trauma
Ocular surgery
Glaucoma
Exposure to irritants/chemicals
Medications:
  bisphosphonates (alendronate, etidronate, palmidronate, risedronate, zoledronic acid) – used to treat osteoporosis
  Zelboraf (vemurafenib) – used to treat melanoma
No particular geographic proclivity is known.

Symptoms

Localization site	Comment
Eye – sclera and conjunctiva	Redness of sclera and conjunctiva that does not improve with gentle pressure on the eye
	Severe eye pain that radiates to eyebrow, jaw, and/or temple. Pain worsens with movement of the eye. Pain is worse at night and may awaken the patient
	Symptoms are subacute in onset
	Photophobia and tearing of eye
	Decreased visual acuity leading to blindness

Secondary Complications

Blindness
Secondary keratitis
Uveitis

Treatment Complications

Corticosteroids: increased risk of infection, hyperglycemia, avascular necrosis of the hip, psychosis, Cushing's disease.

Immunosuppressants: hematopoietic complications with methotrexate are seen in patients not supplemented with folic acid.

Monoclonal antibodies: increased risk of focal leukoencephalopathy with rituximab.

Nonsteroidal anti-inflammatory drugs: increased risk of GI toxicity, such as endoscopic peptic ulcers, bleeding ulcers, perforations, and obstructions.

Bibliography

de Fidelix TS, Vieira LA, de Freitas D, Trevisani VF. Biologic therapy for refractory scleritis: a new treatment perspective. *Int Ophthalmol.* 2015;35(6):903–12.

Sims J. Scleritis: presentations, disease associations and management. *Postgrad Med J.* 2012;88(1046):713–8.

Scleroderma

Epidemiology and Demographics: Scleroderma most commonly first presents between the ages of 20 and 50 years, although any age group can be affected. Women are four to nine times more likely to develop scleroderma than men. Choctaw Native Americans are more likely than Americans of European descent to develop the type of scleroderma that affects internal organs. Scleroderma is less common in the Asian population. In the United States it is slightly more common in African Americans than in Caucasians. Prevalence is estimated at 240 per million and the annual incidence of scleroderma is 19 per million people in the United States. In Germany, the prevalence is between 10 and 150 per million people, and the annual incidence is between 3 and 28 per million people. In South Australia, the annual incidence is 23 per million people, and the prevalence 233 per million people.

Disorder Description: Scleroderma is a chronic systemic autoimmune disease characterized by hardening of the skin. In the more severe form, it also affects internal organs. Scleroderma is classified into limited and diffuse forms. The limited form involves primarily cutaneous manifestations: calcinosis, Raynaud's phenomenon, esophageal dysfunction, sclerodactyly, telangiectasias (CREST syndrome). Diffuse scleroderma is rapidly progressing and affects a large area of the skin and one or more internal organs, frequently the kidneys, esophagus, heart and/or lungs. This form of scleroderma can be quite disabling. Neurologic manifestations of scleroderma include facial pain from trigeminal neuralgia, headache, paresthesias of the hands, and stroke. Neurologic involvement is more commonly seen in those suffering from scleroderma of the craniofacial region. In patients with neurologic involvement, antinuclear antibodies are commonly found, usually in a nucleolar pattern. Subgroups of patients with certain antibodies (i.e., anti-U1RNP and possibly anti-Scl-70 antibodies) may be more prone to neurologic manifestations.

Potential causes include:

Genetic: mutations in HLA genes seem to play a crucial role in the pathogenesis of some cases.

Environmental factors: exposure to silica, aromatic and chlorinated solvents, ketones, trichloroethylene, welding fumes, and terpentine have been linked to the development of scleroderma.

Risk factors include:

Susceptible professions:
Painters
Welders
Glass makers
Chemists
Oil/petroleum industry workers
Miners
Construction workers
Family history of scleroderma.

No particular geographic proclivity is known. However, this disease is less common in the Asian population.

Symptoms

Localization site	Comment
Brain	Stroke/TIA (secondary to central nervous system vasculitis)
	Seizures including intractable epilepsy
	Headaches
	Neuropsychiatric symptoms – behavioral and cognitive deterioration, dementia

Localization site	Comment
Brainstem	Optic neuritis/uveitis
	Trochlear neuropathy (involvement of superior oblique muscle)
	Trigeminal neuralgia
	Glossopharyngeal neuralgia
	Facial neuralgia
	Vestibulocochlear neuropathy (hearing and balance deficits)
Spinal cord	Transverse myelitis
	Myelopathy
	Radiculopathy
	Brachial plexopathy
	Cord compression (cervical and thoracic levels)
Peripheral nerves	Carpal tunnel syndrome
	Ulnar neuropathy
	Mononeuritis multiplex
Muscle	Myopathy manifested as proximal muscle weakness. Muscle histopathology demonstrates primarily polymyositis

Secondary Complications

Most of the secondary complications of scleroderma are related to compressive disease from calcinosis. These include cord compression and various neuropathies including carpal tunnel syndrome, trigeminal neuralgia.

Scleroderma in pregnancy increases the risk to both mother and child. Overall scleroderma is associated with reduced fetal weight for gestational age.

Treatment Complications

Corticosteroids: increased risk of infection, hyperglycemia, avascular necrosis of the hip, psychosis, Cushing's disease.

Immunosuppressants: hematopoietic complications with methotrexate are seen in patients not supplemented with folic acid. Furthermore, medications such as cyclophosphamide, methotrexate, and mycophenolate are teratogenic and hence careful avoidance of such drugs during pregnancy is advised.

Monoclonal antibodies: increased risk of focal leukoencephalopathy with rituximab.

Tyrosine kinase inhibitors: increased risk of imbalance and gait disturbances.

Bibliography

Averbuch-Heller L, Steiner I, Abramsky O. Neurologic manifestations of progressive systemic sclerosis. *Arch Neurol.* 1992;49:1292.

Amaral TN, Peres FA, Lapa AT, Marques-Neto JF, Appenzeller S. Neurologic involvement in scleroderma: a systematic review. *Semin Arthritis Rheum.* 2013;43(3):335–47.

Scoliosis

Epidemiology and Demographics: Scoliosis occurs in about 3% of the population. It is more prevalent in girls. Most commonly picked up between 10 and 20 years of age.

Disorder Description: Scoliosis is defined as sideways curvature of the spine. It may be "S" or "C" shaped. Genetics and environmental factors both play etiologic roles. It may be associated with muscle spasm, cerebral palsy, Marfan syndrome, and tumor such as neurofibromatosis.

Symptoms

Localization site	Comment
Cervical spine	Neck pain, decreased range of motion, cervical radiculopathy, shoulder pain
Lumbosacral spine	LS radiculopathy with decreased range of motion, low back pain, buttock pain
Thoracic spine	Rib prominence, prominent shoulder blade due to rotation of the thoracic cage

Bibliography

Weinstein SL. Zavala DC, Ponseti IV. Idiopathic scoliosis: long-term follow-up and prognosis in untreated patients. *J Bone Joint Surg Am.* 1981;63(5):702–12.

Selective Mutism

Epidemiology and Demographics: Selective mutism is a rare disorder and has generally not been included as a diagnostic category in epidemiological studies of childhood disorders. Based on a small school-based study, it is estimated that selective mutism has a 6-month prevalence of 0.7%. The incidence does not appear to vary by sex or race/ethnicity, and it is more likely seen in young children than in adolescents or adults.

Disorder Description: As stated in DSM-5, selective mutism can be defined as:

A. Consistent failure to speak in specific social situations wherein there is an expectation for speaking (school, for example), despite speaking in other situations.

B. The disturbance interferes with educational or occupational achievement or with social communication.

C. The disturbance in speaking occurs for at least 1 month.

Differential Diagnosis: Differential diagnosis should include communication disorders, neurodevelopmental disorders, schizophrenia and other psychotic disorders, and social anxiety disorder (social phobia).

In communication disorders such as language disorder, speech sound disorder, childhood-onset fluency disorder (stuttering), or pragmatic (social) communication disorder, the speech disturbance is not restricted to a particular situation.

In autism spectrum disorder, schizophrenia and other psychotic disorders, or severe intellectual disability, an individual may have problems in social communication and may not be able to speak properly in social situations. However, for a diagnosis of selective mutism, the individual must display adequate speaking capabilities in at least one social situation (e.g., home).

Secondary Complications: Individuals diagnosed with selective mutism may have social impairment as they may not engage in social interactions with other children. Children with selective mutism may face social isolation as they grow older, and may suffer academic disadvantages as they may be unable to communicate their academic and/or personal needs to teachers.

Treatment Complications: In some trials, selective serotonin reuptake inhibitors (SSRIs) were shown to be no more effective than placebos for children with selective mutism. However, one trial did show efficacy for the SSRI fluoxetine in treatment of selective mutism (in children with a comorbid anxiety disorder). SSRI side effects include nausea, diarrhea, insomnia, headache, anorexia, weight loss, sexual dysfunction, restlessness (akathisia-like), serotonin syndrome (fever diaphoresis, tachycardia, hypertension, delirium, neuromuscular excitability), hyponatremia, seizures (0.2%).

Bibliography

American Psychiatric Association. *Diagnostic and statistical manual of mental disorders: DSM-5.* 5th ed. Washington, DC: American Psychiatric Association; 2013.

Bergman RL, Piacentini J, McCracken JT. Prevalence and description of selective mutism in a school-based sample. *J Am Acad Child Adolesc Psychiatry.* 2002;41(8):938–46.

Dummit ES, Klein RG, Asche B, Martin J, Tancer NK. Fluoxetine treatment of children with selective mutism: an open trial. *J Am Acad Child Adolesc Psychiatry.* 1996;35(5):615–21.

Gray RM, Jordan CM, Ziegler RS, Livingston RB. Two sets of twins with selective mutism: neuropsychological findings. *Child Neuropsychol.* 2002;8(1):41–51.

Kristensen H. Non-specific markers of neurodevelopmental disorder/delay in selective mutism. *Eur Child Adolesc Psychiatry.* 2002;11(2):71–8.

Selenium Deficiency

Epidemiology and Demographics: Dietary sources of selenium include seafood, muscle meat, and cereals. However, the amount of selenium in cereal depends on soil concentration of selenium. Selenium deficiency is seen in countries with low soil concentrations such as Scandinavia, China, and New Zealand. Keshan disease is an endemic disease in regions of China found in children and young women whose dietary intake of selenium is low (<20 µg/day).

In the past, total parenteral nutrition solutions were not supplemented with trace elements such as selenium. Several patients with chronic total parenteral nutrition have been reported to have selenium deficiency.

Disorder Description: Selenium is a component of the glutathione peroxidase enzyme, which serves as antioxidant to proteins, cell membranes, lipids, and nucleic acids. Selenium is also a key component of deiodinase enzymes, important for deiodination of thyroxine to triiodothyronine. Concomitant deficiencies of iodine and selenium may worsen the clinical manifestations of cretinism.

Severe selenium deficiency is associated with skeletal muscle dysfunction and cardiomyopathy and also causes mood disorders and immune function impairment. Selenium deficiency also causes whitened nailbeds.

Keshan disease presents as an endemic cardiomyopathy in children and women of childbearing age in areas of China. The disorder responds to selenium supplements.

Impaired cell-mediated immunity has been demonstrated with depletion of tissue stores of selenium.

Treatment Complications: In patients with autoimmune thyroiditis, selenium supplementation may decrease inflammatory activity and may reduce the risk of postpartum thyroiditis in women who are positive for thyroid peroxidase antibodies.

Selenium toxicity occurs with excess dietary intake or by excessive supplementation. Clinical manifestations of selenium toxicity are nausea, vomiting, diarrhea, hair loss, nail changes, mental status changes, and peripheral neuropathy.

References

Finley JW, Penland JG. Adequacy or deprivation of dietary selenium in healthy men: Clinical and psychological findings. *J Trace Elem Exp Med.* 1998;11:11.

Hawkes WC, Hornbostel L. Effects of dietary selenium on mood in healthy men living in a metabolic research unit. *Biol Psychiatry.* 1996;39:121.

Ishida T, Himeno K, Torigoe Y, et al. Selenium deficiency in a patient with Crohn's disease receiving long-term total parenteral nutrition. *Intern Med.* 2003;42:154.

Kasper DL, Fauci AS, Hauser SL, et al. *Harrison's principles of internal medicine.* 19th ed. New York: McGraw-Hill Education/Medical; 2015.

Mazokopakis EE, Papadakis JA, Papadomanolaki MG, et al. Effects of 12 months treatment with L-selenomethionine on serum anti-TPO levels in patients with Hashimoto's thyroiditis. *Thyroid.* 2007;17:609.

No authors listed. Observations on effect of sodium selenite in prevention of Keshan disease. *Chin Med J (Engl).* 1979;92:471.

Rayman MP. The importance of selenium to human health. *Lancet.* 2000;356:233.

Spallholz JE, Boylan LM, Larsen HS. Advances in understanding selenium's role in the immune system. *Ann N Y Acad Sci.* 1990; 587:123.

Taylor EW, Nadimpalli RG, Ramanathan CS. Genomic structures of viral agents in relation to the biosynthesis of selenoproteins. *Biol Trace Elem Res.* 1997;56:63.

van Rij AM, Thomson CD, McKenzie JM, Robinson MF. Selenium deficiency in total parenteral nutrition. *Am J Clin Nutr.* 1979;32:2076.

Sepsis (Including Septic Shock)

Epidemiology and Demographics: Septic encephalopathy may occur in up to 70% of septic patients.

Disorder Description: Systemic immune response system (SIRS) ≥2 of the following: fever >38°C (>100.4°F), heart rate >90, respiratory rate >20, or PCO_2 <32, WBCs >12,000/mm^3. If a suspected source of infection is present, the patient has sepsis. Sepsis is severe with onset of hypotension. If hypotension is not responsive to fluids, the patient has septic shock.

Septic encephalopathy is the most common neurologic complication of sepsis. Its presence is a poor prognostic indicator.

Symptoms

Localization site	Comment
Cerebral hemispheres	Seizures and status epilepticus
	Vasogenic edema due to systemic inflammation
	Watershed infarction due to hypotension in shock
	Venous infarction due to cerebral vein thrombosis
	Small vessel infarction due to in situ thrombosis
	Meningitis or abscess from direct spread of primary infection
Mental status and psychiatric aspects/complications	Delirium/encephalopathy/coma due to systemic inflammatory response to blood toxins
Brainstem	Infarction due to hypotension in shock
Cerebellum	Infarction due to hypotension in shock
Cranial nerves	Involvement from direct spread of primary infection
Spinal cord	Infarction due to hypotension in shock
	Involvement from direct spread of primary infection

Localization site	Comment
Brachial and lumbar plexus	Due to critical illness
Peripheral neuropathy	Due to critical illness
Neuromuscular junction	Due to neuromuscular blocking agents used to induce coma
Muscle	Due to critical illness

Secondary Complications: Causative infections can directly (e.g., vertebral discitis, sinusitis, otitis) or hematogenously (e.g., fungal infections) spread to the nervous system. Peripheral neuropathy and/or myopathy may occur. Both of these are more common in patients who had septic encephalopathy. Multi-organ failure with organ-specific complications in septic shock. Adult respiratory distress syndrome. Seizures due to abnormal electrolytes, glucose, blood pH, hepatic failure, and uremia. Cerebral vein and deep vein thrombosis.

Treatment Complications: Antibiotics used can have toxic effects on other organs. Sedatives and neuromuscular blocking agents used to treat agitation can have more prolonged sedative effects due to organ dysfunction. Adrenal insufficiency if long-term steroids are needed.

Bibliography

Aminoff MJ, Josephson SA, eds. *Aminoff's neurology and general medicine.* 5th ed. London, UK: Elsevier; 2014.

Bolton CF, Young GB, Zochodne DW. The neurological complications of sepsis. *Ann Neurol.* 1993;33(1):94.

Eidelman LA, Putterman D, Putterman C, Sprung CL. The spectrum of septic encephalopathy. Definitions, etiologies, and mortalities. *JAMA.* 1996;275(6):470.

Septic Embolus

Epidemiology and Demographics: Occurs in 13% to 44% of patients with infective endocarditis.

Disorder Description: Infection of the cardiac valves. Can be complicated by local destruction of valves leading to cardiomyopathy, arrhythmia, perivalvular abscess, and direct spread to nearby structures including the vertebrae, embolic disease to the heart, lung, brain, kidney, intestine, liver, muscles, and extremities.

More aggressive when causative organism is *Staphylococcus aureus* or *Streptococcus bovis*. Risk of embolism increases in setting of left-sided vegetation, large vegetation, older age, diabetes, atrial fibrillation, and antiphospholipid antibodies. Antibiotic treatment lowers risk of embolism.

Best diagnosed with transesophageal echocardiogram and blood cultures.

Silent cerebral infarction in up to 80% of cases, clinically apparent infarction in 35%.

Symptoms

Localization site	Comment
Cerebral hemispheres	Ischemic embolism and infarction with or without septic abscess
	Mycotic aneurysm formation and rupture
	Meningitis
	Seizures due to abscess or hemorrhage
Mental status and psychiatric aspects/complications	Delirium, encephalopathy, and coma
Brainstem	Infarction or meningitis
Cerebellum	Infarction or meningitis
Spinal cord	Infarction
Peripheral neuropathy	Associated with critical illness
Muscle	Infarction and septic abscess

Secondary Complications: Complications include mycotic aneurysm, hydrocephalus related to subarachnoid hemorrhage, complications related to sepsis and hypoperfusion, cardiac arrest.

Treatment Complications

Aminoglycosides can cause ototoxicity and nephrotoxicity, especially when combined with vancomycin.

Central lines can become infected in the setting of bacteremia.

Drug fever.

Intravenous catheter-associated thrombosis.

Anticoagulation is generally contraindicated even if thrombus suspected due to risk of mycotic aneurysm rupture.

Valve surgery is indicated in some cases and can be associated with stroke and typical surgical risk.

Bibliography

Bayer AS. Infective endocarditis. *Clin Infect Dis.* 1993;17:313.

Grabowski M, Hryniewiecki T, Janas J, Stępińska J. Clinically overt and silent cerebral embolism in the course of infective endocarditis. *J Neurol.* 2011;258:1133.

Hoen B, Duval X. Infective endocarditis. *N Engl J Med.* 2013;369:785.

Molavi A. Endocarditis: recognition, management, and prophylaxis. *Cardiovasc Clin.* 1993;23:139.

Serotonin Syndrome

Epidemiology and Demographics: Boyer and Shannon cited a report showing that in 2002 there were 7349 cases of serotonin syndrome, resulting in 93 deaths. It is estimated that 14–16% of those who overdose with selective serotonin reuptake inhibitors display symptoms of serotonin syndrome.

Disorder Description: Serotonin syndrome is a toxic hyperserotonergic state, typically the result of combining serotonergic agents leading to hyperstimulation of brainstem and spinal cord 5-HT_{1A}[1] and 5-HT_{2A} receptors[2].

Serotonin syndrome occurs after the use of serotonergic agents alone or in combination with monoamine oxidase inhibitors. It consists of alteration of mental status, abnormalities of neuromuscular tone, and autonomic hyperactivity. Management involves withdrawal of the offending agent(s), supportive care especially to manage autonomic dysfunction (e.g., hyperthermia), and occasionally the administration of serotonin antagonists.

Serotonin syndrome has many overlapping features with neuroleptic malignant syndrome but may be distinguished by the presence of diarrhea, tremor, and myoclonus rather than the lead pipe rigidity of neuroleptic malignant syndrome.[3]

Symptoms: Serotonin syndrome is characterized by a triad of neuroexcitatory features, including altered mental status, neuromuscular hyperactivity, and autonomic instability.

Post-synaptic $5HT_{1A}$ overstimulation causes hyperactivity, hyperreflexia, and anxiety. Post-synaptic $5HT_{2A}$ overstimulation causes hyperthermia, incoordination, and neuromuscular excitement.[2]

Localization site	Comment
Mental status and psychiatric aspects/ complications	*Altered mental status:* agitation, irritability, anxiety, hypomania, confusion, delirium, hallucinations, drowsiness to coma
Other	*Neuromuscular hyperactivity:* rigidity, hyperreflexia, hypertonia, teeth grinding, myoclonus, clonus, ataxia, tremor
	Autonomic instability: dilated, nonreactive pupils, tachycardia, tachypnea, fever, diarrhea, abdominal pain, flushing, profuse sweating, hypertension or hypotension

Secondary Complications: Patients with severe serotonin syndrome may develop severe hyperthermia (>104°F), rhabdomyolysis (severe creatinine kinase [CK] elevation), generalized tonic–clonic seizures, shock or marked hypertension, renal failure, metabolic acidosis, disseminated intravascular coagulation (DIC, as a consequence of uncontrolled hyperthermia) – multi-organ failure.[2]

Treatment Complications: Mainstay of the treatment is removal of the offending agents and supportive care, which includes cooling, sedation, intubation, muscle paralysis, and management of autonomic instability. Thus, increased morbidity puts patients at higher risk of nosocomial complications. $5HT_{2A}$ receptor antagonists (cyproheptadine, chlorpromazine) have been used in the management of severe serotonin syndrome. Chlorpromazine should not be used routinely to manage serotonin syndrome, especially if the patient is hypotensive and/or neuroleptic malignant syndrome has not been excluded.[2]

References

1. Sternbach H. The serotonin syndrome. *Am J Psychiatry.* 1991;148(6):705–13.
2. Iqbal MM, Basil MJ, Kaplan J, Iqbal T. Overview of serotonin syndrome. *Ann Clin Psychiatry.* 2012;24(4):310–18.
3. Kasper DL, Fauci AS, Hauser SL, et al., eds. *Harrison's principles of internal medicine.* 19th ed. New York: McGraw-Hill Education/Medical; 2015.

Shift Work Disorder

Epidemiology and Demographics: The prevalence of shift work disorder is approximately 2–5% of the general population in industrialized countries in which up to 20% of the population works at night. There is no difference in occurrence between sexes or racial groups.

Disorder Description: Shift work disorder is characterized by insomnia and/or excessive sleepiness with a reduced total sleep time that is associated with a work schedule that overlaps with usual sleep time. The condition is related to circadian misalignment and sleep loss. The symptoms and work schedule must be present for at least 3 months. It is most commonly associated with overnight work, early morning shifts, or rotating shifts. Excessive sleepiness typically occurs during the shift and leads to impaired concentration and alertness, which may impact safety.

Symptoms

Localization site	Comment
Midbrain	Suprachiasmatic nucleus of the hypothalamus (circadian clock)
Mental status and psychiatric aspects/ complications	Increased risk of depression, impaired social function with social isolation and reduced coping skills. Impaired concentration and alertness during wake hours

Secondary Complications: Adverse social consequences may occur when the wake–sleep schedule does not align with others and may lead to impaired social function, depression, and reduced coping skills. Increased risk of errors and accidents, especially in the early morning hours, are associated with excessive sleepiness.

Recent observational studies have shown an association between shift work and adverse health outcomes, including insulin resistance, cardiovascular events, and increased rates of malignancy.

Treatment Complications: A change in work schedule can resolve the disorder and should be considered, if possible, prior to further treatment options.

Behavioral approach includes maintaining a regular sleep schedule, including days off from work, as well as creating an optimal sleep environment that is cool, dark, and quiet. If a more flexible sleep schedule is required because of other daytime obligations, sleep periods can occur bimodally, with the initial 4–5 hours taking place in the early part of the day with a second nap for approximately 2 hours that can occur later in the day.

Pharmacologic management includes short-acting benzodiazepines such as triazolam and temazepam, and short acting nonbenzodiazepine BZ-receptor agonists such as zolpidem have been studied and used with success for initiating sleep and improving subjective measures of sleep; however, they have an increased risk of carry over effect that can contribute to decreased nocturnal alertness. Melatonin at a low dose may also be used; however, it has been shown to minimally improve sleep latency and total sleep time.

Modafinil and armodafinil are also approved for increasing alertness during working hours.

All hypnotics may cause residual somnolence with performance impairment and rebound insomnia after discontinuation. Respiratory suppression may also occur with some hypnotics and can worsen obstructive sleep apnea and hypoventilation. Complex sleep-related behaviors such as somnambulism, sleep-driving, and sleep-eating can occur. Combination with alcohol or other central nervous system depressants can lead to overdose and respiratory depression.

Observational studies have found an association between long-term use of hypnotics and all-cause mortality, although causality has not been established.

The adverse effects of modafinil and armodafinil include dysphoria, tachycardia, and increased blood pressure.

Bibliography

American Academy of Sleep Medicine
International classification of sleep disorders, 3rd ed. Darien, IL: American Academy of Sleep Medicine; 2014.

Boggild H, Knutsson A. Shift work, risk factors and cardiovascular disease. *Scand J Work Environ Health*. 1999;25:85–99.

Knutsson A. Health disorders of shift workers. *Occup Med*. 2003;53:103–8.

Morgenthaler TI, Lee-Chiong T, Alessi C, et al. Practice parameters for the clinical evaluation and treatment of circadian rhythm sleep disorders. An American Academy of Sleep Medicine report. *Sleep*. 2007;30:1445.

Sack RL, Auckley D, Auger RR, et al. Circadian rhythm sleep disorders: Part I, basic principles, shift work and jet lag disorders. *Sleep*. 2007;30:1460–83.

Vyas MV, Garg AX, Iansavichus AV, et al. Shift work and vascular events: systematic review and meta-analysis. *BMJ*. 2012;345:e4800.

Sialidosis

Epidemiology and Demographics: Sialidosis is a rare autosomal recessive disorder. The overall prevalence is unknown. Type I may be more common in people with Italian ancestry. People with type I develop signs and symptoms of sialidosis in their teens or twenties. Type II may present any time from infancy to early childhood.

Disorder Description: A lysosomal storage disease caused by mutations in the NEU1 gene. Deficient enzyme activity results in impaired processing/degradation of sialo-glycoproteins and accumulation of over-sialylated metabolites.

Type I, also referred to as cherry-red spot myoclonus syndrome, is the less severe form. Initially, affected individuals experience gait disturbance and/or reduced visual acuity. Later, type I is characterized by progressive myoclonus, ataxia, leg tremors, and seizures. Type I does not affect intelligence or life expectancy, but results in progressive disability including impaired gait and vision.

Sialidosis type II may present with stillbirth secondary to ascites, hydrops fetalis, hepatosplenomegaly, and dysostosis multiplex. The infantile presentation is less severe, and is also associated with coarse facial features, intellectual disability, and short stature. As children with infantile sialidosis type II get older, they may develop myoclonus and cherry-red spots. Other signs and symptoms include hearing loss, gingival hyperplasia, and widely spaced teeth. Affected individuals may survive into childhood or adolescence.

The juvenile form is the least severe of sialidosis type II. Features of this condition usually appear in late childhood and may include mildly "coarse" facial features, mild bone abnormalities, cherry-red spots, myoclonus, intellectual disability, and angiokeratomas.

Symptoms

Localization site	Comment
Cerebral hemispheres	Myoclonus likely cortical. MRI imaging may show posterior cortical pathway abnormalities
Mental status and psychiatric aspects/complications	Severe intellectual disability in type II
Cerebellum	Ataxia
Cranial nerves	Visual impairment

Secondary Complications: Complications include hepatosplenomegaly, hearing loss, vision loss, bone deformity, coarse facial features.

Treatment Complications: There is no specific therapy for sialidosis. Anti-seizure medications may be used to treat myoclonic seizures and are associated with a wide range of idiosyncratic side effects, most commonly sedation, ataxia, dizziness, headache. Multi-organ issues, and possible cognitive or psychiatric effects, may occur.

Bibliography

d'Azzo A, Machado E, Annunziata I. Pathogenesis, emerging therapeutic targets and treatment in sialidosis. *Expert Opin Orphan Drugs*. 2015;3(5):491–504.

Lu CS, Ng SH, Lai SC, et al. Cortical damage in the posterior visual pathway in patients with sialidosis type 1. *Brain Imaging Behav*. 2016;11(1):214–23.

Sjögren's Syndrome

Epidemiology and Demographics: Occurs in all age groups. The average age of onset is between 40 and 60 years with higher numbers affected with increasing age. Female-to-male ratio is 9:1. No race-related predilection known. Incidence of the syndrome varies between 3 and 6 per 100,000 per year. Prevalence of 500,000 to 2 million people in the United States with some studies reporting that prevalence is 0.1 to 4% of the population.

Disorder Description: Sjögren's syndrome (SS) is a long-term autoimmune disease in which the moisture-producing glands of the body are affected. Individuals with SS present with sicca symptoms, such as xerophthalmia (dry eyes), xerostomia (dry mouth), and parotid gland enlargement. SS can occur as a primary disorder or as a secondary disorder in association with connective tissue disorders, such as rheumatoid arthritis and systemic lupus erythematosus. Central nervous system (CNS) involvement varies widely; however, it is generally regarded to be less frequently involved than the peripheral nervous system (PNS). A pure sensory neuropathy is the most frequent PNS manifestation in which a long-term, insidious course is typically observed. The presence of Anti-Ro (SS-A) antibody has been associated with more severe CNS disease and abnormal angiographic findings.

Potential causes include:

Genetic factors: Studies on the polymorphisms of human leukocyte antigen (HLA)-DR and HLA-DQ gene regions in SS patients show differential susceptibility to the syndrome due to different types of the resulting autoantibody production.

Hormonal factors: Sex hormones, especially estrogen, are believed to affect humoral and cell-mediated immune responses affecting susceptibility to the syndrome. Androgens are generally considered to prevent autoimmunity. Estrogen deficiency stimulates presentation of autoantigens, inducing SS-like symptoms.

Microchimerism factors: Microchimerism of fetal cells (offspring lymphoid cells in maternal circulation) may generate autoimmunity in women who have been previously pregnant. Generation of an autoimmune potential via microchimerism may lead to a switch from a silent form of autoimmunity with age-dependent decrease in self-tolerance.

Environmental factors: Viral proteins, engulfed molecules, or degraded self-structures may initiate autoimmunity by molecular mimicry and increase the chances of SS development. Epstein–Barr virus, hepatitis C, and human T-cell leukemia virus-1 are among the most studied infectious agents in SS. Damaged self-structures targeted for apoptosis may be mistakenly exposed to the immune system, triggering autoimmunity in exocrine glands, which are often prone to autoimmune responses.

Risk factors include:

Female gender.

Age between 40 and 60 years.

History of pregnancy.

Family history of SS.

Prior infection with Epstein–Barr virus, hepatitis C, and/or HTLV-1.

No particular geographic proclivity is known.

Symptoms

Localization site	Comment
Brain	Neuropsychologic abnormalities have included deficits of attention; concentration; verbal intelligence greater than nonverbal intelligence, signifying a subcortical dementia; or dysnomia. Alzheimer's multi-infarct dementia must be excluded
	Affective disorders include hysteria, hypochondriasis, somatization, depression, dysphoria, anxiety, and panic disorders
	CNS involvement of SS may present in a similar way to Behçet's disease and may mimic multiple sclerosis. As with multiple sclerosis, CSF may demonstrate increased IgG synthesis and presence of oligoclonal bands
	Active inhibition of the parasympathetic system at the periaqueductal gray area of the limbic system has been postulated to explain the reduction in lacrimation and alteration in pain sensations in SS
Brainstem	SS can cause numbness or burning of the face, called trigeminal neuralgia. Pain in the back of the throat, which may worsen while swallowing, is called glossopharyngeal neuralgia. Patients with trigeminal or glossopharyngeal neuralgia can have agonizing mouth and facial pain. These neuropathies may co-exist with other neuropathies in different parts of the body
Spinal cord	Subacute or acute transverse myelitis is known to occur secondary to inflammatory ischemic vasculopathy with small vessel angiitis. A specific form of myelitis called neuromyelitis optica is also known to occur
Peripheral nerves	Numbness and coldness in milder forms of SS and burning sensation in more severe forms of SS

Localization site	Comment
Peripheral nerves	Weakness may be present, which is typically greater in the toes and fingers than in the larger muscle groups of the arms and legs
	SS can cause damage to nerves that regulate the coordination of heartbeat, respiration, and gastric motility. Examples of symptoms include lightheadedness when standing, decreased or increased sweating, and feeling full despite eating small meals
	Mononeuritis multiplex: more severe patterns of weakness or clumsiness may cause weakness or paralysis of different muscles
	Specific antibodies: cryoglobulinemia (type II and type III), anti-RF, and low C4
	Multiple mononeuropathies such as carpal tunnel syndrome, ulnar neuropathy, or tarsal tunnel syndrome can occur
Muscle	Individuals with muscle problems may have pain on palpation or spontaneous pain (myalgias). They may be unable to climb stairs or carry things (weakness). Individuals may or may not have symptoms. Individuals may have fever, fatigue, arthralgias, myalgias, or lymphadenopathy. Weakness is more prominent proximally than distally. The course is generally mild and insidious

Secondary Complications

Mononeuritis multiplex

Myelitis: transverse and neuromyelitis optica

Trigeminal neuralgia

Glossopharyngeal neuralgia

Autonomic neuropathy

Peripheral neuropathy: small fiber and long fiber neuropathies

Myopathy

Treatment Complications

Corticosteroids: Increased risk of infection, hyperglycemia, avascular necrosis of the hip, psychosis, Cushing's disease.

Immunosuppression: Hematopoietic complications with methotrexate are seen in patients not supplemented with folic acid. Furthermore, medications such as cyclophosphamide, methotrexate, and mycophenolate are teratogenic and hence careful avoidance of such drugs during pregnancy is advised.

Monoclonal antibodies: Increased risk of focal leukoencephalopathy with rituximab.

Bibliography

Berkowitz AL, Samuels MA. The neurology of Sjogren's syndrome and the rheumatology of peripheral neuropathy and myelitis. *Pract Neurol.* 2014;14(1):14–22.

Chai J, Logigian EL. Neurological manifestations of primary Sjogren's syndrome. *Curr Opin Neurol.* 2010;23(5):509–13.

Sleep-Related Eating Disorder

Epidemiology and Demographics: The prevalence of sleep-related eating disorder (SRED) is 5% in the general population and 9–17% in those with eating disorders; female sex predominance of 60–83%. Age at onset is typically 22–39 years.

Restless leg movement disorder (SRED) can be idiopathic but is commonly associated with a primary sleep disorder (restless leg syndrome [RLS], restless leg movement disorder, obstructive sleep apnea [OSA], and circadian rhythm sleep–wake disorders) or use of a sedative-hypnotic medication (benzodiazepines, benzodiazepine receptor agonists, psychotropic agents [mirtazapine, risperidone, quetiapine, lithium carbonate, anticholinergics]). Onset of SRED has been reported with cessation of smoking/alcohol/substance abuse, acute stress, daytime dieting, and onset of narcolepsy/autoimmune hepatitis/encephalitis and other conditions.

Disorder Description: SRED is characterized by recurrent episodes of nocturnal eating after an arousal with adverse consequences. These episodes are often described as occurring in an involuntary, compulsive, or "out of control" manner with variability in subsequent recall of the episode. Problematic features of this disorder include the consumption of peculiar foods or inedible products, and dysfunctional nocturnal eating often leads to weight gain. There is often inability to return to sleep without eating. Amnestic SRED is often related to sedative-hypnotic medication use, most commonly zolpidem, and is characterized by prolonged episodes with elaborate and sometimes dangerous food preparation. There may be co-existing restless leg syndrome, sleepwalking, and OSA.

Symptoms: See entry for *Confusional Arousals.*

Must be distinguished from night eating syndrome (NES), which is excessive eating between dinner and bedtime and during awakenings with full awareness of the episode. NES is an eating disorder with associated insomnia whereas SRED is classified as a parasomnia often associated with other primary sleep disorders.

Secondary Complications: Complications of weight gain, obesity, precipitation of diabetes mellitus, hypertriglyceridemia, and hypercholesterolemia. Nonrestorative sleep can occur due to fragmentation of sleep. Injuries have been reported including injury from kitchen utensils, burns, poisoning. Secondary depressive disorders may emerge.

Treatment Complications: Treatment includes elimination of precipitating factors, maintaining consistent sleep/wake cycles, and avoidance of sleep deprivation with subsequent increases in homeostatic drive and N3 sleep, which increases the opportunity of parasomnias to occur. Pharmacologic treatment of idiopathic SRED includes selective serotonin reuptake inhibitors (SSRIs). Topiramate and clonazepam are alternative options. SRED related to other sleep disorders should be managed by treating the underlying disorder. For example, RLS-related SRED is treated with dopamine agonists and sleepwalking-related SRED is best managed with low-dose clonazepam.

Bibliography

American Academy of Sleep Medicine. *International classification of sleep disorders*, 3rd ed. Darien, IL: American Academy of Sleep Medicine; 2014.

Auger RR. Sleep-related eating disorders. *Psychiatry (Edgmont).* 2006;3:64–70.

Chiaro G, Caletti MT, Provini F. Treatment of sleep-related eating disorder. *Curr Treat Options Neurol.* 2015;17:361.

Rand CS, Macgregor AM, Stunkard AJ. The night eating syndrome in the general population and among postoperative obesity surgery patients. *Int J Eat Disord.* 1997;22:65–9.

Winkelman JW, Herzog DB, Fava M. The prevalence of sleep-related eating disorder in psychiatric and non-psychiatric populations. *Psychol Med.* 1999;29:1461–6.

Sleep Terrors

Epidemiology and Demographics: The prevalence of sleep terrors in children is 1–6.5% and in adults 2.2%. There is no sex predominance. Age at onset is typically in children 4–12 years of age, but may begin in adulthood. Predisposing factors include sleep deprivation and situational stress.

Disorder Description: Sleep terrors are accompanied by a piercing scream or cry and by behavioral manifestations of intense fear. Signs of autonomic nervous system activation including tachycardia, tachypnea, flushing, diaphoresis, mydriasis, and increased muscle tone are often seen. Often patients are sitting upright but unresponsive to external stimuli. If awakened, they are confused, disoriented, and incoherent. In adults, it can be associated with displacement from bed and running and may be associated with violent behavior.

For uncomplicated, non-injurious parasomnias that present typically, a routine polysomnography (PSG) is not indicated but can show that disorders of arousal typically begin after an arousal from slow wave sleep. PSG may be useful to assess for precipitating causes such as sleep disordered breathing and for evaluation of other potential disorders such as nocturnal seizures. During the PSG, sounds or alarms may be used to induce a sleep terror during N3 sleep to capture the event. The yield of diagnostic PSG was lower in patients on benzodiazepines or antidepressants.

Treatment involves providing reassurance, maintaining safety of the bedroom environment (removal of potentially injurious items, guarding stairways/windows, installation of bed alarms), and avoidance of precipitants. Often sleep terrors are more concerning to family members than to the individual. Pharmacotherapy is typically not indicated but benzodiazepines and tricyclic antidepressants may be effective in cases where sleep terrors are potentially harmful.

Symptoms: See entry for *Confusional Arousals*.

There is an association between sleep terrors and psychiatric disorders including depression, anxiety, obsessive-compulsive and phobic traits.

Secondary Complications: Sleep terrors may result in injury to self or others.

Treatment Complications: Benzodiazepines may result in morning somnolence.

Bibliography

American Academy of Sleep Medicine. *International classification of sleep disorders*, 3rd ed. Darien, IL: American Academy of Sleep Medicine; 2014.

Fois C, Wright MA, Sechi G, Walker MC, Eriksson SH. The utility of polysomnography for the diagnosis of NREM parasomnias: an observational study over 4 years of clinical practice. *J Neurol.* 2015;262:385–93.

Sleepwalking (Somnambulism)

Epidemiology and Demographics: Prevalence varies by age group: a 40% prevalence in 6–16 year olds, 4.3% in adults, and a lifetime prevalence of 18.3%. Both sexes are equally affected. Age at onset can be as early as when a child gains the ability to walk but may begin at any time in life.

Predisposing factors include priming factors of sleep deprivation and situational stress. Hyperthyroidism, migraines, head injury, encephalitis, stroke are rarer potential priming factors.

Precipitating factors include conditions that result in sleep fragmentation or deprivation resulting in increased homeostatic sleep pressure, which increases the opportunity for slow wave sleep parasomnias to arise. Obstructive sleep apnea and other sleep-related respiratory events may be precipitants of disorders of arousal. Other triggers include environmental stimuli (e.g., telephone calls, pagers, electronic devices, noise, light), internal stimuli (distended bladder), travel, sleeping in unfamiliar surroundings, febrile illness in children, physical emotional stress, premenstrual period in women, psychotropic medications (e.g., lithium carbonate, phenothiazines, anticholinergics, sedative/hypnotic agents).

In addition, sedative-hypnotic medications, particularly benzodiazepine receptor agonists (zolpidem, eszoplicone, zaleplon), have been associated with somnabulism. Strong familial predisposition has been noted.

Disorder Description: Sleepwalking is a combination of ambulation with persistence of impaired consciousness after an arousal. Typically, episodes begin as confusional arousals, but can begin by patients immediately becoming displaced from the bed. Behaviors are often inappropriate (e.g., placing car keys in the refrigerator), and patients typically have amnesia regarding the event. The sleepwalking may terminate spontaneously, or the sleepwalker may return to bed and continue to sleep without reaching conscious awareness. The sleepwalker is disoriented, with slow speech, diminished mentation, and blunted response to questioning. Attempting to arouse the person may paradoxically worsen the confusion and disorientation. The individual may appear to be awake during the episode despite diminished external perception and often there is associated anterograde and retrograde memory impairment. Sleepwalking can be dangerous and there have been reports of individuals leaving the house, driving cars, and even discharging firearms although controversy exists regarding ability to perform activities that require complex cognitive processing during parasomnias.

Symptoms: See entry for *Confusional Arousals.*

Secondary Complications: Injury to self or others may ensue as a result of sleepwalking.

Treatment Complications: Treatment involves providing reassurance and avoidance of precipitants. Maintenance of a safe bedroom environment (guarding stairways/windows, installation of bed alarms, and removal of potentially injurious items) is also important. Pharmacotherapy is typically not indicated unless sleepwalking is dangerous to the individual or extremely disruptive to family members in which case benzodiazepines may be effective. There have been reports of paroxetine and trazodone being used successfully. Nonpharmacologic therapy including psychotherapy, progressive relaxation, or hypnosis can be used for long-term management.

Benzodiazepines may result in morning somnolence and may exacerbate underlying sleep disordered breathing.

Bibliography

American Academy of Sleep Medicine. *International classification of sleep disorders*, 3rd ed. Darien, IL: American Academy of Sleep Medicine; 2014.

Attarian H, Zhu L. Treatment options for disorders of arousal: a case series. *Int J Neurosci.* 2013;123: 623–5.

Howell MJ. Parasomnias: an updated review. *Neurotherapeutics.* 2012;9:753–75.

Mahowald M, Cramer Bornemann MA. Non-REM arousal parasomnias. In Kryger M, Roth T, Dement W, eds. *Principles and Practice of Sleep Medicine.* 5th ed. St. Louis: Elsevier Saunders; 2011. pp. 1075–82.

Popat S, William W. While you were sleepwalking: science and neurobiology of sleep disorders & the

enigma of legal responsibilty of violence during parasomnia. *Neuroethics.* 2015;8(2):203–14.

Small Pox Vaccine

Epidemiology and Demographics: Small pox vaccinia virus has been eradicated worldwide so the vaccine is no longer routine. Due to concerns that it can be used as a biologic warfare agent, some countries vaccinate military recruits and first responders.

Disorder Description: The vaccine is composed of the live vaccinia virus. Vaccinia virus is relatively similar to the variola (small pox) virus. When the vaccine is administered it induces a localized infection of vaccinia. Immunity to both vaccinia and variola is achieved.

Symptoms of Illness If Vaccine Not Used

Localization site	Comment
Cerebral hemispheres (unilateral or bilateral, diffuse, cortical, subcortical gray or white matter)	Encephalitis, encephalomyelitis, encephalopathy, meningitis, and seizures
	Microglial encephalitis – widespread demyelination of subcortical white matter
	Postvaccinial encephalopathy – diffuse cerebral edema and perivascular hemorrhages
Mental status and psychiatric aspects/complications	Headache
Vestibular system (and non-specific dizziness)	Syncope, dizziness, and vertigo
Cranial nerves	Bell's palsy, blindness, corneal scarring, keratitis, photophobia
Spinal cord	Myelitis
Muscle	Myalgia, arthralgia, and back pain
Peripheral neuropathy	Paresthesia and Guillain–Barré syndrome

Secondary Complications: Superinfection, accidental inoculation, progressive vaccinia, generalized vaccinia, severe vaccinal skin infections, erythema multiforme major, eczema, myocarditis, myopericarditis, and fetal death.

Treatment Complications: Vaccinia immunoglobulin when administered can cause anaphylaxis/hypersensitivity reactions, aseptic meningitis, hemolysis, infusion reactions, pulmonary edema, and thrombotic events. Extremely rare post-vaccinal encephalitis reported.

Bibliography

Breman JG, Henderson DA. Diagnosis and management of smallpox. *N Engl J Med*. 2002;346:1300.

Casey CG, Iskander JK, Roper MH, et al. Adverse events associated with smallpox vaccination in the United States, January-October 2003. *JAMA*. 2005;294:2734.

Centers for Disease Control and Prevention (CDC). Update: adverse events following civilian smallpox vaccination – United States, 2003. *MMWR Morb Mortal Wkly Rep*. 2004;53:106.

Centers for Disease Control and Prevention (CDC). Supplemental recommendations on adverse events following smallpox vaccine in the pre-event vaccination program: recommendations of the Advisory Committee on Immunization Practices. *MMWR Morb Mortal Wkly Rep*. 2003;52:282.

Miller ER, Moro PL, Cano M, Shimabukuro TT. Deaths following vaccination: What does the evidence show? *Vaccine*. 2015;33(29):3288–92. DOI: 10.1016/j.vaccine.2015.05.023. Epub May 23, 2015.

Moore ZS, Seward JF, Lane JM. Smallpox. *Lancet*. 2006;367:425.

Small Pox Virus

Epidemiology and Demographics: Eradicated by vaccination as of 1979.

Disorder Description: Variola virus infection characterized by fever, rash, and high mortality rate of 30–50% in the severe form and mortality of 1% in the mild form. Shed from vesicles and via upper airway secretions with a long latency period.

Symptoms

Localization site	Comment
Cerebral hemispheres	Encephalitis
Mental status and psychiatric aspects/complications	Delirium, coma

Secondary Complications

Secondary skin infections.
Keratitis and corneal ulcerations leading to blindness
Viral arthritis and osteomyelitis
Bacterial pneumonia
Orchitis
Complications of sepsis
Treatment: Treatment is supportive.

Bibliography

Moore ZS, Seward JF, Lane JM. Smallpox. *Lancet*. 2006;367:425.

WHO. *The global eradication of smallpox: Final report of the global commission for the certification of smallpox eradication*. History of International Public Health, No. 4. Geneva: World Health Organization; 1980.

Sneddon's Syndrome

Epidemiology and Demographics: Very rare disorder with an incidence of ~4/1,000,000 population. Average age range is 20–42 years. Female preponderance. Almost always sporadic but a few familial cases have been reported.

Disorder Description: Non-inflammatory arteriopathy affecting primarily the skin and central nervous system although cardiac manifestations are well described. The main cause of neurologic dysfunction is due to infarction, be it in the form of clinical stroke or insidious small vessel disease.

Symptoms

Localization site	Comment
Cerebral hemispheres	Ischemic strokes cause symptoms appropriate to location but most commonly include hemiplegia, hemianopia, aphasia, and hemisensory deficits
Mental status and psychiatric aspects/complications	Vascular dementia, disorders of concentration and attention
Brainstem	Intranuclear ophthalmoplegia
Cranial nerves	Diplopia/third nerve palsy. Retinal artery occlusion with monocular blindness
Unclear localization	Headache

Secondary Complications: The most obvious is the cutaneous manifestation of livedo racemosa, especially in the trunk and buttocks. Other manifestations include hypertension, heart valve disease, ischemic heart disease, renal failure.

Treatment: There is no accepted treatment although calcium channel blockers help the cutaneous manifestations.

Bibliography

Wu S, Yu Z, Liang H. Sneddon's syndrome: a comprehensive review of the literature. *Orphanet J Rare Dis*. 2014;9:215.

Solvent Inhalant Abuse

Epidemiology and Demographics: Users consist mainly of young children. No race predilection.

Disorder Description: Inhalant abuse – also known as volatile substance abuse, solvent abuse, sniffing, huffing, and bagging. Because of the abuse, i.e. deliberate inhalation of a volatile substance, there is an altered mental state. Individuals from minority and marginalized populations are more common users.

Symptoms

Localization site	Comment
Cerebral hemispheres	Cerebral atrophy (chronic)
	Toxic leukoencephalopathy (chronic)
Mental status and psychiatric aspects/complications	Cognitive impairment (chronic)
	Slurred speech (acute)
Brainstem	Brainstem atrophy (chronic)
	Autonomic instability (acute)
Cerebellum	Cerebellar atrophy (chronic)
Vestibular system (and non-specific dizziness)	Gait disturbance (acute)
Cranial nerves	Cranial neuropathies (acute)
	Nystagmus (acute)
Pituitary gland	Transient central hypothyroidism and hypergonadotropism (chronic)

Localization site	Comment
Mononeuropathy or mononeuropathy multiplex	Neuropathy (chronic)
Peripheral neuropathy	Peripheral neuropathy (chronic)
Muscle	Tremors (chronic)
Neuromuscular junction	Dopaminergic and adrenergic receptor dysregulation

Secondary Complications: Indirectly affects nervous system via:

- Cardiovascular complications: arrhythmias, myocardial infarction resulting in cerebral ischemia
- Respiratory complications: respiratory arrest leading to cerebral ischemia
- Hematologic complications: inhalant abuse, particularly chronic abuse of benzene, may cause aplastic anemia and malignancy multiple myeloma resulting in neurologic symptoms

Bibliography

Baydala L. Inhalant abuse. *Paediatr Child Health*. 2010;15(7):443–8.

Chen HF, Chen SW, Chen P, et al. Chronic glue sniffing with transient central hypothyroidism and hypergonadotropism. *J Chin Med Assoc*. 2003;66(12):747–51.

Hormes JT, Filley CM, Rosenberg NL. Neurologic sequelae of chronic solvent vapor abuse. *Neurology*. 1986;36(5):698–702.

Perry H. Inhalant abuse in children and adolescents. Updated May 9, 2018. Available from www.uptodate.com/contents/inhalant-abuse-in-children-and-adolescents?source=search_result&search=aerosol%20inhalation%20abuse&selectedTitle=2~133.Accessed Sep 18, 2018.

Somatization

(See entries for *Illness Anxiety Disorder [Hypochondriasis]*, *Functional Neurologic Symptom Disorder*, and *Factitious Disorder*)

Epidemiology and Demographics: Somatization is a common condition, with more than 50% of patients in outpatient clinics presenting with a physical complaint that cannot be ascribed to a medical condition. One study, which defined somatization as four or more unexplained symptoms in men, or six or more unexplained symptoms in women, found that somatization was present in 17% of patients in primary care settings and 4% of the general population. Women with this disorder tend to have histories as children of missing, disturbed, or defective parents, and of sexual or physical abuse. The tendency to somatization has been linked to childhood trauma via insecure attachment, and maladaptive patterns of interpersonal relationships.

Disorder Description: Somatization is an overarching term that includes many different illnesses, including somatic symptom disorder, illness anxiety disorder, conversion disorder, psychologic factors affecting other medical conditions, and factitious disorder. Somatization refers to a constellation of symptoms forming a syndrome that leads to substantial distress and psychologic impairment, but not explained by a described general medical condition. It is a chronic syndrome of multiple, recurring somatic symptoms that are not explainable medically and are associated with psychosocial distress and with medical help-seeking behaviors. The DSM-5 does not use the term somatization.

Treatment: Carried out by primary care physicians according to a conservative plan based on being a consistent care provider, preventing unnecessary or dangerous medical procedures, and inquiring in a supportive manner about areas of stress in the patient's life. This can be viewed as a form of supportive psychotherapy. The basic goal is to help the patient cope with the symptoms rather than eliminate them completely. Cognitive-behavioral therapy has also reduced symptoms, ratings of disorder by evaluators, and health care costs. The intervention is focused on stress management, activity regulation, emotional awareness, cognitive restructuring, and interpersonal communication.

Bibliography

American Psychiatric Association. *Diagnostic and statistical manual of mental disorders: DSM-5.* 5th ed. Washington, DC: American Psychiatric Association; 2013.

Creed F, Barsky A. A systematic review of the epidemiology of somatisation disorder and hypochondriasis. *J Psychosom Res.* 2004;56(4):391–408.

Fink P, Ewald H, Jensen J, et al. Screening for somatization and hypochondriasis in primary care and neurological in-patients: a seven-item scale for hypochondriasis and somatization. *J Psychosom Res.* 1999;46(3):261–73.

Lipowski ZJ. Somatization: the concept and its clinical application. *Am J Psychiatry.* 1988;145(11): 1358–68.

Stern T, et al. *Massachusetts General Hospital handbook of general hospital psychiatry.* Philadephia, PA: Saunders; 2010.

Van der Kolk BA, Pelcovitz D, Roth S, Mandel FS. Dissociation, somatization, and affect dysregulation. *Am J Psychiatry.* 1996;153(7):83.

Spasmodic Dysphonia

Epidemiology and Demographics: This condition has been reported as rare, occurring in 1 to 4 people per 100,000[1]; however, recent reports suggest that it is frequently undiagnosed and is more prevalent than previously thought.[2] Spasmodic dysphonia can affect anyone. Women are affected more than men, and the first signs are manifested usually between ages 30 and 50 years, with a mean age of 45 years.[2]

Disorder Description: Spasmodic dysphonia is a neurologic disorder that affects the muscles of the larynx, causing involuntary movements (spasms) that interfere with the ability of the vocal folds to vibrate and produce speech. It is thought to be caused by abnormal functioning in the basal ganglia, an area of the brain that coordinates muscle movement, as well as the brainstem.[1] No genes for isolated spasmodic dysphonia have been identified, but the condition may be an isolated manifestation of a *THAP1* gene mutation that is associated with craniocervical dystonia.[3] Recent research has shown that mutations in the *TUBB4a* gene[3] and *ANO3* gene[3,4] may also influence the development of spasmodic dysphonia.

Spasmodic dysphonia is a form of focal dystonia that causes voice breaks that can occur every few sentences or every other word, depending on the severity. The voice develops a tight, strained quality. Symptoms usually develop gradually. Spasmodic dysphonia has also been associated with tremor, usually of the larynx. The etiology is unclear, but in about half of patients, onset has been associated with viral upper respiratory infection or a major life stressor.[2] The two main types of spasmodic dysphonia are adductor spasmodic dysphonia and abductor spasmodic dysphonia.

Adductor spasmodic dysphonia: The more common type of spasmodic dysphonia, associated with speech that is characterized by choppy, strangled, or strained phonation with intermittent voice offsets on the voicing of vowels. Voice breaks are due to spasmodic hyperadduction (closure) of the vocal folds due to lateral cricoarytenoid and/or transverse and oblique arytenoid muscle contraction that interrupts phonation because the vocal folds cannot vibrate.[1] Voicing takes effort and often sounds strained and hoarse. Patients are generally able to sing, whisper, laugh, cry, and shout without vocal strain, and voicing becomes worse while under emotional stress, talking on the phone, or speaking publically. Fiberoptic laryngoscopy of patients with adductor spasmodic dysphonia shows intermittent, rapid shortening and squeezing of the vocal folds, resulting in quick glottic closure that interrupts airflow and prevents the vocal folds from vibrating appropriately.[1-4]

Abductor spasmodic dysphonia: The less common type of spasmodic dysphonia, characterized by prolonged voiceless consonants due to difficulty with voice onset following voiceless sounds, such as /h/, /s/, /f/, /p/, /t/, and /k/. The vocal folds open too far due to posterior cricoarytenoid muscle contraction and cannot vibrate. Air escapes from the lungs during speech causing the voice to sound weak and breathy, as well as fatigue and sometimes hypoxia.[1] These patients also may exhibit pitch changes, phonatory breaks during vowels, or uncontrolled rise in vowels' fundamental frequency. Fiberoptic laryngoscopy of patients with abductor spasmodic dysphonia shows wide-ranging abduction movements for voiceless consonants that are prolonged and interfere with following vowels.[1-4]

Symptoms

Localization site	Comment
Mental status and psychiatric aspects/complications	Anxiety, depression, and/or attention deficit disorder may be present
Muscle	Posterior cricoarytenoid: abducts vocal folds
	Lateral cricoarytenoid: adducts vocal folds
	Transverse and oblique arytenoids: adduct arytenoid cartilages

Treatment Complications: Adduction spasmodic dysphonia may be treated with intramuscular botulinum toxin injection, causing the muscles to become too weak to close and allowing air to escape from the lungs. This can cause mild to moderate respiratory distress and headaches.

In contrast, spasmodic dysphonia and other focal dystonia may be malingering or somatoform complaints.

References

1. NIH. NIDCD Fact Sheet: Spasmodic Dysphonia. NIH Publication No. 10-4214. Updated Oct 2010.
2. Schweinfurth JM, Billante M, Courey MS. Risk factors and demographics in patients with spasmodic dysphonia. *Laryngoscope.* 2002;112(2):220-3.
3. Jinnah HA, Berardelli A, Comella C, et al. The focal dystonias: current views and challenges for future research. *Mov Disord.* 2013;28(7):926-43.
4. Stamelou M, Charlesworth G, Cordivari C, et al. The phenotypic spectrum of DYT24 due to ANO3 mutations. *Mov Disord.* 2014;29(7):928-34.

Spina Bifida Occulta

Epidemiology and Demographics: Approximately 5% of the population have spina bifida occulta. On average in developed countries it occurs in about 0.4/1000 births. In the United States, it affects about 0.7/1000 births.

Disorder Description: Spina bifida occulta is defined as a neural tube defect that almost always occurs at the base of the spine in the lumbar or sacral region. One or more vertebrae might be involved.

Symptoms

Localization site	Comment
Lumbosacral spine	Hairy patch on the lower back. Hemangioma or lipoma also might be noted. It may occur together with a tethered cord (associated with radicular symptoms, bladder incontinence, frequent urinary tract infection, constipation, scoliosis). Foot deformities are also reported

Secondary Complications: Tethered cord is the most frequent complication, which causes weakness of the lower extremities, numbness, ataxia, and bladder and bowel dysfunction.

Bibliography

Lapsiwala SB, Iskandar BJ. The tethered cord syndrome in adults with spina bifida occulta. *Neurol Res.* 2004;26(7):235–40.

Spinal and Bulbar Muscular Atrophy (Kennedy Disease)

Epidemiology and Demographics: Spinal and bulbar muscular atrophy (SBMA) has an incidence of 3.3/100,000 males. No racial predilection has been reported but has not been reported from individuals of African or Aboriginal background.

Disorder Description: It is a rare, progressive motor neuron disease with multisystem involvement manifesting as androgen insensitivity, diabetes, neuropathy, or autonomic nervous system involvement. Patients present with progressive weakness (limbs, bulbar muscles, respiratory muscles), fasciculations, gynecomastia, and erectile dysfunction. Presents in the 3rd to 5th decade of life.

It is caused by an expansion of an unstable cytosine-adenosine-guanosine (CAG) repeat in a coding sequence of the androgen receptor gene on the long arm of chromosome X. The longer the CAG expansion, the earlier the disease manifests. Fewer than 47 repeats is associated with a sensory-dominant phenotype, whereas more than 47 repeats is associated with a motor-dominant phenotype.

Presents with a perioral tremor or postural weakness. Can be symmetric or asymmetric, can start in lower or upper extremities. Presents also with gynecomastia, cramps, tremor, myalgia.

Symptoms

Localization site	Comment
Brainstem	Involvement of the brainstem motor nuclei results in involvement of the bulbar muscles
Spinal cord	Progressive loss of lower motor neurons (LMN)

Secondary Complications: Asphyxiation from bulbar weakness.

Treatment: Treatment is mostly supportive. Possible mild benefits of antiandrogenic agents.

Bibliography

Finsterer J, Soraru G. Onset manifestations of spinal and bulbar muscular atrophy (Kennedy's disease). *J Mol Neurosci.* 2016;58:321–9.

Spinal Cord Infarct and Foix-Alajouanine

Epidemiology and Demographics: Accounts for approximately 1.2% of all strokes with an incidence of 12/100,000 annually.

Disorder Description: Infarction of spinal cord tissue resulting from atherosclerotic or embolic occlusion of the spinal arteries. The spinal cord has a unique vascular anatomy. Throughout the entire length of the cord, the posterior columns are supplied by a pair of posterior spinal arteries arising at each spinal level. Because of this redundancy, infarcts rarely affect the posterior columns. The anterior two-thirds of the spinal cord is supplied by the anterior spinal arteries. At the cervical level, these are comprised of single arteries arising at every spinal level. As with the posterior segment, there is enough redundant blood supply to make infarcts very rare. In contrast to the above, the anterior segment of the thoracolumbar cord is supplied by a single artery (the artery of Adamkiewicz). This artery is subject not only to atherosclerosis, hypotension, and embolism, but also to occlusion by an abdominal aortic aneurysm or the correction thereof. Symptoms of infarction occur abruptly. In contrast, other patients experience slowly progressive symptoms that are exacerbated by exertion and mimic the claudication seen in spinal stenosis.

Symptoms

Localization site	Comment
Spinal cord	Weakness and loss of sensation below the level of the infarct usually with back pain. The typical lower thoracic location would lead to paraplegia and loss of sensation in both legs. Because the posterior columns are not involved, vibration and position sensations are spared. Urinary incontinence. Symptoms are abrupt in infarct and gradual in Foix-Alajouanine
Anterior horn cells	The anterior horn cells are involved in the ischemic field. This would only be noticeable in the event of a cervical infarction. In that case, there would be atrophy of only the myotome at the site of the infarct

Localization site	Comment
Syndromes with combined upper and lower motor neuron deficits	For the reasons just explained, an infarct of the cervical cord would cause lower motor neuron deficits at the level of the infarct with upper motor neuron deficits at all levels below

Secondary Complications: This is commonly a complication of aortic surgery or of hypotension.

Treatment Complications: Thrombolysis has not been shown to be useful. Elevation of blood pressure may help if this occurs in the setting of hypotension.

Bibliography

Cheshire WP, Santos CC, Massey EW, Howard JF Jr. Spinal cord infarction: etiology and outcome. *Neurology*. 1996;47(2):321–30.

Rigney L, Cappelen-Smith C, Sebire D, Beran RG, Cordato D. Nontraumatic spinal cord ischaemic syndrome. *J Clin Neurosci*. 2015;22(10):1544–9.

Spinal Epidural Abscess

Epidemiology and Demographics: Rare. More common in males. Median age of onset is 50–60 years of age.

Disorder Description: Spinal epidural abscess is defined as a collection of pus between the dura and the bones of the spine. Lumbar and thoracic spine are most commonly affected. It can be due to direct extension of the local infection of vertebral osteomyelitis, psoas muscle abscess, or contiguous soft tissue infection. It may also be due to hematogenous seeding due to septicemia. *Staphylococcus aureus* is the most common organism involved; MRSA is increasingly being identified.

Symptoms

Localization site	Comment
Cervical spine	Neck pain, radicular symptoms, motor weakness, sphincter dysfunction, sensory changes, paralysis, cord compression
Thoracic spine	Mid back pain, sphincter dysfunction, cord compression with difficulty ambulating
Lumbosacral spine	Low back pain, radicular symptoms with radiation, motor weakness, sphincter dysfunction, paralysis, difficulty ambulating

Treatment Complications: Patients with diabetes mellitus, sepsis, infection with MRSA, or aged over 65 years may have incomplete response to medical treatment alone and may warrant surgical intervention.

Bibliography

Sendi P, Bregenzer T, Zimmerli W. Spinal epidural abscess and clinical practice. *QJM*. 2008;101(1): 1–12.

Spinal Epidural Hemorrhage

Epidemiology and Demographics: Estimated incidence is 1/1,000,000 population.

Disorder Description: A collection of blood between the dura and spinal bone. This can occur at any location along the spinal cord and may be traumatic, iatrogenic (after epidural lumbar puncture), or spontaneous. Spontaneous epidural hemorrhage is often seen in association with bleeding diatheses or anticoagulation. Rarely, it is caused by a spinal epidural arteriovenous fistula.

Symptoms

Localization site	Comment
Spinal cord	Weakness and loss of sensation below the level of the infarct. This occurs abruptly and is associated with back pain. Urinary and fecal incontinence are commonly seen

Secondary Complications: This must be distinguished from epidural abscess. The two will have similar complaints, but an abscess should develop more slowly and be associated with systemic signs of infection.

Treatment Complications: The only treatment is surgical and carries the standard risks of surgery including bleeding, infection, and systemic complications of anesthesia.

Bibliography

Hussenbocus SM, Wilby MJ, Cain C, Hali D. Spontaneous spinal epidural hematoma: a case report and literature review. *J Emerg Med*. 2012;42(2):31–4.

Moftakhar P, Hefts SW, Ko NU. Vascular myelopathies. *Semin Neurol*. 2012;32(2):146–53.

Spinal Epidural Lipomatosis

Epidemiology and Demographics: More common in males. Mean age of presentation is in the 40s, but younger ages have been identified in some cases.

Disorder Description: Linked to exogenous steroid use in >75%. Non-steroid-related cases have been reported, including some associated with Cushing disease, Cushing syndrome, hypothyroidism, pituitary prolactinoma, and obesity.

Symptoms

Localization site	Comment
Spinal cord	Myelopathic effects, radicular effects
Dorsal root ganglia	Numbness, paresthesias, or radicular symptoms
Conus medullaris	Sudden/bilateral back pain. Less radicular pain as compared with cauda equina. Motor strength: symmetric, less marked hyperreflexic distal paresis of lower extremities, fasiculations present Sensory: localized numbness to perianal area, symmetric and bilateral Sphincter: early urinary and fecal incontinence. Impotence: frequent
Cauda equina	Gradual and unilateral pain that is radicular in nature. Back pain is not as severe as conus medullaris Motor: more marked asymmetric areflexic paraplegia, atrophy more common Sensory: localized numbness at saddle area, asymmetric and unilateral Sphincter: tend to present late with urinary and fecal incontinence Impotence: less frequent
Unclear localization	Bowel and bladder dysfunction

Bibliography

Rajput D, Srivastava AK, Kumar R. Spinal epidural lipomatosis: An unusual cause of relapsing and remitting paraparesis. *J Pediatr Neurosci.* 2010;5(2):150–2.

Rustom D, Gupta D, Chakrabortty S. Epidural lipomatosis: A dilemma in interventional pain management for the use of epidural steroid. *J Anaesthesiol Clin Pharmacol.* 2013;29(3):410–41. DOI:10.4103/0970-9185.117070.

Spinal Hemangioblastoma

Epidemiology and Demographics: Rare central nervous system tumor that accounts for 2% of all primary spinal tumors, with an annual incidence of 0.014/100,000. Higher incidence in men than in women. Most often presents in the 3rd decade of life. One-third of cases are associated with von Hippel–Lindau disease (see entry for *von Hippel–Lindau Disease*).

Disorder Description: Slow-growing benign vascular tumor. The sporadic form is usually solitary. The presence of multiple tumors or tumors in childhood should raise suspicion for von Hippel–Lindau disease. Microscopically, there is proliferation of abnormal stromal cells alongside normal-appearing capillaries.

Main complications include local mass effect from compression, but hemorrhage of the tumor can result in acute symptoms and carries significant mortality. Hemangioblastomas can be found anywhere in the central or peripheral nervous system, with the posterior fossa being the most common location and the posterior spinal cord representing the second most common.

Symptoms

Localization site	Comment
Spinal cord	Most commonly occurs in the posterior cord, particularly near the dorsal root ganglion. Sensory symptoms are the most frequent finding, followed by motor weakness and pain. Symptomatic tumors are most commonly found in the cervical spine followed by the thoracic spine. Sometimes are associated with syringomyelia
Anterior horn cells	Infrequently involves anterior cord. Anterior involvement is associated with a higher operative risk
Dorsal root ganglia	Very common. Causes radiculopathy
Conus medullaris	Infrequently involves the lumbar spine
Cauda equina	Rare
Specific spinal roots	Most commonly affects the cervical and thoracic spinal roots
Syndromes with combined upper and lower motor neuron deficits	Combined myelopathy and radiculopathy are common

Secondary Complications: Hemorrhage of hemangioblastoma can result in acute paresis and carries a high risk of mortality. Risk of rupture increases with size, especially with tumors greater than 1.5 cm in diameter.

Treatment Complications: Main treatment is surgical resection, with or without embolization. Outcome is generally excellent but there is a risk of recurrence if the tumor is not completely excised. Rare but serious surgical complications include obstructive hydrocephalus and meningitis. Radiation therapy for inaccessible or multiple tumors can halt growth but does not cause tumors to regress.

Bibliography

Conway JE, Chou D, Clatterbuck RE, et al. Hemangioblastomas of the central nervous system in von Hippel-Lindau syndrome and sporadic disease. *Neurosurgery.* 2001;48(1):55–63.

Gläsker S, Van Velthoven V. Risk of hemorrhage in hemangioblastomas of the central nervous system. *Neurosurgery.* 2005;57(1):71–6.

Lonser RR, Oldfield EH. Spinal cord hemangioblastomas. *Neurosurg Clin North Am.* 2006;17(1):37–44.

Lonser RR, Weil RJ, Wanebo JE, Devroom HL, Oldfield EH. Surgical management of spinal cord hemangioblastomas in patients with von Hippel-Lindau disease. *J Neurosurg.* 2003;98(1):106–16.

Spinal Muscular Atrophy (SMA) Type III (Kugelberg–Welander Syndrome)

Epidemiology and Demographics: The incidence of spinal muscular atrophy (SMA) has been estimated at 1/6000–10,000 live births. SMA type III accounts for about 12–30% of cases. Symptoms start between 18 months of age and adulthood. It is associated with a normal lifespan.

Disorder Description: Also known as spinal muscular atrophy (SMA) type III. It is a juvenile form of SMA. It has been subdivided into type IIIA (onset between 18 months and 3 years) and type IIIB (onset after 3 years).

There is progressive proximal weakness of legs and arms and may initially present as difficulty climbing stairs or new onset falling. May have hand tremor or polymyoclonus.

SMA results from homozygous deletions of the "survival of motor neuron" (SMN) gene on chromosome 5q13. Disease is autosomal recessive.

Symptoms

Localization site	Comment
Spinal roots (specific)	SMAs are associated with degeneration of spinal motor neurons
Muscle	Proximal weakness. Legs > arms

Secondary Complications: Sleep disorder and fatigue are common.

Treatment Complications: Potential surgical complications of corrective surgery for scoliosis or hip, if surgery is indicated.

Bibliography

Darras B. Spinal muscular atrophies. *Pediatr Clin North Am.* 2015;62:743–66.

Markowitz JA, Singh P, Darra. BT. Spinal muscular atrophy: a clinical and research update. *Pediatr Neurol.* 2012;46(1):1–12.

Prior TW, Finanger E. Spinal muscular atrophy. Feb 24, 2000. Updated Dec 22, 2016. In Pagon RA, Adam MP, Ardinger HH, et al., eds. *GeneReviews®* [Internet]. Seattle (WA): University of Washington, Seattle; 1993–2018. Available from www.ncbi.nlm.nih.gov/books/NBK1352/. Accessed 5/2017.

Spinal Neoplasm

Epidemiology and Demographics: Spinal tumors make up 5–10% of all central nervous system malignancies. They are divided into the categories of extradural (65% of spinal tumors), intradural extramedullary (30%), and intradural intramedullary (5–10%). Intramedullary tumors are located within the spinal cord while extramedullary tumors are adjacent to the spinal cord.

There is variability in age presentation depending on the type of tumor. Children are more likely to have astrocytomas while adults are more likely to have metastatic spinal tumors. It is estimated that 5–10% of cancer patients will develop symptomatic spinal metastasis. The spine is the third most common site for cancer cells to metastasize (following lung and liver). Elderly patients have an increased frequency of spinal meningiomas with a female-to-male ratio of 4:1.

Disorder Description: Extramedullary tumors include neurofibromas, meningiomas, schwannomas, and metastatic tumors. Neurofibromas and meningiomas can be intradural or extradural. Metastatic tumors are usually extradural. Metastatic tumors are 40 times more common than primary lesions. Metastatic spinal tumors are commonly due to prostate, breast, and lung cancers, lymphomas, and leukemias.

Intradural intramedullary spinal tumors include ependymomas, which are the most common type of intramedullary tumor in adults (50–60%), and gliomas, which are comprised of astrocytomas and high-grade gliomas.

Often, presentation due to spinal cord tumors is slow and progressive. Symptoms can occur after direct compression, ischemia due to vascular infiltration, or invasive infiltration.

Symptoms

Localization site	Comment
Spinal cord	Pain and spinal tenderness often precede neurologic deficits. Motor deficits, paresthesias, numbness often occur. Increased stiffness may be seen below the level of the lesion. Bladder or bowel dysfunction as well as sexual dysfunction may occur. Imbalance with walking occurs when dorsal columns are affected
Anterior horn cells	May be involved in the cases of intradural or intramedullary tumors. Results in muscle weakness, atrophy, and fasciculations
Conus medullaris	Can be compressed by tumor, resulting in lower extremity weakness, numbness, bowel/bladder dysfunction
Cauda equina	Can be compressed by tumor, resulting in lower extremity weakness, numbness, bowel/bladder dysfunction
Specific spinal roots	Spinal roots may be compressed due to spinal tumors resulting in radicular pain as well as weakness and numbness localized to corresponding dermatome and myotome
Syndromes with combined upper and lower motor neuron deficits	Combined myelopathy and radiculopathy is common

Secondary Complications: Spinal tumors can be associated with increased risk of blood clots due to hypercoagulability, especially if they are metastatic tumors. In addition, due to their association with urinary retention from spinal cord compression, patients are at higher risk of urinary tract infections and pyelonephritis.

Treatment Complications: Chemotherapy, radiation, radiosurgery, and radical resection can be considered depending on the type and location of the tumor. Radiation, radiosurgery, and surgery risks include paralysis, bladder incontinence, and urinary retention. Risks of chemotherapy include infection, hair loss, and gastrointestinal discomfort as well as multiple other systemic side effects dependent on the medication.

Bibliography

Hayat MA. *Tumors of the central nervous system: Volume 6, Spinal tumors, Part 1*. Dordrecht: Springer; 2012.

Lumenta CB. *Neurosurgery*. Heidelberg: Springer; 2010.

Spinal Perimedullary Fistula

Epidemiology and Demographics: Most commonly these are small fistulae and occur in older adults. Less commonly, medium-sized fistulae may affect young adults and rarely giant fistulae may affect children. The adult form has a prevalence of 5–10 per million population. The male-to-female ratio is 5:1. Presentation is usually after age 50 years.

Disorder Description: Abnormal connection between a spinal artery and medullary vein. Unlike arteriovenous malformations, these have no intervening nidus. They are present at birth. Symptoms usually develop slowly over time but the childhood giant fistulae may present abruptly and even as subarachnoid hemorrhage.

Symptoms

Localization site	Comments
Spinal cord	Gradual myelopathy consisting of weakness and numbness below the level of the lesion. Progressive urinary and fecal incontinence is also seen
Conus medullaris	The young adult form is often located here and presents with paraplegia and prominent incontinence

Secondary Complications: Some forms are associated with vascular malformations in the skin and brain.

Treatment Complications: Treatment is either by surgical or endovascular repair. Both carry risk of infarction and hemorrhage.

Bibliography

Krings T, Geibprasert S. Spinal dural arteriovenous fistulas. *Am J Neuroradiol.* 2009;30(4):639–48.

Moftakhar P, Hefts SW, Ko NU. Vascular myelopathies. *Semin Neurol.* 2012;32(2):146–53.

Spinal Subarachnoid Hemorrhage

Epidemiology and Demographics: This disorder is extremely rare with few cases reported in the literature.

Disorder Description: Hemorrhage collecting between the arachnoid and pia mater in the spinal cord. This is generally related to trauma or spinal procedures but can also be seen in coagulopathy. Spinal aneurysms are rarely present, with or without spinal perimedullary arteriovenous fistulae. Being in the subarachnoid space, the blood irritates the spinal nerve roots rather than causing compression of the spinal cord itself.

Symptoms

Localization site	Comment
Cauda equina	If the blood collected below L1, then the cauda equina will be compressed causing pain with numbness and weakness affecting all lumbosacral roots
Specific spinal roots	If the blood collects proximally, it may irritate individual nerve roots causing apparent radiculopathy

Secondary Complications: This carries a high risk of permanent weakness and loss of sensation.

Treatment Complications: Most cases are treated surgically with the attendant risks of bleeding, infection, anesthesia, and damage to underlying tissue.

Bibliography

Domenicucci M, Eramieri A, Paolini S, et al. Spinal subarachnoid hemorrhage: our experience and literature review. *Acta Neurochir (Wein).* 2005;147(7):741–50.

Kim JS, Lee SH. Spontaneous spinal subarachnoid hemorrhage with spontaneous resolution. *J Korean Neurosurg Soc.* 2009;45(4):253–5.

Madhugiri VS, Ambekar S, Roopesh Kumar VR, Sasidharan GM, Nanda A. Spinal aneurysms: clinicoradiological features and management paradigms. *J Neurosurg Spine.* 2013;19(1):34–48.

Spondylitis

Epidemiology and Demographics: Incidence is approximately 3 persons per 100,000 per year.

Disorder Description: Spondylitis is defined as inflammation of the vertebrae. Two examples are Pott's disease and ankylosing spondylitis. Ankylosing spondylitis primarily affects the sacroiliac joints.

Symptoms

Localization site	Comment
Cervical spine	Neck pain, radicular symptoms including radiation into shoulders, decreased range of motion
Thoracic spine	Mid back pain
Lumbosacral spine	Low back pain, radicular symptoms, hip pain, buttock pain
Jaw	Temporal mandibular joint pain
Eyes	Iritis or anterior uveitis

Secondary Complications: Cauda equina syndrome can occur in patients with longstanding spondylitis. Urinary retention and/or incontinence, loss of bowel control, sexual dysfunction, and weakness of the lower extremities should raise the possibility of cauda equina syndrome.

Bibliography

Khan MA. Ankylosing spondylitis and related spondyloarthropathies: the dramatic advances in the past decade. *Rheumatology.* 2011;50(4):637–9. https://doi.org/10.1093/rheumatology/keq433.

Wright KA, Crowson CS, Michet CJ, Matteson EL. Time trends in incidence, clinical features and cardiovascular disease in ankylosing spondylitis over 3 decades: a population based study. *Arthritis Care Res.* 2015;67(6):836–41. DOI:10.1002/acr.22512.

Sporothrix schenckii

Epidemiology and Demographics: Typically occurs in people with outdoor occupations.

Disorder Description: Subacute to chronic infection caused by the fungus *Sporothrix schenckii* that involves cutaneous and subcutaneous tissues. Worse in immunocompromised, including diabetes, alcoholism, and chronic obstructive pulmonary disease. Transmitted through soil or other organic material contacting the skin, or through inhalation. Pulmonary disease is tuberculosis-like and is fatal without treatment. Chronic meningitis is a risk in HIV/AIDS or immunosuppression.

Symptoms

Localization site	Comment
Cerebral hemispheres	Meningitis
Mental status and psychiatric aspects/complications	Encephalopathy due to meningitis
Brainstem	Meningitis
Cerebellum	Meningitis
Cranial nerves	Meningitis

Secondary Complications: Skin ulceration and secondary infection by other organisms.

Treatment Complications: Treatment with itraconazole or amphotericin B (nephrotoxicity) in more severe cases, including meningitis. Pulmonary cases may require surgery. Treatment usually needed for up to a year. Immune reconstitution syndrome may occur in AIDS patients and presents with clinical and radiographic worsening in the setting of initiating anti-retroviral therapy.

Bibliography

Freitas DF, de Siqueira Hoagland B, do Valle AC, et al. Sporotrichosis in HIV-infected patients: report of 21 cases of endemic sporotrichosis in Rio de Janeiro, Brazil. *Med Mycol.* 2012;50(2):170–8. Epub Aug 23, 2011.

Hessler C, Kauffman CA, Chow FC. The upside of bias: a case of chronic meningitis due to *Sporothrix schenckii* in an immunocompetent host. *Neurohospitalist.* 2017;7(1):30–34.

Kauffman CA. Sporotrichosis. *Clin Infect Dis.* 1999;29(2):231.

Staphylococcus aureus

Epidemiology and Demographics: Ubiquitous bacterium that colonizes the skin of many individuals.

Disorder Description: Causes a variety of neurologic infections. Infective endocarditis can lead to embolic strokes and mycotic aneurysm; pyomyositis, infection of the skeletal muscle, is possible. *Staphylococcus aureus* bacteremia can cause septic shock and toxic shock syndrome. Meningitis happens in the setting of head trauma or neurosurgery (especially shunts) and rarely due to bacteremia.

Symptoms

Localization site	Comment
Cerebral hemispheres	Meningitis
Mental status and psychiatric aspects/complications	Confusion, lethargy, delirium, coma
Brainstem	Meningitis
Cerebellum	Meningitis
Cranial nerves	Meningitis
Conus medullaris	If infection is due to lumbar puncture
Cauda equina	Infection related to devices and procedures
Plexus	Related to inflammatory state
Peripheral neuropathy	Critical illness polyneuropathy
Muscle	Direct infection

Secondary Complications: Lungs, spleen, joints, bones, and/or skin can all be involved. Spontaneous hemorrhage possible.

Treatment Complications: Resistant strains make polytherapy necessary and, with it are more side effects of antibiotics. Steroids are also used in meningitis.

Bibliography

Aguilar J, Urday-Cornejo V, Donabedian S, et al. Staphylococcus aureus meningitis: case series and literature review. *Medicine (Baltimore).* 2010;89(2):117.

Biller J, Ferro JM, ed. *Neurologic aspects of systemic disease, Part III*. Handbook of Clinical Neurology, Vol 121 (3rd Series). San Diego: Elsevier; 2014.

Status Epilepticus (SE)

Epidemiology and Demographics: The overall incidence of status epilepticus (SE) is 9.9 to 41 per 100,000/year; highest in children and the elderly.

The incidence in Europe is lower (10–16/100,000 population) compared with the United States (18–41/100,000 population). American ethnic minorities have a higher incidence (57/100,000) than whites (20/100,000).

Disorder Description: SE is considered a life-threatening neurologic emergency that requires prompt diagnosis and treatment. Proposed definition by the Internal League Against Epilepsy (ILAE): "Status epilepticus is a condition resulting either from the failure of the mechanisms responsible for seizure termination or from the initiation of mechanisms, which lead to abnormally, prolonged seizures (after time point t1). It is a condition which can have long-term consequences (after time point t2), including neuronal death, neuronal injury, and alteration of neuronal networks, depending on the type and duration of seizures." In the case of convulsive SE, t1 is 5 minutes and t2 is 30 minutes, based on animal models and clinical research. Two main classifications of SE: convulsive and non-convulsive. Convulsive SE includes focal motor SE and generalized myoclonic, tonic, clonic, and tonic–clonic SE.

Mortality associated with SE approaches 20%, with generalized convulsive SE representing about 45–74% of cases. The most important determinant remains the underlying etiology. The most common etiologies include infections, brain injury and epilepsy, withdrawal or changes in antiepileptic drugs, as well as remote symptomatic epilepsy. Autoimmune encephalitis has been recently recognized as an important etiologic consideration.

Treatment involves early and aggressive intervention. General guidelines for generalized SE include benzodiazepines as first line, followed by antiepileptic drugs such as phenytoin, valproic acid, levetiracetam, and phenobarbital. If patients fail to respond, intubation and use of continuous infusion of sedatives such as propofol, midazolam, or pentobarbital are frequently employed. EEG monitoring is important because electrical SE may continue after cessation of motor activity. Anesthetics are typically titrated until EEG shows burst suppression pattern.

Symptoms

Localization site	Comment
Cerebral hemispheres	Generalized tonic, clonic, tonic–clonic, myoclonic, and absence seizures. Focal seizures, which may include subtle clinical motor findings such as facial, eyelid, or limb clonus. Seizures may be subclinical and nonconvulsive with alteration in mentation
	EEG during seizures will show ictal activity, though seizures may occur in an intermittent repetitive fashion or continuously
	CT scan can show decreased attenuation, swelling, loss of gray–white matter differentiation, sulcal effacement, and gyriform patterns of enhancement. MRI findings may show T2 hyperintensity and restricted diffusion, with corresponding low signal on apparent diffusion coefficient (resembling stroke)
Mental status and psychiatric aspects/ complications	Encephalopathy (acute). SE may result in permanent cognitive deficits or slowing. Findings vary with the type of seizures, seizure severity, duration, underlying etiology, and chronologic age of the patient

Secondary Complications: Common complications include respiratory acidosis with or without metabolic acidosis, hypoxia, hyperglycemia and peripheral leukocytosis, arrhythmias, cardiac troponin elevation, and ischemic electrocardiographic patterns. Rhabdomyolysis may result in acute renal failure, myoglobinuria, transaminitis, and disseminated intravascular coagulation. Systemic complications encountered in refractory SE include respiratory failure (about 30% of patients will require tracheostomy), gastrostomy tube placement, venous thrombosis, catheter-associated urinary tract infections, pseudomembranous colitis after repeated antibiotic exposures, sepsis, and infections with multidrug-resistant bacteria. Muscle atrophy and critical illness polyneuropathy can occur as well.

Treatment Complications: Benzodiazepines may suppress level of consciousness and respiratory drive.

Valproic acid can cause platelet dysfunction and hyperammonemia. Fosphenytoin/phenytoin may provoke cardiac arrhythmias and hypotension. Levetiracetam can cause sedation. Propofol is known to cause propofol infusion syndrome and hypotension. Barbiturates can cause prolonged sedation, hypotension, paralytic ileus, immunosuppression, propylene glycol toxicity, hepatic toxicity, pancreatic toxicity, and lingual edema.

Bibliography

Betjemann J, Lowenstein D. Status epilepticus in adults. *Lancet Neurol.* 2015;14(6):615–24.

Helmstaedter C. Cognitive outcome of status epilepticus in adults. *Epilepsia.* 2007;48(8):85–90.

Hocker S. Systemic complications of status epilepticus: an update. *Epilepsy Behav.* 2015;49:83–7.

Stiff Person Syndrome (Glycine Receptor Antibody Syndrome)

Epidemiology and Demographics: Age at presentation varies from 30 to 60 years, but is most frequently seen in patients in their 40s. No gender or race predilection is known. Incidence is 1 per million.

Disorder Description: This is an extremely rare neurologic condition that is characterized by progressive stiffness and rigidity. The stiffness affects primarily the truncal muscles and is accompanied by spasms that cause postural deformities. Initially, stiffness occurs in the thoracolumbar, paraspinal, and abdominal muscles. It later affects the proximal leg and abdominal wall muscles. The stiffness leads to a change in posture, and patients develop a rigid gait. Persistent lumbar hyperlordosis often occurs as it progresses. As the disease progresses, patients sometimes become unable to walk or bend. Patients have chronic pain, but stress, infections, and cold temperature can cause an acute worsening of the pain. The superimposed muscle spasms occur primarily in the proximal limb and axial musculature. The spasms are unpredictable and are extremely sensitive to noise and touch and emotional distress. In rare cases, facial muscles can also be affected. Patients have reported abnormal eye movements and vertigo. Late in the course of the disease, patients are also known to develop hypnogogic myoclonus. The unpredictable nature of the spasms causes

patients to develop psychiatric problems including depression, anxiety, and agoraphobia. Patients with this condition generally have high glutamic acid decarboxylase antibody titers, which are thought to be the cause of the disease.

This disease also occurs secondary to paraneoplastic disease. Paraneoplastic stiff person syndrome tends to affect the neck and arms more than other variations. It progresses very quickly, is more painful, and is more likely to include distal pain than primary stiff person syndrome.

Stiff limb syndrome is a variant of stiff person syndrome. In this condition, stiffness begins in one limb and remains most prominent there. Sphincter and brainstem issues often occur with stiff limb syndrome. Progressive encephalomyelitis with rigidity is another variant of this condition and leads to patients having brainstem and autonomic issues.

Finally, jerking man syndrome or jerking stiff person syndrome is another subtype of the condition. Symptoms begin like primary stiff person syndrome and progress over several years. Patients with this variant develop myoclonus as well as seizures and ataxia.

Potential causes include:

High glutamic acid decarboxylase antibody titers (classical form)

Amphiphysin antibody (paraneoplastic form)

Gephyrin antibody

Breast, ovarian, and/or lung cancer seen in paraneoplastic cause

Genetic: HLA DQB1* 0201 allele

History of type 1 diabetes

Risk factors include:

Presence of HLA DQB1*0201 allele

History of breast, ovarian, and/or lung cancer

Age in 40s

Symptoms

Localization site	Comment
Truncal muscles, abdominal muscles, lumbar muscles	Stiffness and increased tone, proximal arm and leg muscle spasm; slowed movement as quick movement brings on spasm. Patients may walk and sit with an exaggerated upright posture
	Axial musculature involvement is less marked in patients with diabetes
	Skeletal fractures and muscle ruptures may occur during spasms

Localization site	Comment
Brain, brainstem, and cerebellum	Autonomic disturbances, cranial nerve deficits, abnormal eye movements, myoclonus, increased startle response, disturbed sleep secondary to persistent myoclonic jerks; limbic system involvement may lead to spatial memory deficits, sexual arousal abnormalities
Spinal cord	Hyperreflexia
Psychiatric	Anxiety/depression, agoraphobia

Secondary Complications

Skeletal fractures
Depression and anxiety disorders such as agoraphobia
Chronic pain
Epilepsy
Thyroiditis

Treatment Complications

Intrathecal baclofen pump: Device complications are known to occur with the use of intrathecal baclofen pump. The catheter could leak, tear, kink, or become disconnected resulting in an underdose or sudden stop of intrathecal baclofen. An abrupt stop of intrathecal baclofen can lead to: high fever, changed mental status, muscle stiffness, loss of function of many vital organs, or death in rare cases. Pump failures can lead to overdose or underdose of intrathecal baclofen. The signs of an overdose include: drowsiness, lightheadedness, dizziness, difficulty breathing, seizures, loss of consciousness or coma, lower than normal body temperature.

Benzodiazepines: Used as muscle relaxants in this disease process.

Benzodiazepines are:

Habit forming, as such caution should be used in patients with a history of substance abuse. Benzodiazepines also have features of tolerance that may require patients to use higher doses to get the same effect.

Epileptogenic when discontinued abruptly after prolonged usage.

Likely to worsen depression in patients with history of substance abuse. Patients complain of emotional blunting or

inability to feel pleasure or pain with prolonged use of benzodiazepines.

Sedating: commonly cause lethargy.

Paradoxically stimulating, as such patients may complain of insomnia or hyperactivity with prolonged use of nonsteroidal anti-inflammatory drugs.

Intravenous immunoglobulin (IVIG): IVIG can induce reactions in patients with IgA deficiency. This occurs in 1/500–1000 patients. Serious anaphylactoid reactions occur soon after the administration of IVIG. Anaphylaxis associated with sensitization to IgA in patients with IgA deficiency can be prevented by using IgA-depleted immunoglobulin. The presence of IgG anti-IgA antibodies is not always associated with severe adverse reactions to IVIG. As IVIG can lead to thrombosis, it has also been known to cause stroke and acute myocardial infarction. Nephrotoxicity has also been linked to the use of IVIG. IVIG therapy can result in postinfusion hyperproteinemia, increased serum viscosity, and pseudohyponatremia. Aseptic meningitis is also a rare but well-recognized complication of IVIG therapy.

Plasmapheresis (for hyperviscosity syndrome): Hypocalcemia/hypomagnesemia before or after treatment; hypothermia during treatment; transfusion-related reactions are also likely; hypotension may occur in patients taking angiotensin-converting enzyme (ACE) inhibitors, in particular while undergoing column-based plasmapheresis. Thrombocytopenia and hypofibrinogenemia may occur after plasmapheresis (especially if albumin is being used as a replacement product), and patients should be monitored for signs of bleeding

Bibliography

Ciccotto G, Blaya M, Kelley R. Stiff person syndrome. *Neurol Clin.* 2013; 31(1):319–28.

Hadavi S, Noyce AJ, Leslie RD, Giovannoni G. Stiff person syndrome. *Pract Neurol.* 2011;11(5): 272–82.

St. Louis Encephalitis Virus

Epidemiology and Demographics: There are 1000–5000 cases of viral encephalitis per year, 100 of which are St. Louis encephalitis. Largest outbreak was in 1975, with 2800 cases in 31 US states. Mosquito-borne illness found in the United States, Canada, and parts of Central and South America.

Disorder Description: Mosquito-borne flavivirus. Birds are reservoirs for the virus. Eighty percent of infections are asymptomatic. Latency period of 4 to 21 days is followed by flu-like illness. Abrupt onset of mental status deterioration, low-grade headache, and fevers. Diagnosis through antibodies in CSF.

Symptoms

Localization site	Comment
Cerebral hemispheres	47% with seizures, focal or generalized
	Increased intracranial pressure due to cerebral edema
	Myoclonic jerks
Mental status and psychiatric aspects/complications	Confusion, delirium, lethargy
Brainstem	Infection – opsoclonus, nystagmus
Cerebellum	Infection – ataxia
Pituitary gland	Syndrome of inappropriate diuretic hormone (SIADH)

Secondary Complications: Complications include: intellectual disability; recovery over months; 2%–10% mortality, 5%–10% with permanent sequelae; hyponatremia due to SIADH; rarely acute disseminated encephalomyelitis (ADEM); aspiration pneumonia; deep vein thrombosis.

Treatment Complications: Treatment is symptomatic. One small open label trial showed benefit of interferon alfa-2b, but no randomized trials have been performed. Medical therapies for treatment of increased intracranial pressure are needed at times.

Bibliography

Aminoff MJ, Josephson SA, eds. *Aminoff's neurology and general medicine*. 5th ed. London, UK: Elsevier; 2014.

Biller J, Ferro JM, ed. *Neurologic aspects of systemic disease, Part III*. Handbook of Clinical Neurology, Vol 121 (3rd Series). San Diego: Elsevier; 2014.

Rahal JJ, Anderson J, Rosenberg C, Reagan T, Thompson LL. Effect of interferon-alpha2b

therapy on St. Louis viral meningoencephalitis: clinical and laboratory results of a pilot study. *J Infect Dis*. 2004;190(6):1084.

Stokes–Adams Attacks

Disorder Description: A sudden loss of consciousness occurring without regard to body position and without any premonitory warning, followed by flushing. This is usually caused by cardiac arrhythmias.

Symptoms

Localization site	Comment
Cerebral hemispheres	Brief generalized twitching can be caused by global anoxia
Brainstem	Loss of consciousness due to lack of blood flow to the reticular activating centers

Secondary Complications: This is traditionally associated with complete heart block or other ventricular arrhythmias.

Treatment Complications: Mortality is high without treatment.

Bibliography

Harbison J, Newton JL, Seifer C, Kenny RA. Stoke Adams attacks and cardiovascular syncope. *Lancet*. 2002;359(9301):158–60.

O'Rourke RA. Clinical cardiology: the Stoke-Adams syndrome definition and etiology: mechanisms and treatment. *Calif Med*. 1972;117(1):96–9.

Strabismus (Diplopia/Double Vision/Ocular Misalignment)

Epidemiology and Demographics: May affect patients at any age, and it is estimated that about 4% of the US population has strabismus.

Disorder Description: Strabismus refers to misalignment of the eyes so that corresponding images fall on noncorresponding parts of the left and right retinas. The reasons for this misalignment include neuromuscular control of eye movements, and mechanical and neurologic dysfunction.

Strabismus may result in diplopia; however, some patients may suppress one of the two images to avoid diplopia. Poor vision in one eye will also prevent diplopia. Congenital strabismus is most commonly an esotropia, where the eyes are crossed and one or both are facing the nose. It does not have associated neurologic manifestations.

Symptoms

Localization site	Comment
Cerebral hemispheres	High intracranial pressure can cause a sixth nerve palsy (see below) as a false localizing sign. Other symptoms include vision loss from papilledema, headache, and nausea
Brainstem	**Internuclear ophthalmoplegia** is due to dysfunction of the medial longitudinal fasciculus in the brainstem, most commonly due to demyelinating disease or stroke. These patients demonstrate poor adduction of the eye ipsilateral to the lesion, an abducting nystagmus in the contralateral eye and horizontal diplopia
	Skew deviation is a vertical ocular misalignment due to interruption of the vestibular tracts in the brainstem
	Parinaud syndrome (vertical gaze disturbance due to tectal plate compression)
	Mobius syndrome is a congenital disorder resulting from agenesis of the sixth and seventh cranial nerve nuclei. These patients have horizontal ophthalmoplegia and striking facial diplegia resulting in inability to smile
	Duane syndrome is a congenital horizontal ophthalmoplegia
	Raymond syndrome results from a lower medial pons lesion affecting the ipsilateral abducens nerve and undecussated corticobulbar and corticospinal fibers causing ipsilateral ocular abduction palsy and contralateral lower facial palsy and hemiparesis
	Weber syndrome results from a lesion in the ventral midbrain to the cerebral peduncle and the fascicle of the third nerve resulting in a third nerve palsy with contralateral hemiparesis
	Benedikt syndrome results from a lesion of the red nucleus and the fascicle of the third nerve resulting in third nerve palsy with contralateral ataxia and tremor
	Claude syndrome results from a lesion in the dorsal midbrain involving the fascicle of the third nerve and the superior cerebellar peduncle to result in third nerve palsy with contralateral ataxia
Base of skull	Aneurysm of the posterior communicating artery can cause an isolated compressive third nerve palsy (see below) and is a medical emergency

Localization site	Comment
	Processes affecting the cavernous sinuses can affect CN III, IV, and VI in addition to CN V to cause strabismus and facial numbness
Cranial nerves	Isolated injuries to the nerves that supply the extraocular muscles can occur from a wide variety of insults including microvascular ischemia, trauma, and meningeal processes such as tumors
	Oculomotor (CN III) palsy causes deficits in up, down, and inward movement in the eye, along with ptosis and sometimes impaired pupil constriction
	Abducens (CN VI) palsy causes a deficit in abduction (outward) movement of the affected eye to cause horizontal double vision
	Trochlear (CN IV) palsy causes a subtle deficit in downgaze of the affected eye resulting in vertical double vision
	Gradenigo syndrome results from chronic petrous bone inflammation from otitis media or mastoiditis that affects the trigeminal ganglion and abducens nerve that pass through it. It results in ipsilateral abducens (sixth nerve) palsy and facial pain
	Loss of vision in one or both eyes due to optic neuropathy can cause the eyes to drift apart (exotropia) due to loss of binocular sensory input to the brain
Pituitary gland	**Pituitary tumor** invasion of the cavernous sinus can cause any combination of CN III, IV, V1, V2, and VI dysfunction. There may be associated vision loss due to simultaneous compression of the optic nerves/chiasm
Muscle	**Graves' eye disease** classically causes a restrictive eye muscle myopathy. In addition, these patients may have proptosis and eyelid retraction
	Chronic progressive ophthalmoplegia and other mitochondrial myopathies cause slow, usually symmetric weakness of eye movements and eyelids. Rarely the weakness is not symmetric and strabismus develops
	Orbital trauma, surgery, and inflammation can limit movements of individual extraocular muscles either due to weakness or restriction
Neuromuscular junction	**Myasthenia gravis (MG)** is an autoimmune disease that causes variable and fatigable ptosis and strabismus. When generalized, MG may also cause bulbar symptoms and extremity weakness
Unclear localization	Vision loss → sensory strabismus

Secondary Complications: Amblyopia may develop in children under the age of 7 years with strabismus who suppress vision in one eye to mitigate diplopia. These patients should be treated without delay to prevent irreversible vision loss.

Treatment Complications: Treatment of myasthenia gravis or Graves' eye disease with steroids may result in steroid side effects including changes in mood and sleep disturbance.

Bibliography

Bever C, Aquino AV, Penn AS, et al. Prognosis of ocular myasthenia gravis. *Ann Neurol.* 1983;14:516–19.

Sudarshan A, Goldie WD. The spectrum of congenital facial diplegia (Moebius syndrome). *Pediatr Neurol.* 1985;1:180–4.

Thomke F. Brainstem diseases causing isolated ocular motor nerve palsies. *Neuroophthalmology.* 2002;28:53–67.

Zee DS. Internuclear ophthalmoplegia: pathophysiology and diagnosis. *Bailliere's Clin Neurol.* 1992;1:455–70.

Streptococcus Group B

Epidemiology and Demographics: Incidence of *Streptococcus* Group B infection is 4–8/100,000, but increases to 26/100,000 in patients over 65 years old.

Disorder Description: Gram-positive coccus colonizing the genitourinary and gastrointestinal tracts, which causes several types of infections:

1. Neonatal exposure: during vaginal delivery can cause meningitis, sepsis, pneumonia, and bacteremia.
2. Pregnant women: it is a cause of urinary tract infection, endometritis, and chorioamnionitis.
3. Non-pregnant adults: it is a cause of soft tissue and other focal infections, bacteremia, and sepsis.

Symptoms

Localization site	Comment
Cerebral hemispheres	Meningitis
	Seizures
	Infarction

Localization site	Comment
Mental status and psychiatric aspects/complications	Encephalopathy
Brainstem	Meningitis
Cerebellum	Meningitis
Cranial nerves	Meningitis

Secondary Complications: Can have devastating long-term consequences on the infant brain, including death, paralysis, microcephaly, cerebral palsy, intellectual disabilities, and epilepsy.

Treatment Complications: Prophylaxis is used for birth to prevent meningitis.

Bibliography

Phares CR, Lynfield R, Farley MM, et al. Active Bacterial Core Surveillance/Emerging Infections Program Network. Epidemiology of invasive group B streptococcal disease in the United States, 1999–2005. *JAMA.* 2008;299(17):2056.

Schrag SJ, Zywicki S, Farley MM, et al. Group B streptococcal disease in the era of intrapartum antibiotic prophylaxis. *N Engl J Med.* 2000;342(1):15.

Skoff TH, Farley MM, Petit S, et al. Increasing burden of invasive group B streptococcal disease in nonpregnant adults, 1990–2007. *Clin Infect Dis.* 2009;49:85.

Streptococcus Microaerophilic (e.g., *Streptococcus viridans*)

Epidemiology and Demographics: Common normal oral flora in humans.

Disorder Description: Gram-positive bacteria, which can seed into the bloodstream and lead to infective endocarditis (IE). This can happen with dental procedures that involve gingiva and apical teeth (includes teeth cleaning). Prophylaxis is recommended for high-risk groups including patients with: prosthetic heart valves, history of IE, abnormal heart structure in most cases, and abnormal valves in a transplanted heart.

Symptoms

Localization site	Comment
Cerebral hemispheres	Embolic stroke
	Mycotic aneurysm
Mental status and psychiatric aspects/complications	Encephalopathy, delirium, coma
Brainstem	Embolic stroke
Cerebellum	Embolic stroke
Spinal cord	Embolic stoke

Secondary Complications: Bacteremia, other embolism, and other aneurysms.

Treatment Complications: Most strains are sensitive to penicillin, making treatment shorter. Gentamycin, frequently used to cover other organisms, can cause ototoxicity and nephrotoxicity.

Bibliography

Nishimura RA, Otto CM, Bonow RO, et al. 2014 AHA/ACC guideline for the management of patients with valvular heart disease: a report of the American College of Cardiology/American Heart Association Task Force on Practice Guidelines. *J Am Coll Cardiol.* 2014;63(22):e57.

No authors listed. Antibacterial prophylaxis for dental, GI, and GU procedures. *Med Lett Drugs Ther.* 2005;47(1213):59.

Wilson W, Taubert KA, Gewitz M, et al., American Heart Association Rheumatic Fever, Endocarditis, and Kawasaki Disease Committee, American Heart Association Council on Cardiovascular Disease in the Young, American Heart Association Council on Clinical Cardiology, American Heart Association Council on Cardiovascular Surgery and Anesthesia, Quality of Care and Outcomes Research Interdisciplinary Working Group. Prevention of infective endocarditis: guidelines from the American Heart Association: a guideline from the American Heart Association Rheumatic Fever, Endocarditis, and Kawasaki Disease Committee, Council on Cardiovascular Disease in the Young, and the Council on Clinical Cardiology, Council on Cardiovascular Surgery and Anesthesia, and the Quality of Care and Outcomes Research

Interdisciplinary Working Group. *Circulation.* 2007;116(15):1736.

Streptococcus pneumoniae

Epidemiology and Demographics: May infect ages 1 month and older. Incidence in 2–49 age group is much lower than <2 years old and >50 years old. Meningitis represents 6.6% of these infections.

Disorder Description: Common cause of community-acquired meningitis. Immunosuppression (AIDS/transplant) and relative immunosuppression (influenza infection, alcohol abuse, smoking, chronic obstructive pulmonary disease and asthma, multiple myeloma, lupus, pregnancy) are risk factors. Nasopharyngeal colonization or resistant organisms, which is common with long-term administration of antibiotics. Can also cause pneumonia and bacteremia.

Symptoms

Localization site	Comment
Cerebral hemispheres	Meningitis
	Seizure
	Stroke
Mental status and psychiatric aspects/complications	Encephalopathy, stupor, coma
Brainstem	Meningitis
Cerebellum	Meningitis
Cranial nerves	Meningitis

Secondary Complications: Myocardial infarction, cardiac arrhythmia, new or worsening heart failure, and stroke. Pleural effusion, empyema, and pulmonary embolism.

Treatment Complications: Antibiotic resistance to penicillin has made broader spectrum antibiotics necessary in many cases.

Vaccination is recommended for at-risk individuals. The Centers for Disease Control and Prevention (CDC) recommends pneumococcal conjugate vaccine for all babies and children younger than 2 years, all adults >65 years, and people aged 2–64 years with certain medical conditions. Pneumococcal polysaccharide vaccine is recommended for all adults

>65 years, people aged 2–64 years who are at increased risk for disease due to certain medical conditions, and adults aged 19–64 years who smoke cigarettes.

Bibliography

Centers for Disease Control and Prevention (CDC). Active Bacterial Core Surveillance (ABCs) report. Emerging Infections Program Network Streptococcus pneumoniae; 2014. www.cdc.gov/abcs/reports-findings/pubs-strep-pneumo.html. Accessed Jan 29, 2017.

Centers for Disease Control and Prevention (CDC). Vaccines and preventable diseases. Updated Nov 22, 2016. www.cdc.gov/vaccines/vpd/index.html. Accessed Jan 29, 2017.

Thigpen MC, Whitney CG, Messonnier NE, et al. Emerging Infections Programs Network. Bacterial meningitis in the United States, 1998–2007. *N Engl J Med*. 2011;364(21):2016.

Stress

(See entries for *Acute Stress Disorder* and *Posttraumatic Stress Disorder*)

Description: Stress has been defined as the result of conditions in the individual's environment that the person appraises as significantly more taxing than available coping resources. A person will be psychologically vulnerable to a particular situation if he or she does not possess sufficient coping resources to handle it adequately and places considerable importance on the threat implicit in the consequences of this inadequate handling. "Stress" *per se* is not a disorder; however, excessive stress can have psychologic repercussions ranging from exhaustion and burnout to posttraumatic stress disorder, depending on the context and extent. Burnout may be observed as a progressively developed condition resulting from the use of ineffective coping strategies with which professionals try to protect themselves from work-related stress situations. There are three main components of burnout – exhaustion, cynicism, and inefficiency. Exhaustion is the feeling of not being able to offer any more of oneself at work; cynicism represents a distant attitude towards work, those served by it, and colleagues; inefficacy is the feeling of not performing tasks adequately.

Excessive stress can lead to a number of physical ailments including hypertension, hyperlipidemia (and resulting cardiovascular disease), diabetes, irritable bowel syndrome, asthma, pain, depression, and anxiety.

Management: Coping is defined as cognitive and behavioral efforts to manage specific internal and/or external demands that are appraised exceeding the person's resources. There are different ways people cope with stress, such as cognitive or behavioral coping, cognitive or behavioral avoidance, emotion-focused coping, or even substance use. Acceptance and Commitment Therapy (ACT) and Mindfulness based therapies have been shown to be helpful in the management of excessive stress. Psychopharmacologic interventions are not recommended for the management of general stress, exhaustion, or burnout in the absence of other diagnosable psychiatric conditions.

Bibliography

Lazarus R. From psychological stress to the emotions: a history of changing outlooks. *Annu Rev Psychol*. 1993;44:1–21.

Montero-Marin J, Prado-Abril J, Piva Demarzo MM, Gascon S, García-Campayo J. Coping with stress and types of burnout: explanatory power of different coping strategies. *PLoS One*. 2014;9(2):e89090.

Montero-Marín J, García-Campayo J, Mosquera D, López Y. A new definition of burnout syndrome based on Farbers's proposal. *J Occup Med Toxicol*. 2009;4:31.

Sapolsky RM. Stress, glucocorticoids, and damage to the nervous system: the current state of confusion. *Stress*. 1996;1(1):1–19.

Selye H. *The stress of life*. London: Longmans Green and Co; 1957.

Stroke (Ischemic or Hemorrhagic)

Epidemiology and Demographics: Stroke is the second leading cause of death worldwide. In the United States it is the 5th leading cause of death. 2014 statistics, for example, revealed an incidence of 37.6 deaths per 100,000 people. In 2014, 795,000 strokes occurred in the United States. The prevalence was 2.4% in males and 2.9% in females. By race: non-Hispanic white males, 2.2%; non-Hispanic white females, 2.8%; non-Hispanic black males, 3.9%; non-Hispanic black females, 4.0%; Hispanic males, 2.0%; Hispanic females, 2.6%; Asian males, 2.0%; Asian females, 2.5%. By age: males age 20–39, 0.3%; females age 20–39, 0.6%; males age 40–59, 1.6%; females age 40–59, 2.4%; males age 60–79, 6.5%; females age 60–79, 6.1%; males age 80 or over, 13.8%; females age 80 or over, 14.9%. As is evident above, strokes increase with increasing age, are slightly more common in females overall, and are most common in non-Hispanic blacks.

Disorder Description: The term stroke in this context refers to any abnormality involving cerebral tissue and blood, and includes ischemic stroke (87%), intracerebral hemorrhage (10%), and subarachnoid hemorrhage (3%). The symptoms of ischemic stroke and intracerebral hemorrhage are similar and depend on the location of the event. They can only be distinguished by head CT or MRI. Subarachnoid hemorrhages present with a severe headache and have a dedicated entry.

Symptoms: See specific stroke types.

Bibliography

Benjamin EJ, Blaha MJ, Chiuve SE, et al.; on behalf of the American Heart Association Statistics Committee and Stroke Statistics Subcommittee. Heart Disease and Stroke Statistics – 2017 Update: A Report from the American Heart Association. *Circulation.* 2017;135:e146–e603.

Strongyloidiasis

Epidemiology and Demographics: There is no sex predominance and it can afflict all ages. It is endemic worldwide with a worldwide prevalence of approximately 100 million people. It occurs mostly in hot and humid (tropical and subtropical) climates, such as in Latin America and sub-Saharan Africa, although it has also occurred in rural, resource-poor areas of the southeastern United States, Appalachia, and some sections of southern Europe.

Disorder Description: Strongyloidiasis is a parasitic disease caused by the soil-transmitted threadworm *Strongyloides stercoralis*. Larvae are introduced into hosts via exposure to contaminated soil (usually by feces), and directly penetrate intact skin. They then spread hematogenously to the lungs, eventually spreading to the trachea/pharynx, and ultimately resulting in swallowing the larvae, which reach adulthood in the small intestine. This then heralds further transmission and auto-infection (which can result in long-lasting chronic infection).

Those particularly at risk are immunosuppressed or immunocompromised patients, especially those with defective cell-mediated immunity, which increases risk of severe disseminated disease or hyperinfection with multi-organ involvement.

Diagnostic testing consists of stool analysis for larvae.

Symptoms

Localization site	Comment
Cerebral hemispheres	Suppurative meningitis
Mental status and psychiatric aspects/complications	Encephalopathy, ultimately meningitis, and coma
Outside of CNS	Gastrointestinal symptoms (nausea, vomiting, diarrhea), fever, headache, respiratory symptoms (cough, dyspnea, hemoptysis)

Secondary Complications: Secondary complications are often a result of severe infection and migration of larvae systemically into multiple organs. In addition, hematogenous spread and invasion can facilitate polymicrobial infections. Auto-infection results in severe disseminated disease or hyperinfection with multi-organ involvement, which can be potentially fatal.

Treatment Complications: Typical treatment is with anti-helminthic agents, with ivermectin being the treatment of choice, and albendazole being an acceptable alternative but with comparatively lower efficacy. Adverse effects are typically low severity: pruritus, arthralgia, fever, lymphadenitis. Complications of treatment with anti-helminthic agents include rare systemic side effects (edema, tachycardia, gastrointestinal symptoms, liver function test elevations).

Bibliography

Puthiyakunnon S, Boddu S, Li Y, et al. Strongyloidiasis: an insight into its global prevalence and management. *PLoS Negl Trop Dis.* 2014;8(8):e3018. DOI:10.1371/journal.pntd.0003018.

Salvana EMT, Salata RA, King CH. Parasitic infections of the central nervous system. In Aminoff MJ, Josephson SA, eds. *Aminoff's neurology and general medicine.* 5th ed. London: Academic Press; 2014. pp. 947–68.

Schär F, Trostdorf U, Giardina F, et al. Strongyloides stercoralis: global distribution and risk factors. *PLoS Negl Trop Dis.* 2013;7(>7):e2288.

Sturge–Weber Syndrome (Encephalotrigeminal Angiomatosis)

Epidemiology and Demographics: Port wine stains have a frequency of 1/300 live births but Sturge–Weber syndrome is only seen in about 1/50,000. There is no gender preference.

Disorder Description: Disorder of capillary formation involving a port wine stain in the first division of the trigeminal nerve associated with ipsilateral leptomeningeal angiomata in the cerebral cortex and eye, sometimes associated with glaucoma. The cortex underlying the angioma has abnormal intracerebral blood vessels leading to atrophy and cortical dysplasia. As children, patients tend to have a steadily deteriorating course. Symptoms usually stabilize but strokes as adults can lead to late stepwise deterioration.

Symptoms

Localization site	Comment
Cerebral hemispheres	Epilepsy. Migraine-like headache. Stroke-like symptoms, most commonly hemiparesis, hemianopia
Mental status and psychiatric aspects/complications	Developmental delay and cognitive loss
Cranial nerves	Ocular angioma may be associated with glaucoma and vision loss

Secondary Complications: Patients may also have thyroid abnormalities, ENT infections, and obstructive sleep apnea.

Treatment Complications: Seizures may be difficult to control and hemispherectomy may be required. Aspirin is often recommended to maintain blood flow in the abnormal cortical vessels and may lead to bleeding complications.

Bibliography

Comi A. Current therapeutic options in Sturge-Weber syndrome. *Semin Pediatr Neurol.* 2015;22(4):295–301.

Sudarsanam A, Ardorn-Holmes SL. Sturge-Weber syndrome: from the past to the present. *Eur J Paediatr Neurol.* 2014;18(3):257–66.

Subarachnoid Hemorrhage (Nontraumatic)

See also entry for *Aneurysm – Cerebral.*

Epidemiology and Demographics: Incidence ranges from 1 to 16 per 100,000 people worldwide. Incidence is highest in Europe and lowest in Asia, Central America, and South America. In the United States the incidence is 9.7 per 100,000 people. There is a 1.24:1 female-to-male ratio. It is more common in African-Americans and Hispanics than in Caucasians.

Disorder Description: Refers to a sudden release of blood into the space between the arachnoid mater and pia mater. It is associated with aneurysmal rupture approximately 80% of the time. Arteriovenous malformation rupture accounts for about 10% of cases. Other causes include perimesencephalic hemorrhage, mycotic aneurysm, and anticoagulant use (and other bleeding diatheses).

Symptoms

Localization site	Comment
Cerebral hemispheres	Vasospasm can lead to stroke in any territory but most commonly the middle cerebral artery or anterior cerebral artery ipsilateral to the hemorrhage. Symptoms may include aphasia, hemiplegia, hemisensory deficits, and hemianopia. See specific arterial entries for additional details
Mental status and psychiatric aspects/ complications	Long-term effects often include cognitive loss, depression and other mood disorders, and chronic fatigue
Brainstem	Loss of consciousness, bulbar signs, hydrocephalus
Cerebellum	Ataxia, vertigo
Vestibular system	Vertigo, tinnitus, hearing loss
Cranial nerves	Diplopia, pupillary abnormalities, facial palsy, dysarthria, dysphagia
Unclear localization	Severe headache, nausea, emesis, photophobia, neck stiffness, loss of consciousness

Secondary Complications: Issues with cardiac rhythm and cerebral salt wasting/hyponatremia.

Treatment Complications: Vasospasm, stroke, death.

Bibliography

Connolly ES, Rabinstein AA, Carhuapoma JR, et al.; on behalf of the American Heart Association Stroke Council, Council on Cardiovascular Radiology and Intervention, Council on Cardiovascular Nursing, Council on Cardiovascular Surgery and Anesthesia, and Council on Clinical Cardiology. Guidelines for the Management of Aneurysmal Subarachnoid Hemorrhage. A Guideline for Healthcare Professionals from the American Heart Association/American Stroke Association. *Stroke.* 2012;43(6):1711–37.

Subclavian Steal Syndrome

Epidemiology and Demographics: Prevalence is approximately 3–4% but is significantly higher in patients with known peripheral arterial disease.

Disorder Description: High-grade stenosis of the subclavian artery can lead to hypoperfusion of the arm via the axillary artery, the posterior fossa via the vertebral artery, and the heart via the internal mammary artery (only in patients who have had coronary bypass surgery using an internal mammary artery [IMA] graft). The brainstem is normally protected by blood flow from the contralateral vertebral artery through the basilar artery. In severe cases and with exertion of the arm, there may be reversed flow through the vertebral artery leading to brainstem ischemia.

Symptoms

Localization site	Comment
Cerebral hemispheres	Hemianopia
Brainstem	Ataxia, dysarthria, lightheadedness, vertigo
Cerebellum	Cerebellar ataxia
Vestibular system	Vertigo

Secondary Complications: Symptoms involving the affected arm include pain, claudication, ulcers, decreased pulse and blood pressure. In patients with coronary bypass using IMA, there can be diversion of blood from the heart to the arm leading to angina pectoris.

Treatment Complications: Antiplatelet agents may lead to bleeding or peptic ulcer disease. Surgical correction could lead to arterial dissection.

Bibliography

Ochoa VM, Yeghiazarians Y. Subclavian artery stenosis: a review for the vascular medicine practitioner. *Vasc Med.* 2011;16(1):29–34.

Osiro S, Zurada A, Gielecki J, et al. A review of subclavian steal syndrome with clinical correlation. *Med Sci Monit.* 2012;18(5):RA57–63.

Potter BJ, Pinto D. Subclavian steal syndrome. *Circulation.* 2014;129:2320–3.

Subdural Hematoma, Acute Cerebral

Epidemiology and Demographics: Can occur in up to 20% of traumatic brain injuries. Incidence increases with age. Often seen in conjunction with other tissue injury such as skull fracture or contusion. Such concomitant injuries significantly increase mortality.

Disorder Description: A subdural hematoma is a collection of blood between the inner layer of the dura mater and the intact arachnoid mater. Subdural hematomas are usually traumatic with injury to the bridging veins between the cortex and the skull, but can be spontaneous. Acute hemorrhages come from more significant injuries with rapid accumulation of blood and frequently represent a neurosurgical emergency.

Symptoms

Localization site	Comment
Cerebral hemispheres	The initial symptom is worsening headache. Focal symptoms develop from compression of the underlying cortex and may include hemiplegia, hemisensory loss, hemianopia, and aphasia. Seizures are common
Mental status and psychiatric aspects/ complications	The increased cerebral pressure may lead to altered mental status
Brainstem	Bulbar symptoms, dysarthria. In severe cases herniation could lead to pupillary abnormalities, decerebrate/decortical posturing, and coma
Cerebellum	Ataxia
Vestibular system	Vertigo

Secondary Complications: Monitor for the combination of bradycardia and hypertension as this is Cushing's reflex, an early sign of increased intracranial pressure that would mandate surgical intervention.

Treatment Complications: Patients on anticoagulation will need to have the medication reversed and are at risk of thrombosis. Surgical decompression is often required.

Bibliography

Coombs JB, Coombs BL, Chin EJ. Acute spontaneous subdural hematoma in a middle-aged adult: case report and review of the literature. *J Emerg Med.* 2014;47(3):e63–8.

Miller JD, Nader R. Acute subdural hematoma from bridging vein rupture: a potential mechanism for growth. *J Neurosurg.* 2014;120(6):1378–84.

Subdural Hematoma, Chronic Cerebral

Epidemiology and Demographics: Estimates range from 1 to 13 per 100,000 population but incidence is far higher over age 50 years and especially over age 65. There is no gender predilection.

Disorder Description: A subdural hematoma is a collection of blood between the inner layer of the dura mater and the intact arachnoid mater. Subdural hematomas are usually traumatic with injury to the bridging veins between the cortex and the skull, but can be spontaneous. Chronic subdural hematomas appear several weeks after an injury (injuries so mild that they are often not remembered) with symptoms developing slowly over time, in a manner similar to those of a tumor. They occur in the setting of cerebral atrophy, either due to age or alcoholism. This is because the atrophy brings the bridging veins further away from the skull placing them under tension and allowing for easier breakage with lesser trauma.

Symptoms

Localization site	Comment
Cerebral hemispheres	Symptoms develop from compression of the underlying cortex and may include hemiplegia, hemisensory loss, hemianopia, and aphasia. Seizures are common

Localization site	Comment
Mental status and psychiatric aspects/ complications	The increased cerebral pressure may lead to altered mental status
Brainstem	Bulbar symptoms, dysarthria. In severe cases herniation could lead to pupillary abnormalities or coma
Cerebellum	Ataxia
Vestibular system	Vertigo

Secondary Complications: Monitor for the combination of bradycardia and hypertension as this is Cushing's reflex, an early sign of increased intracranial pressure that would mandate surgical intervention.

Treatment Complications: Patients on anticoagulation will need to have the medication held and are at risk of thrombosis. In the absence of severe deficits or herniation, many of these hematomas will resolve without surgery.

Bibliography

Almenawer SA, Farrokhyar F, Hong C, et al. Chronic subdural hematoma management: a systematic review and meta-analysis of 34,829 patients. *Ann Surg.* 2014;259(3):449–57.

Subdural Hematoma, Spinal

Epidemiology and Demographics: May be spontaneous, traumatic, or iatrogenic. All types are extremely rare with only several hundred spontaneous cases and under 20 traumatic cases reported. Spontaneous spinal subdural hematomas have a slight female predominance and can occur at any age, with a mean age of around 60 years.

Disorder Description: A collection of blood between the dura and arachnoid mater of the spinal cord. It can follow trauma or any spinal procedure including surgery, lumbar puncture, and epidural/spinal injections.

Symptoms

Localization site	Comment
Spinal cord	Monoplegia, monoparesis, paraplegia, paraparesis, urinary incontinence, fecal incontinence, back pain, sensory loss below the level of the lesion, spinal shock
Anterior horn cells	Weakness in a myotomal distribution
Dorsal root ganglia	Radiculopathic pain and/or sensory loss in a dermatomal distribution
Conus medullaris	Bilateral leg weakness, urinary incontinence, fecal incontinence
Cauda equina	Cauda equina syndrome
Specific spinal roots	Any root may be affected but the spontaneous form of the disorder is most common in thoracic spine

Secondary Complications: All forms are most common in patients on anticoagulation or with a bleeding diathesis. Spontaneous cases may be seen in association with spinal masses. In traumatic and iatrogenic cases, spinal epidural hematoma coexists.

Treatment Complications: In most cases, this is a surgical emergency.

Bibliography

de Beer MH, Eysink Smeets MM, Koppen H. Spontaneous spinal subdural hematoma. *Neurologist.* 2017;22(1):34–9.

Gordon WE, Kimball BY, Arthur AS. Traumatic lumbar spinal subdural hematoma. *Interdiscip Neurosurg.* 2014;4(1):123–7.

Kim H-J, Cho Y-J, Cho J-Y, Lee D-H, Hong K-S. Acute subdural hematoma following spinal cerebrospinal fluid drainage in a patient with freezing of gait. *J Clin Neurol.* 2009;5(2): 95–6.

Maddali P, Walker B, Fisahn C, et al. Subdural thoracolumbar spine hematoma after spinal anesthesia: a rare occurrence and literature review of spinal hematomas after spinal anesthesia. *Cureus.* 2017;9(2):e1032.

SUNCT/SUNA – Short-Lasting Unilateral Neuralgiform Headache Attacks with Conjunctival Injection and Tearing/Cranial Autonomic Symptoms

Epidemiology and Demographics: Occurs in approximately 10% of African Americans, and in 300 million people throughout the world. Affects males and females equally.

Disorder Description: These types of headaches are characterized by very short-lasting attacks of one-sided severe head pain always associated with cranial autonomic features and triggered by cutaneous stimuli. The International Headache Society describes this condition as having unilateral orbital, supraorbital, or temporal pain. Review of literature suggests that the pain can arise from anywhere in the head. There are two variants on presentation: single stabs, where episodes are short-lived; saw-tooth phenomenon, where attacks are longer and the pain does not fully resolve. When conjunctival injection and tearing are not present, the condition is called SUNA (short-lasting unilateral neuralgiform headache attacks with cranial autonomic symptoms). For the most part, SUNCT (short-lasting unilateral neuralgiform headache attacks with conjunctival injection and tearing) and SUNA are similar conditions on a spectrum.

Symptoms

Localization site	Comment
Cranial nerves	Likely involves trigeminal nerve
Pituitary gland	Some reports suggest a role of pituitary pathology as exhibiting SUNA and SUNCT headaches

Treatment Complications: Previously, SUNA and SUNCT were thought to be untreatable and patients had to endure recurrent attacks. Now, there are at least three medications reported in the literature that have been shown to reduce attack frequency. There are no established treatment guidelines for SUNA and SUNCT. Some reports suggest use of lamotrigine, topiramate, and gabapentin as reducing frequency of attacks. However, given its rarity, there are not enough patients who have been studied and treated to fully understand treatment complications associated with this condition.

Bibliography

Cohen AS, Matharu MS, Goadsby PJ. Suggested guidelines for treating SUNCT and SUNA. *Cephalalgia.* 2005;25:1200.

Cohen AS, Matharu MS, Goadsby PJ. Short-lasting unilateral neuralgiform headache attacks with conjunctival injection and tearing (SUNCT) or cranial autonomic features (SUNA) – a prospective clinical study of SUNCT and SUNA. *Brain.* 2006;129(Pt 10):2746–60.

Goadsby PJ, Cittadini E, Cohen AS. Trigeminal autonomic cephalalgias: paroxysmal hemicrania, SUNCT/SUNA, and hemicrania continua. *Semin Neurol.* 2010;30:186–91.

Sjaastad O. Chronic paroxysmal hemicrania, hemicrania continua and SUNCT: the fate of the three first described cases. *J Headache Pain.* 2006;7(3):151–6.

Superficial Siderosis

Epidemiology and Demographics: Approximately 0.5% of patients over age 65 years. The male-to-female ratio is 3:1.

Disorder Description: A chronic disorder associated with deposition of blood products over the cerebral convexity. The blood is broken down and heme products are free to flow within the CSF. These toxic products cause neuronal damage and demyelination. This is not a specific disease but rather is a syndrome identified by imaging findings and symptoms. It has numerous causes, the most significant one in the elderly being cerebral amyloid angiopathy and in younger people is reversible cerebral vasoconstrictive syndrome. It can also be the consequence of repeated subarachnoid hemorrhages of any cause, e.g., multiple aneurysm ruptures, repeated minor trauma, vasculitis (primary or due to sympathomimetic agents), arteriovenous malformations, dural tumors, etc.

Symptoms

Localization site	Comment
Cerebral hemispheres	Pyramidal weakness, anosmia, sensory loss
Mental status and psychiatric aspects/complications	Dementia

Localization site	Comment
Brainstem	Urinary incontinence
Cerebellum	Ataxia
Vestibular system	Ataxia
Cranial nerves	Sensorineural hearing loss, extraocular palsies
Spinal cord	Myelopathy
Anterior horn cells	Lower motor neuron symptoms (rare)
Specific spinal roots	Sciatica type pain

Secondary Complications: While most cases are spontaneous, it can be seen with hypertension.

Treatment Complications: If a bleeding source is found, it should be corrected surgically with the attendant risks of surgery.

Bibliography

Charidimou A, Linn J, Vernooij MW, et al. Cortical superficial siderosis: detection and clinical significance in cerebral amyloid angiopathy and related conditions. *Brain.* 2015;138(Pt 8): 2126–39.

Fearnley JM, Stevems JM, Rudge P. Superficial siderosis of the central nervous system. *Brain.* 1995;118(Pt 4):1051–66.

Superior Semicircular Canal Dehiscence (SCD)

Epidemiology and Demographics: Superior semicircular canal dehiscence (SCD) is an idiopathic condition affecting the inner ear. It most often occurs in middle-aged individuals, without a female or male predominance. The incidence of symptomatic SCD is unknown but cadaveric studies have found evidence of dehiscent bone over the superior canal in approximately 0.5% of temporal bones.

Disorder Description: Patients with SCD have vertigo and/or oscillopsia, evoked by intense sounds or stimuli that cause changes in middle ear intracranial pressure, such as Valsalva against pinched nostrils, tragal compression, or jugular venous compression.

Some patients with SCD may be asymptomatic and are only diagnosed incidentally after undergoing imaging of the head, while some may suffer from disabling disequilibrium and unsteadiness. The signs of SCD are vertical-torsional nystagmus (in the plane of the superior canal) and vertigo with exposure to loud sounds or maneuvers that change middle ear or intracranial pressure (i.e., Valsalva and pneumatic otoscopy). Patients may also suffer from autophony and may demonstrate a low-frequency conductive hearing loss with bone conduction thresholds less than 0 db. Dehiscence of bone overlying the superior semicircular canal on the affected side is found on computed tomography. Vestibular evoked myogenic potentials occur at a decreased threshold; this is the confirmatory pathophysiologic test.

Symptoms

Localization site	Comment
Inner ear	Dehiscence of bone resulting in a third window phenomenon with vestibular symptoms +/− hearing loss and tinnitus
Cranial nerves	Cochleovestibular nerve is not affected
Central nervous system	Central nervous system is not affected

Secondary Complications: Sudden onset of vertigo in these patients may result in increased risk for injuries or falls. Tinnitus secondary to pulsations of overlying dura may occur. Together with autophony these aural symptoms may cause significant distress to the patient.

Treatment Complications: Treatment of SCD involves a surgical middle cranial fossa approach to plug or resurface the superior canal. A transmastoid approach has also been described.

The craniotomy required for the management of SCD carries significant risks including intracranial hemorrhage, cerebrospinal fluid leak, cerebral edema, and postoperative seizures. Occlusion of the semicircular canal by any route can lead to sensorineural hearing loss and vertigo.

Bibliography

Belden CJ, Weg N, Minor LB, Zinreich SJ. CT evaluation of bone dehiscence of the superior semicircular canal as a cause of sound- and/or pressure-induced vertigo. *Radiology*. 2003;226:337–43.

Beyea JA, Agrawal SK, Parnes LS. Transmastoid semicircular canal occlusion: a safe and highly effective treatment for benign paroxysmal positional vertigo and superior canal dehiscence. *Laryngoscope*. 2012;122:1862–6.

Merchant SN, Rosowski JJ. Conductive hearing loss caused by third-window lesions of the inner ear. *Otol Neurotol*. 2008;29:282–9.

Minor LB. Superior canal dehiscence syndrome. *Am J Otol*. 2000;21:9–19.

Welgampola MS. Evoked potential testing in neuro-otology. *Curr Opin Neurol*. 2008;21:29–35.

Surgical Positioning Neuropathy (Perioperative Peripheral Nerve Injury)

Epidemiology and Demographics: Ihab et al. summarize the predominance of middle-aged men with the condition. Ulnar nerve injuries were the most common, followed by brachial plexopathy, then median neuropathy, and finally, radial neuropathy. In the lower extremities, the peroneal nerve may be compressed, especially in gynecologic procedures.

Disorder Description: Mechanisms of injury include irritation, injury, and infarct of the nerve. The risk factors include changes in body temperature, any electrolyte disturbance, decrease in the supply of oxygen, drop in blood pressure, inadequate hydration, loss of blood, older patient, anesthetic medication used during surgery, diabetes, high blood pressure.

Symptoms

Localization site	Comment
Plexus	Brachial plexopathy
Peripheral neuropathy	Ulnar, median, radial, peroneal neuropathy

Secondary Complications: Motor weakness and subsequent restriction of movement may lead to muscular atrophy. In addition, worsening of the sensory symptoms in the distribution of the nerve may occur.

Bibliography

Gray JE. Nerve injury associated with pelvic surgery. UpToDate. Updated Apr 21, 2017. www .uptodate.com/contents/nerve-injury-associated-with-pelvic-surgery. Accessed Sep 20, 2018.

Ihab K, Rodger B. Positioning patients for spine surgery: avoiding uncommon position-related complications. *World J Orthop*. 2014;5(4):425–43. Published online Sep 18, 2014. DOI: 10.5312/wjo. v5.i4.425.

Susac Syndrome

Epidemiology and Demographics: This is a very rare disorder. Only several hundred cases have been reported and while the true incidence is unknown, the number of reported cases is rising. Many cases are likely being missed due to confusion with diseases such as multiple sclerosis (MS). The female-to-male ratio is 2–3 to 1. It most commonly presents between the ages of 20 and 40 years but can occur at any age.

Disorder Description: A microangiopathy due to immune-mediated endothelial damage limited to the small blood vessels of the cortex, retina, and inner ear. The cause is unknown. This is not a systemic disorder but can be mistaken for other autoimmune disorders affecting the CNS, such as MS and acute disseminated encephalomyelitis.

Symptoms

Localization site	Comment
Cerebral hemispheres	Encephalopathy (behavioral disturbance, memory loss, lethargy, seizures). Migrainous headaches
Mental status and psychiatric aspects/complications	Encephalopathy
Cranial nerves	Vision loss; scintillating scotoma, black spots, photopia. Sensorineural hearing loss

Treatment Complications: Treatment by immune suppression may lead to infections.

Bibliography

Nazari F, Azimi A, Abdi S. What is Susac syndrome? A brief review of articles. *Iran J Neurol*. 2014;13(4):209–14.

Susac JO, Egan RA, Rennebohm RM, Lubow M. Susac's syndrome: 1975–2005 microangiopathy/ autoimmune endotheliopathy. *J Neurol Sci*. 2007;257(1-2):270–2.

Sydenham Chorea (SC)

Epidemiology and Demographics: Sydenham chorea (SC) affects one-third of children who develop an infection with group A beta hemolytic streptococcus, leading to acute rheumatic fever (ARF). Typical age of onset is between 5 and 14 years. Found mainly in females, it generally occurs in the absence of other physical manifestations of ARF, such as arthritis, skin rash, or nodules, typically 1–8 months after an acute episode of ARF. SC can return with a recurrence of ARF; therefore it may be seen in adolescents and young adults. It usually resolves within 6 weeks of onset but sometimes takes up to 6 months.[1]

Disorder Description: SC is an autoantibody-mediated movement disorder that occurs after a prolonged latent period following group A (beta hemolytic) streptococcal infection causing ARF. Carditis is often present in patients with SC, which is probably indicative of a more severe case, and may contribute as a risk factor for a longer lasting duration of choreic symptoms.[2] Antibodies to group A streptococci have affinity for proteins in the neuronal cells causing the chorea.[3] The involvement in SC appears to be selectively in the putamen, caudate nucleus, and globus pallidus.[4]

Symptoms

Localization site	Comment
Basal ganglia	Involuntary motor symptoms such as ballismus, facial grimacing, and hemichorea can occur[5]
Ocular	Central retinal artery occlusion, hypometric saccades, papilledema[5]
Mental status and psychiatric aspects/ complications	Obsessive-compulsive symptoms, increased emotional lability (pseudobulbar affect), motor hyperactivity, irritability, distractibility, age-regressed behavior. Rarely, transient psychosis and learning disabilities[5]
Muscle	Motor impersistence is seen with chorea (milkmaid's grip)

PANDAS (Pediatric Autoimmune Neuro-psychiatric Disorders Associated with Streptococcal infections) closely mimics SC. Investigators noted acute onset of neuro-psychiatric symptoms, particularly obsessive-compulsive disordered (OCD) behavior in patients who had recently suffered a group B streptococcal infection; and in some cases these patients proceeded to develop involuntary movements. There are five essential diagnostic criteria of PANDAS, which include presence of OCD and/or tics, pre-pubertal onset, abrupt onset or episodic course, association with group A streptococcal infection, and neuropsychiatric abnormalities.[6]

Secondary Complications: Seizures, pseudotumor cerebri, and migraine headaches have been recognized as secondary complications to SC.

Treatment Complications: Assorted effects of treatments for secondary complications are possible.

References

1. Marques-Dias MJ, Mercadante MT, Tucker D, Lombroso P. Sydenham's chorea. *Psychiatr Clin North Am.* 1997;20(4):809–20.
2. Cardoso F, Vargas A, Oliveira L, et al. Persistent Sydenham's chorea. *Mov. Disord.* 1999;14:805–7.
3. Church AJ, Dale RC, Cardoso F, et al. CSF and serum immune parameters in Sydenham's chorea: evidence of an autoimmune syndrome? *J Neuroimmunol.* 2003;136(1-2):149–53.
4. Giedd JN, Rapoport JL, Kruesi MJ, et al. Sydenham's chorea: Magnetic resonance imaging of the basal ganglia. *Neurology.* 1995;45:2199–203.
5. Swedo SE, Leonard HL, Schapiro MB, et al. Sydenham's chorea: physical and psychological symptoms of St Vitus dance. *Pediatrics.* 1993;91(4):706–13.
6. Swedo SE, Leckman JF, Rose NR. From research subgroup to clinical syndrome: modifying the PANDAS criteria to describe PANS (pediatric acute-onset neuropsychiatric syndrome). *Pediatr Therapeut.* 2012;2:113.

Syncope and Presyncope

Epidemiology and Demographics: Syncope is an extraordinarily common condition with a prevalence of 42% and incidence of 6%. It occurs most commonly between the ages of 10 and 30 years. At these ages, the etiology is more likely benign. There is a second peak of incidence after age 70. In this age group, more dangerous cardiac and other vascular causes are more likely. There is no gender preference.

Disorder Description: This disorder is characterized by a brief (average 12 seconds) episode of loss of consciousness due to lack of blood flow to either both cerebral hemispheres or to the brainstem reticular activating system. It is most commonly vasovagal in origin but other causes include cardiac, orthostatic (including both neuropathy and hypovolemia), carotid sinus hypersensitivity, and neurologic causes including brainstem stroke, vertebrobasilar insufficiency, and subclavian steal syndrome. Seizure is not a cause of syncope but the two are easily confused. Factors favoring syncope over seizure include short duration of complete loss of consciousness, rapid onset without premonitory neurologic symptoms, and immediate recovery without postictal confusion. Factors favoring seizure include partial loss of consciousness, premonitory focal neurologic deficits, tongue bite, head or limb jerking, and postictal confusion. Urinary incontinence is not useful in distinguishing syncope from seizure.

Symptoms

Localization site	Comment
Cerebral hemispheres	Loss of blood flow to both hemispheres is required for syncope; therefore, carotid artery disease and focal strokes are not likely to be associated with this condition
Mental status and psychiatric aspects/ complications	Brief loss of consciousness without confusion
Brainstem	Loss of blood flow to the brainstem reticular activating system will cause syncope; therefore, vertebrobasilar disease is in the differential of syncope

Secondary Complications: Depends on the etiology. Vasovagal syncope is generally benign but cardiac syncope has a mortality of up to 30%. Neurologic causes are discussed elsewhere in this book.

Bibliography

Brigo F, Nardone R, Bongiovanni LG. Value of tongue biting in the differential diagnosis between epileptic seizure and syncope. *Seizure.* 2012;21(8):568–72.

Brigo F, Nardone R, Ausserer H, et al. The value of urinary incontinence in the differential diagnosis of seizure. *Seizure.* 2013;22(2):85–90.

Da Silva RM. Syncope: epidemiology, etiology, and prognosis. *Front Physiol.* 2014;5:471.

Webb J, Long B, Koyfman A. An emergency medicine-focused review of seizure mimics. *J Emerg Med.* 2017;52(5):645–53.

Syncope, Non-Neurocardiogenic

Epidemiology and Demographics: Syncope has been reported to account for 3% of hospital emergency visits and 1% to 6% of admissions. Although the overall incidence was 6.2 events per 1000 person-years, rates were significantly higher in elderly subjects (17 per 1000 person-years in males and 19 per 1000 person-years in females aged 80 years).

Disorder Description: Almost all cases of neurocardiogenic syncope are postural and occur in the standing position, hence "orthostatic hypotension." Orthostatic hypotension is defined as reduction in systolic blood pressure of at least 20 mmHg or a reduction of diastolic blood pressure of at least 10 mmHg with 3 minutes of standing. Lack of cardiac response or associated tachycardia could indicate that this is neurogenic (non-neurocardiogenic) in nature. Etiology may be central (Parkinson's disease, Lewy body dementia, multi-system atrophy, pure autonomic failure) or peripheral (diabetes mellitus, amyloidosis, spinal cord injury, hypovolemia).

Onset may be abrupt or may rapidly follow warning symptoms like fatigue, nausea, sweating, dizziness, pallor, blurred or graying vision, abdominal discomfort, headache, pins-and-needles, lightheadedness, rapid heart rate, or impaired hearing/tinnitus.

Symptoms

Localization site	Comment
Cerebral hemispheres	Lightheadedness, blurred or graying vision, orthostatic headache, tinnitus, nausea. Passing out can occur due to decreased cerebral perfusion
Mental status and psychiatric aspects/complications	Coexisting cognitive impairment could indicate underlying neurodegenerative disorder related cognitive impairment
Cerebellum	Cerebellar ataxia in multisystem atrophy or alcohol-related autonomic failure
Vestibular system (and nonspecific dizziness)	Tinnitus and dizziness can occur due to increased sensitivity of the CN VIII to hypoperfusion
Spinal cord	Injury to the sympathetic neurons could result in orthostatic hypotension
Peripheral neuropathy	Seen in association with diabetes, ethanol abuse, amyloidosis
Unclear localization	Peripheral autonomic failure can be associated with abnormal sweating Supine hypertension is more likely to indicate a central etiology REM behavior disorder indicates underlying alpha synucleinopathy

Secondary Complications: Orthostatic hypotension, particularly when symptomatic, can cause falling, which has significant associated morbidity, particularly in a frail elderly population. Cognitive decline can occur secondary to cerebral hypoperfusion. Recurrence can occur in about 20% of the patients.

Treatment Complications: Patients develop adaptive habits to avoid fainting; these habits include crossing their legs, walking around instead of standing, frequently tightening their leg muscles, or sitting or lying down when they predict warning symptoms. Walking at nonpeak hours, taking a short cool shower, avoiding hot baths or saunas, and avoiding alcohol and excess caffeine intake are some practical strategies for prevention. All of these can negatively impact quality of life to varying degrees.

Patients are recommended to take increased salt in their diet and adequate hydration. Supine hypertension may co-exist especially if the etiology is central.

Medication treatment alternatives include midrodrine, fludrocortisone, amphetamine/dextroamphetamine (Adderall), or droxidopa.

Bibliography

Chawla J. *Neurocardiogenic syncope.* Medlink Neurology. Updated November 20, 2015. San Diego: Medlink Corporation. Available from www.medlink.com/article/neurocardiogenic_syncope. Accessed Sep 20, 2018.

Grubb BP. Neurocardiogenic syncope. *N Engl J Med.* 2005;352:1004–10.

Syphilis

Epidemiology and Demographics: According to the Centers for Disease Control, primary and secondary syphilis US prevalence rates rose during 2015–2016 to 8.7/100,000 persons. From a low point in 2000, rates have been steadily increasing. While both males and females may be affected, the higher recent numbers are attributed to increasing cases in males, particularly in the gay or bisexual community who have had sex with males.

Disorder Description: Syphilis is due to infection with the spirochete *Treponema pallidum*. Most infected individuals are asymptomatic and are detected through routine blood test screening. Primary syphilis is characterized by the development of a chancre at the local site of infection, typically urogenitally. In the secondary stage, hematogenous spread can lead to involvement of organs throughout the body, including the meninges. While the body's immunity may stop the infection, a subdivision of subjects who are untreated proceed to develop a tertiary form.

There is a high rate of syphilis co-infection with HIV. HIV-associated syphilis is typically a more aggressive form and is discussed under the entry *HIV and AIDS*.

Symptoms

Localization site	Comment
Cerebral hemispheres	Strokes from meningovascular affectation with potential hemiparesis or aphasia. Seizures and myoclonus
Mental status and psychiatric aspects/ complications	Dementia with presentations that can be mistaken as psychiatrically based personality changes
Brainstem	Argyll Robertson pupils are miotic and unreactive to light but reactive to accommodation
Cranial nerves	Optic neuropathy, other cranial neuropathies such as cranial nerve VIII leading to sensorineural hearing deficits, vertigo, and tinnitus. Cranial nerve VII involvement leads to facial palsy
Spinal cord	Tabes dorsalis characterized by involvement of dorsal columns, dorsal roots, and dorsal root ganglia results in diminished position sense with classic gait unsteadiness and slapping gait, lancinating radicular pains, and urinary incontinence. Charcot joints (classically patellar) result from recurrent trauma to lower limbs that fail to experience pain. Transverse myelitis or Brown–Sequard syndrome

Secondary Complications: Diverse complications of increased intracranial pressure such as contribution to developing optic atrophy. Anterior spinal artery involvement with associated anterior spinal cord infarction results in paraplegia and pain and temperature deficits below the lesion level.

Treatment Complications: Penicillin-class drugs, which are usually highly effective, are generally well tolerated and free of neurologic complications.

Bibliography

Centers for Disease Control and Prevention. Syphilis. Updated Sep 25, 2017. www.cdc .gov/std/stats16/Syphilis.htm. Accessed Sep 25, 2018.

Ho EL, Lukehart SA. Syphilis: using modern approaches to understand an old disease. *J Clin Invest*. 2011;121(12):4584–92. https://doi .org/10.1172/JCI57173.

Tuddenham S, Ghanem KG. Neurosyphilis: knowledge gaps and controversies. *Sex Transmit Dis*. 2018;45(3):147–51. DOI: 10.1097/ OLQ.0000000000000723.

Syringobulbia

Epidemiology and Demographics: It is a rare disorder affecting either sex. It is often associated with Chiari malformation type I (CM-1). The average age of onset of symptoms has been reported to be under 15 years.

Disorder Description: It is described as a fluid-filled cavity (syrinx) within the spinal cord that involves the medulla. It often occurs as a slit-like gap within the lower brainstem and can potentially affect one or more of the cranial nerves, leading to facial palsies. Sensory and motor pathways could also be affected. This condition is closely related to syringomyelia, in which the syrinx is within the spinal cord, and the Chiari malformation type I (CM-I). The etiology of syringobulbia is thought to be due to cervical spinal cord tethering, tumors, arachnoiditis, as well as trauma. Syringobulbia has also been reported in association with Chiari malformation type II (CM-II) and myelodysplasia.

Symptoms

Localization site	Comment
Brainstem including medulla	Vertigo, gait instability, nausea, vomiting
Cranial nerve involvement	Nystagmus, loss of pain and temperature sensation in the face, fibrillation of the tongue muscles, as well as stuttering, hearing loss, and tinnitus

Secondary Complications: Syringobulbia introduces a mass effect, and depending on the affected region, it can lead to serious brainstem and cranial nerve deficits, or syringomyelia.

Treatment Complications: Treatment of syringobulbia is usually surgical, which involves using a cerebrospinal fluid (CSF) shunt. This approach is often combined with treating the associated syringomyelia. Hence, all potential neurosurgical complications are applicable here.

Bibliography

Menezes AH, Greenlee JDW, Longmuir RA, Hansen DR, Abode-Lyamah K. Syringohydromyelia in association with syringobulbia and syringocephaly: case report. *J Neurosurg Pediatr.* 2015;15(6):657–61.

National Organization for Rare Disorders. Syringobulbia. https://rarediseases.org/rarediseases/syringobulbia/. Accessed Sep 20, 2018.

Sarikaya S, Acikgoz B, Tekkok IH, Gungen YY. Conus ependymoma with holocord syringohydromyelia and syringobulbia. *J Clin Neurosci.* 2007;14(9):901–4.

Tubbs RS, Bailey M, Barrow WC, et al. Morphometric analysis of the craniocervical juncture in children with Chiari I malformation and concomitant syringobulbia. *Childs Nerv Syst.* 2009;25:689–92.

Systemic Lupus Erythematosus (SLE)

Epidemiology and Demographics: The prevalence of systemic lupus erythematosus (SLE) is highest in women aged 14 to 64 years. SLE does not have an age predilection in males, although it should be noted that in older adults, the female-to-male ratio falls. The female-to-male ratio peaks at 11:1 during the childbearing years. In general, black women have a higher rate of SLE than women of any other race, followed by Asian women and then white women. Estimates of the annual incidence of SLE have ranged from approximately 1 to 10 per 100,000 population, while the prevalence of SLE has been estimated to range from approximately 5.8 to 130 per 100,000 population.

Disorder Description: SLE is a chronic inflammatory condition that can manifest itself in numerous ways and has relapsing–remitting course. It is characterized by an autoantibody response to nuclear and cytoplasmic antigens. SLE is associated with defects in apoptotic clearance and the damaging effects caused by apoptotic debris. The condition is believed to be a type III hypersensitivity response with potential type II involvement. SLE can affect any organ system, but it mainly involves the skin, joints, kidneys, blood cells, and nervous system. Involvement of the central and peripheral nervous systems can result in many different types of neuropsychiatric symptoms. The diagnosis of neuropsychiatric syndromes concurrent with SLE poses a major challenge in the management of SLE because it can involve many different patterns of symptoms, some of which may be mistaken for signs of infectious disease or stroke.

Potential causes include:

Genetic: HLA class I, class II, and class III genes are associated with SLE, but only classes I and II contribute independently to increased risk of SLE. Other genes that contain risk variants for SLE are *IRF5*, *PTPN22*, *STAT4*, *CDKN1A*, *ITGAM*, *BLK*, *TNFSF4*, and *BANK1*.

Drug reaction: Drug-induced SLE is usually a reversible condition that occurs in people being treated for a long-term illness. Drug-induced lupus mimics SLE.

Non-systemic forms of lupus: Discoid (cutaneous) lupus is limited to skin symptoms and is diagnosed by biopsy of rash on the face, neck, scalp, or arms. Approximately 5% of people with DLE progress to SLE.

Risk factors include:

Female gender

Family history

Use of specific medications, the most common being procainamide, isoniazid, hydralazine, quinidine, phenytoin

No particular geographic proclivity is known.

Symptoms

Localization site	Comment
Brain	Headache, cognitive dysfunction, mood disorder, cerebrovascular disease, seizures, anxiety disorder, and psychosis. Diffuse encephalopathies
	Intracranial hypertension syndrome – increased intracranial pressure, papilledema, abducens paresis resulting in double vision
	Movement disorder (chorea)
	Depression affects up to 60% of women with SLE
Brainstem	Most frequent cranial neuropathies involve the eighth nerve followed by the oculomotor set (third, fourth, and sixth), and then the fifth and seventh nerves
Spinal cord	Demyelinating disease
	Myelopathy
Nerve roots	Plexopathy
Peripheral nerves	Mononeuritis multiplex, Guillain–Barré syndrome
Neuromuscular junction	Myasthenia gravis
Muscle	Myositis
	Myopathy (drug induced)

Secondary Complications

Kidney failure

Blood dyscrasias, such as anemia (low red blood cell count), bleeding, or clotting

High blood pressure

Vasculitis (inflammation of the blood vessels)

Memory problems

Behavior changes or hallucinations

Seizures

Stroke

Heart disease or heart attack

Lung conditions, such as pleurisy (inflammation of the chest cavity lining) or pneumonia

Infections

Cancer

Avascular necrosis (death of bone tissue due to a lack of blood supply)

Increased risk of cancer

Treatment Complications

Steroid psychosis.

Immunosuppression from use of corticosteroids may lead to increased risk of infection. Weight gain, easy bruising, thinning bones (osteoporosis), avascular necrosis of the hip, high blood pressure, and diabetes may also occur as a result of prolonged use of corticosteroids.

Retinal damage may occur with the use of antimalarial medications such as hydroxychloroquine.

Long-term use of non-steroidal anti-inflammatory drugs may cause increased risk of gastrointestinal bleeding.

Bibliography

Lisnevskaia L, Murphy G, Isenberg D. Systemic lupus erythematosus. *Lancet.* 2014;384(9957):1878–88.

Tsokos G. Systemic lupus erythematosus. *N Engl J Med.* 2011;365:2110–21.

Vu Lam N, Ghetu M, Bieniek M. Systemic lupus erythematosus: primary care approach to diagnosis and management. *Am Fam Physician.* 2016;94(4):284–94.

Takayasu Arteritis

Epidemiology and Demographics: Rare disorder most commonly found in Asia and India or in those of Asian or Indian descent. In the United States, the incidence is 2.6/million per year. The prevalence is 2.6–6.4/million people. The female-to-male ratio is 4:1 in Asia and 2:1 elsewhere.

Disorder Description: This is a large vessel vasculitis of unknown etiology leading to granulomatous inflammation of the affected vessels. It affects the aorta and its main branches.

Symptoms

Localization site	Comments
Cerebral hemispheres	Stroke (any symptom is possible based on location). Seizure. Headache

Secondary Complications: This is primarily a nonneurologic disorder with symptoms including malaise, arthralgia, fever, weight loss, hypertension, carotid bruit, carotidynia, pericarditis, abdominal pain, Raynaud phenomenon, erythema nodosum, ulcerated subacute nodules, and pyoderma gangrenosum among others.

Treatment Complications: Treatment is by immunosuppression, including monoclonal antibodies, and can lead to infection.

Bibliography

de Souza AW, de Carvalho JF. Diagnostic and classification criteria of Takayasu arteritis. *J Autoimmun.* 2014;48–49:79–83.

Keser G, Direskeneli H, Aksu K. Management of Takayasu arteritis: a systematic review. *Rheumatology (Oxford).* 2014;53(5):793–801.

Tardive Dyskinesia (TD)

Epidemiology and Demographics: Tardive dyskinesia (TD) occurs in middle-aged to elderly people, with females more likely to be affected than males.[1] TD in children is much less common than in adults and older age individuals. TD is mainly a delayed-onset complication of treatment with dopamine-receptor blocking agents (DRBAs), which include antipsychotics and anti-emetics such as metoclopramide.[2] It generally appears 1–6 months after drug exposure.

TD is reported to have existed before the advent of these drugs. Incidence of TD after 3 months of conventional anti-psychotic use is about 3–8%,[3] while in those older than 55 years, incidence increases to approximately 10–20%.[1] The term tardive indicates that it appears late in the course of treatment. With increasing use of second-generation anti-psychotic medication, the incidence is significantly lower.[4]

In two-thirds of people who developed TD after drug exposure, TD lasted for at least 6 months. Remission may occur within months after drug withdrawal or take as long as 1–3 years. Withdrawing the offending drug(s) often exacerbates the severity of the movements. TD symptoms can persist and may even remain permanently.

TD in children is called "withdrawal emergent syndrome." It presents as choreic movements and resembles Sydenham's chorea. The symptoms may appear immediately after anti-psychotic medication is discontinued.

Disorder Description: TD is a movement disorder that occurs as a delayed complication of DRBA use. It is characterized by hyperkinetic movements such as oral, facial, and lingual dyskinesias, which include protruding and rotatory tongue movements, pouting, puckering or smacking lip movements, bulging of the cheeks, chewing movements, excessive blinking, and brow wrinkling. Orofacial hyperkinesia is the prototypical form of neuroleptic-induced TD. Tremors are rare.

Limb dyskinesias may occur and are described as twisting, spreading, and "piano-playing" finger movements, tapping foot movements, and dystonic extensor toe posturing.

Neck and trunk dyskinesias include retro- and torticollis, axial dystonia, shoulder shrugging, rocking, swaying, rotator and thrusting hip movements. Any of these may interfere with gait and mobility. Please see entry for *Tardive Dystonia*.

Respiratory dyskinesias may produce tachypnea, irregular breathing rhythms, and grunting noises.

In addition to female gender and older age, other significant risk factors for developing TD include: traumatic brain injury, dementia, major affective disorder, and diabetes. In terms of medication use, long duration of anti-psychotic medication or use of anti-cholinergic agents also confers risk. Other movement disorders and a history of previous extra-pyramidal reactions to anti-psychotic drugs are also important considerations.

Anti-psychotics have a high affinity for dopamine receptors. Specifically, they block D2 receptors in areas of the brain responsible for fine motor control (basal ganglia and cerebellum), which may lead to tremor, akinesia, spasticity, rigidity, and akathisia. The newer "atypical" neuroleptics have a lower affinity for D2 receptors while readily binding with D1, D3, and D4 dopamine receptors. These newer agents have fewer side effects than the older neuroleptics with a similar therapeutic profile.[5]

Symptoms

Localization site	Comment
Basal ganglia	Oral, facial, lingual, limb, neck, respiratory, and trunk dyskinesias
	Akathisia associated with dyskinesias

Secondary Complications: TD involves movements that are quick, jerky, and repetitive. This condition can impair social interactions and induce feelings of humiliation and chagrin for the person. Another secondary complication of TD may be suicide.[6]

Treatment Complications: Clonazepam and clozapine are commonly used in the treatment of TD. Regular monitoring is essential for patients on clozapine to screen for agranulocytosis, as it can be fatal. Tetrabenazine (TBZ) is considered particularly useful for the dystonic form of TD. Potential adverse effects include depression and suicidality.

References

1. Woerner M, Alvir J, Saltz B, Lieberman J, et al. Prospective study of tardive dyskinesia in the elderly: rates and risk factors. *Am J Psychiatry*. 1998;155(11):1521–8.
2. Tarsy D, Baldessarini R. Tardive dyskinesia. *Annu Rev Med*. 1984;35(1):605–23.
3. Kane J. Tardive dyskinesia. *Arch Gen Psychiatry*. 1982;39(4):473.
4. Gardner D, Baldessarini R, Waraich P. Modern antipsychotic drugs: a critical overview. *CMAJ*. 2005;172(13):1703–11.
5. Seeman P. Atypical antipsychotics: mechanism of action. *Can J Psychiatry*. 2002;47(1):27–38.
6. Yassa R, Jones B. Complications of tardive dyskinesia: A review. *Psychosomatics*. 1985;26(4):305–13.

Tardive Dystonia

Epidemiology and Demographics: The prevalence of tardive dystonia among patients treated with dopamine receptor blocking agents such as antipsychotics and antiemetics is reported to be 2–16%.[1] However, a diagnosis is not always made. In 2007, up to 72% of patients who used atypical antipsychotics had undiagnosed extrapyramidal side effects.[1,2] There is no gender difference noted, but those affected tend to be younger than those with non-dystonic neuroleptic-induced tardive syndromes.[1]

Disorder Description: Tardive dystonia is one of several tardive syndromes that occur with chronic use of dopamine receptor blocking agents. It is characterized by involuntary hyperkinetic movements.[1-4] The dystonia must be present for more than 1 month and must be present during or within 3 months after use of neuroleptics.[1-4] The dystonia may be fixed or action-specific, and is indistinguishable from idiopathic torsion dystonia, except for the concurrent or recent use of neuroleptics or dopamine receptor blocking agents.[1-4] In tardive dystonia, as with idiopathic focal dystonias, the head and neck are the most commonly affected body regions.[1,2] It frequently occurs in the presence of other tardive syndromes.[1,2]

Symptoms

Localization site	Comment
Specific spinal roots	Secondary radiculopathy
Muscle	Painful muscle contractions

Secondary Complications: The main secondary complication of tardive dystonia is pain. Although not clearly a long-term secondary complication of tardive dystonia, craniocervical dystonia may lead to radiculopathy. In cases of truncal or axial tardive dystonia, the result can produce severe scoliosis or opisthotonic posturing. Rarely, antipsychotic-induced dystonia of the laryngeal or pharyngeal muscles causing asphyxia and choking, respectively, has been reported.[2]

Treatment Complications: Treatment options for tardive dystonia are stopping use of the dopaminergic blocking agents (which may lead to exacerbation of psychotic illness) or intramuscular botulinum toxin injections, which may cause weakness or signs and symptoms associated with spread of the toxin outside the intended muscle.

References

1. Bhidayasiri R, Boonyawairoj S. Spectrum of tardive syndromes: clinical recognition and management. *Postgrad Med J*. 2011;87:132e141. DOI:10.1136/pgmj.2010.103234.
2. Haddad PM, Dursun SM. Neurological complications of psychiatric drugs: clinical features and management. *Hum Psychopharmacol Clin Exp*. 2008;23:15–26.
3. Waln O, Jankovic J. An update on tardive dyskinesia: from phenomenology to treatment. *Tremor Other Hyperkinet Mov (NY)*. 2013;3:pii: tre-03-161-4138-1. DOI: 10.7916/D88P5Z71.
4. Hazari N, Kate N, Grover S. Clozapine and tardive movement disorders: A review. *Asian J Psychiatry*. 2013;6:439–51.

Tay–Sachs Disease (Hexosaminidase A Deficiency)

Epidemiology and Demographics: One in 320,000 in the general population with carrier rates as high 1 in 25 in Ashkenazi Jewish populations, Amish, and French Canadians. Autosomal recessive inheritance. Targeted community-based carrier screening has reduced rates in Jews worldwide, such that most cases result from parental consanguinity.

Disorder Description: Tay–Sachs is a rare, lysosomal lipid storage disease, belonging to the GM2 gangliosidoses. Hexosaminidase A is an enzyme required for the normal catabolism of GM2 glycosphingolipid, and deficiency results in a spectrum of neurodegenerative disorders, characterized by accumulation of substrate within neuronal lysosomes. Other GM2 gangliosides include Sandhoff's disease and hexosaminidase activator deficiency.

The typical infant onset variant, known as Tay–Sachs, is characterized by developmental regression with progressive weakness, loss of motor skills, decreased visual attentiveness, and exaggerated and persistent startle beginning between the ages of 3 and 6 months. Progressive neurodegeneration ensues with myoclonic jerks, seizures, blindness, spasticity, and eventual total incapacitation and death usually between ages 2 and 4 years. Progressive acquired macrocephaly is present from 18 months, resulting from reactive cerebral gliosis. A gray–white area around the retinal fovea centralis, due to lipid-laden ganglion cells, leaves a central **"cherry-red" spot**, visible on fundoscopy. Examination also reveals generalized hypotonia with sustained ankle clonus and hyperreflexia. Further deterioration in the second year of life results in decerebrate posturing, difficulties in swallowing, and an eventual vegetative state.

Other forms of the disease include juvenile (onset between 2 and 10 years), chronic, and adult-onset variants, characterized by later onset, slower progression, and variable neurologic findings including progressive dystonia, spinocerebellar degeneration, motor neuron disease, and psychosis in adolescence.

Diagnosis is by demonstration of absent to near-absent beta-hexosaminidase A (HEX A) enzymatic activity in the serum or white blood cells in the setting of normal HEX B enzyme activity. Prenatal diagnosis (preimplantation genetic diagnosis) is available.

Symptoms

Localization site	Comment
Cerebral hemispheres	Deep nuclei
	Extrapyramidal movement disorder
	Dystonia, ataxia, and incoordination in juvenile onset
	Pyramidal involvement – hypotonia with spasticity, hyperreflexia, and clonus in infant onset
	Cognitive/psychosis
	Especially in chronic and adult-onset form
	Psychotic depression, bipolar symptoms, agitation, impaired executive function and memory
	MRI demonstrates non-specific atrophy with hippocampus, and brainstem nuclei affected in adult-onset form
Cranial nerves	Retinal "cherry red" spot

Secondary Complications: Contractures, aspiration.

Treatment Complications: Treatment is mostly supportive. Seizure control can be achieved using conventional antiepileptic drugs, but seizures are often progressive and changing in type and severity. Conventional antipsychotic agents may be used for psychiatric manifestations. Preclinical trials are underway evaluating chaperone therapy to enhance rescue of mutant enzymes to allow some residual enzyme activity.

Bibliography

Hamosh A. OMIM: Tay–Sachs Disease, TSD. Updated May 30, 2013. Johns Hopkins University. Available from www.omim.org/entry/272800. Accessed Jun 8, 2016.

Kaback MM. Hexosaminidase A deficiency. In Pagon RA, Adam MP, Ardinger HH, et al., eds. *GeneReviews®* [Internet]. Seattle (WA): University of Washington, Seattle; 1993–2016.

Temporal Arteritis (Giant Cell Arteritis, Horton's Disease)

Epidemiology and Demographics: Most commonly seen in individuals 55 years and older. Mean age of 71 years. Rarely seen in people less than 55 years old. More common in women compared with men (2:1 female-to-male ratio). More common in individuals of northern European descent, as well those living in higher latitudes. The incidence for temporal arteritis is 15–25 cases/100,000 persons.

Disorder Description: Temporal arteritis is an inflammatory disorder affecting medium- and large-size arteries. There is a predilection for the vertebral arteries, the subclavian arteries, and the extracranial branches of the carotid arteries (i.e., the superficial temporal, ophthalmic, occipital, and posterior ciliary arteries). Temporal arteritis and giant cell aortitis are related etiologies. Inflammation may involve the aortic wall and, rarely, the femoral and coronary arteries. The most common symptoms that occur with this condition include bruits secondary to turbulent blood flow in the carotid artery, fever, severe headache, tenderness or sensitivity of the scalp to light touch, jaw claudication, tongue claudication, reduced visual acuity, diplopia or blindness in severe cases, tinnitus, polymyalgia rheumatica. This is a medical condition that is considered a medical emergency as early and accurate diagnosis is crucial to prevent ischemic vision loss.

A systemic inflammatory response is associated with the vascular manifestations of temporal arteritis and produces a constellation of symptoms. Fever, myalgia, anorexia, weight loss, anemia, and malaise are often encountered. Values for acute-phase reactants (e.g., erythrocyte sedimentation rate [ESR] and C-reactive protein [CRP] level) are typically elevated. The CRP level and thrombocytosis may be stronger predictors of a subsequent positive biopsy than the ESR.

The cause of this condition is multifactorial; however, numerous viruses and bacteria have been proposed. These include:

Varicella zoster
Parvovirus
Parainfluenza
Chlamydia pneumoniae
Mycoplasma pneumoniae

Risk factors include:

Over the age of 55
Female gender
Northern European descent
Genetic: HLA-DR4 haplotype
Viral and/or bacterial infection
Temporal arteritis is primarily seen in western countries.

Symptoms

Localization site	Comment
Vertebral arteries	Dizziness, lightheadedness, vertigo, transient ischemic attack (TIA), stroke most likely involving the posterior circulation of the brain including symptoms such as loss of vision and imbalance
Subclavian, axillary, and proximal brachial artery branches	Arm claudication, absent or asymmetric pulses
Temporal artery	Headache, scalp tenderness, jaw claudication
Ophthalmic/posterior ciliary arteries	Amaurosis fugax: vision loss – partial vision loss in one eye is noted in up to 60% of patients not treated emergently. Blindness results from occlusion of the inflamed ophthalmic or posterior ciliary arteries with resultant ischemia of the optic nerve or tracts; eye pain and hallucinations have also been reported

Localization site	Comment
Aorta	Thoracic aneurysm development, pulsating abdominal mass, aneurysm rupture may lead to death
Systemic	Fever, myalgia, anorexia, weight loss, anemia, and malaise

Secondary Complications:

Vision changes: partial to complete vision loss is possible

Thoracic aneurysm development and/or rupture

Transient ischemic attack

Stroke secondary to intracranial vasculitis

Polymyalgia rheumatica

Treatment Complications:

Steroid psychosis.

Immunosuppression from use of corticosteroids may lead to increased risk of infection. Weight gain, easy bruising, thinning bones (osteoporosis), avascular necrosis of the hip, high blood pressure, and diabetes may also occur as a result of prolonged use of corticosteroids.

Retinal damage may occur with the use of antimalarial medications such as hydroxychloroquine.

Long-term use of non-steroidal anti-inflammatory drugs may cause increased risk of gastrointestinal bleeding.

In cases where dapsone and cyclophosphamide are used patient can also suffer from toxicity effects from the same.

Bibliography

Hoffman GS. Giant cell arteritis. *Ann Intern Med.* 2016;165(9):ITC65-ITC80.

Waldman CW, Waldman SD, Waldman RA. Giant cell arteritis. *Med Clin North Am.* 2013;97(2): 329–35.

Temporal Bone Fracture

Epidemiology and Demographics: Traumatic condition of the temporal bone occurring more frequently in men and younger adults. An extreme lateral force is required to fracture the temporal bone, and these injuries are most commonly seen in vehicular trauma. It is estimated that 30% of head trauma resulting from motor vehicle accidents leads to skull fractures. Of these up to 22% result in temporal bone fractures.

Disorder Description: Temporal bone fractures may be longitudinal (along the long axis of the temporal bone) or transverse (perpendicular to the skull, through the labyrinth), and may result in conductive or sensorineural hearing loss, facial nerve paralysis, cerebrospinal fluid (CSF) leak, and vertigo.

Conductive hearing loss is treated conservatively at first. Hemotympanum usually resolves without treatment. Persistent conductive loss due to ossicular disruption may be treated surgically or with a hearing aid. Sensorineural hearing loss is usually permanent.

Facial nerve paralysis that is complete and immediate in onset should be investigated with electroneuronography (ENOG) in the first 10 days; if degeneration of electrical activity occurs to less than 10% of the normal side, the facial nerve should be surgically explored and repaired.

CSF otorhinorrhea more often than not resolves with conservative measures – bedrest, head elevation, stool softeners, and carbonic anhydrase inhibitors. Persistent CSF leak requires surgical repair.

Vertigo may be due to vestibular concussion or to permanent damage to the vestibule. Most vertigo after temporal bone trauma is self-resolving within 6 to 12 months after central compensation.

Symptoms

Localization site	Comment
Inner ear	Otic capsule may be fractured or contused
Cranial nerves	Cochleovestibular nerve is variably affected
Central nervous system	Central nervous system is not affected

Secondary Complications: Persistent CSF fistula poses the risk of meningitis. Vertigo, facial nerve paralysis, and hearing loss have significant impacts on quality of life. Vestibular impairment may be permanent if central compensation does not occur.

Treatment Complications: A common finding is benign paroxysmal positional vertigo (BPPV) caused by dislodged otoconia, and this is readily treated with Epley maneuver (see above). In other cases, vertigo may be due to posttraumatic endolymphatic hydrops that results from the disturbance of endolymph and perilymph homeostasis. This condition is treated in a similar manner to Meniere's disease. Perilymph fistulae may also form after temporal bone trauma and present with vertigo and nystagmus with positive pressure applied to the inner ear. Treatment is first conservative, and surgical repair if that fails.

Surgery for facial paralysis or CSF leak may result in sensorineural hearing loss. Medical treatment of posttraumatic endolymphatic hydrops with thiazide diuretics or acetazolamide carries the risk of hypotension and electrolyte abnormalities. Repair of perilymph fistula carries a small risk of tympanic membrane perforation or sensorineural hearing loss.

Bibliography

Brodie HA, Thompson TC. Management of complications from 820 temporal bone fractures. *Am J Otol.* 1997;18:188–97.

Johnson FI, Semaan MT, Megerian CA. Temporal bone fracture: evaluation and management in the modern era. *Otolaryngol Clin North Am.* 2008;41(3):597–618.

Temporal Lobe Epilepsy (TLE)

Epidemiology and Demographics: Most common form of focal epilepsy, accounting for 60% of cases.

Disorder Description: Characterized by epileptiform discharges from the temporal lobar regions. Seizures at onset generally present as experiential auras, changes in emotions (fear, euphoria), déjà vu, or perseverative thinking.

Oro-manual automatisms and behavioral arrest are common, and seizures may be bland in appearance. Typically categorized as mesial TLE (more common) and neocortical TLE.

Underlying pathologies most commonly include hippocampal sclerosis (60–70%), cortical dysplasia, low-grade tumors, vascular malformations, and encephalitis. Fifteen to 20% of cases have no detectable structural lesions. Febrile seizures appear to be a risk factor for mesial TLE. Genetic syndromes have been identified such as autosomal dominant lateral temporal epilepsy secondary to mutations in the LGI1 gene.

Interictal EEG may have temporal intermittent rhythmic delta activity and temporal sharp waves. MRI identifies abnormalities in the majority of patients with temporal lobe epilepsy.

Antiepileptic drugs (AEDs) are first line for treatment of TLE. Temporal lobectomy is indicated for medically intractable cases. Vagal nerve or responsive stimulation is an option for non-surgically resectable candidates.

Symptoms

Localization site	Comment
Cerebral hemispheres	Sudden interruption of consciousness. Auras may include deja vu, jamais vu, or fear, gastrointestinal upset (mesial TLE). Auditory hallucinations or distortions, vertigo, or complex visual hallucinations (neocortical TLE)
	Automatisms: lip-smacking, chewing, and fumbling movements of the fingers
Mental status and psychiatric aspects/ complications	Commonly affects cognitive functioning including memory, attention, language, praxis, executive function, judgment, insight, and problem solving
	Social cognitive deficits, such as impairments in facial emotional recognition, or recognition of fear. Theory of mind also shown to be affected
	Dominant TLE associated with greater deficits in verbal memory. Non-dominant TLE associated with more severe deficits in recognition of fear, sadness, and disgust

Secondary Complications: Patients often develop cognitive and social dysfunction secondary to structural changes in the brain, longstanding seizures, use of AEDs, and high rates of psychiatric comorbidity. Prevalence of depression near 30% in patients with TLE overall, higher in patients with prolonged or intractable epilepsy. Suicidality occurs at a much higher rate than expected in this population (up to a 25-fold increase).

Treatment Complications: AEDs are associated with a number of idiosyncratic side effects. Antidepressants, such as selective serotonin reuptake inhibitors, appear to have a relatively low risk of exacerbating seizures, and should be considered in patients with epilepsy if indicated. The risks of dominant temporal lobectomy include memory loss and naming difficulties. Superior quadrantanopsia may occur. Less common effects of surgery may include temporary emotional destabilization and de novo depression or psychosis.

Bibliography

Bora E, Meletti S. Social cognition in temporal lobe epilepsy: A systematic review and meta-analysis. *Epilepsy Behav.* 2016;60:50–7.

Garcia CS. Depression in temporal lobe epilepsy: a review of prevalence, clinical features, and management considerations. *Epilepsy Res Treat.* 2012;2012:809843.

Zhao F, et al. Neuropsychological deficits in temporal lobe epilepsy: A comprehensive review. *Ann Indian Acad Neurol.* 2014;17(4):374–82.

Temporomandibular Joint Syndrome (Consten Syndrome)

Epidemiology and Demographics: Commonly occurs in adults 20–40 years of age; infrequently found in pediatric population. Female-to-male ratio is 4:1. No race predilection is known. Ten million people have the temporomandibular joint (TMJ) syndrome.

Disorder Description: The TMJ is a synovial joint that connects the jaw to the skull. The joint is located just anterior to each ear. The joint allows up/down, side-to-side, protrusion and retraction movements. Pain in this joint is common and can occur because of multiple reasons. Non-joint-related causes include muscle spasm or tension from nocternal jaw clenching or bruxism, and psychologic stress. Joint-related causes from internal derangement of the joint can also cause pain. Finally, arthritic changes caused by degenerative joint disease can also cause the joint to become painful. The trigeminal nerve carries a great degree of enervation to the structures surrounding and making up the TMJ. Irritation of the mandibuar (V3) branch of the trigeminal nerve causes pain locally at the TMJ as well as other V3-associated areas such as scalp, skin, and teeth ipsilateral to the nerve.

The etiology of this condition is thought to be multifactorial. The root causes of this condition are secondary to local damage to the TMJ as well as from systemic diseases.

Risk factors include:

Female gender
Age between 20 and 40
Smoking; female smokers younger than 30 were at especially high risk
History of bruxism
History of neck, shoulder, and back pain
Congenital misalignment of jaw; history of pronounced underbite or overbite
Jaw misalignment secondary to prior jaw/facial trauma
Excessive use of chewing gum
History of rheumatoid arthritis, osteoarthritis, or other types of inflammatory joint diseases
No particular geographic proclivity is known.

Symptoms

Localization site	Comment
Temporomandibular joint	Pain during chewing, ear clicking or popping noise
	Locking of jaw when attempting to open mouth
	Pain that radiates to the ear and jaw typically worsened by eating and chewing
	Palpable spasm of pterygoid and masseter muscle
	Unilateral facial swelling
	Lateral deviation of mandible
	Crepitus may be palpated over joint in advanced disease

Secondary Complications

Failure to thrive/weight loss due to reduced oral intake
Tinnitus
Dental pain
Headaches (tension and/or migraine)
Trigeminal neuralgia

Treatment Complications:

Nonsteroidal anti-inflammatory drugs (NSAIDs) are frequently used for the treatment of this disease process. Excessive use of NSAIDs can cause:

Gastrointestinal disease (e.g., upset stomach, gastric ulcer)
Hypertension
Nephropathy
Cardiomyopathy
Rash

Benzodiazepines are used as muscle relaxants in this disease process, but they are:

> Habit forming, as such caution should be used in patients with a history of substance abuse. Benzodiazepines also have features of tolerance which may require patients to use higher doses to get the same effect.
>
> Epileptogenic when discontinued abruptly after prolonged usage.
>
> Likely to worsen depression in patients with history of substance abuse. Patients complain of emotional blunting or inability to feel pleasure or pain with prolonged use of benzodiazepines.
>
> Sedating; commonly cause lethargy.
>
> Paradoxically stimulating, as such patients may complain of insomnia or hyperactivity with prolonged use of NSAIDs.

Bibliography

American Academy of Family Physicians. Temporomandibular joint (TMJ) pain. *Am Fam Physician*. 2007;76(10):1483–4.

Yule PL, Durham J, Wassell RW. Pain Part 6: Temporomandibular disorders. *Dent Update*. 2016;43(1):39–42, 45–8.

Tension-Type Headache

Epidemiology and Demographics: One population study in the United States estimated a prevalence of 48% over a lifetime. Approximately 40% of patients recall a family member with similar symptoms. Some studies suggest a slight female preference for tension-type headaches over men at a ratio of 5:4. When the headache becomes chronic, the preference for females increases. Most patients with tension-type headache develop symptoms at around age 30 years with peak prevalence at 40–49 years. In children, the mean age of onset is around 7 years, with a prevalence of 31%.

Disorder Description: Previous conventional thinking suggested that tension-type headache is secondary to excess contraction of pericranial and cervical muscles. Many studies suggest an association between emotional distress and these types of headaches. Caffeine excess or withdrawal is associated with tension-type headache; however, no other dietary factors are known to affect this type of headache. The etiology of this condition is still unclear and current thinking suggests that environmental factors play a stronger role than genetics. The International Classification of Headache Disorders Criteria includes the following criteria for diagnosis: bilateral location; mild to moderate intensity that does not affect daily activities; non-pulsating quality; no aggravation with physical activity; no association with nausea or vomiting; association with either photophobia or phonophobia but not both. The chronic form of this condition can be diagnosed if the headache occurs for more than 15 days out of a month for more than 3 months.

Symptoms

Localization site	Comment
Cerebral hemispheres	Possible role of central nervous system nociceptive receptors in the chronic form of this condition. Some studies suggest atrophy of gray matter structures like dorsal rostral and ventral pons, cingulate and insular and orbitofrontal cortex, right posterior temporal lobe, parahippocampus, right cerebellum
Cranial nerves	Involvement of spinal trigeminal nucleus and peripheral nociceptor sensitization
Head and neck muscles	Pericranial and cervical muscle tenderness

Secondary Complications: Tension-type headaches can progress to chronic type, depending on classification and frequency.

Treatment Complications: Conventional therapy for acute headaches involves nonsteroidal anti-inflammatory drugs. However, overuse of these medications can cause gastrointestinal upset. There are no established guidelines or studies on prophylaxis of these types of headaches. However, antiepileptic and antidepressant medications have been prescribed with successful results. Triptans are not recommended for treating acute tension headaches.

Bibliography

Anttila P. Tension-type headache in childhood and adolescence. *Lancet Neurol.* 2006;5(3):268–74.

Kaniecki RG. Migraine and tension-type headache: an assessment of challenges in diagnosis. *Neurology.* 2002;58(9 Suppl 6):S15–S20.

Sacco S, Ricci S, Carolei A. Tension-type headache and systemic medical disorders. *Curr Pain Headache Rep.* 2011;15(6):438–43.

Schwartz BS, Stewart WF, Simon D, Lipton RB. Epidemiology of tension-type headache. *JAMA.* 1998;279(5):381–3.

Testicular Cancer

Epidemiology and Demographics: A relatively rare cancer accounting for 1–1.5% of male cancers with an annual incidence of 5.7/100,000 men. It typically affects men in the third or fourth decades of life. Generally, has excellent cure rate and good prognosis.

Disorder Description: Testicular cancer is a cancer of the testicles, classified into three main categories: germ cell tumors (95%), cord stromal tumors, and miscellaneous germ cell/sex cord stream tumors. Worldwide incidence is lowest in Africa and Asia and highest in European countries. Risk factors include cryptorchidism, personal or family history, infertility, and HIV infection. Metastasis is usually via lymphatic spread, first to the para-aortic lymph nodes, then to mediastinal or supraclavicular lymph nodes.

Symptoms

Localization site	Comment
Cerebral hemispheres	Metastasis (rare)
Mental status and psychiatric aspects/complications	Limbic, brainstem, and hypothalamic encephalitis (associated with anti-Ma1 or 2 antibody)
Brainstem	Brainstem encephalitis as above
Cerebellum	Metastasis (rare)
Spinal cord	Rarely vertebral metastases with spinal cord compression

Secondary Complications: An apical lung metastasis can lead to Pancoast syndrome causing weakness of the intrinsic hand muscles and Horner's syndrome.

Hypercoagulability of malignancy can lead to cerebral venous sinus thrombosis or cerebral infarction.

Treatment Complications

Retroperitoneal lymph node dissection: Can cause ejaculatory dysfunction secondary to damage to nerves exiting the thoracolumbar sympathetic trunk.

Cisplatin: Peripheral neuropathy via damage to the dorsal root ganglion; ototoxicity resulting in tinnitus and hearing impairment.

Ifosfamide: Acute encephalopathy during treatment.

Radiotherapy: Therapeutic irradiation can cause significant injury to the peripheral nerves of the lumbosacral plexus and/or to the spinal cord leading to post-radiation lower motor neuron syndrome, which can present with paresis (rare) and/or transient sensory symptoms.

Bibliography

Albers P, Albrecht W, Algaba F, et al.; European Association of Urology. EAU guidelines on testicular cancer: 2011 update. *Eur Urol.* 2011;60(2):304–19.

Brydøy M, Storstein A, Dahl O. Transient neurological adverse effects following low dose radiation therapy for early stage testicular seminoma. *Radiother Oncol.* 2007;82(2):137–44.

Fung C, Vaughn DJ. Complications associated with chemotherapy in testicular cancer management. *Nat Rev Urol.* 2011;8(4):213–22.

Höftberger R, Rosenfeld MR, Dalmau J. Update on neurological paraneoplastic syndromes. *Curr Opin Oncol.* 2015;27(6):489–95.

Nichols CR. Testicular cancer. *Curr Probl Cancer.* 1998;22(4):187–274. Review. PubMed PMID: 9743088.

Tetanus

Epidemiology and Demographics: As summarized by Brook, the incidence of tetanus varies throughout the world. In the United States, 50–100 cases are reported annually. It is more prevalent in areas with inappropriate hygiene and immunization programs.

Disorder Description: *Clostridium tetani* is an anaerobe that lives in soil. Its toxin causes lowering of inhibition at the nerve endings.

Patients may present with a stiff neck, spasms of the muscles causing backward arching of the head, neck and spine, sustained spasms of the facial muscles, board-like rigid abdomen, trouble swallowing, and respiratory distress.

Symptoms

Localization site	Comment
Cranial nerves	Cranial nerves 7, 6, 3, 4, 12 can cause dysphagia, trismus, focal cranial neuropathies
Muscle	Muscle contraction

Secondary Complications: Respiratory difficulty; the constant contraction of the muscles may cause muscle breakdown and that can lead to renal failure. The paraspinal muscles may contract for prolonged periods and result in compression fractures. The immobility may cause skin breakdown, nutritional deficits, and blood clots.

Treatment Complications: Benzodiazepines may cause altered mental status. Tetanus immunoglobulin may cause hyperthermia.

Bibliography

Brook I. Current concepts in the management of Clostridium tetani infection *Expert Rev Anti Infect Ther*. 2008;6(3):327–36. DOI: 10.1586/14787210.6.3.327.

Sexton DJ. Tetanus. UpToDate. Updated Aug 3, 2018. www.uptodate.com/contents/tetanus. Accessed Sep 20, 2018.

Tethered Cord Syndrome

Epidemiology and Demographics: This disease is usually seen in the pediatric setting but occasionally can also present in adult medical settings. This is a relatively rare disease in the general public.

Disorder Description: The disease is caused by overstretch of the spinal cord and conus. It may relate to intrinsic causes such as growth spurts or pregnancy. Extrinsic causes include injuries.

Patients may present with sensory loss in a dermatomal distribution, loss of reflexes, decreased muscle bulk, lower extremity weakness, urinary incontinence, and lower back pain.

Symptoms

Localization site	Comment
Spinal cord	Altered gait, hyper/hyporeflexia, spasticity
Dorsal root ganglia	Poor sensation or proprioception
Conus medullaris	Urinary incontinence, urgency, frequency, recurrent urinary tract infections
Muscle	Muscular atrophy
Other	Cutaneous lesions, including midline hairy patches, hemangiomas, dermal pits/sinuses, hypertrichosis, subcutaneous lipoma, cigarette burns, lumbosacral appendage and nevi Painless ulcerations of the feet or legs

Secondary Complications: If it manifests early enough, patients may have difficulty meeting milestones during development.

Treatment Complications: Surgical release may cause retethering, blood loss, dural tears, or wound infection.

Bibliography

Jalai CM. Trends in the presentation, surgical treatment, and outcomes of tethered cord syndrome: A nationwide study from 2001 to 2010. *J Clin Neurosci*. 2017;41:92–7. DOI: 10.1016/j.jocn.2017.03.034. Epub Mar 22, 2017.

Khoury C. Closed spinal dysraphism: clinical manifestations, diagnosis, and management UpToDate. Updated Sep 27, 2017. www.uptodate.com/contents/closed-spinal-dysraphism-clinical-manifestations-diagnosis-and-management. Accessed Sep 20, 2018.

O'Neill BR. Use of magnetic resonance imaging to detect occult spinal dysraphism in infants. *J Neurosurg Pediatr*. 2017;19(2):217–26.

White JT. Systematic review of urologic outcomes from tethered cord release in occult spinal dysraphism in children. *Curr Urol Rep*. 2015;16 (11):78. DOI: 10.1007/s11934-015-0550-6.

Thiamine Deficiency

Epidemiology and Demographics: Thiamine deficiency is usually seen as a part of generalized malnutrition. In eastern countries, thiamine deficiency is seen in people eating polished rice (loss of thiamine). In western countries, thiamine deficiency is usually seen in alcoholics. However, conditions such as hyperemesis, starvation, renal dialysis, cancer, AIDS, or gastric surgery also increase the risk of thiamine deficiency either due to poor intake or absorption.[1] Treatment with thiazide diuretics also increases the risk of thiamine deficiency as they increase urinary loss.

Disorder Description: Thiamine deficiency causes beriberi (infantile and adult) and Wernicke–Korsakoff syndrome (see entry for *Wernicke's Disease*).

Infantile beriberi usually presents around age 2–3 months. It presents as severe shortness of breath, cyanosis, cardiomegaly, and heart failure.[2] Neurologic manifestations include aspetic meningitis and seizure.[3] Infants who initially present with apnea or seizures are found to have moderate or severe intellectual disability or epilepsy later in life.[4,5]

Adult beriberi is further divided into dry beriberi and wet beriberi:

Dry beriberi is the term used to describe neurologic manifestation. Symptoms begin with burning pain or mild sensory loss in feet. Over time patient develops length-dependent sensory motor neuropathy. With thiamine replacement, improvement of neurologic symptoms is variable.[1]

Wet beriberi is the term used to describe cardiac manifestation (edema). It is characterized by tachycardia, anemia, and high-output cardiac failure. A possible mechanism for heart failure is reduced peripheral vascular resistance. Thiamine replacement therapy results in marked improvement in heart failure in 12–48 hours.[1]

Symptoms

Localization site	Comment
Mental status and psychiatric aspects/ complications	Disorientation
	Delirium related to ethanol withdrawal
	If the disease is not treated, stupor, coma, and death may ensue
Cerebellum (anterior and superior vermis)	Ataxia

Localization site	Comment
Vestibular system (and non-specific dizziness)	Ataxia
Cranial nerves	Horizontal nystagmus on lateral gaze
	Lateral rectus palsy (usually bilateral)
	Conjugate gaze palsies
	Rarely amblyopia
	Rarely ptosis and miosis
Peripheral neuropathy	Sensory motor peripheral neuropathy
	Autonomic neuropathy

Secondary Complications: Tachycardia and postural hypotension may be related to impaired function of the autonomic nervous system or to the coexistence of cardiovascular beriberi.[1]

Treatment Complications: Immediate administration of high dose of thiamine is used. The dose should be given prior to treatment with intravenous glucose solutions. Glucose infusions may precipitate Wernicke's disease by depleting thiamine stores in a previously unaffected patient or cause a rapid worsening of an early form of the disease. For this reason, thiamine should be administered to all alcoholic patients requiring parenteral glucose.[6,7] Thiamine toxicity syndrome has not been described.

References

1. Kasper DL, Fauci AS, Hauser SL, et al., eds. *Harrison's principles of internal medicine*. 19th ed. New York: McGraw-Hill Education/Medical; 2015.
2. Chaitiraphan S, Tanphaichitr V, Cheng TO. Nutritional heart disease. In Cheng TO, ed. *The international textbook of cardiology*. New York: Pergamon Press; 1986. p .864.
3. Tanphaichitr V. Epidemiology and clinical assessment of vitamin deficiencies in Thai children. In Eeckels RE, Ransome-Kuti O, Kroonenberg CC, eds. *Child health in the tropics*. Dordrecht: Martinus Nijhoff; 1985. p. 157.
4. Fattal-Valevski A, Bloch-Mimouni A, Kivity S, et al. Epilepsy in children with infantile thiamine deficiency. *Neurology*. 2009;73:828.

5. Mimouni-Bloch A, Goldberg-Stern H, Strausberg R, et al. Thiamine deficiency in infancy: long-term follow-up. *Pediatr Neurol*. 2014;51:311.

6. Galvin R, Bråthen G, Ivashynka A, et al. EFNS guidelines for diagnosis, therapy and prevention of Wernicke encephalopathy. *Eur J Neurol*. 2010;17:1408.

7. Malamud N, Skillicorn SA. Relationship between the Wernicke and the Korsakoff syndrome: a clinicopathologic study of seventy cases. *Arch Neurol Psychiat*. 1956;76:586.

Third Ventricle Tumors

Epidemiology and Demographics: Third ventricle tumors represent a rare and heterogeneous group of lesions, varying widely with respect to presentation. There is no clear pattern of sex or geographic predominance in these tumors but they tend to differ dramatically in etiology and clinical presentation based on the age of the patient. In pediatric patients, the tumors are often congenital and present early in life with symptoms related to mass effect or obstruction. They may be associated with an underlying genetic disorder such as neurofibromatosis type 1 or tuberous sclerosis. In adults, tumors may be either acquired or congenital and often remain asymptomatic until incidental discovery later in life. With the exception of colloid cysts and craniopharyngiomas, which each compromise approximately 1–2% of all primary brain tumors, third ventricle tumors are relatively infrequent in the general population.

Disorder Description: Purely intraventricular tumors are rare and when seen typically represent tumors of the choroid plexus. In pediatric patients, these include choroid plexus papillomas and carcinomas whereas in adults they include choroid gliomas and central neurocytomas. More often, third ventricle tumors arise from the walls of the ventricle or from direct extension or seeding from an ectopic site. Third ventricle tumors are thus best broadly categorized based on the location in which they develop within the ventricle.

When tumors arise in the anterior recesses of the ventricle, they are classically sellar–suprasellar or hypothalamic–chiasmatic in origin. In pediatric patients, these include craniopharyngiomas, germinomas, and pilocytic astrocytomas as seen in neurofibromatosis type 1. In adults, these include craniopharyngiomas, lymphoma, pituitary macroadenomas, metastases, and sellar meningiomas.

Tumors of the posterior aspect of the third ventricle are far more common in pediatric patients and often represent extension from the pineal gland, midbrain, or thalamus. They include germinomas, pinealocytomas/blastomas, teratomas, and much rarer glial tumors.

Certain third ventricle tumors characteristically arise at the interventricular foramen. In adults, these commonly represent benign colloid cysts or subependymomas whereas in children, they are caused by subependymal giant cell astrocytomas in association with tuberous sclerosis complex.

Finally, tumors coming up from the floor of the third ventricle are among some of the least common third ventricle tumors and are most frequently caused by hypothalamic hamartomas.

Symptoms

Localization site	Comment
Pituitary gland	Dysfunction of the hypothalamic–pituitary gland axis may result from direct invasion and compression of the sella from tumors in the anterior aspect of the third ventricle and result in diabetes insipidus, adrenal insufficiency, hypothyroidism, hypogonadism, growth retardation, and/or hyperprolactinemia
	Pituitary apoplexy results from local disruption of the arterial blood supply to the pituitary gland and may present acutely as headache, visual loss, diplopia, and altered mentation (rare)
Brainstem	Parinaud syndrome of vertical gaze paresis, pupillary light-near dissociation, and convergence–retraction nystagmus may result from compression of the dorsal midbrain from tumors at the posterior wall of the third ventricle (rare)
Hypothalamus	Tumors arising from the floor of the third ventricle may compress the hypothalamus and result in gelastic epilepsy (uncontrolled laughing seizures) and precocious puberty
Cranial nerves	Hemianopia and diminished visual acuity may stem from anterior extension of third ventricle tumors resulting in compression of the optic chiasm and optic nerves

Localization site	Comment
Mental status and psychiatric aspects/ complications	Non-communicating hydrocephalus can result from an obstructing tumor at any site within the third ventricle but most often is seen in intraventricular tumors or those at the interventricular foramen. Symptoms are nonspecific and include paroxysmal headaches, nausea, vomiting, blurred vision, lethargy, cognitive decline, or behavioral change (irritability, apathy, aggressiveness). Rarely, drop attacks and sudden death can occur
	In pediatric patients, hydrocephalus can present as developmental delay or failure to thrive with macrocephaly

Secondary Complications: Spontaneous intraventricular hemorrhage from third ventricle tumors is a rare but potentially fatal complication due to the high risk of rapidly developing hydrocephalus causing sudden death.

Treatment Complications: Treatment varies widely based on the size, location, and pathology of the tumor. Smaller, benign lesions such as colloid cysts that are not deemed to be at high risk for obstruction can be observed without intervention. Tumors presenting with or at high risk for hydrocephalus often require cerebral shunting, which has numerous potential complications including shunt infection, obstruction, over drainage, or intraventricular hemorrhage. Surgical or endoscopic resection may be warranted in larger, malignant, or rapidly expanding tumors and depending on the approach, several complications may occur. The most common complications are post-operative seizures, intraventricular hemorrhage, CSF leak, venous infarct, or subdural hematoma. Injury to local structures such as the corpus callosum, fornix, and hypothalamus may also occur during surgery resulting in disconnection syndromes, memory impairment, and disturbance of circadian rhythm and core body temperature, respectively.

Bibliography

Diebler C, Dulac O. *Pediatric neurology and neuroradiology: cerebral and cranial diseases.* Berlin/Heidelberg: Springer Berlin Heidelberg; 1987.

Glastonbury CM, Osborn AG, Salzman KL. Masses and malformations of the third ventricle: normal anatomic relationships and differential diagnoses. *Radiographics.* 2011;31(7):1889–905.

Horn EM, Feiz-Erfan I, Bristol RE, et al. Treatment options for third ventricular colloid cysts: comparison of open microsurgical versus endoscopic resection. *Neurosurgery.* 2007;60(4): 613–8; discussion 618–20.

Schiff D, Hsu L, Wen PY. Uncommon brain tumors, skull base tumors, and intracranial cysts. In Samuels M, Feske S, eds. *Office practice of neurology,* 2nd ed. New York: Churchill Livingstone; 2003. p. 1092.

Thoracic Outlet Syndrome (Neurogenic)

Epidemiology and Demographics: As per the listed references, the disease is found more commonly in 20- to 50-year-old females. Occasionally it may present in the pediatric patient.

Disorder Description: Pressure is applied on the nerve bundle above the first rib and behind the clavicle. It may mimic ulnar neuropathy and cervical radiculopathy.

	Thoracic outlet syndrome	Ulnar neuropathy	C8–T1 radiculopathy
Exam		Pain with palpation to the elbow	Pain that radiates down the arm with certain neck maneuvers
Thumb	Thumb abduction is particularly affected	Thumb abduction spared	Thumb abduction may be weak but is as affected as the other C8–T1 innervated muscles
Sensory	Medial forearm	4th and 5th fingers and medial hand	Medial forearm

Symptoms

Localization site	Comment
Plexus	Aching pain, numbness, tingling, weakness in upper extremity in the distribution of the brachial plexus
Mental status and psychiatric aspects/complications	Anxiety and depression from chronic pain

Secondary Complications: Complications include progressive weakness, disabling pain, and paresthesia.

Treatment Complications: Surgical complications include infection, further injury, and recurrence of symptoms.

Bibliography

Brazis PW, et al., eds. Peripheral nerves. In *Localization in clinical neurology*. 6th ed. Philadelphia, PA: Lippincott Williams and Wilkins; 2011. Chapter 2.

Klaassen Z, Sorenson E, Tubbs RS, et al. Thoracic outlet syndrome: A neurological and vascular disorder. *Clin Anat*. 2014;27:724–32. DOI:10.1002/ca.22271.

Köknel Talu G. Thoracic outlet syndrome. *Agri*. 2005;17(2):5–9.

Makhoul RG, Machleder HI. Developmental anomalies at the thoracic outlet: an analysis of 200 consecutive cases. *J Vasc Surg*. 1992:16(4):534.

Thrombocytopenia

Epidemiology and Demographics: Depends on population – in critically ill patients, as many as 40–50% of patients have thrombocytopenia.

Disorder Description: Defined as platelet count less than 150,000/µL, thrombocytopenia can occur from decreased bone marrow production, platelet destruction, consumption, dilution, or sequestration. Decreased platelet counts are associated with hemorrhage, particularly mucosal bleeding. The risk of bleeding is associated not only with absolute platelet number but also with procedure under consideration (such as vascular surgery vs lumbar puncture), quality of circulating platelets, and concurrent coagulopathy (such as in disseminated intravascular coagulation).[1]

Symptoms

Localization site	Comment
Cerebral hemispheres	Particularly with severe thrombocytopenia (<10,000 platelets/µL; disorders with abnormal platelet function may have bleeding at higher absolute numbers), risk of intracranial hemorrhage including lobar, basal ganglia, cerebellar, subdural, and subarachnoid hemorrhages.[2] Can have multiple simultaneous hemorrhages
Mental status and psychiatric aspects/ complications	Intracranial hemorrhages can present as confusion with somnolence or agitation

Secondary Complications: There are often multiple systemic hemorrhages. Thrombocytopenia predisposes to mucocutaneous bleeding.

Treatment Complications: Platelet transfusions carry risk of infection, alloimmunization, allergic reaction, and transfusion-associated reaction. Relationship between dose of prophylactic transfusion and prevention of hemorrhage remains unclear.[3]

References

1. Slichter SJ. Relationship between platelet count and bleeding risk in thrombocytopenic patients. *Transfus Med Rev*. 2004;18:153–67.

2. González-Duarte A, García-Ramos GS, Valdés-Ferrer SI, Cantú-Brito C. Clinical description of intracranial haemorrhage associated with bleeding disorders. *J Stroke Cerebrovasc Dis Off J Natl Stroke Assoc*. 2008;17:204–7.

3. Slichter SJ, Kaufman RM, Assmann SF, et al. Dose of prophylactic platelet transfusions and prevention of haemorrhage. *N Engl J Med*. 2010;362:600–13.

Thrombophilia

Epidemiology and Demographics: Thrombophilias present in >10% of those with venous sinus thrombosis are associated with antiphospholipid antibodies, prothrombin G20210A heterozygosity, Factor V Leiden, and hyperhomocysteinemia.[1]

Disorder Description: A collection of inherited and acquired disorders that increase the risk of thrombosis. For the inherited thrombophilias, the clearest association is with venous thrombosis (including cerebral venous sinus thrombosis) and thromboembolism rather than ischemic stroke.[2] Antiphospholipid antibodies (anti-cardiolipin IgG/IgM, lupus anticoagulant, anti-β2-glycoprotein I IgG/IgM) are associated with both venous and arterial thrombosis.

Symptoms

Localization site	Comment
Cerebral hemispheres	Inherited and acquired thrombophilias are associated with venous sinus thrombosis, which can have focal or diffuse effects (such as by increased intracranial pressure). Arterial ischemic stroke with antiphospholipid antibodies can present as a large-vessel or small-vessel stroke

Secondary Complications: Systemic venous thrombosis and thromboembolism.

Treatment Complications: Anticoagulation, often used long term for treatment of thrombophilia, increases risk of hemorrhage.

References

1. Martinelli I, Passamonti SM, Bucciarelli P. Thrombophilic states. *Handb Clin Neurol.* 2014;120:1061–71.
2. Pahus SH, Hansen AT, Hvas A-M. Thrombophilia testing in young patients with ischemic stroke. *Thromb Res.* 2016;137:108–12.

Thrombotic Thrombocytopenic Purpura (TTP)

Epidemiology and Demographics: Acquired thrombotic thrombocytopenic purpura (TTP) occurs at a rate of 3 per million, usually in adults. Hereditary TTP is very rare, accounting for <5% of cases of TTP. It is more common in women and those of African descent.

Disorder Description: TTP (Moschcowitz syndrome or thrombocytic acroangiothrombosis) is a thrombotic microangiopathy characterized classically by the pentad of microangiopathic hemolytic anemia, thrombocytopenia, fever, renal insufficiency, and neurologic dysfunction. The full presentation is *uncommon* in current times, and most common presenting symptoms are headache/confusion (60%), abdominal discomfort (50%), fever (20%), bleeding (20%), and renal failure (5%).[1] Thrombocytopenia and anemia are present in >80%.

TTP is caused by severe ADAMTS13 (a disintegrin and metalloproteinase with a thrombospondin type 1 motif, member 13) enzymatic deficiency typically because of autoantibody directed against the protein. Autoantibody formation can occur in the context of other autoimmune disorders, infections, drug reactions, or malignancy. In hereditary cases, there is an inherited mutation in the *ADAMTS13* gene. ADAMTS13 protein is a metalloproteinase that cleaves von Willebrand Factor. In its absence, platelets excessively aggregate, leading to microangiopathic occlusions and platelet consumption. This disorder is usually acquired but is rarely genetic.

The acquired cases may be primary or secondary due to malignancy, infection, bone marrow transplantation, pregnancy (especially HELLP syndrome), and medications (e.g., ticlidopine, clopidogrel, acyclovir, quinine, cyclosporine).

Symptoms

Localization site	Comment
Cerebral hemispheres	Diffuse involvement of cortical and subcortical gray and white matter causing ischemic (often lacunar) and hemorrhagic infarcts. On MR imaging, some lesions can be reversible. Imaging can also be consistent with posterior reversible encephalopathy syndrome (PRES).[2] Hallucinations, confusion, delirium may occur
Brainstem	Stroke as per above
Cerebellum	Stroke as per above
Mental status and psychiatric aspects/ complications	Causes an acute confusional state with frequently decreased consciousness. There can be concurrent seizures or more focal findings including hemiparesis, hemisensory deficit, aphasia or ataxia[3]

Secondary Complications: There is a risk of systemic bleeding from microvascular injury and thrombocytopenia. Gastrointestinal symptoms including nausea, vomiting, and diarrhea are frequently seen. Kidney failure is infrequent in TTP.

Treatment Complications: Treatment with plasma exchange requires a large bore central venous catheter with associated infectious, hypotensive, or venous thrombotic risk. Plasma exchange also uses infusion of donor plasma.

References

1. Veyradier A, Meyer D. Thrombotic thrombocytopenic purpura and its diagnosis. *J Thromb Haemost JTH.* 2005;3:2420–7.
2. Bakshi R, Shaikh ZA, Bates VE, Kinkel PR. Thrombotic thrombocytopenic purpura: brain CT and MRI findings in 12 patients. *Neurology.* 1999;52:1285–8.
3. Adams RD, Cammermeyer J, Fitzgerald PJ. The neuropathological aspects of thrombocytic acroangiothrombosis; a clinico-anatomical study of generalized platelet thrombosis. *J Neurol Neurosurg Psychiatry.* 1948;11:27–43.

Suggested Reading

Kessler CS, Khan BA, Lai-Miller K. Thrombotic thrombocytopenic purpura: a hematological emergency. *J Emerg Med*. 2012;43(3):538–44.

Osborn JD, Rodgers GM. Update on thrombotic thrombocytopenic purpura. *Clin Adv Hematol Oncol*. 2011;9(7):531–6.

Thunderclap Headache

Epidemiology and Demographics: The incidence of this condition is unknown as there are multiple etiologies for this presentation. One study reports an incidence of 43/100,000 adults annually. Another case report examining patients in an emergency room showed an incidence of 120/8000 patients.

Disorder Description: A severe type of headache that is sudden in nature and reaches peak, maximum severity within 1 minute. In any presentation of this type of headache, the diagnosis of primary thunderclap headache is one of exclusion. Consideration should be made for subarachnoid hemorrhage, sentinel headache, reversible cerebral vasoconstriction syndrome, arterial dissection, cerebral venous sinus thrombosis, pituitary apoplexy, intracranial hemorrhage, ischemic stroke, reversible posterior leukoencephalopathy, spontaneous intracranial hypotension, colloid cyst, and intracranial infections. CT head, lumbar puncture, and MRI of brain are diagnostic tools that can help differentiate possible etiologies.

Symptoms

Localization site	Comment
Cerebral hemispheres	Involves mostly cerebral hemispheres on either side or bilaterally. The presence of rupture aneurysm, colloid cysts, intracranial abscess, tumors, venous thrombosis can occur anywhere here
Cranial nerves	Depending on location of etiology of thunderclap headache symptom, focal deficits can be seen on cranial nerve exam
Pituitary gland	Pituitary apoplexy is one condition that can present as thunderclap headache

Secondary Complications: Complications from this condition can occur if an etiology is not detected properly. A diagnosis of primary thunderclap headache is of exclusion after extensive imaging, other diagnostic tests, and a thorough history is obtained from the patient.

Treatment Complications: Abortive therapies for thunderclap headaches are similar to those of migraine headaches. However, these therapies should be considered once other possible etiologies are excluded.

Bibliography

Dilli E. Thunderclap headache. *Curr Neurol Neurosci Rep*. 2014;14:437.

Ducros A, Bousser MG. Thunderclap headache. *BMJ*. 2013;8(346):e8557.

Landtblom AM, et al. Sudden onset headache: a prospective study of features, incidence and causes. *Cephalalgia*. 2002;22(5):354–60.

Thyroid Ophthalmopathy

Epidemiology and Demographics: Approximately 20–25% of patients with Grave's disease may have clinically evident ophthalmopathy. The condition is more common in women than men.[1] Cigarette smoking has been confirmed as a risk factor as is autoimmune disease.[2]

Disorder Description: The pathogenesis is understood to be due to increase in the volume of extraocular muscles and retroorbital connective and adipose tissue due to the accumulation of hydrophilic glycosaminoglycans (GAG), which causes a change in osmotic pressure leading to fluid accumulation, muscle swelling, and increase in pressure within the orbit.[1,3]

Symptoms

Localization site	Comment
Cranial nerves	Impairment of extraocular muscles. Diplopia and occasionally vision loss due to severe proptosis

References

1. Burch HB, Wartofsky L. Graves' ophthalmopathy: current concepts regarding pathogenesis and management. *Endocr Rev*. 1993;14:747.

2. Prummel MF, Wiersinga WM. Smoking and risk of Graves' disease. *JAMA*. 1993;269:479.

3. Bahn RS. Graves' ophthalmopathy. *N Engl J Med*. 2010;362:726.

Thyrotoxic Periodic Paralysis

Epidemiology and Demographics: Mainly seen in the Asian population, affecting mostly men.[1] The incidence is believed to be 2% in Asian countries compared with an incidence of 0.1–0.2% in non-Asian countries.[2] Age of onset is generally between 20 and 39 years of age.[3]

Disorder Description: Seen in patients with thyrotoxicosis; increased Na–K ATPase activity is believed to result in severe hypokalemia, which can lead to an acute onset of profound proximal muscle weakness that may progress to paralysis.[2] It is associated with episodic weakness, and it carries the risk of involving respiratory muscles.

Symptoms

Localization site	Comment
Muscle	Weakness proximal > distal. Myalgias. Hyporeflexia/areflexia is common although reflexes may be preserved or increased on occasion. Rarely bulbar weakness

Secondary Complications: Symptoms associated with hyperthyroidism (see entry for *Hyperthyroidism*).

Treatment Complications: Treatments may include potassium orally or emergently through intravenous route. Overshooting may itself result in generalized muscle weakness. A low carbohydrate and low sodium diet may reduce frequency of attacks. Beta-blockers may be used temporarily to attenuate symptoms of hyperthyroidism, and these agents may induce fatigue, generalized weakness, and depression. Treatment of the thyroid gland may be indicated (see entry for *Hyperthyroidism*).

References

1. Lam L, Nair RJ, Tingle L. Thyrotoxic periodic paralysis. *Proc (Bayl Univ Med Cent)*. 2006;19(2):126–9.
2. Lin S-H, Huang C-L. Mechanism of thyrotoxic periodic paralysis. *J Am Soc Nephrol*. 2012;23(6):985–8. DOI:10.1681/ASN.2012010046.
3. Wong P. Hypokalemic thyrotoxic periodic paralysis: a case series. *CJEM* 2003;5:353.

Suggested Reading

Hsieh MJ, Lyu RK, Chang WN, et al. Hypokalemic thyrotoxic periodic paralysis: clinical characteristics and predictors of recurrent paralytic attacks. *Eur J Neurol*. 2008;15:559.

Manoukian MA, Foote JA, Crapo LM. Clinical and metabolic features of thyrotoxic periodic paralysis in 24 episodes. *Arch Intern Med*. 1999;159:601.

Tic Disorders and Gilles de la Tourette Syndrome (Tourette's)

Epidemiology and Demographics: Tic disorders are pediatric illnesses. Adult onset tics are uncommon and are usually secondary to a trauma, encephalitis, or lesion, or are found as an incidental finding in the setting of other neuropsychiatric disease (e.g., Huntington's). Reports of idiopathic tics in adults are rare and, of those, most are discovered to be recurrences of childhood tic disorders. The average ages of onset for motor tics and verbal tics are 7 and 11 years old, respectively. Symptoms tend to decrease in adulthood. The adult incidence of Tourette's is only 0.05%.

Overall prevalence figures vary based on the tic disorder in question. Combined prevalence is 2.82% (4.27% male, 1.78% female). Provisional tic disorder (formerly transient tic disorder) is the most common form of tic disorder and has an incidence of 2.99%. (Despite a slightly higher prevalence in males, gender differences were not statistically significant.)

Persistent (chronic) tic disorder has an incidence of 1.61% (no significant gender discrepancy). There was a 0.69% prevalence of the vocal-only subtype and a 1.65% prevalence of the motor-only subtype.

Tourette syndrome is the most severe of the three defined tic disorders and has an overall incidence of 0.85% in mainstream school populations. Tourette's rates also differ between genders (1.06% in males and 0.25% in females).

Tic disorders occur in higher frequency in special education populations and particularly among children with autism spectrum disorders (prevalence: Tourette's 4.8% and chronic tic disorder 9.0%).

Tourette syndrome is found at similar rates worldwide, except within the Sub-Saharan black African population (where it appears to be absent) and in Afro-Caribbeans, African-Americans, and American Hispanic people (where rates are far lower). This may be a result of sampling bias and cultural effects on reporting rates.

Disorder Description: Tics are fast, sudden, stereotyped, non-rhythmic, suppressible motor movements or vocalizations. While tics may change over time they tend to maintain near identical patterns of movement or speech for an extended period. Motor tics can be simple short single motion movements (eye blink, shoulder shrug) or complex complete behaviors. Vocal or phonic tics can range from throat clearing to speech. Though obscene speech and behaviors (coprolalia and copropraxia) are commonly associated with tic disorders, these symptoms are actually relatively rare. Tics generally first present in young children and peak in severity in the immediate prepubertal period. Tic disorders can be divided up into three main conditions (and two diagnoses for specified and unspecified tic disorders that do not meet criteria for the other three labels). The disorders are hierarchical, with Tourette's as the most severe. If a more severe diagnosis is suggested, a lesser one may not be used. In all cases, the patient must be under 18 years at age of onset and the tics may not be caused by use of any substance or an underlying medical condition.

The disorders are differentiated as follows: Provisional tic disorder has a duration of symptoms of less than 1 year. Persistent (chronic) tic disorder may be either motor OR vocal tic dependent but not both. It must persist for at least 12 months. Finally, Tourette's is characterized by history of both motor and physical tics lasting at least 1 year. The remaining two classifications, other specified and unspecified tic disorder, allow a clinician to still diagnose a tic disorder in cases that don't technically meet the diagnostic requirements.

While not causative of the disorder, certain factors are exacerbatory. They include stress, excitation or exhaustion, maternal smoking in the prenatal period, low birth weight, elderly paternal age at conception and, in the case of Tourette's, a number of specific risk-factor alleles. Tourette's and various tic disorders can, in rare instances, run in families.

Some research supports a connection with 'Pediatric Autoimmune Neuropsychiatric Disorder Associated with Streptococcus' or PANDAS. This condition is associated with development of tics or chorea-like movements and obsessive-compulsive disorder (OCD). This condition is similar to Sydenham chorea but lacks the rheumatic fever related complications. While research on PANDAS is mounting, it is not a ubiquitously accepted condition or etiology and remains a controversial topic.

Tic disorders often present with a range of neuropsychiatric and behavioral concerns. In children, comorbid conditions include attention deficit hyperactivity disorder (ADHD), OCD, and autism spectrum disorder.

In adolescents and adults, comorbid conditions include the aforementioned conditions as well as migraine headache, substance use disorder, and mood disorders such as depression and bipolar disorder. The frequency of comorbidity increases with the severity of the tic disorder (80%–90% of Tourette's patients have non-tic complaints). That said, even mild tics are associated with these conditions.

Tics are thought of as involuntary movements. However, many patients describe some degree of volition and describe the tic as a movement or sound made to satisfy *premonitory urges*. While tics are suppressible, the premonitory urge will often persist until the proper execution of the stereotyped behavior. These sensory tics occur in 90% of patients. This phenomenon appears to be pathognomonic for tic disorders and is not associated with other movement disorders. Because of the frequent comorbidity with OCD, it is often difficult to differentiate complex tics from compulsions.

While tics in general can have many etiologies, primary idiopathic tic disorders present as heterogeneous neuropsychiatric conditions with a plethora of comorbidities. With early intervention, the patient can develop better control of their tics and avoid many of the negative scholastic and social consequences often associated with the condition. Though in most cases the tics are self-limiting with increased age, many of the associated conditions are lifelong disorders in need of treatment.

Symptoms

Localization site	Comment
Cerebral hemispheres	Violent tics may result in vertebral artery occlusion and stroke or concussive cerebral damage
	Deficiency in sensory–motor planning (e.g., increased reactive grip force)
	Decreased motor learning (long-term potentiation and depression of primary motor cortex)
	Decreased volume in pre- and post-central gyrus and caudate nucleus

Localization site	Comment
Mental status and psychiatric aspects/complications	Associated with: depression, anxiety, obsessivity, mildly decreased IQ, ADHD, OCD, substance use disorder, bipolar disorder, and self-injurious behavior
	In addition to coprolalia and copropraxia patients also often display non-obscene, socially inappropriate behavior
Brainstem	Decreased plasticity/habituation of blink-reflex circuit
Cerebellum	Some evidence of dysrhythmia during tics
Spinal cord	Violent tics may cause radiculopathy and myelopathy (particularly in the cervical region)
Unclear localization	Deficient selective-attention (abnormal N1, event-related potential)

Secondary Complications: There have been reports of compressive neuropathy, myelopathy, fractures, and pain associated with violent tics and cerebral damage secondary to head-banging. Additionally, there are cases of vertebral artery occlusion leading to stroke.

Treatment Complications: Mild cases are left untreated or may be treated with behavioral therapy (such as comprehensive behavioral intervention for tics, CBIT).

For patients with severe impairment, pharmaceutical intervention may be warranted. Medication options include anti-psychotics (haloperidol, pimozide), atypical neuroleptics, and α2-agonists.

Central nervous system effects with these drugs include tardive dyskinesia, depression, anxiety, sedation, cognitive blunting, and drug-induced parkinsonism. Physicians should also be on the look out for peripheral effects of these drugs such as dry mouth and hypotension.

Additionally, treatment of comorbid conditions (e.g., ADHD or OCD) may come with a host of other complications and symptoms.

Bibliography

American Psychiatric Association. *Diagnostic and statistical manual of mental disorders: DSM-5*. 5th ed. Washington, DC: American Psychiatric Association; 2013.

Berg D, Steinberger JD, Olanow CW, Naidich TP, Yousry TA. Milestones in magnetic resonance imaging and transcranial sonography of movement disorders. *Mov Disord*. 2011;26(6):979–92.

Chouinard S, Ford B. Adult onset tic disorders. *J Neurol Neurosurg Psychiatry*. 2000;68(6):738–43.

Knight T, Steeves T, Day L, et al. Prevalence of tic disorders: a systematic review and meta-analysis. *Pediatr Neurol*. 2012;47(2):77–90.

Kwak C, Dat Vuong K, Jankovic J. Premonitory sensory phenomenon in Tourette's syndrome. *Mov Disord*. 2003;18:1530–33.

Lehman LL, Gilbert DL, Leach JL, Wu SW, Standridge SM. Vertebral artery dissection leading to stroke caused by violent neck tics of Tourette syndrome. *Neurology*. 2011;77(18):1706–8.

Plessen KJ, Bansal R, Peterson BS. Imaging evidence for anatomical disturbances and neuroplastic compensation in persons with Tourette syndrome. *J Psychosomat Res*. 2009;67:559–73.

Robertson MM. A personal 35 year perspective on Gilles de la Tourette syndrome: prevalence, phenomenology, comorbidities, and coexistent psychopathologies. *Lancet Psychiatr*. 2015:2: 68–87.

Robertson MM. A personal 35 year perspective on Gilles de la Tourette syndrome: assessment, investigations, and management. *Lancet Psychiatry*. 2015;2:88–104.

Suppa A, Marsili L, Di Stasio F, et al. Cortical and brainstem plasticity in Tourette syndrome and obsessive-compulsive disorder. *Mov Disord*. 2014;29(12):1523–31.

Swedo SE, Leckman JF, Rose NR. From research subgroup to clinical syndrome: modifying the PANDAS criteria to describe PANS (pediatric acute-onset neuropsychiatric syndrome). *Pediatr Therapeut*. 2012;2:113.

Wang Z, Maia TV, Marsh R, et al. The neural circuits that generate tics in Tourette's syndrome. *Am J Psychiatry*. 2011;168(12):1326–37.

Tick Paralysis

Epidemiology and Demographics: As summarized by Diaz, in North America, the symptoms usually present in the early spring, and the literature documents more cases in prepubescent girls although cases in both sexes and all ages have been reported.

Disorder Description: The tick species responsible in North America is *Dermacentor andersoni*. The tick must bite for a few hours before releasing the toxin. Initially the patient may feel generalized fatigue. Then she or he may experience motor dysfunction that begins in distal lower extremities. There may be gait unsteadiness. Facial droop is a common finding.

Symptoms

Localization site	Comment
Neuromuscular junction	Motor symptoms as described above

Secondary Complications: The area bitten by the tick may become infected.

Treatment Complications: If the patient's symptoms are severe enough to require intubation, the sedative medications required for intubation may cause changes in mental status. For prevention of the disease, N,N-diethyl-3-methylbenzamide (DEET) can be applied as insect repellant. However, it can rarely cause encephalopathy, especially in children.

Bibliography

Diaz JH. A comparative meta-analysis of tick paralysis in the United States and Australia. *ClinToxicol.* 2015;53(9):874–83.

Patterson SK, et al. Myasthenia gravis and other disorders of the neuromuscular junction. In Brust JCM, ed. *Current diagnosis and treatment: neurology.* 2nd ed. New York: McGraw-Hill; 2002. Chapter 22.

Ropper A, Samuels M. Disorders of the nervous system caused by drugs, toxins, and other chemical agents. In *Adams and Victor's principles of neurology.* 9th ed. New York: McGraw-Hill Education/Medical; 2009. Chapter 43.

Tobacco Use

Epidemiology and Demographics: No gender or race predilection.

Disorder Description: Nicotine derived from tobacco causes most symptoms. Patient usually experiences symptomatology of nicotine withdrawal 30 minutes after their last cigarette use. An individual will experience cravings, sleep disturbance, anxiety, and depressive symptoms, and variation in body temperature. Patients will experience these symptoms at their peak at 2–3 days.

Symptoms

Localization site	Comment
Cerebral hemispheres	Cortical atrophy (chronic)
Mental status and psychiatric aspects/complications	Codependency habits (chronic)
	Depression (chronic)
	Cognitive difficulties (chronic)
	Irritability (chronic)
Brainstem	Disruption of sleep–wake cycle (circadian rhythm) (chronic)
Pituitary gland	Hypothalamic–pituitary–adrenal (HPA) axis dysfunction
Peripheral neuropathy	Paresthesias (chronic)
Muscle	Myalgias (acute)
Neuromuscular junction	Dopamine production decreases, and sensitivity of acetylcholine receptors also decreases (chronic)

Treatment Complications: Varenicline is used as adjunct for people in assistance of quitting smoking. As a result of this treatment, there is a chance of increased suicide ideation in certain individuals. Nicotine replacement agent side effects include insomnia, irritability, headache, dizziness, or paresthesias. Bupropion used to facilitate stopping smoking may be associated with dose-related reduction of the seizure threshold.

Bibliography

Healthline. What is nicotine withdrawal? www
.healthline.com/health/smoking/nicotine-
withdrawal#Symptoms2. Accessed Sep 21, 2018.

Rettner R. Your brain on nicotine: smoking may thin
its outer layer. Live Science. Dec 3, 2010. Available
at www.livescience.com/35222-smoking-thin-
brain-cerebral-cortex-101202.html. Accessed Sep
21, 2018.

Tweed JO, Hsia SH, Lutfy K, Friedman TC. The
endocrine effects of nicotine and cigarette smoke.
Trend Endocrinol Metab. 2012;23(7):334–42.
DOI:10.1016/j.tem.2012.03.006.

Tolosa–Hunt Syndrome

Epidemiology and Demographics: Rare before the age of 20 years. Even distribution in all age groups after the age of 20. Typically occurs around 60 years of age. Affects males and females equally. No race predilection is known. Estimated incidence of one case per million per year.

Disorder Description: Tolosa–Hunt syndrome is a non-caseating granulomatous or nongranulomatous inflammatory process involving the cavernous sinus and superior orbital fissure. This condition causes painful ophthalmoplegia. The ophthalmoplegia is secondary to cranial nerve III, IV, and VI damage from inflammation. Pupillary involvement is often seen with inflammation of the sympathetic fibers around the cavernous portion of the internal carotid artery as well as the parasympathetic fibers that surround the oculomotor nerve. Furthermore, the oculomotor branch (V1) of the trigeminal nerve can also become affected causing sensory changes to the upper part of the face. This condition shares features with a similar disease process called idiopathic orbital pseudotumor. Tolosa–Hunt syndrome carries features similar to Gradenigo syndrome and thus should be differentiated in clinical practice.

The exact cause of this disease process is not known. Pathology demonstrates fibroblastic, lymphocytic, and plasmocytic infiltration of the cavernous sinus.

Recent viral infection is a risk factor.

No particular geographic proclivity is known.

Symptoms

Localization site	Comment
Cavernous sinus/superior orbital fissure	Cranial nerve II: optic nerve – optic disease, edema, obscured/blurred vision to loss of vision
	Cranial nerve III: oculomotor nerve – paralysis of superior, medial, and inferior recti and inferior oblique muscles
	Cranial nerve IV: trochlear nerve – paralysis of the superior oblique muscle
	Cranial nerve V1: ophthalmic branch of the trigeminal nerve – sensory loss to the upper part of the face; loss of ipsilateral corneal reflex
	Cranial nerve VI: abducens nerve – paralysis of lateral rectus muscle
	Sympathetic fibers traveling with internal carotid artery: loss of pupillary light reflex; Horner's syndrome
	Parasympathetic fibers traveling with cranial nerve III: loss of pupillary light reflex
Cerebellopontine angle (rarely)	Hearing loss or diminished hearing ipsilateral to the lesion, wide-based gait, tinnitus, ataxia
Cranial nerve VII: facial nerve (rarely)	Paralysis of facial muscles ipsilateral to the lesion

Secondary Complications

Vision loss
Hearing loss (rarely)
Facial paralysis (rarely)

Treatment Complications

Corticosteroids: Increased risk of infection, hyperglycemia, avascular necrosis of the hip, psychosis, Cushing's disease.

Immunosuppressants: Hematopoietic complications with methotrexate are seen in patients not supplemented with folic acid. Furthermore, medications such as azathioprine and methotrexate are teratogenic and hence careful avoidance of such drugs during pregnancy is advised.

Radiation therapy: Hair loss, fatigue, weakness, skin reaction (itching, blistering, and peeling), dry mouth, mouth sores, jaw stiffness, nausea, lymphedema, tooth decay.

Bibliography

Kline LB, Hoyt WF. The Tolosa-Hunt syndrome. *J Neurol Neurosurg Psychiatry* 2001;71:577.

La Mantia L, Curone M, Rapoport AM, Bussone G, International Headache Society. Tolosa-Hunt syndrome: critical literature review based on IHS 2004 criteria. *Cephalalgia*. 2006;26(7): 772–81.

Tonic Pupil (Large Pupil)

Tonic pupil, Adie's pupil, large pupil, mydriasis, poorly constricting pupil

Epidemiology and Demographics: Large pupils can occur in all races/ethnicities of either sex at any age.

Disorder Description: This entry addresses abnormally large pupils due to efferent dysfunction. This is distinct from pupils that are poorly reactive to light due to dysfunction of the afferent visual pathway (see entry for *Afferent Pupillary Defect*). Unilateral abnormally large pupils are apparent on exam as anisocoria, that is, greater in light compared with dark environments. When the disorder is bilateral, findings can include large pupils that are poorly reactive to light that are not accounted for by poor vision.

Symptoms

Localization site	Comment
Cerebral hemispheres	Benign episodic mydriasis is associated with migraine. Bilateral and unilateral mydriasis are rarely associated with seizure and postictal states
Brainstem	Dorsal midbrain (Parinaud or pretectal) syndrome can include large pupils that are poorly reactive to light, but with intact accommodation (i.e., constriction to a near stimulus). Associated signs include eyelid retraction, limited upgaze, and convergence–retraction "nystagmus"

Localization site	Comment
Cranial nerves	Cranial nerve III palsy causes a large pupil in association with ipsilateral ptosis, upgaze, downgaze, and adduction eye movement deficits. In the case of compressive lesions pupillary dilation can occur prior to development of other signs
	Isolated dysfunction of the ciliary ganglion or short ciliary nerves in the orbit can cause a tonic pupil, which reacts poorly to light, but typically has intact accommodation (i.e., constricts to a near stimulus) with slow redilation. Slit lamp findings include segmental paralysis of the iris with vermiform or "wormlike" iris movements
Dorsal root ganglia	Holmes–Adie syndrome is comprised of tonic pupils and loss of peripheral reflexes, thought to be due to injury to the ciliary and dorsal root ganglia. Onset may be gradual and unilateral. Ross's syndrome is Homes–Adie syndrome with excessive sweating
Peripheral neuropathy	Autonomic neuropathy in diabetic patients, or more rarely dysautonomias or paraneoplastic syndromes, can be associated with poorly reactive pupils
Muscle	Damage to the iris sphincter muscle, for example due to surgery, trauma, or ischemia, can limit pupil reactivity. These findings should be apparent on slit lamp examination
	Angle closure glaucoma is associated with a mid-dilated unreactive pupil due to ischemia. Accompanying symptoms and signs include eye pain, vision changes, and high intra-ocular pressure
	Pharmacologic pupil dilation can be caused by purposeful or inadvertent application of anticholinergic (e.g., tropicamide, scopolamine, atropine) or adrenergic agents (e.g., phenylephrine) to the corneal surface. Rarely, systemic agents with anticholinergic effects (e.g., benzatropine) can impair pupil constriction
Neuromuscular junction	Botulinum toxin inhibits acetylcholine release and activation of the iris sphincter muscle. This occurs in cases of botulism with concurrent symptoms of systemic weakness and autonomic dysfunction. It has been reported following therapeutic administration of botulinum toxin in the extra-ocular muscles
Unclear localization	Argyll Robertson pupils do not react to light, but do react to a near stimulus. They are not typically large at baseline. They are caused by syphilitic damage likely to either the midbrain or the ciliary ganglia

Secondary Complications: Patients may complain of light sensitivity due to more light entering the eye. They may experience blurring of vision at near, if accommodation is affected. This will resolve with either pinhole or reading glasses.

Treatment Complications: For patients who are very sensitive to light, pilocarpine can be used to pharmacologically constrict the large pupil. This is associated with a small pupil and some patients experience brow ache.

Bibliography

Moeller JJ, Maxner CE. The dilated pupil: an update. *Curr Neurol Neurosci Rep.* 2007;7(5):417–22.

Top of the Basilar Syndrome

Disorder Description: Typically embolic event causing occlusion of the distal basilar artery. This causes infarction affecting some or all of the rostral brainstem (basilar perforator arteries), both thalami (thalamic perforators), and both posterior parietal and occipital lobes (posterior cerebral arteries, PCAs). In some cases, only one PCA may be involved, for example, if there is a unilateral fetal PCA origin – see entries on *Posterior Cerebral Artery (PCA), Left Territory Infarction* and *Posterior Cerebral Artery (PCA), Right Territory Infarction.*

Symptoms

Localization site	Comment
Cerebral hemispheres	Balint syndrome (asimultagnosia, optical apraxia, and gaze apraxia), metamorphopsia, memory loss (left or bilateral thalamic), agitated delirium (bilateral thalamic), bilateral hemisensory loss, Anton syndrome (cortical blindness with denial)
Mental status and psychiatric aspects/complications	Somnolence, hallucinations (formed and complex hallucinations unrelated to delirium)
Brainstem	Diplopia, vertical gaze abnormalities, convergence disorders, pupillary abnormalities, skew deviation

Secondary Complications: Central sleep apnea may occur.

Treatment Complications: Treatment is by either thrombolysis or mechanical thrombectomy. Either could precipitate hemorrhagic conversion.

Bibliography

Caplan LR. "Top of the basilar" syndrome. *Neurology.* 1980;30:72–9.

Devuyst G, Bogousslavsky J, Meuli R, et al. Stroke or transient ischemic attack with basilar artery stenosis or occlusion, clinical patterns and outcome. *Arch Neurol.* 2002;59(4): 567–73.

Toxin-Induced Neuropathies

Epidemiology and Demographics: This is a relatively rare condition in the United States.

Disorder Description: The history and social history are important in patients presenting with seemingly unrelated generalized symptoms. It helps raise suspicion when coworkers or other family members have similar complaints. The patient may present to the pediatrician's office with developmental delay or failure to meet milestones. Adult patients may present with burning tingling sensation along with lightheadedness. There are a multitude of potential toxins including heavy metals, and industrial or environmental substances. Taking an occupational and environmental exposure history is crucial.

Symptoms

Localization site	Comment
Mental status and psychiatric aspects/complications	Encephalopathy (e.g., alcohol, lead)
Cerebellum	Dysmetria (alcohol, phenytoin toxicity)
Cranial nerves	Ophthalmoplegia (alcohol)
Spinal cord	Myelopathy (nitrous oxide), corticospinal tract (organophosphate pesticides)

Localization site	Comment
Peripheral neuropathy	Acute inflammatory demyelinating polyneuropathy (arsenic, n-hexane, amiodarone, carbon disulfide, cytosine arabinoside, methyl n-butyl ketone, perhexiline, saxitoxin, suramin, organophosphates, vincristine, vinca alkaloids, nitrofurantoin, dapsone, lead). Thallium can cause a rapidly progressive and painful ascending peripheral neuropathy
Muscle	Myopathy (colchicine)
Neuromuscular junction	Organophosphate esters
Autonomic system	Arsenic, n-hexane, mercury
Other	Lead may cause developmental delay

Secondary Complications: Toxic metabolic encephalopathy from higher concentrations and respiratory failure from certain pesticides.

Treatment Complications: Atropine used in organophosphate toxicity may cause cardiac arrhythmias, altered mental status.

Bibliography

Behse F, et al. Histology and ultrasound of alterations in neuropathy. *Muscle Nerve.* 1978;1(5):368.

London Z, et al. Toxic neuropathies associated with pharmaceutic and industrial agents. *Neurol Clin.* 2007;25(1):257–76.

Transient Global Amnesia

Epidemiology and Demographics: The overall incidence is 4–10/100,000 population per year but the incidence rises to 23.5/100,000 in those over age 50 years. Typical age at presentation is 50–70 years.

Disorder Description: Transient failure of short-term memory encoding (i.e., anterograde amnesia), classically accompanied by repetitive questioning. The patients may have some disorientation but no alteration in mental status. By definition, there cannot be any other signs of cortical dysfunction. The presence of any other stroke-like symptoms (e.g., hemiparesis, sensory loss, hemianopia, vertigo, aphasia, etc.)

should prompt search for an alternative diagnosis. Episodes last at least 4–6 and at most 24 hours and then resolve without treatment. The patients usually will never remember the event. The episode is often precipitated by factors such as stress, Valsalva maneuver, sex, pain, or immersion in water.

Symptoms

Localization site	Comments
Cerebral hemispheres	By definition, no symptoms other than anterograde memory loss may be present
Mental status and psychiatric aspects/complications	Anterograde amnesia. Procedural memory is intact. Retrograde amnesia is rarely present

Secondary Complications: Commonly seen in patients with history of migraines. May be confused with seizures or strokes. Seizures generally have a shorter duration of symptoms and an alteration in consciousness. Strokes generally have other neurologic deficits.

Treatment Complications: None as no treatment is necessary.

Bibliography

Arena JE, Rabinstein AA. Transient global amnesia. *Mayo Clin Proc.* 2015;90(2):264–72.

Szabo K. Transient global amnesia. *Front Neurol Neurosci.* 2014;34:143–9.

Transient Ischemic Attack

Epidemiology and Demographics: Incidence of transient ischemic attack (TIA) is 1.1/1000 population/year in the United States and 0.42/1000/year in the UK. Male-to-female ratio is ~1.4:1. Prevalence is higher in non-Caucasian populations and increases steadily with age.

Disorder Description: An episode of acute focal neurologic deficit lasting under 1 hour and without abnormalities on MR imaging. Rather than a separate disease, this should be considered akin to a stroke that recovered rapidly. The risk of stroke over the subsequent 7 days and especially the next 24 hours may be as high as 11% depending on the patient's medical history and presenting complaints.

Symptoms

Localization site	Comment
Cerebral hemispheres	Hemiparesis. Hemisensory deficit. Hemianopia. Neglect. Aphasia. Lower facial palsy
Mental status and psychiatric aspects/complications	Delirium (rare, limited to thalamic infarcts)
Brainstem	Hemiparesis. Bulbar signs. Crossed sensory deficits. Complete facial palsy
Cerebellum	Ataxia. Vertigo
Vestibular system	Vertigo
Cranial nerves	Any cranial neuropathy may be seen in conjunction with a brainstem TIA

Secondary Complications: Generally found in connection with vascular risk factors such as hypertension, smoking, hyperlipidemia, and diabetes. Early treatment of risk factors and addition of antiplatelet agents may reduce immediate risk of stroke.

Treatment Complications: Antiplatelet agents may lead to bleeding. Antilipemic agents may lead to myopathy/myalgia.

Bibliography

Ranta A, Barber PA. Transient ischemic attack service provision: A review of available service models. *Neurology.* 2016;86:1–7.

Rothwell PM, Giles MF, Chandratheva A, et al.; Early use of Existing Preventive Strategies for Stroke (EXPRESS) study. Effect of urgent treatment of transient ischaemic attack and minor stroke on early recurrent stroke (EXPRESS study): a prospective population-based sequential comparison. *Lancet.* 2007;370(9596):1432–42.

Sehatzadeh S. Is transient ischemic attack a medical emergency? An evidence-based analysis. *Ont Health Technol Assess Ser.* 2015;15(3):1–45.

Trichinosis (Trichinellosis)

Epidemiology and Demographics: There is no sex predominance and it can occur at any age, based on exposure. It is not only endemic to less developed regions (such as parts of Africa and South America) but in fact occurs in 80% of the world, including the United States and Europe (primarily Eastern Europe, such as Romania), as well as western and South East Asia. Other areas that may be uncommonly affected include small islands or small city-states where exposure is limited to potential reservoirs. Worldwide prevalence is unknown but an estimated 10,000 new cases occur each year.

Disorder Description: Trichinosis is a parasitic disease caused by the *Trichinella* genus of nematodes (roundworm), most classically *Trichinella spiralis*, but also including *Trichinella murelli*, and other species worldwide. There are typically two phases: an intestinal/enteral phase and a muscular/parenteral/systemic phase. The first (intestinal) phase occurs within a week of ingestion. In low burden states (<10 larvae), patients can remain asymptomatic, but if larval burden exceeds a few hundred, symptoms (most commonly gastrointestinal as described below) are present. One week after larval ingestion, there may be progression to a second, muscular and/or systemic stage. Here there are symptoms associated with more disseminated disease. These symptoms (due partially to immunological effects) can occur as the subsequent generation of larvae spread hematogenously and lymphatically, with a tropism for highly oxygenated skeletal muscle. In addition to direct tissue damage, the subsequent inflammatory response (largely eosinophilic) plays a part in disease manifestation.

Trichinosis is incurred through consumption by carnivores or omnivores (e.g., ingestion by humans of bears, pigs, hyenas, walruses) of improperly cooked meats.

Diagnosis is achieved through a careful clinical history assessing risk factors and symptomatology, and through serologic testing (ELISA with Western blot is the most common test and largely reliable). Antibody levels are not helpful early in the course, as they are not detectable until approximately 3 weeks subsequent to ingestion and infection. Muscle biopsy can definitively confirm diagnosis, but may have false negatives due to sampling issues. Muscle biopsy yield is enhanced by sampling symptomatic muscles and near a tendinous insertion.

Symptoms

Localization site	Comment
Cerebral hemispheres	Seizures, edema, hemorrhage, emboli, infarctions, and perivascular infiltrates
Mental status and psychiatric aspects/complications	Meningitis/encephalitis
Ocular symptoms	Conjunctival and retinal hemorrhages, periorbital edema, chemosis, visual disturbance, ocular pain
Outside CNS	Gastrointestinal symptoms (nausea, vomiting, diarrhea, abdominal pain) initially
	Fevers and chills, fatigue, headaches, nail bed splinter hemorrhages, cough, dyspnea, dysphagia, rash, arthralgia
Muscle	Myalgia, edema, weakness, rhabdomyolysis
	Myocarditis

Secondary Complications: Due to the immunological response, diverse systemic complications may occur such as cardiac myositis (although cardiac tissue is not commonly affected), renal failure (in part from resultant rhabdomyolysis as direct renal involvement is not common), infarctions, embolic disease, and gastrointestinal symptoms.

Treatment Complications: Depending on disease severity, antiparasitic agents may be prescribed (e.g. mebendazole, albendazole), possibly with corticosteroids. In milder infections treatment may consist of therapy only for symptoms. Treatment complications from antiparasitic agents are uncommon but may include gastrointestinal adverse effects (nausea, vomiting, diarrhea, abdominal pain, decreased appetite). Potential neurologic side effects of steroids are limited given the typically short course regimen that is typically utilized.

Bibliography

Finsterer J, Auer H. Parasitoses of the human central nervous system. *J Helminthol*. 2013;87(3):257–70.

Gottstein B, Pozio E, Nöckler K. Epidemiology, diagnosis, treatment, and control of trichinellosis. *Clin Microbiol Rev*. 2009;22(1):127–45.

Smith DS. Trichinosis (Trichinellosis). Medscape. Updated May 1, 2018. https://emedicine.medscape.com/article/230490-overview. Accessed Oct 11, 2018.

Trichotillomania

Epidemiology and Demographics: The 12-month prevalence of trichotillomania in the US adult population is 1–2%. The female-to-male ratio is approximately 10:1. This gender disparity may be partially due to the differential treatment seeking due to gender. In children, males and females are equally affected (DSM-5).

Disorder Description: As stated in DSM-5, trichotillomania can be defined as:

A. Recurrent pulling out of one's hair, resulting in hair loss.

B. Repeated attempts to cease hair-pulling activity.

C. The hair pulling causes the patient significant clinical distress or impairment in social, occupational, or other areas of functioning.

D. The hair pulling and hair loss are not attributed to another medical condition.

E. The hair pulling is not better explained as a symptom of another mental disorder (for example, the attempt to improve a perceived flaw as in body dysmorphic disorder).

Differential Diagnosis

Normative hair removal/manipulation: Trichotillomania should not be confused with hair removal (plucking, laser, shaving, cutting, etc.) for cosmetic reasons. Hair manipulation, such as twirling, twisting, biting, etc., also should not be diagnosed as trichotillomania.

Other obsessive-compulsive (OCD) and related disorders: Individuals with OCD may pull out hairs as part of their symmetry rituals. Those with body dysmorphic disorder may pull hair in order to remove their perceived bodily defect/flaw.

Neurodevelopmental disorders: In neurodevelopmental disorders, hair pulling may qualify as a stereotypy. Tics, as in Tourette's syndrome, rarely involve hair pulling.

Psychotic disorders: patients may remove hair in response to a delusion or hallucination.

Hair and skin disorders: Organic causes of alopecia such as alopecia areata, androgenic alopecia, telogen effluvium, chronic discoid lupus erythematosus, lichen planopilaris, central centrifugal cicatricial alopecia, pseudopelade, folliculitis decalvans, dissecting folliculitis, and acne keloidalis nuchae should be considered in those who deny hair pulling. Skin biopsy and/or dermoscopy will differentiate between organic and behavioral causes.

Secondary Complications: Trichotillomania may cause significant distress and occupational impairment. It may cause irreversible damage to hair growth and quality. Individuals will often have patches of hair of varying lengths. Though infrequent, medical consequences include digit purpura, musculoskeletal injuries (back, hand, neck, or head pain), blepharitis, and dental damage (due to hair biting). Swallowing of hair (trichophagia) may lead to trichobezoars, with subsequent anemia, abdominal pain, hematemesis, nausea and vomiting, bowel obstruction, and (rarely) perforation

Treatment Complications: Cognitive behavioral therapy is the first-line treatment for trichotillomania. However, some studies have shown efficacy of selective serotonin reuptake inhibitors (SSRIs), clomipramine, and N-acetylcysteine. SSRI side effects include nausea, diarrhea, insomnia, headache, anorexia, weight loss, sexual dysfunction, restlessness (akathisia-like), serotonin syndrome (fever diaphoresis, tachycardia, hypertension, delirium, neuromuscular excitability), hyponatremia, seizures (0.2%). Clomipramine side effects include sedation, weight gain, hypotension, dry mouth, blurred vision, urinary retention, constipation. N-acetyl cysteine is associated with rash, urticaria, and pruritus.

Bibliography

American Psychiatric Association. *Diagnostic and statistical manual of mental disorders: DSM-5.* 5th ed. Washington, DC: American Psychiatric Association; 2013.

Chamberlain SR, Fineberg NA, Blackwell AD, Robbins TW, Sahakian BJ. Motor inhibition and cognitive flexibility in obsessive-compulsive disorder and trichotillomania. *Am J Psychiatry.* 2006;63(7):1282–4.

Flessner CA, Woods DW, Franklin ME, et al. The Milwaukee inventory for subtypes of trichotillomania-adult version (MIST-A): development of an instrument for the assessment of "focused" and "automatic" hair pulling. *J Psychopathol Behav Assess.* 2008;30(1):20–30.

Franklin ME, Flessner CA, Woods DW, et al. The child and adolescent trichotillomania impact project: descriptive psychopathology, comorbidity, functional impairment, and treatment utilization. *J Dev Behav Pediatr.* 2008;29(6):493–500.

O'Sullivan RL, Rauch SL, Breiter HC, et al. Reduced basal ganglia volumes in trichotillomania measured via morphometric magnetic resonance imaging. *Biol Psychiatry.* 1997;42(1):39–45.

Stein DJ, Coetzer R, Lee M, Davids B, Bouwer C. Magnetic resonance brain imaging in women with obsessive-compulsive disorder and trichotillomania. *Psychiatry Res.* 1997;74(3):177–82.

Trigeminal Neuralgia

Epidemiology and Demographics: More commonly found in women, especially over the age of 50 years. When it presents at an earlier age, other diagnoses such as multiple sclerosis should be excluded. The annual incidence is 4 to 13/100,000.

Disorder Description: Patients may present with short duration electric-like pain sensations in the unilateral forehead, cheek, or chin. The causes include idiopathic etiologies, or structural impingements on the trigeminal nerve as may occur with a tumor, a vascular loop, or a plaque associated with multiple sclerosis. Sometimes the simple act of brushing one's teeth may elicit pain.

Symptoms

Localization site	Comment
Mental status and psychiatric aspects	Anxiety and depression
Cranial nerves	Trigeminal nerve

Secondary Complications: Mood disorder and anxiety from chronic pain.

Treatment Complications: Carbamazepine can cause hyponatremia and seizures. Gabapentin can cause sedation. Potential complications from nerve blocks, ablation, or microvascular decompression.

Bibliography

Baad-Hansen L, Benoliel R. Neuropathic orofacial pain: facts and fiction. *Cephalalgia.* 2017;37(7):670–9. DOI: 10.1177/0333102417706310. Epub Apr 12, 2017.

Katusic S, Williams DB, Beard CM. Epidemiology and clinical features of idiopathic trigeminal neuralgia and glossopharyngeal neuralgia: similarities and differences, Rochester, Minnesota, 1945–1984. *Neuroepidemiology*. 1991:10:276.

MacDonald BK, Cockerell OC, Sander JW, Shorvon SD. The incidence and lifetime prevalence of neurological disorders in a prospective community-based study in the UK. *Brain*. 2000;123(Pt 4):665.

Tropical Ataxic Neuropathy

Epidemiology and Demographics: As summarized by Netto et al., a study in Nigeria showed incidence was 64/10,000 individuals. The highest prevalence of 24% was found in people in their 60s. This is a very rare disease in the United States.

Disorder Description: Patients most commonly present with numbness and ataxic gait; occasionally they manifest vision or hearing loss. The causes include malnutrition, either from inadequate amounts of food or difficulty absorbing the nutrients from food, and cyanide or nitrile toxicity (this is especially true in areas of cassava consumption).

Symptoms

Localization site	Comment
Base of skull	Bilateral sensory neural deafness
Cranial nerves	Bilateral optic atrophy
Spinal cord	Posterior column involvement
Anterior horn cells	Pyramidal tract myelopathy
Peripheral neuropathy	Ataxic polyneuropathy

Secondary Complications: Coexistent vitamin A deficiency can occur, which can manifest as night blindness. Risk of falls is high.

Treatment: Vitamin supplementation and diet changes may improve symptoms.

Bibliography

Arul Selvan VL. A case of tropical ataxic neuropathy. *Apollo Med*. 2013;10(3):223–5.

Netto AB, Netto CM, Mahadevan A, Taly AB, Agadi JB. Tropical ataxic neuropathy – a century old enigma. *Neurol India*. 2016;64:1151–9.

Oluwole O, Onabolu A, Link H, Rosling H. Persistence of tropical ataxic neuropathy in a Nigerian community. *J Neurol Neurosurg Psychiatry*. 2000;69(1):96–101. DOI:10.1136/jnnp.69.1.96.

Trypanosomiasis, African

Epidemiology and Demographics: There is no distinct sex predominance or predilection for a specific age group. It is largely seen in Africa with the more acute form (caused by *Trypanosoma brucei rhodesiense*) found more commonly in East Africa, and the more chronic form (caused by *Trypanosoma brucei gambiense*) occurring mainly in Northern, West, and Central Africa. Vigorous efforts have dramatically reduced the frequency of this illness over the years. In 2015, approximately 2800 cases were documented.

Disorder Description: Trypanosomiasis is also known as "African sleeping sickness" and is caused by parasitic protozoans of the *Trypanosoma* genus (*Trypanosoma brucei rhodesiense* and *Trypanosoma brucei gambiense*).

Typically upon ingestion by the tsetse fly, the *Trypanosoma brucei* species develop and divide, spreading to the insect's salivary glands, resulting in transmission to human hosts during the next blood meal. Using a variety of immunologic evasive techniques, they develop further and disseminate in the human host. In the second stage of the human disease, it invades the central nervous system (CNS).

Symptoms

Localization site	Comment
Mental status and psychiatric aspects/ complications	Meningoencephalitis, sleep–wake pattern disruption (day–night reversal), encephalopathy, cognitive difficulties (deficits in concentration or complex tasks), personality changes, psychosis, vegetative or comatose state
Other localizations	Headache, tremor, ataxia, seizure
Outside CNS	Chancre

Secondary Complications: Secondary complications are largely neurological, as noted above, signaling CNS involvement.

Treatment Complications: There are a variety of treatment regimens, but typically pentamidine and suramin are used early on, but in later stages nifurtimox and eflornithine may be utilized. Some regimens include melarsoprol. Complications of antihelminthics include gastrointestinal symptoms, headache, dizziness, fever, and chills. Melarsoprol (a highly toxic arsenical compound) has been associated with encephalopathy.

Bibliography

Finsterer J, Auer H. Parasitoses of the human central nervous system. *J Helminthol.* 2013;87(3): 257–70.

Salvana EMT, Salata RA, King CH. Parasitic infections of the central nervous system. In Aminoff MJ, Josephson SA, eds. *Aminoff's neurology and general medicine.* 5th ed. London: Academic Press; 2014: pp. 947–68.

World Health Organization. Trypanosomiasis, human African (sleeping sickness). Feb 16, 2018. www.who.int/news-room/fact-sheets/detail/trypanosomiasis-human-african-(sleeping-sickness). Accessed Oct 11, 2018.

Tuberculosis (TB)

Epidemiology and Demographics: According to the Centers for Disease Control and Prevention (CDC), up to 25% of the world's population suffer from tuberculosis (TB) infection. In the United States, approximately 2.9 cases/100,000 individuals occurred in 2016, which represented a decline in cases from previous years. Males and females are equally vulnerable to infection. The central nervous system (CNS) is involved in about 1–2% of TB cases.

Disorder Description: TB is caused by the bacillus *Mycobacterium tuberculosis.* HIV and other causes of immunosuppression predispose to TB infection. TB often starts as a pulmonary infection that in a secondary stage of hematogenous spread can affect many body systems. Three main forms of CNS disease are meningitis, intraparenchymal tuberculomas, and arachnoiditis.

Symptoms

Localization site	Comment
Cerebral hemispheres	Meningismus, seizures, headache, diverse focal neurologic deficits
Mental status and psychiatric aspects/complications	Mild to profound alteration in mental status with widely varying time frames of progression and ranging from mild confusion to coma
Cerebellum	Focal deficits from TB abscess
Cranial nerves	Cranial neuropathies
Spinal cord	Arachnoiditis can afflict any level and is associated with painful radiculopathic and compressive myelopathic signs

Secondary Complications: Vasculitis with secondary strokes of the vertebrobasilar or subdivisions of the middle cerebral artery, and vessels that form the circle of Willis, among other possible vascular locations.

Communicating hydrocephalus with diverse complications of increased intracranial pressure.

Treatment Complications: Isoniazid may cause a peripheral neuropathy due to induction of a pyridoxine deficiency, and can be precluded by supplementation with pyridoxine. Optic neuropathy due to ethambutol is unusual at usual doses. Surgical complications may occur if surgery is required to relieve hydrocephalus.

Bibliography

Centers for Disease Control and Prevention. Tuberculosis. Updated Jun 5, 2018. www.cdc.gov/tb/statistics/default.htm. Accessed Sep 25, 2018.

Changal KH, Raina AH. Central nervous system manifestations of tuberculosis: a review article. *J Mycobac Dis.* 2014;4:146. DOI:10.4172/2161-1068.1000146.

Rock RB, Olin M, Baker CA, Molitor TW, Peterson PK. Central nervous system tuberculosis: pathogenesis and clinical aspects. *Clin Microbiol Rev.* 2008;21(2):243–61. DOI:10.1128/CMR.00042-07.

Tuberous Sclerosis (TS; Tuberous Sclerosis Complex, TSC)

Epidemiology and Demographics: Tuberous sclerosis (TS) affects both sexes. TS manifests early with developmental concerns, infantile spasms, and neonatal cardiac rhabdomyomas. Over the course of childhood, other symptoms may become apparent. In adulthood, ongoing monitoring is needed for tumor surveillance. The prevalence of TS is 1/6000 to 1/10,000.

Disorder Description: TS is an autosomal dominant disorder, with about a third of cases inherited from one parent and the remaining two-thirds are *de novo* cases. TS is caused by mutations in either *TSC1* on chromosome 9p34.13, which encodes for hamartin, or *TSC2* on chromosome 16p13.3, which encodes for tuberin. Hamartin and tuberin are regulators in the AKT/mTOR signaling pathway, among others. With mutations in either gene, there is suppression of mTOR, with resultant cell growth and development of hamartomas.

Clinical symptoms of TS are multisystemic and may include: angiofibromas; cardiac rhabdomyoma; cortical dysplasias (tubers); skin lesions including hypopigmented macules/"confetti," Shagreen patch; lymphangioleiomyomatosis; retinal nodular hamartomas; renal angiomyolipoma; subependymal giant cell astrocytoma (SEGA); subependymal nodules; and ungual fibromas. Other features may include dental enamel pits, intraoral fibromas, multiple renal cysts, and nonrenal hamartomas.

Symptoms

Localization site	Comment
Cerebral hemispheres	Central nervous system (CNS) tumors, subependymal nodules, cortical dysplasias, SEGAs; seizures including infantile spasms/hypsarrhythmia
Mental status and psychiatric aspects/ complications	TSC-associated neuropsychiatric disorder (TAND)[1,2]: 1. Autism spectrum disorder (ASD), impaired language pathways,[3] atypical face processing,[4] and global cognitive impairment[5] 2. Attention deficit hyperactivity disorder (ADHD) (dual-task performance), cognitive flexibility, and memory 3. Learning and cognitive impairment (learning disabilities) 4. Disruptive behaviors and emotional problems, aggression, self-injurious behavior, anxiety

Secondary Complications: Brain tumors and renal tumors lead to the higher morbidity and mortality associated with TS. Large/growing renal angiomyolipomas or malignant angiomyolipomas are treated with mTOR inhibitors or other procedures. Renal cell carcinoma is also seen in TSC.

SEGAs which show growth may be treated with mTOR inhibitors or neurosurgery.

Seizures are treated with vigabatrin for infantile spasms or other antiepileptic drugs; removal of tuber if investigation shows one tuber is causing seizures.

Symptomatic cardiac rhabdomyomas are treated surgically or with mTOR inhibitors.

Treatment Complications: Vigabatrin is used for infantile spasms in TS, but requires frequent visual testing due to risk of peripheral visual field restriction.

References

1. de Vries PJ. Neurodevelopmental, psychiatric, and cognitive aspects of tuberous sclerosis complex. In Kwiatkowski DJ, Whittemore VH, Thiele EA, eds. *Tuberous sclerosis complex: genes, clinical features, and therapeutics.* Weinheim, Germany: Wiley-Blackwell; 2010. pp. 229–67.
2. de Vries PJ. Targeted treatments for cognitive and neurodevelopmental disorders in tuberous sclerosis complex. *Neurotherapeutics.* 2010;7:275–82.
3. Lewis WW, Sahin M, Scherrer B, et al. Impaired language pathways in tuberous sclerosis complex patients with autism spectrum disorders. *Cereb Cortex.* 2013;23:1526–32.
4. Spurling Jeste S, Wu JY, Senturk D, et al. Early developmental trajectories associated with ASD in infants with tuberous sclerosis complex. *Neurology.* 2014;83:160–8.
5. Jeste SS, Sahin M, Bolton P, Ploubidis GB, Humphrey A. Characterization of autism in young children with tuberous sclerosis complex. *J Child Neurol.* 2008;23:520–5.

Suggested Reading

Northrup H, Koenig MK, Pearson DA, et al. Tuberous sclerosis complex. Jul 13, 1999. Updated Sep 3, 2015. In Pagon RA, Adam MP, Ardinger HH, et al., eds. *GeneReviews®* [Internet]. Seattle (WA): University of Washington, Seattle; 1993–2016. Available from www.ncbi.nlm.nih.gov/books/NBK1220/ www.omim.org/entry/191100.

Turner Syndrome

Epidemiology and Demographics: Turner syndrome is not exceedingly rare, occurring in 1/2500–3000 live-born girls and affecting only females.

It is a genetic disorder, but can present heterogeneously with respect to severity and age of onset, though usually begins between ages 1 and 3 years with cognitive and behavioral issues. There is no clear geographic distribution.

Disorder Description: Turner syndrome is a sex chromosomal pair disorder, due to loss of one chromosome from the pair (nondisjunction), improper division, or mosaicism.

Turner syndrome is caused by an XO-equivalent sex chromosomal pair, often caused by nondisjunction. Most cases are due to 45 X karyotype (~50%), a minority are due to duplication of the long arm of one X in 46 XXi, while the rest are all mosaics.

Diagnosis begins with identification of clinical features, but is confirmed through karyotyping. Hallmark clinical features for early diagnosis include perinatal edema, hypoplastic left heart, or coarctation of the aorta. However, diagnosis can be made early, in prenatal stages, through ultrasonography (demonstration of fetal edema), maternal serum screening (human chorionic gonadotropin, unconjugated estriol, alpha-fetoprotein), or prenatal karyotyping (often done due to advanced maternal age).

Symptoms

Localization site	Comment
Mental status and psychiatric aspects/complications	Minimal deficits, but can cause learning deficits
Outside CNS	Congenital lymphedema, short stature (most common cause of short stature in otherwise healthy girls), shield chest, gonadal dysgenesis/"streak gonads"

Secondary Complications: Secondary complications are primarily related to multiple non-CNS defects, but females with mosaicism with cells containing a Y chromosome are at increased risk for gonadoblastoma (up to 30%) in their streak gonads. Secondary ovarian failure is also understandably a risk.

Treatment Complications: Treatment is largely symptomatic and supportive. Hormonal therapy (growth hormone and estrogen replacement therapy) is the major symptomatic mainstay. Counseling and fertilization techniques to avoid this issue in offspring can be used. Complications of treatment are largely limited to associated risks for the required supportive care, especially steroid/hormonal therapy.

Bibliography

Sybert VP, McCauley E. Turner's syndrome. *N Engl J Med*. 2004;351(12):1227–38.

Typhoid Fever

Epidemiology and Demographics: Typhoid fever is a common disease throughout the world, with 11–21 million cases occurring each year and with an annual death rate of approximately 200,000 persons. It can afflict males and females equally. While there is no specific age of onset, the majority of infections are in children and young adults rather than in older patients. It is endemic to areas with poor sanitation and unclean water and is mostly seen in southern Asian countries. In areas where water sources are clean, most infections are related to travel and exposure to endemic areas.

Disorder Description: Typhoid fever, which is caused by the *Salmonella enterica* serovar *Salmonella* Typhi, is an enteric baterial infection that is fecal–orally transmitted. Typhoid, together with paratyphoid caused by *Salmonella* Paratyphi A,B, or C, falls under a broader collective term "enteric fever." *Salmonella enterica* infects only humans and produces a typhoid toxin. Risk is based on exposure, but the majority of infections occur in children.

After ingestion, *S. enterica* crosses the intestinal epithelium and spreads to adjacent areas (including liver, spleen, gall bladder, bone marrow), and ultimately spreads systemically. Symptoms usually develop 10–14 days after exposure/ingestion. Fever typically escalates in stepwise fashion, as do systemic symptoms, with a peak usually by the third to fourth weeks, and with subsequent resolution over weeks to months.

If there is clinically related suspicion, blood cultures are typically ordered as the primary diagnostic testing method. However, because the infection can require several days of incubation, false negative results may ensue. Bone marrow culture is the most sensitive testing method, but is rarely performed. A limitation of positive serological testing results, such as those from the Widal test, is the possibility of their indicating prior exposure rather than active disease.

Symptoms

Localization site	Comment
Mental status and psychiatric aspects/complications	Encephalopathy, encephalitis, meningitis, delirium, psychosis and hallucinations, headache, rigidity (rare)
Spinal cord	Myelitis (rare/uncommon)
Other localizations	Hyperreflexia, spasticity, ataxia, parkinsonism (all are rare)
Outside CNS	Fever, gastrointestinal symptoms (nausea, vomiting, diarrhea), hypovolemia, fatigue, hepatosplenomegaly, transaminitis, anemia

Secondary Complications: Secondary complications are typically related to gastrointestinal symptoms and associated hypovolemia as well as from systemic dissemination.

Treatment Complications: Therapeutic choice depends on disease severity, but usually includes fluoroquinolones, cephalosporins (3rd generation), or azithromycin. Drug resistance is not uncommon, so older therapies (ampicillin, TMP-SMX, chloramphenicol) are not often used. If a multidrug-resistant strain is identified, carbapenems may be prescribed. Rare complications of therapeutic agents include changes in mental status and seizures.

Bibliography

Butler T. Treatment of typhoid fever in the 21st century: promises and shortcomings. *Clin Microbiol Infect*. 2011;17(7):959–63.

Johnson R, Mylona E, Frankel G. Typhoidal Salmonella: Distinctive virulence factors and pathogenesis. *Cell Microbiol*. 2018;20(9):e12939.

Tomé AM, Filipe A. Quinolones: review of psychiatric and neurological adverse reactions. *Drug Saf*. 2011;34(6):465–88.

World Health Organization. Typhoid. Updated Sep 11, 2018. www.who.int/immunization/diseases/typhoid/en/. Accessed Oct 11, 2018.

Ulcerative Colitis

Epidemiology and Demographics: The annual incidence of Crohn's disease is about 9 to 12/100,000 persons in North America. The incidence is equal between men and women and among races. The incidence seems to peak in early 20s and is less in smokers or after appendectomy.

Disorder Description: Ulcerative colitis typically presents with hematochezia, diarrhea, and abdominal pain with sudden or gradual onset. Inflammation is limited to the mucosal and submucosal layers of the rectum and can extend to the colon in a contiguous pattern.

Symptoms

Localization site	Comment
Cerebral hemispheres	Thromboembolic events causing transient ischemic attacks or strokes
	Venous sinus thrombosis
	Vasculitis
	Seizures
Mental status and psychiatric aspects/complications	Fatigue, anxiety, depression, sleep disturbances
Cranial nerves	Sensorineural hearing loss
Spinal cord	Autoimmune myelopathy
Peripheral neuropathy	Guillain–Barré syndrome
	Distal symmetric axonal polyneuropathy
Neuromuscular junction	Myasthenia gravis (rare)
Muscle	Polymyositis
Unclear localization	Headache

Secondary Complications: Hypercoagulable state can lead to thromboembolic or venous strokes even when the disease is not clinically active.

Treatment Complications: Biologic treatment and immunosuppression increase the risks of central nervous system infections. Progressive multifocal leukoencephalopathy (PML) is a rare complication of biologic treatment. A case of immunomodulatory therapy-induced lymphoproliferative disorder (ILPD) has been reported in a patient with ulcerative colitis being treated with infliximab.

Bibliography

Casella G, Tontini GE, Bassotti G, et al. Neurological disorders and inflammatory bowel diseases. *World J Gastroenterol.* 2014;20(27):8764–82.

Ferro JM, Oliveira SN, Correia L. Neurologic manifestations of inflammatory bowel diseases. *Handb Clin Neurol.* 2014;120:595–605.

Guinet-Charpentier C, Bilbault C, Kennel A, et al. Unusual association of myasthenia gravis and ulcerative colitis in a 14-year-old boy. *Arch Pediatr.* 2015;22(1):81–3.

Morís G. Inflammatory bowel disease: an increased risk factor for neurologic complications. *World J Gastroenterol.* 2014;20(5):1228–37.

Ulnar Neuropathy

Epidemiology and Demographics: As summarized by Fadel et al., the incidence rate of ulnar neuropathy is 20–25/100,000 person-years and prevalence is 0.6–0.8%.

Disorder Description: This is a relatively common condition that is usually due to inadvertent resting of the elbow on hard surfaces. Many patients do it habitually without even being aware they are doing it. Visual observation can usually point to the diagnosis of ulnar neuropathy.

Muscle innervated by the ulnar nerve	Clinical symptom
Interossei, 3rd and 4th lumbricals	Finger abduction weakness, clawing of 4th and 5th digits (Benediction posture)
Third palmar interosseous	Weakness in adducting the 5th digit (Wartenberg's sign)
Adductor pollicis, flexor pollicis brevis, and interossei	Weakness in grabbing a small item with the index finger and thumb (Froment's sign)
Flexor digitorum profundus to 4th and 5th digits	Weakness in flexion of the distal phalanx of the 4th and 5th digit when making a fist

Deficit According to Localization

Deficit	Ulnar neuropathy at wrist	Ulnar neuropathy at the elbow	Medial cord brachial plexopathy	Lower trunk brachial plexopathy	C8 T1 radiculopathy
Distal 4th and 5th digit flexion	X	X	X	X
Tinel's sign at elbow		X			
Thumb abduction or flexion			X	X	X
Extensor indicis proprius (extension of 2nd digit)				X	X
Medial forearm sensory findings			X	X	X
Radiating neck pain down the upper extremity				X	X
Paraspinal muscle spontaneous activity on EMG					X

X = present.
Adapted from Preston DC, Shapiro BE. Ulnar neuropathy at the elbow. In Electromyography and neuromuscular disorders: clinical-electrophysiologic correlations. 2nd ed. Elsevier Butterworth-Heinemann; 2005. p. 296.

Secondary Complications: Muscle atrophy and limitation of movement may occur.

Treatment Complications: Surgical intervention for ulnar neuropathy at the elbow may rarely cause nerve/tissue injury, blood loss. The surgical anesthesia used may cause altered mental status, especially in the elderly.

Bibliography

Brazis PW, et al., eds. Peripheral nerves. In *Localization in clinical neurology*. 6th ed. Philadelphia, PA: Lippincott Williams and Wilkins; 2011. Chapter 2.

Fadel M. Occupational prognosis factors for ulnar nerve entrapment at the elbow: A systematic review. *Hand Surg Rehabil*. 2017;36(4):244–9.

Uterine Cancer

Epidemiology and Demographics: The most common gynecologic cancer in developed countries, and the second most common in developing countries (cervical is first). Accounts for 6% of all cancers in women. The number of new cases of endometrial cancer is 25.4/100,000 women per year. Average age of diagnosis in the United States is 61 years.

Disorder Description: Uterine cancer is any type of cancer that arises from tissue of the uterus. Adenocarcinoma of the endometrium is the most common site and type of uterine cancer. There are two histologic categories of endometrial carcinomas. Type I include tumors of endometrioid histology that are grade 1 or 2, and comprise approximately 80% of endometrial carcinomas. Type II tumors comprise approximately 10–20% of endometrial carcinomas and include grade 3 endometrioid tumors, as well as tumors of non-endometrioid histology: serous, clear cell, mucinous, squamous, transitional cell, mesonephric, and undifferentiated. The main risk factor for type I is excess estrogen without adequate opposition by progestin (i.e., obesity or post-menopausal estrogen therapy without progestin). Type I endometrioid tumors tend to have a favorable prognosis (90% 5-year survival) and typically present at an early stage with abnormal uterine bleeding. Type II cancers have a less favorable prognosis.

Symptoms

Localization site	Comment
Cerebral hemisphere	Headache, motor weakness, seizures, confusion due to cerebral metastasis (rare)
Cerebellum	Cerebellar ataxia, nystagmus, dysarthria due to paraneoplastic cerebellar degeneration, most often associated with PCA-1 anti-Yo antibody. Cerebellar metastasis may occur (rare)

Localization site	Comment
Spinal cord	Sensorimotor deficits, bowel/bladder dysfunction, pain, due to spinal cord involvement of vertebral metastasis (rare)
Conus medullaris	Sensorimotor deficits, bowel/bladder dysfunction, pain, due to compression of conus medullaris from osseous metastasis (rare)
Cauda equina	Sensorimotor deficits, bowel/bladder dysfunction, pain, due to compression of cauda equina from osseous metastasis (rare)
Peripheral neuropathy	Sensorimotor deficits, paresthesias due to paraneoplastic polyneuropathy (rare)

Secondary Complications: Acute blood loss anemia may occur from heavy uterine bleeding. Endometrial cancer most frequently metastasizes locally to ovaries, fallopian tubes, cervix. The lymphatic system, usually pelvic nodes, may become involved. More distant sites of metastasis involve spread by blood and may include lung, less often liver, brain, and bone.

Treatment Complications: Primary treatment is surgical resection with hysterectomy and unilateral or bilateral salpingo-oophorectomy, radiation therapy, and chemotherapy. Treatment complications include uterine perforation from diagnostic biopsy and post-surgical infection. Adverse effects from pelvic or intravaginal radiation therapy include fatigue, skin reactions, abdominal pain, loose bowel movements. Lower extremity pain, motor–sensory deficits, bowel/bladder dysfunction from radiation-induced pelvic radiculopathy or lumbosacral plexopathy may occur. For intermediate to high risk uterine cancers, commonly used chemotherapy agents are carboplatin and paclitaxel. Carboplatin, a platinum-based agent, may cause peripheral neuropathy and ototoxicity. Paclitaxel, a taxane agent, may cause sensory or motor neuropathy.

Bibliography

Brejt N, Berry J, Nisbet A, Bloomfield D, Burkill G. Pelvic radiculopathies, lumbosacral plexopathies, and neuropathies in oncologic disease: a multidisciplinary approach to a diagnostic challenge. *Cancer Imaging.* 2013;13(4):591–601.

Brock S, Ellison D, Frankel J, Davis C, Illidge T. Anti-Yo antibody-positive cerebellar degeneration associated with endometrial carcinoma: case report and review of the literature. *Clin Oncol (R Coll Radiol).* 2001;13(6):476–9.

Cormio G, Lissoni A, Losa G, et al. Brain metastases from endometrial carcinoma. *Gynecol Oncol.* 1996;61(1):40–3.

Miller DS, Filiaci G, Mannel R, et al. Randomized Phase III Noninferiority Trial of First Line Chemotherapy for Metastatic or Recurrent Endometrial Carcinoma: A Gynecologic Oncology Group Study. LBA2. Presented at the 2012 Society of Gynecologic Oncology Annual Meeting, Austin, TX.

Torre LA, Bray F, Siegel RL, et al. Global cancer statistics, 2012. *CA Cancer J Clin.* 2015;65:87.

Uccella S, Morris JM, Bakkum-Gamez JN, et al. Bone metastasis in endometrial cancer: report on 19 patients and review of the medical literature. *Gynecol Oncol.* 2013;130(3):474–82.

Vasku M, Papathemelis T, Maass N, Meinhold-Heerlein I, Bauerschlag D. Endometrial carcinoma presenting as vasculitic sensorimotor polyneuropathy. *Case Rep Obstet Gynecol.* 2011;2011:968756.

Uterine Mass or Retroflexion (Compressive Neuropathy)

Epidemiology and Demographics: This is a relatively rare disease affecting women.

Disorder Description: When the uterus (most likely retroverted) is enlarged due to pregnancy or tumor (benign such as fibroids), it can compress the sciatic nerve. Most commonly it can present in the early stages with foot drop and numbness at the lateral part of the calf and top of the foot. It can also cause pain that radiates down the back of the thigh, back and side of the calf, and bottom of the foot.

When to consider imaging a patient's pelvis for compression of the sciatic nerve:

symptoms worsened with some positions and not with others;

symptoms are not worsened when patient bears down;

there is no back pain;

on exam, there is gluteal muscle weakness.

Symptoms

Localization site	Comment
Peripheral neuropathy	Sciatic nerve-related compressive symptoms

Secondary Complications: Axonal injury of the sciatic nerve and at the extreme, atrophy and paralysis of muscles involved in knee flexion, ankle flexion, ankle extension, ankle eversion and ankle inversion, toe flexion and extension.

Treatment Complications: Surgical relief of the compression may rarely cause further complications to the nerve and muscles.

Bibliography

Adams R, Victor M. *Principles of neurology.* 5th ed. New York, NY: McGraw-Hill; 1993.

Bodack M. Sciatic neuropathy secondary to a uterine fibroid: a case report. *Am J Phys Med Rehab.* 1999;78(2):157–9.

Brazis PW, et al., eds. Peripheral nerves. In *Localization in clinical neurology.* 6th ed. Philadelphia, PA: Lippincott Williams and Wilkins; 2011. Chapter 2.

Uveitis

Epidemiology and Demographics: Traditionally uveitis is thought to be a disease of young to middle-aged individuals but incidence in older individuals may be higher than previously reported. It is an under-recognized cause of blindness and is believed to cause 10% of cases of legal blindness in the United States.

Disorder Description: Uveitis is inflammation of the uvea, a part of the eye that consists of the iris, ciliary body, and choroid. Uveitis is a broad term to describe a group of conditions in which inflammation primarily affects various components of the uveal tract and secondarily affects other ocular structures. Etiologies include infectious, autoimmune, and conditions in association with systemic inflammatory conditions. A genetic predisposition can also contribute to the development of uveitis. Certain human leukocyte antigen classes are strongly associated with particular uveitic conditions. Approximately 30% of cases of uveitis do not fit into any well-defined diagnostic category and are termed idiopathic. The Standardization of Uveitis Nomenclature consensus conference workshop emphasizes an anatomical approach to classifying uveitis (anterior, intermediate, posterior, pan). The most common form of uveitis is acute anterior uveitis (inflammation of the iris and/or the ciliary body).

Symptoms of uveitis will depend on which anatomical structures of the eye are affected and duration of disease. Anterior uveitis is characterized by pain, redness, photophobia, and blurred vision. Intermediate and posterior uveitis can present with floaters and/or impaired vision and pain. Panuveitis presents with any or all of the above.

Symptoms

Localization site	Comment
Cerebral hemispheres	**Susac's syndrome** is a rare autoimmune disorder characterized by the triad of branch retinal vein occlusions, encephalopathy, and hearing loss. It is thought to be an autoimmune microangiopathy causing infarcts in the brain, cochlea, and retina. The neurologic symptoms predominate with headache being the most frequent presenting complaint. Occlusion of retinal arterioles with normal choroidal circulation in the absence of intraocular inflammation is the characteristic eye finding **Vogt–Koyanagi–Harada disease (VKH)** is a rare multiorgan autoimmune disorder. It is thought to be a T-cell-mediated autoimmune condition directed at an unknown antigen associated with melanocytes. Thus it affects mainly pigmented tissues of the ocular (uvea and retina), auditory, skin, and central nervous systems (leptomeninges). The neurologic symptoms are meningitic in nature and may include fever, headache, nausea, nuchal rigidity. These typically occur in the prodromal phase and thus precede the eye findings. CSF pleocytosis with lymphocytic predominance is a transient finding in 80% of VKH patients. Characteristic eye findings are bilateral panuveitis in the acute phase associated with exudative retinal detachments **Multiple sclerosis (MS)** is an inflammatory disorder affecting the myelin sheaths of neurons in the brain and spinal cord. Optic neuritis is the most frequent ophthalmic complication of MS but uveitis is a known association. MS is most frequently associated with intermediate uveitis (the primary site of inflammation is the vitreous) but can also be associated with anterior uveitis. The visual loss with MS-associated uveitis is generally considered mild

Localization site	Comment
	Sarcoidosis is a multisystem granulomatous disease that can affect almost every organ in the body. The eye is involved in as many as 50% of patients. Any ocular structure can be involved and the orbit is commonly involved. Central nervous system involvement is reported in approximately 5% of patients with sarcoidosis. Any part of the nervous system can be involved although there appears to be a predilection for the basal leptomeninges and cranial nerves
Mental status and psychiatric aspects/ complications	See **Susac syndrome** under cerebral hemispheres. This is associated with encephalopathy
Vestibular system (and nonspecific dizziness)	See **Susac syndrome** entry under cerebral hemispheres. This is associated with hearing loss
Base of skull	See **VKH** under cerebral hemispheres. This affects the leptomeninges
Cranial nerves	See **Sarcoidosis** under cerebral hemispheres. This has a predilection for the cranial nerves
Spinal cord	See **MS** under cerebral hemispheres
Unclear localization	**Behçet's disease** is a rare chronic, relapsing multisystem vasculitis primarily affecting the eyes, mucosa, and skin. Neuro-Behçet's disease is an uncommon but serious manifestation of Behçet's disease. Characteristic clinical presentation patterns have been described by internal consensus recommendations and divide neurologic disease into parenchymal (multifocal/diffuse, brainstem, spinal cord, cerebral, optic neuropathy) and non-parenchymal disease (venous sinus thrombosis, intracranial aneurysm, and acute meningeal syndrome). Ocular involvement is seen in 70% of patients with Behçet's disease. Acutely, patients present with anterior inflammation but the disease course is one of chronic and/ or recurrent inflammation. Posterior segment involvement is characterized by venous and arterial vasculitis and can be blinding
	Acute posterior multifocal placoid pigment epitheliopathy (APMPPE) is a rare bilateral inflammatory condition affecting the choroid and retina. It is characterized by large placoid-like lesions seen on funduscopic examination. The disorder is usually limited to the eye; however, it is often preceded by a viral prodrome and there have been reports of associated neurologic findings. These include neurosensory hearing loss, cerebral vasculitis, stroke, aseptic meningitis. Headache is the most common associated neurologic symptom

Secondary Complications: Left untreated, uveitis can cause a number of complications including glaucoma, cataracts, retinal detachment, cystoid macular edema, optic nerve damage, and hypotony (low eye pressure) from aqueous hyposecretion. Medical and surgical management are available for these sequelae, many of which can result in permanent vision loss.

Treatment Complications: The general paradigm for treating uveitis is to eliminate any infection if present, suppress inflammation, and treat secondary complications of uveitis. Corticosteroids are the first line therapy in most noninfectious uveitis and can be administered either as topical, periocular, intravitreal, or systemic forms. Long-term use of systemic steroids is associated with well-described complications including hyperglycemia, weight gain, loss of bone density, and gastritis. Common ocular complications include cataracts and elevated intraocular pressure. Central serous choroidopathy is a rare side effect that has been reported with any form of corticosteroid use. In patients whose inflammation is not adequately controlled, long-term treatment with steroid-sparing immunomodulatory agents (IMA) is required to reduce the risk of developing unacceptable side effects from steroids. There are a number of medication classes that exist, with a unique side effect profile.

Bibliography

Jabs DA, Nussenblatt RB, Rosenbaum JT; Standardization of Uveitis Nomenclature (SUN) Working Group. Standardization of uveitis nomenclature for reporting clinical data. Results of the first international workshop. *Am J Ophthalmol.* 2005;140(3):509–16.

Valvuloplasty

Epidemiology and Demographics: While there are no readily available statistics on procedural volume for valvuloplasties, generally, the procedure is becoming more common to treat diseased aortic valves, as it has been shown to be an effective bridge to either transcatheter or surgical aortic valve replacement. However, as the rate of rheumatic disease decreases in the developed world, mitral valvuloplasty may be performed less often.

Disorder Description: This procedure may be used when there is a stenotic heart valve. A catheter carrying a balloon is inserted across the valve and then inflated in order to further open the narrowed valve.

Symptoms

Localization site	Comment
Cerebral hemispheres	Focal infarction/emboli/microemboli. Embolic showers may occur
Mental status and psychiatric aspects/complications	Same as above
Brainstem	Same as above
Cerebellum	Same as above
Vestibular system (and nonspecific dizziness)	Same as above
Base of skull	Same as above

Secondary Complications: Emboli can gather on the delivery tool or be scraped off of the aorta or the heart. The procedure may also lead to valvular regurgitation and/or rupture.

Bibliography

Ben-Dor I, Pichard AD, Satler LF, et al. Complications and outcome of balloon aortic valvuloplasty in high-risk or inoperable patients. *JACC Cardiovasc Interv*. 2010;3(11):1150–6.

Hui DS, Shavelle DM, Cunningham MJ, et al. Contemporary use of balloon aortic valvuloplasty. *Tex Heart Inst J*. 2014;41(5):469–76.

Johns Hopkins Medicine Health Library. Valvuloplasty. Available from www.hopkinsmedicine.org/healthlibrary/test_procedures/cardiovascular/valvuloplasty_92,P07990/. Accessed Sep 24, 2018.

Preston-Maher GL, Torii R, Burriesci G. A technical review of minimally invasive mitral valve replacements. *Cardiovasc Eng Technol*. 2015;6(2):174–84.

Vascular Claudication

Epidemiology and Demographics: Vascular claudication is a symptom of the middle stages of peripheral artery disease (PAD). PAD has a prevalence of 12% and an incidence of 2.4%. The prevalence of claudication is 3% at age 40 and 6% at age 60. It is twice as common in males in the 35–45 years age group (0.04% for males and 0.02% for females), but the incidence is equal in males and females (0.6%) over age 65.

Disorder Description: This disorder is caused by insufficient blood flow through the peripheral arteries to supply the metabolic demand of the muscles. It manifests as intermittent but reproducible cramping pain in the lower extremities, usually the calves. This is because the blood flow cannot increase to meet the increased metabolic demand of active muscles. As such, one would not expect pain upon standing, and resting while still standing will relieve the pain. Resting pain occurs in the late stages. The main differential diagnosis is neurogenic claudication. This occurs as a result of temporary compression of the descending cauda equina due to lumbar spinal stenosis and manifests as aching pain and weakness in the back and/or thighs exacerbated by prolonged standing or walking (due to increased stenosis). The patient must either sit or lean forward to relieve the pain as these positions lead to widening of the spinal canal. Resting pain is not expected unless the patient also has concomitant lumbar radiculopathy. Even in those cases, the left pain should be neuropathic and present at all stages of the disease.

Symptoms

Localization site	Comment
Cauda equina	Pain in the back or legs, weakness of the thigh seen in neurogenic but not vascular claudication
Muscle	Pain in the legs, and especially the calves

Secondary Complications: This is commonly seen in addition to cardiac or cerebrovascular disease.

Treatment Complications: Treatment is by antiplatelet agents, which may lead to bleeding, and by controlling risk factors. Treatment with statins is common and may lead to myopathy or neuropathy.

Bibliography

Dua A, Lee C. Epidemiology of peripheral artery disease and critical limb ischemia. *Tech Vasc Interv Radiol*. 2016;19(2):91–5.

Haig AJ, Park P, Henke PK, et al. Reliability of the clinical examination in the diagnosis of neurogenic versus vascular claudication. *Spine J*. 2013;13(12):1826–34.

Ratchford E. Medical management of claudication. *J Vasc Surg*. 2017;66(1):275–80.

Vascular Dementia

Epidemiology and Demographics: This is a disorder of the elderly. A detectable incidence begins at around age 65 and increases exponentially every 5 years thereafter. The prevalence is estimated at 0.98% in ages 70–79, 4.09% in ages 80–89, and 6.1% in ages over 90. There is no gender preference once other risk factors (hypertension, hyperlipidemia, diabetes, and smoking) are accounted for. It is the second most common cause of dementia behind Alzheimer's disease but the two often coexist.

Disorder Description: This is a multi-domain loss of cognitive skills due to vascular disease affecting both the gray and white matter. It may begin after a clinical stroke but may also occur without a single defined clinical vascular event. The memory loss is more often associated with executive dysfunction and mood/behavioral disorders than is Alzheimer's disease. The onset is stepwise rather than progressive and insidious.

Symptoms

Localization site	Comment
Cerebral hemispheres	Dementia; loss of cognitive function across all domains
Mental status and psychiatric aspects/complications	Behavioral and mood disturbances are common

Secondary Complications: Often seen in association with other signs of chronic cerebrovascular disease such as motor/sensory deficits, gait disturbance (including lower body parkinsonism), dysarthria, and dysphagia.

Treatment Complications: There is no specific treatment other than control of risk factors. Antiplatelet agents may lead to bleeding. Statins may lead to myopathy or neuropathy. Acetylcholinesterase inhibitors are sometimes used and may lead to gastrointestinal upset and bradycardia.

Bibliography

McKay E, Counts S. Multi-infarct dementia: a historical perspective. *Dement Geriatr Cogn Dis Extra*. 2017;7:160–71.

Smith EE. Clinical presentation and epidemiology of vascular dementia. *Clin Sci (Lond)*. 2017;131(11):1059–68.

Vascular Insufficiency to Hand

Epidemiology and Demographics: This is more of a category of disorders than a disease. The most common disorder, Raynaud disease, presents between 20 and 50 years of age with a strong female preponderance.

Disorder Description: This refers to any number of disorders that can lead to insufficient blood flow to the hand. Peripheral artery disease is one of those disorders; it is uncommon for it to affect the upper extremity. More likely causes include direct artery trauma, repetitive trauma leading to ulnar or radial artery stenosis, and vasospasm, either primary (Raynaud disease) or secondary (Raynaud phenomenon).

Symptoms

Localization site	Comment
Muscle	Pain, pallor, paresthesia, dysesthesia, and ulcerations in the affected digits. In Raynaud disease, the finger will turn red, white, and/or blue in cold ambient temperatures

Secondary Complications: Repetitive vascular injuries are likely to occur in manual laborers, particularly those who work with vibrating hand tools. Smoking can lead to Berger's disease (thromboangiitis obliterans), although this disorder of small vessel thrombosis usually affects the legs. Secondary vasospasm occurs in the setting of collagen vascular disorders such as rheumatoid arthritis, lupus, and CREST (calcinosis, Raynaud phenomenon, esophageal dysfunction, sclerodactyly, telangiectasias) syndrome.

Treatment Complications: Injuries may be repaired surgically, carrying the risk of infection. Systemic risks of anesthesia. Thrombolytics carry a risk of hemorrhage. Autoimmune disease may be treated with immune suppressants, carrying the risk of infection.

Bibliography

Higgins JP, McClinton MA. Vascular insufficiency of the upper extremity. *J Hand Surg.* 2010;35(9):1545–57.

Vasculitic Neuropathy

Epidemiology and Demographics: The incidence is unknown. It mostly occurs in the 6th through 8th decades.

Disorder Description: Peripheral nervous system involvement caused by vasculitis, classified based on underlying causes or size of involved vessels:

1. Primary systemic vasculitides (giant cell arteritis, polyarteritis nodosa, Churg-Strauss syndrome, microscopic polyangiitis, Wegener's granulomatosis, essential mixed cryoglobulinemia).
2. Secondary systemic vasculitides (drug, malignancy, infection, and connective tissue diseases).
3. Non-systemic vasculitides (non-systemic vasculitic neuropathy).

Symptoms

Localization site	Comment
Cranial nerves	Occurs in 10% of patients
Peripheral neuropathy	Mostly affects both motor and sensory fibers and is painful. There are 3 patterns of presentation: • Mononeuropathy multiplex – 45% • Asymmetric polyneuropathy (individual mononeuropathies overlap) – 35% • Distal symmetric polyneuropathy – 20%

Secondary Complications: Profound weakness can result in joint stiffness and immobility leading to pressure ulcer. Numbness can lead to neuropathic ulcer.

Treatment Complications: Steroids and immunosuppressive drugs are mainstay of treatment. Steroids may cause immunosuppression, hyperglycemia, hypertension, and adrenal suppression.

Bibliography

Gwathmey KG, Burns TM, Collins MP, Dyck PJ. Vasculitic neuropathies. *Lancet Neurol.* 2014;13(1):67–82.

Katirji B, Kaminski HJ, Ruff RL. *Neuromuscular disorders in clinical practice.* 2nd ed. New York: Springer-Verlag New York; 2014.

Venous Angioma

Epidemiology and Demographics: Venous angiomas (developmental venous anomalies) are fairly common with a prevalence of 3%. However, they are almost always benign and asymptomatic with an intracerebral hemorrhage risk of 0.15–0.68% per year. Even in the setting of hemorrhage, almost all patients do very well with little to no morbidity.

Disorder Description: Angiomas consist of an abnormally dilated but otherwise mature vein that converges radially onto either the deep or superficial venous system of the brain. They are commonly seen in association with cavernous malformations. Those malformations have a far higher risk of hemorrhage and morbidity/mortality.

Symptoms

Localization site	Comment
Cerebral hemispheres	Rarely, these lesions lead to a hemorrhage with symptoms appropriate to the location, such as hemiparesis, hemisensory deficits, visual field deficits, etc. Focal deficits could also occur from local mass effect and venous congestion
Brainstem	Rare hemorrhages could lead to bulbar symptoms. Compression of the fourth ventricle could lead to hydrocephalus manifested by headache, nausea, and alteration of consciousness
Cerebellum	There have been a few cases of hemorrhage and venous thrombosis leading to ataxia

Treatment Complications: Even when these lesions are symptomatic, surgical correction should be avoided. If surgery is absolutely necessary, it is usually best to leave the angioma intact and fix the surrounding problems as altering the angioma has a high risk of venous thrombosis. Thrombosed angiomas may be treated with anticoagulation, carrying the risk of bleeding.

Bibliography

Amin-Hanjani S. Venous angiomas. *Curr Treat Options Cardiovasc Med.* 2011;13:240–6.

Amuluru K, Al-Mufti F, Hannaford S, et al. Symptomatic infratentorial thrombosed developmental venous anomaly: case report and review of the literature. *Interv Neurol.* 2016;4(3–4):130–7.

Ventricular Septal Defect

Epidemiology and Demographics: Ventricular septal defects (VSDs) are most commonly a form of acyanotic congenital heart disease. In fact, it is the most common congenital heart disease with an incidence of 2–6/1000 live births. It can be associated with other congenital abnormalities (e.g., Down syndrome) or be isolated. When isolated, it is believed to be related to abnormalities in the *NKX2.5* gene. It can also occur as a consequence of trauma, myocardial infarction, or cardiac surgery. There have been a handful of cases of stroke related to posttraumatic VSD.

Disorder Description: This is a defect in one part of the ventricular septum. The opening can lead to a left to right shunt leading to heart failure and/or pulmonary hypertension. If the pulmonary pressure exceeds the systemic pressure, then the shunt could reverse. This can theoretically lead to paradoxical embolism, but this is rare.

Symptoms

Localization site	Comment
Cerebral hemispheres	Embolic stroke is possible. The symptoms are related to the vascular territory affected by the embolism but may include aphasia, hemiparesis, hemisensory defects, among others
Brainstem	Bulbar signs
Cerebellum	Ataxia

Secondary Complications: Pulmonary hypertension and congestive heart failure are far more likely complications than neurologic ones. Endocarditis has been reported and high-risk individuals may need antibiotic prophylaxis before dental procedures.

Treatment Complications: Although most cases in adults do not need treatment, when treatment is needed, it would require open heart surgery on a bypass machine or transcutaneous closure. Open surgery carries risk of infection, bleeding, stroke, cardiac arrhythmias in addition to the risks of general anesthesia. Transcutaneous closure is safer but does carry a risk of arrhythmias, sometimes requiring permanent pacemaker placement.

Bibliography

Baumgartner H, Bonhoeffer P, De Groot NM, et al.; Task Force on the Management of Grown-up Congenital Heart Disease of the European Society of Cardiology (ESC); Association for European Paediatric Cardiology (AEPC); ESC Committee for Practice Guidelines (CPG). ESC Guidelines for the management of grown-up congenital heart disease (new version 2010). *Eur Heart J.* 2010;31(23):2915–51.

Cinteza EE, Butera G. Complex ventricular septal defects. Update on percutaneous closure. *Rom J Morphol Embryol.* 2016;57(4):1195–205.

De Bruin G, Pereira da Silva R. Stroke complicating traumatic ventricular septal defect. *J Emerg Med.* 2012;43(6):987–8.

Pineda AM, Mihos CG, Singla S, et al. Percutaneous closure of intracardiac defects in adults: state of the art. *J Invasive Cardiol.* 2015;27(12):561–72.

Vertebral Artery Dissection

Epidemiology and Demographics: This accounts for only approximately 2% of all stroke but disproportionately affects younger individuals causing approximately 10–25% of all strokes in those under age 45. It is 2–5 times less common than carotid dissection.

Disorder Description: An injury to the wall of the blood vessel allows blood to enter the intima and separate (dissect) the layers of the wall. The blood located inside the wall will clot. This may lead to an expansion of the wall, stenosis of the artery, and hypoperfusion. A piece of the clot may also reenter the true lumen leading to an embolic stroke. In the case of vertebral arteries, hypoperfusion is rarely an issue since the other vertebral artery will usually supply enough blood to the basilar artery and its branches. However, the posterior inferior cerebellar artery is the one branch off the vertebral artery itself and so is subject to thrombotic stroke as well. Emboli can reach any part of the posterior circulation affecting the posterior cerebral arteries (PCAs), superior cerebellar artery (SCA), or anterior inferior cerebellar artery (AICA). See entries for *Posterior Cerebral Artery (PCA), Left Territory Infarction, Posterior Cerebral Artery (PCA), Right Territory Infarction.*

Symptoms

Localization site	Comment
Cerebral hemispheres	Contralateral homonymous hemianopia due to stroke in the temporo-occipital lobe
Brainstem	Posterior inferior cerebellar artery strokes lead to lateral medullary (Wallenberg) syndrome: Contralateral loss of pain and temperature below the head, ipsilateral loss of sensation in the lower face, dysphagia, dysarthria, ataxia, vertigo, nystagmus, diplopia, palatal myoclonus, Horner's syndrome
Cerebellum	Ataxia and vertigo
Vestibular system	Vertigo

Secondary Complications: These are often idiopathic or related to trauma (including minor trauma such as coughing) but can be seen in the setting of connective tissues disorders such as Ehlers–Danlos syndrome, Marfan syndrome, and fibromuscular dysplasia.

Treatment Complications: Conservative treatment may be with antiplatelet agents or anticoagulants, both of which may lead to cerebral or systemic bleeding. Vertebral artery stenting is also an option and may lead to femoral artery lesion, bleeding, infection, further arterial damage, and intracerebral bleeding.

Bibliography

Ortiz J, Ruland S. Cervicocerebral artery dissection. *Curr Opin Cardiol.* 2015;30(6):603–10.

Tiu C, Terecoasa E, Grecu N, et al. Vertebral artery dissection: a contemporary perspective. *Maedica (Buchar).* 2016;11(2):144–9.

Vertebrobasilar Insufficiency

Epidemiology and Demographics: Extracranial vertebral artery stenosis is more common in Caucasians and in males. It is generally seen after age 45 with an increased prevalence as one ages. Episodes of transient ischemia carry a 30% 5-year stroke risk. Risk factors include hypertension, diabetes, obesity, hyperlipidemia, and smoking,

Disorder Description: This is a transient ischemic event affecting the entire posterior circulation, and as such, it is a form of transient ischemic attack (TIA). It is most commonly due to atherosclerotic narrowing but may also be caused by dissection. See entry for *Vertebral Artery Dissection.*

Symptoms

Localization site	Comment
Cerebral hemispheres	Blindness or hemianopia. Headache
Brainstem	Nausea, vomiting, vertigo (dizziness), diplopia, ataxia, imbalance, weakness on one or both sides of the body, syncope (see entry for *Syncope*), drop attacks
Cerebellum	Ataxia, imbalance
Vestibular system	Vertigo, hearing loss, tinnitus
Cranial nerves	Diplopia (CN III)

Secondary Complications: Untreated, there is a 30% risk of stroke over the next 5 years. Those who fail medical management have an 8–11% risk of stroke over the next year. Commonly seen in association with atherosclerosis in the carotid, coronary arteries, and/or peripheral vascular beds.

Treatment Complications: The main treatment is antiplatelet agents, which have a risk of bleeding. Statins may be used to control hyperlipidemia and may cause myopathy or neuropathy. Stenting is possible but controversial and may lead to bleeding, femoral artery damage, vertebral dissection, TIA, and stroke.

Bibliography

Jenkins JS, Stewart M. Endovascular treatment of vertebral artery stenosis. *Prog Cardiovasc Dis.* 2017; 59(6): 619–25.

Lima Neto AC, Bittar R, Gattas GS, et al.
Pathophysiology and diagnosis of vertebrobasilar insufficiency: a review of the literature. *Int Arch Otorhinolaryngol.* 2017;21(3):302–7.

Vestibular Degeneration (Cochlear Degeneration)

Epidemiology and Demographics: Degenerative changes of the vestibular system in the elderly are common. These result in vestibular symptoms that comprise some of the most common complaints to primary care doctors in patients over 75 years old.

Disorder Description: Vertigo, disequilibrium, and imbalance are common symptoms among the elderly. The cause of vestibular dysfunction in the elderly is multifactorial. Aging results in diffuse degenerative changes to the vestibular system. The number of hair cells in the maculae and cristae decreases with the number of vestibular nerve fibers. Additionally, the number of Purkinje cells in the cerebellar cortex declines with age. The elderly also have decreased sensitivity to vertical and horizontal acceleration due to demineralization of otoconia.

Vestibular testing in the elderly demonstrates bilaterally decreased caloric responses and a decreased sensitivity of the vestibulo-ocular reflex. In addition, posturography demonstrates that the elderly rely much more on visual cues for maintenance of posture. Despite the decline in vestibular function with aging, the elderly still derive benefit from vestibular rehabilitative therapy.

Symptoms

Localization site	Comment
Inner ear	Otoconia demineralize and fragment
	Hair cells degenerate and are replaced with scar
	Reduction in the number of cells in Scarpa's ganglion
Cranial nerves	Reduction in the number of vestibular nerve fibers
Central nervous system	Lipofuscin accumulation within vestibular nuclei
	Decrease in the number of Purkinje cells

Secondary Complications: Falls constitute a major source of morbidity and mortality in the elderly and vestibular dysfunction is a contributing factor in up to half of these patients.

Treatment Complications: Vestibular rehabilitation is generally well tolerated. Commonly used antivertiginous medication such as antihistamines, benzodiazepines, and anticholinergics have an increased side effect profile in the elderly. Notably, these medications can cause mental confusion in the elderly.

Bibliography

Anson E, Jeka J. Perspectives on aging vestibular function. *Front Neurol.* 2016;6:269.

Ishiyama G. Imbalance and vertigo: the aging human vestibular periphery. *Semin Neurol.* 2009;29(5):491–9.

Lalwani AK. Vertigo, dysequilibrium, and imbalance with aging. In Jackler RK, Brackmann DE, eds. *Neurotology.* 2nd ed. Philadelphia: Mosby; 2005. pp. 533–9.

Vestibular Neuritis (Vestibular Neuronitis)

Epidemiology and Demographics: Sporadic disorder, believed to be of viral origin. The etiology may indeed be reactivation of a dormant herpes simplex virus residing in the Scarpa's ganglion of the vestibular nerve. Vestibular neuritis has an annual incidence of 3.5/100,000 in the general population.

Disorder Description: An acute vestibular syndrome (vertigo, nausea, ataxia, and motion intolerance), occurring without hearing loss. The onset is sudden and unexpected, sometimes preceded by a viral syndrome, and the vertigo is continuous and may last for days to weeks. Gait imbalance occurs after the vertigo resolves.

The differential diagnosis is acute labyrinthitis (inflammation of the inner ear of viral, bacterial, or autoimmune origin), sudden sensorineural hearing loss, first onset of Meniere's disease, or any other inner ear disorder that can cause vertigo.

Symptoms

Localization site	Comment
Inner ear	Unaffected, in the classical case
Cranial nerves	Inflammation of the vestibular division of the VIII nerve
Central nervous system	The central nervous system (CNS) is not affected

Secondary Complications: Patients are at risk of injury from falling. Patients with prolonged imbalance may be disabled from physically demanding work.

Treatment Complications: Treatment is supportive – fluids, antiemetics, and benzodiazepines or meclizine. Persistent imbalance may be treated with vestibular physical therapy after the acute phase resolves.

Dehydration can result from intractable vomiting. Vestibular suppressants may cause drowsiness and anticholinergic effects. Benzodiazepines may cause drowsiness and drug dependency.

Bibliography

Hotson JR, Baloh RW. Acute vestibular syndrome. *N Engl J Med.* 1998;339:680–5.

Smouha E. Inner ear disorders. *NeuroRehabilitation.* 2013;32 455–62.

Viral Myelitis

Epidemiology and Demographics: Incidence is between 1 and 8 new cases per million people per year.

Disorder Description: Viral myelitis is defined as an infection or the inflammation of the white matter or gray matter of the spinal cord. The following viruses can be responsible for the myelitis:

Retrovirus (HIV, HTLV) can cause chronic myelitis.

Poliomyelitis (polio virus, enterovirus, echovirus, and coxsackievirus A and B).

Flavivirus (West Nile, Japanese encephalitis, tick-borne encephalitis).

Transverse myelitis or leukomyelitis can be caused by herpes viruses and influenza viruses.

Symptoms

Localization site	Comment
Cerebral hemisphere	Headache, fever, and meningeal signs
Spinal cord	Flaccid weakness of one or more extremities, bowel or bladder dysfunction
Root involvement	Pain and objective sensory loss in perianal region with hyporeflexia or areflexia associated with paresthesias

Secondary Complications: Up to 20% will have recurrent inflammatory episodes within the spinal cord.

Bibliography

Irani DN. Aseptic meningitis and viral myelitis. *Neurol Clin.* 2008;26(3):635–VIII.

Kincaid O, Lipton HL. Viral myelitis: An update. *Curr Neurol Neurosci Rep.* 2006;6:469–75.

Viral Myositis

Epidemiology and Demographics: Viral myositis is common, especially milder forms. There is no sex predominance. It can occur at any age. There is no specific geographic distribution.

Disorder Description: Viral myositis is primarily a sequela of extant viral infection. In adults it is typically mild, but it can progress to rhabdomyolysis, a more serious condition given risk of renal failure. Children have the same severity spectrum, but can present with an intermediate form wherein there is marked pain and tenderness, particularly in the calves, causing the child to refuse to walk at times and refuse even passive dorsiflexion due to pain.

It is thought that viral myositis may be a result of virus-induced myotoxic cytokines acting upon muscle tissue, rather than direct viral invasion (there is little evidence to actively support viral invasion, though it may occur). Self-immune products may play a component as well. Any viral illness can cause viral myositis, but progression to rhabdomyolysis is more common with the following viruses: influenza A and B including H1N1 virus, coxsackievirus, Epstein–Barr virus (EBV), herpes simplex virus (HSV), parainfluenza, adenovirus, echovirus, cytomegalovirus, measles, varicella-zoster, human immunodeficiency virus, dengue. In children, influenza A and B have a predilection to cause the intermediate form, especially occurring as the acute illness subsides, usually 24 to 48 hours after the resolution of the initial symptoms. Chronic myositis may result from echovirus and HIV.

Lab tests may not be overtly abnormal in the case of mild viral myositis. In children experiencing the intermediate form, muscle enzymes may be elevated up to 20 to 30 times normal without rhabdomyolysis or renal failure. In severe viral myositis, there can be progression to rhabdomyolysis (severely elevated creatine [CK]) and ultimately renal failure (increased creatinine, decreased glomerular filtration rate [GFR]). In general, CK can range from <10,000 to in excess of 500,000 IU/L. Myoglobin may or may not be present in urine. Symptoms of systemic viral infection, including increased inflammatory markers or liver function test abnormalities, are possible. Muscle biopsy may be normal, or show inflammatory myopathy in the case of chronic myositis.

Symptoms

Localization site	Comment
Muscle	Myalgias, especially back and proximal extremities. May not have weakness. Tenderness, erythema
Outside CNS	Fever, GI symptoms

Secondary Complications: Secondary complications can include severe myositis to the point it transitions to rhabdomyolysis, which can lead to renal failure.

Treatment Complications: Treatment is largely supportive and to treat the underlying viral infection in milder cases. Advanced cases with rhabdomyolysis would require IV fluids to reduce risk of progression to renal failure. In chronic viral myositis, IV gammaglobulin may improve clinical outcome.

Intravenous immunoglobulin can cause mild coagulopathy. Otherwise there are no specific complications of treatment except fluid overload from IV fluids.

Bibliography

Crum-Cianflone NF. Bacterial, fungal, parasitic, and viral myositis. *Clin Microbiol Rev.* 2008;21(3):473–94.

Vitamin A Deficiency

Epidemiology and Demographics: Vitamin A deficiency is rarely seen in the United States and other developed countries. However, it is still the third most common cause of nutritional deficiency in the world.[1] Vitamin A is a fat-soluble vitamin. In developed countries vitamin A deficiency is usually seen in patients with fat malabsorption disorders such as cystic fibrosis, celiac disease, cholestatic liver disease such as primary biliary cholangitis, small bowel Crohn's disease, and pancreatic insufficiency.

Disorder Description: Vitamin A is very important for the mucous membranes as it is needed for production of mucopolysaccharides, which help to protect against infections. If vitamin A is deficient, the wetness of the mucous membranes will decrease and the membranes will become dry. This can be seen in the eyes as xerophthalmia. Vitamin A is used in the rods for phototransduction. Patients with vitamin A deficiency are not able to see in low light intensity and develop night blindness.

Vitamin A deficiency also causes nonspecific skin problems, such as hyperkeratosis, phrynoderma (follicular hyperkeratosis), destruction of hair follicles and their replacement with mucus-secreting glands and poor bone growth.[1]

Impairment of the humoral and cell-mediated immune system via direct and indirect effects on the phagocytes and T cells has been noted with vitamin A deficiency.[1]

Secondary Complications: Vitamin A plays an important role in maintaining immunity. Vitamin A treatment appears to reduce complications of measles and mortality in children in developing countries. Supplementation with vitamin A is recommended in developing countries by the World Health Organization.[1-3]

Treatment Complications: Excessive dietary vitamin A intake has been a long-known cause of idiopathic intracranial hypertension.[4] Other retinoids used in the treatment of acne and cancer therapy, all-trans-retinoic acid, retinol, isotretinoin, etretinate, and tretinoin, have also been reported to be associated with idiopathic intracranial hypertension.[4,5] Ingestion of large quantities of bear liver by hunters is another source of vitamin A intoxication and underlying idiopathic intracranial hypertension.

Reports have suggested a role for vitamin A in the pathogenesis of idiopathic intracranial hypertension.[4] Elevated serum vitamin A, retinol, and retinol binding protein levels have been reported in some patients with idiopathic intracranial hypertension.[6,7] Patients with idiopathic intracranial hypertension have been found to have higher CSF vitamin A, retinol, and retinol binding protein levels compared with controls.[8,9] The significance of these findings remains unknown. A hypothesis suggests that excess retinol or retinol binding protein in the CSF interferes with CSF resorption.

Vitamin A deficiency affects photoreceptors (rods) in the retina and causes night blindness.

Retinoic acid has been known to be very teratogenic in pregnancy, particularly in the first trimester, leading to spontaneous abortions and fetal malformations such as microcephaly and cardiac anomalies.[10]

Acute toxicity occurs in adults when an excessive amount of vitamin A is ingested as single dose. Symptoms include nausea, vomiting, vertigo, and blurry vision.[11] In very high doses, drowsiness, malaise, and recurrent vomiting can follow the initial symptoms listed above.

Chronic toxicity causes nonspecific symptoms such as dry skin, nausea, headache, fatigue, irritability, hepatomegaly, alopecia, hyperostosis. Cirrhosis and veno-occlusive disease have been described also.[12]

References

1. Williams SR. *Nutrition and diet therapy*. 8th ed. St. Louis: Mosby; 1997. p. 159.
2. Moskowitz Y, Leibowitz E, Ronen M, Aviel E. Pseudotumor cerebri induced by vitamin A combined with minocycline. *Ann Ophthalmol*. 1993;25:306.
3. Bello S, Meremikwu MM, Ejemot-Nwadiaro RI, Oduwole O. Routine vitamin A supplementation for the prevention of blindness due to measles infection in children. *Cochrane Database Syst Rev*. 2014;1:CD007719.
4. Friedman DI. Medication-induced intracranial hypertension in dermatology. *Am J Clin Dermatol*. 2005;6:29.
5. Fraunfelder FW, Fraunfelder FT, Corbett JJ. Isotretinoin-associated intracranial hypertension. *Ophthalmology*. 2004;111:1248.
6. Selhorst JB, Kulkantrakorn K, Corbett JJ, et al. Retinol-binding protein in idiopathic intracranial hypertension (IIH). *J Neuroophthalmol*. 2000;20:250.
7. Warner JE, Bernstein PS, Yemelyanov A, et al. Vitamin A in the cerebrospinal fluid of patients with and without idiopathic intracranial hypertension. *Ann Neurol*. 2002;52:647.
8. Tabassi A, Salmasi AH, Jalali M. Serum and CSF vitamin A concentrations in idiopathic intracranial hypertension. *Neurology*. 2005;64:1893.
9. Warner JE, Larson AJ, Bhosale P, et al. Retinol-binding protein and retinol analysis in cerebrospinal fluid and serum of patients with and without idiopathic intracranial hypertension. *J Neuroophthalmol*. 2007;27:258.
10. Soprano DR, Soprano KJ. Retinoids as teratogens. *Annu Rev Nutr*. 1995;15:111.
11. Biesalski HK. Comparative assessment of the toxicology of vitamin A and retinoids in man. *Toxicology*. 1989;57:117.
12. Geubel AP, De Galocsy C, Alves N, et al. Liver damage caused by therapeutic vitamin A administration: estimate of dose-related toxicity in 41 cases. *Gastroenterology*. 1991;100:1701.

Suggested Reading

Alemayehu W. Pseudotumor cerebri (toxic effect of the "magic bullet"). *Ethiop Med J*. 1995;33:265.
Colucciello M. Pseudotumor cerebri induced by all-trans retinoic acid treatment of acute promyelocytic leukemia. *Arch Ophthalmol*. 2003;121:1064.
Huiming Y, Chaomin W, Meng M. Vitamin A for treating measles in children. *Cochrane Database Syst Rev*. 2005;4:CD001479.
Sharieff GQ, Hanten K. Pseudotumor cerebri and hypercalcemia resulting from vitamin A toxicity. *Ann Emerg Med*. 1996;27:518.
Yeh YC, Tang HF, Fang IM. Pseudotumor cerebri caused by all-trans-retinoic acid treatment for acute promyelocytic leukemia. *Jpn J Ophthalmol*. 2006;50:295.

Vitamin B12 – Cobalamin Deficiency

Epidemiology and Demographics: Common causes of vitamin B12 deficiency include poor absorption from the stomach or intestines, decreased intake, and increased requirements.[1,2]

Pernicious anemia is the most common cause of cobalamin deficiency: selective impaired absorption of vitamin B12 due to intrinsic factor deficiency. This may be caused by either loss of gastric parietal cells in chronic atrophic gastritis or may result from surgical resection of stomach or from rare hereditary causes of impaired synthesis of intrinsic factor. Cobalamin deficiency in pernicious anemia is thought to result directly from an autoimmune attack on gastric intrinsic factor (IF).[1] There are two types of anti-IF antibodies: one that blocks the attachment of cobalamin to IF and the other that blocks attachment of the cobalamin–intrinsic factor complex to ileal receptors.[1,2] The net result of these anti-IF antibodies is to prevent absorption of dietary cobalamin, leading to cobalamin deficiency.

Vegans and vegetarians are also at risk for B12 deficiency due to inadequate dietary intake of B12. Vitamin B12 occurs mainly in animal products (eggs, meat, milk). Alcoholics and patients with malnutrition are at high risk for the development of folate and/or vitamin B12 deficiency.

Vitamin B12 gets absorbed from the small bowel, mainly the terminal ileum. Surgical removal of the small bowel (e.g., in Crohn's disease), inflammatory bowel disease, or bacterial overgrowth can interfere with vitamin B12 absorption and lead to deficiency.

Hydrochloric acid is needed to split B12 from food proteins and salivary binding proteins. Forms of achlorhydria (including that artificially induced by drugs such as proton pump inhibitors and histamine 2 receptor antagonists) can cause B12 malabsorption from foods.

Metformin also interferes with vitamin B12 absorption.[3]

Nitrous oxide (N_2O) inactivates vitamin B12 and its use in anesthesia may precipitate rapid neuropsychiatric deterioration in vitamin B12-deficient individuals.[4,5] Patients contemplating N_2O anesthesia should be checked for vitamin B12 deficiency and treated prior to such exposure. Similarly, inhalant abuse of N_2O may cause neuropsychiatric problems, even in vitamin B12-sufficient subjects.

Vitamin B12 and folate deficiency often coexist and are not easily differentiated on a clinical basis. Patients with megaloblastic anemia should be evaluated for both deficiencies.

Disorder Description: Vitamin B12 (cobalamin) deficiency usually affects brain, spinal cord, peripheral nerves, and optic nerves. The spinal cord is usually affected first and often exclusively. The term *subacute combined degeneration* (SCD) is reserved for myelopathy associated with vitamin B12 deficiency, and it distinguishes it from other types of spinal cord diseases that also involve the posterior and lateral columns. Peripheral neuropathy is also seen commonly with vitamin B12 deficiency. Whether peripheral neuropathy is primarily related to nerve damage or results from damage to the posterior root fibers at entry to the dorsal cord has been debated, but the available pathologic evidence favors spinal cord involvement.[1,2]

Early in the course of the illness, the only symptom is paresthesia. Complaints of numb hands typically appear before or with lower extremity paresthesia.[1,2] Later, the patient develops signs of involvement of the posterior and lateral columns of the spinal cord. Loss of vibration and position sense is seen mostly and it is more pronounced in the feet and legs than in the hands and arms, and frequently involves the trunk. The motor signs include mild symmetric loss of strength in proximal limb muscles, spasticity, enhanced tendon reflexes, clonus, and extensor plantar responses from lateral column involvement. Initially the patellar and Achilles reflexes are diminished but with development of myelopathy they are increased.

Neuropsychiatric symptoms range from irritability, apathy, somnolence, suspiciousness, emotional instability, to confusional state, depression, and psychosis. Lindenbaum and coworkers have reported cases in which neuropsychiatric symptoms were present without spinal cord or peripheral nerve abnormalities.[2,6] Vitamin B12 deficiency is one of the reversible causes of dementia, and it is routinely checked as a part of dementia workup.

Vitamin B12 deficiency causes optic atrophy and vision loss. That visually evoked potentials may be abnormal in vitamin B12-deficient patients without clinical signs of visual impairment suggests that the visual pathways are affected more often than is evident from the neurologic examination alone.[1]

Vitamin B12 is measured in blood by radioassay. Serum B12 level below 100 pg/mL is usually associated with neurologic signs and symptoms. Serum B12 levels of 200 to 300 pg/mL may still be associated with vitamin B12 deficiency in about 5–10% of cases. High serum concentrations of methylmalonic acid and homocysteine (cobalamin metabolites) are additional reliable indicators of vitamin B12 deficiency and should be used to corroborate the diagnosis in cases of low- to midrange B12 levels.[2,7]

Electrophysiologic studies reveal distal sensory motor axonal peripheral neuropathy and abnormal somatosensory and visual evoked potential latencies. Anemia and macrocytosis are absent in about 40% of patients with vitamin B12 deficiency.[6] Intrinsic factor antibodies are present in approximately 60% and antiparietal cell antibodies are present in about 90% of patients with pernicious anemia.[1]

Symptoms

Localization site	Comment
Cerebral hemispheres	Dementia
Mental status and psychiatric aspects/complications	Irritability
	Apathy
	Somnolence
	Suspiciousness
	Emotional instability
	Marked confusional state
	Depression
	Psychosis
Cranial nerves	Optic atrophy
Peripheral neuropathy	Sensory motor axonal neuropathy
Autonomic system	Urinary sphincter symptoms
	Impotence
Spinal cord (posterior and lateral column involvement)	Myelopathy

Treatment Complications: One treatment regimen for pernicious anemia patients consists of 1000 μg cyanocobalamin intramuscular injection weekly for 1 month and monthly thereafter. Patients with malabsorption syndrome can absorb free cobalamin and therefore can be treated with oral cobalamin supplementation. About 50% of patients who have been treated for cobalamin deficiency exhibit some permanent neurologic deficit.[1]

A common mistake by clinicians is to treat megaloblastic anemia by giving folic acid; this corrects the anemia but may worsen or even evoke the spinal cord lesions due to underlying vitamin B12 deficiency.

References

1. Kasper D, Fauci A, Hauser S, et al. Vitamin and trace mineral deficiency and excess. In Kasper, DL, Fauci AS, Hauser SL, et al., eds. *Harrison's principles of internal medicine*. 19th ed. New York: McGraw-Hill Education/Medical; 2015.
2. Ropper A, Samuels M, Klein J. Diseases of the nervous system caused by nutritional deficiency. In *Adams and Victor's principles of neurology*. 10th ed. New York: McGraw-Hill Education/Medical; 2014. Chapter 41.
3. Zhao-Wei Ting R, Szeto C, Ho-Ming Chan M, Ma K, Chow K. Risk factors of vitamin B12 deficiency in patients receiving metformin. *Arch Intern Med*. 2006;166(18).
4. Doran M, Rassam SS, Jones LM, Underhill S. Toxicity after intermittent inhalation of nitrous oxide for analgesia. *BMJ*. 2004;328:1364.
5. Hadzic A, Glab K, Sanborn KV, Thys DM. Severe neurologic deficit after nitrous oxide anesthesia. *Anesthesiology*. 1995;83:863.
6. Lindenbaum J, Healton EB, Savage DG, et al. Neuropsychiatric disorders caused by cobalamin deficiency in the absence of anemia or macrocytosis. *N Engl J Med*. 1988;318:1720.
7. Allen RH, Stabler SP, Savage DG, Lindenbaum J. Diagnosis of cobalamin deficiencies: I. Usefulness of serum methylmalonic acid and total homocysteine concentrations. *Am J Hematol*. 1990;34:90.

Suggested Reading

Flippo TS, Holder WD Jr. Neurologic degeneration associated with nitrous oxide anesthesia in patients with vitamin B12 deficiency. *Arch Surg*. 1993;128:1391.
Schilling RF. Is nitrous oxide a dangerous anesthetic for vitamin B12-deficient subjects? *JAMA*. 1986;255:1605.

Vitamin D Deficiency

Epidemiology and Demographics: Vitamin D deficiency has been reported with increasing frequency in children in the United States and several other developed nations since the mid 1980s.[1-4]. The prevalence of vitamin D deficiency or insufficiency (25-hydroxyvitamin D [25(OH)D] <20 ng/mL [50 nmol/L]) in the pediatric population in the United States is about 15%.[5-7]

Vitamin D insufficiency appears to be common amongst several other populations[8-11] including those who are dark skinned, obese, taking medications that accelerate the metabolism of vitamin D (such as phenytoin), hospitalized on a general medical ward, or pregnant, and those who have limited effective sun exposure due to protective clothing or consistent use of sun screens, osteoporosis, malabsorption (including inflammatory bowel disease and celiac disease), chronic kidney disease, or coexisting primary hyperparathyroidism.

Disorder Description: Patients with moderate to mild vitamin D deficiency (serum 25(OH)D between 15 and 20 ng/mL) are mostly asymptomatic. Severe vitamin D deficiency leads to reduced intestinal absorption of calcium and phosphorus, which leads to the state of hypocalcemia. Hypocalcemia causes secondary hyperparathyroidism and finally demineralization of bones. Vitamin D deficiency manifests most commonly as rickets in children and osteomalacia in adults.

Vitamin D may act like a neurosteroid hormone during cerebral development and may play a role in the areas of neurotransmission, neuroprotection, and neuroimmunomodulation. Vitamin D deficiency has been associated with neurologic and psychiatric disorders. Vitamin D deficiency has been associated with neuromuscular disorders and dementia in adults.[12]

Myopathy is commonly seen in osteomalacia. Proximal muscle weakness is the initial symptom in about 30% of cases with vitamin D deficiency. Patients complain of proximal limb pain, which may be partly myopathic and partly of bone origin.

Symptoms

Localization site	Comment
Cerebral hemispheres	Seizure[13–14]
	Dementia[15]
	Multiple sclerosis[16–18]
Mental status and psychiatric aspects/complications	Schizophrenia[19]
	Anxiety[20]
	Depression[20]
Peripheral neuropathy	Sensory motor neuropathy[21]
Muscle	Proximal myopathy 30%[21]

Secondary Complications: Prenatal vitamin D deficiency could be a risk factor for schizophrenia according to a neurodevelopmental hypothesis. McGrath et al. have described a decreased incident risk of long-term schizophrenic psychosis in 9114 subjects supplemented with vitamin D over the first year of life.[19] Clinical trials support the hypothesis of the efficacy of vitamin D supplementation in mood disorders.[20]

In rachitic children seizures are observed with low levels of calcium and vitamin D. Long-term vitamin D supplementation led to a reduced incidence of these symptoms. Vitamin D deficiency is seen with the use of antiepileptic medications. This could be partly explained by the observation that antiepileptic medications induce cytochrome P450 enzyme, which leads to an increase in the catabolism of 25(OH)D2 to the inactive metabolite 24,25-dihydroxyvitamin.[22]

Epidemiological data suggest that low serum 25(OH)D2 concentrations are associated with a high incidence of multiple sclerosis.[16,18]

Epidemiological data revealed that low serum 25(OH)D2 concentrations are seen in subjects with Alzheimer's disease.

Elderly patients are at heightened risk for vitamin D deficiency, which may lead to secondary hyperparathyroidism and bone mineralization defects.

Treatment Complications: Symptoms of acute vitamin D intoxication are due to hypercalcemia and include confusion, polyuria, polydipsia, anorexia, vomiting, and muscle weakness. Chronic intoxication may cause renal stones, bone demineralization, and pain.

References

1. Weisberg P, Scanlon KS, Li R, Cogswell ME. Nutritional rickets among children in the United States: review of cases reported between 1986 and 2003. *Am J Clin Nutr.* 2004;80:1697S.
2. McAllister JC, Lane AT, Buckingham BA. Vitamin D deficiency in the San Francisco Bay Area. *J Pediatr Endocrinol Metab.* 2006;19:205.
3. Mylott BM, Kump T, Bolton ML, Greenbaum LA. Rickets in the Dairy State. *WMJ.* 2004;103:84.
4. Shah M, Salhab N, Patterson D, Seikaly MG. Nutritional rickets still afflicts children in north Texas. *Tex Med.* 2000;96:64.
5. Mansbach JM, Ginde AA, Camargo CA Jr. Serum 25-hydroxyvitamin D levels among US children aged 1 to 11 years: do children need more vitamin D? *Pediatrics.* 2009;124:1404.
6. Saintonge S, Bang H, Gerber LM. Implications of a new definition of vitamin D deficiency in a multiracial US adolescent population: the National Health and Nutrition Examination Survey III. *Pediatrics.* 2009;123:797.
7. Gordon CM, Feldman HA, Sinclair L, et al. Prevalence of vitamin D deficiency among healthy infants and toddlers. *Arch Pediatr Adolesc Med.* 2008;162:505.

8. Thomas MK, Lloyd-Jones DM, Thadhani RI, et al. Hypovitaminosis D in medical inpatients. *N Engl J Med*. 1998;338:777.

9. Van der Meer IM, Karamali NS, Boeke AJ, et al. High prevalence of vitamin D deficiency in pregnant non-Western women in The Hague, Netherlands. *Am J Clin Nutr*. 2006;84:350.

10. Yu CK, Sykes L, Sethi M, et al. Vitamin D deficiency and supplementation during pregnancy. *Clin Endocrinol (Oxf)*. 2009;70:685.

11. Compher CW, Badellino KO, Boullata JI. Vitamin D and the bariatric surgical patient: a review. *Obes Surg*. 2008;18:220.

12. Annweiler C, Schott A, Berrut G, et al. Vitamin D and ageing: neurological issues. *Neuropsychobiology*. 2010;62:139–50.

13. Ali FE, Al-Bustan MA, Al-Busairi WA, Al-Mulla F. Loss of seizure control due to anticonvulsant-induced hypocalcemia. *Ann Pharmacother*. 2004;38:1002–5.

14. Christiansen C, Rodbro P, Sjo O. 'Anticonvulsant action' of vitamin D in epileptic patients? A controlled pilot study. *Br Med J*. 1974;2:258–9.

15. Rondanelli M, Trotti R, Opizzi A, Solerte SB. Relationship among nutritional status, pro/antioxidant balance and cognitive performance in a group of free-living healthy elderly. *Minerva Med*. 2007;98:639–45.

16. Torkildsen O, Knappskog PM, Nyland HI, Myhr KM. Vitamin D-dependent rickets as a possible risk factor for multiple sclerosis. *Arch Neurol*. 2008;65:809–11.

17. Kampman MT, Wilsgaard T, Mellgren SI. Outdoor activities and diet in childhood and adolescence relate to MS risk above the Arctic Circle. *J Neurol*. 2007;254:471–7.

18. Munger KL, Zhang SM, O'Reilly E, et al. Vitamin D intake and incidence of multiple sclerosis. *Neurology*. 2004;62:60–5.

19. McGrath J, Saari K, Hakko H, et al. Vitamin D supplementation during the first year of life and risk of schizophrenia: a Finnish birth cohort study. *Schizophr Res*. 2004;67:237–45.

20. Gloth FM 3rd, Alam W, Hollis B. Vitamin D versus broad spectrum phototherapy in the treatment of seasonal affective disorder. *J Nutr Health Aging*. 1999;3:5–7.

21. Skaria J, Katiyar BC, Srivastava TP, Dube B. Myopathy and neuropathy associated with osteomalacia. *Acta Neurol Scand*. 1975;51:37–58.

22. Pack A. Bone health in people with epilepsy: is it impaired and what are the risk factors? *Seizure*. 2008;17:181–6.

Vitamin E Deficiency

Epidemiology and Demographics: Vitamin E deficiency is rarely seen in healthy adults. Vitamin E deficiency occurs mainly in two circumstances: either a defect in intestinal absorption of vitamin E or inherent hepatic enzyme deficiency that blocks incorporation of vitamin E into lipoprotein. Populations with increased risk of developing vitamin E deficiency include those with cirrhosis, cholestatic liver disease, cystic fibrosis, small bowel bacterial overgrowth, pancreatic insufficiency, celiac disease, and Crohn's disease. Certain hereditary disorders are also associated with vitamin E deficiency.[1–2]

Disorder Description: Ataxia with vitamin E deficiency (AVED) is an autosomal recessive disease caused by mutations in the alpha tocopherol transfer protein gene on chromosome 8q13.1. Impairment of function of alpha tocopherol transport protein results in inability to retain and use dietary vitamin E.[3–5] It usually presents as a slowly progressive ataxia and neuropathy.[6–7] Treatment is usually high doses of vitamin E, though complete recovery from neurologic symptoms is uncommon.[8] The absence of dysarthria and skeletal or cardiac muscle involvement helps to differentiate it from Friedreich ataxia.

Abetalipoproteinemia (Bassen–Kornzweig disease) is another autosomal recessive disorder, caused by mutations in microsomal triglyceride transfer protein (MTTP).[9–12] This protein is essential for the formation and secretion of beta-lipoproteins. Beta-lipoproteins are essential for absorption of fat and fat-soluble vitamins A, D, E, and K. Early in life, vitamin E deficiency presents as diarrhea, steatorrhea, and failure to thrive. Neurologic symptoms are mainly related to vitamin E deficiency and present as progressive ataxia. Patients also develop retinitis pigmentosa due to concurrent vitamin A deficiency. Characteristic acanthocytes (spiculated red blood cells) are seen on peripheral blood smears. Neuropathologic changes affect posterior columns and spinocerebellar tracts.[12]

Some studies suggest that there may be some association between development of Alzheimer's disease and vitamin E deficiency.[13] In randomized trials, vitamin E supplementation does not affect the risk of cognitive impairment or dementia,[14] but may possibly slow the progression of Alzheimer's disease.

There are some suggestions that vitamin E supplementation may protect against worsening of tardive dyskinesia but does not improve symptoms.[15–16]

Symptoms

Localization site	Comment
Cerebral hemispheres	? Alzheimer's dementia
Cerebellum	Ataxia
	Dysarthria
	Tremors
Cranial nerves	Ophthalmoplegia
	Pigmented retinopathy
	Night blindness
Basal ganglia	? Tardive dyskinesia
Spinal cord	Myelopathy
Peripheral neuropathy	Large fiber axonal neuropathy
Muscle	Myopathy

Secondary Complications: Vitamin E deficiency reduces the lifespan of red blood cells. Hemolytic anemia is seen in premature infants with vitamin E deficiency.[17] Thalassemia, sickle cell anemia, and other chronic hemolytic anemias may be associated with low vitamin E plasma levels. Oral therapy with vitamin E supplementation may be beneficial.[18–20]

Treatment Complications: No syndrome of acute vitamin E toxicity has been described. In premature infants, high-dose vitamin E may increase the risk for sepsis. Chronic intake of an excessive amount of vitamin E has been associated with increased risk of mortality.[21]

References

1. Ropper A, Samuels M, Klein J. *Adams and Victor's principles of neurology.* 10th ed. New York: McGraw-Hill Education/Medical; 2014.

2. Kasper DL, Fauci AS, Hauser SL, et al., eds. *Harrison's principles of internal medicine.* 19th ed. New York: McGraw-Hill Education/Medical; 2015.

3. Ouahchi K, Arita M, Kayden H, et al. Ataxia with isolated vitamin E deficiency is caused by mutations in the alpha-tocopherol transfer protein. *Nat Genet.* 1995;9:141.

4. Gotoda T, Arita M, Arai H, et al. Adult-onset spinocerebellar dysfunction caused by a mutation in the gene for the alpha-tocopherol-transfer protein. *N Engl J Med.* 1995;333:1313.

5. Kono N, Ohto U, Hiramatsu T, et al. Impaired α-TTP-PIPs interaction underlies familial vitamin E deficiency. *Science.* 2013;340:1106.

6. Yokota T, Shiojiri T, Gotoda T, et al. Friedreich-like ataxia with retinitis pigmentosa caused by the His101Gln mutation of the alpha-tocopherol transfer protein gene. *Ann Neurol.* 1997;41:826.

7. Mariotti C, Gellera C, Rimoldi M, et al. Ataxia with isolated vitamin E deficiency: neurological phenotype, clinical follow-up and novel mutations in TTPA gene in Italian families. *Neurol Sci.* 2004;25:130.

8. Schuelke M, Mayatepek E, Inter M, et al. Treatment of ataxia in isolated vitamin E deficiency caused by alpha-tocopherol transfer protein deficiency. *J Pediatr.* 1999;134:240.

9. Wetterau JR, Aggerbeck LP, Bouma ME, et al. Absence of microsomal triglyceride transfer protein in individuals with abetalipoproteinemia. *Science.* 1992;258:999.

10. Sharp D, Blinderman L, Combs KA, et al. Cloning and gene defects in microsomal triglyceride transfer protein associated with abetalipoproteinaemia. *Nature.* 1993;365:65.

11. Shoulders CC, Brett DJ, Bayliss JD, et al. Abetalipoproteinemia is caused by defects of the gene encoding the 97 kDa subunit of a microsomal triglyceride transfer protein. *Hum Mol Genet.* 1993;2:2109.

12. Rampoldi L, Danek A, Monaco AP. Clinical features and molecular bases of neuroacanthocytosis. *J Mol Med (Berl).* 2002;80:475.

13. Sokol RJ. Vitamin E deficiency and neurological disorders. In Packer L, Fuchs J, eds. *Vitamin E in health and disease.* New York: Marcel Dekker; 1993. p. 815.

14. Kumar N. Nutritional neuropathies. *Neurol Clin.* 2007;25:209.

15. Lohr JB, Caligiuri MP. A double-blind placebo-controlled study of vitamin E treatment of tardive dyskinesia. *J Clin Psychiatry.* 1996;57:167.

16. Soares KV, McGrath JJ. Vitamin E for neuroleptic-induced tardive dyskinesia. *Cochrane Database Syst Rev.* 2001;4:CD000209.

17. Oski FA, Barness LA. Vitamin E deficiency: a previously unrecognized cause of hemolytic anemia in the premature infant. *J Pediatr.* 1967;70:211.

18. Ray D, Deshmukh P, Goswami K, Garg N. Antioxidant vitamin levels in sickle cell disorders. *Natl Med J India.* 2007;20:11.

19. Rachmilewitz EA, Shifter A, Kahane I. Vitamin E deficiency in beta-thalassemia major: changes in hematological and biochemical parameters after a therapeutic trial with alpha-tocopherol. *Am J Clin Nutr.* 1979;32:1850.

20. Jaja SI, Aigbe PE, Gbenebitse S, Temiye EO. Changes in erythrocytes following supplementation with alpha-tocopherol in children suffering from sickle cell anaemia. *Niger Postgrad Med J.* 2005;12:110.

21. Miller ER 3rd, Pastor-Barriuso R, Dalal D, et al. Meta-analysis: high-dosage vitamin E supplementation may increase all-cause mortality. *Ann Intern Med.* 2005;142:37.

Vitamin K Deficiency

Epidemiology and Demographics: Vitamin K deficiency is rarely seen in healthy adults. Newborns are at high risk of developing vitamin K deficiency because of low fat stores, low levels of vitamin K in breast milk, sterile intestinal tract, immature liver, and poor placental transport of vitamin K.[1] In adults, vitamin K deficiency may be seen in patients with chronic small-intestinal disease (e.g., celiac disease, Crohn's disease) or obstructed biliary tracts, or after small-bowel resection. Broad-spectrum antibiotic treatment can precipitate vitamin K deficiency by reducing numbers of gut bacteria, which synthesize vitamin K, and by inhibiting the metabolism of vitamin K.[1,2] Warfarin inhibits conversion of vitamin K to its active form.[1-2] Antiepileptic drugs also interfere with vitamin K metabolism and cause vitamin K deficiency.[1-2]

Disorder Description: Vitamin K is required for carboxylation of glutamic acid, which is necessary for calcium binding to γ-carboxylated proteins such as prothrombin, factors VII, IX and X, protein C, and protein S. Warfarin inhibits γ-carboxylation by preventing the conversion of vitamin K to its active form.[1]

Symptoms: In adults the second most common cause of cerebral hemorrhage after hypertension is use of anticoagulant treatment. The hemorrhages are mainly located in the lobes of the brain. Cerebral hemorrhage, which is precipitated by warfarin therapy, is treated with fresh-frozen plasma and vitamin K, and sometimes with prothrombin complex concentrate, which contains clotting factors.[2]

If a newborn with vitamin K deficiency is not treated urgently, they are at risk for vitamin K deficient bleeding (VKDB), previously known as hemorrhagic disease of the newborn. Classic VKDB develops within the first week of life and is characterized by bleeding from gastrointestinal, umbilical, and circumcision sites or cutaneous bleeding. Early-onset VKDB develops within the first 24 hours of life and is likely associated with maternal vitamin K deficiency (such as in anticonvulsant medication use). About 25% of newborns develop intracranial hemorrhage.[3] Late-onset VKDB typically develops between 3 weeks and 8 months of age and also has a high frequency of intracranial hemorrhage. Late-onset VKDB and associated intracranial hemorrhage appear to be increasing in the United States as a result of parental refusal of vitamin K prophylaxis at birth and with exclusive breast feeding.[4,5]

Antiepileptic medications (phenytoin) interfere with vitamin K metabolism. For that reason, pregnant women taking phenytoin (and some other antiepileptic drugs) should be given vitamin K before delivery, and the newborn infant also should receive vitamin K to prevent bleeding.[2]

Spinal extramedullary hematomas are seen in patients with anticoagulant therapy. Vitamin K should be considered in patients who present with acute spinal cord and cauda equina compression without trauma.[6,7]

Secondary Complications: Clinical signs and symptoms of vitamin K deficiency include easy bruisability, mucosal bleeding, splinter hemorrhages, melena, and hematuria. In severe cases, hemorrhagic shock and death can occur.

Treatment Complications: Toxicity from dietary vitamin K use has not been described. High doses of vitamin K can impair the actions of oral anticoagulants.[8]

References

1. Ropper A, Samuels M, Klein J. *Adams and Victor's principles of neurology.* 10th ed. New York: McGraw-Hill Education/Medical; 2014.

2. Kasper DL, Fauci AS, Hauser SL, et al., eds. *Harrison's principles of internal medicine.* 19th ed. New York: McGraw-Hill Education/Medical; 2015.

3. Volpe JJ. Intracranial hemorrhage in early infancy: renewed importance of vitamin K deficiency. *Pediatr Neurol.* 2014;50:545.

4. Centers for Disease Control and Prevention. Notes from the field: Late vitamin K deficiency bleeding in infants whose parents declined vitamin K prophylaxis – Tennessee, 2013. *MMWR Morb Mortal Wkly Rep.* 2013;62:901.

5. Schulte R, Jordan LC, Morad A, et al. Rise in late onset vitamin K deficiency bleeding in young infants because of omission or refusal of prophylaxis at birth. *Pediatr Neurol.* 2014;50:564.

6. Morandi X, Riffaud L, Chabert E, Brassier G. Acute nontraumatic spinal subdural hematomas in three patients. *Spine.* 2001;26(23):E547–1.

7. Mattle H, Sieb JP, Rohner M, Mumenthaler M. Nontraumatic spinal epidural and subdural hematomas. *Neurology.* 1987;37(8):1351.

8. Schurgers LJ, Shearer MJ, Hamulyák K, et al. Effect of vitamin K intake on the stability of oral anticoagulant treatment: dose-response relationships in healthy subjects. *Blood.* 2004;104:2682.

Vitreous Hemorrhage (Sudden ICP Elevation)

Epidemiology and Demographics: The annual incidence of acute onset vitreous hemorrhage (VH) is about 7/100,000. Common causes of vitreous hemorrhage include proliferative diabetic retinopathy, trauma, retinal break, proliferative retinopathy after retinal vein occlusion, posterior vitrous detachment without retinal tear, and neovascular age-related macular degeneration. It can be spontaneous. In a study of 169 eyes with vitreous hemorrhage of unknown etiology prior to vitrectomy surgery, patients tended to be 50–70 years old without sex predilection. Hypertension was a frequently associated risk factor.

Terson's syndrome is a rare cause of vitreous hemorrhage associated with intracranial hemorrhage. The incidence of vitreous hemorrhage in subarachnoid hemorrhage varies widely from 8% to 44%. It is thought to be underreported as patients with more severe intracranial hemorrhage are at increased risk of intraocular hemorrhage, and highest risk patients are unlikely to complain of visual symptoms.

Disorder Description: Vitreous hemorrhage occurs when there is extravasation of blood into the potential spaces within and around the vitreous body. Vitreous hemorrhage associated with intracranial, subdural, and subarachnoid hemorrhage is termed Terson's Syndrome. The mechanism of the intraocular bleeding is unclear, but the prevailing theory is that the sudden rise in intracranial pressure is transmitted down the optic nerve sheath leading to venous hypertension and bleeding in the retinal vessels. Another proposed mechanism is that there is direct extension of blood into the subarachnoid space within the optic nerve sheath through small perivascular subarachnoid channels to the retina. Incidence of intraocular hemorrhage in intracranial hemorrhage reported in the literature varies widely.

Symptoms

Localization site	Comment
Varying localization	**Subarachnoid hemorrhage** refers to blood in the subarachnoid space between the pia and arachnoid membranes. Head trauma is a common cause, but spontaneous subarachnoid hemorrhage most commonly occurs after rupture of a cerebral aneurysm followed by arteriovenous malformation. As described above, Terson's syndrome is a potentially underreported complication
	Visual symptoms include acute visual disturbance with descriptions of hazy vision, floaters, smoke signals, cobwebs, and shadows

Secondary Complications: Epiretinal membrane is the most common intraocular complication of vitreous hemorrhage in Terson's syndrome. Proliferative vitreoretinopathy, retinal folds, retinal detachment, and amblyopia in younger patients are other reported complications. Ghost cell glaucoma, a condition in which de-hemoglobinized red blood cells block the aqueous outflow structures of the eye, is also a concern in Terson's syndrome. Elevated intracranial pressure leading to papilledema can lead to permanent vision loss. Neurologic complications of subarachnoid hemorrhage include rebleed, hydrocephalus, vasospasm, and seizures.

Permanent vision loss is possible, particularly when seen as part of diabetic retinopathy.

Treatment Complications: In most patients, vitreous hemorrhage resolves within 12 months but vitrectomy surgery can expedite this process, especially in cases of non-clearing hemorrhage. In a report of 36 patients treated with vitrectomy, most patients experienced visual recovery after removal of vitreous hemorrhage. Younger patients and shorter time to surgery were predictors of better visual recovery. Four patients in the study developed late complication of proliferative vitreoretinopathy associated retinal detachment.

Bibliography

Garweg JG, Koerner F. Outcome indicators for vitrectomy in Terson syndrome. *Acta Ophthalmol.* 2009;87(2):222–26. DOI:10.1111/j.1755-3768.2008.01200.x.

Kim DY, Soo Geun J, Seunghee B, et al. Acute-onset vitreous hemorrhage of unknown origin before vitrectomy: causes and prognosis. *J Ophthalmol.* 2015;2015: Article ID 429251. DOI:10.1155/2015/429251.

Lee GI, Choi KS, Han MH, et al. Practical incidence and risk factors of Terson's syndrome: a retrospective analysis in 322 consecutive patients with aneurysmal subarachnoid hemorrhage. *J Cerebrovasc Endovas Neurosurg.* 2015;17(3): 203–8. DOI:10.7461/jcen.2015.17.3.203.

Spraul CW, Grossniklaus HE. Vitreous hemorrhage. *Surv Ophthalmol.* 1997;42(1):3–39.

Vogt–Koyanagi–Harada Syndrome

Epidemiology and Demographics: Predominant age of presentation is 3–89 years, with the maximum frequency in persons in their 30s. Females are more commonly affected than males; the female-to-male ratio in most large series is 2:1. Seen in Eastern and Southeastern Asian, Middle Eastern, Hispanic, and Native American populations. The disorder is extremely uncommon in Caucasians and Africans. Exact incidence and prevalence are not known.

Disorder Description: This condition is an autoimmune disease that affects melanin-containing tissues. Although this is a multisystem disease, the most prominent manifestation causes bilateral, diffuse uveitis with pain, redness, and blurring of vision. Auditory manifestations can lead patient to have tinnitus, hyperacusis, and vertigo. Neurologic involvement of the meninges causes patients to have stiffness of neck and back. Patients also develop cranial nerve palsies, hemiparesis, transverse myelitis, and ciliary ganglionitis. Dermatologic manifestations cause alopecia and vitiligo. Vitiligo is most prominent in the sacral region.

This condition occurs in four phases:

Prodromal phase: No symptoms to mild flu-like symptoms. Symptoms include fever, headache, nausea, neck stiffness, discomfort from loud noises, tinnitus and/or vertigo, orbital pain, light sensitivity, and tearing from eyes. Patient may complain of touch sensitivity to skin and hair. Some patients have also presented with optic neuritis and cranial nerve palsies.

Acute uveitic phase: This phase typically lasts a couple of weeks. Patients present with bilateral panuveitis resulting in blurred vision. Patient can demonstrate optic nerve hyperemia and papillitis on funduscopic exam. Patient can also present with bullous serous retinal detachments.

Convalescent phase: Patients demonstrate gradual tissue depigmentation and alopecia. Funduscopic exam demonstrates depigmentation resulting in orange–red discoloration and clumping of the retinal pigment epithelium.

Chronic recurrent phase: Patient has repeated bouts of uveitis that are associated with cataracts, glaucoma, and ocular hypertension.

Potential causes include:

Viral infection or skin or eye trauma.

Abnormal T-cell-mediated immune response directed against self-antigens, located on melanocytes.

Risk factors include:

Females between 20 and 50 years of age.

Asian, Latino, Middle Eastern, American Indian, or Mexican Mestizo origin.

HLA-DR4 and DRB1/DQA1 allele; HLA-DRB1*0405 plays a large role in susceptibility.

Secondary Complications

- Vision loss
- Optic atrophy
- Cataracts

- Glaucoma
- Permanent skin changes

Treatment Complications

Steroids: Methylprednisolone and prednisone are commonly used to treat this condition. The use of methylprednisolone causes an increased risk of infection, hyperglycemia, avascular necrosis of the hip, psychosis, Cushing's disease, and osteoporosis.

Immunomodulators: Cyclosporine, tacrolimus, mycophenolate mofetil, azathioprine, cyclophosphamide, or chlorambucil are also utilized when patients do not respond to systemic steroids. Cyclophosphamide has been known to cause hemorrhagic cystitis, neutropenia or lymphoma, premature menopause, infertility in men and women. Cyclophosphamide is carcinogenic and therefore increases the risk for developing lymphomas, leukemia, skin cancer, transitional cell carcinoma of the bladder, and multiple myeloma. Furthermore, azathioprine is teratogenic and careful avoidance of such drugs during pregnancy is advised. Azathioprine can cause patients to develop progressive multifocal leukoencephalopathy, lymphoma, and other possible malignancies. Cyclosporine can lead to the development of pancreatitis, enlargement of gums, convulsions, nephrotoxicity, and hepatotoxicity. It is nephrotoxic, neurotoxic, increases the risk of squamous cell carcinoma and infections, and often causes hypertension due to renal vasoconstriction and increased sodium reabsorption. Most immunomodulators carry an increased risk of cancer.

Bibliography

Andreoli CM, Foster CS. Vogt-Koyanagi-Harada disease. *Int Ophthalmol Clin.* 2006;46(2):111–22.

Rajendram R, Evans M, Rao NA. Vogt-Koyanagi-Harada disease. *Int Ophthalmol Clin.* 2005;45(2):115–34.

Voltage-Gated Potassium Channel Antibody Syndrome (Limbic Encephalitis)

Epidemiology and Demographics: Mean age of presentation is about 60 years (range 30–80 years). Group of patients with anti-LGI1 antibody associated limbic encephalitis have a male predominance. No race predilection is known. The incidence of this condition worldwide is not known. In Denmark, the incidence has been reported to be 1.1 cases per million.

Disorder Description: Limbic encephalitis is a rare neurologic disorder characterized by amnesia, seizures, and psychiatric disturbances, associated with anti-neuronal antibodies that can target either intracellular or neuronal cell surface antigens such as voltage-gated potassium channels (VGKCs). Limbic encephalitis is the second most common non-prion diagnostic of rapidly progressive dementia. VGKC is a complex linked to the neuronal cell surface. Syndromes associated with antibodies against VGKC are typical limbic encephalitis and Morvan's syndrome, defined by the association of psychiatric symptoms, hallucinations, peripheral nerve hyperexcitability, hyperhidrosis, and other symptoms of autonomic dysfunction. This condition has been associated with blood disorders such as Hodgkin's and non-Hodgkin's lymphomas and acute myeloid leukemia. This condition is also associated with Charcot–Marie–Tooth disease. It is now acknowledged that most VGKC antibodies are instead directed towards associated/complexed proteins. The VGKC, like other ion channels, belong to a multiprotein complex. Some of the proteins that associate to the channel directly/indirectly include, but are not limited to, LGI1, CASPR2, Contactin2, DPPX, ADAM22, and ADAM23. The majority of patients improve with immunosuppressant treatment but recovery is often incomplete, and most are left with mild disability. Death occurs in less than 10%, but up to 20% go on to develop relapses.

Exact cause of this condition is unknown though there is some association with tumors: history of thymoma and history of tumor.

Risk factors include:
- Male
- Age between 30 and 80 years
- Thymoma or history of other kind of a tumor

No particular geographic proclivity is known.

Symptoms

Localization site	Comment
Brain: mesial temporal lobes	Signs and symptoms vary based on the type of receptor affected: – Initial symptoms include forgetfulness, drowsiness, and withdrawal from activities. Patient may also develop depression, bizarre thoughts and/or behaviors – *Anti-LGI-1 encephalitis manifestations:* Amnesia/confusion, hallucinations, myoclonus/dyskinesia, sleep disorders such as REM sleep behavior disorder, hypersomnia or insomnia and ataxia. Tonic seizures, with movements of the leg, arm or face, refractory to treatment with antiepileptic drugs – *Anti-CASPR2 nervous system manifestations:* Patients with anti-CASPIR2 antibodies develop symptoms from the central nervous system and/or the peripheral nervous system. The classic presentation is with Morvan's syndrome, a disease with the features of neuromyotonia (i.e., peripheral hyperexcitability) and limbic encephalitis. Other patients present with isolated neuromyotonia or limbic encephalitis MRI brain demonstrates that the patient has T2 signal hyperintensity in the mesial temporal lobes (insular cortex and hippocampus) EEG usually shows interictal foci of epileptiform activity or slowing over antero-temporal or mid-temporal (sometimes also frontal) regions and ictal activity in the same areas

Secondary Complications

Seizures

Memory problems/difficulty with concentration

Behavioral and psychiatric/psychologic conditions

Inability to live or function independently or without supervision

Treatment Complications

Corticosteroids: Increased risk of infection, hyperglycemia, avascular necrosis of the hip, psychosis, Cushing's disease.

Intravenous immunoglobulin (IVIG): IVIG can induce reactions in patients with IgA deficiency. This occurs in 1/500–1000 patients. Serious anaphylactoid reactions occur soon after the administration of IVIG. Anaphylaxis associated with sensitization to IgA in patients with IgA deficiency can be prevented by using IgA-depleted immunoglobulin. The presence of IgG anti-IgA antibodies is not always associated with severe adverse reactions to IVIG. As IVIG can lead to thrombosis, IVIG has also been known to cause stroke and acute myocardial infarction. Nephrotoxicity has also been linked to the use of IVIG. IVIG therapy can result in postinfusion hyperproteinemia, increased serum viscosity, and pseudohyponatremia. Aseptic meningitis is also a rare but well-recognized complication of IVIG therapy.

Plasmapheresis: Hypocalcemia/hypomagnesemia before or after treatment, hypothermia during treatment, transfusion-related reactions are also likely, hypotension may occur in patients taking angiotensin-converting enzyme (ACE) inhibitors, in particular while undergoing column-based plasmapheresis. Thrombocytopenia and hypofibrinogenemia may occur after plasmapheresis (especially if albumin is being used as a replacement product) and patient should be monitored for signs of bleeding.

Immunosuppressants: Rituximab and cyclophosphamide are commonly used to treat this condition. Rituximab is a monoclonal antibody medication that carries the risk of cardiac arrest, tumor lysis syndrome, progressive multifocal leukoencephalopathy (PML), immunotoxicity, cytokine release syndrome, pulmonary toxicity, and bowel obstruction/perforation. It has also been known to reactivate hepatitis B infection and other viral infections. Cyclophosphamide has been known to cause hemorrhagic cystitis, neutropenia or lymphoma, premature menopause, infertility in men and women. Cyclophosphamide is carcinogenic and therefore increases the risk for developing lymphomas, leukemia, skin cancer, transitional cell carcinoma of the bladder, and multiple myeloma.

Bibliography

Day B, Eisenman L, Black J, Maccotta L, Hogan R. A case study of voltage-gated potassium channel antibody-related limbic encephalitis with PET/MRI findings. *Epilepsy Behav Case Rep.* 2015;4:23–6.

Merchut MP. Management of voltage-gated potassium channel antibody disorders. *Neurol Clin.* 2010;28(4):941–59.

Vincent A, Buckley C, Schott JM, et al. Potassium channel antibody-associated encephalopathy: A potentially immunotherapy-responsive form of limbic encephalitis. *Brain.* 2004;127:701–12.

Volume Depletion

Epidemiology and Demographics: Volume depletion is one cause of orthostatic hypotension. Orthostatic hypotension is the second most common cause of syncope and has a prevalence of 5% under age 50 and 30% over age 70, although most of those cases are due to other causes such as cardiac disease, antihypertensive use, and autonomic disease.

Disorder Description: A drop in total blood volume due to hemorrhage, diarrhea, vomiting, or dehydration will lead to a drop in blood pressure. This hypotension is exacerbated by standing.

Symptoms

Localization site	Comment
Cerebral hemispheres	Lightheadedness, dizziness, visual blurring, syncope
Brainstem	Lightheadedness, dizziness, visual blurring, syncope

Secondary Complications: May be due to failure to drink enough water but is usually seen in combination with systemic bleeding, diarrhea, or emesis.

Treatment Complications: None for water repletion in the setting of diarrhea or emesis. If the volume depletion is due to bleeding, then a transfusion may be needed, carrying the risk of blood-borne pathogen infection and transfusion reaction.

Bibliography

Ntusi NA, Coccia CB, Cupido BJ, Chin A. An approach to the clinical assessment and management of syncope in adults. *S Afr Med J.* 2015;105(8):690–3.

Ricci F, De Caterina R, Fedorowski A. Orthostatic hypotension: epidemiology, prognosis, and treatment. *J Am Coll Cardiol.* 2015;66(7):848–60.

von Hippel–Lindau Disease

Epidemiology and Demographics: Incidence of 1/36,000 births worldwide. Equal incidence in males and females of all ethnicities. Most commonly presents in third decade but can present at any age.

Disorder Description: Autosomal dominant syndrome characterized by tumors in the nervous system, kidney, pancreas, adrenal glands, and adnexal organs.

Uncontrolled angiogenesis is the result of a mutation in the VHL gene, which encodes a protein that in normal conditions regulates hypoxia inducible factor. Hemangioblastomas can grow anywhere in the nervous system with predilection for the posterior fossa and posterior spinal cord. They are the most common lesions associated with VHL disease. The inner ear is subject to the locally invasive endolymphatic sac tumor (ELST). Other tumor types include retinal angioma, clear cell renal cell carcinoma, pheochromocytoma, serous cystadenoma and neuroendocrine tumors of the pancreas, and papillary cystadenoma of the epididymis and broad ligament. Families with VHL disease have been divided into two types based upon the likelihood of developing pheochromocytoma (type 2 is high risk).

Symptoms

Localization site	Comment
Mental status	Anxiety and behavioral changes, particularly short-temperedness, can result from associated pheochromocytoma
Brainstem	Brainstem involvement of hemangioblastoma is common and presents with numbness, gait ataxia, and dysphagia
Cerebellum	The cerebellum is the most common location of hemangioblastoma. Most common symptoms are headache and ataxia. Dysmetria and hydrocephalus are regularly seen
Vestibular system (and nonspecific dizziness)	Tinnitus and hearing loss are the most common symptoms of endolymphatic sac tumors, which are often bilateral
Cranial nerves	Facial paralysis can result from endolymphatic sac tumor. Cranial nerve hemangioblastoma is rare
Spinal cord	Spinal hemangioblastoma can lead to numbness, weakness, gait ataxia, hyperreflexia, and pain. The cervical and thoracic cord are common locations for hemangioblastoma
Anterior horn cells	Hemangioblastomas less frequently involve the anterior cord
Dorsal root ganglia	Radiculopathy from hemangioblastoma is common
Conus medullaris	Hemangioblastoma can infrequently cause symptoms of conus medullaris

Localization site	Comment
Cauda equina	Hemangioblastoma can rarely cause cauda equina syndrome
Specific spinal roots	Cervical and thoracic spinal nerve roots are commonly affected by hemangioblastoma
Plexus	Rare location for hemangioblastoma
Peripheral neuropathy	Rare location for hemangioblastoma

Secondary Complications: Renal cell carcinoma presents with hematuria and is the leading cause of mortality. Hemorrhagic hemangioblastoma is another common cause of mortality. Visual loss from optic hemangioblastoma is common. Untreated endolymphatic sac tumors can lead to drop metastasis. Pheochromocytoma can lead to episodic hypertension.

Treatment Complications: Primary treatment for both hemangioblastoma and ELST is resection. For hemangioblastomas that appear in clusters or are not amenable to surgery, radiation therapy can halt growth but does not decrease their size. Cochlear implantation is a consideration for deafness after resection of ELST.

Bibliography

Butman JA, Linehan WM, Lonser RR. Neurologic manifestations of von Hippel-Lindau disease. *JAMA.* 2008;300(11):1334–42.

Lonser RR, Glenn GM, Walther M, et al. von Hippel-Lindau disease. *Lancet.* 2003;361(9374):2059–67.

Megerian CA, Semaan MT. Evaluation and management of endolymphatic sac and duct tumors. *Otolaryngol Clin North Am.* 2007;40(3):463–78.

Waldenström's Macroglobulinemia (Lymphoplasmacytic Lymphoma)

Epidemiology and Demographics: Median age of onset of Waldenström's macroglobulinemia (WM) is between 60 and 65 years, with some cases occurring in late teens. Male predominance (60%). In the United States this condition is more common among Caucasians, with people of African descent representing only 5% of all patients. In the United Kingdom, the annual incidence of the disease is 10.3 per million. Rare condition with 1400 to 1600 cases annually in the United States.

Disorder Description: WM is a chronic, indolent B-cell lymphoproliferative disorder that has features that are similar to non-Hodgkin's lymphomas. It is characterized by the presence of a high level of a macroglobulin (immunoglobulin M [IgM]), elevated serum viscosity, and the presence of a lymphoplasmacytic infiltrate in the bone marrow. The clinical presentation is similar to that of multiple myeloma except that organomegaly is common in WM and is uncommon in multiple myeloma, and lytic bony disease and renal disease are uncommon in WM but are common in multiple myeloma. Peripheral neuropathy occurs in nearly half of patients with this condition, and hyperviscosity-related nervous system disorders are encountered in up to a third. Other neurologic complications, such as encephalopathy or myelopathy caused by direct tumor infiltration, paraprotein deposition or autoimmune phenomena, are rare. WM can present with central nervous system (CNS) symptoms, either as a result of serum hyperviscosity or direct tumor infiltration of CNS. The latter phenomenon is known as Bing–Neel syndrome (BNS). BNS is usually suspected in patients with WM who exhibit CNS symptoms and abnormal brain magnetic resonance imaging (MRI), which can be further confirmed with cerebrospinal fluid (CSF) analysis and/or biopsy.

Potential causes include:

Mutation of the MYD88 gene (90% of patients)
Mutation of the CXCR4 gene (27% of patients)
Chromosomal abnormalities: deletions of 6q23 and 13q14, and gains of 3q13–q28, 6p and 18q

Overexpression of Src tyrosine kinase and FGFR3
Risk factors include:
First-degree relative with WM
Male gender
Personal history of autoimmune disease with autoantibodies
History of liver inflammation
History of HIV
History of rickettsiosis
Exposure to farming
Pesticide exposure
Wood dust exposure
Organic solvent exposure

No specific areas in the world are thought to have higher proclivity.

Symptoms

Localization site	Comment
Brain	– Confusion, slurred speech, headache, fatigue, ataxia, memory problems, nausea, vomiting, diplopia, nystagmus, and extremity numbness (Bing–Neel syndrome) – Dizziness, headache, hearing and visual problems (hyperviscosity syndrome) – Cranial nerve palsies (CN II, CN VII, and CN VIII) – Stroke – Seizures
Peripheral nervous system	– Discomfort and sensory loss in the legs – Diminished vibratory sense – Loss of pinprick sensation – EMG/nerve conduction studies can demonstrate sensory or sensorimotor axonal loss – Gait abnormalities secondary to sensory loss in lower extremities

Secondary Complications

- Cardiac failure
- Hyperviscosity syndrome
- Visual disturbances secondary to hyperviscosity syndrome
- Increased incidence of lymphomas, myelodysplasia, and leukemias
- Amyloidosis of the heart, lungs, liver, kidney, and joints
- Diarrhea and malabsorption secondary to gastrointestinal (GI) involvement

- Bleeding dyscrasias secondary to platelet dysfunction
- Coagulation factor and fibrinogen abnormalities due to interaction with plasma IgM
- Raynaud phenomenon secondary to cryoglobulinemia
- Increased predisposition to infection due to B-cell dysfunction
- Increased incidence of lymphomas, myelodysplasia, and leukemias
- Renal disease (less common)

Treatment Complications

- Nucleoside analogs: T-cell dysfunction.
- Plasmapheresis (for hyperviscosity syndrome): Hypocalcemia/hypomagnesemia before or after treatment, hypothermia during treatment, transfusion-related reactions are also likely, hypotension may occur in patients taking angiotensin-converting enzyme (ACE) inhibitors, in particular while undergoing column-based plasmapheresis. Thrombocytopenia and hypofibrinogenemia may occur after plasmapheresis (especially if albumin is being used as a replacement product) and patient should be monitored for signs of bleeding.
- Immunosuppressants: Rituximab and cyclophosphamide are commonly used to treat this condition. Rituximab is a monoclonal antibody medication that carries the risk of cardiac arrest, tumor lysis syndrome, progressive multifocal leukoencephalopathy (PML), immunotoxicity, cytokine release syndrome, pulmonary toxicity, and bowel obstruction/perforation. It has also been known to reactivate hepatitis B infection and other viral infections. Cyclophosphamide has been known to cause hemorrhagic cystitis, neutropenia or lymphoma, premature menopause, infertility in men and women. Cyclophosphamide is carcinogenic and therefore increases the risk for developing lymphomas, leukemia, skin cancer, transitional cell carcinoma of the bladder, and multiple myeloma.
- Nitrogen mustards: Bendamustine is commonly used in combination with the immunosuppressants. Usage of this medication can cause nausea, fatigue, vomiting, diarrhea, fever, constipation, loss of appetite, cough, headache, unintentional weight loss, difficulty breathing, rashes, and stomatitis, as well as immunosuppression, anemia, and low platelet counts.
- Proteasome inhibitor: Bortemozib is also known to be effective in treating this condition. Bortezomib is associated with peripheral neuropathy, which in some cases can be painful. Patients suffering from pre-existing peripheral neuropathy may experience an exacerbation of their symptoms. This medication is also associated with the development of shingles, which can be mitigated with prophylactic acyclovir. Acute interstitial nephritis has also been reported.
- Steroids: Dexamethasone is commonly used concurrently with chemotherapy to counteract the side effects of antitumor treatments. The use of dexamethasone causes an increased risk of infection, hyperglycemia, avascular necrosis of the hip, psychosis, Cushing's disease.

Bibliography

Baehring JM, Hochberg EP, Raje N, Ulrickson M, Hochberg FH. Neurological manifestations of Waldenström macroglobulinemia. *Nat Clin Pract Neurol*. 2008;4(10):547–56.

Fonseca R, Hayman S. Waldenström macroglobulinaemia. *Br J Haematol*. 2007;138:700.

Wernicke's Disease (Component of Wernicke–Korsakoff Syndrome)

Epidemiology and Demographics: In the United States, Wernicke's disease is most commonly seen in alcoholics though patients with malnutrition due to hyperemesis, starvation, renal dialysis, cancer, AIDS, or gastric surgery are also at risk.[1,2] Alcohol interferes with the absorption of thiamine and also increases urinary excretion. Patients receiving chronic diuretic therapy are also at risk of thiamine deficiency due to increased loss of urinary thiamine. Autopsy studies reveal a higher incidence of Wernicke's disease than that predicted by clinical studies.[3,4] While cases of Wernicke's disease in men outnumber those in women, women appear to be more susceptible to developing disease than men.[3,4]

Disorder Description: Wernicke's disease is due to acute deficiency of thiamine. Thiamine is a cofactor of several enzymes, including transketolase, pyruvate dehydrogenase, and α-ketoglutarate dehydrogenase. Thiamine deficiency produces diffuse cerebral glucose utilization, mitochondrial damage, and glutamate excitotoxicity. Carl Wernicke described this syndrome as a triad of ophthalmoplegia, ataxia, and global confusion. But only one-third of patients with Wernicke's disease present with the classic clinical triad.[5]

Acute cases of Wernicke's disease reveal periventricular lesions surrounding the third ventricle, aqueduct, and fourth ventricle, with petechial hemorrhages on pathology.[3,6]

Chronic cases reveal atrophy of the mammillary bodies.[3,7,8]

Amnestic defect is due to lesions in the dorsal medial nuclei of the thalamus.[6]

Differential Diagnosis. Etiologies of acute delirium or acute ataxia, structural diseases in the medial thalami, hippocampi or inferior medial temporal lobes such as top-of-the-basilar stroke, hypoxic–ischemic encephalopathy, herpes simplex encephalitis, and third ventricular tumors, etc.[2]

Symptoms

Localization site	Comment
Mental status and psychiatric aspects/complications	Disorientation Delirium related to ethanol withdrawal If the disease is not treated, stupor, coma, and death may ensue
Cerebellum (anterior and superior vermis)	Ataxia
Vestibular system (and non-specific dizziness)	Ataxia
Cranial nerves	Horizontal nystagmus on lateral gaze Lateral rectus palsy (usually bilateral) Conjugate gaze palsies Rarely amblyopia Rarely ptosis and miosis
Peripheral neuropathy	Sensory motor peripheral neuropathy Autonomic neuropathy

Secondary Complications: Tachycardia and postural hypotension may be related to impaired function of the autonomic nervous system or to the coexistence of cardiovascular beriberi.[1] As the symptoms recede, an amnestic state with impairment in recent memory and learning may become more apparent, known as Korsakoff's syndrome.

Treatment Complications: Immediate administration of a high dose of thiamine is used. The dose should be given prior to treatment with intravenous glucose solutions. Glucose infusions may precipitate Wernicke's disease by depleting thiamine stores in a previously unaffected patient or cause a rapid worsening of an early form of the disease. For this reason, thiamine should be administered to all alcoholic patients requiring parenteral glucose.[9–10] Thiamine toxicity syndrome has not been described.

References

1. Ropper A, Samuels M, Klein J. *Adams and Victor's principles of neurology.* 10th ed. New York: McGraw-Hill Education/Medical; 2014.
2. Kasper DL, Fauci AS, Hauser SL, et al., eds. *Harrison's principles of internal medicine.* 19th ed. New York: McGraw-Hill Education/Medical; 2015.
3. Victor M, Adams RA, Collins GH. *The Wernicke-Korsakoff syndrome and related disorders due to alcoholism and malnutrition.* Philadelphia: FA Davis; 1989.
4. Harper C. The incidence of Wernicke's encephalopathy in Australia: a neuropathological study of 131 cases. *J Neurol Neurosurg Psychiatry.* 1983;46:593.
5. Galvin R, Bråthen G, Ivashynka A, et al. EFNS guidelines for diagnosis, therapy and prevention of Wernicke encephalopathy. *Eur J Neurol.* 2010;17:1408.
6. Malamud N, Skillicorn SA. Relationship between the Wernicke and the Korsakoff syndrome: a clinicopathologic study of seventy cases. *Arch Neurol Psychiat.* 1956;76:586.
7. Torvik A. Two types of brain lesions in Wernicke's encephalopathy. *Neuropathol Appl Neurobiol.* 1985;11:179.
8. Park SH, Kim M, Na DL, Jeon BS. Magnetic resonance reflects the pathological evolution of Wernicke encephalopathy. *J Neuroimaging.* 2001;11:406.
9. Wrenn KD, Murphy F, Slovis CM. A toxicity study of parenteral thiamine hydrochloride. *Ann Emerg Med.* 1989;18:867.
10. Agabio R. Thiamine administration in alcohol-dependent patients. *Alcohol Alcohol.* 2005;40:155.

Whipple's Disease

Epidemiology and Demographics: Whipple's disease is a rare disorder with an estimated incidence of 1/1,000,000. There is a male predominance with a male-to-female ratio of 3 to 1. Whipple's disease is more common in Caucasians with an average age of onset of 50 years.

Disorder Description: Whipple's disease is a malabsorption syndrome caused by *Tropheryma whippelii* infection, which is a weakly gram-positive actinomycete. Whipple's disease is a multisystem infection with the GI tract being the most affected site, causing steatorrhea, diarrhea, weight loss, and abdominal pain. Fever, arthralgia, and lymphadenopathy are among other presentations. Neurologic symptoms occur in 4–11% of the patients.

Symptoms

Localization site	Comment
Cerebral hemispheres	Dementia
	Seizure
	Parkinsonism
	Supranuclear ocular palsy
	Conjugate gaze paresis
	Oculomasticatory myorhythmia and oculofacial–skeletal myorhythmia
Mental status and psychiatric aspects	Dementia
	Confusion
	Personality changes
Brainstem	Polydipsia
	Hyperphagia
	Hypersomnolence
Cerebellum	Cerebellar ataxia
Cranial nerves	Optic neuritis
Spinal cord	Myelopathy
Peripheral neuropathy	Axonal polyneuropathy
Muscle	Myopathy

Secondary Complications: Malabsorption can lead to deficiency of vitamins and essential micronutrients. Confusion, memory changes, numbness, weakness, and gait ataxia can occur as a result of malabsorption in addition to the Whipple's disease itself. Neuropathy, myelopathy, and optic neuropathy can occur with other nutritional deficiencies such as vitamin B12.

Bibliography

Anderson M. Neurology of Whipple's disease. *J Neurol Neurosurg Psychiatry*. 2000;68:2–5.

Compain C, Sacre K, Puéchal X, et al. Central nervous system involvement in Whipple disease: clinical study of 18 patients and long-term follow-up. *Medicine (Baltimore)*. 2013;92:324–30.

Fenollar F, Lagier JC, Raoult D. Tropheryma whipplei and Whipple's disease. *J Infect*. 2014;69(2):103–12.

Lynch T, Fahn S, Louis ED, Odel JG. Oculofacial-skeletal myorhythmia in Whipple's disease. *Mov Disord*. 1997;12:625–6.

Marth T, Raoult D. Whipple's disease. *Lancet*. 2003;361(9353):239–46.

Panegyres PK, Edis R, Beaman M, Fallon M. Primary Whipple's disease of the brain: characterization of the clinical syndrome and molecular diagnosis. *QJM*. 2006;99:609–23.

X-Linked Dystonia–Parkinsonism

Epidemiology and Demographics: X-linked dystonia–parkinsonism (XDP), also known as Lubag syndrome, is a rare genetic syndrome found worldwide (due to immigration), and particularly affects those from the Philippines. Even in the Philippines, overall, incidence is at most 0.31/100,000. However, on the island of Panay, from which it is thought to originate, the incidence is 5.74/100,000; more specifically the province of Capiz has the highest frequency at more than 23/100,000. Males are overwhelmingly affected, with the most recent male-to-female ratio at 100:1, and affected females having affected male siblings. XDP typically manifests in a broad range of ages, most commonly at middle age (late 30s to early 40s), though the range of ages has spanned from 12 to mid-60s. Typically, disease progresses on average for 16 years, and the average patient dies in their 50s.

Disorder Description: XDP is an X-linked progressive neurodegenerative disease affecting mainly male Filipinos. Presentation usually starts with focal dystonia that generalizes and can be accompanied by parkinsonism.

XDP is an X-linked disorder, with DYT3 and TAF1 as the causative genes, resulting in caudate/putaminal atrophy/degeneration, though underlying mechanisms are still unknown.

Diagnosis is primarily based on clinical features, but is confirmed through cytogenetic testing to find aforementioned genetic deficits. Monitoring of development, feeding, growth, hearing, and vision, as well as for cardiac, renal, and dental anomalies, especially in the first year of life, is most helpful since prenatal growth can be normal.

Symptoms

Localization site	Comment
Cerebral hemispheres	Caudate and/or putaminal atrophy, resulting in focal dystonia (mostly lower extremities and craniofacial), generalizes to parkinsonism (micrographia, slow periodic resting tremor, hypomimia, shuffling gait, bradykinesia)
Mental status and psychiatric aspects/ complications	Depression, anxiety, sleep dysfunction
Outside CNS	Variable, but distinctive, facial features: arched brows, down slanted palpebral fissures, low hanging columella, high palate, grimacing smile, and talon cusps. Also, coloboma and cataracts are possible
	Broad and often angulated thumbs and great toes, short stature, and weight gain
	Congenital heart defects, urinary and renal abnormalities, as well as cryptorchidism

Secondary Complications: Secondary complications are primarily related to the aforementioned extra-CNS symptoms.

Treatment Complications: Data are sparse, but the only effective treatment so far has been zolpidem and there is only partial response to dopaminergic therapy, similar to use in Parkinson disease. Levodopa/carbidopa as well as haloperidol have shown only partial response, and only in the minority of cases. Zolpidem has been more effective in reducing parkinsonian symptoms in these cases, but data are not comprehensive.

Complications of treatment are largely limited to lack of efficacy, or side effects of medications, such as hallucinations, impulsivity, arrhythmias, psychomotor symptoms for dopaminergic drugs, as well as sedation for zolpidem.

Bibliography

Rosales RL. X-linked dystonia parkinsonism: clinical phenotype, genetics and therapeutics. *J Mov Disord.* 2010;3(2):32–8.

Z

Zika Virus

Epidemiology and Demographics: As of May 2017, 48 countries and territories in the Caribbean and North, Central, and South Americas had confirmed mosquito-born transmission of Zika virus. Five countries have reported sexually transmitted Zika cases. In the United States, mosquito-borne transmission had occurred in Florida and Texas; however, none in 2017. Other infection has been reported in travelers in other cities.[1]

Disorder Description: Zika is a single-stranded RNA arthropod-borne flavivirus that is primarily transmitted by infected *Aedes* mosquitoes, which is the most common mode; however, other modes include sexual transmission, maternal–fetal transmission, and laboratory acquisition. Other potential modes of transmission include breastfeeding and blood transfusions.

Clinical manifestations occur in 20–25% of infected individuals, and may include flu-like symptoms such as fever, rash, headache, joint pain, and myalgias. Most patients recover in 5–7 days. Infection during pregnancy may be teratogenic and may cause certain birth defects.

Serum and urine may be sent for PCR testing.

Symptoms

Localization site	Comment
Cerebral hemispheres	Malformations of cortical development[2]
	Meningoencephalitis[2]
	Microcephaly[2]
	Intracranial calcifications[2]
	Ventriculomegaly[2]
Mental status and psychiatric aspects/complications	Encephalopathy
Brainstem	Hypoplasia[2]
Cerebellum	Hypoplasia[2]
Base of skull	Enlargement of cisterna magna[2]
Cranial nerves	Miller–Fisher syndrome
	Sensorineural hearing loss

Localization site	Comment
Spinal cord	Myelitis
Specific spinal roots	Guillain–Barré syndrome
Peripheral neuropathy	Sensory polyneuropathy
Unclear localization	Ophthalmologic abnormalities

Secondary Complications: Guillain–Barré syndrome has been reported. Myocarditis, thrombocytopenic purpura, and thrombocytopenia have been reported.

Treatment Complications: There is no vaccine or medication for Zika virus. Supportive care is recommended. NSAIDs should be avoided until dengue has been ruled out.

References

1. World Health Organization. Regional Zika Epidemiological update (Americas). Available from www.paho.org/hq/index.php?option=com_content&view=article&id=11599&Itemid=41691&lang=en. Accessed May 27, 2017.
2. De Fatima Vasco Aragao M, van der Linden V, Brainer-Lima AM, et al. Clinical features and neuroimaging (CT and MRI) findings in presumed Zika virus related congenital infection and microcephaly: retrospective case series study. *BMJ*. 2016;353:i1901. DOI:10.1136/bmj.i1901.

Zinc Deficiency

Epidemiology and Demographics: Inadequate dietary intake of zinc is an important cause of zinc deficiency in children in developing countries.[1] Breast milk and the complementary foods (high in phytates, which reduce zinc absorption) provided to children in developing countries are a poor source of zinc supplement.[2] Alcoholics and pregnant patients are also at risk for developing zinc deficiency.[3]

Patients receiving chronic total parenteral nutrition solutions lacking adequate zinc supplementation or with conditions causing zinc losses, such as diarrhea and inflammatory bowel disease, are also at risk of developing zinc deficiency.[4]

Chronic diseases such as malnutrition, malabsorption syndromes, necrotizing enterocolitis in preterm infants, and gastric bypass also affect zinc absorption and increase risk of deficiency.[5–6]

Diabetes increases the risk of zinc deficiency by increasing urinary loss.[7] Medications such as thiazides, loop diuretics, and angiotensin receptor blockers increase urinary loss of zinc and increase the risk of zinc deficiency, particularly in patients with poor intake.

Acrodermatitis enteropathica is an autosomal recessive inherited disorder resulting from mutations in the SLC39A4 gene on chromosome 8q24.3, which encodes a protein that appears to be involved in zinc transportation. Partial defect in intestinal zinc absorption results in zinc deficiency.[8–9]

Zinc depletion in sickle cell patients appears to be related to increased urinary excretion caused by a renal tubular defect and perhaps chronic hemolysis or impaired absorption.[10–11]

Wilson's disease, also known as hepatolenticular degeneration, is a genetic disorder that occurs in approximately 1/33,000 individuals. Characterized by complications of excessive copper accumulation in the liver, brain, and other organs, it is due to a genetic mutation leading to abnormal copper transport from the gastrointestinal tract. Diverse neurologic presentations especially with assorted movement abnormalities as well as psychiatric symptoms such as psychosis are common. It is associated with a classic triad of a low ceruloplasmin, high levels of urinary copper, and the Kayser–Fleischer ring. Zinc deficiency may also occur since copper and zinc are competitively absorbed from the gastrointestinal tract, and because a treatment for Wilson's disease (penicillamine) may itself lead to zinc deficiency.[1]

Disorder Description: Mild chronic zinc deficiency can cause impaired growth in children, delayed sexual maturation, decreased taste sensation, hair loss, and impaired immune function. Severe chronic zinc deficiency causes hypogonadism, oligospermia, growth retardation, hypopigmented hair, hair loss, and poor immunity.

Clinical features of acrodermatitis enteropathica include diarrhea, alopecia, muscle wasting, depression, irritability, and a characteristic rash involving the extremities and around the orifices. The rash is vesicular and pustular crusting with scaling and erythema. Thymic hypoplasia has also been described.

A serum zinc level <12 μmol/L is diagnostic of zinc deficiency.[1]

Zinc deficiency appears to contribute to the risk of developing diarrhea and pneumonia in children in developing countries. Zinc (20 mg/day until recovery) supplementation may be an effective adjunctive therapy for diarrhea and pneumonia in children ≥6 months of age.[1]

Intestinal absorption of copper is inhibited by zinc. Thus, chronic excessive intake of zinc may be associated with copper deficiency. Copper deficiency can present as fragile, abnormally formed hair, depigmentation of the skin, edema, anemia and hepatosplenomegaly, and osteoporosis. The neurologic manifestations include ataxia, neuropathy, myelopathy, and cognitive deficits that can mimic vitamin B12 deficiency.[12–13] Intranasal zinc preparations may lead to irreversible damage to the nasal mucosa and anosmia.

Acute zinc toxicity (inhalation of fumes from welding or after oral ingestion) causes nausea, vomiting, fever, respiratory distress, excessive salivation, sweating, and headache.

References

1. Kasper DL, Fauci AS, Hauser SL, et al., eds. *Harrison's principles of internal medicine.* 19th ed. New York: McGraw-Hill Education/Medical; 2015.

2. Hambidge KM, Krebs NF. Zinc deficiency: a special challenge. *J Nutr.* 2007;137:1101.

3. Vallee BL, Wacker WE, Bartholomay AF, Hoch FL. Zinc metabolism in hepatic dysfunction. II. Correlation of metabolic patterns with biochemical findings. *N Engl J Med.* 1957;257:1055.

4. King JC. Assessment of techniques for determining human zinc requirements. *J Am Diet Assoc.* 1986;86:1523.

5. Ruz M, Carrasco F, Rojas P, et al. Zinc absorption and zinc status are reduced after Roux-en-Y gastric bypass: a randomized study using 2 supplements. *Am J Clin Nutr.* 2011;94:1004.

6. Jakubovic BD, Zipursky JS, Wong N, et al. Zinc deficiency presenting with necrolytic acral erythema and coma. *Am J Med.* 2015;128:e3.

7. Walter RM Jr, Uriu-Hare JY, Olin KL, et al. Copper, zinc, manganese, and magnesium status and complications of diabetes mellitus. *Diabet Care.* 1991;14:1050.

8. Küry S, Dréno B, Bézieau S, et al. Identification of SLC39A4, a gene involved in acrodermatitis enteropathica. *Nat Genet.* 2002;31:239.

9. Wang K, Pugh EW, Griffen S, et al. Homozygosity mapping places the acrodermatitis enteropathica gene on chromosomal region 8q24.3. *Am J Hum Genet.* 2001;68:1055.

10. Phebus CK, Maciak BJ, Gloninger MF, Paul HS. Zinc status of children with sickle cell disease: relationship to poor growth. *Am J Hematol.* 1988;29:67.

11. Yuzbasiyan-Gurkan VA, Brewer GJ, Vander AJ, et al. Net renal tubular reabsorption of zinc in healthy man and impaired handling in sickle cell anemia. *Am J Hematol.* 1989;31:87.

12. Kumar N, Gross JB Jr, Ahlskog JE. Copper deficiency myelopathy produces a clinical picture like subacute combined degeneration. *Neurology.* 2004;63:33.

13. Kumar N. Copper deficiency myelopathy (human swayback). *Mayo Clin Proc.* 2006;81:1371.

SECTION 2 **Medication Adverse Effects**

Cardiovascular and Renal Medications

Jeff Freund, PharmD, BCACP Froedtert Health
Heather LaRue, PharmD UW Health University Hospital
Greta Nemergut, PharmD, BCCCP UW Health University Hospital

Angiotensin-Converting Enzyme (ACE) Inhibitors

Class Members: benazepril (Lotension®), captopril, enalapril (Vasotec®), fosinopril, lisinopril (Prinivil®, Zestril®), moexipril (Univasc®), perindopril (Aceon®), quinapril (Accupril®), ramipril (Altace®), trandolapril (Mavik®)

Typical Uses: hypertension, heart failure, kidney disease

Potential Neurologic or Psychiatric Medication Adverse Effects: The adverse effect profile of angiotensin-converting enzyme (ACE) inhibitors is similar among agents used to treat hypertension in this class. The most common neurologic adverse effect (>10%) is dizziness, which is due to blood pressure lowering effect. Common adverse effects (1–10%) include depression, headache, somnolence, and insomnia/sleep disturbances. As a medication class, ACE inhibitors are generally well tolerated, with neurologic and psychiatric adverse effects usually being mild and transient.

Further Reading

DiPiro JT. *Pharmacotherapy: a pathophysiologic approach.* New York: McGraw-Hill Medical; 2008.
Enalapril. In *DRUGDEX® System (electronic version).* Greenwood Village, CO: Truven Health Analytics, Inc. www.micromedexsolutions.com/. Accessed Dec 10, 2015.
Zestril (lisinopril) package insert. Wilmington, DE: AstraZeneca Pharmaceuticals LP; Jun 2014.

Angiotensin Receptor Blockers (ARBs)

Class Members: azilsartan (Edarbi®), candesartan (Atacand®), eprosartan (Teveten®), irbesartan (Avapro®), losartan (Cozaar®), olmesartan (Benicar®), telmisartan (Micardis®), valsartan (Diovan®)

Typical Uses: hypertension, heart failure, diabetic nephropathy

Potential Neurologic or Psychiatric Medication Adverse Effects: The adverse effect profile of angiotensin receptor blockers (ARBs) is similar among agents used to treat hypertension in this class. The most common neurologic adverse effect (>10%) is dizziness, which is dose related and due to the blood pressure lowering effect of the medications. Dizziness was reported with higher frequencies (17%) in short-term heart failure trials, and it is recommended to start ARBs at lower doses in patients with heart failure to reduce dizziness. Other neurologic effects found in postmarketing studies include headache and asthenia.

Further Reading

Candesartan. In *DRUGDEX® System (electronic version).* Greenwood Village, CO: Truven Health Analytics, Inc. www.micromedexsolutions.com/. Accessed Dec 10, 2015.
Cozaar (losartan potassium) package insert. Whitehouse Station, NJ: Merck & Co; Jan 2014.
DiPiro JT. *Pharmacotherapy: a pathophysiologic approach.* New York: McGraw-Hill Medical; 2008.

Antiarrhythmics

Amiodarone

Class Members: amiodarone (Cordarone®), dronedarone (Multaq®)

Typical Uses: atrial fibrillation, ventricular arrhythmia

Potential Neurologic or Psychiatric Medication Adverse Effects: Common neurologic effects of amiodarone include gait problems, tremor, involuntary movements, and peripheral neuropathy. Less frequent neurologic effects observed with amiodarone therapy include headache, insomnia, fatigue, dizziness, proximal muscle weakness, paresthesia, and altered sense of smell. Visual impairment, even **blindness,** as a result of optic neuritis and optic neuropathy have been rarely reported. Thyroid toxicity can occur in the form of either **hyperthyroidism** or **hypothyroidism.** Hyperthyroidism may present with personality changes, including psychosis, agitation, and depression, as well as cognitive impairment or confusion. Hypothyroidism presentation can range from fatigue to myxedema coma. **Angioedema** and **anaphylaxis** have been rarely reported. **Teratogenic effects** may occur, including both neurodevelopmental (e.g., speech and motor delays) and neurologic (e.g., ataxia) effects. The majority of the neurologic effects observed with amiodarone are not seen with dronedarone; however, altered taste and asthenia have been rarely reported with dronedarone use.

Further Reading

Amiodarone. In *DRUGDEX® System (electronic version).* Greenwood Village, CO: Truven Health Analytics, Inc. www.micromedexsolutions.com/. Accessed on Dec 20, 2015.

Ross DS. Overview of the clinical manifestations of hyperthyroidism in adults. In Cooper DS, ed. *UpToDate.* Waltham, MA: UpToDate. www.uptodate.com/contents/overview-of-the-clinical-manifestations-of-hyperthyroidism-in-adults. Accessed Dec 20, 2015.

Sampson KJ, Kass RS. Anti-arrhythmic drugs. In Brunton LL, Chabner BA, Knollmann BC, eds. *Goodman & Gilman's the pharmacological basis of therapeutics.* 12th ed. New York, NY: McGraw-Hill; 2011. Chapter 29.

Digoxin (Lanoxin®)

Typical Uses: atrial fibrillation, heart failure

Potential Neurologic or Psychiatric Medication Adverse Effects: Neurologic adverse effects are frequently reported with digoxin; these include weakness, confusion, dizziness, headache, anxiety, and depression. **Encephalopathy, seizures,** hallucinations, and nightmares have been reported with supratherapeutic digoxin concentrations. Nausea is a frequently reported adverse effect. Visual effects, such as blurred vision, halos around bright objects, and disturbed color vision, can occur at therapeutic concentrations, with increased likelihood at toxic concentrations.

Disturbed color vision can present as either reduced color discrimination or yellow vision.

Further Reading

Digoxin. In *DRUGDEX® System (electronic version).* Greenwood Village, CO: Truven Health Analytics, Inc. www.micromedexsolutions.com/. Accessed Dec 20, 2015.

Sampson KJ, Kass RS. Anti-arrhythmic drugs. In Brunton LL, Chabner BA, Knollmann BC, eds. *Goodman & Gilman's the pharmacological basis of therapeutics.* 12th ed. New York, NY: McGraw-Hill; 2011. Chapter 29.

Procainamide (Pronestyl®)

Typical Uses: ventricular arrhythmias, atrial arrhythmias

Potential Neurologic or Psychiatric Medication Adverse Effects: Procainamide can commonly cause nausea, which is typically a dose-related side effect. Musculoskeletal effects of procainamide have been reported rarely, including muscle weakness, myasthenia gravis, and myopathy. Ataxia, dizziness, tremor, neuropathy, mania, and psychosis have also been rarely reported. Hypersensitivity may occur after administration. Systemic lupus erythematosus has been reported in patients on long-term procainamide, with series reports ranging from 0.2% up to 30%.

Further Reading

Procainamide. In *DRUGDEX® System (electronic version).* Greenwood Village, CO: Truven Health Analytics, Inc. www.micromedexsolutions.com/. Accessed Dec 20, 2015.

Sampson KJ, Kass RS. Anti-arrhythmic drugs. In Brunton LL, Chabner BA, Knollmann BC, eds. *Goodman & Gilman's the pharmacological basis of therapeutics,* 12th ed. New York, NY: McGraw-Hill; 2011. Chapter 29.

Other Antiarrhythmics

Class Members: dofetilide (Tikosyn®), sotalol (Betapace®), lidocaine (Xylocaine®)

Typical Uses: atrial fibrillation, ventricular arrhythmia, other dysrhythmias, anesthesia, and pain control (lidocaine)

Potential Neurologic or Psychiatric Medication Adverse Effects: Syncope, lightheadedness, and dizziness are commonly reported with antiarrhythmic use; however, these adverse effects are typically equally seen in placebo groups and may be a result of arrhythmias rather than a medication adverse effect. Headache is also commonly seen in antiarrhythmic trials, although no more commonly than in the placebo groups. Adverse effects commonly reported with sotalol include nausea, asthenia, sleep problems, paresthesias, anxiety or depression, reduced libido, and very commonly fatigue. Central nervous system effects of lidocaine typically represent toxicity, including anxiety, dizziness, tinnitus, tremors, blurred vision, nystagmus, dysarthria, and drowsiness. This may lead to worsening toxicity such as seizures, loss of consciousness, and respiratory arrest. Toxicity is rarely seen with lidocaine topical application, although case reports of anxiety and dizziness have occurred with the lidocaine patch.

Further Reading

Lidocaine. In *DRUGDEX® System [Internet database]*. Greenwood Village, CO: Thomson Micromedex. Updated periodically.

Sampson KJ, Kass RS. Anti-arrhythmic drugs. In Brunton LL, Chabner BA, Knollmann BC, eds. *Goodman & Gilman's the pharmacological basis of therapeutics*, 12th ed. New York, NY: McGraw-Hill; 2011. Chapter 29.

Sotalol. In *DRUGDEX® System (electronic version)*. Greenwood Village, CO: Truven Health Analytics, Inc. www.micromedexsolutions.com/. Accessed Dec 20, 2015.

Anticoagulants

Class Members: warfarin (Coumadin®), dabigatran (Pradaxa®), rivaroxaban (Xarelto®), apixaban (Eliquis®), edoxaban (Savaysa®)

Typical Uses: atrial fibrillation, thromboembolism treatment and prevention

Potential Neurologic or Psychiatric Medication Adverse Effects: Increased risk of bleeding is seen with all oral anticoagulants and can result in neurologic symptoms depending on the location of the bleeding (e.g., intracranial, epidural, spinal, subdural). Hypersensitivity (angioedema, flushing) has been reported rarely. Drug interactions can lead to elevated levels of all oral anticoagulants, which

may increase risk of bleeding. Anticoagulant effects of warfarin are increased by antibiotics, in particular sulfamethoxazole–trimethoprim may lead to significant INR elevation. Levels of dabigatran, rivaroxaban, and apixaban are all increased by p-glycoprotein inhibitors such as amiodarone and ketoconazole; rivaroxaban and apixaban levels are also increased by CYP3A4 inhibitors such as the azole antifungals, protease inhibitors (e.g., ritonavir), and non-dihydropyridine calcium channel blockers (e.g., diltiazem).

Further Reading

Apixaban. In *DRUGDEX® System (electronic version)*. Greenwood Village, CO: Truven Health Analytics, Inc. www.micromedexsolutions.com/. Accessed Dec 20, 2015.

Dabigatran. In *DRUGDEX® System (electronic version)*. Greenwood Village, CO: Truven Health Analytics, Inc. www.micromedexsolutions.com/. Accessed Dec 20, 2015.

Rivaroxaban. In *DRUGDEX® System (electronic version)*. Greenwood Village, CO: Truven Health Analytics, Inc. www.micromedexsolutions.com/. Accessed Dec 20, 2015.

Warfarin. In *DRUGDEX® System (electronic version)*. Greenwood Village, CO: Truven Health Analytics, Inc. www.micromedexsolutions.com/. Accessed Dec 20, 2015.

Antiplatelets

Class Members: aspirin (Aspergum®, Norwich®, Bayer®, St. Joseph®, Ecotrin®, Halfprin®, Genacote®, Easprin®, Zorprin®), clopidogrel (Plavix®), prasugrel (Effient®), ticagrelor (Brilinta®)

Typical Uses: coronary artery disease, myocardial infarction prevention and treatment, peripheral artery disease, stroke prevention. Aspirin may also be used for atrial fibrillation, headache, fever, and pain.

Potential Neurologic or Psychiatric Medication Adverse Effects: Increased risk of bleeding is seen with all of the antiplatelet agents and can result in neurologic symptoms depending on location (e.g., intracranial, intraocular, epidural). This risk is increased in certain patient populations, including those on concomitant anticoagulants or nonsteroidal anti-inflammatory drugs (NSAIDs), the elderly, and those with a history of bleeding. Hypersensitivity (angioedema, flushing) and serum sickness (fever, arthralgias, myalgias) can also occur. Aspirin hypersensitivity is more common in patients with history of asthma, atopic dermatitis, and/or rhinitis. High doses of aspirin can lead to salicylism; presenting symptoms include headaches, confusion, and tinnitus. Rare side effects of clopidogrel have been reported including taste disorder and confusion.

Further Reading

Aspirin. In *DRUGDEX® System (electronic version)*. Greenwood Village, CO: Truven Health Analytics, Inc. www.micromedexsolutions.com/. Accessed Dec 20, 2015.

Clopidogrel. In *DRUGDEX® System (electronic version)*. Greenwood Village, CO: Truven Health Analytics, Inc. www.micromedexsolutions.com/. Accessed Dec 20, 2015.

Ticagrelor. In *DRUGDEX® System (electronic version)*. Greenwood Village, CO: Truven Health Analytics, Inc. www.micromedexsolutions.com/. Accessed Dec 20, 2015.

Beta-Blockers

Class Members: acebutolol (Sectral®), atenolol (Tenormin®), betaxolol (Kerlone®), bisoprolol (Zebeta®), carteolol (Ocupress®), carvedilol (Coreg®), esmolol (Brevibloc®), labetalol (Trandate®), metoprolol (Lopressor®, Toprol-XL®), nadolol (Corgard®), nebivolol (Bystolic®), penbutolol (Levatol®), pindolol (Visken®), propranolol (Inderal®), sotalol (Betapace®), timolol (Betimol®)

Typical Uses: hypertension, angina, myocardial infarction, atrial fibrillation, congestive heart failure, migraine prophylaxis (propranolol)

Potential Neurologic or Psychiatric Medication Adverse Effects: The adverse effect profile of beta-blockers is similar among agents used to treat hypertension in this class. The most common neurologic and psychiatric adverse effects (>10%) include dizziness, fatigue, and asthenia. These effects are usually temporary, occurring at the onset of therapy and then diminishing over time. Beta-blockers have been associated with headache, insomnia, confusion, and short-term memory loss during controlled trials, but at low rates (1–10%). Lastly, abrupt cessation of beta-blockers may precipitate withdrawal symptoms, which can include neurologic adverse effects of headache and diaphoresis.

When discontinuing beta-blockers, it is important to taper gradually and/or use prolonged administration of small doses prior to completely stopping to avoid withdrawal symptoms.

Further Reading

COREG (carvedilol) package insert. Research Triangle Park, NC: GlaxoSmithKline; Oct 2015.

DiPiro JT. *Pharmacotherapy: a pathophysiologic approach*. New York: McGraw-Hill Medical; 2008.

Toprol-XL (metoprolol succinate) package insert. Wilmington, DE: AstraZeneca Pharmaceuticals LP; May 2014.

Calcium Channel Blockers

Dihydropyridines

Class Members: amlodipine (Norvasc®), felodipine (Plendil®), isradipine (DynaCirc®), nicardipine (Cardene®), nifedipine (Procardia®, Adalat®), nisoldipine (Sular®)

Typical Uses: hypertension, angina, coronary artery disease, Raynaud's phenomenon

Potential Neurologic or Psychiatric Medication Adverse Effects: The adverse effect profile of non-dihydropyridine calcium channel blockers is similar among agents used to treat hypertension in this class. From a neurologic and psychiatric adverse effect standpoint, the dihydropyridine calcium channel blockers are well tolerated. The most common adverse effects (>10%) include dizziness, headache, and lightheadedness. Dizziness is due to the lowering of blood pressure and is more common when initiating therapy. Starting the medication with lower initial doses may reduce dizziness. Common adverse effects (1–10%) include asthenia, parasthesias, and fatigue. These effects are usually temporary, occurring at the onset of therapy and then diminishing over time.

Further Reading

DiPiro JT. *Pharmacotherapy: a pathophysiologic approach*. New York: McGraw-Hill Medical; 2008.

Nifedipine. In *DRUGDEX® System (electronic version)*. Greenwood Village, CO: Truven Health Analytics, Inc. www.micromedexsolutions.com/. Accessed Dec 10, 2015.

Norvasc (amlodipine) package insert. New York, NY: Pfizer Labs; Mar 2015.

Nondihydropyridines

Class Members: verapamil (Calan®), diltiazem (Cardizem®, Taztia®, Tiazac®)

Typical uses: hypertension, angina, atrial fibrillation, supraventricular tachycardia, migraine prophylaxis (verapamil), pulmonary hypertension (diltiazem)

Potential Neurologic or Psychiatric Medication Adverse Effects: The adverse effect profile of nondihydropyridine calcium channel blockers is similar among agents used to treat hypertension in this class. The most common adverse effects (>10%) include dizziness and headache. Dizziness is due to peripheral vasodilation and resulting blood pressure lowering. Common adverse effects (1–10%) include headache and asthenia and are more common with diltiazem than verapamil. Less frequent (<1%) neurologic and psychiatric adverse effects include abnormal dreams, amnesia, fatigue, nervousness, drowsiness, depression, personality change, insomnia, tinnitus, tremor, hallucinations, paresthesias, gait abnormalities, and confusion.

Further Reading

Calan (verapamil tablets) package insert. New York, NY: GD Searle LLC; Oct 2013.

Cardizem CD (diltiazem) package insert. Bridgewater, NJ: Biovail Corporation; Nov 2010.

DiPiro JT. *Pharmacotherapy: a pathophysiologic approach.* New York: McGraw-Hill Medical; 2008.

Diuretics

Loop Diuretics

Class Members: bumetanide (Bumex®), ethacrynic acid (Edecrin®), furosemide (Lasix®), torsemide (Demedex®)

Typical Uses: congestive heart failure, edema, hypertension

Potential Neurologic or Psychiatric Medication Adverse Effects: The adverse effect profile of loop diuretics is similar among agents used to treat hypertension in this class. The most common neurologic adverse effect (>10%) is dizziness, which is due to the blood pressure lowering effect of these medications. Dizziness is more common during initiation of therapy, and elderly patients may be more sensitive to the adverse effects.

Thus, it is important to start at a lower dose when initiating loop diuretics for geriatric patients. Additionally, because their mechanism of action relies on the inhibition of sodium and chloride reabsorption in the ascending loop of Henle in the kidneys, loop diuretics can cause significant hyponatremia, hypokalemia, and hypochloremia. These electrolyte imbalances can lead to adverse effects including mental confusion, fatigue, faintness, muscle cramps, headache, paresthesia, thirst, anorexia, nausea, and vomiting.

Further Reading

Bumetanide In *DRUGDEX® System (electronic version).* Greenwood Village, CO: Truven Health Analytics, Inc. www.micromedexsolutions.com/. Accessed 12 Oct, 2015.

DiPiro JT. *Pharmacotherapy: a pathophysiologic approach.* New York: McGraw-Hill Medical; 2008.

Lasix (furosemide) package insert. Bridgewater, NJ: Aventis Pharmaceuticals; Mar 2012.

Potassium-Sparing Diuretics

Class Members: amiloride, triamterene (Dyrenium®), eplerenone (Inspra®), spironolactone (Aldactone®)

Typical Uses: hypertension, heart failure, edema

Potential Neurologic or Psychiatric Medication Adverse Effects: Potassium-sparing diuretics are well tolerated, with few neurologic or psychiatric adverse effects associated with them. The adverse effect profile is similar among agents used to treat hypertension in this class. The most common neurologic adverse effect is dizziness (1–3%). This is usually dose related and due to the blood pressure lowering effect of the medications. Less common adverse effects of potassium-sparing diuretics include headache, dizziness, drowsiness, lethargy, ataxia, and mental confusion. Additionally, because their mechanism of action may lead to increased potassium, muscle weakness and confusion may be due to drug-induced hyperkalemia. If hyperkalemia is suspected or confirmed, the medication should be discontinued.

Further Reading

Aldactone (spironolactone) package insert. New York, NY: G.D. Searle LLC Division of Pfizer Inc; Jun 2013.

DiPiro JT. *Pharmacotherapy: a pathophysiologic approach.* New York: McGraw-Hill Medical; 2008.

Eplerenone. In *DRUGDEX® System (electronic version).* Greenwood Village, CO: Truven Health Analytics, Inc. www.micromedexsolutions.com/. Accessed Dec 10, 2015.

Thiazide and Thiazide-Like Diuretics

Class Members: chlorthalidone (Thalitone®), hydrochlorothiazide, metolazone (Zaroxolyn®)

Typical Uses: hypertension, edema

Potential Neurologic or Psychiatric Medication Adverse Effects: The adverse effect profile of thiazide diuretics is similar among agents used to treat hypertension in this class. The most common neurologic adverse effect (>10%) is dizziness, which is due to the blood pressure lowering effect. Common adverse effects (1–10%) include headache, parasthesias, and restlessness. Additionally, because the mechanism of action relies on blocking the reabsorption of sodium and chloride in the distal tubule of the kidneys, thiazide diuretics can cause significant hyponatremia, hypokalemia, and hypochloremia. These electrolyte imbalances can lead to adverse effects including mental confusion, fatigue, faintness, muscle cramps, headache, paresthesia, thirst, anorexia, nausea, or vomiting.

Further Reading

Chlorthalidone. In *DRUGDEX® System (electronic version).* Greenwood Village, CO: Truven Health Analytics, Inc. www.micromedexsolutions.com/. Accessed Dec 10, 2015.

DiPiro JT. *Pharmacotherapy: a pathophysiologic approach.* New York: McGraw-Hill Medical; 2008.

Hydrochlorothiazide tablet package insert. Cranberry, NJ: Aurobindo Pharma USA, Inc; Oct 2011.

Lipid Lowering

Bile Acid Sequestrants

Class Members: cholestyramine (Prevalite®, Questran®, Questran Light®), colesevelam (Welchol®), colestipol (Colestid®)

Typical Uses: primary hypercholesterolemia, pruritus, diarrhea due to bile acids or *Clostridium difficile,* heterozygous familial hypertriglyceridemia and type 2 diabetes (colesevelam only), digitalis toxicity, generalized atherosclerosis

Potential Neurologic or Psychiatric Medication Adverse Events: The adverse effect profile is similar among bile acid sequestrant agents. Common adverse effects (1–10%) include headache, fatigue, and asthenia. Other adverse effects include anxiety, dizziness, drowsiness, neuralgia, paresthesia, vertigo, insomnia, anorexia, and light-headedness. Cholestyramine and colestipol can bind to many other medications and reduce their efficacy and should be dosed 4 to 6 hours before or 1 hour after other medications.

Further Reading

Bile acid sequestrants. *Drug Facts and Comparisons. Facts & Comparisons [database online].* St. Louis, MO: Wolters Kluwer Health, Inc; 2015.

Cholestyramine, colesevelam, colestipol. In *Lexi-Drugs. Lexicomp.* Hudson, OH: Wolters Kluwer Health, Inc. http://online.lexi.com. Accessed Dec 20, 2015.

Drug comparison (cholestyramine, colesevelam, colestipol). In *Micromedex 2.0.* Greenwood Village, CO: Truven Health Analytics, Inc. http://micromedexsolutions.com. Accessed Dec 20, 2015.

Ezetimibe (Zetia®)

Typical Uses: hyperlipidemia, homozygous familial hypercholesterolemia, homozygous sitosterolemia, carotid atherosclerosis, cardiac prophylaxis after acute coronary syndrome

Potential Neurologic or Psychiatric Medication Adverse Events: Common adverse effects (1–10%) include headache and fatigue. Postmarketing adverse effects include depression, dizziness, headache, and parasthesia.

Further Reading

Ezetimibe. *Drug Facts and Comparisons. Facts & Comparisons [database online].* St. Louis, MO: Wolters Kluwer Health, Inc; 2015.

Ezetimibe. In *Micromedex 2.0.* Greenwood Village, CO: Truven Health Analytics, Inc. http://micromedexsolutions.com. Accessed Dec 1, 2015.

Ezetimibe. In *Lexi-Drugs. Lexicomp.* Hudson, OH: Wolters Kluwer Health, Inc. http://online.lexi.com. Accessed Dec 1, 2015.

Fibric Acid Derivatives

Class Members: fenofibrate (Fenoglide®, Lipofen®, Lofibra®, Tricor®, Triglide®), fenofibrate (micronized) (Antara®, Lofibra®), fenofibric acid (Fibricor®), choline fenofibrate (Trilipix®), gemfibrozil (Lopid®)

Typical Uses: hypertriglyceridemia, hypercholesterolemia, dyslipidemia, prevention of cardiovascular disease (gemfibrozil)

Potential Neurologic or Psychiatric Medication Adverse Events: The adverse effect profile is similar among most fibric acid derivative products. Headache is a very common adverse effect (>10%) in patients taking fenofibric acid and choline fenofibrate. Common adverse effects (1–10%) include dizziness, fatigue, vertigo, insomnia, pain, and headache (for fenofibrate and fenofibrate micronized). Other adverse effects for gemfibrozil include decreased libido, impotence, depression, hypesthesia, paresthesia, peripheral neuritis, somnolence, confusion, intracranial hemorrhage, seizure, and syncope. Other adverse effects for other fibric acid derivatives include asthenia, mood disorders, cognitive disorders, sleep disorders, perception disorders, lethargy, malaise, somnolence, and tiredness.

Further Reading

Drug comparison (fenofibrate, fenofibrate micronized, fenofibric acid, choline fenofibrate, gemfibrozil) In *Micromedex 2.0*. Greenwood Village, CO: Truven Health Analytics, Inc. http://micromedexsolutions .com. Accessed Dec 20, 2015.

Fenofibrate, fenofibrate micronized, fenofibric acid, choline fenofibrate, gemfibrozil. In *Lexi-Drugs*. *Lexicomp*. Hudson, OH: Wolters Kluwer Health, Inc. http://online.lexi.com. Accessed Dec 20, 2015.

Fibric acid derivatives. *Drug Facts and Comparisons*. *Facts & Comparisons [database online]*. St. Louis, MO: Wolters Kluwer Health, Inc; 2015.

HMG CoA Reductase Inhibitors (Statins)

Class Members: atorvastatin (Lipitor®); fluvastatin (Lescol®, Lescol XL®); lovastatin (Mevacor®); pitavastatin (Livalo®); pravastatin (Pravachol®); rosuvastatin (Crestor®); simvastatin (Zocor®)

Typical Uses: primary prevention of cardiovascular disease in high-risk patients including reduction in risk of: angina, myocardial infarction, stroke, revascularization procedures, and cardiovascular mortality; secondary prevention of cardiovascular event in patients with coronary heart disease including reduction in risk of: myocardial infarction, stroke, revascularization procedures, hospitalization for congestive heart failure, angina, progression of coronary atherosclerosis, coronary death; hypercholesterolemia including primary (heterozygous familial and nonfamilial), homozygous familial hypercholesterolemia, mixed dyslipidemia, hypertriglyceridemia, primary dysbetalipoproteinemia

Potential Neurologic or Psychiatric Medication Adverse Events: Reports of side effects of statins varies, with pitavastatin having the lowest reported adverse effects. Very common adverse effects (>10%) include headache (atorvastatin only). Common adverse effects (1–10%) include asthenia, depression, dizziness, headache, insomnia, parasthesia, vertigo, fatigue, and hemorrhagic cerebral infarction (atorvastatin only). Irritability, dream disorder, dysphasia, neuropathy, sexual dysfunction, and cognitive impairment, including memory loss, forgetfulness and memory impairment, have been reported with use of statins. Amnesia has been reported with the use of atorvastatin, simvastatin, and pravastatin. Other adverse effects are drug specific. Facial paralysis, hyperkinesia, hypertonia, hypesthesia, incoordination, somnolence, and torticollis were seen with atorvastatin. Additional side effects with fluvastatin and lovastatin include attention and motor control disorder, anxiety, dysfunction of cranial nerves, peripheral nerve palsy, and psychic disturbances. Tremor was seen with the use of fluvastatin, lovastatin, and pravastatin. Atorvastatin may increase the effects of intravenous midazolam and patients should be monitored for respiratory depression and prolonged sedation.

Further Reading

Blood cholesterol management. In *Lexi-Drugs*. *Lexicomp*. Hudson, OH: Wolters Kluwer Health, Inc. http://online.lexi.com. Accessed Dec 20, 2015.

Class comparison (statins). In *Micromedex 2.0*. Greenwood Village, CO: Truven Health Analytics, Inc. http://micromedexsolutions.com. Accessed Dec 20, 2015.

Drug comparison (atorvastatin, fluvastatin, lovastatin, pitavastatin, pravastatin, rosuvastatin, simvastatin). In *Micromedex 2.0*. Greenwood Village, CO: Truven Health Analytics, Inc. http://micromedexsolutions.com. Accessed Dec 20, 2015.

HMG-CoA reductase inhibitors. *Drug Facts and Comparisons. Facts & Comparisons [database online]*. St. Louis, MO: Wolters Kluwer Health, Inc; 2015.

Niacin ER (Niaspan®), Niacin (Niacor®)

Typical Uses: slow progression of atherosclerotic disease, dyslipidemia, hypertriglyceridemia, secondary prevention of myocardial infarction, pellagra

Potential Neurologic or Psychiatric Medication Adverse Events: Very common adverse events (>10%) include headache; however, this side effect varied and only reached >10% incidence in patients taking 1500 mg of niacin ER daily. Common adverse effects (1–10%) include headache at all other doses of niacin ER studied. When starting treatment with niacin products, headache is often associated with flushing, itching, and tingling, which is transient. Other adverse events reported with niacin products are dizziness, insomnia, migraine, chills, nervousness, and pain.

Further Reading

Niacin. *Drug Facts and Comparisons. Facts & Comparisons [database online]*. St. Louis, MO: Wolters Kluwer Health, Inc; 2015.

Niacin. In *Micromedex 2.0*. Greenwood Village, CO: Truven Health Analytics, Inc. http://micromedexsolutions.com. Accessed Dec 20, 2015.

Niacin. In *Lexi-Drugs. Lexicomp*. Hudson, OH: Wolters Kluwer Health, Inc. http://online.lexi.com. Accessed Dec 20, 2015.

Methyldopa (Aldomet®)

Typical Uses: hypertension

Potential Neurologic or Psychiatric Medication Adverse Effects: The neurologic and psychiatric adverse effect profile for methyldopa is significant. Drowsiness is the most common adverse effect (15%), which occurs within the first 48–72 hours of initiation or dose increase and is usually transient. If a dose increase is warranted, it is recommended to increase the evening dose first to take advantage of the adverse effect. Dizziness due to orthostatic hypotension is also a very common side effect (>10%). Additionally, larger doses (> 1 gram per day) of methyldopa have been shown to impair concentration and decrease mental acuity. Lastly, common side effects (1–10%) include nightmares, mild psychosis, vertigo, headache, parasthesias, and asthenia. These side effects are more common at larger doses and are usually temporary, occurring at the onset of therapy and then diminishing over time.

Further Reading

Aldomet (methyldopa) package insert. West Point, PA: Merck & Co., Inc.; Jul 1998.

Methyldopa In DRUGDEX® System (electronic version). Greenwood Village, CO: Truven Health Analytics, Inc. www.micromedexsolutions.com/. Accessed Oct 12, 2015.

Orlistat (Xenical®)

Typical Uses: obesity management, including weight loss and weight management, in patients with a BMI of at least 30 kg/m² or 27 kg/m² and other risk factors (e.g., hypertension, diabetes, dyslipidemia)

Potential Neurologic or Psychiatric Medication Adverse Events: Headache is the only very common adverse effect (>10%). Common adverse effects (1–10%) include fatigue, sleep disorder, dizziness, anxiety, and depression. Depression did not occur in the first year of treatment; it only began in year 2 of treatment. Headache and dizziness occurred in the first year of treatment, but were not present in the second year of treatment. Concomitant use with antiepileptic medications can reduce the efficacy of the antiepileptic and result in increased frequency or severity of seizures.

Further Reading

Orlistat. *Drug Facts and Comparisons. Facts & Comparisons [database online]*. St. Louis, MO: Wolters Kluwer Health, Inc; 2015.

Orlistat. In *Micromedex 2.0*. Greenwood Village, CO: Truven Health Analytics, Inc. http://micromedexsolutions.com. Accessed Dec 1, 2015.

Orlistat. In RxList®. WebMD, LLC. www.rxlist.com. Accessed Dec 1, 2015.

Reserpine

Typical Uses: hypertension

Potential Neurologic or Psychiatric Medication Adverse Effects: The psychiatric adverse effect profile of reserpine is significant. The most common adverse effect is severe depression (6–30%), and is more common when used in higher doses (>0.25 mg/day). Depression is often severe enough to require hospitalization or result in suicide attempts and can last for several months following discontinuation. Reserpine should be used with caution in patients with a history of depression and should be discontinued if signs of depression occur. Additional neurologic side effects include dizziness, headache, paradoxical anxiety, nervousness, nightmares, pseudoparkinsonism, and drowsiness.

Further Reading

Reserpine tablets package insert. Princeton, NJ: Sandoz Inc.; Mar 2010.

Vasodilators

Endothelin Receptor Antagonists and Prostanoids

Class Members: endothelin receptor antagonists: ambrisentan (Letairis®); bosentan (Tracleer®); macitentan (Opsumit®); **prostanoids:** epoprostenol (Flolan®); treprostinil (Orenitram®, Remodulin®, Tyvaso®); iloprost (Ventavis®)

Typical Uses: pulmonary arterial hypertension, acute vasodilator testing for pulmonary arterial hypertension (epoprostenol), prevention of digital ulcers and Raynaud's phenomenon (bosentan)

Potential Neurologic or Psychiatric Medication Adverse Events: Epoprostenol has the highest rate of adverse effects, which is likely related to its use in more severe stages of pulmonary hypertension. Very common adverse effects (>10%) include headache. Other very common adverse effects include agitation, anxiety, chills, dizziness, hyperesthesia, hypoesthesia, nervousness, pain, paresthesia, and tremor (epoprostenol only). Common adverse effects (1–10%) include syncope, insomnia, and dizziness. Other reported adverse effects that occurred less frequently include asthenia, fatigue, and restlessness.

Further Reading

Ambrisentan, bosentan, macitentan, epoprostenol, treprostinil, iloprost. In *Lexi-Drugs. Lexicomp.* Hudson, OH: Wolters Kluwer Health, Inc. http://online.lexi.com. Accessed Dec 22, 2015.

Drug comparison (ambrisentan, bosentan, macitentan, epoprostenol, treprostinil, iloprost). In *Micromedex 2.0.* Greenwood Village, CO: Truven Health Analytics, Inc. http://micromedexsolutions.com. Accessed Dec 22, 2015.

Vasodilators. *Drug Facts and Comparisons. Facts & Comparisons [database online].* St. Louis, MO: Wolters Kluwer Health, Inc; 2015.

Nitrates and Peripheral Vasodilators

Class Members: nitrates: isosorbide dinitrate IR and ER (Isordil®, Dilatrate SR®, IsoDitrate ER®), isosorbide mononitrate IR and ER (Imdur®, Monoket®), nitroglycerin: oral (Nitrostat®, Nitrolingual®, NitroMist®), topical ointment (Nitro-Bid®), topical patch (Nitro-Dur®, Minitran®), rectal (Rectiv®), intravenous (Nitronal®); **peripheral vasodilators:** hydralazine

Typical Uses: nitrates: angina, heart failure, Raynaud's phenomenon, anal fissure (topical application only), prevention or treatment of gastrointestinal varices, osteoporosis, erectile dysfunction, prinzmetal angina, acute myocardial infarction (nitroglycerin only), intra- and perioperative hypertension, and cocaine-induced coronary syndrome (intravenous nitroglycerin only); **hydralazine:** hypertension, heart failure, severe aortic insufficiency after valve replacement

Potential Neurologic or Psychiatric Medication Adverse Events: Very common adverse effects (>10%) include headache, with incidences of >50% for nitrates. The headache can be severe and occur with each dose. Common adverse effects (1–10%) include dizziness, lightheadedness, syncope, fatigue, emotional lability, and parasthesia. Other reported adverse effects occurring less frequently include: neuritis, anxiety, tremor, and weakness. Depression, disorientation, chills, and psychotic reaction were reported with hydralazine. Isosorbide mononitrate was associated with additional adverse effects including hypothesia, migraine, paresis, ptosis, impaired concentration, confusion, decreased libido, impotence, insomnia, nervousness, paroniria, somnolence, asthenia, malaise, depression, nightmares, restlessness, and vertigo, all reported at 5% or less. Use of intravenous nitroglycerin and hydralazine has been associated with increased intracranial pressure.

Further Reading

Drug comparison (isosorbide dinitrate, isosorbide mononitrate, nitroglycerin, hydralazine). In *Micromedex 2.0*. Greenwood Village, CO: Truven Health Analytics, Inc. http://micromedexsolutions .com. Accessed Dec 22, 2015.

Isosorbide dinitrate, isosorbide mononitrate, nitroglycerin, hydralazine. In *Lexi-Drugs. Lexicomp*. Hudson, OH: Wolters Kluwer Health, Inc. http://online.lexi.com. Accessed Dec 22, 2015.

Vasodilators. *Drug Facts and Comparisons. Facts & Comparisons [database online]*. St. Louis, MO: Wolters Kluwer Health, Inc; 2015.

Medications to Treat Diabetes

Curtis L. Triplitt, PharmD, CDE Texas Diabetes Institute, Department of Medicine, Division of Diabetes, University of Texas Health Science Center at San Antonio

Alpha-Glucosidase Inhibitors (AGIs)

Class Members: acarbose (Precose®), miglitol (Glyset®)

Typical Uses: type 2 diabetes mellitus, type 1 diabetes mellitus, prevention of diabetes mellitus

Potential Neurologic or Psychiatric Medication Adverse Effects: Neurologic and psychiatric adverse effects have not been observed. AGIs have mostly gastrointestinal side effects, including gas, bloating, urgency, and diarrhea. Drug interactions are rare, although there is a case report of a 10-year-old patient who had a 40% reduction in valproate levels upon initiation of acarbose. Rechallenge resulted in recurrence.

Further Reading

Serrano JS, et al. May acarbose impair valproate bioavailability? *Meth Find Exp Clin Pharmacol.* 1996;18(Suppl C):98.

Amylinomimetics

Class Members: pramlintide (Symlin®)

Typical Uses: type 1 or 2 diabetes mellitus in conjunction with prandial insulin

Potential Neurologic or Psychiatric Medication Adverse Effects: Nausea and vomiting are common side effects with rates of 28–48% and vomiting rates of 6–11% versus placebo. Patients with type 1 diabetes mellitus experience more side effects versus type 2 diabetes mellitus. Anorexia/weight loss may occur as pramlintide is an analog of the hormone amylin, which decreases food intake via a central nervous system mechanism. In addition fatigue (3% versus placebo) and dizziness (1–2% versus placebo) may occur. Black box warnings include an early in therapy risk of severe hypoglycemia. Prandial insulin should be reduced by 30–50% upon initiation. Delayed gastric emptying via vagal afferent nerve pathways is possible and anticholinergic medications may worsen this effect.

Further Reading

Lee NJ, Norris SL, Thakurta S. Efficacy and harms of the hypoglycemic agent pramlintide in diabetes mellitus. *Ann Fam Med.* 2010;8:542–9.

Mietlicki Baase EG, Hayes MR. Amylin activates distributed CNS nuclei to control energy balance. *Physiol Behav.* 2014;136:39–46.

Biguanides

Class Members: metformin (Glucophage®, Riomet®), metformin extended release (Glucophage XR®, Glumetza®, Fortamet®)

Typical Uses: type 2 diabetes mellitus, gestational diabetes, polycystic ovary syndrome, prevention of type 2 diabetes mellitus

Potential Neurologic or Psychiatric Medication Adverse Effects: Worsening peripheral neuropathy may occur secondary to metformin-induced intestinal malabsorption of vitamin B12. Worsening diabetic peripheral neuropathy has been noted in some patients. Oral or subcutaneous supplementation of vitamin B12 may overcome the malabsorption. A black box warning for lactic acidosis is present for all products. OCT2 renal tubular excretion inhibitors such as lamotrigine or bupropion may increase metformin concentrations. Topiramate may decrease bicarbonate concentrations, which could complicate the clinical picture if lactic acidosis is suspected with metformin.

Further Reading

Contrave (naltrexone HCl/buproprion HCl) package insert. Deerfield, IL/La Jolla, CA: Takeda Pharmaceuticals American, Inc./Orexigen Therapeutics, Inc.; 2014.

Wile DJ, Toth C. Association of metformin, elevated homocysteine, and emthylmalonic acid levels and clinically worsened diabetic peripheral neuropathy. *Diabet Care*. 2010;33:156–61.

Dipeptidyl Peptidase-4 Inhibitors (DPP-4 inhibitors)

Class Members: sitagliptin (Januvia*), saxagliptin (Onglyza*), linagliptin (Tradjenta*), alogliptin (Nesina*), vildagliptin

Typical Uses: type 2 diabetes mellitus, type 1 diabetes mellitus

Potential Neurologic or Psychiatric Medication Adverse Effects: Alogliptin is the only DPP-4 inhibitor that had a higher incidence of headache than placebo in controlled trials (alogliptin 4.2% vs placebo 2.5%, sitagliptin 5.8% vs placebo 5.5%, saxagliptin 6.5% vs placebo 5.9%, linagliptin 3.1% vs placebo 3.3% in placebo-controlled trials). No dose–response or other characteristics that predispose were reported. Drug–drug interactions have been reported with saxagliptin and conivaptan when used for hyponatremia from syndrome of inappropriate antidiuretic hormone (SIADH). Saxagliptin levels will be higher, but no known adverse effects from higher levels have been documented. Sitagliptin, linagliptin, and alogliptin have no significant drug interactions with neurologic or psychiatric medications.

Further Reading

Lehrke M, Marx N, Patel S, et al. Safety and tolerability of linagliptin in patients with type 2 diabetes: a comprehensive pooled analysis of 22 placebo-controlled studies. *Clin Ther*. 2014;36:1130–46.

Richard KR, Shelburne JS, Kirk JK. Tolerability of dipeptidyl peptidase-4 inhibitors: a review. *Clin Ther*. 2011;33:1609–29.

Willams-Herman D, Engel SS, Round E, et al. Safety and tolerability of sitagliptin in clinical studies: a pooled analysis of data from 10,246 patients with type 2 diabetes. *BMC Endocr Disord*. 2010;10:7.

Glucagon-Like Peptide-1 Receptor Agonists (GLP-1RA)

Class Members: exenatide (Byetta*, Bydureon*), liraglutide (Victoza*, Saxsenda*), albiglutide (Tanzeum*), dulaglutide (Trulicity*), lixisenetide (Lyxumia*)

Typical Uses: type 2 diabetes mellitus, weight loss (liraglutide)

Potential Neurologic or Psychiatric Medication Adverse Effects: Nausea/vomiting is a class effect (exenatide 25–35%, exenatide weekly 10–25%, liraglutide 20–30% at doses up to 1.8 mg daily, albiglutide 10%, dulaglutide 16–28%). Mechanisms involve delayed gastric emptying and may also involve vagal afferent nerve pathways. Anorexia and weight loss as class effects may also occur. GLP-1RAs decrease food intake and food-reward central nervous system (CNS) responses when compared with placebo. Albiglutide and possibly dulaglutide may not penetrate CNS as well due to molecular size, which may result in less weight loss. There is a black box warning for thyroid C-cell tumors for long-acting medications (does not include exenatide [Byetta] or lixisenatide). Do not use in patients with a history of medullary thyroid carcinoma (MTC) or with a history of multiple endocrine neoplasia type 2 (MEN 2). Rodents, at GLP-1 stimulation levels considered attainable in humans, had higher rates of MTC. Significance is unknown in humans. Humans have very few, if any, GLP-1 receptors on the C-cells located on the thyroid, but when MTC is surgically removed, approximately a third of tissue samples may express GLP-1 receptors. To date, no increased incidence has been reported.

Further Reading

Smits MM, van Raalte DH, Tonneijck L, et al. GLP-1 based therapies: clinical implications for gastroenterologists. *Gut*. 2016;65:702–11.

Trujillo JM, Nuffer W, Ellis SL. GLP-1 receptor agonists: a review of head-to-head clinical trials. *Adv Endocrinol Metab*. 2015;6:19–28.

Van Bloemendall L, IJzerman RG, Ten Kulve JS, et al. GLP-1 receptor activation modulates appetite and reward-related brain areas in humans. *Diabetes*. 2014;63:4186–96.

Waser B, Blank A, Karamitopoulou E, Perren A, Reubi JI. Glucagon-like-peptide-1 receptor expression in normal and diseased human thyroid and pancreas. *Mod Pathol*. 2015;28:391–402.

Sodium Glucose Cotransporter-2 Inhibitors (SGLT2 Inhibitors)

Class Members: canagliflozin (Invokana®), dapagliflozin (Farxiga®), empagliflozin (Jardiance®)

Typical Uses: type 2 diabetes mellitus

Potential Neurologic or Psychiatric Medication Adverse Effects: Orthostatic dizziness/hypotension/syncope (1–2%) from intravascular volume depletion/lowering of blood pressure may be seen. This is a class effect and more common in the elderly, with concomitant loop diuretic use, and estimated glomerular filtration rate (eGFR) <60 mL/minute/1.73 m². A positive urine glucose test will always be present due to the mechanism of SGLT2 inhibitors. Canagliflozin levels may be reduced by strong inducers of glucuronidation (e.g., carbamazepine, phenobarbital, St. John's wort); consider the 300 mg dose.

Further Reading

Invokana package insert. Titusville, NJ: Janssen Pharmaceuticals, 2013.

Sulfonylureas and Other Secretagogues (Meglitinides)

Class Members: sulfonylureas: glipizide (Glucotrol®, Glucotrol XL®), glyburide (Micronase®, Diabeta®), glimepiride (Amaryl®), chlorpropamide (Diabinese®), acetohexamide, tolbutamide, glicazide, gliquidone; **meglitinides:** repaglinide (Prandin®), nateglinide (Starlix®)

Typical Uses: type 2 diabetes mellitus

Potential Neurologic or Psychiatric Medication Adverse Effects: Central nervous system side effects are thought to be directly related to hypoglycemia or the glucose-lowering effect, which has been shown to result in adrenergic symptoms of hypoglycemia in some patients. Drug–drug interactions include: (1) naltrexone C_{max} and AUC increased by 2-fold by glyburide, significance unknown; (2) inducers of CYP2C9 (e.g., carbamazepine, St. John's wort) may decrease efficacy of sulfonylureas; and (3) strong inhibitors or inducers of CYP2C8 may alter repaglinide levels; gemfibrozil has documented cases of severe hypoglycemia.

Further Reading

Contrave® package insert. Deerfield, IL/La Jolla, CA: Takeda Pharmaceuticals American, Inc./ Orexigen Therapeutics, Inc.; 2014.

Niemi M, Backman JT, Neuvonen M, et al. Effects of gemfibrozil, itraconazole, and their combination on the pharmacokinetics and pharmacodynamics of repaglinide: potentially hazardous interaction between gemfibrozil and repaglinide. *Diabetologia.* 2003;46:347–51.

Xu H, Williams KM, Liauw WS, et al. Effects of St John's wort and CYP2C9 genotype on the pharmacokinetics and pharmacodynamics of gliclazide. *Br J Pharmacol.* 2008;153:1579–86.

Thiazolidinediones (TZDs)

Class Members: pioglitazone (Actos®), rosiglitazone (Avandia®)

Typical Uses: type 2 diabetes mellitus, non-alcoholic fatty liver disease/non-alcoholic steatohepatitis, restenosis reduction after cardiac stent placement, prevention of stroke, prevention of type 2 diabetes mellitus

Potential Neurologic or Psychiatric Medication Adverse Effects: Weight gain (2–4 kg) is a class effect that is dose and time dependent. Half of weight gain is due to excess fluid retention, and the other half is due to true weight gain. Black box warning states that TZDs may cause or exacerbate congestive heart failure as they increase plasma volume. Monitor for signs and symptoms of heart failure and weight. Use cautiously in any heart failure patient. Consider alternative therapy in patients with New York Heart Association class III or IV heart failure. Gabapentin, pregabalin, pramipexole, and/or dihydropyridine calcium channel blockers may contribute to TZD-induced peripheral edema. Strong inducers of CYP2C8 (e.g., carbamazepine) may decrease pioglitazone or possibly rosiglitazone efficacy.

Further Reading

Horita S, Makamura M, Satoh N et al. Thiazolidinediones and edema: recent advances in the pathogenesis of thiazolidinediones-induced renal sodium retention. *PPAR Res.* 2015;2015: Article ID 646423.

Triplitt C, Cersosimo E, DeFronzo R. Pioglitazone and alogliptin combination therapy in type 2 diabetes. A pathophysiologically sound treatment. *Vasc Health Risk Manag.* 2010;6:671–90.

Hormones and Medications to Treat Endocrine and Bone Disorders

Emily Zimmerman, PharmD, BCPS UW Health University Hospital
Casey Gallimore, PharmD, MS University of Wisconsin-Madison School of Pharmacy

Alpha Receptor Blockers

Class Members: alpha-1 selective antagonist: prazosin (Minipress®), doxazosin (Cardura®), terazosin (Hytrin®), alfuzosin (Uroxatral®); **alpha-1$_A$ and alpha-1$_D$ selective antagonist:** tamsulosin (Flomax®), silodosin (Rapaflo®)

Typical Uses: benign prostatic hyperplasia, hypertension, urinary tract symptoms, sleep quality and reduced nightmares (prazosin only)

Potential Neurologic or Psychiatric Medication Adverse Effects: The adverse effect profile is similar among agents within the class. Very common adverse effects (>10%) include dizziness and headache. Common adverse effects (1–10%) include somnolence, lethargy, and asthenia. Prazosin is the only alpha antagonist that has been demonstrated to improve sleep quality in patients with posttraumatic stress disorder who report nightmares.

Further Reading

Ahmadpanah M, Sabzeiee P, Hosseini SM, et al. Comparing the effect of prazosin and hydroxyzine on sleep quality in patients suffering from posttraumatic stress disorder. *Neuropsychobiology*. 2014;69:235–42.

Prazosin hydrochloride. In *Micromedex 2.0*. Greenwood Village, CO: Truven Health Analytics, Inc. http://micromedexsolutions.com. Accessed Jan 2, 2016.

Westfall TC, Westfall DP. Adrenergic agonists and antagonists. In Brunton LL, Chabner BA, Knollmann BC, eds. *Goodman & Gilman's the pharmacological basis of therapeutics*, 12th ed. New York, NY: McGraw-Hill; 2011. Chapter 12.

Androgenic Anabolic Steroids

Class Members: testosterone (Androderm®, AndroGel®, AndroGel Pump®, Aveed®, Axiron®, Depo-Testosterone®, First-Testosterone®, First-Testosterone MC®, Fortesta®, Natesto®, Striant®, Testim®, Testopel®, Vogelxo®, Vogelxo Pump®), danazol (Danocrine®), fluoxymesterone (Androxy®), methyltestosterone (Android®, Methitest®, Testred®), oxandrolone (Oxandrin®), oxymetholone (Anadrol®)

Typical Uses: testosterone, fluoxymesterone (delayed puberty, hypogonadism, replacement therapy, metastatic breast cancer), danazol (endometriosis, fibrocystic breast disease, hereditary angioedema), oxandrolone (adjunct for weight loss), oxymetholone (anemias secondary to deficient red cell production)

Potential Neurologic or Psychiatric Medication Adverse Effects: The most common adverse effects of androgenic steroids are endocrine effects including hirsutism, voice changes, weight gain, edema, flushing, sweating, nervousness, emotional lability, and libido changes. The specific frequency of adverse effects has not been defined for danazol, fluoxymesterone, methyltestosterone, oxandrolone, and oxymetholone; however, potential psychiatric and neurologic effects include anxiety and depression. In addition headache and paresthesia are possible with fluoxymesterone and methyltestosterone, and excitation and insomnia with oxandrolone and oxymetholone. Common adverse effects (1–10%) of testosterone include aggressiveness, irritability, mood swings, headache, fatigue, insomnia, taste disorder, arthralgia, back pain, joint pain and swelling, paresthesia, tremor, and weakness. Oxandrolone and oxymetholone have black box warnings for peliosis hepatitis, liver cell tumors, and blood lipid changes such as decreased high-density lipoprotein (HDL) and increased low-density lipoprotein (LDL). Black box warnings for danazol include increased risk of thromboembolic events, peliosis hepatitis and hepatic adenoma, and intracranial hypertension. Use of androgenic anabolic steroids is contraindicated in pregnancy.

Further Reading

Androgens. In *AHFS Drug Information STAT!Ref Online Electronic Medical Library*. Bethesda, MD: American Society of Health-System Pharmacists. http://online.statref.com/document.aspx? fxid=1&docid=497. Accessed Jan 18, 2016.

Testosterone, danazol, fluoxymesterone, methyltestosterone, oxandrolone, oxymetholone. In *Lexi-Drugs. Lexicomp*. Hudson, OH: Wolters Kluwer Health, Inc. http://online.lexi.com. Accessed Jan 18, 2016.

Bisphosphonates

Class Members: alendronate sodium (Fosamax®), etidronate disodium (Didronel®), ibandronate sodium (Boniva®), pamidronate disodium (Aredia®), risedronate sodium (Actonel®, Actonel® with Calcium), zoledronic acid (Zometa®, Reclast®)

Typical Uses: treatment and prevention of osteoporosis, treatment of Paget disease of the bone, treatment of moderate or severe hypercalcemia associated with malignancy (pamidronate, zoledronic acid), treatment of osteolytic bone metastases of breast cancer or solid tumors and osteolytic lesions of multiple myeloma (pamidronate, zolendronic acid), prevention and treatment of heterotopic ossification due to spinal cord injury or after total hip replacement (etidronate)

Potential Neurologic or Psychiatric Medication Adverse Effects: Flu-like symptoms are common with intravenous bisphosphonate use. They typically occur within 24–72 hours after the infusion and may manifest as a low-grade fever, myalgias, and arthralgias. Additional very common (>10%) or common (1–10%) adverse neurologic and psychiatric effects of intravenous bisphosphonates include headache, weakness, back pain, and bone pain. Common adverse effects of oral bisphosphonates include headache, musculoskeletal pain, and muscle cramps or spasms. Rarely patients experience severe musculoskeletal pain (bone, joint, and/or muscle pain) that requires discontinuation of the bisphosphonate. Such pain can develop within days to years (mean onset about 3 months) after starting a bisphosphonate.

Further Reading

Alendronate, etidronate, ibandronate, pamidronate, risedronate, zoledronic acid In: *Lexi-Drugs. Lexicomp*. Hudson, OH: Wolters Kluwer Health, Inc. http://online.lexi.com. Accessed Jun 28, 2016.

Bone resorption inhibitors. In: *AHFS Drug Information STAT!Ref Online Electronic Medical Library*. Bethesda, MD: American Society of Health-System Pharmacists. http://online.statref .com/document.aspx?fxid=1&docid=497. Accessed Jun 28, 2016.

Calcitonin (Miacalcin®, Fortical®)

Typical Uses: adjunctive therapy for hypercalcemia, treatment of symptomatic Paget disease of bone, treatment of osteoporosis

Potential Neurologic or Psychiatric Medication Adverse Effects: Calcitonin is generally well tolerated with only mild and infrequent adverse effects. Reports of adverse effects are more common with the parenteral preparation compared with the nasal spray formulation. Transient nausea occurring within 30 minutes of administration is the most common adverse effect (10%) related to parenteral calcitonin. Nausea with intranasal calcitonin is less frequent (1–3%). Common (1–10%) neurologic and psychiatric effects reported with intranasal calcitonin use include depression (1–3%), dizziness (1–3%), paresthesia (1–3%), back pain (5%), and myalgia (1–3%).

Further Reading

Calcitonin. In *Lexi-Drugs. Lexicomp*. Hudson, OH: Wolters Kluwer Health, Inc. http://online.lexi .com. Accessed Jun 29, 2016.

Calcitonin. In *AHFS Drug Information STAT!Ref Online Electronic Medical Library*. Bethesda, MD: American Society of Health-System Pharmacists. http://online.statref.com/document.aspx? fxid=1&docid=497. Accessed Jun 29, 2016.

Cinacalcet (Sensipar®)

Typical Uses: treatment of primary hyperparathyroidism, treatment of secondary hyperparathyroidism with chronic kidney disease (CKD) on dialysis, treatment of hypercalcemia with parathyroid carcinoma

Potential Neurologic or Psychiatric Medication Adverse Effects: Cinacalcet reduces serum calcium concentrations, which places patients at increased risk of hypocalcemia and associated symptoms including paresthesias, myalgias, cramping, tetany, and seizures due to a decreased seizure threshold. It is important to monitor serum calcium concentrations during treatment with cinacalcet and if it drops below 8.4 mg/dL, cinacalcet should be discontinued and appropriate measures taken to increase the serum calcium concentration. Across all indications for cinacalcet use, the most common adverse effects experienced by patients are nausea (30–66%) and vomiting (26–52%). Among dialysis patients, adverse neurologic and psychiatric effects reported with cinacalcet use in at least 5% of patients and at a higher rate compared to placebo-treated patients included dizziness, weakness, noncardiac chest pain, and myalgia.

Further Reading

Cinacalcet. In *Lexi-Drugs. Lexicomp.* Hudson, OH: Wolters Kluwer Health, Inc. http://online.lexi.com. Accessed Jun 29, 2016.

Cinacalcet. In *AHFS Drug Information STAT!Ref Online Electronic Medical Library.* Bethesda, MD: American Society of Health-System Pharmacists. http://online.statref.com/document.aspx?fxid=1&docid=497. Accessed Jun 29, 2016.

Hormonal Contraceptives

Class Members: estrogen–progestin combinations: drospirenone and ethinyl estradiol, levonorgestrel and ethinyl estradiol, norethindrone and ethinyl estradiol, desogestrel and ethinyl estradiol, norgestrel and ethinyl estradiol, ethynodiol diacetate and ethinyl estradiol, norgestimate and ethinyl estradiol, cyproterone ethinyl estradiol, ethynodiol diacetate and ethinyl estradiol, norethindrone and mestranol, dienogest and estradiol valerate, norelgestromin and ethinyl estradiol, etonogestrel and ethinyl estradiol; **progestin-only:** norethindrone

Typical Uses: contraception, acne vulgaris, premenstrual dysphoric disorder, endometriosis, dysfunctional uterine bleeding

Potential Neurologic or Psychiatric Medication Adverse Effects: Hormonal contraceptives are available as estrogen–progestin combinations and progestin-only products. Available routes of administration include oral, intravaginal, and transdermal. The adverse effect profile is similar across hormonal contraceptive agents, but exact frequency may vary depending on hormonal dose and route of administration. Potential neurologic and psychiatric adverse effects include mood changes and depression. Occurrence of depression appears to be more frequent in patients with a history of depression. Additional adverse effects that have been reported with hormonal contraceptive use include dizziness, fatigue, insomnia, anxiety or nervousness, aggressiveness, emotional lability, irritability, changes in libido, and premenstrual syndrome. If recurrent, persistent or severe headache or migraine headache occurs, hormonal contraception should be discontinued. Estrogen-progestin combinations have a black box warning for increased risk of cardiovascular events with concurrent cigarette smoking, especially in women over the age of 35. In addition, the transdermal contraceptive patch has a warning for increased risk of venous thromboembolism compared to oral and transvaginal products.

Further Reading

Contraceptives. In *AHFS Drug Information STAT!Ref Online Electronic Medical Library.* Bethesda, MD: American Society of Health-System Pharmacists. http://online.statref.com/document.aspx?fxid=1&docid=497. Accessed Jan 27, 2016.

Martin KA, Douglas PS. Risks and side effects associated with estrogen-progestin contraceptives. In Post TW, ed. *UpToDate.* Waltham, MA: UpToDate; 2016.

Hormone Replacement Therapy (HRT)

Class Members: estradiol, esterified estrogen, estropipate, conjugated equine estrogen, conjugated synthetic estrogen, conjugated equine estrogen and medroxyprogesterone, estradiol and norgestimate, estradiol and norethindrone acetate, ethinyl estradiol and norethindrone, estradiol and drospirenone.

Typical Uses: vasomotor symptoms associated with menopause, vulvar and vaginal atrophy associated with menopause, osteoporosis prevention (estrogen–progestin preparations only), acne vulgaris (ethinyl estradiol and norethindrone)

Potential Neurologic or Psychiatric Medication Adverse Effects: Hormone therapy for management of vasomotor symptoms can be separated into estrogen preparations and estrogen–progestin combinations, and is available in multiple forms (oral, transdermal, topical gels and lotions, intravaginal creams and tablets, and vaginal rings). Potential adverse effects are similar across most agents. The hormonal changes of menopause may complicate ability to distinguish between adverse effects of HRT and underlying menopausal symptoms. Exact frequency of adverse effects varies across agents, but in general very common adverse effects (>10%) observed with HRT include headache, breast pain and back pain, and potentially common adverse effects (1–10%) include depression, anxiety, emotional lability, dizziness, migraine, arthralgia, weakness, myalgia, leg cramps, and dysmenorrhea. Hormone replacement therapies have a black box warning for increased risk of endometrial cancer, breast cancer, cardiovascular disease, and dementia.

Further Reading

Estrogens and estrogen angonist–antagonists. In: *AHFS Drug Information STAT!Ref Online Electronic Medical Library*. Bethesda, MD: American Society of Health-System Pharmacists. http://online.statref.com/document.aspx?fxid=1&docid=497. Accessed Jan 27, 2016.

Martin KA, Barbieri RL. Preparations for menopausal hormone therapy. In Post TW, ed. *UpToDate*. Waltham, MA: UpToDate; 2016.

Parathyroid Hormone

Class Members: teriparatide (Forteo®)

Typical Uses: osteoporosis (postmenopausal women, men, glucocorticoid induced)

Potential Neurologic or Psychiatric Medication Adverse Effects: A very common adverse effect (>10%) of parathyroid hormone is transient hypercalcemia 4 to 6 hours post dose; however, rarely <1% of patients have sustained hypercalcemia values greater than 13 mg/dL. The package insert for Forteo® does note that a higher

percentage of patients experienced depression while on teriparatide therapy compared to placebo (4.1% vs 2.7%). Other psychiatric side effects are minimal and not reported in the literature.

Further Reading

Forteo (teriparatide) package insert. Indianapolis, IN: Eli Lilly & Co; 2011.

Teriparatide. In *Lexi-Drugs. Lexicomp*. Hudson, OH: Wolters Kluwer Health, Inc. http://online.lexi.com. Accessed Jan 2, 2016.

Phosphodiesterase-5 (PDE-5) Inhibitors

Class Members: sildenafil (Viagra®, Revatio®), vardenafil (Levitra®), tadalafil (Cialis®, Adcirca®), avanafil (Stendra®)

Typical Uses: erectile dysfunction (ED), benign prostatic hyperplasia (Cialis®), pulmonary hypertension (Revatio®, Adcirca®)

Potential Neurologic or Psychiatric Medication Adverse Effects: The adverse effect profiles for the PDE-5 inhibitors are similar except for sildenafil, in which visual disturbances have been reported. The most common adverse effect (>10%) is headache, which is likely related to vasodilatory properties of these medications, and is dose related. Common (1–10%) adverse effects include insomnia and dizziness. In patients with antidepressant-related ED, these medications may be an effective strategy for treatment. Patients with depression and concurrent ED had improvement in those depression symptoms when receiving treatment for ED.

Further Reading

McCabe MP, Althof SE. A systematic review of the psychosocial outcomes associated with erectile dysfunction: does the impact of erectile dysfunction extend beyond a man's inability to have sex? *J Sex Med*. 2014;11:347–63.

Sildenafil. In *DRUGDEX® System (electronic version)*. Greenwood Village, CO: Truven Health Analytics, Inc. www.micromedexsolutions.com/. Accessed Jan 2, 2016.

Taylor MJ. Strategies for managing antidepressant-induced sexual dysfunction: a review. *Curr Psychiatry Rep*. 2006;8:431–6.

Thyroid Supplement

Class Members: levothyroxine (Synthroid®, Levoxyl®, Levothroid®), liothyronine (Cytomel®) T3, liotrix (Thyrolar®), desiccated thyroid (Armour Thyroid®).

Typical Uses: hypothyroidism

Potential Neurologic or Psychiatric Medication Adverse Effects: Imbalances in endogenous or exogenous thyroid hormone can present as psychologic disturbances. An overabundance of thyroid hormone can cause restlessness, insomnia, anxiety, decreased appetite, and weight loss. A lack of thyroid hormone can present as fatigue, lethargy, depression, and psychomotor retardation. Most clinicians recommend monitoring thyroid-stimulating hormone (TSH) and T4 when patients present with symptoms of either imbalance. It is recommended to monitor TSH at least 4 weeks after initiation and any change in dose. The adverse effect profile of thyroid supplements is due to the in vivo imbalance of thyroid hormone, which supports the need for monitoring.

Further Reading

Garber JR, Cobin RH, Gharib H, et al. Clinical practice guidelines for hypothyroidism in adults: cosponsored by the American Association of Clinical Endocrinologists and the American Thyroid Association. *Endocr Pract.* 2012;18: 988–1028.

Gastrointestinal Medications

Christi Ann Albert, PharmD, BCPS UW Health University Hospital
Casey Gallimore, PharmD, MS University of Wisconsin-Madison School of Pharmacy

Antacids

Class Members: calcium carbonate (Mylanta® Children's Upset Stomach Relief, Titralac® Regular, Tums® Antacid/Calcium Supplement, Titralac® Extra Strength, Tums® E-X Antacid/Calcium Supplement, Alka-Mints®, Maalox® Quick Dissolve® Chewables, Maalox® Quick Dissolve® Chewables Maximum Strength), aluminum hydroxide (Alu-Cap®, Amphojel®, ALternaGEL®, Amphojel®, Alu-Tab®), magnesium hydroxide (Milk of Magnesia, Phillips'® Milk of Magnesia, Phillips'® Milk of Magnesia Concentrate), magnesium oxide (Uro-Mag®, Magnesium Oxide Tablets, Mag-Ox® 400)

Typical Uses: adjunct treatment of peptic ulcers; relief of esophageal reflux, acid indigestion, heartburn, dyspepsia, and sour stomach; prevention of stress ulceration and GI bleeding; reduce the risk associated with gastric aspiration; management of hyperphosphatemia

Potential Neurologic or Psychiatric Medication Adverse Effects: Gastrointestinal adverse effects such as constipation and diarrhea are the main concern with the use of antacids, while adverse neurologic and psychiatric effects tend to be less problematic. Headache is a common adverse effect (1–10%) of calcium carbonate. Aluminum and magnesium accumulation are rare, but can occur in patients with certain risk factors for reduced excretion, and may result in neurologic/psychiatric effects. Aluminum and magnesium may accumulate in the bones, lungs, and nerve tissue of patients with severe chronic kidney disease (glomerular filtration rate [GFR] <30 mL/minute per 1.73 m²) due to a decreased renal excretion. Aluminum toxicity may manifest as bone and muscle pain, proximal muscle weakness, osteomalacia, iron-resistant microcytic anemia, hypercalcemia, and slowly progressive dementia. Symptoms of aluminum-related dementia include dysarthria, myoclonus, mental changes, hallucinations, and seizures. The clinical manifestations of hypermagnesemia are predictable based on the plasma magnesium concentration, and involve neuromuscular and cardiovascular effects, and hypocalcemia. Neuromuscular effects at a plasma concentration of 4–6 meq/L are headache, lethargy, drowsiness, and diminished deep tendon reflexes; at 6–10 meq/L symptoms progress to somnolence and absent deep tendon reflexes; and at concentrations over 10 meq/L, muscle paralysis may occur.

Further Reading

Antacids and adsorbents. In *AHFS Drug Information STAT!Ref Online Electronic Medical Library.* Bethesda, MD: American Society of Health-System Pharmacists. http://online.statref.com/document.aspx?fxid=1&docid=497. Accessed Jun 27, 2016.

Calcium carbonate, aluminum hydroxide, magnesium hydroxide, magnesium oxide. In *Lexi-Drugs. Lexicomp.* Hudson, OH: Wolters Kluwer Health, Inc. http://online.lexi.com. Accessed Jun 27, 2016.

H₂ Antagonists

Class Members: cimetidine (Tagamet®), famotidine (Pepcid®), nizatidine (Axid®), ranitidine (Zantac®)

Typical Uses: anaphylaxis adjunct therapy, dyspepsia, duodenal ulcer, erosive esophagitis, esophagitis, gastric ulcer, gastroesophageal reflux disease, heartburn, *Helicobacter pylori* eradication, hypersecretory conditions, indigestion, stress ulcer prophylaxis in ICU patients, systemic mast cell disease, nonsteroidal anti-inflammatory drug (NSAID)-induced ulcer prophylaxis, Zollinger–Ellison syndrome

Potential Neurologic or Psychiatric Medication Adverse Effects: The most common neurologic adverse effect of H$_2$ antagonists is headache, reported at an incidence ranging from 2 to 16%. Other common adverse effects (1–10%) include agitation, anxiety, dizziness, disorientation, delirium, drowsiness, confusion, hallucinations, insomnia, irritability, malaise, somnolence, and vertigo, all of which are more common in elderly and debilitated patients, and/or patients with poor renal or liver function. Adverse neurologic effects are more likely with cimetidine than other agents due to its metabolite, cimetidine sulfoxide. There have been case reports of cimetidine dosed inappropriately in renal disease having rarely caused psychosis, depression, and seizures. There have been case reports of aseptic meningitis at typical doses, and unresponsiveness, central nervous system depression, and death at toxic dosages of cimetidine.

Further Reading

Drug Facts and Comparisons. Facts & Comparisons [database online]. St. Louis, MO: Wolters Kluwer Health, Inc; Mar 2005.

Lexi-Drugs. Lexicomp. Hudson, OH: Wolters Kluwer Health, Inc. http://online.lexi.com. Accessed Jan 10, 2016.

Micromedex 2.0. Greenwood Village, CO: Truven Health Analytics, Inc. http://micromedexsolutions .com. Accessed Jan 10, 2016.

Metoclopramide (Reglan®)

Typical Uses: gastroparesis, gastroesophageal reflux, nausea and vomiting prevention for chemotherapy, post-operative nausea and vomiting, paralytic ileus, post-pyloric feeding tube placement, increase lactation in breast feeding mothers, acute migraine

Potential Neurologic or Psychiatric Medication Adverse Effects: Central nervous system (CNS) toxicities are a dose-limiting factor in metoclopramide therapy. Very common adverse effects (>10%) include asthenia, restlessness, drowsiness, and fatigue. Incidence of acute reversible extrapyramidal symptoms can vary from 2 to 30% and can include bradykinesia, dysphagia, dystonias, facial spasms, opisthotonos, torticollis, trismus, and other tetanus-like reactions and are dose related. Acute extrapyramidal symptoms, particularly acute dystonias, can be reversed with benztropine or intravenous diphenhydramine. Rarely, acute dystonias can be fatal if not treated. Common adverse effects (1–10%) include dizziness, headache, lassitude, and sedation. Depression and suicidal ideation have been reported with and without a prior history of depression. While not common, metoclopramide carries a boxed warning for irreversible tardive dyskinesias with prolonged or high exposures. Rare, but potentially fatal cases of neuroleptic malignant syndrome have been reported. Pediatric, elderly, and patients with severe renal disease are more sensitive to the CNS toxicities of metoclopramide. Parkinson disease can be exacerbated by metoclopramide and parkinsonian-like symptoms have been reported in patients without underlying Parkinson disease. Metoclopramide can reduce the seizure threshold and should be used cautiously in epilepsy. A discontinuation syndrome may occur with abrupt cessation of metoclopramide; symptoms include dizziness, nervousness, and/or headache.

Further Reading

Metoclopramide. In *Drug Facts and Comparisons. Facts & Comparisons [database online].* St. Louis, MO: Wolters Kluwer Health, Inc; Mar 2005.

Metoclopramide. In *Lexi-Drugs. Lexicomp.* Hudson, OH: Wolters Kluwer Health, Inc. http://online .lexi.com. Accessed Jan 10, 2016.

Metoclopramide. In *Micromedex 2.0.* Greenwood Village, CO: Truven Health Analytics, Inc. http:// micromedexsolutions.com. Accessed Jan 10, 2016.

Proton Pump Inhibitors (PPIs)

Class Members: lansoprazole (Prevacid®, Prevacid Solutab®), dexlansoprazole (Dexilant®, Kapidex®), pantoprazole (Protonix®), omeprazole (Prilosec®, Zegerid®), esomeprazole (Nexium®), rabeprazole (Aciphex®)

Typical Uses: Barrett's esophagitis, duodenal ulcer disease, dyspepsia, erosive esophagitis, heartburn, esophageal stricture, gastric ulcers, gastroesophageal reflux disease, *Helicobacter pylori* gastrointestinal infection, NSAID-induced ulcer prophylaxis, peptic ulcer disease, stress ulcer prophylaxis in ICU patients, Zollinger–Ellison syndrome

Potential Neurologic or Psychiatric Medication Adverse Effects: The adverse effect profile is similar among agents within the PPI class. Headache is the most commonly reported neuropsychiatric adverse effect with a reported incidence of 2–12%. Other common adverse effects (1–10%) include dizziness and fatigue, and less commonly reported asthenia and somnolence. Paresthesias and seizures have rarely occurred in the setting of hypocalcemia or hypomagnesemia as the result of long-term PPI exposure (generally >1 year). Use of PPIs for >3 years can also rarely result in cyanocobalamin deficiency secondary to hypo- or achlorhydria, which can manifest with the following symptoms: dementia, depression, acute psychosis, paresthesias, numbness, weakness, and autonomic neuropathies.

Further Reading

Drug Facts and Comparisons. Facts & Comparisons [database online]. St. Louis, MO: Wolters Kluwer Health, Inc; March 2005.

Lexi-Drugs. Lexicomp. Hudson, OH: Wolters Kluwer Health, Inc. http://online.lexi.com. Accessed Jan 10, 2016.

Micromedex 2.0. Greenwood Village, CO: Truven Health Analytics, Inc. http://micromedexsolutions.com. Accessed Jan 10, 2016.

Scopolamine (Transderm Scop®)

Typical Uses: prevention of post-operative nausea and vomiting, prevention of nausea and vomiting associated with motion sickness, decrease intestinal motility, mydriasis induction

Potential Neurologic or Psychiatric Medication Adverse Effects: Adverse effects are more profound with oral, IV, IM, or SQ administration in comparison to transdermal. Although systemic exposure is low when administered ophthalmically, systemic adverse effects have been reported. Very common adverse effects (>10%) include dry mouth, dizziness, and drowsiness. Common adverse effects (1–10%) include agitation, blurred vision, confusion, mydriasis, restlessness, somnolence, and urinary retention. The following idiosyncratic reactions have been reported: acute toxic psychosis, agitation, speech disorder, hallucinations, paranoia, and delusions. A discontinuation syndrome may occur if prolonged use of scopolamine is stopped abruptly. Symptoms include abdominal cramping, bradycardia, dizziness, disturbances of equilibrium, headache, hypotension, mental confusion, muscle weakness, nausea, sweating, and vomiting. Scopolamine should be used cautiously in patients with underlying renal or hepatic disease or elderly patients because they are more sensitive to its central nervous system toxicities.

Further Reading

Scopolamine. In *Drug Facts and Comparisons. Facts & Comparisons [database online]*. St. Louis, MO: Wolters Kluwer Health, Inc; Mar 2005.

Scopolamine. In *Lexi-Drugs. Lexicomp*. Hudson, OH: Wolters Kluwer Health, Inc. http://online.lexi.com. Accessed Jan 10, 2016.

Scopolamine. In *Micromedex 2.0*. Greenwood Village, CO: Truven Health Analytics, Inc. http://micromedexsolutions.com. Accessed Jan 10, 2016.

Vitamins and Minerals

Chris Hulstein, PharmD UW Health University Hospital
Casey Gallimore, PharmD, MS University of Wisconsin-Madison School of Pharmacy

Iron Preparations

Class Members: ferric carboxymaltose (Injectafer®), ferumoxytol (Feraheme®), iron dextran (Dexferrum®, INFeD®), iron sucrose (Venofer®), sodium ferric gluconate (Ferrlecit®), ferrous fumarate (Ircon®, Hemocyte®, Nephro-Fer®, Feostat®), ferrous gluconate (Fergon®), ferrous sulfate (Fer-Gen-Sol® Drops, Mol-Iron®, Feratab®, Feosol®, Slow FE®), carbonyl iron (Icar® Pediatric, Feosol® Caplets), and polysaccharide-iron complex (Ferrex®-150, Fe-Tinic® 150, Hytinic®, Niferex®-150, Niferex® Elixir, Niferex®)

Typical Uses: treatment and prevention of iron deficiency anemia

Potential Neurologic or Psychiatric Medication Adverse Effects: Iron is available in oral and intravenous preparations. Neurologic or psychiatric adverse effects are rare with oral iron preparations. In contrast, gastrointestinal effects such as stomach cramping, constipation, nausea, vomiting, dark stools, gastrointestinal irritation, and epigastric pain are very common. Among intravenous agents, headache with iron sucrose, and dizziness and cramps with sodium ferric gluconate are very commonly (>10%) occurring adverse neurologic and psychiatric effects. Common adverse effects (1–10%) of individual intravenous agents include **iron sucrose**: dizziness (1–7%), limb pain (3–6%), arthralgia (1–4%), myalgia (≤4%), weakness (1–3%), back pain (1–2%); **sodium ferric gluconate**: headache (7%), pain (10%), fatigue (6%), leg cramps (10%), weakness (7%), paresthesias (6%), arm pain, arthralgia, back pain, myalgia, agitation, chills, decreased consciousness, lightheadedness, malaise, rigors, and somnolence; **ferric carboxymaltose**: nausea, hypertension, dizziness, and headache; and **ferumoxytol**: dizziness. Frequency of adverse effects with iron dextran has not been defined, but possible neurologic and psychiatric adverse effects include chills, disorientation, dizziness, headache, malaise, seizure, unconsciousness, unresponsiveness, arthralgia, arthritis/arthritis exacerbation, back pain, myalgia, paresthesia, and weakness. Additionally, a delayed reaction manifesting with arthralgia, backache, myalgia, adenopathy, moderate to high fever, backache, chills, dizziness, headache, malaise, nausea, and/or vomiting may onset within 24–48 hours after administration of iron dextran. Generally delayed reactions subside within 3–7 days. Patients with rheumatoid arthritis or other inflammatory diseases and patients receiving large doses are at increased risk for delayed reactions. Serious hypersensitivity reactions are rare (0.2–3% for iron dextran, <1% all other agents), but possible with all intravenous agents. Such reactions commonly occur within 30 minutes after completion of infusion, and may manifest as shock, clinically important hypotension, loss of consciousness, and/or collapse.

Further Reading

Iron preparations. In *AHFS Drug Information STAT!Ref Online Electronic Medical Library*. Bethesda, MD: American Society of Health-System Pharmacists. http://online.statref.com/document.aspx?fxid=1&docid=497. Accessed Jun 27, 2016.

Isotretinoin (Absorica®, Accutane®, Amnesteem®, Claravis®, Myorisan®, Sotret®, Zenatane®)

Typical Uses: isotretinoin is FDA-labeled for severe recalcitrant nodular acne. Off-label uses include moderate acne, psoriasis neuroblastoma, cutaneous T-cell lymphoma (mycosis fungoides and Sézary syndrome), squamous cell skin cancers, and prevention of acne in high-risk patients

Potential Neurologic or Psychiatric Medication Adverse Effects: The most commonly reported psychiatric adverse effect is depression. Some have reported that depression subsided with discontinuation of therapy and recurred with reinstitution of therapy. Psychosis may also occur (incidence undefined). Sad mood, hopelessness, feelings of guilt, worthlessness or help-lessness, loss of pleasure or interest in activities, diffi-culty concentrating, changes in sleep patterns, changes in weight or appetite, restlessness, or acting on dan-gerous impulses may also be related to treatment with isotretinoin. Rare side effects include suicidal ideation, suicide attempts, suicide, aggressive and/or violent behavior, pseudotumor cerebri, dizziness, drowsiness, headache, insomnia, lethargy, malaise, nervousness, paresthesias, seizures, stroke, syncope, weakness, and emotional instability. A brochure titled *Recognizing Psychiatric Disorders in Adolescents and Young Adults: A Guide for Prescribers of Isotretinoin* is available from the manufacturer detailing the recognition of the above psychiatric-related side effects. Visual distur-bances such as blurred vision, tunnel vision, tempo-rary loss of vision, double vision, photophobia, color vision disorders, and difficulty seeing have also been reported. Hearing impairment and tinnitus have been noted in patients taking isotretinoin though causality has not yet been determined. It should be noted that isotretinoin is part of a Risk Evaluation and Mitigation Strategy (REMS) program due to potential adverse effects relating to a developing fetus.

Further Reading

Isotretinoin package insert. Nutley, NJ: Roche; Jan 2010.
Isotretinoin. In *DRUGDEX® System (electronic version)*. Greenwood Village, CO: Truven Health Analytics, Inc. www.micromedexsolutions.com/. Accessed Jan 29, 2016.

Vitamin A

Class Members: retinol, retinal, retinoic acid, beta-carotene

Typical Uses: The only FDA-labeled indication for vitamin A is vitamin A deficiency. Off-label use of vitamin A is extensive including supplementation in patients at high risk for deficiency (such as those living in populations where vitamin A deficiency is a public health concern), macular degeneration,

erythropoietic protoporphyria, infection, dermato-logic maladies, cardiovascular disease, and cancer, to name a few.

Potential Neurologic or Psychiatric Medication Adverse Effects: Side effects resulting from long-term use may include irritability, drowsiness, dizziness, delirium, coma, headache, swelling of the optic disk, bulg-ing eyeballs, visual disturbances, fatigue, malaise, lethargy, and psychiatric changes mimicking severe depression or schizophrenic disorder. Acute toxicity may cause headache, increased cerebrospinal fluid pressure, vertigo, blurred vision, muscular incoor-dination, and a bulging fontanelle in infants. These effects typically resolve and are more common in young children. Some dosage forms may contain benzyl alcohol, which, at large amounts (99 mg/kg/day or more), has been associated with a potentially fatal toxicity known as gasping syndrome in neo-nates. Gasping syndrome may cause convulsions or intracranial hemorrhage. Vitamin A may cause a number of fetal defects, which may include central nervous system malformations such as cranial neural crest defects following high doses of vitamin A in the pregnant female.

Further Reading

Vitamin A. In *DRUGDEX® System (electronic version)*. Greenwood Village, CO: Truven Health Analytics, Inc. www.micromedexsolutions.com/. Accessed Jan 29, 2016.
Vitamin A. In *Natural Medicines Comprehensive Database*. Stockton, CA: Therapeutic Research Faculty. http://naturaldatabase .therapeuticresearch.com/. Accessed Jan 29, 2016.
Vitamin A. In *AHFS Drug Information STAT!Ref Online Electronic Medical Library*. Bethesda, MD: American Society of Health-System Pharmacists. http://online.statref.com/document .aspx?fxid=1&docid=497. Accessed Dec 15, 2015).

Vitamin B Complex

Class Members: folic acid, pyridoxine hydrochloride (vitamin B6), riboflavin (vitamin B2), thiamine hydro-chloride (vitamin B1), cyanocobalamin and hydroxo-cobalamin (vitamin B12)

Typical Uses: dietary supplementation, treatment of vitamin B deficiencies

Potential Neurologic or Psychiatric Medication Adverse Effects: The vitamin B complexes are generally considered non-toxic and well tolerated; however, the specific frequency of adverse effects has not been defined. Reported psychiatric and neurologic effects vary slightly by agent, dosage, and duration of use. Administration of large dosages of **pyridoxine** (>2 grams per day) for an extended period (≥2 months) can cause peripheral neuropathy or neuronopathy syndromes that may manifest as an impaired sense of position and vibration of the distal limbs, gradual and progressive sensory ataxia, and diminished or absent deep tendon reflexes. Altered sleep patterns, difficulty concentrating, irritability, overactivity, excitement, mental depression, confusion, impaired judgment, and general malaise have been reported rarely in patients receiving 15 mg of **folic acid** daily for at least 1 month. Parenteral administration of single, large doses (100–500 mg) of **thiamine** is usually non-toxic; however, adverse effects, including psychiatric and neurologic effects such as feelings of warmth, tingling, pain, weakness, sweating, and restlessness, have been occasionally reported following repeat intravenous administration of the drug. **Vitamin B12** is also usually nontoxic even in large doses; however, abnormal gait, anxiety, ataxia, dizziness, headache, hypoesthesia, nervousness, pain, paresthesia, arthritis, back pain, myalgia, and weakness have been reported with its use. No toxic effects have been reported with riboflavin use.

Further Reading

Vitamin B complex. In *AHFS Drug Information STAT!Ref Online Electronic Medical Library*. Bethesda, MD: American Society of Health-System Pharmacists. http://online.statref.com/document.aspx?fxid=1&docid=497. Accessed Jun 28, 2016.

Vitamin D

Class Members: doxercalciferol (Hectorol®), ergocalciferol (Drisdol®, Calciferol® Drops, Calciferol®, Calcidol), paricalcitol (Zemplar®), calcitriol (Rocaltrol®, Calcijex®), dihydrotachysterol (Hytakerol®, DHT® Intensol, DHT®)

Typical Uses: prevention or treatment of rickets or osteomalacia, management of hypocalcemia associated with hypoparathyroidism or pseudohypoparathyroidism

Potential Neurologic or Psychiatric Medication Adverse Effects: Very common adverse effects (>10%) of doxercalciferol include headache (28%), malaise (28%), and dizziness (12%). Common adverse effects (1–10%) of individual agents include **doxercalciferol:** sleep disorder (3%) and arthralgia (5%); **paricalcitol:** pain (4% to 8%), dizziness (5% to 7%), chills (5%), insomnia (5%), vertigo (5%), headache (3% to 5%), anxiety (3%), depression (3%), fatigue (3%), malaise (3%), arthralgia (5%), arthritis (5%), weakness (3% to 5%), leg cramps (3%), and muscle spasm (3%); **calcitriol:** headache. Frequencies of adverse neurologic and psychiatric effects of dihydrotachysterol and ergocalciferol have not been defined. Rarely, vitamin D analogs can precipitate hypercalcemia, which may manifest in central nervous system (CNS) toxicity. Early neurologic and psychiatric manifestations of such toxicity include weakness, headache, somnolence, muscle or bone pain, and metallic taste. Late manifestations include photophobia, decreased libido, and rarely overt psychosis.

Further Reading

Vitamin D. In *AHFS Drug Information STAT!Ref Online Electronic Medical Library*. Bethesda, MD: American Society of Health-System Pharmacists. http://online.statref.com/document.aspx?fxid=1&docid=497. Accessed Jun 27, 2016.

Vitamin E

Typical Uses: Vitamin E is primarily used as a dietary supplement to treat vitamin E deficiency, one that may lead to peripheral neuropathy. The list of indications other than primary vitamin E deficiency is extensive, but most lack significant evidence to support its use. Vitamin E has been utilized in the treatment and prevention of cardiovascular disease and cancer; however, its use as a preventative agent in these settings is not recommended. Relating to the skin, vitamin E may be used for aging skin, sunburn, and dermatitis. Though data are lacking, vitamin E has been utilized in the setting of Alzheimer's disease and other dementias, night cramps, restless leg syndrome, fatigue, chronic fatigue syndrome, tardive dyskinesia, neuromuscular disorders, Huntington's disease, chronic progressive hereditary chorea, myotonic dystrophy, prevention of intraventricular hemorrhage in premature neonates, postherpetic neuralgia (use is not supported), retinitis pigmentosa, and as an adjunct in the treatment of epilepsy.

Potential Neurologic or Psychiatric Medication Adverse Effects: Vitamin E may cause fatigue, headache, weakness, blurred vision, emotional disturbances, and may increase the risk of hemorrhagic stroke, though data are conflicting.

Further Reading

Vitamin E. In *Natural Medicines Comprehensive Database*. Stockton, CA: Therapeutic Research Faculty. http://naturaldatabase .therapeuticresearch.com/. Accessed Jan 29, 2016.

Vitamin E. In *AHFS Drug Information STAT!Ref Online Electronic Medical Library*. Bethesda, MD: American Society of Health-System Pharmacists. http://online.statref.com/document .aspx?fxid=1&docid=497. Accessed Dec 15, 2015.

Zinc

Typical Uses: Zinc is most often used as a supplement when taken systemically or as a protectant to promote healing when applied topically to chapped or irritated skin, and is FDA labeled for Wilson's disease. Commonly, zinc is also taken to reduce symptom severity and duration of the common cold and other respiratory infections. Though this practice was supported by a recent Cochrane review, the review was withdrawn in April of 2015 due to potential errors in data analysis. Zinc may improve wound healing in those who are zinc deficient and is commonly found in diaper rash creams. Ophthalmic preparations containing zinc are used as astringents for ocular irritation and angular conjunctivitis. Zinc may shorten the duration of acute diarrhea by approximately 1 day in pediatric patients with a zinc deficiency. In men, zinc has been used in the setting of benign prostatic hyperplasia, male infertility, impotence, and to boost athletic performance. It should be noted that zinc is co-formulated in many lotions, creams, multivitamins, and pharmaceuticals including certain preparations of insulin and total parenteral nutrition.

Potential Neurologic or Psychiatric Medication Adverse Effects: Dizziness, headache, lethargy, fatigue, and neuropathy have all been reported. Intranasal formulations may cause a partial or complete loss of smell that may be permanent. Case reports have linked zinc-containing denture adhesives to sensory disturbances, numbness, tingling, limb weakness, and difficulty walking if the denture adhesive was applied multiple times daily for several years. Fatigue is a potential symptom of metal fume fever, an occupational hazard for those working with or around zinc oxide fumes.

Further Reading

Singh M, Das RR. Zinc for the common cold. *Cochrane Database Syst Rev*. 2013;6:CD001364.

Zinc. In *Micromedex 2.0*. Greenwood Village, CO: Truven Health Analytics, Inc. http:// micromedexsolutions.com. Accessed Jan 29, 2016.

Zinc. In *Natural Medicines Comprehensive Database*. Stockton, CA: Therapeutic Research Faculty. http://naturaldatabase.therapeuticresearch.com/. Accessed Jan 29, 2016.

Medications to Treat Asthma and Allergies

Megan Bauer, PharmD 2500 Overlook Terrace, Madison WI
Christi Ann Albert, PharmD, BCPS UW Health University Hospital

Anticholinergic Bronchodilators

Class Members: aclidinium (Tudorza® Pressair®), ipratropium (Atrovent® HFA), tiotropium (Spiriva® HandiHaler®)

Typical Uses: asthma/bronchospasm, asthma exacerbation, chronic obstructive pulmonary disease (COPD), exercise-induced bronchospasm

Potential Neurologic or Psychiatric Medication Adverse Effects: Common side effects include headache (4–7%), dizziness (<1–3%), and falling (1%). Depression and insomnia have been reported with tiotropium use (≤4%).

Further Reading

Antimuscarinics/antispasmodics. In *AHFS Drug Information STAT!Ref Online Electronic Medical Library*. Bethesda, MD: American Society of Health-System Pharmacists. http://online .statref.com/document.aspx?fxid=1&docid=497. Accessed Jan 16, 2016.

DRUGDEX® System (electronic version). Greenwood Village, CO: Truven Health Analytics, Inc. www .micromedexsolutions.com/. Accessed Jan 16, 2016.

Lexi-Drugs. Lexicomp. Hudson, OH: Wolters Kluwer Health, Inc. http://online.lexi.com. Accessed Jan 16, 2016.

Antihistamines

Class Members: 1st generation antihistamines: chlorpheniramine (ChlorTrimeton®), cyproheptadine (Periactin®), diphenhydramine (Benadryl®, Unisom®), dimenhydrinate (Dramamine®), doxylamine (Unisom®), hydroxyzine (Vistaril®); **2nd generation antihistamines:** loratadine (Claritin®), desloratadine (Clarinex®), cetirizine (Zyrtec®), levocetirizine (Xyzal®), fexofenadine (Allegra®); **topical antihistamines:** azelastine (Astelin®), olopatadine (Patanol®, Pataday®), ketotifen (Zaditor®, Alaway®)

Typical Uses: allergic asthma, allergic conjunctivitis, anaphylaxis adjunct therapy, hypersensitivity reactions, insomnia, motion sickness, parkinsonism, pregnancy-related nausea and vomiting, pruritus, rhinitis, urticaria

Potential Neurologic or Psychiatric Medication Adverse Effects: Systemic neuropsychiatric adverse effects with ophthalmically or nasally applied antihistamines are not common. Adverse effects are more prevalent and profound with 1st generation, in comparison to 2nd generation, antihistamines. The incidence of drowsiness/sedation/somnolence and malaise with 1st generation antihistamines is >10%, whereas it is 1–10% for 2nd generation antihistamines. Of all the antihistamines, diphenhydramine is the most sedating. Headaches are also very common for both 1st and 2nd generation antihistamines. Other common adverse effects (1–10%) include asthenia, disturbed coordination, dizziness, fatigue, impaired reaction time and performance, and lassitude. Young children may commonly, more rarely in adults, experience paradoxical reactions including confusion, excitation, emotional lability, euphoria, hallucinations, hyperactive behavior, insomnia, irritability, nervousness, restlessness, and tremor. Overdosages have been reported that result in psychotic symptoms including agitation, ataxia, confusion, delirium, hallucinations, hysteria, inattentiveness, and restlessness.

Further Reading

Drug Facts and Comparisons. Facts & Comparisons [database online]. St. Louis, MO: Wolters Kluwer Health, Inc; Mar 2005.

Lexi-Drugs. Lexicomp. Hudson, OH: Wolters Kluwer Health, Inc. http://online.lexi.com. Accessed Jan 10, 2016.

Micromedex 2.0. Greenwood Village, CO: Truven Health Analytics, Inc. http://micromedexsolutions .com. Accessed Jan 10, 2016.

Decongestants

Class Members: pseudoephedrine (Sudafed®), phenylephrine (Neo-Synephrine®), oxymetolazine (Afrin®), naphazoline (Naphcon-A®)

Typical Uses: nasal decongestant

Potential Neurologic or Psychiatric Medication Adverse Effects: These agents are sympathomimetics and act as agonists of the sympathetic nervous system. Frequency of adverse effects is not consistently defined. Topical agents (oxymetazoline and naphazoline) can be absorbed systemically and cause headache, nervousness, nausea, dizziness, insomnia, and weakness. Common side effects of systemic agents (pseudoephedrine and phenylephrine) include insomnia, restlessness, tremor, anxiety, hallucinations, seizures, fear, nervousness, excitability, dizziness, weakness, headache, drowsiness, euphoria, dysphoria, and paresthesia. Large doses may cause lightheadedness, nausea, and/or vomiting. Hyperactivity reports range from 6.9% to 12.8%. Geriatric patients may be more sensitive to sympathomimetic agents. A case report of myoclonic jerking and bizarre behavior was reported in a dialysis patient taking 60 mg of pseudoephedrine four times daily. Pseudoephedrine and phenylephrine have been reported to induce mania. They are also contraindicated with monoamine oxidase inhibitor (MAOI) therapy due to risk of hypertensive crisis. Sales of pseudoephedrine are monitored in the United States because it can be used for synthesis of methamphetamine and methcathinone, which have a great potential for abuse and habituation. These medications can yield a false positive on a urine drug screen.

Further Reading

DRUGDEX® System (electronic version). Greenwood Village, CO: Truven Health Analytics, Inc. www .micromedexsolutions.com/. Accessed Jan 16, 2016.

Goodman LS, et al. *Goodman & Gilman's the pharmacological basis of therapeutics.* 12th ed. New York: McGraw-Hill Medical; 2011.

Katzung BG, Masters SB, Trevor AJ. *Basic and clinical pharmacology.* 12th ed. New York, NY: McGraw-Hill Companies Inc.; 2010.

Lexi-Drugs. Lexicomp. Hudson, OH: Wolters Kluwer Health, Inc. http://online.lexi.com. Accessed Jan 16, 2016.

Vasoconstrictors. In *AHFS Drug Information STAT!Ref Online Electronic Medical Library.* Bethesda, MD: American Society of Health-System Pharmacists. http://online.statref.com/document .aspx?fxid=1&docid=497. Accessed Jan 16, 2016.

Leukotriene Antagonists

Class Members: montelukast (Singulair®), zafirlukast (Accolate®)

Typical Uses: allergic rhinitis, asthma, exercise-induced bronchoconstriction; off-label: urticaria

Potential Neurologic or Psychiatric Medication Adverse Effects: The adverse effect profile is similar between montelukast and zafirlukast. A very common adverse effect (>10% incidence) is headache (18% with montelukast and 13% with zafirlukast). Common adverse effects (1–10%) include dizziness and asthenia/fatigue. Concerns for neuropsychiatric events have occurred in the post marketing period and include depression, anxiety, agitation, aggressive behavior, irritability, dream abnormalities, hallucinations, depression, disorientation, insomnia, restlessness, attention and memory impairment, somnambulism, tremor, suicidal ideation and behavior, and prompted the FDA to perform a safety review. This revealed a 0.01% incidence of suicidal ideation, which may be drug-induced. Clinicians should counsel patients to report any of these side effects. Rare reports of peripheral neuropathy have been reported and diagnosed as Churg–Strauss syndrome and is likely explained as an underlying eosinophilic infiltrative disorder prior to initiating a leukotriene antagonist. Post marketing reports of hypoesthesia and seizures have also been reported.

Further Reading

DRUGDEX® System (electronic version). Greenwood Village, CO: Truven Health Analytics, Inc. www .micromedexsolutions.com/. Accessed Jan 16, 2016.

Goodman LS, et al. *Goodman & Gilman's the pharmacological basis of therapeutics.* 12th ed. New York: McGraw-Hill Medical, 2011.

Katzung BG, Masters SB, Trevor AJ. *Basic and clinical pharmacology*. 12th ed. New York, NY: McGraw-Hill Companies Inc.; 2010.

Leukotriene modifiers. In *AHFS Drug Information STAT!Ref Online Electronic Medical Library*. Bethesda, MD: American Society of Health-System Pharmacists. http://online.statref.com/document.aspx?fxid=1&docid=497. Accessed Jan 16, 2016.

Lexi-Drugs. Lexicomp. Hudson, OH: Wolters Kluwer Health, Inc. http://online.lexi.com. Accessed Jan 16, 2016.

Long-Acting Beta Agonists (LABA)

Class Members: arformoterol (Brovana®), formoterol (Foradil® Aerolizer® Inhaler), salmeterol (Serevent® Diskus®)

Typical Uses: asthma/bronchospasm, asthma exacerbation, chronic obstructive pulmonary disease (COPD), exercise-induced bronchospasm

Potential Neurologic or Psychiatric Medication Adverse Effects: Side effects among different long-acting beta agonists are similar, the most common (>10%) being headache and neuromuscular pain. Common adverse effects include dizziness (4%), sleep disturbances, paresthesia, anxiety, and migraine (all ranging from 1% to 3%). Rare side effects (<1%) include restlessness, depression, vertigo, agitation, and aggression. Tremor (1.9–8.6%) and insomnia (1.5–2.4%) have been reported with formoterol. Nonspecific pain (8%), back pain (6%), paralysis and paresthesia (<2%) have been reported with arformoterol.

Further Reading

DRUGDEX® System (electronic version). Greenwood Village, CO: Truven Health Analytics, Inc. www.micromedexsolutions.com/. Accessed Jan 16, 2016.

Lexi-Drugs. Lexicomp. Hudson, OH: Wolters Kluwer Health, Inc. http://online.lexi.com. Accessed Jan 16, 2016.

Selective β2-adrenergic agonists. In *AHFS Drug Information STAT!Ref Online Electronic Medical Library*. Bethesda, MD: American Society of Health-System Pharmacists. http://online.statref.com/document.aspx?fxid=1&docid=497. Accessed Jan 16, 2016.

Methylxanthines

Class Members: theophylline (Theo-24®, Elixophyllin®, Theolair®, Quibron®, Theochron®, Uniphyl®, Unicontin®), aminophylline (Aminophylline DF®)

Typical Uses: asthma/bronchospasm, asthma exacerbation, chronic obstructive pulmonary disease (COPD), exercise-induced bronchospasm

Potential Neurologic or Psychiatric Medication Adverse Effects: Many adverse effects can occur with this drug class at therapeutic doses, but frequencies are not defined. Side effects include headache, insomnia, tremor, irritability, restlessness, seizure. Rapid IV administration of aminophylline may cause dizziness. Theophylline-induced nonconvulsive status epilepticus has been reported and should be considered in patients with CNS abnormalities.

Further Reading

DRUGDEX® System (electronic version). Greenwood Village, CO: Truven Health Analytics, Inc. www.micromedexsolutions.com/. Accessed Jan 16, 2016.

Lexi-Drugs. Lexicomp. Hudson, OH: Wolters Kluwer Health, Inc. http://online.lexi.com. Accessed Jan 16, 2016.

Respiratory smooth muscle relaxants. In *AHFS Drug Information STAT!Ref Online Electronic Medical Library*. Bethesda, MD: American Society of Health-System Pharmacists. http://online.statref.com/document.aspx?fxid=1&docid=497. Accessed Jan 16, 2016.

Short-Acting Beta Agonists (SABA)

Class Members: albuterol (VoSpire® ER, ProAir® HFA, Ventolin® HFA, AccuNeb®), levalbuterol (Xopenex®)

Typical Uses: asthma/bronchospasm, asthma exacerbation, chronic obstructive pulmonary disease (COPD), exercise-induced bronchospasm

Potential Neurologic or Psychiatric Medication Adverse Effects: Agents in this class exhibit characteristics of sympathomimetic agents and their effects are typically dose related. Emotional hypersensitivity has been reported in up to 20% of patients. Common adverse effects include nervousness (7%), tremor and headache (5–7%), dizziness (2–7%), insomnia and weakness (2%).

These medications are often associated with anxiety; however, a specific incidence has not been reported.

Further Reading

Albuterol sulfate, levalbuterol hydrochloride, levalbuterol tartrate. In: *AHFS Drug Information STAT!Ref Online Electronic Medical Library.* Bethesda, MD: American Society of Health-System Pharmacists. http://online.statref.com /document.aspx?fxid=1&docid=497. Accessed Jan 16, 2016.

DRUGDEX® System (electronic version). Greenwood Village, CO: Truven Health Analytics, Inc. www .micromedexsolutions.com/. Accessed Jan 16, 2016.

Lexi-Drugs. Lexicomp. Hudson, OH: Wolters Kluwer Health, Inc. http://online.lexi.com. Accessed Jan 16, 2016.

Antimicrobial Medications

Susanne G. Barnett, PharmD, BCPS University of Wisconsin-Madison School of Pharmacy
Jennifer C. Dela-Pena, PharmD, BCPS Advocate Health Care
Tyler Liebenstein, PharmD, BCPS-AQ ID UW Health University Hospital
Eileen Shannon, PharmD UW Health University Hospital

Aminoglycosides

Class Members: amikacin, gentamicin, tobramycin, streptomycin

Typical Uses: bone and joint infections, respiratory tract infections, endocarditis, intra-abdominal infections, urinary tract infections

Potential Neurologic or Psychiatric Medication Adverse Effects: Aminoglycosides have a black box warning for neurotoxicities, which include ototoxicity, optic nerve dysfunction, peripheral neuritis, arachnoiditis, and encephalopathy. These effects are more pronounced in patients with renal dysfunction, advanced age, and concomitant use of nephrotoxic and neurotoxic agents. Ototoxicity is irreversible and is associated with higher dosing and prolonged therapy. Additionally, aminoglycosides have a black box warning for causing neuromuscular blockade and respiratory paralysis when administered soon after anesthesia or muscle relaxants.

Further Reading

Amikacin. In *Lexi-Drugs. Lexicomp*. Hudson, OH: Wolters Kluwer Health, Inc. http://online.lexi .com. Accessed Dec 7, 2015.
Gentamicin. In *In-Depth Answers*. Ann Arbor, MI: Truven Health Analytics. www .micromedexsolutions.com. Accessed Dec 7, 2015.
Tobramycin package insert. Lake Forest, IL: Hospira, Inc.; 2008.

Amphotericin B – multiple formulations (conventional amphotericin B, AmBisome®, Abelcet®)

Typical Uses: candidiasis, aspergillosis, histoplasmosis, blastomycosis, cryptococcosis

Potential Neurologic or Psychiatric Medication Adverse Effects: Rates of neurologic adverse effects are similar among amphotericin formulations. Very common adverse effects (>10%) include headache. Common adverse effects (1–10%) include anxiety, confusion, insomnia, and paresthesia. All amphotericin formulations are associated with infusion reactions (fever, chills) although these are less frequent with the lipid formulations (AmBisome®, Abelcet®) than conventional amphotericin B.

Further Reading

Abelcet® (amphotericin B) package insert. Gaithersburg, MD: Sigma-Tau Pharmaceuticals, Inc; 2013.
AmBisome® (amphotericin B) package insert. Northbrook, IL: Astellas Pharmac US, Inc; 2012.
Lexicomp Online®. Hudson, OH: Lexi-Comp, Inc. http://online.lexi.com/. Accessed Jan 5, 2016.
Micromedex 2.0. Greenwood Village, CO: Truven Health Analytics, Inc. http:// micromedexsolutions.com. Accessed Jan 5, 2016.

Antivirals

Class Members: acyclovir (Zovirax®, Sitavig®), valacyclovir (Valtrex®), famciclovir (Famvir®), ganciclovir (Cytovene®, Zirgan®), valgancyclovir (Valcyte®)

Typical Uses: treatment of herpes-viruses type 1 (HSV-1), type 2 (HSV-2), varicella-zoster virus (VZV) (acyclovir only), cytomegalovirus (CMV), and HSV (ganciclovir only)

Potential Neurologic or Psychiatric Medication Adverse Effects: Adverse reactions associated with all antiviral medications include headache (very common, >10%), and fatigue, dizziness (common, >1%). Common

(>1%) adverse effects of acyclovir include tremors, myoclonus, extrapyramidal signs, confusion, hallucinations, agitation, autonomic instability, seizure, coma. Rare but serious include aggressive behavior, encephalopathy, and psychosis. Common (>1%) adverse effects of valacyclovir include depression and arthralgia. Rare but serious include seizures, encephalopathy, aggressive behavior, coma, decreased consciousness, mania, psychosis, and aseptic meningitis. A common (>1%) adverse effect of famciclovir use is paresthesia; a rare but serious side effect is hallucinations. Very common (>10%) adverse effects associated with ganciclovir include anorexia, neuropathy, behavioral changes, convulsions, and coma. Rare but serious include abnormal dreams, anxiety, depression, seizures, abnormal thinking, encephalopathy, hallucinations, extrapyramidal reactions, stroke, and intracranial hypertension. Very common (>10%) adverse reactions associated with valganciclovir include insomnia, tremor, peripheral neuropathy, and paresthesia. Common (>1%) include anorexia, behavioral changes, agitation, confusion, depression, hallucinations, psychosis, and seizure. Rare but serious include convulsion and coma.

Further Reading

Acyclovir. In *In-Depth Answers*. Ann Arbor, MI: Truven Health Analytics. www .micromedexsolutions.com. Accessed Nov 5, 2015.

Acyclovir package insert. Greenville, NC: GlaxoSmithKline; 2003.

Aoki FY. Antiviral drugs (other than antiretrovirals). In Mandell GL, Bennett JE, Dolin R, eds. *Mandell, Douglas, and Bennett's principles and practice of infectious diseases*. 7th ed. Philadelphia: Churchill Livingstone Elsevier; 2010. pp. 569–84.

Azole Antifungals

Class Members: fluconazole (Diflucan®), itraconazole (Sporanox®), voriconazole (Vfend®), posaconazole (Noxafil®), isavuconazonium sulfate (Cresemba®)

Typical Uses: candidiasis, histoplasmosis, blastomycosis, aspergillosis, mucormycosis, cryptococcosis, invasive mold prophylaxis

Potential Neurologic or Psychiatric Medication Adverse Effects: Very common adverse effects (>10%) include headache. Common adverse effects (1–10%) include dizziness, fatigue, tremor, somnolence, confusion, insomnia, and peripheral neuropathy. Voriconazole has a unique adverse effect among the azoles of visual disturbances, manifested as altered visual perception, blurred vision, color vision changes, and/or photophobia. These visual disturbances may occur irrespective of voriconazole serum concentration. Voriconazole is also associated with hallucinations and encephalopathy, which are more common with supratherapeutic voriconazole serum concentrations (>5.5 mg/L), as well as concomitant CYP2C19 inhibitors such as omeprazole.

Further Reading

Andes D, Pascual A, Marchetti O. Antifungal therapeutic drug monitoring: established and emerging indications. *Antimicrob Agents Chemother*. 2009;53:24–34.

Cresemba® package insert. Northbrook, IL: Astellas Pharma US, Inc.; 2015.

Diflucan® (fluconazole) package insert. New York, NY: Pfizer Inc.; 2014.

Lexicomp Online®. Hudson, OH: Lexi-Comp, Inc. http://online.lexi.com/. Accessed: Jan 5, 2016.

Micromedex® 2.0 (electronic version). Greenwood Village, CO: Truven Health Analytics, Inc. www .micromedexsolutions.com/. Accessed Jan 5, 2016.

Noxafil® (posaconazole) package insert. Whitehouse Station, NJ: Merck & Co. Inc.; 2014.

Sporanox® (itraconazole) package insert. Titusville, NJ: Janssen Pharmaceuticals, Inc.; 2014.

Vfend® (voriconazole) package insert. New York, NY: Pfizer Inc.; 2015.

Aztreonam (Azactam®, Cayston®)

Typical Uses: gram negative infections, including *Pseudomonas aeruginosa*, generally safe in patients with a history of beta-lactam allergy (exception: ceftazidime)

Potential Neurologic or Psychiatric Medication Adverse Effects: Aztreonem is generally well tolerated. The most frequently encountered adverse events include seizure (<1%) and fever (<1%).

Further Reading

Azactam® (aztreonam) package insert. Princeton, NJ: Bristol-Myers Squibb; 2013.

Aztreonam. In *In-Depth Answers*. Ann Arbor, MI: Truven Health Analytics; 2016. www .micromedexsolutions.com. Accessed Sep 22, 2015.

Chambers HF. Carbapenems and monobactams. In Mandell GL, Bennett JE, Dolin R, eds. *Mandell, Douglas, and Bennett's principles and practice of infectious diseases*. 7th ed. Philadelphia: Churchill Livingstone Elsevier; 2010. pp. 341–5.

Beta-Lactam/Beta-Lactamase Inhibitors

Class Members: amoxicillin/clavulanate (Augmentin®), ampicillin/sulbactam (Unasyn®), ceftazidime/avibactam (Avycaz®), ceftolozane/tazobactam (Zerbaxa®), piperacillin/tazobactam (Zosyn®), ticarcillin/clavulanate (Timentin®)

Typical Uses: amoxicillin/clavulanate, ampicillin/sulbactam: lower respiratory tract infections, oitis media, sinusitis, skin and skin structure infections; **ceftazidime/avibactam, ceftolozane/tazobactam:** complicated urinary tract infections including pyelonephritis, complicated intra-abdominal infections (in combination with metronidazole); **piperacillin/tazobactam, ticarcillin/clavulanate:** intra-abdominal infections, complicated and uncomplicated skin and skin structure infections, bone and joint infections, complicated urinary tract infections including pyelonephritis, endometritis or pelvic inflammatory disease, nosocomial infections including pneumonia, and sepsis

Potential Neurologic or Psychiatric Medication Adverse Effects: In general, the beta-lactam/beta-lactamase inhibitors are well tolerated. Amoxicillin/clavulanate, ampicillin/sulbactam, and ticarcillin/clavulanate do not commonly cause neurologic and psychiatric adverse effects. Ceftazidime/avibactam, however, is very commonly (>10%) associated with anxiety and dizziness. Ceftolozane/tazobactam is commonly (1–10%) associated with headache. Pipercillin/tazobactam has been reported to commonly (1–10%) cause headache, insomnia, dizziness, fever, agitation, pain, and anxiety.

Further Reading

Amoxicillin/clavulanate potassium. In *In-Depth Answers*. Ann Arbor, MI: Truven Health Analytics. www.micromedexsolutions.com. Accessed Oct 12, 2015.

Augmentin® (amoxicillin/clavulanate) package insert. Bridgewater, NJ: Dr. Reddy's Laboratories Inc.; 2013.

Chambers HF. Penicillins and β-lactam inhibitors. In Mandell GL, Bennett JE, Dolin R, eds. *Mandell,*

Douglas, and Bennett's principles and practice of infectious diseases. 7th ed. Philadelphia: Churchill Livingstone Elsevier; 2010. pp. 309–22.

Carbapenems

Class Members: doripenem (Doribax®), ertapenem (Invanz®), imipenem/cilastatin (Primaxin®), meropenem (Merrem®)

Typical Uses: mixed aerobic/anaerobic infections, intra-abdominal infections, infections caused by extended-spectrum beta-lactamase (ESBL)-producing organisms; **doripenem, imipenem/cilastatin, and meropenem (excluding ertapenem):** nosocomial infections including those caused by *Pseudomonas aeruginosa*

Potential Neurologic or Psychiatric Medication Adverse Effects: The adverse effect profile is similar among carbapenem agents. Common adverse effects (1–10%) include headache and nausea. Seizures is a common (1–10%) adverse effect in neonates and infants <3 months of age associated with meropenem and imipenem/cilastatin administration. Altered mental status is a common (1–10%) adverse effect associated with ertapenem. Although rare in adults (<1%), all carbapenems have been associated with seizures, with imipenem having the highest epileptogenic potential. Seizures occur most often in individuals with pre-existing contributing factors (brain lesions, history of seizures or strokes, concomitant administration of medications that decrease the seizure threshold, bacterial meningitis, or decreased renal function). Dose adjustment is recommended in patients with decreased renal function in order to avoid medication accumulation and increased risk of seizures. Co-administration of carbapenems with valproic acid or divalproex sodium will result in decreased valproic acid serum concentrations and a possible increased risk of breakthrough seizures. Alternative antimicrobials should be considered in a patient whose seizures are well controlled on valproic acid or divalproex sodium. Probenecid interferes with active tubular secretion of carbapenems and concomitant administration can result in increased antibiotic concentrations.

Further Reading

Chambers HF. Carbapenems and monobactams. In Mandell GL, Bennett JE, Dolin R, eds. *Mandell, Douglas, and Bennett's principles and practice of infectious diseases*. 7th ed. Philadelphia: Churchill Livingstone Elsevier; 2010. pp. 341–5.

Meropenem. In *In-Depth Answers*. Ann Arbor, MI: Truven Health Analytics. www .micromedexsolutions.com. Accessed Oct 28, 2015.

Merrem® (meropenem) package insert. Wilmington, DE: AstraZeneca Pharmaceuticals LP; 2006.

Cephalosporins

Class Members: first generation: cefazolin (Ancef®, Kefzol®), cephalexin (Keflex®), cephapirin (Cefadyl®), cephradine (Anspor®, Velosef®), cefadroxil (Duricef®); **second generation**: cefaclor (Ceclor®), cefuroxime (Ceftin®, Zinacef®), cefoxitin (Mefoxin®), cefonicid (Monocid®), cefprozil (Cefzil®), cefotetan (Cefotan®); **third generation**: ceftriaxone (Rocephin®), ceftazidime (Fortaz®, Tazicef®), cefpodoxime (Vantin®), ceftibuten (Cedax®), cefditoren (Spectracef®), cefdinir (Omnicef®), cefixime (Suprax®), cefotaxime (Claforan®), cefoperazone (Cefobid®), ceftizoxime (Cefizox®); **fourth generation**: cefepime (Maxipime®); **fifth generation**: ceftaroline (Teflaro®)

Typical Uses: first generation: endocarditis, skin and soft tissue infection, otitis media, streptococcal pharyngitis, respiratory tract infections, urinary tract infections, bone and joint infections; **second generation**: intra-abdominal infections, pelvic inflammatory disease, respiratory tract infections, bone and joint infections, urinary tract infections; **third generation**: acute otitis media, bacteremia secondary to gram-negative species (extended-spectrum beta-lactamase negative), meningitis, endocarditis, skin and soft tissue infections, intra-abdominal infections, Lyme's disease, pelvic inflammatory disease, gonorrhea, urinary tract infections; **fourth generation**: nosocomial infections due to *Pseudomonas aeruginosa*, febrile neutropenia, endocarditis, respiratory tract infections, skin and soft tissue infections, urinary tract infections; **fifth generation**: community-acquired respiratory tract infection, skin and soft tissue infection

Potential Neurologic or Psychiatric Medication Adverse Effects: Seizures (<1%) have been associated with cephalosporins, especially in patients with renal failure. Drug therapy should be discontinued if seizure is suspected secondary to cephalosporin administration and an anticonvulsant may be used if clinically indicated. Common (1–10%) adverse effects include confusion, headache, insomnia, and fever. Ceftriaxone is associated with kernicterus in neonates and should be avoided in this patient population.

Further Reading

Cefazolin. In *Lexi-Drugs. Lexicomp*. Hudson, OH: Wolters Kluwer Health, Inc. http://online.lexi .com. Accessed Dec 7, 2015.

Cefepime. In *In-Depth Answers*. Ann Arbor, MI: Truven Health Analytics. www .micromedexsolutions.com. Accessed Dec 7, 2015.

Rocephin® (ceftriaxone) package insert. South San Francisco, CA: Genentech USA, Inc.; 2015.

Clindamycin (Cleocin®)

Typical Uses: bone and joint infections, lower respiratory tract infections, gynecologic infections, intra-abdominal infections, skin and skin structure infections

Potential Neurologic or Psychiatric Medication Adverse Effects: Clindamycin is not associated with common neurotoxicity and psychiatric adverse events. Although rare, cases of polyarthritis have been reported.

Further Reading

Clindamycin. In *In-Depth Answers*. Ann Arbor, MI: Truven Health Analytics. www .micromedexsolutions.com. Accessed Dec 7, 2015.

Clindamycin. In *Lexi-Drugs. Lexicomp*. Hudson, OH: Wolters Kluwer Health, Inc. http://online.lexi .com. Accessed Dec 7, 2015.

Clindamycin package insert. Lake Forest, IL: Akorn, Inc.; 2012.

Daptomycin (Cubicin®)

Typical Uses: complicated skin and skin structure infections, bacteremia secondary to vascular access and endocarditis, septic arthritis, osteomyelitis, severe infections due to methicillin-resistant *Staphylococcus aureus* and vancomycin-resistant *Enterococcus*

Potential Neurologic or Psychiatric Medication Adverse Effects: Daptomycin is commonly (1–10%) associated with creatinine kinase (CPK) elevation and the development of myopathy, especially in renal failure and with concomitant use of HMG-CoA reductase inhibitors. CPK should be monitored weekly or more frequently if patients are at increased risk of myopathy. Daptomycin should be discontinued if patients develop signs and symptoms of myopathy with CPK greater than 1000 U/L or in asymptomatic patients with CPK greater than 2000 U/L. Other common adverse events include insomnia, dizziness, headache, and anxiety.

Further Reading

Cubicin® (daptomycin) package insert. Lexington, MA: Cubist Pharmaceuticals, Inc.; 2003.

Daptomycin. In *In-Depth Answers*. Ann Arbor, MI: Truven Health Analytics. www .micromedexsolutions.com. Accessed Dec 7, 2015.

Daptomycin. In *Lexi-Drugs. Lexicomp*. Hudson, OH: Wolters Kluwer Health, Inc. http://online.lexi .com. Accessed Dec 7, 2015.

Echinocandins

Class Members: micafungin (Mycamine®), caspofungin (Cancidas®), anidulafungin (Eraxis®)

Typical Uses: candidemia, aspergillosis

Potential Neurologic or Psychiatric Medication Adverse Effects: The adverse effect profile is similar among agents within the echinocandin class. Very common adverse effects (>10%) include headache, insomnia, anxiety, and dizziness. Common adverse effects (1–10%) include fatigue, rigors, depression, confusion, intracranial hemorrhage, delirium, and seizure.

Further Reading

Cancidas® (caspofungin) package insert. Northbrook, IL: Astellas Pharma US, Inc.; 2013.

Eraxis® (anidulafungin) package insert. New York, NY: Pfizer Inc.; 2013.

Lexicomp Online®. Hudson, OH: Lexi-Comp, Inc. http://online.lexi.com/. Accessed: Jan 2, 2016.

Micromedex 2.0. Greenwood Village, CO: Truven Health Analytics, Inc. http:// micromedexsolutions.com. Accessed Jan 2, 2016.

Mycamine® (micafungin) package insert. Whitehouse Station, NJ: Merck & Co, Inc.; 2015.

Ethambutol (Myambutol®)

Typical Uses: tuberculosis, *Mycobacterium avium* infection

Potential Neurologic or Psychiatric Medication Adverse Effects: Common adverse effects (1–10%) include confusion, disorientation, dizziness, hallucinations, mania, headache, and peripheral neuritis. Ethambutol may cause decreases in visual acuity due to optic neuritis. Symptoms may include decreased acuity, scotoma, color blindness, and visual defects. These effects may be related to dose and duration of treatment. Optic neuritis is generally reversible upon discontinuation of ethambutol, although irreversible blindness has been reported. Testing of visual acuity should be performed before initiating ethambutol therapy and periodically during drug administration.

Further Reading

Ethambutol. *Micromedex 2.0*. Greenwood Village, CO: Truven Health Analytics, Inc. http:// micromedexsolutions.com. Accessed Jan 2, 2016.

Ethambutol. *Lexicomp Online®*. Hudson, OH: Lexi-Comp, Inc. http://online.lexi.com/. Accessed Jan 2, 2016.

Myambutol® (ethambutol) package insert. Toronto, Ontario, Canada: Patheon Inc.; 2007.

Fidaxomicin (Dificid®)

Typical uses: *Clostridium difficile* infections

Potential Neurologic or Psychiatric Medication Adverse Effects: Due to minimal systemic absorption, fidaxomicin is not associated with common neurologic or psychiatric adverse effects.

Further Reading

Dificid™ (fidaxomicin) package insert. San Diego, CA: Optimer Pharmaceuticals, Inc.; 2011.

Fidaxomicin. In *In-Depth Answers*. Ann Arbor, MI: Truven Health Analytics. www .micromedexsolutions.com. Accessed Oct 12, 2015.

Fluoroquinolones

Class Members: ciprofloxacin (Cipro®), delafloxacin (Baxdela®), gemifloxacin (Factive®), levofloxacin (Levaquin®), moxifloxacin (Avelox®)

Typical Uses: bone and joint infections, respiratory tract infections, intra-abdominal infections, urinary tract infections, acute bacterial skin and skin structure infections including those caused by methicillin-resistant *Staphylococcus aureus* and *Pseudomonas aeruginosa* (delafloxacin)

Potential Neurologic or Psychiatric Medication Adverse Effects: Fluoroquinolones have black box warnings for tendon rupture and myasthenia gravis. Risk of tendinitis is increased with concomitant use of corticosteroids, advanced age, and in lung, heart and kidney transplant patients. Exacerbation of myasthenia gravis is associated with fluoroquinolones and it is recommended to avoid their use in patients with known history of myasthenia gravis. Common (1–10%) adverse effects include headache ($\leq$4%), dizziness (3%), insomnia (2%), nervousness (<2%), and somnolence (<2%). Other common adverse effects for delafloxacin include nausea. Concomitant use of fluoroquinolones with anticonvulsants (phenytoin), antipsychotics (aripiprazole, clozapine, haloperidol, iloperidone, olanzapine, paliperidone, quetiapine, risperidone, thioridazine), and antidepressants (escitalopram, imipramine, nortriptyline, paroxetine, sertraline, venlafaxine) can increase the risk of QT prolongation and close monitoring is warranted. Delafloxacin does not appear to increase the risk of QT prolongation when used alone or in combination with other QT prolonging medications.

Further Reading

Baxdela® (delafloxacin) package insert. Lincolnshire, IL: Melinta Therapeutics, Inc.; 2017.

Cipro® (ciprofloxacin) package insert. Wayne, NJ: Bayer HealthCare Pharmaceuticals Inc.; 2009.

Levofloxacin. In *In-Depth Answers*. Ann Arbor, MI: Truven Health Analytics. www.micromedexsolutions.com. Accessed Dec 7, 2015.

Moxifloxacin. In *Lexi-Drugs. Lexicomp*. Hudson, OH: Wolters Kluwer Health, Inc. http://online.lexi.com. Accessed Dec 7, 2015.

Fosfomycin (Monurol®)

Typical Uses: treatment of uncomplicated urinary tract infections, specifically those caused by susceptible strains of *Escherichia coli* and *Enterococcus faecalis*

Potential Neurologic or Psychiatric Medication Adverse Effects: A very common (>10%) adverse effect associated with fosfomycin use is headache. Common (>1%) adverse effects include asthenia, dizziness, and pain.

Further Reading

Amsden GW. Tables of Antimicrobial Agent Pharmacology. In Mandell GL, Bennett JE, Dolin R, eds. *Mandell, Douglas, and Bennett's principles and practice of infectious diseases*. 7th ed. Philadelphia: Churchill Livingstone Elsevier; 2010. pp. 706–9.

Fosfomycin. In *In-Depth Answers*. Ann Arbor, MI: Truven Health Analytics. www.micromedexsolutions.com. Accessed Nov 5, 2015.

Fosfomycin tromethamine package insert. Cadempino, Switzerland: Zambon Switzerland Ltd.; 2011.

Glycopeptides

Class Members: dalbavancin (Dalvance®), oritavancin (Orbactiv®), telavancin (Vibativ®), vancomycin (Vancocin®)

Typical Uses: acute bacterial skin and skin structure infections

Potential Neurologic or Psychiatric Medication Adverse Effects: Common (1–10%) adverse effects associated with the glycopeptides class include headache and dizziness. Very common (>10%) adverse effects associated with telavancin include insomnia and psychiatric disturbances. Common (1–10%) oritavancin adverse effects include myalgia and tenosynovitis. Paresthesia and rigors have been reported as common (1–10%) adverse effects associated with dalbavancin. Vancomycin is commonly associated with ototoxicity especially in patients with renal dysfunction, underlying hearing loss, and concomitant use of ototoxic agents such as aminoglycosides. Serum trough monitoring is recommended to minimize vancomycin-induced ototoxicity.

Further Reading

Dalbavancin. In *Lexi-Drugs. Lexicomp*. Hudson, OH: Wolters Kluwer Health, Inc. http://online.lexi.com. Accessed Dec 7, 2015.

Oritavancin. In *In-Depth Answers*. Ann Arbor, MI: Truven Health Analytics. www.micromedexsolutions.com. Accessed Dec 7, 2015.

Vancomycin package insert. Princeton, NJ: Sandoz Inc.; 2015.

Isoniazid (Nydrazid®)

Typical Uses: tuberculosis

Potential Neurologic or Psychiatric Medication Adverse Effects: Very common adverse effects (>10%) include peripheral neuropathy. Peripheral neuropathy is dose-related, occurs most commonly in the malnourished and in those predisposed to neuritis (e.g., alcoholics and diabetics), and is usually preceded by paresthesias of the feet and hands. Concomitant pyridoxine therapy is recommended for those with risk factors for neuropathy. Common adverse effects (1–10%) include convulsions, dizziness, lethargy, memory impairment, and toxic psychosis. Isoniazid carries a black box warning for hepatotoxicity, which in severe cases may present with encephalopathy. The risk of hepatotoxicity is higher in patients concomitantly receiving other anti-tubercular agents associated with hepatotoxicity, such as rifampin and pyrazinamide.

Further Reading

Isoniazid. In *Micromedex 2.0*. Greenwood Village, CO: Truven Health Analytics, Inc. http://micromedexsolutions.com. Accessed Jan 2, 2016.

Isoniazid. In *Lexi-Drugs. Lexicomp*. Hudson, OH: Wolters Kluwer Health, Inc. http://online.lexi.com. Accessed Jan 2, 2016.

Isoniazid package insert. Eatontown, NJ: West-Ward Pharmaceutical Corp.; 2015.

Macrolides

Class Member: azithromycin (Zithromax®), erythromycin (Eryc®, PCE®, Ery-Tab®, E.E.S.®, Eryped®, Pediamycin®, Erythrocin®), clarithromycin (BIaxin®)

Typical Uses: upper and lower respiratory tract infections, *Chlamydial trachomatis*, atypical mycobacterial infections, traveler's diarrhea (azithromycin)

Potential Neurologic or Psychiatric Medication Adverse Effects: Macrolides have few associated neurologic or psychiatric adverse effects. Common (1–10%) azithromycin adverse effects include dizziness and headache. Common (1–10%) clarithromycin adverse effects include headache, insomnia, and vertigo. Few neurologic or psychiatric adverse effects have been reported for erythromycin. Caution should be used when administering macrolides with other medications known to prolong the QT interval (examples include amitriptyline, escitalopram, and trazodone) due to a potential for additive QT interval effects and increased risk of serious cardiovascular adverse effects. Consideration of QT interval monitoring may be clinically warranted.

Further Reading

Azithromycin. In *In-Depth Answers*. Ann Arbor, MI: Truven Health Analytics. www.micromedexsolutions.com. Accessed Oct 28, 2015.

Sivapalasingam S, Steigbigel NH. Macrolides, clindamycin, and ketolides. In Mandell GL, Bennett JE, Dolin R, eds. *Mandell, Douglas, and Bennett's principles and practice of infectious diseases*. 7th ed. Philadelphia: Churchill Livingstone Elsevier; 2010. pp. 427–48.

Zithromaz® (azithromycin) package insert. New York, NY: Pfizer Labs; 2013.

Metronidazole (Flagyl®)

Typical Uses: treatment or prevention of infections caused by anaerobic bacteria, treatment of parasitic infections

Potential Neurologic or Psychiatric Medication Adverse Effects: A very common (>10%) adverse effect associated with metronidazole use is headache. Dizziness is a common (>1%) adverse effect. The following neurologic side effects are rare but serious: central nervous system (CNS) lesions seen on MRI (reversible), aseptic meningitis, cerebellar toxicity, encephalopathy, seizure, depression, psychosis, and behavior changes.

CNS adverse effects are generally reversible within days to weeks upon discontinuation of metronidazole. Metronidazole should be used with caution in patients with a history of seizure or other central nervous system disorders. Dose-related, reversible peripheral neuropathy is another rare but significant neurologic side effect. Peripheral neuropathy occurs when high doses are used for long periods (e.g., patients taking 1.5 grams daily or more for >30 days). Plasma levels of lithium may be increased with concomitant metronidazole use and plasma lithium concentrations, serum creatinine, and serum electrolytes should be monitored. Phenytoin may cause increased elimination of metronidazole resulting in reduced plasma levels and possible reduced effectiveness of the antibiotic. Alcoholic beverages and drugs containing alcohol should be avoided during therapy and for at least 1 day after the last dose of metronidazole due to the possibility of a disulfiram-like reaction (flushing, vomiting, and tachycardia). Use of oral metronidazole has been associated with psychotic reactions in alcoholic patients concurrently using disulfiram. Avoid metronidazole use in patients who have taken disulfiram in the last 2 weeks.

Further Reading

Metronidazole. In *In-Depth Answers*. Ann Arbor, MI: Truven Health Analytics. www .micromedexsolutions.com. Accessed Nov 5, 2015.

Metronidazole package insert. New York (NY): Pfizer Labs., 2015.

Salvatore M. Metronidazole. In Mandell GL, Bennett JE, Dolin R, eds. *Mandell, Douglas, and Bennett's principles and practice of infectious diseases.* 7th ed. Philadelphia: Churchill Livingstone Elsevier; 2010. pp. 419–26.

Neuraminidase Inhibitors

Class Members: oseltamivir (Tamiflu®), zanamivir (Relenza®)

Typical Uses: influenza (Type A and B) prophylaxis and treatment

Potential Neurologic or Psychiatric Medication Adverse Effects: Common adverse effects (1–10%) associated with zanamivir therapy are arthralgia, rheumatic arthritis, dizziness, and fever. Rare adverse effects for the neuraminidase inhibitor class from post-marketing surveillance reports include agitation, confusion, anxiety, delirium, hallucinations, and seizures.

Further Reading

Oseltamivir. In *In-Depth Answers*. Ann Arbor, MI: Truven Health Analytics. www .micromedexsolutions.com. Accessed Dec 7, 2015.

Tamiflu® (oseltamivir) package insert. South San Francisco, CA: Genentech, Inc.; 2014.

Zanamivir. In *Lexi-Drugs. Lexicomp*. Hudson, OH: Wolters Kluwer Health, Inc. http://online.lexi .com. Accessed Dec 7, 2015.

Nitrofurantoin (Furadantin®, Macrobid®, Macrodantin®)

Typical Uses: treatment and prophylaxis of uncomplicated cystitis in patients with adequate renal function

Potential Neurologic or Psychiatric Medication Adverse Effects: Although rare (<1%), peripheral neuropathies associated with numbness, weakness, paresthesias, dysesthesia, and muscular atrophy have been reported. Neuropathies may be severe and/or irreversible. Increased risk occurs with impaired renal function, high-dose therapy, anemia, diabetes, electrolyte imbalances, vitamin B deficiency, and/or debilitating diseases. Concomitant administration of uricosuric drugs, such as probenecid, can inhibit renal tubular secretion resulting in increased serum levels, increased toxicities, and decreased efficacy.

Further Reading

Hooper DC. Urinary tract agents: nitrofurantoin and methenamine. In Mandell GL, Bennett JE, Dolin R, eds. *Mandell, Douglas, and Bennett's principles and practice of infectious diseases.* 7th ed. Philadelphia: Churchill Livingstone Elsevier; 2010. pp. 515–20.

Macrobid® (nitrofurantoin) package insert. North Norwich, NY: Norwich Pharmaceuticals, Inc.; 2009.

Nitrofurantoin. In *In-Depth Answers*. Ann Arbor, MI: Truven Health Analytics. www .micromedexsolutions.com. Accessed Sep 22, 2015.

Oxazolidinones

Class Members: linezolid (Zyvox®), tedizolid (Sivextro®)

Typical Uses: skin and skin structure infections, pneumonia, meningitis, osteomyelitis, vancomycin-resistant *Enterococcus faecium* infections

Potential Neurologic or Psychiatric Medication Adverse Effects: The adverse effect profile is similar among agents within the oxazolidinone class. Common adverse effects (1–10%) include headache, dizziness, facial paralysis, hypoesthesia, insomnia, and paresthesia. Linezolid is a weak monoamine oxidase inhibitor (MAOI). Caution should be exercised in patients taking medications with serotonergic properties (e.g., many antidepressants) due to the risk of serotonin syndrome. Linezolid is contraindicated in patients taking other MAOIs or within 2 weeks of taking an MAOI. Tedizolid does not carry this same warning because it is not an MAOI. In rare cases, linezolid has been associated with peripheral and optic neuropathy (<2%). This has primarily been reported in patients treated for longer than 28 days. Tedizolid has also been associated with peripheral and optic neuropathy in clinical trials. However, tedizolid has only been studied for 6 days' duration and no data are available beyond 6 days.

Further Reading

Lexicomp Online®. Hudson, OH: Lexi-Comp, Inc. http://online.lexi.com/. Accessed Jan 5, 2016.

Micromedex 2.0. Greenwood Village, CO: Truven Health Analytics, Inc. http:// micromedexsolutions.com. Accessed Jan 5, 2016.

Sivextro® (tedizolid) package insert. Whitehouse Station, NJ: Merck & Co., Inc.; 2015.

Zyvox® (linezolid) package insert. New York, NY: Pfizer Inc.; 2015.

Penicillins

Class Members: natural: penicillin G (Bicillin®, Permapen®, Pfizerpen®), penicillin V; **aminopenicillins:** amoxicillin (Amoxil ®, Larotid ®, Moxatag ®), ampicillin; **antistaphylococcal:** dicloxacillin, nafcillin, oxacillin

Typical Uses: natural: *Streptococcus pyogenes* (strep throat), *Treponema pallidum* (syphilis and neurosyphilis); **aminopencillins:** *Streptococcus pyogenes* (strep throat), otitis media; **antistaphylococcal:** methicillin-susceptible staphylococcal infections including skin and skin structure and wound infections, cellulitis, osteomyelitis, and pneumonia; penicillin-susceptible streptococci strains including *Streptococcus pneumoniae*

Potential Neurologic or Psychiatric Medication Adverse Effects: All penicillins are associated with rash, hypersensitivity reactions, and anaphylaxis. Although rare (<1%), agitation, anxiety, confusion, dizziness, headache, insomnia, and seizures have been reported. Neurotoxicity, including seizures, is associated with administration of high doses and in patients with renal dysfunction. Caution should be used when administering penicillins with other medications that substantially decrease the seizure threshold (e.g., bupropion). Phenytoin levels should be monitored closely in patients concomitantly receiving dicloxacillin (an antistaphylococcal penicillin) as co-administration may lead to a reduction in phenytoin levels. Theoretical drug interactions exist between nafcillin (an antistaphylococcal penicillin) and clozapine, mirtazapine, and selegiline, which may result in decreased neurologic/psychiatric medication exposure and efficacy.

Further Reading

Chambers HF. Penicillins and beta-lactam inhibitors. In Mandell GL, Bennett JE, Dolin R, eds. *Mandell, Douglas, and Bennett's principles and practice of infectious diseases.* 7th ed. Philadelphia: Churchill Livingstone Elsevier; 2010. pp. 309–22.

Penicillin. In *In-Depth Answers*. Ann Arbor, MI: Truven Health Analytics. www .micromedexsolutions.com. Accessed Oct 12, 2015.

Penicillin G Sodium package insert. Kundl, Austria: Teva Pharmaceutical Industries Ltd.; 2008.

Pyrazinamide

Typical Uses: tuberculosis

Potential Neurologic or Psychiatric Medication Adverse Effects: Common adverse effects (1–10%) include fever, photosensitivity, and porphyria. Pyrazinamide may cause hepatotoxicity, which in severe cases may present with encephalopathy. The risk of hepatotoxicity is higher in patients concomitantly receiving other antitubercular agents associated with hepatotoxicity, such as rifampin and isoniazid. Pyrazinamide is also associated with arthralgia, which is most commonly due to hyperuricemia, rather than neurologic causes. Serum uric acid levels typically return to normal upon cessation of pyrazinamide.

Further Reading

Pyrazinamide. In: *Micromedex 2.0.* Greenwood Village, CO: Truven Health Analytics, Inc. http:// micromedexsolutions.com. Accessed Jan 2, 2016.

Pyrazinamide. In *Lexicomp Online®*. Hudson, OH: Lexi-Comp, Inc. http://online.lexi.com/. Accessed Jan 2, 2016.

Pyrazinamide package insert. Atlanta, GA: Mikart, Inc.; 2012.

Rifampin (Rifadin®)

Typical Uses: tuberculosis, prosthetic joint infections

Potential Neurologic or Psychiatric Medication Adverse Effects: Common adverse effects (1–10%) include headache, confusion, dizziness, somnolence, visual changes, behavioral changes, and psychosis. Rifampin is associated with hepatotoxicity, which in severe cases may present with encephalopathy.

The risk of hepatotoxicity is higher in patients concomitantly receiving other anti-tubercular agents associated with hepatotoxicity, such as isoniazid and pyrazinamide.

Further Reading

Rifampin. In *Micromedex 2.0*. Greenwood Village, CO: Truven Health Analytics, Inc. http://micromedexsolutions.com. Accessed Jan 2, 2016.

Rifampin. In *Lexicomp Online*®. Hudson, OH: Lexi-Comp, Inc. http://online.lexi.com/. Accessed Jan 2, 2016.

Rifadin® (rifampin) package insert. Bridgewater, NJ: Sanofi-aventis US LLC; 2013.

Sulfamethoxazole–Trimethoprim (Bactrim®, Septra®)

Typical Uses: urinary tract infections, skin and skin structure infections, pneumocystis pneumonia

Potential Neurologic or Psychiatric Medication Adverse Effects: Common adverse effects (1–10%) include headache, fatigue, insomnia, peripheral neuritis, and aseptic meningitis.

Further Reading

Bactrim® (sulfamethoxazole-trimethoprim) package insert. Philadelphia, PA: AR Scientific; 2005.

Sulfamethoxazole-trimethoprim. In *Micromedex 2.0*. Greenwood Village, CO: Truven Health Analytics, Inc. http://micromedexsolutions.com. Accessed Jan 5, 2016.

Sulfamethoxazole-trimethoprim. In *Lexicomp Online*®. Hudson, OH: Lexi-Comp, Inc. http://online.lexi.com/. Accessed Jan 5, 2016.

Tetracyclines

Class Members: tetracycline (Doryx®, Oracea®, Achromycin®, Sumycin®), minocycline (Minocin®, Solodyn®, Arestin®, Dynacin®), doxycycline (Monodox®, Oracea®, Vibramycin®, Atridox®, Doryx®, Doxteric®, Aticlate®)

Typical Uses: susceptible respiratory infections, atypical organisms, *Rickettsia*, spirochetes (including *Helicobacter pylori*), and *Plasmodium* species

Potential Neurologic or Psychiatric Medication Adverse Effects: Two rare but serious adverse effects associated with the use of all three tetracycline agents are intracranial hypertension (known as IH or pseudotumor cerebri) and bulging fontanelle (in infants). Symptoms of IH include severe headache, blurred vision, diplopia, and vision loss. Women of childbearing age who are overweight or have a history of IH are at a greater risk for developing tetracycline-associated IH. Risk of IH increases with concomitant use of tetracyclines with isotretinoin. Tetracycline common (>1%) adverse effects include headache, dizziness, and blurry vision. Rare but serious side effects include neuromuscular blockade and neuritis (with topical formulation). Tetracycline is renally cleared; use with caution in patients with renal dysfunction. A minocycline-associated very common (>10%) adverse effect is headache. Common (>1%) adverse effects of minocycline use include malaise, fatigue, and drowsiness. Vertigo is a common side effect unique to minocycline. Vertigo typically begins on the second or third day of therapy and has been reported more frequently in women than in men. Concomitant use of ergot alkaloids and minocycline increases risk of ergotism. Doxycycline common (>1%) adverse effects include headache, anxiety, and insomnia. Chronic ethanol ingestion, carbamazepine, phenytoin, and barbiturates decrease the half-life of doxycycline and worsen side effects.

Further Reading

Doxycycline. In *In-Depth Answers*. Ann Arbor, MI: Truven Health Analytics. www.micromedexsolutions.com. Accessed Nov 5, 2015.

Doxycycline package insert. Salisbury South, South Australia: FH Faulding & Co. Ltd.; 2005.

Salvatore M. Tetracyclines and chloramphenicol. In Mandell GL, Bennett JE, Dolin R, eds. *Mandell, Douglas, and Bennett's principles and practice of infectious diseases*. 7th ed. Philadelphia: Churchill Livingstone Elsevier; 2010. pp. 385–94.

Antiretroviral Medications

Anthony T. Podany, PharmD Antiviral Pharmacology Laboratory, University of Nebraska Medical Center
Caroline Jamison, PharmD Antiviral Pharmacology Laboratory, University of Nebraska Medical Center
Uriel Sandkovsky, MD MS, FIDSA North Infectious Diseases Consultants

Entry Inhibitors (Chemokine Receptor Inhibitors and Fusion Inhibitors)

Class Members: enfuvirtide (Fuzeon®), maraviroc (Selzentry®)

Typical Uses: HIV treatment (experienced patients)

Potential Neurologic or Psychiatric Medication Adverse Effects: Enfuvirtide and maraviroc do not exhibit a large degree of neuropsychiatric adverse effects. In phase III clinical trials peripheral neuropathy was associated with enfuvirtide use (RR 1.2 versus placebo). Maraviroc use is associated with dizziness (8.2%) as well as disturbances in initiating and maintaining sleep (7%). Depressive symptoms were reported in 3.5% of patients randomized to receive maraviroc treatment in phase III clinical trials.

Further Reading

Abers MS, Shandera WX, Kass JS. Neurological and psychiatric adverse effects of antiretroviral drugs. *CNS Drugs.* 2014;28:131–45.

Integrase Strand Transfer Inhibitors

Class Members: raltegravir (Isentress®), elvitegravir (Vitekta®), dolutegravir (Tivicay®), fixed dose combination products (Stribild®, Genvoya®, Triumeq®)

Typical Uses: HIV; HIV post-exposure prophylaxis

Potential Neurologic or Psychiatric Adverse Effects: The integrase strand transfer inhibitor class of antiretroviral agents seldom cause neuropsychiatric manifestations on their own. However, agents in this class are often, if not always, given in combination with other antiretroviral drugs, often as a fixed dose combination (FDC) tablet. The FDC products contain nucleoside reverse transcriptase inhibitors, which have been associated with a mild to moderate amount of neuropsychiatric adverse effects. Adverse effects of the nucleoside reverse transcriptase inhibitors are covered in a separate monograph within this chapter. Large phase III clinical trails have demonstrated a low risk for neuropsychiatric adverse effects with raltegravir dosed at 400 mg twice daily in adults. Reported adverse events included headache (4%), dizziness (2%), and insomnia (4%). A recent meta-analysis of raltegravir use reported similar rates, with the addition of vertigo (3%) and abnormal dreams (2.5%), as well as depression and suicidality (up to 2.5%). Clinical trials involving the use of elvitegravir (in combination with two nucleoside reverse transcriptase inhibitors) in over 350 patients have reported a 4% rate of nausea and 3% rate of headache. Of note, elvitegravir is concomitantly dosed with a pharmacokinetic booster (typically cobicistat) in the treatment of HIV. Pharmacokinetic boosters are potent inhibitors of cytochrome P450 enzymes and may greatly increase plasma drug concentrations of other concomitantly administered medications. Numerous case reports have been published detailing off target inhibition of metabolism of concomitantly dosed drugs, leading to increased adverse effects associated with these drugs. Dolutegravir use has been associated with minimal rates of neuropsychiatric adverse effects. In clinical trials of dolutegravir (in combination with two nucleoside reverse transcriptase inhibitors) insomnia (3–7%), depression (1%), abnormal dreams (<1%), dizziness (<1%), and headache (2%) have all been reported.

Further Reading

Rockstroh JK, DeJesus E, Lennox JL, et al. Durable efficacy and safety of raltegravir versus efavirenz when combined with tenofovir/emtricitabine in treatment-naive HIV-1–infected patients: final 5-year results from STARTMRK. *J Acquir Immune Defic Syndr.* 2013;63:77–85.

Teppler H, Brown DD, Leavitt RY, et al. Long-term safety from the raltegravir clinical development program. *Curr HIV Res.* 2011;9:40–53.

Non-Nucleotide Reverse Transcriptase Inhibitors (NNRTIs)

Class Members: efavirenz (Sustiva®), nevirapine (Viramune®), etravirine (Intelence®), delavirdine (Rescriptor®), rilpivirine (Edurant®), fixed dose combination products (Atripla®, Complera®)

Typical Uses: HIV; HIV post-exposure prophylaxis

Potential Neurologic or Psychiatric Medication Adverse Effects: Common class adverse effects include headache, fatigue, dizziness, and anxiety, with incidence ranging from 1% to 20%, depending on the medication. Depression has been reported with efavirenz (≤19%), delavirdine (10–15%), rilpivirine (5–9%), and nevirapine (3%). Neuropsychiatric events are very common with efavirenz use, in up to 68% of patients, and often lead to treatment interruption or discontinuation. Dizziness, lightheadedness, sleep disturbances, vivid dreams, nervousness, and irritability can be seen within the first month of efavirenz therapy and usually resolve within 6–8 weeks. Several reports have described headache, decreased concentration, and mood changes months to years after efavirenz therapy initiation. Efavirenz may worsen neurocognitive impairment and has been associated with less improvement in HIV-associated neurocognitive impairment than other antiretrovirals. In a study of over 3000 patients on efavirenz-based antiretroviral therapy, initial treatment with an efavirenz-based HIV regimen was associated with a 2-fold increase in suicidality compared with patients receiving non-efavirenz-based HIV therapy. Case reports have described similar neuropsychiatric adverse effects with nevirapine use, including visual hallucinations, persecutory delusions, mood changes, nightmares, and vivid dreams, although to a lesser extent than efavirenz. Abnormal dreams, nightmares, and insomnia were reported in clinical trials associated with rilpivirine use.

Further Reading

Abers MS, Shandera WX, Kass JS. Neurological and psychiatric adverse effects of antiretroviral drugs. *CNS Drugs.* 2014;28:131–45.

Mollan KR, Smurzynski M, Eron JJ, et al. Association between efavirenz as initial therapy for HIV-1 infection and increased risk for suicidal ideation or attempted or completed suicide: an analysis of trial data. *Ann Intern Med.* 2014;161:1–10.

Nucleoside Reverse Transcriptase Inhibitors (NRTIs)

Class Members: abacavir (Ziagen®), tenofovir (Viread®), emtricitabine (Emtriva®), lamivudine (Epivir®), stavudine (Zerit®), zidovudine (Retrovir®), didanosine (Videx®) *Note: These drugs are often in fixed dose combination products with different trade names*

Typical Uses: HIV; HIV post-exposure prophylaxis; tenofovir/emtricitabine (Truvada) is also approved for pre-exposure prophylaxis for prevention of HIV infection in uninfected high-risk individuals

Potential Neurologic or Psychiatric Medication Adverse Effects: The most common class adverse effect of nucleoside reverse transcriptase inhibitors (NRTIs) is headache, with incidence of greater than 10% for all medications with the exception of didanosine; zidovudine and stavudine reported incidence greater than 40%. Other neuropsychiatric side effects associated with several NRTIs include depression, anxiety, insomnia, dizziness, fatigue, and weakness, with incidence varying greatly among medications and adverse reactions (<1% to >20%). Peripheral neuropathy is also common, particularly with stavudine (15–30%) and didanosine (15–25%). Neuropathy is also seen with tenofovir (1–5%), emtricitabine (4%), zidovudine (≥5%), and lamivudine (<1%). Compared with HIV-induced peripheral neuropathy, NRTI-induced neuropathy tends to present more abruptly and will resolve with therapy discontinuation. NRTI-induced neuropathy typically occurs within the first 3 months of therapy initiation and is described as distal and symmetric, with the lower extremities typically involved first. There have been multiple case reports of headache, paresthesias, confusion, irritability, and insomnia in patients who switched from lamivudine- to emtricitabine-based therapy. Depression, nightmares, hallucinations, mood changes, mania, anxiety, and psychosis have been reported with abacavir use. Hearing loss associated with NRTI use has been reported in the literature. Case reports and post-marketing data report several neuropsychiatric adverse effects with zidovudine, including confusion, loss of mental acuity, mania, paresthesia, photophobia, seizures, somnolence, syncope, taste perversion, and tremor. Several case reports have linked NRTI therapy with the unmasking of Leber's hereditary optic neuropathy in patients with a genetic predisposition to the disease.

Further Reading

Abers MS, Shandera WX, Kass JS. Neurological and psychiatric adverse effects of antiretroviral drugs. *CNS Drugs*. 2014;28:131–45.

Protease Inhibitors

Class Members: darunavir (Prezista®), ritonavir (Norvir®), lopinavir, atazanavir (Reyataz ®), fixed dose combination products (Prezcobix®, Kaletra®, Evotaz®); **older non-widely used agents:** amprenavir, indinavir, tipranavir (Aptivus®), fosamprenavir (Lexiva®), nelfinavir (Viracept ®)

Typical Uses: HIV; HIV post-exposure prophylaxis

Potential Neurologic or Psychiatric Medication Adverse Effects: Protease inhibitors may cause central nervous system (CNS) toxicity on their own as well as potentiate the neurotoxicity of other antiretroviral agents. Metabolic abnormalities and atherogenesis are both class effects of protease inhibitors. With long-term use of protease inhibitors patients may be at an increased risk for stroke and other cardiovascular adverse effects. Protease inhibitors as a class strongly inhibit cytochrome P450 activity; by doing so, protease inhibitors have the ability to potentiate the metabolism of concomitantly used medications that undergo cytochrome P450 metabolism. Clinicians must carefully evaluate the effect of concomitant protease inhibitor therapy in individuals receiving medications in addition to antiretrovirals. The newest member of the protease inhibitor class, darunavir, appears to be associated with the lowest occurrence of neuropsychiatric adverse effects among the class. In clinical trials evaluating darunavir efficacy in HIV treatment naïve individuals, headaches (7%) and abnormal dreams (<2%) were both reported. In evaluation of darunavir in HIV treatment experienced adults, rates of headache associated with darunavir use dropped to 3%. Ritonavir, a protease inhibitor strictly used as a pharmacokinetic boosting agent, is one of the biggest culprits of CNS adverse effects within the class. Ritonavir neuropsychiatric effects typically occur early in treatment (within first month) and include such things as circumoral paresthesias (25%), peripheral paresthesias (7%), and taste alterations (12%). CNS adverse effects of ritonavir appear to occur less often at the lower pharmacokinetic boosting dose than when ritonavir was used at a higher dose in treatment of HIV; nonetheless its adverse effects may still present when used as part of a multidrug regimen for HIV. Adverse effects related to ritonavir typically resolve completely upon discontinuation of use. Tipranavir, an older protease inhibitor not widely used in current practice, carries a black box warning for increased risk of intracranial hemorrhage.

Further Reading

Abers MS, Shandera WX, Kass JS. Neurological and psychiatric adverse effects of antiretroviral drugs. *CNS Drugs*. 2014;28:131–45.

Immunosuppressive Medications

Heather J. Johnson, PharmD, BCPS University of Pittsburgh School of Pharmacy

Alemtuzumab (Campath®, Lemtrada®)

Typical Uses: prevention or treatment of solid organ transplant rejection, B-cell chronic lymphocytic leukemia, relapsing–remitting multiple sclerosis

Potential Neurologic or Psychiatric Medication Adverse Effects: Very common adverse effects (>10%) include anxiety, headache, insomnia, and fatigue. Common adverse effects (1–10%) include anxiety, asthenia, somnolence, and paresthesias. Rare adverse effects (<1%) include depression, memory impairment, migraine, suicidal ideation. Progressive multifocal leukoencephalopathy (PML) is a rare adverse event related to the immunosuppressive activity of alemtuzumab. It is characterized by apathy, ataxia, cognitive deficiency, confusion, and hemiparesis.

Further Reading

Campath® (alemtuzumab) package insert. Cambridge, MA: Genzyme Corporation; 2009.
Lemtrada® (alemtuzumab) package insert. Cambridge, MA: Genzyme Corporation; 2014.

Antithymocyte Globulin

Class Members: antithymocyte globulin (rabbit) (rATG) (Thymoglobulin®), antithymocyte globulin (equine) (eATG) (ATGAM®)

Typical Uses: treatment of acute allograft rejection (kidney, heart, liver), prevention of acute allograft rejection

Potential Neurologic or Psychiatric Medication Adverse Effects: Very common adverse effects (>10%) include asthenia, headache, and malaise. Common adverse effects include dizziness.

Further Reading

Micromedex 2.0. Greenwood Village, CO: Truven Health Analytics, Inc. http://micromedexsolutions.com. Accessed Jan 15, 2016.

Azathioprine (Imuran®)

Typical Uses: prevention of solid organ transplant rejection, treatment of rheumatoid arthritis, Crohn's disease, dermatomyositis, chronic refractory immune thrombocytopenia, ulcerative colitis, autoimmune hepatitis

Potential Neurologic or Psychiatric Medication Adverse Effects: Neurologic or psychiatric adverse effects have not been reported with azathioprine. However, like any long-term immunosuppressive agent, azathioprine has been associated with rare cases of progressive multifocal leukoencephalopathy (PML), a rare adverse event characterized by apathy, ataxia, cognitive deficiency, confusion, and hemiparesis.

Further Reading

Azathioprine. In *Micromedex 2.0.* Greenwood Village, CO: Truven Health Analytics, Inc. http://micromedexsolutions.com. Accessed Jan 15, 2016.

Basiliximab (Simulect®)

Typical Uses: prevention of acute allograft rejection (heart, kidney, liver transplantation), treatment of refractory acute graft-versus-host disease

Potential Neurologic or Psychiatric Medication Adverse Effects: Very common adverse effects (>10%) include headache, tremor, and insomnia. Common adverse effects (1–10%) include agitation, anxiety, depression, dizziness, fatigue, hypoesthesia, and malaise. It should be noted that these adverse effects were similar in patients receiving placebo and that all patients received a calcineurin inhibitor and corticosteroid sometimes in combination with azathioprine or mycophenolate mofetil.

Further Reading

Simulect® (basiliximab) package insert. East Hanover, NJ: Novartis Pharmaceuticals Corporation; 2016.

Calcineurin Inhibitors

Class Members: cyclosporine (Sandimmun®, Neoral®, Gengraf®), tacrolimus (Prograf®, Astagraf®, Envarsus®)

Typical Uses: prevention of allograft rejection, treatment of psoriasis, rheumatoid arthritis, prevention of acute graft-versus-host disease, treatment of focal segmental glomerulosclerosis, interstitial cystitis, nephrotic syndrome, lupus nephritis, ulcerative colitis

Potential Neurologic or Psychiatric Medication Adverse Effects: Very common adverse effects (>10%) include headache, tremors, and paresthesias. While these occur with both cyclosporine and tacrolimus, the frequency is higher with tacrolimus. Common adverse effects (1–10%) include seizures, dizziness, depression, insomnia, nervousness, anxiety, confusion, neuropathy, malaise, paranoia, and migraine. Rare adverse events: abnormal dreams, amnesia, flaccid paralysis, nightmares, quadriparesis, impaired writing, neuralgia, and mutism. A rare, but serious manifestation of calcineurin neurotoxicity is PRES (posterior reversible encephalopathy syndrome), which can occur any time after transplantation, but often presents in the first months. Calcineurin inhibitor blood levels do not necessarily correlate with the development of PRES, but are often elevated. Hypertension, hypomagnesemia, hypocholesterolemia, and concomitant steroids have been implicated as risk factors. Clinical symptoms of PRES include seizures, acute encephalopathy, headache, and visual disturbances. Both cyclosporine and tacrolimus are medications with a narrow therapeutic range, and elevated concentrations may result in increased likelihood of adverse effects. Both are subject to numerous drug–drug interactions that may precipitate increased exposure. As substrates of cytochrome P450, increased calcineurin inhibitor concentrations may result with concomitant administration of azole antifungals, macrolide antibiotics, as well as non-dihydropyridine calcium channel blockers. Additionally, the proliferation signal inhibitors sirolimus and everolimus also compete for the same metabolizing enzymes and concentrations of both may increase.

Further Reading

Chen S, Hu J, Xu L et al. Posterior reversible encephalopathy syndrome after transplantation: a review. *Mol Neurobiol.* 2016;53:6897–9.

Heinrich TW, Marcangelo M. Psychiatric issues in solid organ transplantation. *Har Rev Psychiatry.* 2009;17:398–406.

Micromedex 2.0. Greenwood Village, CO: Truven Health Analytics, Inc. http://micromedexsolutions.com. Accessed Jan 15, 2016.

Corticosteroids

Class Members: prednisone (Deltasone®), methylprednisolone (Solu-Medrol®)

Typical Uses: allergic states, dermatologic diseases, endocrine disorders, gastrointestinal diseases, hematologic disorders, neoplastic diseases, nervous system, ophthalmic diseases, renal diseases, respiratory diseases, rheumatic disorders

Potential Neurologic or Psychiatric Medication Adverse Effects: Reported adverse effects include dementia, extrapyramidal symptoms, meningitis, neuropathy, paralytic syndrome, pseudotumor cerebri, seizures, mood disturbances, psychosis, acute myopathy, depression, euphoria, insomnia, mood swings, personality changes, emotional instability, headache, psychic derangements, seizure, and vertigo. The frequency with which these occur is not classified. Psychosis and mood disturbances may be more prevalent with high doses even of short duration, whereas other adverse effects may develop over long-term use of corticosteroids.

Further Reading

Micromedex 2.0. Greenwood Village, CO: Truven Health Analytics, Inc. http://micromedexsolutions.com. Accessed Jan 15, 2016.

Mycophenolic Acid Derivatives

Class Members: mycophenolate mofetil (CellCept®), mycophenolate sodium (Myfortic®)

Typical Uses: prevention of organ transplant rejection, treatment of autoimmune hepatitis, lupus nephritis, myasthenia gravis, and psoriasis

Potential Neurologic or Psychiatric Medication Adverse Effects: Very common adverse effects (>10%) include asthenia, headache, tremor, insomnia, dizziness, anxiety, and paresthesias. Common side effects (1–10%) include agitation, confusion, delirium, depression, emotional lability, hallucinations, malaise, nervousness, psychosis, seizure, somnolence, and abnormal thinking. It is important to keep in mind that the above-mentioned adverse effects were reported with mycophenolic acid derivatives administered against a background of other immunosuppressive medications including corticosteroids and calcineurin inhibitors. The rates of these adverse effects were not different between the mycophenolate and azathioprine arms. Very rarely progressive multifocal leukoencephalopathy (PML) has been associated with mycophenolic acid derivatives. It is characterized by apathy, ataxia, cognitive deficiency, confusion, and hemiparesis.

Further Reading

CellCept® (mycophenolate mofetil) package insert. South San Francisco, CA: Genentech USA, Inc; 2015.

Mycophenolate. In *Lexi-Drugs. Lexicomp*. Hudson, OH: Wolters Kluwer Health, Inc. http://online .lexi.com. Accessed Jan 31, 2016.

Myfortic® (mycophenolate sodium) package insert. East Hanover, NJ: Novartis Pharmaceuticals Corporation; 2013.

Proliferation Signal Inhibitors (Mammalian Target of Rapamycin Inhibitors)

Class Members: everolimus (Zortress®, Affinitor®), sirolimus (Rapamune®)

Typical Uses: prophylaxis of solid organ transplant rejection, treatment of pulmonary lymphangioleiomyomatosis, angiomyolipoma of kidney, breast cancer, neuroendocrine tumor of pancreas, renal cell carcinoma, subependymal giant cell astrocytoma, Waldenstrom macroglobulinemia

Potential Neurologic or Psychiatric Medication Adverse Effects: Very common adverse effects (>10%) include headache, and insomnia. Common adverse effects (1–10%) and include dizziness, somnolence, agitation, anxiety, depression, migraine, hallucination, seizure, and tremor. Rare adverse events include PRES (posterior reversible encephalopathy syndrome), characterized by seizures, acute encephalopathy, and visual disturbances, and progressive multifocal leukoencephalopathy (PML). Progressive multifocal leukoencephalopathy is a rare adverse event related to the immunosuppression. It is characterized by apathy, ataxia, cognitive deficiency, confusion, and hemiparesis.

Further Reading

Everolimus. In *Lexi-Drugs. Lexicomp*. Hudson, OH: Wolters Kluwer Health, Inc. http://online.lexi .com. Accessed Jan 31, 2016.

Sirolimus. In *Lexi-Drugs. Lexicomp*. Hudson, OH: Wolters Kluwer Health, Inc. http://online.lexi .com. Accessed Jan 31, 2016.

Oncology and Hematology Medications

Latha Radhakrishnan, PharmD, BCPS, BCOP   University of Illinois at Chicago College of Pharmacy

Scott M. Wirth, PharmD, BCOP   University of Illinois at Chicago College of Pharmacy

Blinatumomab (Blincyto®)

Typical Uses: acute lymphoblastic leukemia (ALL)

Potential Neurologic or Psychiatric Medication Adverse Effects: Blinatumomab, a bispecific T-cell engager that binds to CD19 and CD3, has been associated with severe neurologic toxicities that can be life-threatening or fatal. Neurotoxicity has occurred in half of all patients receiving blinatumomab in clinical trials. Neurotoxicity was severe (grade 3 or higher) in about 15% of these patients. Patients may experience loss of consciousness, syncope, aphasia, confusion, coordination disorders, encephalopathy, and/or seizures while receiving therapy. Psychiatric disorders have also been reported in clinical trials. Therapy should be withheld for severe neurotoxicity and discontinued for seizure disorders or delayed resolution (more than 7 days) of severe neurotoxicity after holding therapy. Current prescribing information has a black box warning for monitoring neurologic toxicities while on therapy with blinatumomab.

Further Reading

Blincyto® (blinatumomab) package insert. Thousand Oaks, CA: Amgen Inc.; 2014.

Topp MS, Gökbuget N, Zugmaier G et al. Phase II trial of the anti-CD19 bispecific T cell-engager blinatumomab shows hematologic and molecular remissions in patients with relapsed or refractory B-precursor acute lymphoblastic leukemia. *J Clin Oncol.* 2014;32:4134.

Topp MS, Gökbuget N, Stein AS, et al. Safety and activity of blinatumomab for adult patients with relapsed or refractory B-precursor acute lymphoblastic leukaemia: a multicentre, single-arm, phase 2 study. *Lancet Oncol.* 2015;16:57–66.

Cytarabine (Ara-C) (Intravenous) (Cytosar-U®)

Typical Uses: acute myeloid leukemia (AML), acute lymphocytic leukemia (ALL), chronic myeloid leukemia (CML), meningeal leukemia

Potential Neurologic or Psychiatric Medication Adverse Effects: Cytarabine therapy may result in neurotoxicity that is primarily cerebellar and occurs at high doses (≥ 3 grams/m^2 IV every 12 hours). Standard, lower doses (~ 100 mg/m^2) rarely cause neurotoxicity. Neurotoxicity primarily occurs within 3 to 8 days of therapy, and in some cases may be permanent. Clinical signs of cerebellar toxicity include nystagmus, ataxia, dysarthria, dysdiadochokinesia, and/or dysmetria. Cerebral toxicity may also occur following therapy, potentially resulting in seizures, somnolence, confusion, memory loss, cognitive dysfunction, and/or coma. The overall incidence of neurologic toxicity with high-dose cytarabine is 8% to 25%. Patients with renal impairment are especially at risk with the incidence reported as high as 55%. Other risk factors include patient age greater than 50 years, total dose greater than or equal to 20 grams/m^2, and abnormal pretreatment liver function. Patients with any signs of cerebral or cerebellar dysfunction should have cytarabine discontinued immediately.

Further Reading

Cytarabine injection package insert. Rockford, IL: Mylan Institutional LLC; 2014.

Herzig RH, Hines JD, Herzig GP, et al. Cerebellar toxicity with high-dose cytosine arabinoside. *J Clin Oncol.* 1987;5:927–32.

Jolson HM, Bosco L, Bufton MG, et al. Clustering of adverse drug events: analysis of risk factors for cerebellar toxicity with high-dose cytarabine. *J Natl Cancer Inst.* 1992;84:500.

Smith GA, Damon LE, Rugo HS, Ries CA, Linker CA. High-dose cytarabine dose modification reduces the incidence of neurotoxicity in patients with renal insufficiency. *J Clin Oncol*. 1997;15:833.

Erythropoiesis-Stimulating Agents

Class Members: darbepoetin alfa (Aranesp®), epoetin alfa (Epogen®, Procrit®)

Typical Uses: treatment of anemia associated with chronic kidney disease (CKD), treatment of chemotherapy-induced anemia in patients with non-myeloid malignancies, treatment of anemia associated with zidovudine therapy in patients with HIV infection (epoetin alfa), perioperatively to reduce the need for allogeneic red blood cell transfusions in anemic patients (epoetin alfa)

Potential Neurologic or Psychiatric Medication Adverse Effects: Adverse effects reported with erythropoiesis-stimulating agent (ESA) use are thought to be mainly attributed to the correction of the underlying anemia or to the patient's disease rather than to the medication itself. Seizures have been reported in patients with CKD receiving an ESA. It is believed that seizures in this setting are the result of an overly rapid correction of hematocrit that subsequently causes an elevation in blood pressure, or the increased risk of seizures in the CKD population. Headache has also been reported with ESAs, and once again is thought to be attributable to an increase in blood pressure with use. The greatest risk with ESA use is an increased risk of death and serious and life-threatening cardiovascular events (myocardial infarction, stroke, venous thromboembolism, vascular access thrombis) observed in clinical trials when ESAs were administered to target hemoglobin levels >11 g/dL. A flu-like syndrome presenting with diaphoresis, chills, shivering, malaise, feeling of cold or warmth, myalgia, bone pain and arthralgia of the limbs and pelvis, generalized aches and pains, fever, paresthesias, and/or abdominal pain/cramps has been reported within 90–120 minutes of initiating an epoetin alfa intravenous infusion. Symptoms are transient and generally resolve within 2–12 hours.

Further Reading

Darbepoetin alfa. In *Lexi-Drugs. Lexicomp*. Hudson, OH: Wolters Kluwer Health, Inc. http://online .lexi.com. Accessed Jun 28, 2016.

Epoetin alfa. In *Lexi-Drugs. Lexicomp*. Hudson, OH: Wolters Kluwer Health, Inc. http://online.lexi .com. Accessed Jun 28, 2016.

Hematopoietic agents. In *AHFS Drug Information STAT!Ref Online Electronic Medical Library*. Bethesda, MD: American Society of Health-System Pharmacists. http://online.statref.com/ document.aspx?fxid=1&docid=497. Accessed Jun 28, 2016.

Fluoropyrimidine Antimetabolites

Class Members: fluorouracil (Adrucil®); capecitabine (Xeloda®)

Typical Uses: breast cancer, colon cancer, rectal cancer, pancreatic cancer, gastric cancer

Potential Neurologic or Psychiatric Medication Adverse Effects: Neurologic side effects are relatively rare with fluoropyrimidine therapy. However, both fluorouracil and capecitabine (an oral prodrug of fluorouracil) can cause cerebellar toxicity manifesting as ataxia, nystagmus, and/or dysmetria. Symptoms can be delayed (weeks after therapy initiation) and most often resolve after discontinuation of the agent. Both agents can also rarely cause encephalopathy resulting in confusion, agitation, seizure, nausea, headaches, and/or memory loss. Encephalopathy has been correlated with hyperammonemia, particularly with high-dose fluorouracil therapy. Other neurologic effects including peripheral neuropathy have also been reported. Patients should be monitored for neurologic effects during and following therapy with fluoropyrimidines.

Further Reading

Pirzada NA, Imram IA, Dafer RM. Fluorouracil induced neurotoxicity. *Ann Pharmacother*. 2000;34:35–8.

Renoir D, Gill S. Capecitabine-induced cerebellar toxicity. *Clin Colorectal Cancer*. 2006; 6:70.

Said MW, Wood TE, McGee PJ, et al. Peripheral neuropathy associated with capecitabine. *Anti-Cancer Drugs*. 2004;15:767–71.

Videnovic A, Semenov I, Chua-Adajar R, et al. Capecitabine-induced multifocal leukoencephalopthy: a report of five cases. *Neurology*. 2005;65:1792.

Yeh KH, Cheng AL. High-dose 5-fluorouracil infusional therapy is associated with hyperammonemia, lactic acidosis and encephalopathy. *Br J Cancer*. 1997;75:464–5.

Granulocyte Colony-Stimulating Factors (G-CSF) and Granulocyte–Macrophage Colony-Stimulating Factors (GM-CSF)

Class Members: filgrastim (Neupogen˚), Tbo-filgrastim (Granix˚), filgrastim-sndz (Zarxio˚), pegfilgrastim (Neulasta˚), sargramostim (Leukine˚)

Typical Uses: decrease the duration of severe neutropenia and incidence of infection in patients receiving myelosuppressive treatment; increase survival in patients acutely exposed to myelosuppressive doses of radiation; mobilization of autologous hematopoietic progenitor cells into the peripheral blood for apheresis collection; reduce the incidence and duration of neutropenic complications in symptomatic patients with congenital, cyclic, or idiopathic neutropenia

Potential Neurologic or Psychiatric Medication Adverse Effects: The granulocyte colony-stimulating factor (G-CSF) and granulocyte–macrophage colony-stimulating factor (GM-CSF) agents are generally well tolerated. Mild to moderate medullary bone pain is the adverse effect most commonly reported across these agents (filgrastim 5–33%, pegfilgrastim 31%, sargramostim 21%). The frequency of bone pain appears to be dependent on the dose and/or route of administration. While other adverse neurologic and psychiatric effects have been reported at a fairly high frequency with G-CSF and GM-CSF agents, a causal relationship between these agents and these adverse effects is not clear for several reasons. First, these agents are used to treat patients with serious underlying disease, and second, adverse effects that have been reported in patients receiving these medications have also occurred in patients not receiving the medication. Very common adverse effects (>10%) reported in patients receiving pegfilgrastim or filgrastim include fatigue, anorexia, skeletal pain, headache, myalgia, abdominal pain, arthralgia, generalized weakness, and dizziness. However, these adverse effects generally were attributed to the underlying malignancy or to concomitant cytotoxic chemotherapy. Similarly, very common (>10%) adverse effects reported with sargramostim use include malaise (57%), headache (26%), chills (25%), anxiety (11%), insomnia (11%), weakness (66%), arthralgia (11–21%), and myalgia (18%).

Further Reading

Filgrastim. In *Lexi-Drugs. Lexicomp*. Hudson, OH: Wolters Kluwer Health, Inc. http://online.lexi .com. Accessed Jun 28, 2016.

Hematopoietic Agents. In *AHFS Drug Information STAT!Ref Online Electronic Medical Library*. Bethesda, MD: American Society of Health-System Pharmacists. http://online.statref.com/ document.aspx?fxid=1&docid=497. Accessed Jun 28, 2016.

Pegfilgrastim. In *Lexi-Drugs. Lexicomp*. Hudson, OH: Wolters Kluwer Health, Inc. http://online.lexi .com. Accessed Jun 28, 2016.

Sargramostim. In *Lexi-Drugs. Lexicomp*. Hudson, OH: Wolters Kluwer Health, Inc. http://online .lexi.com. Accessed Jun 28, 2016.

Interferon

Class Members: interferon alpha-2b (Intron˚ A), peginterferon alfa-2b (Sylatron˚)

Typical Uses: melanoma (interferon alpha-2b, peginterferon alfa-2b); interferon alpha-2b has also been used in AIDS-related Kaposi's sarcoma, follicular lymphoma, hairy cell leukemia

Potential Neurologic or Psychiatric Medication Adverse Effects: The adverse effect profile is similar between both interferon agents. Black box warnings of life-threatening neuropsychiatric disorders exist for both formulations. Severe or worsening symptoms warrant permanent discontinuation. Depressed mood and impaired cognitive dysfunction is considered to be a chronic and common toxicity of high-dose interferon therapy. A previous history of depression or other psychiatric disorders is considered a risk factor. Patients may display anxiety, mood changes, and episodes of mania. Psychiatric disorders are dose- and duration-related. Selective serotonin reuptake inhibitors (SSRIs) have been studied prophylactically to reduce the development of depression. Additional studies are needed to prophylactically prescribe an SSRI prior to the start of treatment. Impaired cognitive dysfunction presents as short-term memory, psychomotor slowing, poor coordination and performance. This toxicity appears to be reversible when therapy is discontinued.

Further Reading

Intron® A (interferon alpha-2b injection, solution) package insert. Whitehouse Station, NJ: Merck & Co., Inc.; Feb 2016.

Kirkwood JM, Bender C, Agarwala S. Mechanisms and management of toxicities associated with high-dose interferon alfa-2b therapy. *J Clin Oncol.* 2002;20:3703–18.

Sylatron® (peginterferon alpha-2b injection, powder, lyophilized, for solution) package insert. Whitehouse Station, NJ: Merck & Co., Inc.; Feb 2016.

Intrathecal Chemotherapy

Class Members (common): methotrexate, cytarabine (Ara-C), liposomal cytarabine (DepoCyt®)

Typical Uses: lymphomatis meningitis, meningeal leukemia

Potential Neurologic or Psychiatric Medication Adverse Effects: Direct instillation of chemotherapy into the intrathecal space can result in severe neurologic side effects. Though most common with methotrexate, all agents have the potential to cause chemical arachnoiditis when given intrathecally. Patients can present with symptoms such as headache, back pain, nuchal rigidity, and fever. Liposomal cytarabine, a formulation of cytarabine that results in prolonged cerebrospinal concentrations of the medication, has recommendations to give glucocorticoids for 5 days beginning on the day of administration to minimize these effects. More severe reactions, such as transverse myelopathy, have also occurred with these agents, resulting in sensory loss and/or paraplegia due to spinal cord dysfunction. Patients should also be monitored for the incidence of leukoencephalopathy manifesting as confusion, irritability, somnolence, ataxia, dementia, seizures, and/or coma. Neurotoxicity from these agents can be progressive and even fatal. Patients should be monitored closely for early signs of neurotoxicity (headache, nausea, fever) and dose reductions and/or discontinuation should be considered.

Further Reading

Cytarabine injection package insert. Rockford, IL: Mylan Institutional LLC; Sep 2014.

DepoCyt® (cytarabine injection, lipid complex) package insert. Gaithersburg, MD: Sigma-Tau Pharmaceuticals, Inc.; Dec 2014.

Dunton SF, Nitschke R, Spruce WE, et al. Progressive ascending paralysis following administration of intrathecal and intravenous cytosine arabinoside. A Pediatric Oncology Group study. *Cancer.* 1986;57:1083.

Methotrexate sodium injection, solution package insert. Rockford IL: Mylan Institutional LLC; Sep 2014.

Ipilimumab (Yervoy®)

Typical Uses: melanoma

Potential Neurologic or Psychiatric Medication Adverse Effects: Ipilimumub, an antibody that binds CTLA-4, has been associated with rare severe neuropathy that is immune mediated. Neuropathy may occur within months or be delayed as long as 2 years after initiation of treatment. Severe (grade 3 or worse) neuropathy occurs in 1% to 2% of patients and may present as weakness, paresthesias, or other sensory complications. Peripheral motor neuropathy as well as enteric and central neuropathy (encephalitis) have also been reported. Due to the severity of these symptoms and the reported incidence of fatal Guillain–Barré syndrome in clinical trials, the current prescribing information includes a black box warning for immune-mediated neuropathies. Therapy should be withheld and/or discontinued for moderate to severe neurotoxicity. Initiation of systemic corticosteroids should also be considered in order to reverse immune-mediated effects.

Further Reading

Bhatia S, Huber BR, Upton MP, et al. Inflammatory enteric neuropathy with severe constipation after ipilimumab treatment for melanoma: A case report. *J Immunother.* 2009;32:203–5.

Wilgenhof S, Neyns B. Anti-CTLA-4 antibody-induced Guillain-Barré syndrome in a melanoma patient. *Ann Oncol.* 2011;22:991–3

Yervoy® (ipilimumab injection) package insert. Princeton, NJ: E.R. Squibb & Sons, LLC; Mar 2017.

Ixabepilone (Ixempra®)

Typical Uses: breast cancer

Potential Neurologic or Psychiatric Medication Adverse Effects: One of the most common side effects of ixabepilone is neurotoxicity, which presents as peripheral neuropathy. The incidence for severe neuropathy ranges from 1% to 40% in breast cancer patients depending on whether patients were untreated versus heavily pretreated. This toxicity manifests as a sensory neuropathy; however, motor neuropathy has also been reported at a lower rate. The neurotoxicity is dose-dependent, cumulative, and reversible. Dose reductions are an acceptable method of managing the symptoms. Patients start to experience this side effect after 3–4 cycles of ixabepilone administration. Studies have shown that the median onset to improvement of symptoms may range from 4 to 6 weeks in patients experiencing severe toxicity. The common symptoms are paresthesias, muscle weakness, and numbness in extremities. One study showed an increased incidence of neurotoxicity was correlated with a higher response rate in non-curative breast cancer patients.

Further Reading

Durando X, Dalenc F, Abrial C, et al. Neurotoxicity as a prognostic factor in patients with metastatic breast cancer treated with ixabepilone as a first-line therapy. *Oncology.* 2015;88:180–8.

Kushlaf HA. Emerging toxic neuropathies and myopathies. *Neurol Clin.* 2011;29:679–87.

Vahdat LT, Roche HH, Hortobagyi GN, et al. Ixabepilone-associated peripheral neuropathy: data from across the phase II and III clinical trials. *Support Care Cancer.* 2012;20:2661–8.

Nelarabine (Arranon®)

Typical Uses: T-cell acute lymphoblastic leukemia, T-cell acute lymphoblastic lymphoma

Potential Neurologic or Psychiatric Medication Adverse Effects: Nelarabine has been associated with neurotoxicity in clinical trials and currently has a black box warning for severe neurologic adverse events. Neurotoxicity is dose limiting and may manifest as peripheral neuropathy, seizures, loss of consciousness, ataxia, and/or paralysis. Severe neurotoxicity may be similar in presentation to Guillain–Barré syndrome (status epilepticus, craniospinal demyelination, ascending neuropathy). Those receiving concurrent intrathecal therapy, or those with previous craniospinal irradiation may have increased risk for neurotoxicity. Current prescribing information recommends discontinuing nelarabine for any incidence of grade 2 or greater neurologic toxicity. However, toxicity may not always resolve following discontinuation of therapy.

Further Reading

Arranon® (nelarabine injection) package insert. Research Triangle Park, NC: GlaxoSmithKline LLC; Dec 2014.

Cooper TM. Role of nelarabine in the treatment of T-cell acute lymphoblastic leukemia and T-cell lymphoblastic lymphoma. *Ther Clin Risk Manag.* 2007;3:1135–41.

DeAngelo DJ, Yu D, Johnson JL, et al. Nelarabine induces complete remissions in adults with relapsed or refractory T-lineage acute lymphoblastic leukemia or lymphoblastic lymphoma: Cancer and Leukemia Group B study 19801. *Blood.* 2007;109:5136.

Nitrosoureas

Class Members: carmustine (BiCNU®; Gliadel® Wafer), lomustine (Gleostine®)

Typical Uses: brain tumors, non-Hodgkin's lymphoma, Hodgkin's lymphoma, multiple myeloma

Potential Neurologic or Psychiatric Medication Adverse Effects: Nitrosoureas have been shown to cause multiple neurologic effects. Lomustine, which is only available in an oral formulation, has been shown to cause disorientation, dysarthria, visual disturbances (including blindness), lethargy, and ataxia. Though it is often difficult to determine an association with the medication for these effects, patients should be monitored closely and considered for discontinuation if causality is determined. Carmustine can produce similar effects, particularly when given at high doses to facilitate hematopoietic stem cell transplantation. Neurologic toxicity in this setting can present as altered mental status, seizures, quadriparesis, confusion, ocular toxicity, and/or ataxia. Intracarotid administration has also been shown to cause similar effects. Patients receiving the Gliadel® Wafer implant have been shown to have increased risk of seizures. Patients should be monitored closely for seizures, and anti-seizure medications should be considered for initiation prior to surgery.

Further Reading

BiCNU® (carmustine) package insert. Eatontown, NJ: Heritage Pharmaceuticals Inc.; Mar 2017.

Burger PC, Kamenar E, Schold SC, et al. Encephalomyelopathy following high-dose BCNU therapy. *Cancer.* 1980;48:1318.

Gleostine® (lomustine, capsule gel coated) package insert. Miami, FL: NextSource Biotechnology, LLC; Jan 2016.

Gliadel® (carmustine wafer) package insert. Atlanta, GA: Arbor Pharmaceuticals, LLC; Nov 2014.

Mahaley MS Jr, Whaley RA, Blue M, Bertsch L. Central neurotoxicity following intracarotid BCNU chemotherapy for malignant gliomas. *J Neurooncol*. 1986;3:297–314.

Oxazaphosphorines

Class Members: ifosfamide (Ifex®), cyclophosphamide (Cytoxan®)

Typical Uses: gynecologic cancers (ifosfamide), germ cell tumors of the ovaries and testis (ifosfamide), lymphomas (ifosfamide), osteosarcoma (ifosfamide), neuroblastoma (ifosfamide, cyclophosphamide), multiple myeloma (ifosfamide, cyclophosphamide), testicular cancer (ifosfamide), breast cancer (cyclophosphamide), leukemias (cyclophosphamide), lymphomas (cyclophosphamide), ovarian cancer (cyclophosphamide), retinoblastoma (cyclophosphamide)

Potential Neurologic or Psychiatric Medication Adverse Effects: Neurotoxicity is more commonly seen with ifosfamide than its structurally similar alkylating agent, cyclophosphamide. However, neurotoxicity can manifest with the administration of high-dose IV cyclophosphamide. Neurotoxicity is listed as a black box warning for ifosfamide. These signs and symptoms can range from confusion and dizziness to encephalopathy and coma. High single doses of ifosfamide can contribute to the neurotoxicity seen with this agent. The incidence of ifosfamide neurotoxicity is 10–40% of patients. Reported signs and symptoms are ataxia, delirium, visual disturbances, hallucinations, encephalopathy, and coma. The incidence of encephalopathy is broad and ranges between 5% and 60% of patients receiving ifosfamide. Neurotoxicity is more common when given as a large bolus dose or continuous infusion. Risk factors for developing ifosfamide-induced neurotoxicity include low serum albumin, presence of pelvic disease, and elevated serum creatinine. Patients that display these risk factors should receive ifosfamide at fractionated schedules. The use of methylene blue for the treatment of ifosfamide-induced neurotoxicity has been extensively studied. Peripheral neuropathy has a low incidence of occurrence.

Further Reading

Fleming RA. An overview of cyclophosphamide and ifosfamide pharmacology. *Pharmacotherapy*. 1997;17:146S–54S.

Ifosfamide injection, solution package insert. Deerfield IL: Baxter Healthcare Corporation; Aug 2014.

Klastersky J. Side effects of ifosfamide. *Oncology*. 2003;65(Suppl 2):7–10.

Patel PN. Methylene blue for management of ifosfamide-induced encephalopathy. *Ann Pharmacother*. 2006;40:299–303.

Platinum Analogs

Class Members: cisplatin (Platinol-AQ®), carboplatin (Paraplatin®), oxaliplatin (Eloxatin®)

Typical Uses: esophageal cancer (cisplatin), anal cancer (cisplatin), cancer of unknown origin (cisplatin), cervical cancer (cisplatin), cervical cancer (cisplatin), gastric cancer (cisplatin), ovarian cancer (cisplatin, carboplatin), head and neck cancer (cisplatin), testicular cancer (cisplatin, carboplatin), non-Hodgkin's lymphoma (cisplatin, carboplatin), lung cancer (cisplatin, carboplatin), retinoblastoma (cisplatin), bladder cancer (cisplatin), sarcoma (cisplatin), colorectal cancer (oxaliplatin), stomach cancer (oxaliplatin), pancreatic cancer (oxaliplatin)

Potential Neurologic or Psychiatric Medication Adverse Effects: Neurotoxicity is prevalent with the platinum analogs and can be dose-limiting. Cisplatin and oxaliplatin are more commonly associated with these complications. However, such toxicities can occur with high doses of carboplatin used in hematopoietic cell transplantation. At standard doses, peripheral neuropathy can develop with both cisplatin and oxaliplatin. This typical presentation of neuropathy occurs after cumulative doses have been reached. There are two types of neuropathy that can occur with oxaliplatin administration. Acute neuropathy occurs in 85–95% of patients treated. The symptoms include cold-induced paresthesias and dysesthesias as well as jaw stiffness. These symptoms can be infusion-rate related, occur hours post administration, and continue for a few days. Delayed neuropathy occurs later and presents as sensory neuropathy after cumulative doses. Cisplatin ototoxicity can occur in roughly 30% of patients. Ototoxicity can present as hearing loss and tinnitus. Less common toxicities associated with the platinum agents are vestibulopathy and encephalopathy.

Further Reading

Amptoulach S, Tsavaris N. Neurotoxicity caused by the treatment with platinum analogues. *Chemother Res Pract.* 2011;2011:843019.

Avan A, Postma TJ, Ceresa C, et al. Platinum-induced neurotoxicity and preventive strategies: past, present, and future. *Oncologist.* 2015;20:411–32.

Miltenburg NC, Boogerd W. Chemotherapy-induced neuropathy: a comprehensive survey. *Cancer Treat Rev.* 2014;40:872–82.

Proteasome Inhibitors

Class Members: bortezomib (Velcade®), carfilzomib (Kyprolis®), ixazomib (Ninlaro®)

Typical Uses: multiple myeloma, mantle cell lymphoma

Potential Neurologic or Psychiatric Medication Adverse Effects: All three available proteasome inhibitors have been reported to cause peripheral neuropathy. Neurotoxicity seems to be most common with bortezomib, resulting in grade 3 or worse neuropathy occurring in 16% of patients receiving twice weekly intravenous therapy. The incidence may be reduced to 6% when bortezomib is given subcutaneously instead of intravenously. Bortezomib has also been known to cause motor neuropathy (weakness in lower extremeties) and autonomic neuropathy (constipation or diarrhea) in some patients. Carfilzomib and ixazomib seem to cause less peripheral neuropathy than bortezomib. Grade 3 or worse peripheral neuropathy has been reported in 1% or less of patients receiving intravenous carfilzomib and in about 2% of patients receiving the novel oral proteasome inhibitor ixazomib. Therapy with proteasome inhibitors may need to be discontinued for neurotoxicity, and toxicity may resolve in a majority of patients. Dose adjustments for ixazomib and bortezomib are available in the prescribing information if peripheral neuropathy occurs.

Further Reading

Kyprolis® (carfilzomib injection, powder, lyophilized, for solution) package insert. Thousand Oaks, CA: Onyx Pharmaceuticals, Inc.; May 2017.

Moreau P, Pylypenko H, Grosicki S, et al. Subcutaneous versus intravenous administration of bortezomib in patients with relapsed multiple myeloma: a randomised, phase 3, non-inferiority study. *Lancet Oncol.* 2011;12:431.

Ninlaro® (ixazomib citrate capsule) package insert. Cambridge, MA: Millennium Pharmaceuticals, Inc.; Nov 2015.

Velcade® (bortezomib injection, powder, lyophilized, for solution) package insert. Cambridge, MA: Millennium Pharmaceuticals, Inc.; Sep 2015.

Vij R, Wang M, Kaufman JL, et al. An open-label, single-arm, phase 2 (PX-171-004) study of single-agent carfilzomib in bortezomib-naive patients with relapsed and/or refractory multiple myeloma. *Blood.* 2012;119:5661.

Selective Serotonin Receptor Modulators

Class Members: tamoxifen (Nolvadex®), raloxifene (Evista®)

Typical Uses: breast cancer (tamoxifen, raloxifene), endometrial cancer (tamoxifen), osteoporosis (raloxifene)

Potential Neurologic or Psychiatric Medication Adverse Effects: The incidence of tamoxifen-related depression ranges from 1% to 15% in various studies. It is considered dose-dependent. A past history of mood disorders may be a risk factor for developing tamoxifen-induced depression. Symptoms of depression include abrupt mood changes, loss of interest, insomnia, hypersomnia, and changes in activities of daily life. Loss of appetite, increases in appetite, weight gain, and weight loss are also possible side effects. Patients have reported suicidal ideations. Studies have shown these depressive symptoms perhaps have led to non-adherence and discontinuation of hormonal therapy. There also could be neuropsychologic side effects that present with cognitive changes such as inability to concentrate. Treatment includes the use of selective serotonin receptor inhibitors (SSRIs). There is the concern of significant drug–drug interactions between tamoxifen and many of the SSRIs, which can result in decreased exposure of tamoxifen metabolites. This may lead to lower cure rates in patients diagnosed with breast cancer. Venlafaxine has also been studied for the treatment of tamoxifen-induced depression. Trials looking at raloxifene and its effects on depression, cognitive symptoms, and sexual dysfunction are inconclusive.

Some studies show that raloxifene may improve symptoms of depression and sexual function.

Further Reading

Bourque A, Karama S, Looper K, et al. Acute tamoxifen-induced depression and its prevention with venlafaxine. *Psychosomatics*. 2009;50: 162–5.

Thompson DS, Spanier CA, Vogel VG. The relationship between tamoxifen, estrogen, and depressive symptoms. *Breast J*. 1999;5:375–82.

Yang ZD, Yu J, Zhang Q. Effects of raloxifene on cognition, mental health, sleep, and sexual function in menopausal women. *Maturitas*. 2013;75:341–8.

Taxanes

Class Members: paclitaxel (Taxol®), paclitaxel protein-bound (Abraxane®), docetaxel (Taxotere®), cabazitaxel (Jevtana®)

Typical Uses: breast cancer (paclitaxel, packitaxel protein-bound, docetaxel), cancer of unknown origin (paclitaxel), bladder cancer (paclitaxel), gastric cancer (paclitaxel, docetaxel), head and neck cancer (paclitaxel, docetaxel), lung cancer (paclitaxel, paclitaxel protein-bound, docetaxel), ovarian cancer (paclitaxel, paclitaxel protein-bound, docetaxel), testicular cancer (paclitaxel), pancreatic cancer (paclitaxel protein-bound), prostate (docetaxel, cabazitaxel)

Potential Neurologic or Psychiatric Medication Adverse Effects: Neurotoxicity presents primarily as sensory axonal neuropathy when higher and cumulative doses have been administered. It is considered a dose-limiting toxicity for all class agents. All taxanes can cause paresthesias and dysesthesias in the extremities. The paclitaxel solvent, Cremophor®, has been thought to increase the neurotoxicity potential. Paclitaxel-induced neuropathy occurs in roughly 30% of patients. It is unclear from the clinical trials if the incidence of neuropathy is similar with the use of nab-paclitaxel as compared with solvent-based paclitaxel. Neuropathy is seen less with the use of docetaxel. Cabazitaxel, which is approved for the treatment of hormone-refractory metastatic prostate cancer, has also been shown to cause peripheral neuropathy in 13% of patients treated. Grades 3 and 4 neuropathy had an incidence of less than 1%.

Further Reading

Abraxane® (paclitaxel injection, powder, lyophilized, for suspension) package insert. Summit, NJ: Abraxis BioScience, LLC; Jul 2015.

Gorenstein E, Schwarz TL. The paradox of paclitaxel neurotoxicity: mechanisms and unanswered questions. *Neuropharmacology*. 2014;76:175–83.

Jevtana® (cabazitaxel injection, solution) package insert. Bridgewater, NJ: Sanofi-aventis US LLC; May 2017.

Kudlowitz D, Muggia F. Nanoparticle albumin-bound paclitaxel (nab-paclitaxel): extending its indications. *Expert Opin Drug Metab Toxicol*. 2014;13:681–5.

Thalidomide Analogs

Class Members: thalidomide (Thalomid®), lenalidomide (Revlimid®), pomalidomide (Pomalyst®)

Typical Uses: multiple myeloma, myelodysplastic syndrome, mantle cell lymphoma, erythema nodosum leprosum

Potential Neurologic or Psychiatric Medication Adverse Effects: Neurotoxicity from thalidomide analogs most often presents as peripheral neuropathy, but also somnolence and dizziness have been reported. The representative agent in this class, thalidomide, has the highest potential of all agents with an incidence of peripheral neuropathy that is over 50%. Patients on thalidomide should be monitored monthly during treatment for at least 3 months, then periodically. Practitioners should also consider measuring the sensory nerve action potential (SNAP) amplitudes at baseline and every 6 months according to prescribing information. For any incidence of peripheral neuropathy, therapy should be discontinued. Lenalidomide and pomalidomide seem to cause significantly less peripheral neuropathy than thalidomide. Lenalidomide treatment causes neuropathy in about 5% of patients (depending on indication), with less than 1% of patients having severe symptoms in those treated for multiple myeloma. Pomalidomide, which is currently approved for relapsed or refractory multiple myeloma, also seems to have a lower incidence of neurotoxicity. When given in combination with low-dose dexamethasone, only 15% of patients on pomalidomide have any incidence of peripheral neuropathy, with only about 1% being severe (grade 3 or higher). Due to toxicity risk (including embryo–fetal toxicity), all three agents currently have Risk Evaluation and Mitigation Strategy (REMS) programs for preventing and reporting adverse effects.

Further Reading

Dimopoulos MA, Chen C, Spencer A, et al. Long-term follow-up on overall survival from the MM-009 and MM-010 phase III trials of lenalidomide plus dexamethasone in patients with relapsed or refractory multiple myeloma. *Leukemia*. 2009;23:2147.

Pomalyst® (pomalidomide capsule) package insert. Summit, NJ: Celgene Corporation; Jun 2016.

Revlimid® (lenalidomide capsule) package insert. Summit, NJ: Celgene Corporation; Jan 2017.

San Miguel J, Weisel K, Moreau P, et al. Pomalidomide plus low-dose dexamethasone versus high-dose dexamethasone alone for patients with relapsed and refractory multiple myeloma (MM-003): a randomised, open-label, phase 3 trial. *Lancet Oncol*. 2013;14:1055.

Thalomid® (thalidomide capsule) package insert. Summit, NJ: Celgene Corporation; Jan 2017.

Vascular Endothelial Growth Factor (VEGF) Signaling Inhibitors

Class Members: bevacizumab (Avastin®), ramucirumab (Cyramza®), ziv-Aflibercept (Zaltrap®)

Typical Uses: colorectal cancer (bevacizumab, ramucirumab, ziv-aflibercept), non-small cell lung cancer (bevacizumab, ramucirumab), gastric cancer (ramucirumab), glioblastoma (bevacizumab), cervical cancer (bevacizumab), ovarian cancer (bevacizumab)

Potential Neurologic or Psychiatric Medication Adverse Effects: Intravenous anti-VEGF inhibitors are not commonly neurotoxic, but careful monitoring for serious neurologic effects should be performed throughout therapy. As a class, these agents may all cause reversible posterior leukoencephalopathy syndrome (RPLS) manifesting in symptoms such as confusion, seizures, fatigue/lethargy, headache, visual changes (including blindness), and other neurologic disturbances. These effects are reported in less than 1% of patients in clinical trials but may result in death or long-term impairment. Discontinue these agents for any of the above neurologic effects and confirm with magnetic

resonance imaging (MRI). Symptoms typically resolve within days of discontinuation.

Further Reading

Cyramza® (ramucirumab solution) package insert. Indianapolis, IN: Eli Lilly and Company; Mar 2017.

Avastin® (bevacizumab injection, solution) package insert. South San Francisco, CA: Genentech, Inc.; Dec 2016.

Ozcan C, Wong SJ, Hari P. Reversible posterior leukoencephalopathy syndrome and bevacizumab. *N Engl J Med*. 2006;354:980–2.

Zaltrap® (ziv-aflibercept solution) package insert. Bridgewater, NJ: Sanofi-aventis US LLC; Jun 2016.

Vinca Alkaloids

Class Members: vincristine (Oncovin®), vinorelbine (Navelbine®), vinblastine (Velban®), vindesine (Eldisine®)

Typical Uses: leukemias (vincristine), lymphomas (vincristine, vinblastine), neuroblastoma (vincristine), breast cancer (vinorelbine, vinblastine), cervical cancer (vinorelbine), lung cancer (vinorelbine, vinblastine), ovarian cancer (vinorelbine), bladder cancer (vinblastine), prostate cancer (vinblastine), germ cell tumors (vinblastine), melanoma (vinblastine), renal cancer (vinblastine)

Potential Neurologic or Psychiatric Medication Adverse Effects: Neurotoxicity is a dose-limiting toxicity for all the vinca alkaloids. As a class, neuropathy typically presents in the extremities. However, neuropathies occur at a higher incidence with vincristine. Neuropathy can occur with increased single doses, with threshold doses of $>2–6$ mg/m^2. For this reason, doses are usually capped at 2 mg regardless of the patient's height and weight. Vincristine can cause both sensory (35% to 45%) and motor neuropathies. This can further present as autonomic and cranial neuropathies. Autonomic neuropathies can manifest as gastrointestinal side effects such as constipation and abdominal pain. For this reason, patients receiving vincristine infusions should be initiated on a bowel regimen. In addition, as azole-based therapy can exacerbate these toxicities, it is recommended that they not be co-administered with vincristine. Symptoms of cranial neuropathy are characterized as vision loss and facial weakness.

Neurotoxicity can be seen with vinorelbine, vinblastine, and vindesine; however, at a lower incidence than vincristine. The neuropathies experienced with vinca alkaloids are reported as highly reversible.

Further Reading

Magge R, DeAngelis LM. The double-edged sword: neurotoxicity of chemotherapy. *Blood Rev.* 2015;29:93–100.

Park SB, Goldstein D, Krishnan AV, et al. Chemotherapy-induced peripheral neurotoxicity: a critical analysis. *CA Cancer J Clin.* 2013;63: 419–37.

Vinblastine sulfate injection, solution package insert. Lake Zurich, IL: Fresenius Kabi USA, LLC; Jan 2017.

Vincristine sulfate injection, solution package insert. Lake Forest, IL: Hospira, Inc.; Jan 2017.

Vinorelbine injection, solution package insert. Parsippany, NJ: Actavis Pharma, Inc.; May 2015.

Disease-Modifying Antirheumatic Medications (DMARDs)

Daniel J. Langenburg, PharmD Portland VA Medical Center
Rebecca R. Fiore, PharmD Rockford VA Community Based Outpatient Clinic

Abatacept (Orencia®)

Typical Uses: FDA-labeled indications include treatment of rheumatoid arthritis (RA) and juvenile idiopathic arthritis; off-label uses include uveitis for children or adolescents

Potential Neurologic or Psychiatric Medication Adverse Effects: A frequent central nervous system side effect (>10%) seen in patients is headache. Less than 10% of patients experience dizziness. From the controlled trials that were submitted to the FDA, the most common central nervous system effects from abatacept use also include dizziness and headache. There may be drug interactions associated with this medication that require specific dose adjustments. Many of these interactions are associated with the increased risk of infection and malignancy (as the manufacturer does not recommend use with anakinra or TNF-inhibitors); however, caution should be taken when initiating a new medication when a patient is using abatacept as certain medications may increase the risk of adverse reactions. There are no black box warnings associated with this medication.

Further Reading

Orencia® (abatacept) package insert. Princeton, NJ: Bristol-Myers Squibb; Jun 2015.
Sweet B. Abatacept. *Am J Health-Syst Pharm.* 2006;63:2065–77.

Hydroxychloroquine (Plaquenil®)

Typical Uses: rheumatoid arthritis, acute malaria, systemic lupus erythematosus (SLE), Q fever (non-FDA approved)

Potential Neurologic or Psychiatric Medication Adverse Effects: The frequency of adverse effects with long-term use is not well defined between hydroxychloroquine and other 4-aminoquinoline anti-malarial medications (amodiaquine and chloroquine). Possible adverse effects include irritability, nervousness, emotional changes, nightmares, psychosis, headache, dizziness, vertigo, tinnitus, nystagmus, nerve deafness, convulsions, and ataxia. Potentially irreversible visual changes and retinal damage can occur with hydroxychloroquine use. This can present as blurred vision, photophobia, halos around light, visual field defects, reading difficulty, and flashing lights. The risk of retinal toxicity is typically small at low hydroxychloroquine doses and increases when the daily dose exceeds 6.5 mg/kg of ideal body weight. Eye examinations should be performed prior to starting hydroxychloroquine and annually thereafter to monitor for changes in vision. Hydroxychloroquine should be discontinued if visual disturbances occur and the patient should be closely monitored. Note that these changes may progress even after hydroxychloroquine has been discontinued.

Further Reading

Hydroxychloroquine In *Lexi-Drugs. Lexicomp.* Hudson, OH: Wolters Kluwer Health, Inc. http://online.lexi.com. Accessed Oct 2, 2016.
Plaquenil® (hydroxychloroquine) package insert. Bridgewater, NJ: Sanofi-aventis US LLC; Apr 2012.

IL-1 Inhibitors

Class Members: anakinra (Kineret®), canakinumab (Ilaris®)

Typical Uses: anakinra is FDA approved for neonatal-onset multisystem inflammatory disease and rheumatoid arthritis, off-label uses include juvenile idiopathic arthritis and recurrent pericarditis; canakinumab is FDA approved for cryopyrin-associated periodic syndromes and systemic juvenile idiopathic arthritis

Potential Neurologic or Psychiatric Medication Adverse Effects: The side effect profile for both IL-1 inhibitors is similar. The most frequent central nervous system effects for this class include headache (<15%); canakinumab also has an adverse drug event of vertigo. There are drug interactions associated with this medication that require specific dose adjustments, including those that may increase the risk of general adverse drug reactions, as well as an increased risk of infection and malignancy. A literature review was also completed in 2012, which reviewed the effect of immunologic influences on schizophrenia. There has been evidence that indicates at least some cases of schizophrenia have an immunologic component. Anakinra has been studied in this context, which has shown conflicting results. There is no black box warning associated with anakinra or canakinumab use.

Further Reading

Ilaris® (canakinumab) package insert. East Hanover, NJ: Novartis Pharmaceuticals; Jul 2016.

Kineret® (anakinra) package insert. Stockholm, Sweden: Swedish Orphan Biovitrum AB; May 2016.

Richard M, et al. Schizophrenia and the immune system: Pathophysiology, prevention and treatment. *Am J Health Syst Pharm.* 2012;69:757–66.

Leflunomide (Arava®)

Typical Uses: rheumatoid arthritis, cytomegalovirus treatment in transplant patients resistant to standard antivirals (non-FDA approved), prevention of solid organ transplant rejection (non-FDA approved)

Potential Neurologic or Psychiatric Medication Adverse Effects: Common adverse effects (1–10%) include headache, dizziness, pain, anxiety, depression, fever, insomnia, malaise, migraine, sleep disorders, vertigo, weakness, and paresthesia. Leflunomide is considered teratogenic and known to cause embryo lethality. All sexually active male and female patients taking leflunomide should use appropriate contraception to prevent pregnancy. If a female patient becomes pregnant during use, accelerated drug elimination should occur until the plasma teriflunomide (active metabolite of leflunomide) level is <0.02 mg/L.

Further Reading

Arava® (leflunomide) package insert. Bridgewater, NJ: Sanofi-aventis US LLC; Feb 2016.

Leflunomide. In *Lexi-Drugs. Lexicomp.* Hudson, OH: Wolters Kluwer Health, Inc. http://online.lexi .com. Accessed Oct 2, 2016.

Methotrexate (Otrexup®, Rasuvo®, Rheumatrex®, Trexall®)

Typical Uses: nononcology uses include treatment of psoriasis and rheumatoid arthritis; off-label uses include Crohn's disease, acute graft-versus-host disease (prophylaxis), dermatomyositis/polymyositis, multiple sclerosis, systemic lupus erythematosus, and adult uveitis

Potential Neurologic or Psychiatric Medication Adverse Effects: There are several different types of effects this medication can have on the central nervous system. No specific incidence of side effects was disclosed; however, pertinent effects include cognitive dysfunction, drowsiness, fatigue, mood changes, and neurologic symptoms (at high doses, including confusion, transient blindness, seizures, and coma). Due to methotrexate being a substrate of p-glycoprotein, medications that affect the metabolism of p-glycoprotein may affect methotrexate levels in a patient, and increase the risk of side effects. Methotrexate has been reported to cause fetal death and/or congenital anomalies and should be avoided for women of childbearing age. There is currently a black box warning for central nervous system effects with methotrexate use in pregnancy, so it should only be used if the benefit of use clearly outweighs the risk. In addition, methotrexate has been found to have higher rates of toxicity in children with Down syndrome, and in patients treated for acute lymphoblastic leukemia. It should also be used with caution and monitored closely in the elderly due to increased risk of toxicity. Methotrexate may cause **neurotoxicity** related to leukoencephalopathy, which may be progressive and fatal. In one case report a patient started on methotrexate for rheumatoid arthritis developed increased intracranial pressure. The patient presented with psychosis, including auditory and visual hallucinations, as well as disturbed sleep. These symptoms resolved after discontinuation.

Further Reading

Buitenkamp TD, Mathôt RA, de Haas V, Pieters R, Zwaan CM. Methotrexate-induced side effects are not due to differences in pharmacokinetics in children with Down syndrome and acute lymphoblastic leukemia. *Hematologica*. 2010;95:1106–13.

Methotrexate tablet package insert. Morgantown, WV: Mylan Pharmaceuticals; May 2013.

Sur S, Chauhan A. Methotrexate-induced pseudotumor cerebri and psychosis in a case of rheumatoid arthritis. *J Neuropsychiatry Clin Neurosci*. 2012;24:E18.

Sulfasalazine (Azulfidine®)

Typical Uses: FDA-labeled indications for rheumatoid arthritis and ulcerative colitis; off-label uses include Crohn's disease, psoriasis, ankylosing spondylitis, and psoriatic arthritis

Potential Neurologic or Psychiatric Medication Adverse Effects: The most frequent central nervous system effect seen in patients taking this medication is headache (<10%). Less frequent neurologic effects from sulfasalazine (<1%) include depression, drowsiness, hallucination, peripheral neuropathy, and seizures. No specific drug interactions were noted that would increase the risks of psychiatric medication adverse effects, and there is no black box warning associated with this medication. However, there is a precaution for central nervous system effects, due to death from irreversible neuromuscular and central nervous system changes. There is no clear risk of psychoses for patients being treated with sulfasalazine. There are cases of patients experiencing mood disturbances and psychoses when sulfasalazine is combined with chloroquine, but none found to be related to sulfasalazine only.

Further Reading

Azulfidine® (sulfasalazine) package insert. Kalamazoo, MI: Pharmacia & Upjohn; Feb 2014.

Jajić Z, Jajić I. Acute psychoses in patients with psoriatic arthritis during treatment with sulfasalazine. *Reumatizam*. 1998;46:43–4.

Tumor Necrosis Factor-Alpha (TNF-α) Inhibitors

Class Members: adalimumab (Humira®), certolizumab pegol (Cimzia®), etanercept (Enbrel®), golimumab (Simponi®), infliximab (Remicade®)

Typical Uses: rheumatoid arthritis, ankylosing spondylitis, psoriatic arthritis, plaque psoriasis (adalimumab, etanercept, infliximab), Crohn's disease (adalimumab, certolizumab pegol, infliximab), ulcerative colitis (adalimumab, golimumab, infliximab), hidradenitis suppurativa (adalimumab), uveitis (adalimumab)

Potential Neurologic or Psychiatric Medication Adverse Effects: Non-CNS adverse effect profiles of TNF-α inhibitors are similar among class members. Very common neurologic adverse effects (>10%) include headache (adalimumab, infliximab). Common adverse effects (1–10%) include paresthesia (adalimumab, golimumab), headache (certolizumab pegol, etanercept), confusion (adalimumab), fatigue/weakness (certolizumab pegol, etanercept, infliximab), pain (adalimumab, infliximab), myasthenia (adalimumab), tremor (adalimumab), anxiety (certolizumab), bipolar mood disorder (certolizumab), suicidal tendencies (certolizumab), dizziness (golimumab), and chills (infliximab). Post-marketing surveillance has revealed the potential for new onset or worsening demyelinating central nervous system diseases with TNF-α inhibitor use. These include optic neuritis, multiple sclerosis, systemic vasculitis, and Guillain–Barré syndrome. Any patient developing these neurologic side effects with a TNF-α inhibitor should discontinue therapy and consider use of an alternative agent.

Further Reading

Adalimumab. In *Lexi-Drugs. Lexicomp*. Hudson, OH: Wolters Kluwer Health, Inc. http://online.lexi.com. Accessed Oct 3, 2016.

Certolizumab. In *Lexi-Drugs. Lexicomp*. Hudson, OH: Wolters Kluwer Health, Inc. http://online.lexi.com. Accessed Oct 3, 2016.

Etanercept. In *Lexi-Drugs. Lexicomp*. Hudson, OH: Wolters Kluwer Health, Inc. http://online.lexi.com. Accessed Oct 3, 2016.

Golimumab. In *Lexi-Drugs. Lexicomp*. Hudson, OH: Wolters Kluwer Health, Inc. http://online.lexi.com. Accessed Oct 3, 2016.

Infliximab. In *Lexi-Drugs. Lexicomp*. Hudson, OH: Wolters Kluwer Health, Inc. http://online.lexi.com. Accessed Oct 3, 2016.

Medications to Treat Neurodegenerative Diseases

Angela M. Hill, PharmD, BCPP, CPh University of South Florida Byrd Alzheimer's Institute
Jasmine B. R. Cutler, PharmD, CPh University of South Florida Byrd Alzheimer's Institute
Kristin Robinson, PharmD Florida A&M University College of Pharmacy and Pharmaceutical Sciences

Amantadine (Symmetrel®)

Typical Uses: idiopathic Parkinson's disease, postencephalitic parkinsonism, symptomatic parkinsonism (due to carbon monoxide intoxication), drug-induced extrapyramidal reactions, influenza A prophylaxis and treatment, Parkinson's disease dementia, chorea of Huntington's disease, multiple sclerosis-related fatigue, restless legs syndrome, traumatic brain injury, Lewy body dementia

Potential Neurologic or Psychiatric Medication Adverse Effects: The most frequent adverse effects associated with amantadine (1–10%) include headache, dizziness, drowsiness, fatigue, confusion, abnormal dreams, agitation, irritability, anxiety, nervousness, insomnia, ataxia (uncontrolled body movements), delirium, hallucinations, and depression. Additional adverse effects include xerostomia (dry mouth), gastric distress (e.g., nausea), anorexia, constipation, and diarrhea. Patients should not operate heavy machinery or perform tasks that require mental alertness until they know how amantadine affects their physical and mental capabilities. Amantadine should be used with caution in patients with a history of psychosis, seizure disorder, cardiovascular disease, and hepatic and renal impairment. Patients with untreat angle closure glaucoma should avoid the use of amantadine due to its anticholinergic-like side effects. Doses of amantadine should be divided and administered twice daily to elderly patients to decrease the risk of central nervous system effects. Prescribers should monitor behaviors associated with impulse control disorders such as pathologic gambling, hypersexuality, and/or binge eating. Benefits from amantadine therapy in Parkinson's disease decrease over time (e.g., several months); however, abrupt discontinuation of amantadine is strongly discouraged to avoid neuroleptic malignant syndrome (NMS). NMS is characterized by fever or hyperthermia, muscle rigidity, altered consciousness, involuntary movements, altered mental status, tachycardia, and hyper- or hypotension. Additional laboratory findings may indicate NMS such as leukocytosis and CPK elevation. Prescribers are advised to slowly taper doses with caution to avoid agitation, delirium, hallucinations, paranoia, parkinsonian crisis, slurred speech, or stupor. Prescribers are also advised to monitor for potential drug–drug interactions that may decrease the therapeutic effect of amantadine, increase the risk of anticholinergic effects, or increase the risk of QTc-prolongation.

Further Reading

Amantadine. *Clinical Pharmacology [Internet]*. Tampa, FL: Elsevier. 2017. Available from www.clinicalpharmacology.com. Accessed Aug 14, 2017.

Chen JJ, Dashtipour K. Parkinson disease. In DiPiro JT, Talbert RL, Yee GC, et al., eds. *Pharmacotherapy: a pathophysiologic approach*. 10th ed. New York, NY: McGraw-Hill; 2017: p. 895. http://accesspharmacy .mhmedical.com.ezproxy.hsc.usf.edu/content .aspx?bookid=1861&sectionid=134127873. Accessed Aug 14, 2017.

Lexicomp Online, Lexi-Drugs Online. Hudson, OH: Wolters Kluwer Clinical Drug Information, Inc.; Aug 14, 2017.

Spritzer SD, Kinney CL, Condie J, et al. Amantadine for patients with severe traumatic brain injury: a critically appraised topic. *Neurologist*. 2015;19:61–4.

Stinton C, McKeith I, Taylor JP, et al. Pharmacological management of Lewy body dementia: a systematic review and meta-analysis. *Am J Psychiatry*. 2015;172:731–42.

Symmetrel® (amantadine hydrochloride) package
    insert. Chadds Ford, PA. Endo Pharmaceuticals
    Inc.; Jan 2009.

Anticholinergics

Class Members: atropine, benztropine (Cogentin®),
trihexyphenidyl (Artane®), oxybutynin (Ditropan®,
Gelnique®, Oxytrol®), tolterodine (Detrol®), darifenacin (Enablex®), solifenacin (Vesicare®), tiotropium
(Spiriva®), ipratropium (Atrovent®), meclizine, promethazine (Phenergan®), cyproheptadine, diphenhydramine (Benadryl®)

Typical Uses: Parkinson's disease, drug-induced extrapyramidal disorders, overactive bladder, hypersensitivity reactions, allergic rhinitis, asthma, chronic
obstructive pulmonary disease (COPD), nausea and
vomiting, motion sickness, insomnia, benign prostatic
hyperplasia

**Potential Neurologic or Psychiatric Medication Adverse
Effects:** The adverse effect profile is similar among
agents within the anticholinergic class, yet various
agents possess differing degrees of anticholinergic
properties. The most frequently encountered adverse
effects (>10%) include dry mouth, dry skin, dental
problems, constipation, blurred vision, hyperpyrexia
(overheating), confusion, sedation, and dementia-
like symptoms (especially with long-term use). These
adverse effects are dose dependent, and concomitant
use of multiple agents with anticholinergic properties
simultaneously increases the overall anticholinergic
burden scale and adverse side effects. Anticholinergic
side effects are more pronounced in the elderly population, and may increase the risk for falls and injury. This
occurs because clearance of medications is reduced in
advanced age, and tolerance develops when anticholinergics are used for insomnia. The use of medications
with strong anticholinergic effects increases the cumulative risk of cognitive impairment and mortality, especially in the elderly. Darifenacin and solifenacin are
uroselective agents and are preferred in patients who
are intolerant to anticholinergic adverse effects. Use of
transdermals, like Gelnique, or extended release formulations may also lower incidence of anticholinergic
adverse effects. Other less common but noteworthy
adverse effects include nervousness, exacerbation of
preexisting psychotic symptoms, increased anxiety,
disorientation, depression, visual hallucinations,
numbness of fingers, dysphonia (difficulty in speaking),

mydriasis (dilation of the pupil), cycloplegia (paralysis
of accommodation), tachycardia, cardiac arrhythmias,
rapid, shallow breathing, nausea, increased intraocular
pressure, and urinary retention.

Further Reading

American Geriatrics Society. Updated Beers criteria
    for potentially inappropriate medication use in
    older adults. *J Am Geriatr Soc.* 2015;63:2227–46.

Cai X, Campbell N, Khan B, et al. Long-term
    anticholinergic use and the aging brain.
    Alzheimers Dement. 2013;9:377–85.

Fox C, Richardson K, Maidment ID, et al.
    Anticholinergic medication use and cognitive
    impairment in the older population: the Medical
    Research Council Cognitive Function and Aging
    Study. *J Am Geriatr Soc.* 2011;59:1477–83.

Haft S, Farquhar D, Carey R, Mirza N. Anticholinergic
    use is a major risk factor for dysphonia. *Ann Otol
    Rhinol Laryngol.* 2015;124:797–802.

Kara Ö, Arik G, Kizilarslanoglu MC, et al. Potentially
    inappropriate prescribing according to the
    STOPP/START criteria for older adults. *Aging
    Clin Exp Res.* 2016;28:761–8.

Mintzer J, Burns A. Anticholinergic side-effects of
    drugs in elderly people. *J R Soc Med.* 2000;93:
    457–462.

Salahudeen MS, Duffull SB, Nishtala PS.
    Anticholinergic burden quantified by
    anticholinergic risk scales and adverse outcomes
    in older people: a systematic review. *BMC Geriatr.*
    2015;15:31.

Catechol-O-Methyl Transferase (COMT) Inhibitors

Class Members: entacapone (Comtan®), tolcapone
(Tasmar®)

Typical Uses: Parkinson's disease

**Potential Neurologic or Psychiatric Medication Adverse
Effects:** Hallucinations, confusion, tremors, muscle
pain, dizziness, drowsiness, insomnia, or dreaming
more than usual can occur. The most common side
effects with this class of medications include diarrhea,
elevated liver transaminases, discoloration of urine,
and rhabdomyolysis. Because of the risk of liver disease, treatment with tolcapone should be discontinued
within 3 weeks of initiation if no clinical benefit is seen.

Tolcapone should be discontinued if individual liver transaminases (SGOT or SGPT) exceed two times the upper limit of normal or if clinical signs and symptoms suggest the onset of hepatic dysfunction (i.e., nausea, fatigue, lethargy, anorexia, jaundice, dark urine, pruritus, and/or right upper quadrant tenderness). When these agents are used with levodopa/carbidopa, dyskinesias may occur.

Further Reading

Burn D. Parkinson's disease: treatment. *The Pharmaceutical Journal*. 2000;264:476–9.

Chen JJ, Swope D. Parkinson's disease. In DiPiro JT, Talbert RL, Yee GC, et al., eds. *Pharmacotherapy: a pathophysiologic approach*. 9th ed. New York: McGraw-Hill Education/Medical; 2014: Chapter 43.

Entacopone. In *Lexi-Drugs. Lexicomp*. Hudson, OH: Wolters Kluwer Health, Inc. http://online.lexi .com. Accessed Feb 26, 2016.

Jankovic J, Aguillar L. Current approaches to the treatment of Parkinson's disease. *Neuropsychiatr Dis Treat*. 2008;4:743–57.

Müller T. Catechol-O-methyltransferase inhibitors in Parkinson's disease. *Drugs*. 2015;75:157–74.

Tolcapone. In *Lexi-Drugs. Lexicomp*. Hudson, OH: Wolters Kluwer Health, Inc. http://online.lexi .com. Accessed Feb 26, 2016.

Cholinesterase Inhibitors

Class Members: donepezil (Aricept*), memantine/donepezil (Namzaric*), rivastigmine (Exelon*), galantamine (Razadyne*, Reminyl*)

Typical Uses: Alzheimer's disease and other dementias, rivastigmine is FDA-approved for Parkinson's disease dementia

Potential Neurologic or Psychiatric Medication Adverse Events: The adverse effect profile is similar among the agents within the cholinesterase inhibitor class. Very common adverse effects (>10%) include nausea, vomiting, diarrhea, loss of appetite, tired feeling, or sleep problems. Muscle cramps, vivid dreams, or nightmares are commonly seen with donepezil. Stevens–Johnson syndrome and acute generalized exanthematous pustulosis have been reported in patients taking galantamine. Patients taking cholinesterase inhibitors are at risk for seizures and impaired cardiac conduction.

Allergic dermatitis may occur with the rivastigmine transdermal patch. Clinicians are encouraged to inform patients to administer this class with food to minimize gastric distress, and to protect the sleep quality by administering the once-a-day products in the morning with meals.

Further Reading

Agboton C, Mahdavian S, Singh A, Ghazvini P, Hill A, et al. Impact of nighttime donepezil administration on sleep in the older adult population: a retrospective study. *Mental Health Clinician*. 2014;4:95.

Alzheimer's Disease. Pharmacotherapy. A Pathophysiologic Approach. 2014. McGraw Hill Companies.

Birks J. Cholinesterase inhibitors for Alzheimer's disease. *Cochrane Database Syst Rev*. 2006;25:CD005593.

Chitnis S, Rao J. Rivastigmine in Parkinson's disease dementia. *Expert Opin Drug Metab Toxicol*. 2009;5:941–55.

Dwolatzky T, Clarfield A. Cholinesterase inhibitors and memantine in more advanced Alzheimer's disease. The debate continues. *Aging Health*. 2012;8:233–7.

Emre M, Aarsland D, Albanese A, et al. Rivastigmine for dementia associated with Parkinson's disease. *N Engl J Med*. 2004;351:2509–18.

Howard R, McShane R, Lindesay J, et al. Donepezil and memantine for moderate-to-severe Alzheimer's disease. *N Engl J Med*. 2012;366:893–903.

Lockhart I, Mitchell S, Kelly S. Safety and tolerability of donepezil, rivastigmine and galantamine for patients with Alzheimer's disease: systemic review of the "real-world" evidence. *Dement Geriatr Cogn Disord*. 2009;28:389–403.

Dopamine Agonists

Class Members: bromocriptine (Parlodel*), carbergoline (Dostinex*), pergolide (Permax*), pramipexole (Mirapex*), ropinorole (Requip*), apomorphine (Apokyn*), rotigitine (Neupro*), quinagolide (Norprolac*)

Typical Uses: Parkinson's disease, restless leg syndrome, hyperprolactinemia, acromegaly

Potential Neurologic or Psychiatric Medication Adverse Effects: Potential neuropsychiatric adverse effects include hallucinations, headache, confusion, light-headedness, seizures, exacerbation of dyskinesias (twitching, twisting, uncontrolled repetitive movements of the tongue, lips, face, arms, or legs), dizziness, mood or mental changes, and sudden drowsiness. Other side effects that can occur include postural hypotension, chest pain, discomfort, or pressure, chills, cold sweats, and swelling. Pleuropulmonary fibrosis can occur with the ergoline derivatives (i.e., bromocriptine, cabergoline, pergolide). Application site reactions (i.e., burning, itching, redness, skin rash, swelling, or soreness) can occur with rotigitine. Some patients experience new or unusual or increased urges while taking bromocriptine.

Further Reading

Burn D. Parkinson's disease: treatment. *Pharm J.* 2000;264:476–9.

Chen JJ, Swope D. Parkinson's disease. In DiPiro JT, Talbert RL, Yee GC, et al., eds. *Pharmacotherapy: a pathophysiologic approach.* 9th ed. New York: McGraw-Hill Education/Medical; 2014. Chapter 43.

Jankovic J, Aguillar L. Current approaches to the treatment of Parkinson's disease. *Neuropsychiatr Dis Treat.* 2008;4:743–57.

Moore T, Glenmullen J, Mattison D. Reports of pathological gambling, hypersexuality, and compulsive shopping associated with dopamine receptor agonist drugs. *JAMA Intern Med.* 2014;174:1930–3.

Pérez-Pérez J, Pagonabarraga J, Martínez-Horta S, et al. Head-to-head comparison of the neuropsychiatric effect of dopamine agonists in Parkinson's disease: a prospective, cross-sectional study in non-demented patients. *Drugs Aging.* 2015;32(5):401–7.

Weiss H, Pontone G. Dopamine receptor agonist drugs and impulse control disorders. *JAMA Intern Med.* 2014;174(12):1935–7.

Dopamine Precursors

Class Members: levodopa/carbidopa (Sinemet®, Sinemet CR®, Duopa®, Rytary®), levodopa/carbidopa/entacapone (Stalevo®)

Typical Uses: Idiopathic Parkinson's disease, postencephalitic parkinsonism associated with cerebral arteriosclerosis, symptomatic parkinsonism (due to carbon monoxide intoxication and/or manganese intoxication), restless leg syndrome (RLS), amblyopia

Potential Neurologic or Psychiatric Medication Adverse Effects: Patients diagnosed with Parkinson's disease can be prescribed levodopa (or other affiliated formulations) as the disease progresses. Doses should be started low and slowly titrated according to symptom control and patient tolerability. The most frequent adverse effects associated with dopamine precursors (>10%) include dyskinesias (on–off episodes) and involuntary movements, orthostatic hypotension, syncope, hypotension, dizziness, headache, gastric distress, depression with suicidal ideations, insomnia, anxiety, confusion, abnormal dreams and nightmares, and polyneuropathy. Additional adverse effects (1–10%) include hallucinations, agitation, somnolence, hypersexuality, and impulse behaviors (e.g., pathologic gambling). Motor fluctuations or "on–off "episodes develop over time with an estimated risk of 10% per year of levodopa use; however, motor fluctuations may develop within 5 to 6 months of therapy. Abrupt discontinuation of all levodopa-containing agents is strongly discouraged to avoid neuroleptic malignant syndrome (NMS). NMS is characterized by fever or hyperthermia, muscle rigidity, altered consciousness, involuntary movements, altered mental status, tachycardia, and hyper- or hypotension. Additional laboratory findings may indicate NMS such as leukocytosis and CPK elevation. Prescribers are advised to slowly taper doses with caution to avoid agitation, delirium, hallucinations, paranoia, parkinsonian crisis, slurred speech or stupor. Levodopa-containing agents should be used with caution in patients with a history of psychosis, seizure disorder, cardiovascular disease, and hepatic and renal impairment.

Further Reading

Chen JJ, Dashtipour K. Parkinson disease. In DiPiro JT, Talbert RL, Yee GC, et al. eds. *Pharmacotherapy: a pathophysiologic approach.* 10th ed. New York, NY: McGraw-Hill; 2017: p. 895. http://accesspharmacy .mhmedical.com.ezproxy.hsc.usf.edu/content .aspx?bookid=1861&sectionid=134127873. Accessed Aug 14, 2017.

Jankovic J, Aguillar L. Current approaches to the treatment of Parkinson's disease. *Neuropsychiatr Dis Treat.* 2008;4:743–57.

Lexicomp Online, Lexi-Drugs Online. Hudson, OH: Wolters Kluwer Clinical Drug Information, Inc. Accessed Aug 14, 2017.

Sinemet® (carbidopa levodopa tablets) package insert. Morgantown, WV: Mylan Pharmaceuticals Inc.; Jul 2014.

Stalevo® (carbidopa, levodopa and entacapone tablets) package insert. East Hanover, New Jersey. Novartis Pharmaceuticals Inc.; Feb 2016.

Thanvi B, Lo N, Robinson T. Levodopa-induced dyskinesia in Parkinson's disease: clinical features, pathogenesis, prevention and treatment. *Postgrad Med J*. 2007;83:384–8.

Memantine (Namenda®, Namenda XR®), Memantine/Donepezil (Namzaric®)

Typical Uses: Alzheimer's disease, mild to moderate vascular dementia, depression, schizophrenia, obsessive-compulsive disorder, substance abuse, pervasive development disorders, bipolar disorder, acquired pendular nystagmus, and binge eating disorder

Potential Neurologic or Psychiatric Medication Adverse Effects: The most frequent adverse effects (>5%) include dizziness, headache, confusion, constipation, agitation, somnolence, amnesia, anxiety, sedation, insomnia, hyperactivity, and increased sexual interest and arousal. Additional adverse effects (<5%) include depression, hallucinations, hypertension, influenza-like symptoms/upper respiratory infections, and peripheral edema. Administration with a morning meal to avoid insomnia and gastric distress is advised. Memantine should be used with caution in patients with existing cardiovascular disease (e.g., angina, bradycardia), renal and hepatic impairment, and seizure disorders. Should be used with extreme caution in patients who report a hypersensitivity to memantine or an allergy to any of its derivatives (e.g., amantadine).

Further Reading

Albrecht H, Dieterich M, Pöllmann W, Starck M, Straube A. Drug therapy for acquired pendular nystagmus in multiple sclerosis. *J Neurol*. 1996;244:9–16.

Lexicomp Online, Lexi-Drugs Online. Hudson, Ohio: Wolters Kluwer Clinical Drug Information, Inc.; Aug 14, 2017.

Matsunaga S, Kishi T, Iwata N. Memantine monotherapy for Alzheimer's disease: a systematic review and meta-analysis. *PloS One*. 2015;10:e0123289.

Memantine. *Clinical Pharmacology [Internet]*. Tampa, FL: Elsevier; 2017. Available from: www.clinicalpharmacology.com. Accessed Aug 14, 201.

Namenda (memantine hydrochloride) extended release capsule package insert. New York City, NY: Forest Pharmaceuticals, Inc.; Jun 2016.

Robinson DM, Keating GM. Memantine: a review of its use in Alzheimer's disease. *Drugs*. 2006;66:1515–34.

Shi X, Lin X, Hu R, Sun N, Hao J, Gao C. Toxicological differences between NMDA receptor antagonists and cholinesterase inhibitors. *Am J Alzheimers Dis Other Demen*. 2016;31:405–12.

Zdanys K, Tampi RR. A systematic review of off-label uses of memantine for psychiatric disorders. *Prog Neuropsychopharmacol Biol Psychiatry*. 2008;32:1362–74.

Natalizumab (Tysabri®)

Typical Uses: multiple sclerosis, Crohn's disease

Potential Neurologic or Psychiatric Medication Adverse Effects: The most frequent adverse effects associated with natalizumab (>10%) include headache, fatigue, depression, neuromuscular effects (e.g., arthralgia, extremity pain, and back pain), rash, infusion-related reactions, influenza or flu-like syndrome, nausea, gastroenteritis, abdominal discomfort, and respiratory and urinary tract infections. Additional adverse effects (1–10%) include vertigo, dysesthesia (impairment of sensitivity – touch), syncope, somnolence, muscle cramps, tremors, rigors, joint swelling, night sweats, peripheral edema, and menstrual irregularities. Natalizumab, a monoclonal antibody, is an immunosuppressive agent, which may increase the risk of opportunistic and severe herpes infections. Natalizumab is also associated with hepatotoxicity and a rare, yet severe inflammatory response, due to immune system recovery, known as immune reconstitution inflammatory syndrome (IRIS). All potential candidates should receive a full workup and be assessed for human immunodeficiency virus (HIV), treponema, hepatitis B and C, cytomegalovirus (CMV), and tuberculosis prior to initiating therapy. Tysabri® has a boxed warning for progressive multifocal leukoencephalopathy (PML), a disabling and potentially fatal opportunistic viral infection of the brain. Signs and symptoms associated with PML include cognitive impairment, visual deficits, apraxia (inability to execute movements although one is physically capable of executing them), and seizures. Risk factors for PML include prolonged used of natalizumab (>2 years), history of immuno-suppressive therapy, and anti-JC virus antibodies. The risk of developing PML ranges from <1/1000 in patients who are anti-JCV antibody-negative, have no history of immunosuppressive therapy, and treatment with natalizumab less than 24 months to up to 13/1000 in patients who are anti-JCV antibody-positive, have a history of immunosuppressive therapy, and treatment with natalizumab greater than 24 months. There are currently no interventions that may prevent or treat PML. Although discontinuation of natalizumab in the presence of PML is advised, PML has been reported following the discontinuation of Tysabri®. Routine monitoring of lab tests (e.g., liver function, CBC, ELISA, CSF), imaging (e.g., MRI), and signs and symptoms of PML for at least 6 months is strongly advised. Tysabri® is only available through the TOUCH® Prescribing Program to registered patients, prescribers, and select pharmacies and infusion centers.

Further Reading

Coles A. Newer therapies for multiple sclerosis. *Ann Indian Acad Neurol.* 2015;18(Suppl 1):S30–34.

Fabis-Pedrini MJ, Xu W, Burton J, et al. Asymptomatic progressive multifocal leukoencephalopathy during natalizumab therapy with treatment. *J Clin Neurosci.* 2016;25:145–7.

Lexicomp Online, Lexi-Drugs Online. Hudson, Ohio: Wolters Kluwer Clinical Drug Information, Inc.; Aug 14, 2017.

Natalizumab. *Clinical Pharmacology [Internet].* Tampa, FL: Elsevier; 2017. www.clinicalpharmacology .com. Accessed Aug 14, 2017.

Plavina T, Subramanyam M, Bloomgren G, et al. Anti-JC virus antibody levels in serum or plasma further define risk of natalizumab-associated progressive multifocal leukoencephalopathy. *Ann Neurol.* 2014;76:802–12.

Rommer PS, Dudesek A, Stuve O, et al. Monoclonal antibodies in treatment of multiple sclerosis. *Clin Exp Immunol.* 2014;175:373–84.

Tysabri® (natalizumab) injection package insert. Cambridge, MA: Biogen, Idec Inc.; May 2016.

Riluzole (Rilutek®)

Typical Uses: Riluzole is FDA-approved for amyotrophic lateral sclerosis (ALS); however, there are case reports and off-label use of riluzole in refractory depression, obsessive-compulsive disorder, generalized anxiety disorder, and chorea of Huntington's disease.

Potential Neurologic or Psychiatric Medication Adverse Effects: Very common adverse effects include asthenia (abnormal physical weakness or lack of energy), vertigo, somnolence, dizziness, malaise, anorexia, and circumoral paresthesias (abnormal sensation around the mouth). Asthenia, circumoral paresthesia, anorexia, dizziness, somnolence, and vertigo are thought to be dose-related. Additional common adverse effects include nausea, abdominal pain, vomiting, and constipation. Other less common adverse effects include agitation, hostility, and tremor (at least 1%). Dizziness occurs more often in women (11%) than men (4%).

Further Reading

Armstrong MJ, Miyasaki JM. Evidence-based guideline: pharmacologic treatment of chorea in Huntington disease: report of the guideline development subcommittee of the American Academy of Neurology. *Neurology.* 2012;79: 597–603.

Coric V, Taskiran S, Pittenger C, et al. Riluzole augmentation in treatment-resistant obsessive–compulsive disorder: an open-label trial. *Biol Psych.* 2005;58:424–8.

Miller R, Jackson C, Kasarskis E, et al. Practice parameter update: the care of the patient with amyotrophic lateral sclerosis: drug, nutritional, and respiratory therapies (an evidence-based review). Report of the quality standards subcommittee of the American Academy of Neurology. *Neurology.* 2009;73:1218–26.

Phuken J, Hardiman O. The management of amyotrophic lateral sclerosis. *J Neurol.* 2009;256:176–86.

Pollack M. Refractory generalized anxiety disorder. *J Clin Psych.* 2009;70(Suppl 2):32–8.

Rilutek (riluzole) tablet [product information]. Laval, Quebec: Sanofi-aventis Canada, Inc; May 2010.

Rilutek. *In RxList®.* WebMD, LLC. www.rxlist.com. Accessed Jan 28, 2016.

Sanacora G, Kendell S, Levin Y, et al. Preliminary evidence of riluzole efficacy in antidepressant-treated patients with residual depressive symptoms. *Biol Psychiatry.* 2007;61:822–5.

Tetrabenazine (Xenazine®)

Typical Uses: tetrabenazine is FDA-approved for chorea associated with Huntington disease; however, there are case reports of off-label use of tetrabenazine in the treatment of tardive dyskinesia, and to a lesser extent in the treatment of tics associated with Tourette's syndrome, dystonia, and myoclonus

Potential Neurologic or Psychiatric Medication Adverse Effects: The most frequently encountered adverse effects (>10%) include sedation/somnolence, depression, anxiety, insomnia, akathisia (agitation and restlessness), fatigue, and nausea. Other less common adverse effects include parkinsonism, bradykinesia (slowness of movement), extrapyramidal disorder, hypertonia (abnormal increase in muscle tension), balance difficulty, falls, and dysphagia (difficulty swallowing). All these side effects appear to be dose related and have higher incidence when used concomitantly with selective serotonin reuptake inhibitors (SSRIs), mood-stabilizing antiepileptic drugs, or antipsychotics. If combined with an SSRI, fluoxetine and paroxetine should be avoided. Other potential side effects associated with tetrabenazine include prolongation of the QT interval, orthostatic hypotension, and neuroleptic malignant syndrome (NMS). Adverse reactions such as QT interval prolongation, NMS, and extrapyramidal disorders may be increased with concomitant use of dopamine antagonists. Several post-marketing adverse events reported include tremors, confusion, and worsening aggression. Tetrabenazine possesses a black box warning for increasing the risk compared with placebo of suicidal thinking and depression in patients with Huntington's disease.

Further Reading

DiPiro JT. *Pharmacotherapy: a pathophysiologic approach*. 9th ed. New York: McGraw-Hill Medical; 2014.

Kertesz DP, Swartz MV, Tadger S, et al. Tetrabenazine for tardive tremor in elderly adults: a prospective follow-up study. *Clin Neuropharmacol*. 2015;38:23–5.

Margolis RL. Tetrabenazine, depression and suicide: good news. *J Huntingtons Dis*. 2014;3:137–8.

Mehanna R, Hunter C, Davidson A, et al. Analysis of CYP2D6 genotype and response to tetrabenazine. *Mov Disord*. 2013;28:210–15.

Xenazine® (tetrabenazine tablets) package insert. Washington, DC: Prestwick Pharmaceuticals; May 2008.

Xenazine. In *RxList®*. WebMD, LLC. www.rxlist.com. Accessed Feb 3, 2016.

Medications to Treat Epilepsy

Jeannine Conway, PharmD, BCPS University of Minnesota College of Pharmacy

Brivaracetam (Briviact®)

Typical Uses: adjunctive treatment for focal seizures for patients 16 years of age and older

Potential Neurologic or Psychiatric Medication Adverse Events: Very common adverse events (>10%) include dizziness, somnolence, and sedation. Common adverse events (1–10%) include fatigue, gait disturbance, balance disorder, and irritability. Only somnolence and sedation were determined to be dose-related adverse reactions. Suicidal behavior and ideation is a warning for all antiseizure medications. Patients should be monitored regularly for changes in mood and suicidal thoughts. Hypersensitivity reactions have been reported including bronchospasm and angioedema. Brivaracetam is secondarily metabolized by CYP 2C19 and poor metabolizers may require lower doses. Brivaracetam did not provide any additional therapeutic benefit when added to levetiracetam treatment. Slow titration is recommended particularly with elderly patients.

Further Reading

Briviact (brivaracetam) package insert. Smyrna, GA: UCB, Inc.; Mar 2016.

Carbamazepine (and Related Agents Like Oxcarbazepine, Eslicarbazepine)

Class Members: carbamazepine (Tegretol®, Tegretol XR®, Carbatrol®, Equetro®), oxcarbazepine (Trileptal®, Oxtellar XR®), eslicarbazepine acetate (Aptiom®)

Typical Uses: trigeminal neuralgia, bipolar 1 acute manic or mixed episodes, focal onset seizures with or without secondary generalization.

Potential Neurologic or Psychiatric Medication Adverse Events: Very common adverse events (>10%) include ataxia, dizziness, somnolence, nystagmus, and headache. Common adverse events (1–10%) include asthenia, trouble with speech, paresthesia, tremor, vertigo, impairment of balance, insomnia, anxiety, and mood swings. Specific to carbamazepine and its tricyclic structure, monoamine oxidase inhibitor (MAOI) medications should be avoided within 14 days of taking carbamazepine and caution with concomitant tricyclic antidepressants is warranted. Patients of Asian descent should be considered for testing for the HLA-B*1502 allele, which has been found to be associated with a higher risk of toxic epidermal necrolysis and Stevens–Johnson syndrome. Additionally, the HLA-A*3101 allele is associated with an increased risk of serious rash in patients with European, Korean, and Japanese ancestry. Drug reaction with eosinophilia and systemic symptoms (DRESS) including Stevens–Johnson syndrome and toxic epidermal necrolysis has been reported. Rashes should be examined and discontinuation of the medication should be considered. The presence of a fever, elevated liver function tests, and eosinophilia should be evaluated for suspected DRESS. Suicidal behavior and ideation is a warning for all antiseizure medications. Patients should be monitored regularly for changes in mood and suicidal thoughts. Hyponatremia can occur during the use of any of these medications and may present with lethargy, confusion, malaise, or obtundation. Cross-sensitivity can occur between carbamazepine and oxcarbazepine/eslicarbazepine requiring close patient monitoring for signs of hypersensitivity. Carbamazepine causes significant liver enzyme induction resulting in the potential for numerous drug–drug interactions. Special attention should be paid to patients' concomitant medications when carbamazepine is added to or removed from a patient's medication regimen.

Further Reading

Aptiom (eslicarbazepine acetate) package insert. Marlborough, MA: Sunovion Pharmaceuticals Inc.; Sep 2016.

Tegretol (carbamazepine) package insert. East Hanover, NJ: Novartis Pharmaceuticals Corporation; Jan 2014.

Trileptal (oxcarbazepine) package insert. East Hanover, NJ: Novartis Pharmaceuticals Corporation; April 2017.

Ethosuximide (Zarontin®)

Typical Uses: absence seizures

Potential Neurologic or Psychiatric Medication Adverse Events: Very common adverse effects (>10%) include fatigue and headache. Common adverse effects (1–10%) include hyperactivity, attention problems, hostility, decreased concentration, personality changes, sleep problems, depression, memory problems, dizziness, and apathy. Drug reaction with eosinophilia and systemic symptoms (DRESS) including Stevens–Johnson syndrome and toxic epidermal necrolysis has been reported. Rashes should be examined and discontinuation of the medication should be considered. The presence of a fever, elevated liver function tests, and eosinophilia should be evaluated for suspected DRESS. Suicidal behavior and ideation is a warning for all antiseizure medications. Patients should be monitored regularly for changes in mood and suicidal thoughts.

Further Reading

Glauser TA, Cnaan A, Shinnar S, et al. Ethosuximide, valproic acid, and lamotrigine in childhood absence epilepsy: Initial monotherapy outcomes at 12 months. *Epilepsia.* 2013;51:141–55.

Zarontin (ethosuximide capsule) package insert. New York, NY: Parke-Davis Div of Pfizer Inc.; May 2016.

Felbamate (Felbatol®)

Typical Uses: refractory patients with seizures where the potential benefits of treatment outweigh the risk of aplastic anemia or liver failure; focal onset seizures in adults as monotherapy and adjunctive treatment and in children with Lennox–Gaustaut

Potential Neurologic or Psychiatric Medication Adverse Events: Very common adverse effects (>10%) include headache, somnolence, dizziness, and insomnia. Common adverse effects (1–10%) include anxiety, tremor, depression, paresthesia, ataxia, nervousness, emotional lability, and agitation. Felbamate should be reserved for refractory patients due to the risk of aplastic anemia and liver failure. Patients who have elevated liver enzyme tests should not take felbamate. The optimal method for patient monitoring is unclear because of the low number of reports of aplastic anemia and hepatic failure. However, at baseline and frequently during treatment, complete blood counts with a differential and serum transaminase levels should be monitored. Suicidal behavior and ideation is a warning for all antiseizure medications. Patients should be monitored regularly for changes in mood and suicidal thoughts.

Further Reading

Felbatol (felbamate tablet) package insert. Somerset, NJ: Meda Pharmaceuticals Inc.; July 2011.

Pellock JM, Faught E, Leppik IE, Shinnar S, Zupanc ML. Felbamate: Consensus of current clinical experience. *Epilepsy Res.* 2006;71:89–101.

Gabapentin (Neurontin®, Gralise®), Gabapentin Enacarbil (Horizant®)

Typical Uses: restless leg syndrome, postherpetic neuralgia, adjunctive treatment of focal seizures, neuropathic pain

Potential Neurologic or Psychiatric Medication Adverse Events: Very common adverse events (>10%) include dizziness, somnolence, sedation, headache, and ataxia. Common adverse events (1–10%) include nystagmus, tremor, depression, dysarthria, abnormal thinking, incoordination, asthenia, hostility, and emotional lability. Gabapentin is completely eliminated via the kidney and has very minimal drug interactions making it a desirable choice for patients on multiple medications. Patients may abuse gabapentin and withdrawal symptoms, including anxiety, insomnia, nausea, pain, and sweating, upon abrupt discontinuation have been reported. Drug reaction with eosinophilia and systemic symptoms (DRESS) including Stevens–Johnson syndrome and toxic epidermal necrolysis has been reported. Rashes should be examined and discontinuation of the medication should be considered. The presence of a fever, elevated liver function tests, and eosinophilia should be evaluated for suspected DRESS. Suicidal behavior and ideation is a warning for all antiseizure medications. Patients should be monitored regularly for changes in mood and suicidal thoughts.

Further Reading

Horizant (gabapentin enacarbil tablet, extended release) package insert. Atlanta, GA: Arbor Pharmaceuticals; Oct 2016.

Neurontin (gabapentin capsule) package insert. New York, NY: Parke-Davis Div of Pfizer Inc; Mar 2017

Lacosamide (Vimpat®)

Typical Uses: adjunctive and monotherapy treatment for focal seizures for patients 17 years of age and older

Potential Neurologic or Psychiatric Medication Adverse Events: Very common adverse events (>10%) include dizziness and headache. Common adverse events (1–10%) include fatigue, gait disturbance, asthenia, ataxia, somnolence, tremor, nystagmus, balance disorder, memory impairment, and depression. The risk for dizziness and ataxia increases above doses of 400 mg per day and they are most likely to occur during titration. Concomitant use of other sodium channel blockers, including carbamazepine, oxcarbazepine, lamotrigine, and phenytoin, increases the risk of side effects as the dose increases. Suicidal behavior and ideation is a warning for all antiseizure medications. Patients should be monitored regularly for changes in mood and suicidal thoughts. Drug reaction with eosinophilia and systemic symptoms (DRESS) including Stevens–Johnson syndrome and toxic epidermal necrolysis has been reported. Rashes should be examined and discontinuation of the medication should be considered. The presence of a fever, elevated liver function tests, and eosinophilia should be evaluated for suspected DRESS. Lacosamide is relatively free of drug–drug interactions, but slow titration is recommended particularly with elderly patients.

Further Reading

Vimpat (lacosamide) package insert. Smyrna, GA: UCB, Inc.; Mar 2017.

Lamotrigine (Lamictal®, Lamictal® XR)

Typical Uses: adjunctive and monotherapy for focal seizures, primarily generalized seizures, and juvenile myoclonic epilepsy. Maintenance treatment of bipolar disorder

Potential Neurologic or Psychiatric Medication Adverse Events: Very common adverse events (>10%) include dizziness, ataxia, somnolence, diplopia, and blurred vision. Common adverse events (1–10%) include headache, incoordination, insomnia, tremor, depression, anxiety, irritability, and trouble with concentration. Rash is one of the greatest concerns when prescribing lamotrigine. Cautious, conservative dosing when concomitant valproate is being used is recommended. Valproate reduces the clearance of lamotrigine resulting in a doubling of half-life, and a much smaller dose of lamotrigine will be required. Drug reaction with eosinophilia and systemic symptoms (DRESS) including Stevens–Johnson syndrome and toxic epidermal necrolysis has been reported. Rashes should be examined and discontinuation of the medication should be considered. The presence of a fever, elevated liver function tests, and eosinophilia should be evaluated for suspected DRESS. Suicidal behavior and ideation is a warning for all antiseizure medications. Patients should be monitored regularly for changes in mood and suicidal thoughts. Cases of aseptic meningitis have been reported. Patients presenting with meningitis symptoms require evaluation of other causes for meningitis to ensure appropriate treatment. Upon rechallenge of lamotrigine, aseptic meningitis may quickly recur.

Further Reading

Lamictal (lamotrigine tablet) package insert. Research Triangle Park, NC: GlaxoSmithKline LLC; May 2016.

Levetiracetam (Keppra®, Keppra XR®)

Typical Uses: FDA approved for adjunctive treatment of focal seizures (for patients 1 month of age and older), primary generalized seizures (for patients 6 years of age and older), and juvenile myoclonic epilepsy (for patients 12 years of age and older); there is evidence that for focal seizures monotherapy is also appropriate

Potential Neurologic or Psychiatric Medication Adverse Events: Very common adverse events (>10%) include asthenia, somnolence, and headache. Common adverse events (1–10%) include dizziness, depression, ataxia, vertigo, anxiety, emotional lability, hostility, aggressiveness, and paresthesia. Interestingly, there does not appear to be a relationship between dose and the rates of somnolence, fatigue, irritability, and dizziness. Somnolence and asthenia most frequently occur within the first 4 weeks of treatment. Behavioral abnormalities including aggression, agitation, anger, anxiety, and depression are possible and may require treatment discontinuation for symptom resolution. Psychotic symptoms including paranoia may occur and treatment discontinuation may be necessary. Suicidal behavior and ideation is a warning for all antiseizure medications. Patients should be monitored regularly for changes in mood and suicidal thoughts. Levetiracetam is virtually devoid of drug–drug interactions making it a first choice in medically complicated patients on high-risk medications such as warfarin and immunosuppressants.

Further Reading

Keppra (levetiracetam tablet) package insert. Smyrna, GA: UCB Farchim SA; April 2010.

Verrotti A, Prezioso G, Di Sabatino F, et al. The adverse event profile of levetiracetam: A meta-analysis on children and adults. *Seizure*. 2015;31:49–55.

Perampanel (Fycompa®)

Typical Uses: adjunctive treatment of focal and generalized seizures for patients aged 12 years and older

Potential Neurologic or Psychiatric Medication Adverse Events: Very common adverse events (>10%) include dizziness, somnolence, headache, and irritability. Common adverse events (1–10%) include fatigue, falls, ataxia, vertigo, dysarthria, anxiety, gait disturbance, hypersomnia, and insomnia. As the dose increases the rates of anxiety, aggression, and anger increase particularly at the dose of 12 mg per day, and patients may require a dose reduction. Serious psychiatric and behavioral reactions were reported during the clinical trials and in post-marketing monitoring including hostility, aggression, belligerence, agitation, physical assault, homicidal ideation, and/or threats. Suicidal behavior and ideation is a warning for all antiseizure medications. Patients should be monitored regularly for changes in mood and suicidal thoughts. Neurologic warnings include risks of dizziness, gait disturbance, somnolence, and fatigue, which led to treatment discontinuation in 2–3% of patients in clinical trials. Falls occurred in 5–10% of patients, which, in some cases, resulted in serious injury.

Further Reading

Ettinger AB, LoPresti A, Yang H, et al. Psychiatric and behavioral adverse events in randomized clinical studies of the noncompetitive AMPA receptor antagonist perampanel. *Epilepsia*. 2015;56:1252–63.

Fycompa® (perampanel tablet) package insert. Woodcliff Lake, NJ: Eisai Inc.; April 2016.

Phenytoin (Dilantin®, Phenytek®)

Typical Uses: generalized tonic–clonic and focal onset seizures, prevention and treatment of seizures during and after neurosurgery

Potential Neurologic or Psychiatric Medication Adverse Events: Phenytoin has been available for use since 1938. As a result, details about rates of side effects are difficult to find. Common neurologic side effects are usually dose related and include nystagmus, ataxia, somnolence, confusion, slurred speech, dizziness, vertigo, insomnia, paresthesias, and decreased coordination. Due to the non-linearity of the dose–response relationship potentially resulting in small dose increases causing significant side effects, smaller dose adjustment is generally recommended. Long-term use of phenytoin has been associated with cerebellar damage, which may be irreversible. Suicidal behavior and ideation is a warning for all antiseizure medications. Patients should be monitored regularly for changes in mood and suicidal thoughts. Drug reaction with eosinophilia and systemic symptoms (DRESS) including Stevens–Johnson syndrome and toxic epidermal necrolysis has been reported. Rashes should be examined and discontinuation of the medication should be considered. The presence of a fever, elevated liver function tests, and eosinophilia should be evaluated for suspected DRESS.

Further Reading

Dilantin (phenytoin sodium capsule, extended release) package insert. New York, NY: Parke-Davis Div of Pfizer Inc; Feb 2017.

Pregabalin (Lyrica®)

Typical Uses: adjunctive therapy for adults with focal seizures, fibromyalgia, neuropathic pain due to diabetic peripheral neuropathy and associated with spinal injury, and postherpetic neuralgia

Potential Neurologic or Psychiatric Medication Adverse Events: Very common adverse events (>10%) include dizziness and somnolence. Common adverse events (1–10%) include neuropathy, ataxia, vertigo, confusion, amnesia, asthenia, headache, tremor, incoordination, abnormal gait, impairment of balance, difficulty with concentration, diplopia, insomnia, nervousness, and euphoria. Abrupt discontinuation is not recommended as withdrawal symptoms may occur. It is speculated that abuse of pregabalin may be possible due to the euphoric effect, and patients who have previously abused benzodiazepine or alcohol should be closely monitored. Suicidal behavior and ideation is a warning for all antiseizure medications. Patients should be monitored regularly for changes in mood and suicidal thoughts.

Further Reading

Lyrica (pregabalin capsule) package insert. New York, NY: Parke-Davis Div of Pfizer Inc; Jan 2017.

Toth C. Pregabalin: latest safety evidence and clinical implications for the management of neuropathic pain. *Ther Adv Drug Saf.* 2014;5:38–56.

Rufinamide (Banzel®)

Typical Uses: adjunctive therapy for treatment of seizures due to Lennox–Gastaut syndrome in patients 1 year of age and older

Potential Neurologic or Psychiatric Medication Adverse Events: Very common adverse events (>10%) include somnolence and headache. Common adverse events (1–10%) include fatigue, dizziness, ataxia, diplopia, psychomotor hyperactivity, aggression, and disturbance in attention. Status epilepticus has been reported but it is unclear if it is due to the medication or underlying seizure disorder. Drug reaction with eosinophilia and systemic symptoms (DRESS) including Stevens–Johnson syndrome and toxic epidermal necrolysis has been reported. Rashes should be examined and discontinuation of the medication should be considered. The presence of a fever, elevated liver function tests, and

eosinophilia should be evaluated for suspected DRESS. **Suicidal behavior and ideation** is a warning for all antiseizure medications. Patients should be monitored regularly for changes in mood and suicidal thoughts.

Further Reading

Banzel (rufinamide tablet, film coated) package insert. Woodcliff Lake, NJ: Eisai Inc.; Jun 2015.

Tiagabine (Gabitril®)

Typical Uses: adjunctive therapy for focal seizures for patients 12 years of age and older

Potential Neurologic or Psychiatric Medication Adverse Events: Very common adverse events (>10%) include dizziness, asthenia, feeling nervous, tremor, and somnolence. Common adverse events (1–10%) include difficulty with concentration, disturbance in speech, insomnia, ataxia, confusion, difficulty with memory, paresthesia, depression, emotional lability, abnormal gait, hostility, nystagmus, and agitation. Tiagabine should not be used in patients without seizures due to the risk of new onset seizures and status epilepticus that has been reported. Additionally, status epilepticus has been reported in patients with seizures but it is unclear if it is due to the medication or underlying seizure disorder. Suicidal behavior and ideation is a warning for all antiseizure medications. Patients should be monitored regularly for changes in mood and suicidal thoughts. Cognitive and neuropsychiatric adverse events also include EEG abnormalities including generalized spike and wave activity and reports of status epilepticus in patients with seizures.

Further Reading

Gabitril (tiagabine hydrochloride tablet, film coated) package insert. North Wales, PA: Cephalon, Inc.; Aug 2016.

Topiramate (Topamax®, Trokendi Xr®, Qudexy XR®)

Typical Uses: monotherapy and adjunctive therapy for patients 2 years of age and older with focal or primarily generalized seizures, migraine prophylaxis

Potential Neurologic or Psychiatric Medication Adverse Events: Very common adverse events (>10%) include dizziness, ataxia, word finding difficulties, speech impairment, paresthesia, nystagmus, somnolence, fatigue, nervousness, psychomotor slowing, difficulty with memory, confusion, depression, difficulty with concentration and anorexia. Common adverse events (1–10%) include asthenia, vertigo, tremor, abnormal gait, mood problems, emotional lability, agitation, impaired cognition, insomnia, aggressive behavior, depression, and anxiety. Suicidal behavior and ideation is a warning for all antiseizure medications. Patients should be monitored regularly for changes in mood and suicidal thoughts. Hyperammonemic encephalopathy resulting in lethargy and altered mental status can occur with topiramate alone or in combination with valproate treatment. Teratogenicity risks include primarily cleft lip and/or palate. Significant cognitive and neuropsychiatric adverse effects are reported with topiramate and are the most likely cause of treatment discontinuation. Cognitive related dysfunction can occur with rapid dose escalation. Gradually increasing the dose can improve tolerability.

Further Reading

Topamax (topiramate tablet, coated) package insert. Titusville, NJ: Janssen Pharmaceuticals, Inc.; May 2017.

Valproate Products

Class Members: valproic acid (Depakene®), valproate sodium (Depacon®), divalproex sodium (Depakote, Depakote® ER)

Typical Uses: monotherapy and adjunctive therapy for focal, absence, primary generalized seizures including juvenile myoclonic epilepsy, migraine prophylaxis, manic episodes associated with bipolar disorder

Potential Neurologic or Psychiatric Medication Adverse Events: Very common adverse events (>10%) include asthenia, somnolence, dizziness, insomnia, headache, and tremor. Common adverse events (1–10%) include diplopia, ataxia, paresthesia, nystagmus, depression, mood swings, and anxiety. Valproate products have several warnings related to serious adverse reactions. Teratogenicity risks include primarily neural tube defects. Additionally, infants exposed in utero have reduced IQ scores at age 6 as compared to children not exposed to valproate products. Women of childbearing potential should only receive valproate

products if the risks of not treating outweigh the risks. Hyperammonemia encephalopathy resulting in lethargy, altered mental status can occur with valproate alone or in combination with topiramate treatment. Drug reaction with eosinophilia and systemic symptoms (DRESS) including Stevens–Johnson syndrome and toxic epidermal necrolysis has been reported. Rashes should be examined and discontinuation of the medication should be considered. The presence of a fever, elevated liver function tests, and eosinophilia should be evaluated for suspected DRESS. Suicidal behavior and ideation is a warning for all antiseizure medications. Patients should be monitored regularly for changes in mood and suicidal thoughts.

Further Reading

Depakote (divalproex sodium tablet, delayed release) package insert. North Chicago, IL: AbbVie Inc.; May 2017.

Nanau R, Neuman MG. Adverse drug reactions induced by valproic acid. *Clin Biochem*. 2013;46:1323–38.

Vigabatrin (Sabril®)

Typical Uses: adjunctive medication for refractory focal seizures in patients 10 years of age and older, monotherapy for infantile spasms in infants 1 month to 2 years of age

Potential Neurologic or Psychiatric Medication Adverse Events: Very common adverse events (>10%) include headache, somnolence, dizziness, nystagmus, tremor, fatigue, and blurred vision. Common adverse events (1–10%) include confusion, aggressive behavior, diplopia, memory impairment, abnormal coordination, disturbance in attention, paresthesia, irritability, depression, anxiety, depressed mood, and peripheral neuropathy. Vigabatrin is only available through a Risk Evaluation and Mitigation Strategy program (REMS) requiring prescribers to be certified, patients to consent, and pharmacies to also be certified to comply with the REMS requirements and only to dispense to enrolled patients. The clinical use of vigabatrin is significantly limited due to the risk of permanent vision loss, which can occur at any time including after discontinuation. If no clinical benefit is seen within 3 months for complex partial seizures or 2–4 weeks for infantile spasms, the medication should be discontinued. Vision must be assessed by an ophthalmic professional with visual field assessments at baseline, every 3 months while on therapy, and every 3–6 months after discontinuation. Magnetic resonance imaging abnormalities including increased T2 signal and restricted diffusion involving the thalamus, basal ganglia, brainstem, and cerebellum have been reported in up to 22% of infants. The clinical correlation of abnormalities with symptoms has not been established. These abnormalities do not occur in patients older than 3 years. Suicidal behavior and ideation is a warning for all antiseizure medications. Patients should be monitored regularly for changes in mood and suicidal thoughts.

Further Reading

Ferrie CD, Robinson RO, Panayiotopoulos CP. Psychotic and severe behavioural reactions with vigabatrin: a review. *Acta Neurol Scand.* 1996;93(1):1–8.

Vigabatrin (vigabatrin tablet, film coated) package insert. Deerfield, IL: Lundbeck Pharmaceuticals LLC; April 2017.

Zonisamide (Zonegran®)

Typical Uses: adjunctive medication for focal seizures and initial monotherapy in adults with focal seizures

Potential Neurologic or Psychiatric Medication Adverse Events: Very common adverse effects (>10%) include headache, dizziness, weight loss/lack of appetite, and somnolence. Common adverse effects (1–10%) include difficulty concentrating, difficulty with memory, confusion, mental slowing, nausea, ataxia, nystagmus, paresthesia, agitation/irritability, insomnia, anxiety, and nervousness. Kidney stones are also a common adverse effect and may be related to metabolic acidosis, which also may present with symptoms of confusion or lethargy. Measurement of serum bicarbonate is recommended before treatment and periodically during treatment. Drug reaction with eosinophilia and systemic symptoms (DRESS) including Stevens–Johnson syndrome and toxic epidermal necrolysis has been reported. Rashes should be examined and discontinuation of the medication should be considered. The presence of a fever, elevated liver function tests, and eosinophilia should be evaluated for suspected DRESS. Suicidal behavior and ideation is a warning for all antiseizure medications. Patients should be monitored regularly for changes in mood and suicidal thoughts. Status epilepticus has been reported but it is unclear if it is due to the medication or underlying seizure disorder.

Further Reading

Verrotti A, Loiacono G, Di Sabatino F, Zaccara G. The adverse event profile of zonisamide: a meta-analysis. *Acta Neurol Scand.* 2013;128(5):297–304.

Zonegran (zonisamide capsule) package insert. St. Michael, Barbados: Concordia Pharmaceuticals Inc.; April 2016.

Medications to Treat Headache and Migraine

F. Michael Cutrer, MD Mayo Clinic College of Medicine
Aaron A. Bubolz, DO Aurora Health Care Medical Group

Antiemetics

Typical Uses: nausea, emesis/vomiting including that related to acute migraine

Cannabinoids

Class Members: nabilone (Cesamet®), dronabinol (Marinol®)

Potential Neurologic or Psychiatric Medication Adverse Effects: Nabilone is a closely related tetrahydrocannabinol (THC) analog that has been available in other countries and is now approved for use in the United States. Dronabinol has sympathomimetic activity which may often produce central nervous system and psychiatric adverse effects including conjunctival injection, euphoria, somnolence, detachment, depersonalization, temporal deterioration, dizziness, anxiety, nervousness, panic, paranoid reactions, thinking abnormalities, irritability, insomnia, restlessness, vertigo, dysphoria, hallucinations, increased appetite and orthostatic hypotension, and abuse.

Further Reading

Dronabinol, In *Micromedex 2.0*. Greenwood Village, CO: Truven Health Analytics, Inc. http://micromedexsolutions.com. Accessed Jan 22, 2016.

Gutierrez K. Pharmacotherapeutics. In *Clinical reasoning in primary care*. 2nd ed. St. Louis, MO: Saunders Elsevier; 2007. pp. 894–902.

Katzung B, Trevor A. In *Basic & clinical pharmacology*. 13th ed. New York, McGraw-Hill Publishing; 2015. pp. 1068–71, 1080.

Longstreth GF, Hesketh PJ. Characteristics of antiemetic drugs. In Post TW, ed. *UpToDate*. Waltham, MA: UpToDate; 2016.

Nabilone. In *Micromedex 2.0*. Greenwood Village, CO: Truven Health Analytics, Inc. http://micromedexsolutions.com. Accessed Jan 22, 2016.

Dopamine Receptor Antagonists

Class Members: phenothiazines: chlorpromazine, prochlorperazine, perphenazine, promethazine, thiethylperazine; **butyrophenones:** droperidol, haloperidol; **benzamides:** metoclopramide, trimethobenzamide, domperidone

Potential Neurologic or Psychiatric Medication Adverse Effects: Phenothiazines also have M1-muscarinic and H1-histamine blocking effects. Adverse effects include extrapyramidal reactions (dystonia, tardive dyskinesia, pseudoparkinsonism, akathisia, neuroleptic malignant syndrome), exacerbation of parkinsonism symptoms, reduced seizure threshold, orthostatic hypotension, and sedation. The butyrophenones subclass of the dopamine receptor antagonists are major tranquilizers that potentiate the actions of opioids and have an antiemetic effect when used alone. Their main adverse effects include QT prolongation, torsades de pointes, hypotension, alpha blockade, acute dystonia, and extreme sedation. Overall they have less extrapyramidal symptoms and orthostatic hypotension than the phenothiazines. Benzamides may also have serotonergic and/or cholinergic effects at specific doses. As blood–brain barrier permeability is subject to metoclopramide many central nervous system and psychiatric side effects may be expected such as anxiety, restlessness, depression, akathisia, dizziness, dystonia, dystonic reactions (torticollis, oculogyric crisis), parkinsonism, sedation, and tardive dyskinesia. Overall extrapyramidal symptom frequency is 4% but may be as high as 30% in men under the age of 30 years. Reversal drugs include diphenhydramine, benztropine, and diazepam. Domperidone does not cross the blood–brain barrier and therefore avoids most neurologic side effects. Metoclopramide has a black box warning from the US Food and Drug Administration related to risks of irreversible tardive dyskinesia with higher dosing and long-term use.

Further Reading

Brunton LL, Laurence L, Chabner BA, Knollmann BC. *Goodman & Gilman's the pharmacological basis of therapeutics.* 12th ed. New York: McGraw-Hill Publishing; 2011. pp. 1341–6.

Gutierrez K. Pharmacotherapeutics. In *Clinical reasoning in primary care.* 2nd ed. St. Louis, MO: Saunders Elsevier; 2007. pp. 894–902.

Katzung B, Trevor A. *Basic & clinical pharmacology.* 13th ed. New York: McGraw-Hill Publishing; 2015. pp. 1068–1071, 1080.

Longstreth GF, Hesketh PJ. Characteristics of antiemetic drugs. In Post TW, ed. *UpToDate.* Waltham, MA: UpToDate; 2016.

Micromedex 2.0. Greenwood Village, CO: Truven Health Analytics, Inc. http://micromedexsolutions.com. Accessed Jan 22, 2016.

Neurokinin Receptor Antagonists

Class Members: aprepitant (Emend®), fosaprepitant (Emend®), rolapitant (Varubi®), netupitant (Akynzeo®)

Potential Neurologic or Psychiatric Medication Adverse Effects: Neurokinin-1 (NK1) receptor antagonists are moderate inhibitors of the CYP3A4 or CYP2D6 (rolapitant) metabolic pathways and cause central blockade at the area postrema. These receptor are agonized by substance P and can be antagonized by the medications in this class listed above. These NK1 receptor antagonists do indeed cross the blood–brain barrier and they have no affinity for serotonin, dopamine, or corticosteroid receptors. Adverse effects are relatively minimal including fatigue and dizziness.

Further Reading

Brunton LL, Laurence L, Chabner BA, Knollmann BC. *Goodman & Gilman's the pharmacological basis of therapeutics.* 12th ed. New York: McGraw-Hill Publishing; 2011. pp. 1341–6.

Gutierrez K. Pharmacotherapeutics. In *Clinical reasoning in primary care.* 2nd ed. St. Louis, MO: Saunders Elsevier; 2007. pp. 894–902.

Katzung B, Trevor A. *Basic & clinical pharmacology.* 13th ed. New York: McGraw-Hill Publishing; 2015. pp. 1068–1071, 1080.

Longstreth GF, Hesketh PJ. Characteristics of antiemetic drugs. In Post TW, ed. *UpToDate.* Waltham, MA: UpToDate; 2016.

Micromedex 2.0. Greenwood Village, CO: Truven Health Analytics, Inc. http://micromedexsolutions.com. Accessed Jan 22, 2016.

Serotonin Receptor Antagonists

Class Members: ondansetron (Zofran®), granisetron (Kytril®), dolasetron (Anzemet®), and palonosetron (Aloxi®)

Potential Neurologic or Psychiatric Medication Adverse Effects: Oral formulations are comparable in efficacy to intravenous dosing. 5-HT3-receptor antagonists are metabolized by P-450 2D6 and do not inhibit dopamine or muscarinic receptors. Headache is the most frequent adverse event (24%) followed by dizziness (10%) and asthenia (5%). Other adverse events include fatigue (13%), malaise, weakness, somnolence, agitation, anxiety, central nervous system stimulation, pain, shivering, orthostatic hypotension, and syncope. 5-HT3 receptor antagonists have been less associated with cognitive, psychomotor, or affective disturbances than the dopamine antagonists or the antihistamines. The dose of ondansetron should be reduced with the presence of concomitant hepatic disease.

Further Reading

Brunton LL, Laurence L, Chabner BA, Knollmann BC. *Goodman & Gilman's the pharmacological basis of therapeutics.* 12th ed. New York: McGraw-Hill Publishing; 2011. pp. 1341–6.

Gutierrez K. Pharmacotherapeutics. In *Clinical reasoning in primary care.* 2nd ed. St. Louis, MO: Saunders Elsevier; 2007. pp. 894–902.

Katzung B, Trevor A. *Basic & clinical pharmacology.* 13th ed. New York: McGraw-Hill Publishing; 2015. pp. 1068–1071, 1080.

Longstreth GF, Hesketh PJ. Characteristics of antiemetic drugs. In Post TW, ed. *UpToDate.* Waltham, MA: UpToDate; 2016.

Micromedex 2.0. Greenwood Village, CO: Truven Health Analytics, Inc. http://micromedexsolutions.com. Accessed Jan 22, 2016.

Botulinum Toxin A Injections

Class Members: onabotulinum toxin A (Botox®, Botox cosmetic®)

Typical Uses: chronic migraine, bladder dysfunction, blepharospasm, cervical dystonia, spasticity, strabismus, wrinkles

Potential Neurologic or Psychiatric Medication Adverse Effects: A very common adverse effect (>10%) is cervical dystonia (11%); common adverse effects (1–10%) include primary axillary hyperhidrosis (3% to 10%). Other less common adverse effects of botulinum toxin A include excessive weakness in neck extensor muscles, eyelid ptosis, brow ptosis, diplopia, dysphagia, dysphonia, blurred vision, neck pain, and seizure. Black box warning: botulinum toxin products may spread from the area of injection to produce symptoms hours to weeks after injection consistent with botulinum toxin effects. Swallowing and breathing difficulties can be life threatening, and there have been reports of death. Children treated for spasticity likely have the greatest risk, but symptoms can also occur in adults. Cases of spread of effect have occurred at doses comparable to those used to treat cervical dystonia and upper limb spasticity, and at lower doses.

Further Reading

Brunton LL, Laurence L, Chabner BA, Knollmann BC. *Goodman & Gilman's the pharmacological basis of therapeutics.* 12th ed. New York: McGraw-Hill Publishing; 2011. p. 1792.

Gutierrez K. Pharmacotherapeutics. In *Clinical reasoning in primary care.* 2nd ed. St. Louis, MO: Saunders Elsevier; 2007. p. 381.

Post TW, ed. *UpToDate.* Waltham, MA: UpToDate. Accessed Jan 22, 2016.

OnabotulinumtoxinA. In *Micromedex 2.0.* Greenwood Village, CO: Truven Health Analytics, Inc. http://micromedexsolutions.com. Accessed Jan 22, 2016.

Butalbital

Class Members: butalbital, caffeine, and acetaminophen (Fioricet®, Esgic); butalbital, caffeine, and aspirin (Fiorinal®); butalbital and acetaminophen (Phrenilin®)

Typical Uses: tension or muscle contraction headache, migraine

Potential Neurologic or Psychiatric Medication Adverse Effects: Very common adverse effects (>10%) include dizziness, lightheadedness, drowsiness, and "hangover" effect. Common adverse effects (1–10%) include confusion, mental depression, unusual excitement, nervousness, faint feeling, headache, insomnia, nightmares, fatigue, and weakness. Other reported side effects include a shaky feeling, tingling, agitation, heavy eyelids, high energy, hot spells, numbness, sluggishness, dry mouth, hyperhidrosis, and seizure. Mental confusion, depression, or excitement can also occur due to intolerance, particularly in elderly or debilitated patients, or due to overdosage of butalbital. It should also be noted that in patients treated with warfarin, butalbital decreases the anticoagulation effect thereby lowering INR. Butalbital may be habit forming and can be associated with a withdrawal syndrome characterized by restlessness, convulsions, and hallucinations. Butalbital may cause central nervous system depression, which may impair physical or mental abilities; patients must be cautioned about performing tasks that require mental alertness.

Further Reading

DailyMed. Bethesda, MD: US National Library of Medicine. https://dailymed.nlm.nih.gov/dailymed/index.cfm. Accessed Jan 22, 2016.

Micromedex 2.0. Greenwood Village, CO: Truven Health Analytics, Inc. http://micromedexsolutions.com. Accessed Jan 22, 2016.

Post TW, ed. *UpToDate.* Waltham, MA: UpToDate; 2016.

Caffeine

Class Members: oral caffeine (Cafcit®, Keep Alert, No Doz®, Stay Awake, Vivarin®)

Typical Uses: central nervous system stimulant, augmentation of seizure induction during electroconvulsive therapy (ECT) (caffeine and sodium benzoate); spinal puncture headache (caffeine and sodium benzoate); central nervous system stimulant, diuretic (caffeine and sodium benzoate)

Potential Neurologic or Psychiatric Medication Adverse Effects: Central nervous system stimulation, agitation, delirium, confusion, dizziness, hallucination, headache, insomnia, irritability, psychosis, restlessness, anxiety, nervousness, panic, tremor or worsening of tremor, tinnitus, sensitivity to pain or touch, fasciculations, seizures/lowering of seizure threshold, convulsions, medullary stimulation. Decreased reaction time to both visual and auditory events. Decline in delicate muscular coordination, accurate timing, and arithmetic skills. Withdrawal presents as fatigue, sedation, headaches, nausea, and weakness. Acute or chronic exposure causally related to headache. Rebound headaches if overused and withdrawal headaches if stopped.

Further Reading

Gutierrez K. Pharmacotherapeutics. In *Clinical reasoning in primary care*. 2nd ed. St. Louis, MO: Saunders Elsevier; 2007: p. 164.

Helms RA, Quan DJ, Herfindal ET, Gourley GK. *Textbook of therapeutics: drug and disease management*. 8th ed. Philadelphia, PA: Lippincott Williams and Wilkins; 2007. p. 445.

Katzung B, Trevor A. *Basic & clinical pharmacology*. 13th ed. New York: McGraw-Hill Publishing; 2015: pp. 257, 341–342, 1092.

Micromedex 2.0. Greenwood Village, CO: Truven Health Analytics, Inc. http:// micromedexsolutions.com. Accessed Jan 22, 2016.

Post TW, ed. *UpToDate*. Waltham, MA: UpToDate; 2016.

Ergotamines

Dihydroergotamine (D.H.E. 45®, Migranal® Nasal Spray)

Typical Uses: migraine, status migrainosus, cluster headache

Potential Neurologic or Psychiatric Medication Adverse Effects: Very common adverse effects (>10%) include nausea (72%). Common adverse effects (1–10%) include taste disorder (nasal spray) (8%), dizziness (4%), drowsiness (3%), stiffness (1%), weakness (1%). Uncommon adverse effects (<1%) include cerebral hemorrhage, cerebrovascular accident, numbness, subarachnoid hemorrhage. Other reported side effects in which percentages are not specified include paresthesia, dizziness, anxiety, dyspnea, headache, flushing, diarrhea, increased sweating, and pleural and retroperitoneal fibrosis after long-term use of dihydroergotamine. Black box warning: serious

and/or life-threatening peripheral ischemia has been associated with the coadministration of dihydroergotamine with potent CYP3A4 inhibitors including protease inhibitors and macrolide antibiotics. Because CYP3A4 inhibition elevates the serum levels of dihydroergotamine, the risk for vasospasm leading to cerebral ischemia and/or ischemia of the extremities is increased. Hence, concomitant use of these medications is contraindicated.

Further Reading

Bajwa ZH, Smith JH. Acute treatment of migraine in adults. In: Post TW, ed. *UpToDate*. Waltham, MA: UpToDate; 2016.

Brunton LL, Laurence L, Chabner BA, Knollmann BC. *Goodman & Gilman's the pharmacological basis of therapeutics*. 12th ed. New York: McGraw-Hill Publishing; 2011. pp. 347–8.

DailyMed. Bethesda, MD: US National Library of Medicine. https://dailymed.nlm.nih.gov/ dailymed/index.cfm. Accessed Jan 22, 2016.

Dihydroergotamine mesylate In *Micromedex 2.0*. Greenwood Village, CO: Truven Health Analytics, Inc. http://micromedexsolutions.com. Accessed Jan 22, 2016.

DiPiro JT, Talbert RL, Yee GC, et al. In *Pharmacotherapy: a pathophysiologic approach*. 9th ed. New York: McGraw-Hill; 2014. p. 951.

Gutierrez K. Pharmacotherapeutics. In *Clinical reasoning in primary care*. 2nd ed. St. Louis, MO: Saunders Elsevier; 2007; pp. 393–401.

Katzung B, Trevor A. *Basic & clinical pharmacology*. 13th ed. New York: McGraw-Hill Publishing; 2015. pp. 286–91.

Ergotamine (Ergomar®, Cafergot®, Wigraine®)

Typical Uses: migraine

Potential Neurologic or Psychiatric Medication Adverse Effects: The adverse effect profile is similar among agents within the ergotamine class. Common CNS-mediated adverse effects (1–10%) include nausea/vomiting (10%). Other reported side effects include vertigo, numbness, paresthesia, weakness, delirium, auditory hallucinations, rebound/withdrawal headache, numbness, tingling of fingers and toes, extremity muscle pain, precordial pain, transient tachycardia, pruritus, ischemic neuropathy, fatigue, and abdominal pain. Black box warning: ergot alkaloids are contraindicated in combination with strong inhibitors of CYP3A4 (includes protease inhibitors, azole antifungals, and some macrolide antibiotics). Serotonin syndrome is an uncommon disorder that may occur when there is excess synaptic serotonin activity within the central nervous system as a result of an overdose of a single or a combination of several serotonergic drugs. The ergotamines, triptans, second generation antidepressants, tramadol, meperidine, ondansetron, and selective serotonin reuptake inhibitors are all implicated in serotonin syndrome. The symptoms include hypertension, hyperthermia, diarrhea, hyperreflexia, tremor, agitation, and coma. It should be considered when using combinations of multiple serotonin modulatory agents when treating migraine.

Further Reading

Bajwa ZH, Smith JH. Acute treatment of migraine in adults. In: Post TW, ed. *UpToDate*. Waltham, MA: UpToDate; 2016.

Brunton LL, Laurence L, Chabner BA, Knollmann BC. *Goodman & Gilman's the pharmacological basis of therapeutics*. 12th ed. New York: McGraw-Hill Publishing; 2011. pp. 347–8.

DailyMed. Bethesda, MD: US National Library of Medicine. https://dailymed.nlm.nih.gov/dailymed/index.cfm. Accessed Jan 22, 2016.

DiPiro JT, Talbert RL, Yee GC, et al. In *Pharmacotherapy: a pathophysiologic approach*. 9th ed. New York: McGraw-Hill; 2014. p. 951.

Gutierrez K. Pharmacotherapeutics. In *Clinical reasoning in primary care*. 2nd ed. St. Louis, MO: Saunders Elsevier; 2007; pp. 393–401.

Katzung B, Trevor A. *Basic & clinical pharmacology*. 13th ed. New York: McGraw-Hill Publishing; 2015. pp. 286–91.

Micromedex 2.0. Greenwood Village, CO: Truven Health Analytics, Inc. http://micromedexsolutions.com. Accessed Dec 20, 2015.

Isometheptene Mucate

Class Members: acetaminophen, isometheptene, and caffeine (Prodrin®); acetaminophen, isometheptene, and dichloralphenazone (Midrin®)

Typical Uses: migraine, tension-type headache

Potential Neurologic or Psychiatric Medication Adverse Effects: Dizziness and central nervous system depression, which may impair physical or mental abilities. When using isometheptene mucate in a patient with frequent headaches, care must be exercised in patients who also receive prophylactic headache treatment with a tricyclic antidepressant such as amitriptyline as the combination increases the likelihood of tachycardia and palpitations.

Further Reading

Micromedex 2.0. Greenwood Village, CO: Truven Health Analytics, Inc. http://micromedexsolutions.com. Accessed Jan 22, 2016.

Post TW, ed. *UpToDate*. Waltham, MA: UpToDate; 2016.

Muscle Relaxants

Class Members: tizanidine (Zanaflex®), cyclobenzaprine (Flexeril®), orphenadrine (Norflex®)

Typical Uses: tension headache, muscle spasm in neck and back that triggers or exacerbates headache

Potential Neurologic or Psychiatric Medication Adverse Effects: The adverse effect profile is similar among agents within the skeletal muscle relaxant class. Very common adverse effects (>10%) include dry mouth (49–88%), somnolence/drowsiness/sedation (48–92%), dizziness (16–45%), and weakness/asthenia (41–78%). Common adverse effects (1–10%) include fatigue, headache (5%), nervousness (3%), speech disorder (3%), visual hallucinations/delusions (3%), anxiety (1%), depression (1%), fever (1%), dyskinesia (3%), back pain (1%), myasthenia (1%), paresthesia (1%), confusion/disorientation (1–3%), dysarthria (1%), and abnormal EEG (1%). The following side effects are reported in <1% of patients: abnormal dreams, abnormal thinking, deafness, dementia, depersonalization, hemiplegia, neuralgia, optic neuritis, paralysis, psychotic-like symptoms, seizure, suicide attempt, syncope, vertigo, tremor, ataxia, Bell's palsy, insomnia, neuroleptic malignant syndrome, peripheral neuropathy, lightheadedness, syncope, euphoria, and dilation of pupils. Tizanidine is a substrate of CYP1A2 (major) and should not be used in combination with ciprofloxacin or fluvoxamine (potent CYP1A2 inhibitors) as dangerous potentiation of hypotensive and sedative effects may result.

Further Reading

Brunton LL, Laurence L, Chabner BA, Knollmann BC. *Goodman & Gilman's the pharmacological basis of therapeutics.* 12th ed. New York: McGraw-Hill Publishing; 2011. pp. 297, 1828.

Chisholm-Burns MA, Wells BG, Schwinghammer TL, et al. *Pharmacotherapy principles and practice.* 3rd ed. New York: McGraw-Hill; 2013. p. 906.

Cyclobenzaprine hydrochloride. In *Micromedex 2.0.* Greenwood Village, CO: Truven Health Analytics, Inc. http://micromedexsolutions.com. Accessed Jan 22, 2016.

DailyMed. Bethesda, MD: US National Library of Medicine. https://dailymed.nlm.nih.gov/dailymed/index.cfm. Accessed Jan 22, 2016.

Katzung B, Trevor A. *Basic & clinical pharmacology.* 13th ed. New York: McGraw-Hill Publishing; 2015. pp. 145, 150, 469.

Post TW, ed. *UpToDate.* Waltham, MA: UpToDate; 2016.

Nonsteroidal Anti-inflammatory Drugs (NSAIDs)

Class Members: naproxen sodium (Aleve [OTC], All Day Pain Relief [OTC], All Day Relief [OTC], Anaprox, Anaprox DS, EC-Naprosyn, EnovaRX-Naproxen, Equipto-Naproxen, Flanax Pain Relief [OTC], Mediproxen [OTC], Naprelan, Naprosyn, Naproxen Comfort Pac, Naproxen DR, Naproxen Kit); **ibuprofen** (Addaprin [OTC], Advil Junior Strength [OTC], Advil Migraine [OTC], Advil [OTC], Caldolor, Children's Advil [OTC], Children's Ibuprofen [OTC], Children's Motrin Jr Strength [OTC], Children's Motrin [OTC], Dyspel [OTC], EnovaRX-Ibuprofen, Genpril [OTC], HyVee Ibuprofen Children's [OTC], I-Prin [OTC], IBU-200 [OTC], Ibuprofen Children's [OTC], Ibuprofen Comfort Pac, Ibuprofen Junior Strength [OTC], Infants' Advil [OTC], Infants' Ibuprofen [OTC], KS Ibuprofen [OTC], Motrin IB [OTC], Motrin Infants' Drops [OTC], Motrin Junior Strength [OTC], Motrin [OTC], NeoProfen, Provil [OTC]); **ketorolac** (Toradol®; Toradol® IM); **indomethacin** (Indocin; Tivorbex)

Typical Uses: migraine, headache, pain, inflammation, primary dysmenorrhea related headache, autonomic cephalalgias, arthritis

Potential Neurologic or Psychiatric Medication Adverse Effects: The adverse effect profile is similar among agents within the NSAID class. Very common adverse effects (>10%) include headache (17% for ketorolac). Common adverse effects (1–10%) include dizziness (≤9%), drowsiness (3–9%), malaise (<3%), depression (<3%), vertigo (<3%), nervousness (1–3%), tinnitus (3–9%), somnolence (3–9%), lightheadedness, and sweating. The following side effects are reported in <1% of patients: aseptic meningitis, psychosis, hallucinations, cognitive dysfunction, fuzziness, confusion, visual disturbance, seizures, hearing loss, paresthesias, sweating, and blurred vision. Black Box warning: NSAIDs may cause an increased risk of serious cardiovascular thrombotic events, myocardial infarction, and stroke, which can be fatal.

Further Reading

Brunton LL, Laurence L, Chabner BA, Knollmann BC. *Goodman & Gilman's the pharmacological basis of therapeutics.* 12th ed. New York: McGraw-Hill Publishing; 2011. pp. 973–6.

DailyMed. Bethesda, MD: US National Library of Medicine. https://dailymed.nlm.nih.gov/dailymed/index.cfm. Accessed Jan 22, 2016.

Naproxen sodium. In *Micromedex 2.0.* Greenwood Village, CO: Truven Health Analytics, Inc. http://micromedexsolutions.com. Accessed Jan 22, 2016.

Solomon DH. Nonselective NSAIDs: overview of adverse effects. Post TW, ed. *UpToDate.* Waltham, MA: UpToDate; 2016.

Opiates/Opioids

Class Members: oxycodone (Oxaydo®, Oxecta®, Roxicodone®, Oxycontin®), morphine (Avinza®, Kadian®, Oramorph® SR, MS Contin®)

Typical Uses: severe acute pain, cancer pain

Potential Neurologic or Psychiatric Medication Adverse Effects: Opiates cross the blood–brain barrier and activate receptors in the medulla producing central nervous system side effects. As dose determines the response, adverse effects of opiate therapy are more common and severe with increased doses of this class of medications. The binding of opiate receptors in the central nervous system may result in drowsiness, sleep, unconsciousness, decreased mental and physical activity, changes in mood, emotional lability, apathy, tranquility, excessive sweating, feelings of floating, headache, dizziness, confusion, dysphoria, unusual dreams, hallucinations, delirium, and decreased ability to make accurate judgments. Further effects include opioid-induced hyperalgesia/ nociceptive sensitization (allodynia), increased risk of suicide, chronic neuropathic pain states, intensified tone in the large trunk muscles (truncal rigidity), motor un-coordination, weakness, abnormal homeostatic regulation of body temperature, hyperpyrexic coma, decreased stage 3 and 4 sleep, sleep-disordered breathing, central sleep apnea, and seizures (tramadol). Specific percentages as they pertain to two typical opiate adverse effects profiles are provided here. Morphine: dizziness (6%), headache (less than 2% to greater than 10%), lightheadedness, somnolence (3% or greater), miosis, urinary retention (oral, less than 5%; epidural/intrathecal, 15–70%), myoclonus, orthostatic hypotension, syncope, coma (less than 5%), raised intracranial pressure, seizure (less than 5%), drug dependence, and drug withdrawal. Oxycodone: syncope (less than 1%), asthenia (controlled-release, 6%; immediate-release, 3% or greater), dizziness (adults, controlled-release, 13%; immediate-release, 3% or greater; pediatrics, 9%), headache (adults, 3% or greater; pediatrics, 14%), somnolence (controlled-release, 23%; immediate-release, 3% or greater), opioid withdrawal (1–5%). One of the leading causes of death in the United States results from opiate overdose, and methadone causes a severe disproportionate amount of opiate-associated deaths compared with other opiates.

Further Reading

Brunton LL, Laurence L, Chabner BA, Knollmann BC. *Goodman & Gilman's the pharmacological basis of therapeutics*. 12th ed. New York: McGraw-Hill Publishing; 2011. pp. 491–8.

Gutierrez K. Pharmacotherapeutics. In *Clinical reasoning in primary care*. 2nd ed. St. Louis, MO: Saunders Elsevier; 2007. pp. 226–9.

Helms RA, Quan DJ, Herfindal ET, Gourley GK. *Textbook of therapeutics: drug and disease management*. 8th ed. Philadelphia, PA: Lippincott Williams and Wilkins; 2007. pp. 1676–7.

Katzung B, Trevor A. *Basic & clinical pharmacology*. 13th ed. New York: McGraw-Hill Publishing; 2015. pp. 531–51.

Micromedex 2.0. Greenwood Village, CO: Truven Health Analytics, Inc. http://micromedexsolutions.com. Accessed Jan 22, 2016.

Post TW, ed. *UpToDate*. Waltham, MA: UpToDate; 2016.

Salicylates

Class Member: aspirin (Ascriptin Maximum Strength [OTC], Ascriptin Regular Strength [OTC], Aspercin [OTC], Aspir-low [OTC], Aspirtab [OTC], Bayer Aspirin Extra Strength [OTC], Bayer Aspirin Regimen Adult Low Strength [OTC], Bayer Aspirin Regimen Children's [OTC], Bayer Aspirin Regimen Regular Strength [OTC], Bayer Genuine Aspirin [OTC], Bayer Plus Extra Strength [OTC], Bayer Women's Low Dose Aspirin [OTC], Buffasal [OTC], Bufferin Extra Strength [OTC], Bufferin [OTC], Buffinol [OTC], Ecotrin Arthritis Strength [OTC], Ecotrin Low Strength [OTC], Ecotrin [OTC], Halfprin [OTC], St Joseph Adult Aspirin [OTC], Tri-Buffered Aspirin [OTC])

Typical Uses: treatment of mild-to-moderate pain, headaches, inflammation, and fever

Potential Neurologic or Psychiatric Medication Adverse Effects: The following potential side effects may occur with salicylates but the frequency of occurrence is not available: agitation, cerebral edema, coma, confusion, dizziness, fatigue, headache, hyperthermia, insomnia, lethargy, nervousness, Reye's syndrome, hearing loss, tinnitus, dimness of vision, and weakness.

Further Reading

Brunton LL, Laurence L, Chabner BA, Knollmann BC. *Goodman & Gilman's the pharmacological basis of therapeutics*. 12th ed. New York: McGraw-Hill Publishing; 2011: pp. 979–81.

Gutierrez K. Pharmacotherapeutics. In *Clinical reasoning in primary care*. 2nd ed. St. Louis, MO: Saunders Elsevier; 2007; 247, 253.

Post TW, ed. *UpToDate*. Waltham, MA: UpToDate. Accessed Jan 22, 2016.

Serotonin 1D/1B Selective Agonists (Triptans)

Class Members: sumatriptan (PO, SC, NS, transdermal) (Imitrex®), zolmitriptan (PO, NS) (Zomig®), naratriptan (Amerge®), rizatriptan (Maxalt®), almotriptan (Axert®), eletriptan (Relpax®), and frovatriptan (Frova®)

Typical Uses: migraine, triptans are first tier pharmacologic options for treatment of acute migraine as a result of 5-HT$_{1D/1B}$ heteroreceptor activation on presynaptic trigeminal nerve endings to inhibit the release of vasodilating peptides (calcitonin gene-related peptide, substance P, and neurokinin A) thereby resulting in vasoconstriction preventing stretching of pain endings

Potential Neurologic or Psychiatric Medication Adverse Effects: Subcutaneous sumatriptan has the highest incidence of adverse events, while the adverse effects of all oral triptans are relatively similar in overall incidence. Sumatriptan, and thus triptans as a class, have more adverse events than aspirin with metoclopramide. There are generally worse side effects with parenteral than oral formulations. Side effects include dizziness, vertigo, atypical sensations (warm tingling sensation), paresthesia, chest heaviness and tightness, feelings of pressure (4%) or pain in the chest, neck, and jaw, drowsiness, anxiety, malaise, fatigue, weakness, throat and sinus discomfort, alterations in vision, abdominal discomfort, dysphagia, nausea, and sweating. An additive effect is seen in combination with other vasoconstrictors. Triptans are contraindicated in patients at risk for or with history of ischemic heart disease (myocardial infarctions), vasospastic coronary artery disease (Prinzmetal's angina), uncontrolled hypertension, stroke, transient ischemic attacks, peripheral vascular disease, hemiplegic or basilar migraines. Avoid in patients with ischemic bowel disease, diabetes mellitus, and migraines with prolonged aura. Caution in pregnancy, lactation, or use in children under the age of 18.

Almotriptan, rizatriptan, sumatriptan, and zolmitriptan are contraindicated in patients who have taken a monoamine oxidase inhibitor within the preceding 2 weeks, and all triptans are contraindicated in patients with near-term prior exposure to ergot alkaloids or other 5-HT agonists. More specifically, do not use triptans within 24 hours of administration of ergot alkaloids, methysergide, or another triptan. Less than 10% of patients receiving zolmitriptan, naratriptan,

or rizatriptan discontinue treatment after a year as a result of adverse events. **Black box warning:** serotonin syndrome results from too much serotonin in the brain and presents as weakness, hyperreflexia, and loss of coordination. Agitation, restlessness, confusion, tremors, elevated blood pressure, and diaphoresis may also be seen. Frovatriptan and naratriptan are more likely than other triptans to be responsible for serotonin syndrome. The vast majority of the literature and the common consensus among headache professionals would be that there is no increased risk of serotonin syndrome from other triptans. Indeed, some experts doubt that this syndrome even occurs. Serotonin syndrome may rarely occur when triptans are combined with selective serotonin reuptake inhibitor (SSRI) or serotonin–norepinephrine reuptake inhibitor (SNRI) therapy but the risk is felt to be very low to nonexistent. Triptan therapy (except naratriptan) should not commence sooner than 2 weeks after discontinuation of a monoamine oxidase inhibitor. Thus, many headache experts suggest that triptans in combination with SSRIs or SNRIs can be used in most cases where both are needed as long as the risks and benefits are discussed and patients are monitored for symptoms of serotonin syndrome.

Eletriptan: The incidence of minor side effects was also dose related, but all adverse effects were transient and reversible. Reported side effects include asthenia (4–10%), somnolence (3–7%), stroke, and seizures. Eletriptan is contraindicated in patients with severe hepatic, renal, or peripheral vascular disease. Eletriptan interacts with CYP3A4 inhibitors and thus should not be used within 72 hours of treatment with other drugs that are potent CYP3A4 inhibitors such as ketoconazole, itraconazole, nefazodone, troleandomycin, clarithromycin, ritonavir, and nelfinavir.

Naratriptan: Adverse event rates with naratriptan therapy are similar to placebo and do not appear to be dose related. Side effects with this triptan include dizziness (up to 2%), paresthesia (up to 2%), somnolence (up to 2%), and stroke. Naratriptan is contraindicated in patients with severe hepatic, renal, or peripheral vascular disease impairing their overall function. Oral contraceptives increase plasma naratriptan concentrations, whereas smoking decreases plasma naratriptan concentrations.

Rizatriptan: The most common adverse effects with rizatriptan therapy are dizziness (4–10%), asthenia/fatigue

(4–7%), nausea, and somnolence (4–10%). Other side effects include medication overuse headache and stroke. It should be used with caution in patients with renal or hepatic disease but is not contraindicated. Concentrations of rizatriptan are increased when used concomitantly with propranolol.

Sumatriptan: Side effects with sumatriptan administration are most significant when using the subcutaneous formulation. Overall, side effects from nasal spray or oral formulations are felt to be much more moderate. Overall, common side effects with sumatriptan therapy include injection site reactions, chest pressure or heaviness, flushing, weakness, drowsiness, dizziness (oral 2%/subQ 12%), malaise, a feeling of warmth or burning sensation (oral 2%/subQ 7%), numbness (1–5%), and paresthesias (oral, 5%/subQ, 7.8–42%). Most of these reactions occur soon after administration and resolve spontaneously within 30 minutes. The most common side effect of intranasal sumatriptan is an unpleasant taste. More serious side effects seen when using sumatriptan include intracranial hemorrhage, stroke, and seizures.

Zolmitriptan: There is a dose–response relationship in terms of both efficacy and adverse effects when using zolmitriptan. The most common side effects reported include nausea, dizziness (oral 8%/nasal spray 4%), somnolence (oral 7%/nasal spray 3%), paresthesia (7%), asthenia (6%), hyperesthesia (nasal spray 3%), sensation of hot or cold (6%), fatigue, and tightness in the throat or chest. The incidence of unpleasant taste is lower with intranasal zolmitriptan when compared with intranasal sumatriptan. Again, more serious side effects include cerebral hemorrhage and stroke.

Zolmitriptan is contraindicated in patients with Wolff–Parkinson–White syndrome and serum levels will increase if used in parallel with propranolol.

Almotriptan: The side effects most commonly seen with almotriptan include dizziness (4%), paresthesia (1%), and somnolence (5%). Cerebral hemorrhage and stroke have also been reported, especially in patients with underlying cerebrovascular disease.

Frovatriptan: Therapy with frovatriptan may be frequently complicated by dizziness (8%). Frovatriptan is contraindicated in patients with peripheral vascular disease.

Further Reading

Brunton LL, Laurence L, Chabner BA, Knollmann BC. *Goodman & Gilman's the pharmacological basis of therapeutics*. 12th ed. New York: McGraw-Hill Publishing; 2011. pp. 345–7.

Gutierrez K. Pharmacotherapeutics. In *Clinical reasoning in primary care*. 2nd ed. St. Louis, MO: Saunders Elsevier; 2007. pp. 391–3

Katzung B, Trevor A. *Basic & clinical pharmacology*. 13th ed. New York: McGraw-Hill Publishing; 2015. pp. 283–5, 290–1.

Micromedex 2.0. Greenwood Village, CO: Truven Health Analytics, Inc. http://micromedexsolutions.com. Accessed Jan 22, 2016.

Rizatriptan. In Post TW, ed. *UpToDate*. Waltham, MA: UpToDate; 2016.

Zolmitriptan. In Post TW, ed. *UpToDate*. Waltham, MA: UpToDate; 2016.

Medications to Treat Mental Health and Substance Abuse Disorders

Mei T. Liu, PharmD, BCPP Ernest Mario School of Pharmacy
Kelly N. Gable, PharmD, BCPP SIUE School of Pharmacy
Megan Maroney, PharmD, BCPP Ernest Mario School of Pharmacy

Acamprosate (Campral®)

Typical Uses: maintenance of abstinence from alcohol in patients with alcohol dependence

Potential Neurologic or Psychiatric Medication Adverse Effects: Common adverse effects (1–10%) include asthenia, anxiety, depression, dizziness, dry mouth, nausea, insomnia, and paresthesia. Other adverse reactions such as headache, syncope, somnolence, decreased libido, amnesia, abnormal thinking, and tremor have also been reported. Acamprosate is mainly excreted by the kidney. It is contraindicated in patients with severe renal impairment (creatinine clearance less than 30 mL/minute). Dosage adjustment is recommended in patients with a creatinine clearance of 30–50 mL/minute to lessen the risk of adverse reactions due to drug accumulation. Elderly patients are more likely to have decreased renal function, and renal function monitoring is helpful with proper dose selection. Warnings exist for symptoms of suicidality and depression in patients who take acamprosate and monitoring of these symptoms is recommended. Although suicide attempts and suicidal ideation had been reported in the clinical trials, there are insufficient data to determine whether the risk was increased due to the medication.

Further Reading

Campral® (acamprosate calcium) package insert. St. Louis, MO: Forest Pharmaceuticals, Inc; Jan 2012.

Jonas DE, Amick HR, Feltner C, et al. Pharmacotherapy for adults with alcohol use disorders in outpatient settings: a systematic review and meta-analysis. *JAMA*. 2014;311: 1889–900.

Alpha-2 Adrenergic Agonists

Class Members: clonidine (Catapres®, Kapvay®), dexmedetomidine (Precedex®), guanfacine (Intuniv®, Tenex®), tizanadine (Zanaflex®)

Typical Uses: hypertension, attention deficit hyperactivity disorder (ADHD) (clonidine and guanfacine), motor or vocal tics (clonidine and guanfacine), opioid withdrawal, muscle spasticity and acute low back pain (tizanidine), intensive care unit or procedural sedation (dexmedetomidine)

Potential Neurologic or Psychiatric Medication Adverse Effects: The most common adverse effects (>10%) with the alpha-2 agonists include drowsiness, xerostomia, headache, fatigue, dizziness, insomnia (guanfacine), muscle weakness (tizanidine), and agitation (dexmedetomidine). Clonidine is typically more sedating than guanfacine. Sedation is dose-dependent and often transient, typically subsiding after 2–3 weeks of treatment. Sedation and anticholinergic adverse effects are more troublesome in the elderly. Other common adverse effects (1–10%) include lethargy, irritability, sleep disturbances such as nightmares, vivid dreams and insomnia, emotional disturbances, anxiety, nervousness, depression (dose-dependent), erectile dysfunction, decreased libido, behavioral changes such as aggressive behavior or agitation, delirium, delusions, hallucinations, dyskinesia, speech disorder, malaise, paresthesia, restlessness, parotid pain, weakness, muscle and joint pain, accommodation disturbances, blurred vision, crying, and fever. The incidence of adverse events may be less with the transdermal form of clonidine due to the lower peak/trough plasma ratio. Warnings exist for risk of suicidal thoughts and behavior including attempts and completed suicide with clonidine and guanfacine, although there is little evidence to directly suggest causation. Warnings regarding sedation and drowsiness recommend that patients not operate heavy machinery or drive after taking an alpha-2 agonist. Sedation may also be potentiated when used with other CNS-depressing medications or alcohol. Tizanidine has been associated with visual hallucinations or delusions and should be used with caution in patients with psychiatric disorders. Abrupt cessation may lead to withdrawal symptoms such as nervousness, agitation, headache, and tremor. It is recommended to gradually taper alpha-2 agonists upon discontinuation.

Further Reading

Clonidine. In *Lexi-Drugs. Lexicomp*. Hudson, OH: Wolters Kluwer Health, Inc. http://online.lexi .com. Accessed Jul 26, 2017.

Doering PL, Li R. Substance-related disorders II: alcohol, nicotine, and caffeine. In DiPiro JT, Talbert RL, Yee GC, et al., eds. *Pharmacotherapy: a pathophysiologic approach*. 9th ed. New York, NY: McGraw-Hill; 2014. Chapter 49.

Saseen JJ, MacLaughlin EJ. Hypertension. In DiPiro JT, Talbert RL, Yee GC, et al., eds. *Pharmacotherapy: a pathophysiologic approach*. 9th ed. New York, NY: McGraw-Hill; 2014. Chapter 3.

Antidepressants

Amoxapine (Asendin®)

Typical Uses: treatment of depression accompanied by anxiety or agitation, treatment of depression in patients with neurotic or reactive depressive disorder, treatment of endogenous or psychotic depression

Potential Neurologic or Psychiatric Medication Adverse Effects: Very common adverse effects (>10%) include drowsiness and fatigue. Common adverse effects (1–10%) include anxiety, insomnia, restlessness, nervousness, palpitations, tremor, confusion, excitement, nightmares, ataxia, alterations in EEG patterns, dizziness, headache, and nausea. Other less common neurologic and psychiatric adverse effects such as seizure, hypomania, incoordination, paresthesia of the extremities, numbness, and disorientation have been reported. Patients with bipolar disorder are at increased risk of experiencing hypomania/mania with antidepressant use. Amoxapine possesses a black box warning for increasing the risk compared with placebo

of suicidal thinking and behavior in children, adolescents, and young adults (18–24 years old) in short-term studies of major depressive disorder (MDD) and other psychiatric disorders. It is contraindicated in patients who have hypersensitivity to dibenzoxazepine, and it is not recommended for use in patients in acute recovery phase post myocardial infarction. It is also contraindicated to use amoxapine concurrently with other tricyclic antidepressants and monoamine oxidase inhibitors due to the risk of serotonin syndrome. Amoxapine may increase the response to alcohol, barbiturates, and other central nervous system (CNS) depressants. Amoxapine should be used with caution in patients with a history of urinary retention, angle-closure glaucoma, increased intraocular pressure, cardiovascular disorders, or seizure disorders. Due to its neuroleptic activity, patients should be monitored for extrapyramidal symptoms, tardive dyskinesia, or neuroleptic malignant syndrome. Amoxapine should be discontinued if these adverse reactions occur. Amoxapine can cause symptoms of grand mal convulsions, status epilepticus, central nervous system depression, and coma in overdose. Small quantities of amoxapine should be prescribed to lower the risk of overdose. Elderly patients may be more sensitive to the adverse reactions and amoxapine should be used with caution in this population and starting at a lower dose.

Further Reading

Amoxapine package insert. Tulsa, OK: Physicians Total Care, Inc; Jun 2009.

Amoxapine. In *Micromedex 2.0*. Greenwood Village, CO: Truven Health Analytics, Inc. www .micromedexsolutions.com. Accessed Jul 25, 2017.

Bupropion (Wellbutrin®, Zyban®)

Typical Uses: depression (with or without seasonal pattern), smoking cessation, attention deficit hyperactivity disorder (ADHD) (off-label)

Potential Neurologic or Psychiatric Medication Adverse Effects: Due to the dopamine re-uptake inhibition and enhanced dopaminergic effect, bupropion most frequently causes insomnia and wakefulness. Other more frequent adverse effects include headache, restlessness/agitation, tremor, and anxiety. It can negatively impact sleep and trigger insomnia, especially if a dose is taken later in the day, generally past 4 PM. Rarely, bupropion can cause paresthesia, abnormal movements (twitching), and abnormal dreams. Bupropion has a dose-dependent impact on the seizure threshold (total daily dose >450 mg) and should be avoided in patients at a higher risk for seizure (active eating disorder, alcohol use disorder, epilepsy). Due to its dopamine-enhancing impact, it is possible that bupropion could rarely induce psychosis (hallucinations, delusions) or mania. There is a black box warning regarding increase in suicidal ideation in children, adolescents, and young adults (18–24 years of age) treated for depression. Monitor patients closely for suicidal thinking and behavior, clinical worsening, or unusual changes in behavior.

Further Reading

American Psychiatric Association. *Practice guideline for the treatment of patients with major depressive disorder*. 3. Arlington: American Psychiatric Association; 2010.

Bupropion. In *Lexi-Drugs. Lexicomp*. Hudson, OH: Wolters Kluwer Health, Inc. http://online.lexi .com. Accessed May 22, 2017.

Bupropion. In *Micromedex 2.0*. Greenwood Village, CO: Truven Health Analytics, Inc. http:// micromedexsolutions.com. Accessed May 22, 2017.

Dopheide JA, Stimmel GL. Depression treatment: more ups than downs. *The Rx Consultant*. Jun 2012;XXI:6.

Stahl SM. *Stahl's essential psychopharmacology: Neuroscientific basis and practical applications*. 4th ed. Cambridge, UK: Cambridge University Press; 2013.

Mirtazapine (Remeron®)

Typical Uses: depression, posttraumatic stress disorder (PTSD); due to mirtazapine's appetite stimulating and sedative properties, it is often used to treat depression in the elderly and depression as a result of chronic disease states (cancer, HIV/AIDS)

Potential Neurologic or Psychiatric Adverse Effects: The most frequently encountered adverse effects of mirtazapine include drowsiness (may experience higher sedation at lower doses of 15 and 30 mg) and dizziness. Less frequent but possible adverse effects are abnormal dreaming, apathy, agitation, and paresthesia. Antidepressant-induced akathisia is more likely to occur within the first few weeks of starting treatment. There is a black box warning regarding increase

in suicidal ideation in children, adolescents, and young adults (18–24 years of age) treated for depression. Monitor patients closely for suicidal thinking and behavior, clinical worsening, or unusual changes in behavior. Serotonin syndrome (agitation, mental status changes, delirium, tachycardia, diaphoresis, tremor, myoclonus) is also a risk when mirtazapine is given along with other serotonin-enhancing medications (selective serotonin reuptake inhibitors [SSRIs], serotonin–norepinephrine reuptake inhibitors [SNRIs], tramadol, triptans).

Further Reading

American Psychiatric Association. *Practice guideline for the treatment of patients with major depressive disorder*. 3. Arlington: American Psychiatric Association; 2010.

Dopheide JA, Stimmel GL. Depression treatment: more ups than downs. *The Rx Consultant*. Jun 2012;XXI:6.

Mirtazapine. In *Lexi-Drugs. Lexicomp*. Hudson, OH: Wolters Kluwer Health, Inc. http://online.lexi .com. Accessed May 22, 2017.

Mirtazapine. In *Micromedex 2.0*. Greenwood Village, CO: Truven Health Analytics, Inc. http:// micromedexsolutions.com. Accessed May 22, 2017.

Stahl SM. *Stahl's essential psychopharmacology: Neuroscientific basis and practical applications*. 4th ed. Cambridge, UK: Cambridge University Press; 2013.

Monoamine Oxidase Inhibitors (MAOIs)

Class Members: isocarboxazid (Marplan®), phenelzine (Nardil®), tranylcypromine (Parnate®)

Typical Uses: depression (often utilized for treatment refractory depression), anxiety

Potential Neurologic or Psychiatric Medication Adverse Effects: More frequently encountered adverse effects include dizziness and ataxia (orthostasis), drowsiness, and headache. MAOIs may induce hyperreflexia, twitching, and rarely seizures. When combined with foods/beverages containing tyramine, there is an increased risk for the development of a hypertensive crisis (severe headache, nausea/vomiting, photophobia, neck stiffness, and sweating). There have been several reports of transient increases in blood pressure shortly (30 minutes to 2 hours) after ingestion of MAOIs. MAOIs may result in severe central nervous system excitation and increased sympathetic outflow, which can be manifested by neuromuscular irritability, hyperthermia, hypertension or hypotension, and arrhythmias. Overdose is potentially fatal and requires close observation and supportive care. MAOIs should not be co-administered with other serotonin-enhancing medications (selective serotonin reuptake inhibitors [SSRIs], serotonin–norepinephrine reuptake inhibitors [SNRIs], tramadol, triptans) due to serotonin syndrome risk and toxicity. There is a black box warning regarding increase in suicidal ideation in children, adolescents, and young adults (18–24 years of age) treated for depression. Monitor patients closely for suicidal thinking and behavior, clinical worsening, or unusual changes in behavior.

Further Reading

Davidson J, Turnbill C. Isocarboxazid: Efficacy and tolerance. *J Affect Disord.* 1983;5:183–9.

Dopheide JA, Stimmel GL. Depression treatment: more ups than downs. *The Rx Consultant.* Jun 2012;XXI:6.

Lexi-Drugs. Lexicomp. Hudson, OH: Wolters Kluwer Health, Inc. http://online.lexi.com. Accessed May 22, 2017.

Micromedex 2.0. Greenwood Village, CO: Truven Health Analytics, Inc. http://micromedexsolutions .com. Accessed May 22, 2017.

Stahl SM. *Stahl's essential psychopharmacology: Neuroscientific basis and practical applications.* 4th ed. Cambridge, UK: Cambridge University Press; 2013.

Serotonin–Norepinephrine Reuptake Inhibitors (SNRIs)

Class Members: venlafaxine (Effexor®), desvenlafaxine (Pristiq®), duloxetine (Cymbalta®), levomilnacipran (Fetzima®), milnacipran (Savella®)

Typical Uses: depression, anxiety (GAD, panic disorder, social anxiety disorder), neuropathic pain syndromes, obsessive-compulsive disorder (OCD), posttraumatic stress disorder (PTSD), attention deficit hyperactivity disorder (ADHD) (off-label), and hot flashes

Potential Neurologic or Psychiatric Medication Adverse Effects: The most frequently encountered adverse

effects of SNRIs include headache, insomnia, and dizziness. Less frequent tolerability concerns include initial worsening of anxiety, drowsiness, abnormal dreams, yawning, paresthesia, and depersonalization. As a class, SNRIs are more likely to increase blood pressure and heart rate due to their norepinephrine reuptake inhibition. Due to their serotonergic activity, serotonin syndrome is also a risk when SNRIs are given along with other serotonin-enhancing medications (selective serotonin reuptake inhibitors [SSRIs], tricyclic antidepressants [TCAs], tramadol, triptans). There is a black box warning regarding increase in suicidal ideation in children, adolescents, and young adults (18–24 years of age) treated for depression. Monitor patients closely for suicidal thinking and behavior, clinical worsening, or unusual changes in behavior.

Further Reading

American Psychiatric Association. *Practice guideline for the treatment of patients with major depressive disorder.* 3. Arlington: American Psychiatric Association; 2010.

Dopheide JA, Stimmel GL. Depression treatment: more ups than downs. *The Rx Consultant.* Jun 2012;XXI:6.

Lexi-Drugs. Lexicomp. Hudson, OH: Wolters Kluwer Health, Inc. http://online.lexi.com. Accessed May 22, 2017.

Micromedex 2.0. Greenwood Village, CO: Truven Health Analytics, Inc. http:// micromedexsolutions.com. Accessed May 22, 2017.

Stahl SM. *Stahl's essential psychopharmacology: Neuroscientific basis and practical applications.* 4th ed. Cambridge, UK: Cambridge University Press; 2013.

Selective Serotonin Reuptake Inhibitors (SSRIs)

Class Members: citalopram (Celexa®), escitalopram (Lexapro®), fluoxetine (Prozac®), fluvoxamine (Luvox®), paroxetine (Paxil®), sertraline (Zoloft®)

Typical Uses: major depressive disorder, anxiety disorders, bulimia nervosa, premenstrual dysphoric disorder, obsessive-compulsive disorder, posttraumatic stress disorder

Potential Neurologic or Psychiatric Medication Adverse Effects: The adverse effect profile is similar among agents within the SSRI class. Very common adverse effects (>10%) include somnolence or insomnia, headache, dizziness, sexual dysfunction, nervousness, and asthenia. Although somnolence or insomnia can occur with any SSRI, somnolence is most common with paroxetine and fluvoxamine. Sexual dysfunction is considered a chronic side effect and may include reduced libido in women and men, anorgasmia in women, erectile dysfunction in men, and increased ejaculation latency in men. Common adverse effects (1–10%) include fatigue, anxiety, agitation, yawning, amnesia, paresthesia, tremor, myalgia, and abnormal dreams. Dizziness, insomnia, somnolence, tremor, yawning, fatigue, paresthesia, asthenia, anxiety, and nervousness are thought to be dose-related. Patients with bipolar disorder are at increased risk of experiencing hypomania/mania with antidepressant use. All SSRIs possess a black box warning for increasing the risk compared with placebo of suicidal thinking and behavior in children, adolescents, and young adults (18–24 years old) in short-term studies of major depressive disorder (MDD) and other psychiatric disorders. A discontinuation syndrome may occur if an SSRI is stopped abruptly. Symptoms include nausea, headache, chills, insomnia, and dizziness.

Further Reading

American Psychiatric Association. *Practice guideline for the treatment of patients with major depressive disorder*. 3. Arlington: American Psychiatric Association; 2010.

Dopheide JA, Stimmel GL. Depression treatment: more ups than downs. *The Rx Consultant*. Jun 2012;XXI:6.

Lexi-Drugs. Lexicomp. Hudson, OH: Wolters Kluwer Health, Inc. http://online.lexi.com. Accessed May 22, 2017.

Micromedex 2.0. Greenwood Village, CO: Truven Health Analytics, Inc. http://micromedexsolutions.com. Accessed May 22, 2017.

Stahl SM. *Stahl's essential psychopharmacology: Neuroscientific basis and practical applications*. 4th ed. Cambridge, UK: Cambridge University Press; 2013.

Trazodone (Oleptro®)

Typical Uses: depression, insomnia (off-label but most common use), chronic pain syndromes, anxiety

Potential Neurologic or Psychiatric Medication Adverse Effects: The most frequently encountered adverse effects include sedation, headache, dizziness, and ataxia (syncope/orthostasis). Less common include confusion, disorientation, abnormal dreams, night sweats, tinnitus, slurred speech, hallucinations, and seizure risk (<1%). Priapism (sustained, painful, and extended erection) is a rare, yet more serious potential adverse effect of trazodone due to its more potent alpha-1 antagonist activity. There is a black box warning regarding increase in suicidal ideation in children, adolescents, and young adults (18–24 years of age) treated for depression with trazodone. Monitor patients closely for suicidal thinking and behavior, clinical worsening, or unusual changes in behavior.

Further Reading

American Psychiatric Association. *Practice guideline for the treatment of patients with major depressive disorder*. 3. Arlington: American Psychiatric Association; 2010.

Dopheide JA, Stimmel GL. Depression treatment: more ups than downs. *The Rx Consultant*. Jun 2012;XXI:6.

Stahl SM. *Stahl's essential psychopharmacology: Neuroscientific basis and practical applications*. 4th ed. Cambridge, UK: Cambridge University Press; 2013.

Trazodone. In *Lexi-Drugs. Lexicomp*. Hudson, OH: Wolters Kluwer Health, Inc. http://online.lexi.com. Accessed May 22, 2017.

Trazodone. In *Micromedex 2.0*. Greenwood Village, CO: Truven Health Analytics, Inc. http://micromedexsolutions.com. Accessed May 22, 2017.

Tricyclic Antidepressants (TCAs)

Class Members: secondary amine TCAs: nortriptyline (Pamelor®), desipramine (Norpramin®), protriptyline (Vivactyl®); **tertiary amine TCAs:** amitriptyline (Elavil®), doxepin (Sinequan®), clomipramine (Anafranil®), imipramine (Tofranil®)

Typical Uses: depression, neuropathic pain syndromes (secondary amine TCAs), migraine prophylaxis, anxiety, posttraumatic stress disorder (PTSD), obsessive-compulsive disorder (OCD) (clomipramine), insomnia

Potential Neurologic or Psychiatric Medication Adverse Effects: The most frequent tolerability concerns associated with tertiary amine TCA include anticholinergic adverse effects (blurred vision, confusion, and delirium), sedation/drowsiness, dizziness, and ataxia (orthostasis). Cognitive dysfunction and disorientation can result from excessive sedation. All TCAs can induce initial worsening of anxiety, irritability, and restlessness (akathisia). Rarely, TCAs may induce changes in EEG patterns, cause abnormal dreams, and induce mania or hallucinations. As a class, TCAs are more likely to increase blood pressure and heart rate due to their norepinephrine reuptake inhibition. Due to their serotonergic activity, serotonin syndrome is also a risk when TCAs are given along with other serotonin-enhancing medications (selective serotonin reuptake inhibitors [SSRIs], serotonin–norepinephrine reuptake inhibitors [SNRIs], tramadol, triptans). There is a black box warning regarding increase in suicidal ideation in children, adolescents, and young adults (18–24 years of age) treated for depression. Monitor patients closely for suicidal thinking and behavior, clinical worsening, or unusual changes in behavior. TCAs should be used with caution in patients with known cardiovascular disease due to their propensity to induce cardiac conduction abnormalities. All TCAs also lower the seizure threshold. An overdose with a TCA medication is considered toxic and lethality is high due to seizure and cardiovascular risk.

Further Reading

American Psychiatric Association. *Practice guideline for the treatment of patients with major depressive disorder*. 3. Arlington: American Psychiatric Association; 2010.

Dopheide JA, Stimmel GL. Depression treatment: more ups than downs. *The Rx Consultant*. Jun 2012;XXI:6.

Lexi-Drugs. Lexicomp. Hudson, OH: Wolters Kluwer Health, Inc. http://online.lexi.com. Accessed May 22, 2017.

Micromedex 2.0. Greenwood Village, CO: Truven Health Analytics, Inc. http://micromedexsolutions.com. Accessed May 22, 2017.

Stahl SM. *Stahl's essential psychopharmacology: Neuroscientific basis and practical applications*. 4th ed. Cambridge, UK: Cambridge University Press; 2013.

Vilazodone (Viibryd®)

Typical Uses: depression, anxiety

Potential Neurologic or Psychiatric Adverse Effects: Tolerability concerns that arise with vilazodone are similar to those that occur with selective serotonin reuptake inhibitors (SSRIs) and buspirone. The most frequent tolerability concerns include headache, dizziness, and insomnia. Less frequent may include restlessness, jitteriness, akathisia, abnormal dreams, somnolence, and paresthesia. Due to its serotonergic activity, serotonin syndrome is also a risk when vilazodone is given along with other serotonin-enhancing medications (SSRIs, serotonin–norepinephrine reuptake inhibitors [SNRIs], tramadol, triptans). There is a black box warning regarding increase in suicidal ideation in children, adolescents, and young adults (18–24 years of age) treated for depression. Monitor patients closely for suicidal thinking and behavior, clinical worsening, or unusual changes in behavior.

Further Reading

Dopheide JA, Stimmel GL. Depression treatment: more ups than downs. *The Rx Consultant*. Jun 2012;XXI:6.

Laughren TP, Gobburu J, Temple RJ, et al. Vilazodone: clinical basis for the US Food and Drug Administration's approval of a new antidepressant. *J Clin Psychiatry*. 2011;72(9):1166–73.

Stahl SM. *Stahl's essential psychopharmacology: Neuroscientific basis and practical applications*. 4th ed. Cambridge, UK: Cambridge University Press; 2013.

Vilazodone. In *Lexi-Drugs. Lexicomp*. Hudson, OH: Wolters Kluwer Health, Inc. http://online.lexi.com. Accessed May 22, 2017.

Vilazodone. In *Micromedex 2.0*. Greenwood Village, CO: Truven Health Analytics, Inc. http://micromedexsolutions.com. Accessed May 22, 2017.

Vortioxetine (Trintellix®)

Typical Uses: depression (specific focus on cognitive dysfunction associated with depression)

Potential Neurologic or Psychiatric Medication Adverse Effects: The most frequent tolerability concerns with vortioxetine include dizziness and abnormal dreams.

Sexual dysfunction (anorgasmia, erectile dysfunction, and/or decreased libido) has been reported in >10% of patients taking vortioxetine. Rarely, this medication has the potential to induce hyponatremia and seizures or worsen angle-closure glaucoma. Hypomania/mania can occur upon taking this medication in individuals with a diagnosis or history of bipolar disorder. Due to its serotonergic activity, serotonin syndrome is also a risk when vortioxetine is given along with other serotonin-enhancing medications (selective serotonin reuptake inhibitors [SSRIs], serotonin–norepinephrine reuptake inhibitors [SNRIs], tramadol, triptans). There is a black box warning regarding increase in suicidal ideation in children, adolescents, and young adults (18–24 years of age) treated for depression. Monitor patients closely for suicidal thinking and behavior, clinical worsening, or unusual changes in behavior.

Further Reading

Dopheide JA, Stimmel GL. Depression treatment: more ups than downs. *The Rx Consultant*. Jun 2012;XXI:6.

Stahl SM. *Stahl's essential psychopharmacology: Neuroscientific basis and practical applications.* 4th ed. Cambridge, UK: Cambridge University Press; 2013.

Vortioxetine. In *Lexi-Drugs. Lexicomp*. Hudson, OH: Wolters Kluwer Health, Inc. http://online.lexi.com. Accessed May 22, 2017.

Vortioxetine. In *Micromedex 2.0*. Greenwood Village, CO: Truven Health Analytics, Inc. http://micromedexsolutions.com. Accessed May 22, 2017.

Antipsychotics

First-Generation (Typical) Antipsychotics (FGAs)

Class Members: chlorpromazine (Thorazine®), thioridazine (Mellaril®), loxapine (Loxitane®), perphenazine (Trilafon®), trifluoperazine (Stelazine®), thiothixene (Navane®), fluphenazine (Prolixin®), haloperidol (Haldol®)

Typical Uses: psychosis, schizophrenia, Tourette syndrome, acute agitation/aggression

Potential Neurologic or Psychiatric Medication Adverse Effects: Lower potency agents (chlorpromazine, thioridazine) more commonly induce dizziness and ataxia (orthostasis), sedation/hypersomnia, and anticholinergic (blurred vision, delirium risk) adverse effects. Higher potency agents (fluphenazine, haloperidol) more commonly induce extrapyramidal side effects such as dystonia, akathisia (restlessness, insomnia), pseudoparkinsonism (rigidity/stiffness, resting tremor, unsteady gait), and tardive dyskinesia. Other less common adverse effects associated with the class of first-generation antipsychotics include agitation, altered temperature regulation, sweating, and headache. Neuroleptic malignant syndrome (NMS) is a rare and potentially life-threatening adverse effect of antipsychotics. Patients with NMS may present with altered mental status, fever, rigidity, hypertension, and tachycardia. All antipsychotics lower the seizure threshold, with chlorpromazine exhibiting the highest risk among the FGAs. All antipsychotics also have a warning associated with an increased risk of death when used for the treatment of elderly patients with dementia-related psychosis.

Further Reading

Buchanan RW, et al. The 2009 schizophrenia PORT psychopharmacology treatment recommendations and summary statements. *Schizophr Bull*. 2010;36:71–93.

Lexi-Drugs. Lexicomp. Hudson, OH: Wolters Kluwer Health, Inc. http://online.lexi.com. Accessed May 22, 2017.

Micromedex 2.0. Greenwood Village, CO: Truven Health Analytics, Inc. http://micromedexsolutions.com. Accessed May 22, 2017.

Stahl SM. *Stahl's essential psychopharmacology: Neuroscientific basis and practical applications*. 4th ed. Cambridge, UK: Cambridge University Press; 2013.

Second-Generation (Atypical) Antipsychotics (SGAs)

Class Members: clozapine (Clozaril®), risperidone (Risperdal®), olanzapine (Zyprexa®), quetiapine (Seroquel®), ziprasidone (Geodon®), aripiprazole (Abilify®), paliperidone (Invega®), asenapine (Saphris®), iloperidone (Fanapt®), lurasidone (Latuda®), brexpiprazole (Rexulti®), cariprazine (Vraylar®)

Typical Uses: schizophrenia, schizoaffective disorder, bipolar disorder, depression, adjunctive therapy (aripiprazole, brexpiprazole, quetiapine), acute agitation/aggression, irritability associated with autism (aripiprazole, risperidone)

Potential Neurologic or Psychiatric Medication Adverse Effects: Tolerability concerns differ greatly among the SGAs. As a class, SGAs are all associated with weight gain, dyslipidemia, and hyperglycemia; however, these are much more common with the use of clozapine, olanzapine, and quetiapine. Hypersomnia, sedation, and headache occur more frequently with quetiapine, risperidone/paliperidone, olanzapine, and clozapine. Wakefulness, insomnia, restlessness, and akathisia are more common with aripiprazole and lurasidone. Hyperprolactinemia most frequently occurs with risperidone and paliperidone. All antipsychotics have the potential to induce extrapyramidal side effects such as dystonia, akathisia (restlessness, insomnia), pseudoparkinsonism (rigidity/stiffness, resting tremor, unsteady gait), and tardive dyskinesia. Neuroleptic malignant syndrome (NMS) is a rare and potentially life-threatening adverse effect of antipsychotics. Patients with NMS may present with altered mental status, fever, rigidity, hypertension, and tachycardia. All antipsychotics lower the seizure threshold, with clozapine exhibiting the highest risk among the SGAs. All antipsychotics also have a warning associated with an increased risk of death when used for the treatment of elderly patients with dementia-related psychosis. There is a black box warning regarding increase in suicidal ideation in children, adolescents, and young adults (18–24 years of age) treated for depression with an antipsychotic. Monitor patients closely for suicidal thinking and behavior, clinical worsening, or unusual changes in behavior.

Further Reading

Buchanan RW, et al. The 2009 schizophrenia PORT psychopharmacology treatment recommendations and summary statements. *Schizophr Bull.* 2010;36:71–93.

Lexi-Drugs. Lexicomp. Hudson, OH: Wolters Kluwer Health, Inc. http://online.lexi.com. Accessed May 22, 2017.

Micromedex 2.0. Greenwood Village, CO: Truven Health Analytics, Inc. http://micromedexsolutions.com. Accessed May 22, 2017.

Stahl SM. *Stahl's essential psychopharmacology: Neuroscientific basis and practical applications.* 4th ed. Cambridge, UK: Cambridge University Press; 2013.

Atomoxetine (Strattera®)

Typical Uses: attention deficit hyperactivity disorder (ADHD)

Potential Neurologic or Psychiatric Medication Adverse Effects: Due to its norepinephrine activity, atomoxetine is more likely to induce insomnia and should be dosed earlier in the day. The most frequently encountered adverse effects include headache and insomnia. Patients may also describe feeling jittery, disrupted sleep, anxiety, and rarely agitation. New-onset psychosis, aggression, and mania in children/adolescents has been described after initial onset of treatment with atomoxetine, and treatment should be discontinued if this occurs. There is a black box warning regarding increase in suicidal ideation in children and adolescents treated in the short-term with atomoxetine. Monitor patients closely for suicidal thinking and behavior, clinical worsening, or unusual changes in behavior. Atomoxetine is metabolized by CYP2D6, and its levels may be increased with the concomitant use of CYP2D6 inhibitors.

Further Reading

American Academy of Pediatrics. ADHD: clinical practice guideline for the diagnosis, evaluation, and treatment of attention-deficit/hyperactivity disorder in children and adolescents. *Pediatrics.* 2011;128:1007–22.

Atomoxotine. In *Lexi-Drugs. Lexicomp.* Hudson, OH: Wolters Kluwer Health, Inc. http://online.lexi.com. Accessed May 22, 2017.

Atomoxetine. In *Micromedex 2.0.* Greenwood Village, CO: Truven Health Analytics, Inc. http://micromedexsolutions.com. Accessed May 22, 2017.

Santosh PJ, Sattar S, Canagaratnam M. Efficacy and tolerability of pharmacotherapies for attention-deficit hyperactivity disorder in adults. *CNS Drugs.* 2011;25:737–63.

Benzodiazepines

Class Members: clonazepam (Klonopin®), alprazolam (Xanax®), lorazepam (Ativan®), diazepam (Valium®), clorazepate (Tranxene®), chlordiazepoxide (Librium®), oxazepam (Serax®), temazepam (Restoril®), triazolam (Halcion®), flurazepam (Dalmane®)

Typical Uses: insomnia, seizure disorder, muscle relaxation (diazepam), anxiety (clonazepam, alprazolam), alcohol withdrawal (diazepam, chlordiazepoxide, lorazepam), akathisia (clonazepam)

Potential Neurologic or Psychiatric Medication Adverse Effects: The most frequently encountered adverse effects include sedation, ataxia, headache, and slurred speech. The more lipophilic benzodiazepines (alprazolam, diazepam, clorazepate) produce a much quicker onset of calmness and sedation and have a higher abuse potential. Amnesia, confusion, or short-term memory loss is more common with triazolam or flurazepam. Rarely, a paradoxical reaction leading to aggression, agitation, anxiety, hallucinations, or stimulation can occur and is more common in children and adolescents. Benzodiazepines should be used with caution or avoided completely in combination with other CNS-depressing medications such as opioids due to increased risk of respiratory depression and death. Benzodiazepines with identified longer half-lives (diazepam, chlordiazepoxide) should be used with caution in patients with impaired hepatic function or in the elderly. Alternatively, lorazepam, oxazepam, and temazepam are considered safer to use when hepatic function is impaired due to less extensive liver metabolism.

Further Reading

Lexi-Drugs. Lexicomp. Hudson, OH: Wolters Kluwer Health, Inc. http://online.lexi.com. Accessed May 22, 2017.

Micromedex 2.0. Greenwood Village, CO: Truven Health Analytics, Inc. http://micromedexsolutions.com. Accessed May 22, 2017.

Stahl SM. *Stahl's essential psychopharmacology: Neuroscientific basis and practical applications.* 4th ed. Cambridge, UK: Cambridge University Press; 2013.

Buprenorphine

Class Members: buprenorphine (Buprenex®, Butrans®, Probuphine®, Subutex®), buprenorphine/naloxone (Suboxone®, Zubsolv®, Bunavail®)

Typical Uses: treatment of opioid dependence, moderate to severe pain

Potential Neurologic or Psychiatric Medication Adverse Effects: The most frequent adverse effect of buprenorphine injection (up to 66%) is sedation. The most common adverse effects (>10%) with the tablet and buccal film include headache, nausea, insomnia, pain, withdrawal syndrome, anxiety, and depression. The most common adverse effects (>10%) with the implant were implant-site pain, pruritus, and erythema. Common adverse effects (1–10%) with the implant include headache, depression, nausea, vomiting, fatigue, asthenia, dizziness, and somnolence. The transdermal patch is associated with headache, dizziness, and drowsiness (all >10%), but appears to have a lower incidence (1–10%) of anxiety, depression, insomnia, and pain. The patch is also associated with fatigue, hypoesthesia or paresthesia, and migraine (1–10%). Common adverse effects (1–10%) with the injection include dizziness, headache, and respiratory depression and with the tablet include chills, flu-like symptoms, nervousness, drowsiness, and dizziness. Patients taking buprenorphine should be cautioned against performing tasks that require mental alertness. The buccal film and transdermal patch carry a boxed warning for the potential to cause life-threatening respiratory depression, especially during initiation or dose escalation. Misuse or abuse of the contents of the buccal film or transdermal patch by chewing, swallowing, snorting, or injection poses a significant risk of overdose and death. Accidental exposure by children to even one dose can result in a fatal overdose. Patients with oral mucositis may be more prone to toxicity or overdose with the buccal film. Insertion and removal of implants are associated with the risk of implant migration, protrusion, expulsion, and nerve damage resulting from the procedure. Buprenorphine should be used with caution in patients with impaired hepatic function, head trauma, toxic psychosis, central nervous system (CNS) depression, coma, or a history of seizure disorder. Elderly patients may be more sensitive to the adverse effects of buprenorphine. Prolonged use during pregnancy may lead to life-threatening opioid withdrawal syndrome in the neonate. Abrupt discontinuation of buprenorphine following prolonged use is not recommended due to the risk of withdrawal symptoms. Concomitant use with benzodiazepines or other CNS depressants should be avoided.

Further Reading

Buprenorphine. In *Lexi-Drugs. Lexicomp*. Hudson, OH: Wolters Kluwer Health, Inc. http://online .lexi.com. Accessed July 25, 2017.

Probuphine® (buprenorphine) package insert. Princeton, NJ: Braeburn Pharmaceuticals, Inc; May 2016.

Suboxone® (buprenorphine/naloxone) package insert. Richmond, VA: Invidior Inc; Feb 2017.

Buspirone (BuSpar®)

Typical Uses: generalized anxiety disorder (GAD), treatment-resistant depression (adjunctive therapy)

Potential Neurologic or Psychiatric Medication Adverse Effects: The most frequently encountered adverse effects include dizziness, nausea, headache, and somnolence. Other less common effects include paresthesia, abnormal dreams, tremor, and confusion. If used concurrently with other serotonergic medications (selective serotonin reuptake inhibitors [SSRIs], serotonin–norepinephrine reuptake inhibitors [SNRIs], tramadol, triptans), there is an increased risk for serotonin syndrome development. Use along with a CYP3A4 inhibitor increases this risk. Rarely, use of buspirone has induced dopamine-related movement disorders such as dystonia, akathisia, and pseudoparkinsonism. Buspirone is widely viewed as an alternative anxiolytic agent to the use of benzodiazepines, as it is less sedating and is not associated with abuse or dependence. Buspirone is not effective when used "as needed" or for situational anxiety, and patients should be advised to take it daily for best efficacy.

Further Reading

Buspirone. In *Lexi-Drugs. Lexicomp*. Hudson, OH: Wolters Kluwer Health, Inc. http://online.lexi .com. Accessed May 22, 2017.

Buspirone. In *Micromedex 2.0*. Greenwood Village, CO: Truven Health Analytics, Inc. http:// micromedexsolutions.com. Accessed May 22, 2017.

Dopheide JA, Stimmel GL. Depression treatment: more ups than downs. *The Rx Consultant*. Jun 2012;XXI:6.

Stahl SM. *Stahl's essential psychopharmacology: Neuroscientific basis and practical applications*. 4th ed. Cambridge, UK: Cambridge University Press; 2013.

Disulfiram (Antabuse®)

Typical Uses: alcoholism, cocaine dependence, contact dermatitis due to nickel

Potential Neurologic or Psychiatric Medication Adverse Effects: Transient adverse effects include mild drowsiness, fatigue, impotence, and headache. Vertigo, irritability, agitation, disorientation, delirium, behavioral or personality changes, and psychoses have been reported with disulfiram. Seizure, optic or peripheral neuritis, polyneuritis, or peripheral neuropathy also may occur. The severity of the neuropathy is directly related to dose and duration of exposure. Disulfiram has a black box warning that it should never be administered to patients in a state of alcohol intoxication or without the patient's full knowledge. Disulfiram is contraindicated in patients with psychoses. It should be used with caution in patients with epilepsy or cerebral damage as disulfiram may aggravate preexisting EEG abnormalities. Hepatic failure resulting in transplantation or death has been reported. Liver function tests should be monitored at baseline and 10 to 14 days after initiation of disulfiram. Patients should notify their physicians if they have symptoms of hepatitis such as fatigue, weakness, nausea, anorexia, jaundice, or dark urine. Metronidazole, paraldehyde, or alcohol-containing items such as cough syrups, mouth wash, or aftershave can interact with disulfiram and cause symptoms of throbbing headache, flushing, nausea, syncope, vertigo, anxiety, and confusion. The intensity of the reaction usually is dose-related to the amounts of alcohol ingested and may occur up to 14 days after the last dose of disulfiram. Symptoms of severe disulfiram reaction may include respiratory depression, unconsciousness, convulsions, and death. The duration of the reaction ranges from 30 minutes to several hours or as long as there is alcohol in the blood. Disulfiram can increase phenytoin concentrations and lead to phenytoin intoxication. Phenytoin levels should be monitored at baseline and after initiation of disulfiram. Concurrent use with isoniazid can cause unsteady gait or changes in mental status and disulfiram should be discontinued if these occur.

Further Reading

Anatbuse® (disulfiram) package insert. Sellersville, PA: Teva Women's Health, Inc; Feb 2013.

Chick J. Safety issues concerning the use of disulfiram in treatment alcohol dependence. *Drug Saf*. 1999;20:427–35.

Disulfiram. In *Micromedex 2.0*. Greenwood Village, CO: Truven Health Analytics, Inc. www .micromedexsolutions.com. Accessed Jul 25, 2017.

Lithium Carbonate (Lithobid®)

Typical Uses: bipolar disorder (acute mania, depression, and maintenance), treatment-refractory depression (adjunctive therapy)

Potential Neurologic and Psychiatric Adverse Effects: More frequently encountered adverse effects with lithium include ataxia, drowsiness, headache, lethargy, mild to moderate intentional tremor, and vertigo. Less reported but notable and more concerning are hyperactive deep tendon reflex, restlessness, muscular weakness, lack of coordination, slowed intellectual functioning, confusion, and slurred speech. More severe central nervous system (CNS) depression and confusion may be indicative of lithium toxicity and could lead to seizure development or coma. Of note, patient-reported lethargy, slowed speech, and confusion may be related to lithium-induced hypothyroidism or lithium toxicity. Coupled with the above listed tolerability concerns, renal impairment may increase lithium tolerability concerns and toxicity risk. Lithium levels may increase when it is concomitantly administered with angiotensin converting enzyme (ACE) inhibitors, angiotensin II receptor blockers (ARBs), diuretics, and nonsteroidal anti-inflammatory drugs (NSAIDs). Due to its serotonergic activity, serotonin syndrome is also a risk when lithium is given along with other serotonin-enhancing medications (selective serotonin reuptake inhibitors [SSRIs], serotonin–norepinephrine reuptake inhibitors [SNRIs], tramadol, triptans). Lithium has a narrow therapeutic window, and 12-hour post-dose serum levels should be evaluated every 1 to 3 months or as clinically indicated, with a goal therapeutic range of 0.5 to 1.2 mEq/L. Toxicity is often identified when serum levels are above 1.5 mEq/L. Accompanying signs and symptoms of toxicity include more severe tremor, nausea/vomiting, diarrhea, nystagmus, confusion, ataxia, and coma or death.

Further Reading

Dopheide JA, Stimmel GL. Depression treatment: more ups than downs. *The Rx Consultant*. Jun 2012;XXI:6.

Ellis P, Wheeler A. Lithium in general practice. *Best Pract*. 2007;Issue 3:16–27.

Lithium. In *Lexi-Drugs. Lexicomp*. Hudson, OH: Wolters Kluwer Health, Inc. http://online.lexi .com. Accessed May 22, 2017.

Lithium. In *Micromedex 2.0*. Greenwood Village, CO: Truven Health Analytics, Inc. http:// micromedexsolutions.com. Accessed May 22, 2017.

Lorcaserin (Belviq®, Belviq XR®)

Typical Uses: adjunct to diet and exercise for weight management in adults

Potential Neurologic or Psychiatric Medication Adverse Effects: The only very common adverse effect (>10%) reported is headache. Common adverse effects (1–10%) include cognitive impairment such as impairments in attention and memory, confusion, nausea, prolactin elevation, fatigue, dizziness, anxiety, insomnia, stress, and depression. Patients should be cautious when operating machinery due to impaired cognitive function. Priapism is a potential adverse effect and lorcaserin should be used with caution in men with anatomical deformation of the penis or who have conditions that might predispose them to priapism such as sickle cell anemia. Prolactin should be measured in patients with signs or symptoms of hyperprolactinemia. Warnings exist for symptoms of euphoria, hallucinations, sedation, and dissociation at supratherapeutic doses (40 mg and 60 mg), and the total daily dose of lorcaserin should not exceed 20 mg. Patients should be monitored for the emergence or worsening of depression, suicidal thoughts or behavior, and any unusual changes in mood or behavior. The use of lorcaserin is contraindicated during pregnancy due to the risk of weight loss and may result in fetal harm. It should be used with caution when combined with other medications indicated for erectile dysfunction. Risk of serotonin syndrome or neuroleptic malignant syndrome is increased when used with other serotonergic medications such as selective serotonin reuptake inhibitors, serotonin–norepinephrine reuptake inhibitors, tricyclic antidepressants, monoamine oxidase inhibitors, bupropion, lithium, tramadol, triptans, dextromethorphan, St. John's wort, antipsychotics, or other dopamine antagonists. Symptoms include mental status changes, tachycardia, labile blood pressure, hyperthermia, hyperreflexia, incoordination, chills, tremor, and hyperhidrosis.

Further Reading

Belviq®/BelviqXR® (lorcaserin) package insert. Woodcliff Lake, NJ: Eisai Inc; May 2017.

Melatonin Receptor Agonists

Class Members: ramelteon (Rozerem®), tasimeltron (Hetlioz®)

Typical Uses: insomnia, non-24 hour sleep–wake disorder

Potential Neurologic or Psychiatric Medication Adverse Effects: Very common adverse effects (>10%) include headache, nightmare, and abnormal dreams for tasimelteon and prolactin level increase for ramelteon. Common adverse effects (1–10%) of ramelteon include somnolence, fatigue, dizziness, nausea, and insomnia exacerbation. Complex behaviors such as "sleep-driving," hallucinations, bizarre behavior, agitation, and mania have been reported with ramelteon. Decreased testosterone levels and increased prolactin levels have been reported with ramelteon, and patients should be monitored for symptoms of hyperprolactinemia such as amenorrhea or galactorrhea. Angioedema has been reported in patients after taking ramelteon and patients who have a history of angioedema after taking ramelteon should not be rechallenged with the drug. Strong cytochrome P450 1A2 inhibitors such as fluvoxamine can increase the concentration of melatonin receptor agonists and increase the risk of adverse effects while strong cytochrome P450 3A4 inducers such as rifampin can reduce the efficacy. Patients should not consume alcohol or take other CNS depressants while taking melatonin receptor agonists to avoid additive CNS depressant effects. Patients should avoid driving, operating machinery, or engaging in any hazardous activity after taking melatonin receptor agonists.

Further Reading

Hetlioz® (tasimelteon) package insert. Washington, DC: Vanda Pharmaceuticals Inc; Dec 2014.
Rozerem® (rameltron) package insert. Deerfield, IL: Takeda Pharmaceuticals America, Inc; Nov 2010.

Nicotine Replacement Therapy

Class Members: nicotine gum, inhaler (Nicotrol®), lozenges, nasal spray, transdermal patch (Habitrol®, NicodermCQ®)

Typical Uses: smoking cessation

Potential Neurologic or Psychiatric Medication Adverse Effects: The most frequent adverse effects (>10%) include headache (nasal spray/inhaler). Other common adverse effects (1–10%) with the nasal spray and inhaler include dizziness, anxiety, sleep disorder, depression, fatigue, back pain, arthralgia, jaw and neck pain, dependence and withdrawal symptoms, influenza-like symptoms, and fever (inhaler). Headache is also a common and seemingly dose-related adverse effect with the lozenges. Other adverse effects with the gum, lozenge, and/or transdermal systems include impaired concentration, depression, dizziness, headache, insomnia, abnormal dreams/nightmares, somnolence, nervousness, tinnitus (gum), diaphoresis (transdermal), and pain. The intranasal spray has also been associated with headache, back pain, confusion, aphasia, amnesia, migraine, and numbness. The risk of adverse effects may be increased in those who continue to smoke or use other nicotine products along with nicotine replacement therapy (NRT) or in those who exceed the recommended dosage. Chewing the nicotine gum too rapidly may result in lightheadedness. Strenuous physical activity may increase the risk of nicotine toxicity with the transdermal patch. Sustained use of NRT (i.e., more than 6 months) should be discouraged because chronic consumption of nicotine in any form may result in intoxication and dependence. NRT is usually contraindicated in women who are or may become pregnant. NRT may pose less risk to the fetus than cigarette smoking because plasma nicotine concentrations are similar to or lower than those produced by cigarette smoking (except for the inhaler) and do not expose the mother or fetus to carbon monoxide or other hazardous substances.

Further Reading

Nicotine. In *Lexi-Drugs. Lexicomp.* Hudson, OH: Wolters Kluwer Health, Inc. http://online.lexi .com. Accessed Jul 26, 2017.
Nicotine. In *AHFS® Drug Information.* Bethesda, MD: American Society of Health-System Pharmacists, Inc. http://factsandcomparisons.com. Accessed Jul 27, 2017.

Opioid Antagonists

Class Members: naltrexone (Revia®, Vivitrol®), naloxone (Narcan®, Evzio®)

Typical Uses: naltrexone: alcohol dependence, opioid dependence, cholestatic pruritus; **naloxone:** opioid overdose, septic shock, opioid-induced pruritus

Potential Neurologic or Psychiatric Medication Adverse Effects: Frequent adverse effects (>10%) include headache, insomnia, dizziness, anxiety, decreased energy, and nervousness. Other common adverse effects (1–10%) include suicidal ideation, depression, somnolence, fatigue, chills, increased energy, feeling down, and irritability. In neonates, opioid withdrawal symptoms may include convulsions, seizures, excessive crying, and hyperactive reflexes. Naltrexone may precipitate withdrawal in patients who are physically dependent on opiates. To minimize this risk, patients should remain free from opiates for at least 7–10 days prior to starting naltrexone. To be certain of a patient's abstinence, a naloxone challenge test may be performed. Administration of large doses of opiates to attempt to overcome the antagonist activity of naltrexone may produce acute opiate overdose. Signs and symptoms of overdose may occur with administration of smaller doses of opiates long after the last naltrexone dose. Excessive doses of naloxone in post-operative patients may cause agitation. Death, coma, and encephalopathy have been reported with use of naloxone in the post-operative setting. Naloxone crosses the placenta and may precipitate withdrawal in a fetus.

Further Reading

Evzio® (naloxone) package insert. Richmond, VA: Kaleo, Inc; 2014.

Naltrexone. In *Lexi-Drugs. Lexicomp*. Hudson, OH: Wolters Kluwer Health, Inc. http://online.lexi .com. Accessed Jan 23, 2016.

Naltrexone. In *AHFS® Drug Information*. Bethesda, MD: American Society of Health-System Pharmacists, Inc. http://factsandcomparisons .com. Accessed Jan 23, 2016.

Sedative Hypnotics Non-Benzodiazepine Type

Class Members: zolpidem (Ambien®, Ambien CR®, Zolpimist®, Edluar®, Intermezzo®), zaleplon (Sonata®), eszopiclone (Lunesta®)

Typical Uses: insomnia

Potential Neurologic or Psychiatric Medication Adverse Effects: Very common adverse effects (>10%) include headache, dizziness, and somnolence. Common adverse effects (1–10%) include drowsiness, lethargy, feeling "drugged," lightheadedness, depression, abnormal dreams, amnesia, and paresthesia. Complex behaviors such as sleep-driving or sleep-eating have been reported, and they are more likely to occur if a non-benzodiazepine hypnotic is combined with alcohol or other central nervous system (CNS) depressants. Although rare, adverse effects such as decreased inhibition, visual or auditory hallucinations, bizarre behavior, agitation, depersonalization, amnesia, and anxiety have been reported. Next-day psychomotor impairment can occur and abrupt discontinuation of medications may cause transient rebound insomnia. CNS depressant effects of non-benzodiazepine hypnotics are additive when combined with alcohol or other CNS-depressant drugs. Use with caution in the elderly, patients with depression, compromised respiratory function, or hepatic impairment. Women appear to be more susceptible to the next-day impairment due to slower elimination of zolpidem, and lower dose of zolpidem is recommended for women. Patients should avoid driving, operating machinery, or engaging in any hazardous activity after taking non-benzodiazepine hypnotics. Non-benzodiazepine hypnotics are schedule IV controlled substances and they have been associated with abuse, dependence, and withdrawal. Withdrawal symptoms with these medications are usually less severe compared with benzodiazepines and patients may experience insomnia, delirium, drug cravings, anxiety, tremor, and palpitations.

Further Reading

Gunja N. The clinical and forensic toxicology of Z-drugs. *J Med Toxicol*. 2013;9:155–62.

Wilson SJ, Nutt DJ, Alford C, et al. British Association for Psychopharmacology consensus statement on evidence-based treatment of insomnia, parasomnias and circadian rhythm disorders. *J Psychopharmacol*. 2010;24:1577–601.

Zammit G. Comparative tolerability of newer agents for insomnia. *Drug Saf*. 2009;32:735–48.

Sodium Oxybate (Xyrem®)

Typical Uses: cataplexy in narcolepsy, excessive daytime sleepiness in narcolepsy, fibromyalgia, alcohol withdrawal syndrome, and maintenance of alcohol abstinence

Potential Neurologic or Psychiatric Medication Adverse Effects: Very common adverse effects (>10%) include dizziness and dose-related nausea. Common dose-related adverse effects (1–10%) include feeling drunk, paresthesia, sleepwalking, sleep paralysis, irritability, disorientation, and confusion. Other common adverse effects (1–10%) include somnolence, tremor, depression, and anxiety. Sodium oxybate has a black box warning for respiratory depression. It is a schedule III controlled substance and the sodium salt gamma hydroxybutyrate (GHB) is a schedule I controlled substance. Sodium oxybate is associated with abuse, misuse, central nervous system (CNS) adverse effects such as seizure, respiratory depression, decreased consciousness, coma, and death. Other neuropsychiatric adverse effects such as hallucinations, paranoia, psychosis, and agitation have also been reported. Sodium oxybate should be used with caution in patients with depression, sleep-related breathing disorders, or substance use disorders. Lower starting doses should be used in geriatric patients, patients with hepatic impairment, or in patients who are on divalproex sodium. Sodium oxybate is a CNS depressant and the concurrent use of alcohol or sedative hypnotics is contraindicated. It is also contraindicated in patients with succinic semialdehyde dehydrogenase deficiency. Additionally, the use of sedating antidepressants or antipsychotics, sedating antiepileptic medications, or muscle relaxants may increase the risk of respiratory depression, profound sedation, syncope, and death. Sodium oxybate is only available through a restricted distribution program and prescribers and patients must enroll in the Xyrem Risk Evaluation and Mitigation Strategy (REMS) Program. It has a rapid onset of action and patients should take the medication while in bed and lie down immediately to decrease the risk of falls. Patients should avoid driving, operating machinery, or engaging in any hazardous activity for at least 6 hours after taking the second dose, or until they are able to tolerate the adverse effects.

Further Reading

Busardo FP, Kyriakou C, Napoletano S, et al. Clinical applications of sodium oxybate (GHB): from narcolepsy to alcohol withdrawal syndrome. *Eur Rev Med Pharmacol Sci.* 2015;19: 4654–63.

Xyrem® (sodium oxybate) package insert. Palo Alto, CA: Jazz Pharmaceuticals, Inc; Jul 2017.

Stimulants

Class Members: methylphenidate (Ritalin IR/SR/LA®, Metadate ER/CD®, Concerta®, Quillivant XR®, Daytrana® patch), dexmethylphenidate (Focalin IR/XR®), mixed amphetamine salt (Adderall IR/XR®), dextroamphetamine (Dexedrine IR®, ProCentra®), lisdexamfetamine (Vyvanse®)

Typical Uses: attention deficit hyperactivity disorder (ADHD), treatment-refractory depression

Potential Neurologic or Psychiatric Adverse Effects: The most frequently encountered adverse effects include headache, insomnia, irritability, restlessness, emotional lability, and anxiety. Less commonly reported effects are tics, agitation, paresthesia, fatigue, hypervigilance, anger outbursts, and psychosis. When dosed too high, stimulants can induce a "zombie-like" effect, which may appear as apathy, staring, or preoccupation. All stimulants are listed as DEA controlled substances (C-II) in the United States. Misuse, dependency, and diversion are possible. They should be cautiously prescribed in a patient with a history of a substance use disorder. Stimulants may also exacerbate symptoms of underlying psychiatric conditions, such as mania or psychosis. Patients should be screened for bipolar disorder prior to initiating treatment with a stimulant. Stimulant medications should be discontinued if symptoms of psychosis (paranoia/delusions, auditory/visual hallucinations) develop during treatment. All stimulants have the potential to lower the seizure threshold and should be used with caution in a patient with a known seizure disorder. All stimulants also have the potential to increase blood pressure and heart rate. In patients with pre-existing structural cardiac abnormalities, the cardiac adverse effect of stimulants may be associated with stroke, myocardial infarction, or sudden death.

Further Reading

American Academy of Pediatrics. ADHD: clinical practice guideline for the diagnosis, evaluation, and treatment of attention-deficit/hyperactivity disorder in children and adolescents. *Pediatrics.* 2011;128:1007–22.

Lexi-Drugs. Lexicomp. Hudson, OH: Wolters Kluwer Health, Inc. http://online.lexi.com. Accessed May 22, 2017.

Micromedex 2.0. Greenwood Village, CO: Truven Health Analytics, Inc. http://micromedexsolutions.com. Accessed May 22, 2017.

Santosh PJ, Sattar S, Canagaratnam M. Efficacy and tolerability of pharmacotherapies for attention-deficit hyperactivity disorder in adults. *CNS Drugs.* 2011;25:737–63.

Suvorexant (Belsomra®)

Typical Uses: insomnia characterized by difficulties with sleep onset and/or sleep maintenance

Potential Neurologic or Psychiatric Medication Adverse Effects: Common adverse effects (1–10%) include somnolence, headache, dizziness, abnormal dreams, and fatigue. Rare (<1%) adverse effects include complex behavior such as "sleep-driving," excessive daytime sleepiness, amnesia, anxiety, sleep paralysis, hypnagogic/hypnopompic hallucinations, worsening depression, suicidal ideation, and mild cataplexy. Women and obese patients, particularly obese women, are at an increased risk of exposure-related adverse effects. Suvorexant can impair driving skills and increase the risk of falling asleep while driving. Risk of impaired alertness and motor coordination increases with dose. Patients should take suvorexant within 30 minutes before bedtime with at least 7 hours remaining before the planned time of awakening to reduce the risk of next-day impairment. Co-administration with other central nervous system (CNS) depressants or cytochrome P450 3A4 inhibitors may increase the risk of CNS depression, and patients should avoid consuming alcohol while taking suvorexant. Suvorexant is contraindicated in patients with narcolepsy and it is not recommended for patients with severe hepatic impairment. Suvorexant is a schedule IV controlled substance, and it should be used with caution in patients with substance use disorder.

Further Reading

Belsomra® (suvorexant) package insert. Whitehouse Station, NJ: Merck & Co., Inc; May 2016.

Citrome L. Suvorexant for insomnia: a systematic review of the efficacy and safety profile for this newly approved hypnotic – what is the number needed to treat, number needed to harm and likelihood to be helped or harmed? *Int J Clin Pract.* 2014;68:1429–41.

Varenicline Tartrate (Chantix®)

Typical Uses: smoking cessation

Potential Neurologic or Psychiatric Medication Adverse Effects: Case reports and post-marketing pharmacovigilance data first identified a possible association of varenicline use with neuropsychiatric adverse effects including depression, mania, psychosis, hallucinations, paranoia, delusions, homicidal ideation, hostility, agitation, aggression, anxiety, panic, and suicidal or self-injurious behavior in patients both with and without pre-existing psychiatric illness. In 2009 the FDA required a black box warning on varenicline products warning of the potential risk for neuropsychiatric side effects. In contrast, large observational studies, randomized controlled trials, and meta-analyses have not shown an increased risk of neuropsychiatric effects when varenicline is used for smoking cessation compared with placebo or other smoking cessation therapies. A large, manufacturer-conducted, randomized, double-blind, placebo- and active-controlled study examined the neuropsychiatric safety of varenicline versus active comparator or placebo in 8000 smokers with or without a history of psychiatric disorders. Patients were stratified based on presence of psychiatric history and randomized to varenicline, extended-release bupropion, transdermal nicotine, or placebo for 12 weeks. No significant differences in the proportion of patients who experienced moderate to severe neuropsychiatric adverse events were observed between treatment and placebo groups. Adverse events were more common for patients with psychiatric diagnoses compared with no psychiatric history, but overall rates were low for both groups. The authors concluded that varenicline use results in moderate to severe neuropsychiatric adverse events at a rate no higher than 1.5% in smokers without a psychiatric disorder and no higher than 4% in smokers with a pre-existing psychiatric disorder. Subsequently, in 2016 the FDA elected to remove the black box warning for neuropsychiatric effects; however, if patients do experience any behavioral changes and/or psychiatric symptoms after starting varenicline it should be discontinued.

Further Reading

Anthenelli RM, Benowitz NL, West R, et al. Neuropsychiatric safety and efficacy of varenicline, bupropion, and nicotine patch in smokers with and without psychiatric disorders (EAGLES): a double-blind, randomised, placebo-controlled clinical trial. *Lancet*. 2016;387:2507–20.

Varenicline. In *Lexi-Drugs. Lexicomp*. Hudson, OH: Wolters Kluwer Health, Inc. http://online.lexi .com. Accessed Jul 10, 2017.

Varenicline. In *AHFS Drug Information STAT!Ref Online Electronic Medical Library*. Bethesda, MD: American Society of Health-System Pharmacists. http://online.statref.com/document .aspx?fxid=1&docid=497. Accessed Jul 10, 2017.

Index

abacavir, 749–750
abatacept, 764
abdominal aortic aneurysm repair, 35
abdominal migraine (cyclic vomiting
    syndrome), 137–138
abducens nerve (CN VI)
    diabetic neuropathy, 151–152
    double vision, 624
    Gradenigo syndrome, 236, 624
abetalipoproteinemia, 410–411, 573, 690
abscesses
    intracranial
        Bacteroides, 54–55
        fungal, 222
        hemorrhage into, 247–248
        nocardiosis, 422–423
    psoas muscle, 540
    spinal epidural, 614
absence seizures, 3, 317
    atypical, 3
ACA (anterior cerebral artery)
        infarction, 28, 331–332
acamprosate, 790
acanthocytosis, 409–410
    with abetalipoproteinemia, 410–411
acarbose, 719
ACE inhibitors, 496, 709
acetazolamide, 100, 243, 297
acetazolamide-responsive myotonia,
    513–514
AChA (anterior choroidal artery)
        infarction, 28–29
acoustic neuroma (vestibular
        schwannoma), 595
acquired hepatocerebral degeneration, 4
acrodermatitis enteropathica, 705
acromegaly, 492
actinomycosis, 4
acute brachial neuritis (Parsonage–
        Turner syndrome), 5, 417
acute disseminated encephalomyelitis
        (ADEM), 5–6
    post-immunization, 503–505
    post-infectious, 146, 178, 364,
        505–507

acute inflammatory demyelinating
        polyneuropathy, *see* Guillain–
        Barré syndrome
acute kidney injury, 568–569, 577
acute necrotizing encephalopathy, 301
acute postasthmatic amyotrophy
        (Hopkins syndrome), 273–274
acute posterior multifocal placoid
        pigment epitheliopathy, 677
acute respiratory distress syndrome
        (ARDS), 294
acute stress disorder, 7–8
acyclovir, 264, 266, 738–739
adalimumab, 766
ADAMTS13 deficiency, 655–656
Addison's disease, 10–11
ADEM, *see* acute disseminated
        encephalomyelitis
adenovirus, 8
adenylosuccinate lyase (ASL)
        deficiency, 9
ADH, *see* antidiuretic hormone
ADHD, *see* attention deficit hyperactivity
        disorder
Adie's pupil, 662–663
adjustment disorder, 10, 354, 511
adrenal gland
    hyperadrenalism, 277–278
    insufficiency, 10–11
    pheochromocytoma, 484–485
adrenoleukodystrophy, 11–12
adrenomyeloneuropathy, 11–12
advanced sleep–wake phase disorder, 12
AEDs, *see* antiepileptic drugs
aerosol inhalation abuse
    nitrous oxide, 421–422, 687
    solvents, 13, 234–235, 267, 610
afferent pupillary defect, 13–14
age-related macular degeneration,
        352–353
AION (anterior ischemic optic
        neuropathy), 41, 423, 501
air embolism, 14
akinetic (atonic) seizures, 45
albiglutide, 720

albuterol (salbutamol), 736–737
alcohol abuse, 14–16
    abstinence medication, 790, 799–800
    Korsakoff syndrome, 323–324, 537
    Marchiafava–Bignami disease, 363
    Wernicke disease, 537, 651, 700–701
    withdrawal, 16–17
aldosterone excess, 277–278
alemtuzumab, 751
Alice in Wonderland syndrome, 192
alien limb phenomenon, 50
almotriptan, 788, 789
alogliptin, 720
Alpers disease (Alpers–Huttenlocher
        syndrome), 17–18
alpha-2 adrenergic agonists, 785, 790–791
alpha-galactosidase A deficiency
        (Fabry disease), 198–199
alpha-glucosidase inhibitors, 719
alpha-receptor blockers (alpha-1
        adrenergic receptor antagonists),
        421, 512, 722
ALS–parkinsonism–dementia complex
        (ALS-PDC), 21–23
altitude, central sleep apnea, 99–100
aluminum toxicity, 153–154, 570, 727
alveolar echinococcosis, 170
Alzheimer's disease, 18–19, 690–691
amantadine, 767
amaurosis fugax, 20, 644
amblyopia, 551, 625
American trypanosomiasis (Chagas
        disease), 113
aminoacidopathies
    biotinidase deficiency, 62–64
    homocysteinemia, 272–273, 281
    homocystinuria, 273
    maple syrup urine disease, 362–363
    phenylketonuria, 484
    pyridoxine-dependent seizures,
        553–554
aminoglycosides, 738
amiodarone, 709–710
ammonium ions (hyperammonemia),
        278–279, 779

adenylosuccinate lyase deficiency, 9
amnesia
    dissociative (psychogenic), 159–161
    Korsakoff syndrome, 323–324, 537
    transient global, 664
amniotic fluid embolism, 108
amoebiasis, 20
amoxapine, 791
amphetamines, 803–804
    ecstasy, 173–174
    methamphetamine, 373–374
amphotericin B, 42, 79, 222, 269, 738
amylinomimetics, 719
amyloid
    Alzheimer's disease, 18
    amyloidosis, 21
    cerebral amyloid angiopathy, 105
        familial, 205
amyotrophic lateral sclerosis (ALS),
        219–220
    ALS–parkinsonism–dementia com-
        plex, 21–23
anabolic steroids, 323, 358, 722–723
anakinra, 764–765
analgesics
    medication-overuse headache, 366
    NSAIDs, 786
    opioids, 786–787, 798–799
    salicylates, 787
anaplastic astrocytoma, 43
ANCAs (antineutrophil cytoplasmic
        antibodies), 237–238
Andersen–Tawil syndrome, 23, 477
Anderson–Fabry disease, 198–199
androgens, 323, 358, 722–723
anemia
    erythropoiesis-stimulating agents,
        755
    hemolytic–uremic syndrome, 247
    iron deficiency, 310–311, 730
    paroxysmal nocturnal hemoglobin-
        uria, 471–472
    vitamin B12 deficiency (pernicious
        anemia), 226, 686, 688
    vitamin E deficiency, 691
anesthesia
    and aminoglycosides, 738
    and hyperkalemic periodic paralysis,
        281
    malignant hyperthermia, 358–359
    nitrous oxide, 421–422, 687
aneurysms
    aortic aneurysm repair, 35
    carotid artery, 87–88

intracranial
    cerebral, 23–24
    mycotic, 398–399
    in pregnancy, 107
angel dust (phencyclidine), 483
Angelman syndrome, 24–25, see also
        Prader–Willi syndrome
angioma, 94–95, 680–681
angiomatosis (Sturge–Weber syndrome),
        232, 571, 629
angiostrongyliasis, 25–26
angiotensin-converting enzyme (ACE)
        inhibitors, 496, 709
angiotensin receptor blockers (ARBs), 709
angle closure glaucoma, 231–232
anorexia nervosa, 26–27, 486
anoxic encephalopathy, 27–28
antacids, 727
anterior cerebral artery (ACA)
        infarction, 28, 331–332
anterior choroidal artery (AChA)
        infarction, 28–29
anterior interosseous nerve syndrome, 533
anterior ischemic optic neuropathy
        (AION), 41, 423, 501
anterior spinal artery (ASA) occlusion, 29
antiarrhythmic drugs, 709–711
anti-asthma drugs, 734, 735–737
antibiotics, 340, 738, 739–747, see also
        antifungal drugs; antiviral drugs
    resistance, 181
anticholinergic drugs, 768
    bladder care, 275
    bronchodilators, 734
    poisoning, 29
    to prevent dystonic reaction, 168
anticoagulants, 377, 711, 783, see also
        antiplatelet drugs
    in atrial fibrillation, 46
    HIT, 250–251
    in pregnancy, 108
antidepressant drugs, 355, 427, 480, 547,
        791–796
    in bipolar I/II disorders, 64, 65
    in factitious disorder, 204
    in PTSD, 512
    seizure risk, 77, 355
    serotonin syndrome, 601–602
        MAIOs, 355, 480
        other drugs, 792, 793, 795, 796
    sexual dysfunction, 357, 794, 795–796
    suicide risk, 791, 792, 793, 794, 795, 796
antidiuretic hormone (ADH)
    deficiency, 492

excess (SIADH), 174, 292, 543
antiemetic drugs, 728, 729, 781–782
antiepileptic drugs (AEDs), 189, 774–780
    absence seizures, 3
    atonic seizures, 45
    BECTS (rolandic epilepsy), 58
    MERRF, 199
    for mood stabilization, 64, 307
    in pregnancy/postpartum, 190–191,
        692, 779
    for radiation-induced peripheral
        neuropathy, 560
    tonic–clonic seizures, 228
    and vitamin D deficiency, 689
antifungal drugs, 42, 79, 222, 269, 738,
        739, 742
antihelminthic drugs, 26, 432
antihistamines, 734
anti-Hu syndrome, 30
antihypertensive drugs, 496, 709,
        712–713, 716, 717
    beta-blockers, 196, 290, 516, 712
    in pre-eclampsia, 516
anti-MAG demyelinating polyneuropa-
        thy, 30–31, 418–419
antimicrobials, 738–747, see also antibi-
        otics; antifungal drugs; antiviral
        drugs
antiparkinsonian drugs, 338, 468–469,
        767–771
    dopa-responsive dystonia, 163
    in pregnancy, 384
    and psychosis, 545
antiplatelet drugs, 711–712, see also
        anticoagulants
antipsychotic drugs, 305, 565, 589–590,
        591–592
    in catatonia (contraindicated), 93
    in delirium, 144, 305
    in dementia, 19, 338
    dystonic reaction, 168
    first generation (typical), 781–782, 796
    neuroleptic malignant syndrome, 590,
        767, 770, 796, 797
    in Parkinson's disease, 545
    in pregnancy, 116
    in PTSD, 512
    rabbit syndrome, 555–556
    second-generation (atypical), 592,
        796–797
    tardive dyskinesia, 555, 589–590,
        641–642
    tardive dystonia, 642–643
antiretroviral drugs, 269, 271, 748–750

antirheumatic drugs (DMARDs), 579,
764–766
antisocial personality disorder, 306
antithrombin deficiency, 31
antithymocyte globulin, 751
anti-VEGF drugs, 352, 762
antiviral drugs, 140, 256, 738–739
for herpesviruses, 264, 266, 276
for HIV, 269, 271, 748–750
for influenza, 301, 745
Anton syndrome, 103
anxiety disorders, *see also* illness anxiety
disorder
due to another medical condition,
31–32, 454
generalized anxiety disorder, 227–228
hyperventilation syndrome, 287–288
panic disorder, 455–457
selective mutism, 598–599
anxiolytic drugs, 799, *see also* hypnotic drugs
benzodiazepines, 32, 567, 622, 648,
797–798
aorta
arteritis, 32–33
coarctation, 33
dissection, 33–34
surgical procedures, 35–36
Takayasu arteritis, 641
trauma, 36–37
aortic valve
regurgitation, 34
stenosis, 35, 678
aortography, 36
aphasia
Broca's area lesions, 377
Landau–Kleffner syndrome, 330
primary progressive, 219, 525–526
logopenic variant, 18
Wernicke, 376
apraxia of eyelid opening, 550
aprepitant, 782
aqueductal stenosis, 37–38
arachnoid cysts, 38, 491
arachnoiditis, 38–39
ARDS (acute respiratory distress syndrome), 294
arformoterol, 736
argininosuccinate (adenylosuccinate)
lyase deficiency, 9
Argyll Robinson pupil, 662
armodafinil, 316, 322
arteries, intra-arterial injections, 308, 345
arteriopathy
arteritis
aortic, 32–33

giant-cell, 32, 41, 501, 644–645
polyarteritis nodosa, 255, 395–396
Takayasu, 641
non-inflammatory
fibromuscular dysplasia, 212
moyamoya disease, 385
Sneddon's syndrome, 609–610
arteriovenous malformations (AVMs)
cerebral, 40–41, 441–443
fistula, 39–40, 89–90, 617–618
orbital, 438
hereditary hemorrhagic telangiectasia, 442–443
pulmonary, 441, 443
arteritic anterior ischemic optic neuropathy (AAION), 41, 501
arthritis, *see also* spondylosis
cervical spine, 109
DMARDs, 579, 764–766
osteoarthritis, 443
reactive, 563–564
rheumatoid, 578–579
ASA (anterior spinal artery) occlusion, 29
ASD, *see* atrial septal defect; autism
spectrum disorder
aspergillosis, 41–42
aspirin, 711–712, 787
asthma
acute postasthmatic amyotrophy,
273–274
drugs, 734, 735–737
astrocytoma, 42
cerebellar, 43–44
grade I (pilocytic), 42–43
grade II (diffuse), 43
grade III (anaplastic), 43
grade IV (glioblastoma), 43
ataxia
coenzyme Q$_{10}$ deficiency, 520
Friedreich's ataxia, 216–218
FXTAS, 216
vestibulocerebellar syndrome, 207
vitamin E deficiency, 690
atherosclerosis
carotid artery, 88–89
claudication, 307–308, 678–679
intracranial, 308–309
atlantoaxial subluxation, 44–45
atomoxetine, 797
atonic seizures, 45
atrial fibrillation, 45–46
atrial septal defect (ASD), 46–47
attention deficit hyperactivity disorder
(ADHD), 47, 307, 353–354, 547
treatment, 47, 797, 803–804

atypical facial pain, 47–48
atypical parkinsonism, 48–51
ALS-PDC, 21–23
CBD, 49–50, 128–129
LBD, 48, 50, 337
MSA, 48, 49, 50, 391–393
PSP, 48, 49, 197, 529
autism spectrum disorder, 51–52, *see also*
fragile X syndrome
autobiographical memory, 159–160
autoimmune disorders
ADEM, 5–6, 146, 178, 364, 503–507
anti-Hu syndrome, 30
anti-MAG Abs, 30–31, 418–419
autonomic neuropathy,
paraneoplastic, 461
CANOMAD syndrome, 81
celiac disease, 96–97
CIDP, 116–118
cryoglobulinemia type III, 134–135
encephalitis, 6, 177–178, 276,
462–463, 695–696
encephalomyelitis, 461–462
GAD Ab syndromes, 235–236
GALOP syndrome, 224
granulomatosis with polyangiitis,
237–238
Guillain–Barré syndrome, 6–7, 78,
254, 255, 757
Hashimoto's thyroiditis, 241
LEMS, 329–330, 463, 550
multiple sclerosis, 389–390,
436, 676
myasthenia gravis, 396–397, 463–464,
550, 624, 743
neuromyelitis optica, 414, 605
neuromyotonia, 414–415
opsoclonus–myoclonus
syndrome, 464
pernicious anemia, 686
reactive arthritis, 563–564
retinopathy, 465
rheumatoid arthritis, 578–580
scleroderma, 530, 596–598
sensory neuronopathy, 465–466
Sjögren's syndrome, 604–606
stiff person syndrome, 621–622
sulfatide antibodies, 419
Susac syndrome, 635, 676
Sydenham chorea, 635–636
systemic lupus erythematosus,
639–640
TTP, 655–656
Vogt–Koyanagi–Harada
disease, 676, 694

autonomic nervous system, *see also* syncope
  central alveolar hypoventilation syndrome, 126
  diabetic neuropathy, 150–151
  paraganglioma, 458–459
  paraneoplastic neuropathy, 461
  parasympathetic blockade, 29
  postural orthostatic tachycardia syndrome, 512–513
  pure autonomic failure, 551
  Sjögren's syndrome, 605
  and vincristine, 762
AVMs, *see* arteriovenous malformations
avoidant/restrictive food intake disorder, 52–53
axis (C2)
  atlantoaxial subluxation, 44–45
  odontoid fracture, 111–112
axonal polyneuropathy, 500
azathioprine, 238, 695, 751
azole antifungals, 739
aztreonam, 739

babesiosis, 54
back pain
  degenerative disc disease, 142, 342
  discitis, 157
  herniated discs, 261
  lumbar stenosis, 344
  radiculopathy, 560
back strain/sprain, 54, 343–344
baclofen pump, intrathecal, 622
bacterial infections
  actinomycosis, 4
  aortitis, 32–33
  Bacteroides spp., 54–55
  brucellosis, 75–76
  Campylobacter enteritis, 78
  cat scratch disease, 93–94
  Citrobacter spp., 119–120
  Clostridium spp., 120–121
    tetanus, 120, 121, 649–650
  diphtheria, 155–156
  ehrlichiosis, 174–175
  Enterobacteriaceae, 119–120, 181–182
  Fusobacterium spp., 222–223
  Haemophilus influenzae type B, 240
  infective endocarditis, 299–300, 600–601, 625–626
  leprosy, 334
  leptospirosis, 335
  Listeria monocytogenes, 339–340
  Lyme disease, 347–348

Mycoplasma pneumoniae, 397–398
mycotic aneurysm, 398–399
necrotizing fasciitis, 91, 207, 208
Neisseria meningitis, 407–409
nocardiosis, 422–423
osteomyelitis, 156–157, 447
pertussis, 156, 482–483
Pseudomonas aeruginosa, 538–539
pyomyositis, 552–553
Rocky Mountain spotted fever, 579–580
sepsis, 600
Staphylococcus aureus, 619
Streptococcus spp.
  group A (rheumatic fever), 116, 379, 577–578, 635–636
  group B, 625
  microaerophilic, 625–626
  PANDAS, 635–636, 658
  S. pneumoniae, 626–627
syphilis, 32, 271, 637–638, 662
tuberculosis, 271, 669
typhoid, 671–672
Whipple's disease, 702
Bacteroides spp., 54–55
balance problems, *see* vertigo
Balint syndrome, 55–56
Bardet–Biedl syndrome, 573
bariatric surgery complications, 56
Bartonella henselae (cat scratch disease), 93–94
basal ganglia
  calcification, 206–207
  copper deposition (Wilson's disease), 92, 383, 384
  MCA occlusion, 376
  and movement disorders, 384
  neurodegeneration with brain iron accumulation, 409–410, 411
basilar artery
  locked-in syndrome, 341, 481
  top of the basilar syndrome, 663
basilar invagination, 56–57
basiliximab, 751–752
Bassen–Kornzweig syndrome (abetalipoproteinemia), 410–411, 573, 690
Batten's disease (neuronal ceroid lipofuscinoses), 528, 573
B cell disorders, *see also* lymphoma
  multiple myeloma, 389
  plasma cell dyscrasias, 492–493
  Waldenström's macroglobulinemia, 699–700
Becker muscular dystrophy, 57

Beck's syndrome (ASA occlusion), 29
BECTS (benign epilepsy of childhood with centro-temporal spikes), 58
behavioral variant frontotemporal dementia (bv-FTD), 219
Behçet's disease, 677
Bell's palsy (facial nerve), 200–201, 265
  inability to close eyelids, 319
  parotid cancer, 469
  in pregnancy, 417
bendamustine, 700
Benedikt syndrome, 624
benign acute childhood myositis, 301
benign epilepsy of childhood with centro-temporal spikes (BECTS), 58
benign familial infantile convulsions and choreoathetosis (ICCA), 58–59
benign familial neonatal infantile seizures (BFNIS), 59
benign familial neonatal seizures (BFNS), 59
benign fasciculation syndrome, 59–60
benign hereditary chorea (essential chorea), 193–194
benign paroxysmal positional vertigo (BPPV), 60–61
benzamides, 728, 781, 782
benzodiazepines, 32, 567, 622, 648, 797–798
beriberi, 537, 651
beta-blockers, 196, 290, 516, 712
beta-lactam/beta-lactamase inhibitors, 181, 740
bevacizumab, 762
BFNIS (benign familial neonatal infantile seizures), 59
BFNS (benign familial neonatal seizures), 59
Bickers–Adams–Edwards syndrome, 37
Bickerstaff encephalitis, 6
biguanides, 719–720
bile acid sequestrants, 714
bilirubin-induced neurologic dysfunction (kernicterus), 319–320, 741
binge eating disorder, 61, *see also* bulimia nervosa
Bing–Neel syndrome, 699
Binswanger's disease, 61–62, 312
biotinidase deficiency, 62–64
bipolar I disorder, 64, 800
bipolar II disorder, 65, 800
bipolar and related disorder due to another medical condition, 66

bisphosphonates, 723
black widow spider venom, 66–67
bladder cancer, 67–68
blastomycosis, 68
blepharospasm, 68–69, 367–368
blinatumomab, 754
blindness, *see* vision, loss of
blood hyperviscosity, 288, 505, 507, 622, 699–700
blood pressure, *see* hypertension; orthostatic hypotension
body dysmorphic disorder, 69–70
bone, *see also entries at* osteo-
    Paget's disease, 451
    tumors, 230–231, 445, 447–448
borderline personality disorder, 204
Borrelia burgdorferi (Lyme disease), 347–348
bortezomib, 700, 760
botulinum toxin injections, 69, 110, 368, 783
botulism, 70, 120, 550
bovine spongiform encephalopathy (BSE), 70–71
BPPV (benign paroxysmal positional vertigo), 60–61
brachial plexopathy, 71
    acute neuritis, 5, 417
    burner syndrome, 71–72
    after cardiac surgery, 86
    crutch use neuropathy, 134
    neoplasm-related, 72
    radiation neuropathy, 559–560
    root avulsion, 580–581
Bradbury–Eggleston syndrome, 551
brain–lung–thyroid spectrum disorder, 193–194
brainstem
    central pontine myelinolysis, 97–98, 292, 570
    concussion, 73
    encephalitis, 172, 182
    lacunar stroke, 328
    locked-in syndrome, 341, 481
    ophthalmoplegia, 624
    Parinaud syndrome, 197, 467, 652
breast cancer, 73–74
    brachial plexopathy, 72
    chemotherapy, 757–758, 760–761
    meningitis, 83
brief psychotic disorder, 74–75
brivaracetam, 774
Broca's area, 377
bronchodilators, 734, 736–737

brucellosis, 75–76
BSE (bovine spongiform encephalopathy), 70–71
buckthorn fruit poisoning, 76
bulimia nervosa, 76–77, *see also* binge eating disorder
buprenorphine, 798–799
bupropion, 77, 357, 791–792
Burkitt lymphoma, 77
burner syndrome, 71–72
burnout, 627
buspirone, 799
butalbital, 783
butyrophenones (haloperidol), 168, 781, 796

cabazitaxel, 761
CADASIL, 105, 312
caffeine, 783–784
Calabar swelling, 342
calcineurin inhibitors, 695, 752
calcitonin, 723
calcium
    hypercalcemia, 389, 568, 689
    hypocalcemia, 288–289
calcium channel blockers, 712–713
Campylobacter enteritis, 78
canagliflozin, 721
canakinumab, 764–765
candidiasis, 78–79, 221–222
cannabinoids, medicinal, 781
cannabis, 79–80
    withdrawal, 80–81
CANOMAD syndrome, 81
capecitabine, 755
capillary telangiectasia, 81–82
carbamazepine, 64, 191, 774–775
carbapenems, 740
    resistance, 181
carbon dioxide (hypercarbia/hypercapnia), 118–119, 279
carbon disulphide toxicity, 82
carbon monoxide poisoning, 82
carboplatin, 759–760
carcinoid tumors, 82–83
carcinomatous meningitis, 83–84
cardiac surgery, 85–86
cardioembolic stroke, 46, 85, 375
cardiogenic syncope, 86–87
cardiovascular disorders
    aorta, *see* aorta
    aortic valve regurgitation, 34
    aortic valve stenosis, 35, 678
    arrhythmias, 84–85

Andersen–Tawil syndrome, 23, 477
atrial fibrillation, 45–46
    medication, 709–711
    orthostatic tachycardia, 512–513
    prolonged QT syndrome, 533, 743, 744
    Stoke Adams attacks, 623
    and TCAs, 795
atrial septal defect, 46–47
congestive heart failure, 101–102, 126–127
diabetic autonomic neuropathy, 151
hypertrophic cardiomyopathy, 287
infective endocarditis, 299–300, 600–601, 625–626
mitral prolapse, 380–381
mitral regurgitation, 379–380
mitral stenosis, 380, 678
myocardial infarction, 399–400
patent ductus arteriosus, 472
patent foramen ovale, 472–473
prosthetic valves, 536
rheumatic fever, 116, 379, 577–578
ventricular septal defect, 681
carfilzomib, 760
caries, 147
carmustine, 758–759
carnitine deficiency, 518–519
carotid artery
    aneurysm, 87–88
    carotid–cavernous fistula, 89–90
    dissection, 88
    endarterectomy/stenting, 88–89
carotid sinus hypersensitivity, 90
carpal tunnel syndrome, 90–91, 417, 418, 533
cartilage (relapsing polychondritis), 565–566
cassava root poisoning, 91
catamenial neuropathy, 180
cataplexy, 405, 406, 802–803
cataracts, 91–93
catatonia, 93, 160
cat scratch disease, 93–94
cauda equina syndrome, 94, 618
cavernous angioma, 94–95
cavernous sinus, *see also* venous sinus thrombosis
    carotid–cavernous fistula, 89–90
    thrombophlebitis, 95
    thrombosis, 95–96
    Tolosa–Hunt syndrome, 661–662
    tumor, 96
CBD (corticobasal degeneration), 49–50, 128–129

celiac disease, 96–97
central pontine myelinolysis, 97–98, 292, 570
central retinal artery occlusion, 98, 416
central retinal vein occlusion, 98–99
central serous choroidopathy, 99
central sleep apnea
    Cheyne–Stokes respiration, 101–102, 114
    high altitude, 99–100
    medications/substance abuse, 100–101
    primary, 519–520
central visual impairment, 102–103
centronuclear myopathy, 103–104
cephalosporins, 741
cerebellum
    astrocytoma/glioma, 43–44
    coenzyme Q_{10} deficiency, 520
    Dandy–Walker syndrome, 141
    drug-induced tremors, 166
    Lhermitte–Duclos disease, 338–339
    medulloblastoma, 367
    MSA-C, 49, 393–394
    vestibulocerebellar ataxia, 207
cerebral amyloid angiopathy, 105, see also lobar hemorrhage
    familial, 205
cerebral palsy, 106
cerebral venous thrombosis, see venous sinus thrombosis
cerebrospinal fluid leaks, 297, 645
cerebrotendinous xanthomatosis, 107
cerebrovascular disease, see stroke
certolizumab pegol, 766
cervical arthritis, 109
cervical disc disorders, 109–110
    degenerative disease, 142
    herniation, 260
cervical dystonia, 110
cervical facet syndrome, 110–111
cervical instability (atlantoaxial subluxation), 44–45
cervical myofascial pain syndrome, 111
cervical odontoid fracture, 111–112
cervical radiation myelopathy, 558
cervical spondylosis, 112
cervical trauma, 111, 112–113
cervical tumors, 406–407
Chagas disease, 113
channelopathies
    Andersen–Tawil syndrome, 23, 477
    BFNIS, 59
    BFNS, 59
    Dravet syndrome, 164–165

familial hemiplegic migraine, 205–206
    hyperkalemic periodic paralysis, 281–282, 477
    hypokalemic periodic paralysis, 291, 476–477
    LEMS, 329–330, 463, 550
    limbic encephalitis, 695–696
    myotonia syndromes, 414–415, 477, 513–514
Charcot–Marie–Tooth disease
    type 1, 258
    type 3, 258–259
CHARGE syndrome, 374
Charles Bonnet syndrome, 92, 103, 352, 436
chemotherapy, 230, 337, 754–763
    intrathecal, 77, 757
    PCV, 432
    radiochemotherapy, 557, 559
cherry-red spot myoclonus syndrome (sialidosis type I), 603
Cheyne–Stokes respiration, 101–102, 114
child abuse, 114–115, 204
children, see also metabolic disorders; neonates; neurodevelopmental disorders
    ADEM/encephalomyelitis, 5–6, 178, 364, 503–507
    adenovirus, 8
    adrenoleukodystrophy (cerebral form), 11–12
    Alpers disease, 17–18
    amblyopia, 551, 625
    aqueductal stenosis, 37
    bone tumors, 445–446
    brain tumors, 43, 183, 652
        glioma, 43–44
        medulloblastoma, 367
    central visual loss, 103
    centronuclear myopathy, 103–104
    cerebral palsy, 106
    cyclic vomiting syndrome, 137–138
    disruptive mood dysregulation disorder, 158–159
    dopa-responsive dystonia, 163
    epilepsy
        absence, 3, 317
        BECTS (rolandic), 58
        BFNIS, 59
        BFNS, 59
        cortical dysplasia, 128
        Doose syndrome, 162–163
        Dravet syndrome, 164–165

early myoclonic encephalopathy, 169
        ESES, 175–176
        folinic acid-responsive, 214
        GABA transaminase deficiency, 224
        ICCA, 58–59
        infantile spasms, 299
        juvenile myoclonic, 318, 528–529
        Landau–Kleffner syndrome, 330
        Lennox–Gastaut syndrome, 332–333, 778
        Ohtahara syndrome, 430–431
        progressive myoclonic, 528–529
        pyridoxine-dependent, 553–554
        Rasmussen encephalitis, 562–563
        temporal lobe, with febrile convulsions, 210
    febrile seizures, 210–211
    GAMT deficiency, 238
    GLUT1 deficiency, 236
    Haemophilus influenzae type B, 240
    Hand–Schuller–Christian disease, 240–241
    hemolytic–uremic syndrome, 247
    HHV-6, 275–276
    Hopkins syndrome, 273–274
    influenza-associated encephalopathy, 301
    measles, 364–365
    meningitis
        coxsackie virus, 129–130
        echovirus, 171–172
        meningococcal, 407–409
    Menkes disease, 370–371
    mitochondrial disorders, 332, 404–405
    muscular dystrophy
        Becker, 57
        Duchenne, 57
        facioscapulohumeral, 202
    nightmare disorder, 420–421
    otitis media, 117, 236, 363–364
    radiotherapy side effects, 184
    retinoblastoma, 440
    selective mutism, 598–599
    spinal muscular atrophy type III, 616
    Sydenham chorea, 635–636
    tic disorders, 201–202, 657–659
    tuberous sclerosis, 571, 670
chlorpromazine, 796
cholesteatoma, 117, 118
cholesterol embolism, 115
cholinesterase inhibitors, 19, 769

chorea
  chorea gravidarum, 115–116, 383
  essential, 193–194
  hemiballism, 244–245
  Huntington's, 277, 383, 384, 773
  orofacial dyskinesia, 441
  Sydenham, 635–636
choreoathetosis, 58–59
chorioretinopathy, 99
chromosomal abnormalities, *see also*
    trinucleotide repeat disorders
  Angelman syndrome, 24–25
  Down syndrome, 44–45, 163–164,
    765
  Klinefelter syndrome, 322–323
  Prader–Willi syndrome, 514–515
  ring chromosome 20 syndrome, 580
  Turner syndrome, 671
chronic (congestive) heart failure,
    101–102, 126–127
chronic inflammatory demyelinating
    polyneuropathy (CIDP)/
    chronic idiopathic sensory
    polyneuropathy, 116–117
  multifocal, 387
chronic kidney disease, 569–570
chronic otitis media, 117–118
chronic progressive external ophthalmo-
    plegia, 550, 624
chronic respiratory failure, 118–119
ciguatera (fish) poisoning, 119
cimetidine, 727–728
cinacalcet, 724
circadian rhythm disorders
  advanced sleep–wake phase disorder, 12
  delayed sleep–wake phase disorder,
    142–143
  fatal familial insomnia, 209
  irregular sleep–wake rhythm disorder,
    311–312
  jet lag, 316–317
  shift work disorder, 602–603
cirrhosis, 4, 256
cisplatin, 759–760
Citrobacter spp., 119–120
CJD (Creutzfeldt–Jakob disease), 130–131
  variant form, 70–71
Claude syndrome, 624
claudication, 307–308, 678–679
clindamycin, 741
clonazepam, 567, 797–798
clonidine, 790–791
Clostridium botulinum/botulism, 70, 120,
    550

Clostridium perfringens, 120–121
Clostridium tetani/tetanus, 120, 121,
    649–650
clozapine, 592, 796–797
cluster headache, 121
CMV (cytomegalovirus), 139–140, 271
coagulopathy, 122
  hypercoagulability, *see* thrombophilia
  hypocoagulability
    thrombocytopenia, 297–298, 654,
      655–656
    vitamin K deficiency, 692–693
cobalamin (B12) deficiency, 226, 537,
    686, 732
cocaine, 122–123
Coccidioides immitis, 123–124, 221
cochlear degeneration, 683
coenzyme Q_{10} deficiency, 520–521
  Leigh disease, 332
  NADH CoQ reductase deficiency,
    404–405
coma, 481
complex regional pain syndrome, 124
compression fractures, vertebral,
    124–125
COMT inhibitors, 469, 768–769
concussion
  brainstem, 73
  post-concussion syndrome, 187
conduct disorders, 157–158
  intermittent explosive disorder,
    306–307
confusional arousal, 125–126
congenital central alveolar hypoventila-
    tion syndrome, 126
congestive heart failure, 101–102,
    126–127
Consten syndrome (temporomandibular
    joint syndrome), 647–648
continuous spikes and waves during
    sleep syndrome, 175–176
contraceptives, 724
conversion disorder, 204, 220–221, 511
  loss of vision, 221
convulsions, *see also* epilepsy
  eclampsia, 172–173, 190–193, 397
  febrile, 210–211
copper
  deficiency, 127–128, 705
  Menkes disease, 370–371
  Wilson's disease, 92, 384
cornea (keratitis), 319
corpus callosum necrosis (Marchiafava–
    Bignami disease), 363

cortical dysplasia, 128
cortical visual impairment, 102–103
corticobasal degeneration (CBD), 49–50,
    128–129
corticosteroids, 91, 238, 391, 752
  critical illness myopathy, 131–132
cortisol
  Addison's disease, 10–11
  hypercortisolism, 136–137, 277–278
    Cushing disease, 491, 492
cough headache, 523
coxsackie virus, 129–130
cramp, 395–396
cranial nerves, *see also individual nerves*
  diphtheric polyneuropathy, 155
  radiation neuropathy, 559–560
  Tolosa–Hunt syndrome, 661–662
craniofacial tremor, 130
craniopharyngioma, 490, 491
creatine deficiency, 238
Creutzfeldt–Jakob disease (CJD),
    130–131
  variant form, 70–71
critical illness myopathy, 131–132
critical illness neuropathy/
    polyneuropathy, 132–133
Crohn's disease, 133–134
crutch use neuropathy, 134
cryoglobulinemia, 134–135, 257
cryptococcal meningitis, 135–136, 271
crystal meth (methamphetamine),
    373–374
Cuban epidemic neuropathy, 136
Cushing syndrome, 136–137,
    277–278
  Cushing disease, 491, 492
cyanide (cassava root) poisoning, 91
cyclic vomiting syndrome, 137–138
cyclophosphamide, 237, 566, 759
cyclosporine, 695, 752
cyclothymic disorder, 138–139
cystic echinococcosis, 170
cysticercosis with myositis, 139
cytarabine (ara-C), 754
  intrathecal, 77, 757
cytomegalovirus (CMV), 139–140, 271

danazol, 722–723
Dandy–Walker syndrome, 141
daptomycin, 741–742
darbepoetin alfa, 755
Darlings disease (histoplasmosis),
    268–269
darunavir, 750

deafness, *see* hearing loss
decompression sickness, 141–142
decongestants, 735
deep brain stimulation, 110, 247, 401
deep territory MCA ischemia, 375, 376
Dejerine–Sottas disease, 258–259
delayed sleep–wake phase disorder, 142–143
delirium, 143–144, 306, 548
    febrile, 301
    ICU psychosis, 305
delirium tremens, 16
delusional disorder, 144–145
dematiaceous fungi, 145–146
dementia
    ALS-PDC, 21–23
    Alzheimer's disease, 18–19, 690–691
    antipsychotic drug use, 19, 338
    CJD/vCJD, 70–71, 130–131
    dialysis-related, 153–154, 570
    frontotemporal, 219–220, 529
    HIV, 270
    Lewy body, 48, 50, 337–338
    medications for, 769, 771
    primary progressive aphasia, 219, 525–526
    vascular, 388–389, 679
        Binswanger's disease, 61–62, 312
    workup, 18
dengue, 146–147, 213
dental disease, 147–148
dentatorubral-pallidoluysian atrophy (DRPLA), 148, 528
depakote, *see* valproate
depersonalization/derealization disorder, 149
depression, *see also* antidepressants
    bipolar disorders, 64, 65
    cyclothymic disorder, 138–139
    major depressive disorder, 353–356, 511
    medication-associated, 717, 731, 749, 760–761
    persistent depressive disorder, 479–480
    psychotic, 546, 589
    and seizures, 354, 355
de Quervain's tenosynovitis, 149–150
dermatomyositis, 150, 255, 498–499
developmental disorders, *see* neurodevelopmental disorders
dexamethasone, 700
dexmedetomidine, 790–791
diabetes insipidus, 492, 543

diabetes mellitus, 92
    autonomic neuropathy, 150–151
    CIDP, 116–117
    cranial mononeuropathy, 151–152
    distal symmetric polyneuropathy, 153
    hyperglycemia, 280
    hypoglycemia, 290
    ketoacidosis, 152
    oral hypoglycemic agents, 719–721
    peripheral mononeuropathy, 152
    polyradiculopathy, 153
    retinopathy, 416, 572
dialysis-related disorders, 569–570
    dementia, 153–154, 570
    disequilibrium syndrome, 154, 570
3,4-diaminopyridine (DAP), 329
diamorphine (heroin)
    toxicity, 261–262
    withdrawal, 262–263
didanosine, 749–750
diffuse astrocytoma, 43
diffuse idiopathic skeletal hyperostosis (DISH), 154–155
digoxin, 710
dihydroergotamine, 784
dipeptidyl peptidase-4 inhibitors, 720
diphtheria, 155–156
diplopia, 623–625
discitis, 156–157
discs, *see* intervertebral discs
disease-modifying antirheumatic drugs (DMARDs), 579, 764–766
disequilibrium syndrome, 154, 570
DISH (diffuse idiopathic skeletal hyperostosis), 154–155
disorders of sex development (Klinefelter syndrome), 322–323
disruptive, impulse-control, and conduct disorders, 157–158, 306–307
disruptive mood dysregulation disorder, 158–159, 306
dissociative disorders, 511
    depersonalization/derealization disorder, 149
    dissociative identity disorder, 160, 161–162
    psychogenic amnesia, 159–161
distal spinal muscular atrophy, 162
distal symmetric polyneuropathy, 153
disulfiram, 799–800
diuretics, 281, 713–714
diving (decompression sickness), 141–142
dizziness, *see* vertigo

DLB (dementia with Lewy bodies), 48, 50, 337–338
docetaxel, 761
dolutegravir, 748
domperidone, 781–782
donepezil, 19, 769
Doose syndrome, 162–163
dopamine precursors, 163, 338, 384, 468, 770–771
dopamine receptor agonists, 384, 468–469, 769–770
dopamine receptor antagonists, 781–782, *see also* antipsychotic drugs
    dystonic reactions, 168, 591, 728
        oculogyric crisis, 430
        tardive dystonia, 642–643
dopa-responsive dystonia, 163
dorsal midbrain (Parinaud) syndrome, 197, 467, 652
double vision, 623–625
Down syndrome, 44–45, 163–164, 765
doxycycline, 747
Dravet syndrome, 164–165
dronabinol, 781
dronedarone, 709–710
drop attacks
    atonic seizures, 45
    in elderly women, 165
DRPLA (dentatorubral-pallidoluysian atrophy), 148, 528
drug abuse, *see* substance abuse
drug-induced tremors, 165–167
drug reaction with eosinophilia and systemic symptoms (DRESS), 774, 775–776, 777, 778, 779, 780
Duchenne muscular dystrophy, 167
dulaglutide, 720
dyskinesia
    orofacial, 441
    paroxysmal, 470–471
    tardive, 555, 589–590, 641–642
dysphagia
    botulinum toxin, 110, 783
    psychogenic, 540–541
dysphonia, spasmodic, 611–612
dysthymia (persistent depressive disorder), 479–480, *see also* major depressive disorder
dystonia
    cervical, 110
    dopa-responsive, 163
    dystonic reaction to dopamine antagonists, 168, 591, 728

oculogyric crisis, 430
tardive dystonia, 642–643
Meige syndrome, 69, 367–368
myoclonus dystonia, 401
in pregnancy, 383
primary torsion dystonia, 526–527
rapid onset dystonia–parkinsonism,
561–562
repetitive hand use, 570–571
X-linked dystonia parkinsonism, 703

ear
BPPV, 60–61
Meniere's disease, 369
otitis externa, 538–539
otitis media
chronic, 117–118
Gradenigo syndrome, 236, 624
mastoiditis, 363–364
otosclerosis, 448–449
ototoxic drugs, 738, 743, 747, 759
perilymphatic fistula, 473–474
semicircular canal dehiscence,
633–634
temporal bone fracture, 645–646
vestibular degeneration, 683
vestibular neuritis, 683–684
early infantile epileptic encephalopathy,
430–431
early myoclonic encephalopathy, 169
eastern equine encephalitis virus,
169–170
eating disorders
anorexia nervosa, 26–27, 486
avoidant/restrictive food intake
disorder, 52–53
binge eating, 61
bulimia nervosa, 76–77
pica, 486–487
sleep-related eating disorder, 606
echinocandins, 742
echinococcosis, 170–171
echovirus, 171–172
eclampsia, 108, 172–173, 190–191, 397,
see also pre-eclampsia
ecstasy (MDMA), 173–174
ectopia lentis (lens subluxation),
333–334
efavirenz, 749
Ehler–Danlos syndrome, 174
ehrlichiosis, 174–175
elbow (epicondylitis), 185
electrical status epilepticus in sleep
(ESES), 175–176

electroconvulsive therapy, 176–177, 545,
547
eletriptan, 788
elimination disorders
encopresis, 179
enuresis, 183
elvitegravir, 748
embolism
air, 14
amniotic fluid, 108
cardioembolic, 46, 85, 375
cholesterol, 115
fat, 209–210
gas (decompression sickness),
141–142
septic, 600–601
empty sella syndrome, 177
emtricitabine, 749–750
encephalitis, 177–178, see also encephalomyelitis
amebic, 20
autoimmune
Bickerstaff, 6
limbic, 177–178, 276, 462–463,
695–696
brainstem (enterovirus), 172, 182
cysticercosis, 139
dengue, 146–147, 213
eastern equine encephalitis, 169–170
flaviviruses (in general), 212–214
hepatitis A, 254
HIV-associated, 271
HSV-I, 263–264
HSV-II
adult, 264, 265
neonatal, 264
Japanese encephalitis virus, 213,
315–316
La Crosse virus, 327
measles, 364–365
MERS, 301, 460
mumps, 394–395
Mycoplasma pneumoniae, 397–398
rabies, 556
Rasmussen, 562–563
St. Louis encephalitis virus, 622–623
encephalitis lethargica, 179
encephalomyelitis
ADEM, 5–6
post-immunization, 503–505
post-infectious, 146, 178, 364,
505–507
Lyme disease, 348
paraneoplastic, 461–462

encephalomyopathy, 520
encephalopathy, see also encephalitis
anoxic, 27–28
bilirubin, 319–320, 741
BSE, 70–71
dengue, 146, 213
in eclampsia, 108, 172
epileptic
Dravet syndrome, 164–165
early myoclonic encephalopathy,
169
folinic acid-responsive, 214
GABA transaminase deficiency, 224
Ohtahara syndrome, 430–431
hepatic, 251–252
with cirrhosis, 4, 256
medication-associated, 744,
746–747
hypercapneic, 118–119
hypertensive (PRES), 285, 501–503,
575–576
in HUS, 247
medication-associated, 502, 509,
570, 752, 753, 762
in pregnancy, 108, 172, 416
influenza, 301
maple syrup urine disease, 362–363
PLERM, 432
post-transplant, 508–509
renal failure-associated, 569–570
septic, 600
Wernicke, 537, 569–570, 651,
700–701
Korsakoff syndrome, 323–324, 537
encephalotrigeminal angiomatosis
(Sturge–Weber syndrome), 232,
571, 629
encopresis, 179
endocarditis
infective, 299–300, 600–601,
625–626
mycotic aneurysm, 398–399
endocrine myopathies, 179–180
endometrial cancer, 674–675
endometriosis (ectopic tissue), 180
endothelin receptor antagonists, 717
enfuvirtide, 748
entacapone, 469, 768–769
enteritis (Campylobacter), 78
Enterobacteriaceae, 119–120, 181–182
enteroviruses, 182–183
coxsackie, 129–130
echovirus, 171–172
poliovirus, 182, 494–495

enuresis, 183
eosinophilic meningitis
	(angiostrongyliasis), 25–26
eosinophils, hypereosinophilic
	syndrome, 279–280
ependymoma, 183–184
ephedra/ephedrine, 184–185
epicondylitis, 185
epidermoid tumors, 185–186
epidural abscesses, 614
epidural hematoma (intracranial),
	186–188
epidural hemorrhage (spinal), 614
epidural lipomatosis, 615
epidural neoplasms (spinal metastases),
	188
epilepsy, 189, see also antiepileptic drugs
	absence seizures, 3, 317
		atypical, 3
	amnesia, 160
	atonic seizures, 45
	BECTS (rolandic), 58
	BFNIS, 59
	BFNS, 59
	cortical dysplasia, 128
	and depression, 354, 355
	Doose syndrome, 162–163
	Dravet syndrome, 164–165
	early myoclonic encephalopathy, 169
	folinic acid-responsive, 214
	frontal lobe, 218–219
	GABA transaminase deficiency, 224
	ICCA, 58–59
	infantile spasms, 299
	juvenile absence epilepsy, 3, 317
	juvenile myoclonic epilepsy, 318
	Landau–Kleffner syndrome, 330
	Lennox–Gastaut syndrome, 332–333,
		778
	medication-associated seizures, 736,
		740, 741, 758, 792
	occipital lobe, 428–429
	Ohtahara syndrome, 430–431
	parietal lobe, 466–467
	in pregnancy, 189–191
	progressive myoclonic epilepsy,
		528–529
		DRPLA, 148, 528
		Lafora disease, 328–329, 528
		MERRF, 400–401, 528
	pyridoxine-dependent, 553–554
	Rasmussen encephalitis, 562–563
	ring chromosome 20 syndrome, 580
	status epilepticus, 620–621

epilepsia partialis continua,
	191–192
	ESES, 175–176
	nonconvulsive, 424, 736
	temporal lobe, 646–647
		with febrile convulsions, 210
		mesial temporal sclerosis, 371–372
	tonic–clonic seizures, 228
Epley maneuver, 60
epoetin alfa, 755
epoprostenol, 717
Epstein–Barr virus, 192, 349
erectile disorder, 192–193, 725
ergotamine/dihydroergotamine, 784–785
erythrocytes
	acanthocytosis, 409–411
	polycythemia vera, 496–497
erythromelalgia, 195
erythropoiesis-stimulating agents, 755
ESES (electrical status epilepticus in
	sleep), 175–176
eslicarbazepine, 774–775
essential chorea, 193–194
essential myoclonus, 194–195
essential palatal myoclonus, 451, 452
essential thrombocythemia, 195
essential tremor, 195–196
estrogens
	contraceptives, 724
	HRT, 724–725
etanercept, 766
ethambutol, 742
ethanol, see alcohol abuse
ethosuximide, 3, 775
ethylene oxide poisoning, 196
everolimus, 753
exenatide, 720
exertional headache, 524
extradural hematoma, 186–188
eye, see also optic nerve; vision, loss of;
	afferent pupillary defect, 13–14
	amaurosis fugax, 20, 644
	AV fistula, 438
	cataracts, 91–93
	diabetic autonomic neuropathy, 151
	eye worm infestation, 342
	gaze abnormalities
		frontal eye field ischemia, 377
		ocular apraxia, 55
		ophthalmoplegia, 550, 623–625,
			661–662
		Parinaud syndrome, 197, 467, 652
		PSP, 529
	glaucoma, 231–232

inflammation, 439–440
	keratitis, 319
	lens subluxation, 333–334
	macular degeneration, 352–353
	microphthalmos, 374–375
	miosis, 378–379
	oculogyric crisis, 430
	onchocerciasis, 432–433
	orbital hemorrhage, 438–439
	paraneoplastic retinopathy, 465
	pregnancy-associated conditions,
		415–417
	retinal detachment, 99, 571–572
	retinitis pigmentosa, 573–574
	scleritis, 595–596
	strabismus/diplopia, 623–625
	thyroid ophthalmopathy, 197, 439,
		624, 656
	tonic pupil, 662–663
	tumors, 440–441
	uveitis, 676–677, 694
	vitreous hemorrhage, 693–694
eyedrops (in glaucoma), 232
eyelids
	Bell's palsy, 319
	blepharospasm, 68–69, 367–368
	ptosis, 549–551
	retraction, 196–197, 319
ezetimibe, 714

Fabry disease, 198–199
facet syndrome, cervical, 110–111
facial chorea, 441
facial myoclonus, 199–200
facial nerve (CN VII)
	hemifacial spasm, 69, 245–246
	palsy (Bell's palsy), 200–201, 265
		inability to close eyelids, 319
		parotid cancer, 469
		in pregnancy, 417
	trauma, 201, 645
	tumors, 200
facial pain
	atypical, 47–48
	glossopharyngeal neuralgia, 233–234,
		605
	Gradenigo syndrome, 236
	Raeder's paratrigeminal neuralgia,
		560–561
	trigeminal neuralgia, 605, 667–668
facial tics, 201–202
facial tremor, 130
facioscapulohumeral muscular dystro-
	phy, 202

factitious disorder, 160, 202–204, 486
factor V Leiden, 204
fainting, *see* syncope
famcyclovir, 739
familial cerebral amyloid angiopathy, 205
familial hemiplegic migraine, 205–206
familial idiopathic basal ganglia
    calcification, 206–207
familial vestibulocerebellar syndrome,
    207
fasciculation (benign fasciculation syn-
    drome), 59–60
fasciitis, 207–208
fascioliasis, 208
fatal familial insomnia, 209
fat embolism, 209–210
fatty acid-related disorders
    adrenoleukodystrophy, 11–12
    carnitine deficiency, 518–519
    Refsum disease, 259, 573
febrile delirium, 301
febrile seizures, 210–211
    with temporal lobe epilepsy, 210
fecal soiling (encopresis), 179
felbamate, 775
female sexual interest/arousal disorder,
    211
femoral neuropathy, 211–212, 418, 570
    psoas hemorrhage, 540
fenofibrate, 715
fibric acid derivatives, 715
fibromuscular dysplasia, 212
fidaxomicin, 742
filbanserin, 211
filgrastim, 756
flaccid paralysis
    postasthmatic, 273–274
    viral, 182, 315
flaviviruses, 212–214
    dengue, 146–147, 213
    Japanese encephalitis, 213, 315–316
    St. Louis encephalitis, 622–623
    Zika, 704
fluoropyrimidine antimetabolites, 755
fluoroquinolones, 742–743
fluorouracil, 755
focal cortical dysplasia, 128
folic acid/folate
    deficiency, 214, 537
    supplements, 190, 732
folinic acid-responsive seizures, 214
food poisoning
    botulism, 70, 120, 550
    Campylobacter enteritis, 78

ciguatera (in fish), 119
    hepatitis A, 253–255
    Listeria, 339–340
foot drop, 152, 418, 478–479
formoterol, 736
foscarnet, 276
fosfomycin, 743
fragile X syndrome, 214–216
fragile X tremor ataxia syndrome
    (FXTAS), 216
Friedreich's ataxia, 216–218
frontal eye fields, 377
frontal lobe epilepsy, 218–219
frontal lobe ischemia (MCA occlusion),
    376–377
frontal variant of Alzheimer's disease, 18
frontotemporal dementia, 219–220
    primary progressive aphasia, 219,
    525–526
    PSP, 529
frovatriptan, 789
functional neurologic symptom disorder
    (conversion disorder), 204,
    220–221, 511
    loss of vision, 221
fungal infections
    aspergillosis, 41–42
    blastomycosis, 68
    candidiasis, 78–79, 221–222
    Coccidioides immitis, 123–124, 221
    cryptococcal meningitis, 135–136,
    271
    dematiaceous fungi, 145–146
    histoplasmosis, 268–269
    meningitis (in general), 221–222
    mucormycosis, 386–387
    Paracoccidioides brasiliensis, 457–458
    Pseudallescheria boydii, 538
    spinal, 222
    Sporothrix schenckii, 619
Fusobacterium spp., 222–223
FXTAS (fragile X tremor ataxia syn-
    drome), 216

gabapentin/gabapentin enacarbil, 560,
    775–776
GABA transaminase deficiency, 224
GAD (glutamic acid decarboxylase) Ab
    syndromes, 235–236, 621–622
galactosylceramidase deficiency (Krabbe
    disease), 325
GALOP syndrome (gait disorder autoan-
    tibody late-age onset polyneu-
    ropathy), 224

gamma knife surgery, 196, 370
GAMT (guanidinoacetate methyltrans-
    ferase) deficiency, 238
gancyclovir, 739
ganglioglioma, 224–225
ganglion cyst, 225
gastrointestinal system
    Campylobacter enteritis, 78
    Crohn's disease, 133–134
    diabetic autonomic neuropathy, 151
    medications, 727–729
    tumors
        carcinoid, 82–83
        metastatic, 225–226
    ulcerative colitis, 673
Gaucher disease, 528
gaze abnormalities
    frontal eye field ischemia, 377
    ocular apraxia, 55
    ophthalmoplegia, 550, 623–625,
    661–662
    Parinaud syndrome, 197, 467, 652
    PSP, 529
GBS, *see* group B *Streptococcus*; Guillain–
    Barré syndrome
gender dysphoria, 226–227
generalized anxiety disorder, 227–228
generalized non-convulsive seizures
    (absence seizures), 3, 317
generalized tonic–clonic seizures, 228
genital herpes (HSV-II), 264–265, 381
germ cell tumors, 228–230, 491, 649
German measles (rubella), 582
Gerstmann's syndrome, 376
giant-cell arteritis, 32, 644–645
    AION, 41, 501
giant cell tumor of bone, 230–231
glandular fever (infectious mononucle-
    osis), 192
glaucoma, 231–232
glioblastoma (grade IV astrocytoma), 43
glioma
    astrocytoma, *see* astrocytoma
    ependymoma, 183–184
    oligodendroglioma, 431–432
    optic tract, 436
gliomatosis cerebri, 232–233
glipizide, 721
globus pallidus degeneration, 551–552
glomus jugulare tumor, 233
glossopharyngeal neuralgia, 233–234,
    605
glucagon-like peptide-1 receptor ago-
    nists, 720

glucocorticoids, *see* corticosteroids
glucose
    hyperglycemia, 280
    hypoglycemia, 290
glue sniffing, 13, 234–235, 267, 610
GLUT1 deficiency syndrome, 236
glutamic acid decarboxylase antibody
        (GAD Ab) syndromes, 235–236,
        621–622
gluten intolerance, 96–97
glyburide, 721
glycogen storage disease type V (McArd-
        le's disease), 402
glycopeptides, 743
golfer's elbow, 185
golimumab, 766
Gradenigo syndrome, 236, 624
granulocyte colony-stimulating factors
        (G-CSF), 756
granuloma, fungal, 222
granulomatosis with polyangiitis (Wege-
        ner's granulomatosis), 237–238
granulomatous amebic encephalitis, 20
grass pea toxicity (neurolathyrism), 413
Graves' eye disease, 197, 439, 624, 656,
        see also hyperthyroidism
grief, 353
Grisel syndrome, 44
group B *Streptococcus* (GBS), 625
growth hormone excess, 492
Guam (ALS–parkinsonism–dementia
        complex), 21–23
guanfacine, 790–791
guanidinoacetate methyltransferase
        (GAMT) deficiency, 238
Guillain–Barré syndrome (GBS), 6–7
    Campylobacter, 78
    hepatitis A, 254
    hepatitis B, 255
    medication-associated, 757
gynecologic cancers, 238–239
    ovarian, 228, 229–230, 449–450
    uterine, 674–675

H$_2$ antagonists, 727–728
Haemophilus influenzae type B, 240
hair pulling (trichotillomania), 486,
        666–667
Hallevorden–Spatz syndrome (PKAN),
        410, 457
hallucinations
    Charles Bonnet syndrome, 92, 103,
        352, 436
    and depression, 546

in parkinsonism, 50, 337, 544
    peduncular hallucinosis, 473
    and tizanidine, 791
hallucinogenic drugs
    ketamine, 320–321
    LSD, 349–350
    mescaline, 371
    phencyclidine, 483
    psilocybin, 539
haloperidol, 168, 781, 796
hand
    repetitive use, 570–571
    vascular insufficiency, 679–680
hand foot and mouth disease, 182
Hand–Schuller–Christian disease,
        240–241
Hashimoto's thyroiditis, 241
headache, *see also* migraine
    carotid artery disease, 87, 88, 89
    cluster, 121
    cough, 523
    exertional, 524
    hemicrania continua, 245
    ice pick, 295
    medication-overuse, 366
    occipital neuralgia, 429–430
    paroxysmal hemicrania, 470
    post-lumbar puncture, 242, 243,
        507–508
    in pregnancy, 241–243
    sexual activity, 524–525
    SUNCT/SUNA, 632–633
    tension, 242, 648–649
    thunderclap, 575, 656
    venous sinus thrombosis, 108
head injuries
    amnesia, 160
    brainstem concussion, 73
    carotid–cavernous fistula, 89–90
    cervical spine, 111–113
    extradural hematoma, 186–188
    persistent vegetative state, 480–482
    in PTSD, 511
    subdural hematoma, 630–631
    temporal bone fracture, 645–646
hearing loss
    Meniere's disease, 369
    otitis media, 117–118, 363–364
    otosclerosis, 448–449
    ototoxic drugs, 738, 743, 759
    temporal bone fracture, 645
    vestibular schwannoma, 595
heart disease, *see* cardiovascular disor-
        ders

heart surgery, 85–86
heavy metal poisoning
    lead, 330–331
    manganese, 359–360
heel (plantar fasciitis), 207
hemangioblastoma, 243–244, 697–698
    retinal, 571
    spinal, 615–616
hematomyelia, 244
hemiballism, 244–245
hemicrania continua, 245, *see also* parox-
        ysmal hemicrania
hemifacial spasm, 69, 245–246
hemimasticatory spasm, 246
hemiparkinsonism–hemiatrophy
        syndrome, 246–247
hemiplegic migraine, 205–206
hemolytic–uremic syndrome (HUS), 247
hemorrhage
    AVM rupture, 40–41
    epidural (extradural) hematoma,
        186–188
    hemorrhagic transformation of isch-
        emic stroke, 248–249
    into abscesses, 247–248
    into brain tumors, 249
    intraventricular, 310, 340–341
    lobar, 340–341
    orbital, 438–439
    in pregnancy, 107–108
    psoas muscle, 540
    subarachnoid, 23–24, 108, 629–630,
        693
    spinal, 618
    thrombocytopenia, 654
    vitreous, 693–694
hemorrhagic disease of the newborn
        (vitamin K deficiency), 692
Henoch–Schönlein purpura, 249–250
heparin, 31, 108, 377
heparin-induced thrombocytopenia
        (HIT), 250–251
hepatic disease, *see* liver disease
hepatitis, viral
    acute, 252–253
    HAV, 253–255
    HBV, 255–256, 257
        chronic, 253
    HCV, 256–257
        chronic, 253
        cryoglobulinemia, 134–135, 257
    neuropathy, 257–258
hereditary hemorrhagic telangiectasia,
        442–443

hereditary motor sensory neuropathy type 1 (Charcot–Marie–Tooth disease), 258

hereditary motor sensory neuropathy type 3 (Dejerine–Sottas disease), 258–259

hereditary motor sensory neuropathy type 4 (Refsum disease), 259, 573

hereditary spastic paraplegia, 259–260

Hering's phenomenon, 197

heroin
    toxicity, 261–262
    withdrawal, 262–263

herpesviruses
    Epstein–Barr, 192, 349
    herpes/varicella zoster, 265–266, 503
    HHV-6, 275–276
    HSV-I, 263–264
    HSV-II, 264–265, 381

hexane toxicity, 267

hexosaminidase A deficiency (Tay–Sachs disease), 643–644

HHV-6 (human herpesvirus 6), 275–276

highly active antiretroviral therapy (HAART), 269, 271

hip pathology/surgery, 267–268

histiocytosis (Rosai–Dorfman disease), 581

Histoplasma capsulatum, 268–269

HIT (heparin-induced thrombocytopenia), 250–251

HIV-positive patients, 269–271
    antiretroviral drugs, 271, 748–750
        IRIS, 269, 271
    cryptococcal meningitis, 135–136, 271
    histoplasmosis, 268, 269
    HSV-II, 265
    neurocognitive disorder, 270
    PML, 271, 527

HMG CoA reductase inhibitors (statins), 715

hoarding disorder, 272

homocysteinemia, 272–273, 281

homocystinuria, 273

Hopkins syndrome, 273–274

hormone replacement therapy (HRT), 724–725

Horner syndrome, 378–379, 407, 550

HSV-I (herpes simplex virus I), 263–264

HSV-II (herpes simplex virus II), 264–265, 381

HTLV-1 associated myelopathy, 274–275

human ewingii ehrlichiosis (HEE), 174, 175

human granulocytic anaplasmosis/ehrlichiosis (HGA/HGE), 174, 175

human monocytotropic ehrlichiosis (HME), 174–175

humerus, fracture, 276–277

Hunter syndrome, 350–351

Huntington's chorea, 277, 383, 384, 773

Huntington's disease-like 2 (HDL2), 409–410

HUS (hemolytic–uremic syndrome), 247

hydralazine, 717–718

hydrocephalus, 37–38, 221–222, 653

hydroxychloroquine, 764

5-hydroxytryptamine (5-HT), *see entries at* serotonin

hyperadrenalism, 277–278, *see also* hypercortisolism; pheochromocytoma

hyperammonemia, 278–279, 779
    adenylosuccinate lyase deficiency, 9

hyperbaric oxygen therapy, 141–142

hyperbilirubinemia (kernicterus), 319–320, 741

hypercalcemia, 389, 568, 689

hypercarbia/hypercapnia, 118–119, 279

hypercortisolism, 136–137, 277–278
    Cushing disease, 491, 492

hypereosinophilic syndrome, 279–280

hyperglycemia, 280

hyperhomocysteinemia, 281

hyperkalemic periodic paralysis, 281–282, 477

hyperlordosis, 282

hypermagnesemia, 282, 727

hypernatremia, 282–283

hyperparathyroidism, 283–284

hyperperfusion syndrome, 89

hyperprolactinemia, 284, 532

hypersomnia, *see also* narcolepsy
    idiopathic, 295–296
    Kline–Levine syndrome, 301, 321–322

hypertension
    antihypertensive drugs, 709, 712–713, 716, 717
    chronic, 284–285
    hypertensive crisis, 285–286, 355, 480
    lobar hemorrhage, 340–341
    in pregnancy
        eclampsia, 108, 172–173, 190–191, 397
        pre-eclampsia, 515–516

hypertensive encephalopathy, *see posterior reversible encephalopathy syndrome (PRES)*

hyperthermia, malignant, 358–359

hyperthyroidism, 286–287
    Graves' eye disease, 197, 439, 624, 656
    thyrotoxic periodic paralysis, 477, 657

hypertrophic cardiomyopathy, 287

hypertrophic polyneuropathy (hereditary motor sensory neuropathy type 3), 258–259

hyperventilation syndrome, 287–288

hyperviscosity syndrome, 288, 505, 507, 622, 699–700

hypnotic drugs, 302–303, 304, 603, *see also* anxiolytic drugs
    melatonin receptor agonists, 801
    non-benzodiazepine, 316, 802
    suvorexant, 804

hypoactive sexual desire disorder
    female, 211
    male, 357–358

hypocalcemia, 288–289

hypochondriasis (illness anxiety disorder), 298–299

hypoglossal nerve (CN XII), 289–290

hypoglycemia, 290

hypokalemia, 281

hypokalemic periodic paralysis, 291, 476–477

hypomagnesemia, 291–292

hypomania, 261
    bipolar disorders, 65, 66
    cyclothymic disorder, 138–139

hyponatremia, 292, 774
    polydipsia, 542–543

hypoparathyroidism, 292–293
    therapy, 725

hypophosphatemia, 293

hypotension, orthostatic, 551, 637, 697

hypothermia, therapeutic, 27

hypothyroidism, 241, 726

hypoventilation syndromes
    central alveolar hypoventilation syndrome, 126
    obesity hypoventilation syndrome, 425

hypovolemia, 697

hypoxia, 293–294

ibuprofen, 786

ICCA (infantile convulsions and choreoathetosis), 58–59

ice pick headache, 295

idiopathic cranial dystonia (Meige syndrome), 69, 367–368

idiopathic hypersomnia, 295–296

idiopathic intracranial hypertension
(IIH), 296–297
in pregnancy, 242, 243
tetracycline use, 747
vitamin A excess, 685–686
idiopathic thrombocytopenic purpura
(ITP), 297–298
ifosfamide, 759
IgA vasculitis (Henoch–Schönlein purpura), 249–250
IIH, *see* idiopathic intracranial hypertension
illness anxiety disorder, 298–299
immune reconstitution inflammatory
syndrome (IRIS), 269, 271
immunization, *see* vaccines
immunoglobulins
anti-MAG polyneuropathy, 30–31,
418–419
cryoglobulinemia, 134–135, 257
IgM macroglobulinemia, 699–700
IVIG therapy, 7, 505, 506–507, 622,
696
MGUS, 383
plasma cell dyscrasias, 492–493
immunosuppressive drugs, 237–238, 509,
570, 695, 696, 751–753, 771–772
in pregnancy, 397, 695
impotence (erectile disorder), 192–193,
725
impulse-control disorders, 157–158
intermittent explosive disorder,
306–307
inborn errors of metabolism, *see* metabolic disorders
inclusion body myositis, 498–499
incontinence
encopresis, 179
enuresis, 183
indomethacin, 245, 470
infantile convulsions and choreoathetosis
(ICCA), 58–59
infantile severe myoclonic epilepsy (Dravet syndrome), 164–165
infantile spasms, 299
infections, *see* bacterial infections; fungal
infections; parasitic infections;
protozoal infections; viral
infections
infectious mononucleosis, 192
infective endocarditis, 299–300, 600–601,
625–626
mycotic aneurysm, 398–399
inflammatory bowel disease

Crohn's disease, 135
ulcerative colitis, 673
infliximab, 766
influenza, 300–302, 745
inhalant abuse
nitrous oxide, 421–422, 687
solvents, 13, 234–235, 267, 610
insomnia
chronic, 302–303
fatal familial insomnia, 209
short-term, 303–304
treatment, 302–303, 304, 801, 802,
804
insufficient sleep syndrome, 304
insular cortex, 376
integrase strand transfer inhibitors, 748
intensive care unit (ICU) patients
myopathy, 132–133
neuropathy, 132–133
psychosis, 305
PTSD/PICS, 511–512
interferon, 256, 257, 275, 756–757
interleukin-1 (IL-1) inhibitors, 764–765
intermittent claudication, 307–308,
678–679
intermittent explosive disorder, 306–307
internal iliac artery stenosis, 307–308
internuclear ophthalmoplegia, 624
intervertebral discs
cervical, 109–110, 142, 260
degenerative disease, 142, 342
discitis, 156–157
herniation, 260–261
lumbar, 142, 261, 342
intoxication, *see* substance abuse; toxins/
toxicity
intra-aortic balloon assistance, 36
intra-arterial injections, 308, 345
intracranial hypertension, 296–297
in pregnancy, 242, 243
tetracycline use, 747
vitamin A excess, 685–686
intrathecal pharmacotherapy, 77, 622,
757
intravascular malignant lymphomatosis,
309–310
intraventricular hemorrhage, 310,
340–341
ipilimumab, 757
iron
deficiency, 310–311
neurodegeneration with brain iron
accumulation
neuroferritinopathy, 411

PKAN, 410, 457
supplements, 730
irregular sleep–wake rhythm disorder,
311–312
Isaacs syndrome (neuromyotonia),
414–415
ischemic demyelination, 312–313
ischemic monomelic neuropathy, 313,
345
ischemic stroke
ACA infarction, 28, 331–332
AChA infarction, 28–29
atherosclerosis, intracranial, 308–309
cardioembolic, 46, 85, 375
carotid artery endarterectomy/stent-
ing, 88–89
depression following, 354
hemorrhagic transformation,
248–249
lacunar, 327–328
MCA infarction, 375–377
moyamoya disease, 385–386
PCA infarction, 500–501
in pregnancy, 107–108
spinal, 29, 313–314, 613–614
TIAs, 385, 664–665, 683
top of the basilar syndrome, 663
vertebral artery dissection, 681–682
isometheptene mucate, 785
isoniazid, 743–744
isotretinoin, 730–731
ITP (idiopathic thrombocytopenic purpura), 297–298
ivermectin, 432
IVIG (intravenous immunoglobulin), 7,
505, 506–507, 622, 696
ixabepilone, 757–758
ixazomib, 760

Japanese encephalitis virus, 213,
315–316
Jarisch–Herxheimer reaction, 335
jaw
hemimasticatory spasm, 246
temporomandibular joint syndrome,
647–648
JC virus, 271, 527
jerking stiff person syndrome, 621
jet lag sleep disorder, 316–317
juvenile absence epilepsy, 3, 317
juvenile myoclonic epilepsy, 318
juvenile xanthogranuloma, 232

Kennedy disease, 613

keratitis, 319
kernicterus, 319–320, 741
Keshan disease (selenium deficiency), 599–600
ketamine, 320–321
ketoacidosis, diabetic, 152
ketogenic diet, 163, 236
kidney disease
    action myoclonus–renal failure syndrome, 528
    acute renal failure, 568–569, 577
    cancer, 567–568
    chronic renal failure, 569–570
    HUS, 247
kindling, 16
kinky hair disease (Menkes disease), 370–371
Kleine-Levin syndrome, 301, 321–322
Klinefelter syndrome, 322–323
konzo (cassava root poisoning), 91
Korsakoff syndrome, 323–324, 537
Krabbe disease, 325
Kugelberg–Welander syndrome, 616
kwashiorkor, 536–537
kyphosis, 326

lacosamide, 776
lacrimal gland inflammation, 439
La Crosse encephalitis virus, 327
lacunar stroke, 327–328
Lafora disease, 328–329, 528
Lambert–Eaton myasthenic syndrome (LEMS), 329–330, 463, 550
lamivudine, 749–750
lamotrigine, 190, 776
Landau–Kleffner syndrome, 330
LARIAT® device, 46
late-onset multiple carboxylase deficiency, 62–64
lateral/sigmoid sinus thrombosis, 364
lathyrism, 413
latrotoxin (black widow spider venom), 66–67
LBD (Lewy body dementia), 48, 50, 337–338
lead toxicity, 330–331
Leber's hereditary optic atrophy, 331
leflunomide, 765
Leigh disease, 332
Lemierre syndrome, 223
LEMS (Lambert–Eaton myasthenic syndrome), 329–330, 463, 550
lenalidomide, 761
Lennox–Gastaut syndrome, 332–333, 778
lens subluxation, 333–334

leprosy, 334
leptomeningeal carcinomatosis, 83–84
leptospirosis, 335
Lesch–Nyhan syndrome, 335–336
leukemia, 336–337, 754, 758
leukoencephalopathy
    adrenoleukodystrophy, 11–12
    Binswanger's disease, 61–62, 312
    CADASIL, 105, 312
    in eclampsia, 172
    ischemic, 312–313
    metachromatic leukodystrophy, 372–373
    PML, 271, 527, 752, 753
    PRES, see posterior reversible encephalopathy syndrome
leukotriene antagonists, 735
levetiracetam, 776–777
Levine–Critchley syndrome, 409–410
levodopa, 163, 338, 384, 468, 770–771
levothyroxine, 565, 726
Lewis–Sumner syndrome, 387
Lewy body dementia (LBD), 48, 50, 337–338
Lhermitte–Duclos disease, 338–339
Lhermitte's sign, 391, 558
lidocaine, 711
ligament ossification (DISH), 154–155
lightning strike, 339
limbic (autoimmune) encephalitis, 177–178, 276, 462–463, 695–696
linagliptin, 720
linezolid, 745–746
lipid-lowering agents, 714–716
lipid metabolism disorders
    abetalipoproteinemia, 410–411, 573, 690
    adrenoleukodystrophy, 11–12
    carnitine deficiency, 518–519
    Refsum disease, 259, 573
lipomatosis, spinal, 615
liraglutide, 720
Listeria monocytogenes, 339–340
lithium, 64, 361, 590, 800
liver disease
    acquired hepatocerebral degeneration, 4
    acute liver failure, 251
    alcoholic, 16
    chronic liver failure, 251–252
    drug toxicity
        amphetamines, 173, 373
        anti-tubercular drugs, 744, 746–747

COMT inhibitors, 768–769, 799
    disulfiram, 799
echinococcosis, 170–171
viral hepatitis
    acute, 252–253
    chronic, 253
    HAV, 253–255
    HBV, 253, 255–256
    HCV, 134–135, 253, 256–257
    neuropathy, 257–258
liver flukes (fascioliasis), 208
lixisenetide, 720
lobar hemorrhage, 340–341
locked-in syndrome, 341, 481, see also persistent vegetative state
logopenic variant of primary progressive aphasia (lvPPA), 18
loiasis, 342, 432
lomustine, 758–759
long-acting beta agonists (LABAs), 736
long QT syndrome, 533, 743, 744
loop diuretics, 281, 713
lorcaserin, 800
lordosis, 282
loss of consciousness, see also locked-in syndrome
    medication-associated, 754, 758
    persistent vegetative state, 480–482
    syncope, 636–637
        cardiogenic, 86–87
        carotid sinus hypersensitivity, 90
        Stokes–Adams attacks, 623
lower limb, see also lumbosacral plexopathy
    claudication, 307–308, 678–679
    distal symmetric polyneuropathy, 153
    femoral neuropathy, 211–212, 418, 540, 570
    GALOP syndrome, 224
    hereditary spastic paraplegia, 259–260
    ischemic monomelic neuropathy, 313, 345
    peroneal neuropathy (foot drop), 152, 418, 478–479
    plantar fasciitis, 207
    sciatic neuropathy
        hip pathology/surgery, 267–268
        piriformis syndrome, 489
        in pregnancy, 418
        uterine mass compression, 675–676
LSD (lysergic acid), 349–350
lumbar puncture, headache after, 242, 243, 507–508

lumbar spine
  degenerative disc disease, 142, 342
  disc herniation, 261
  hyperlordosis, 282
  radiation myelopathy, 558
  spondylolisthesis, 343
  spondylolysis, 343
  spondylosis, 343
  sprain, 343–344
  stenosis, 344
lumbosacral plexopathy
  immune, 344
  intra-arterial injections, 345
  ischemic, 345
  in pregnancy, 346, 417
  radiation neuropathy, 559–560, 649,
    675
  root avulsion, 580–581
  traumatic, 346
  tumors, 229
lumbosacral radiculopathy, 265, 270, 560
lung
  AVMs, 441, 443
  cancer, 72, 346–347
    LEMS, 329–330, 463
  paragonimiasis (lung fluke), 459–460
Lyme disease, 347–348
lymphocytic choriomeningitis virus,
  348–349
lymphoma
  Burkitt, 77
  intravascular lymphomatosis,
    309–310
  orbital, 440
  primary CNS, 270–271, 521–523
  Waldenström's macroglobulinemia,
    699–700
lymphomatoid granulomatosis, 349
lysergic acid (LSD), 349–350
lysosomal storage diseases, 350
  Fabry disease, 198–199
  Gaucher disease, 528
  Hunter syndrome, 350–351
  Krabbe disease, 325
  metachromatic leukodystrophy,
    372–373
  neuronal ceroid lipofuscinoses, 528,
    573
  Sanfilippo syndrome, 584
  sialidosis, 528, 603–604
  Tay–Sachs disease, 643–644

macrolides, 744
macular degeneration, 352–353

mad cow disease, 70–71
magnesium
  for eclampsia/pre-eclampsia, 173,
    397, 416–417, 516
  hypermagnesemia, 282, 727
  hypomagnesemia, 291–292
major depressive disorder, 353–356, 511,
    see also persistent depressive
    disorder
  with psychotic features, 546–548, 589
malaria, 356–357, 764
male hypoactive sexual desire disorder,
    357–358
malignant hyperthermia, 358–359
malignant MCA syndrome, 377
malingering, 160, 203–204, 359
malnutrition, 536–537, see also trace
    elements; vitamins
  refeeding syndrome, 27, 53
  tropical ataxic neuropathy, 668
manganese toxicity, 359–360
mania/manic episodes, 360–362, 546
  bipolar disorders, 64, 65, 66
MAOIs (monoamine oxidase inhibitors),
    792–793
  hypertension, 355
  serotonin syndrome, 355, 356, 480,
    601–602
maple syrup urine disease, 362–363
marasmus, 536–537
maraviroc, 748
Marchiafava–Bignami disease, 363
Marcus Gunn jaw wink syndrome, 197
Marcus Gunn pupil, 13–14
Marfan's syndrome, 334
marijuana, 79–80
  withdrawal, 80–81
mastoiditis, 363–364
MCA (middle cerebral artery) infarction,
    375–377
McArdle's disease, 402
McLeod syndrome, 409–410
MDMA (ecstasy), 173–174
measles, 364–365
measles, mumps and rubella (MMR)
    vaccine, 365–366
median nerve
  carpal tunnel syndrome, 90–91,
    417, 418, 533
  diabetic neuropathy, 152
medication-overuse headache, 366
medulloblastoma, 367
meglitinides, 721
Meige syndrome, 69, 367–368

melanoma, 368, 757
melatonin, 567
melatonin receptor agonists, 801
memantine, 771
memory loss, see amnesia; dementia
Meniere's disease, 369
meningioma, 369–370, 440, 491
meningitis
  angiostrongyliasis, 25–26
  carcinomatous, 83–84
  Citrobacter, 119–120
  coxsackie virus, 129–130
  cryptococcal, 135–136, 271
  echovirus, 171–172
  enteroviruses, 182
  fungal (in general), 221–222
  histoplasmosis, 268
  HSV-II, 264, 381
  lamotrigine, 777
  Lyme disease, 348
  lymphocytic choriomeningitis virus,
    348–349
  meningococcal, 407–409
  Mollaret, 381–382
  mumps, 394–395
  paragonimiasis, 459
meningoencephalitis
  amebic, 20
  hepatitis A, 254
Menkes disease, 370–371
menstrual psychosis, 564–565, see also
    premenstrual dysphoric disorder
meralgia paresthetica, 418
MERRF (myoclonic epilepsy with ragged
    red fibers), 400–401, 528
mescaline, 371
mesial temporal sclerosis, 371–372
metabolic acidosis, 780
metabolic disorders
  adenylosuccinate lyase deficiency, 9
  aminoacidopathies
    biotinidase deficiency, 62–64
    homocysteinemia, 272–273, 281
    homocystinuria, 273
    maple syrup urine disease, 362–363
    phenylketonuria, 484
    pyridoxine-dependent seizures,
      553–554
  creatine deficiency, 238
  glycogen storage disease type V, 402
  of lipid metabolism
    abetalipoproteinemia, 410–411,
      573, 690
    adrenoleukodystrophy, 11–12

carnitine deficiency, 518–519
Refsum disease, 259, 573
lysosomal storage diseases, 350
Fabry disease, 198–199
Gaucher disease, 528
Hunter syndrome, 350–351
Krabbe disease, 325
metachromatic leukodystrophy, 372–373
Sanfilippo syndrome, 584
sialidosis, 528, 603–604
Tay–Sachs disease, 643–644
of purine metabolism
Lesch–Nyhan syndrome, 335–336
molybdenum cofactor deficiency, 382–383
metachromatic leukodystrophy, 372–373
metformin, 719–724
methadone, 263
methamphetamine, 373–374
methotrexate, 237–238, 374, 765
intrathecal, 77, 757
methyldopa, 716
methylprednisolone, 238, 390, 752
methylxanthines, 736
metoclopramide, 728, 782
metronidazole, 744–745
MGUS (monoclonal gammopathy of uncertain significance), 383
microangiopathy, see also diabetes mellitus
HUS, 247
Susac syndrome, 635, 676
TTP, 655–656
micronutrients, see trace elements; vitamins
microphthalmos, 374–375
middle cerebral artery (MCA) infarction, 375–377
migraine, see also abdominal migraine
with aura, 377–378
hemiplegic, 205–206
medications for, 784–785, 788–789
ophthalmoplegic, 733
in pregnancy, 242
in PTSD, 510
retinal, 572–573
mild encephalitis/encephalopathy with a reversible splenial lesion (MERS), 301, 460
Miller Fisher syndrome, 6, see also Guillain–Barré syndrome
minimally conscious state, 482
minocycline, 747

miosis, 378–379
mirtazapine, 792
mitochondrial disorders
Alpers disease (DNA depletion syndrome), 17–18
chronic progressive external ophthalmoplegia, 550, 624
coenzyme Q_{10} deficiency, 520–521
Leber's hereditary optic atrophy, 331
Leigh disease, 332
MERRF, 400–401, 528
NADH CoQ reductase deficiency, 404–405
mitral valve
prolapse, 380–381
regurgitation, 379–380
stenosis, 380, 678
MMR vaccine, 365–366
Mobius syndrome, 624
modafinil, 316, 322
Mollaret meningitis, 381–382
molybdenum cofactor deficiency, 382–383
monoamine oxidase inhibitors, see MAOIs
monoclonal gammopathy (paraproteinemia)
anti-MAG polyneuropathy, 30–31, 418–419
cryoglobulinemia, 134–135
MGUS, 383
plasma cell dyscrasias, 492–493
mononeuropathy multiplex, 152, 254, 257, 270
CIDP, 387
montelukast, 735
mood disorders, see bipolar disorders; depression; mania
morphine, 786–787
motor neuron diseases
amyotrophic lateral sclerosis, 219–220
hereditary spastic paraplegia, 259–260
LEMS, 329–330, 463, 550
myasthenia gravis, 396–397, 463–464, 550, 624, 743
primary lateral sclerosis, 525
radiation-induced, 558
SBMA, 613
spinal muscular atrophy, 162, 616
moyamoya disease, 385–386
MSA (multiple system atrophy), 48, 49, 50, 391–393
MSA-C, 49, 393–394

mTOR inhibitors, 753
mucopolysaccharidosis type II (Hunter syndrome), 350–351
mucopolysaccharidosis type III (Sanfilippo syndrome), 584
mucormycosis, 386–387
multifocal demyelinating CIDP (MADSAM), 387
multifocal motor neuropathy (with conduction block), 387–388
multi-infarct (vascular) dementia, 388–389
Binswanger's disease, 61–62, 312
multiple myeloma, 389
multiple personality disorder (dissociative identity disorder), 160, 161–162
multiple sclerosis, 389–390, 427, 436, 676
in pregnancy, 390–391
multiple system atrophy (MSA), 48, 49, 50, 391–393
MSA-C, 49, 393–394
mumps, 394–395
Munchausen's syndrome/Munchausen's syndrome by proxy (factitious disorder), 160, 202–204, 486
muscle cramps, 395–396
muscle relaxants, 785–786
muscular dystrophy
Becker, 57
Duchenne, 167
facioscapulohumeral, 202
myotonic dystrophy, 92, 402–403
mushrooms, magic, 539
mutism, 598–599
myasthenia
LEMS, 329–330, 463, 550
myasthenia gravis, 396–397, 463–464, 550, 624, 743
Mycobacterium leprae (leprosy), 334
mycophenolic acid derivatives, 753
Mycoplasma pneumoniae encephalitis, 397–398
mycotic aneurysm, 398–399
mydriasis, 13–14, 662–663
myelin-associated glycoprotein (MAG) autoantibodies, 30–31, 418–419
myelitis, see also encephalomyelitis
transverse, 254
neuromyelitis optica, 414, 605
viral, 182, 254, 264, 684
herpes zoster, 265–266
polio, 182, 494
myocardial infarction, 399–400

myoclonic epilepsy, 528–529
Doose syndrome, 162–163
Dravet syndrome, 164–165
DRPLA, 148, 540
juvenile, 318
Lafora disease, 328–329, 528
MERRF, 400–401, 528
myoclonus
dystonia, 401
early myoclonic encephalopathy, 169
essential, 194–195
facial, 199–200
opsoclonus–myoclonus syndrome, 464
palatial, 451–452
propriospinal, 534–535
myofascial pain, cervical, 111
myopathy, *see also* myositis
centronuclear, 103–104
critical illness, 131–132
daptomycin, 741–742
endocrinopathy, 179–180
hepatitis B, 256
nemaline rod, 409
rhabdomyolysis, 301, 576–577, 684
sarcoid, 584–585
myophosphorylase deficiency (McArdle's
disease), 402
myositis
acute, 584–585
cysticercosis, 139
dermatomyositis, 150, 255, 498–499
orbital, 439
polymyositis, 255, 274, 498–499
pyomyositis, 552–553
viral, 684–685
influenza, 301
myotonia
neuromyotonia, 414–415
paramyotonia congenita, 477
potassium-aggravated, 513–514
myotonic dystrophy
cataracts, 92
type 1, 402–403
type 2, 403
myotubular (centronuclear) myopathy,
103–104

nabilone, 781
NADH CoQ reductase deficiency, 404–405
naltrexone, 801–802
nanophthalmos, 374–375
naproxen, 786
naratriptan, 788
narcolepsy, 405–406

nasopharyngeal cancer, 406
natalizumab, 771–772
neck, *see entries at* cervical
necrotizing fasciitis, 207, 208
Neisseria meningitis, 407–409
nelarabine, 758
nemaline rod myopathy, 409
nematodes
angiostrongyliasis, 25–26
loiasis, 342, 432
onchocerciasis, 432–433
strongyloidosis, 628–629
trichinosis, 665–666
neonates
BFNIS, 59
BFNS, 59
centronuclear myopathy, 103–104
congenital heart defects
ASD, 46–47
PDA, 472
PFO, 472–473
VSD, 681
early myoclonic encephalopathy, 169
folinic acid-responsive seizures, 214
GABA transaminase deficiency, 224
herpes encephalitis, 264
kernicterus, 319–320, 741
maple syrup urine disease, 362–363
molybdenum cofactor deficiency,
382–383
myasthenia, 397
vitamin K deficiency, 692
neural tube defects, 612–613
neuraminidase inhibitors, 301, 745
neuroacanthocytosis, 409–410
with abetalipoproteinemia, 410–411
PKAN, 410, 457
neuroaxonal dystrophy, 485–486
neuroblastoma, 440
neurocardiogenic syncope, 86–87
neurocysticercosis, 139
neurodegenerative disorders, 767–773,
see also individual disorders
neurodevelopmental disorders
ADHD, 307, 353–354, 547, 797,
803–804
Angelman syndrome, 24–25
autism spectrum disorder, 51–52
Lesch–Nyhan syndrome, 335–336
Prader–Willi syndrome, 514–515
Rett syndrome, 574
neuroendocrine tumors, *see also* neurofibromatosis type 1; von Hippel–
Lindau disease

carcinoid, 82–83
neuroblastoma, 440
paraganglioma, 458–459
pheochromocytoma, 484–485
schwannoma, 200, 595
neuroferritinopathy, 411
neurofibromatosis type 1 (NF1), 231,
411–412, 440
neurofibromatosis type 2 (NF2),
412–413, 440
neurokinin receptor antagonists, 782
neurolathyrism, 413
neuroleptic malignant syndrome, 590,
767, 770, 796, 797
neuromuscular junction disorders
LEMS, 329–330, 463, 550
myasthenia gravis, 396–397, 463–464,
550, 624, 743
neuromyelitis optica, 414, 605
neuromyotonia (Isaacs syndrome),
414–415
neuronal ceroid lipofuscinoses, 528, 573
neurosyphilis, 32, 271, 637–638
neurotoxins, *see* toxins/toxicity
neutropenia, 756
nevirapine, 749
niacin, 716
deficiency (pellagra), 419–420, 537
nicotine dependency, 660–661
nicotine replacement therapy, 801
varenicline, 804–805
night eating syndrome, 606
nightmare disorder, 420–421
nitrofurantoin, 745
nitrates (vasodilators), 717–718
nitrogen mustards, 700, 758–759
nitrosoureas, 758–759
nitrous oxide, 421–422, 687
nocardiosis, 422–423
nodding syndrome, 432
nodular myopathy, 585
non-arteritic anterior ischemic optic
neuropathy (NAION), 423, 501
nonconvulsive status
epilepticus, 424, 736
non-nucleotide reverse transcriptase
inhibitors (NNRTIs), 749
non-steroidal anti-inflammatory drugs
(NSAIDs), 786
Norrie's disease, 571
'North Sea' progressive myoclonus epilepsy, 528
nucleoside reverse transcriptase inhibitors (NRTIs), 749–750

nutrition, *see also* trace elements; vitamins
  malnutrition, 536–537, 668
  refeeding syndrome, 27, 53
  tropical ataxic neuropathy, 668

obesity hypoventilation syndrome, 425
obesity management
  bariatric surgery, 56
  drugs, 716, 800
obsessive-compulsive disorder (OCD), 425–428, 511, 589, 635–636
  body dysmorphic disorder, 69–70
  hoarding disorder, 272
  trichotillomania, 486, 666–667
obstructive sleep apnea, 428
  obesity hypoventilation syndrome, 425
obturator neuropathy, 418
occipital lobe epilepsy, 428–429
occipital neuralgia, 429–430
OCD (obsessive-compulsive disorder), 425–428, 511, 589, 635–636
ocular apraxia, 55
oculogyric crisis, 430
oculomotor nerve (CN III)
  diabetic neuropathy, 151–152
  Marcus Gunn jaw wink syndrome, 197
  palsy, 550, 624
oculopharyngeal dystrophy, 550
odontoid fracture, 111–112
Ohtahara syndrome, 430–431
olanzapine, 796–797
oligodendroglioma, 431–432
olivopontocerebellar atrophy (MSA-C), 49, 393–394
onchocerciasis, 432–433
oncology drugs, *see* chemotherapy
open angle glaucoma, 231–232
ophthalmic nerve, 319, 560–561
ophthalmoplegia, 550, 623–625
  Tolosa–Hunt syndrome, 661–662
ophthalmoplegic migraine, 433
opioid antagonists, 801–802
opioids
  buprenorphine, 798–799
  central sleep apnea, 100–101
  heroin, 261–263
  toxicity, 261–262, 433–434, 786–787
  withdrawal, 262–263, 434–435
oppositional defiant disorder, 307
opsoclonus–myoclonus syndrome, 464
optic ataxia, 55

optic nerve (CN II)
  AION, 41, 423, 501
  atrophy, 435–436
  compression, 437–438
  glaucoma, 231–232
  glioma, 436
  Leber's hereditary optic atrophy, 331
  neuritis, 416, 436–437, 465, 503–504, 742
  neuromyelitis optica, 414, 605
  perineuritis, 475
oral contraceptives, 724
oral hypoglycemic agents, 719–721
orbital arteriovenous fistula, 438
orbital hemorrhage, 438–439
orbital inflammation (pseudotumor), 439–440
orbital tumors, 440–441
orbito-rhino-cerebral and skull base syndrome, 222
orlistat, 716
orofacial dyskinesia, 441
orthostatic hypotension, 551, 637, 697
orthostatic tachycardia syndrome, 512–513
orthostatic tremor, 442
Osler–Weber–Rendu syndrome, 442–443
osmotic demyelination syndrome (central pontine myelinolysis), 97–98, 292, 570
osteoarthritis, 443, *see also* spondylosis
osteoblastoma, 444–445
osteochondroma, 445–446
osteoma, 446
osteomalacia, 446
osteomyelitis, 156–157, 447
osteoporosis, 447, 723, 725
osteosarcoma, 447–448
otitis externa, 538–539
otitis media
  chronic, 117–118
  Gradenigo syndrome, 236, 624
  mastoiditis, 363–364
otosclerosis, 448–449
ototoxic drugs, 738, 743, 747, 759
ovarian cancer, 228, 229–230, 238–239, 449–450
oxaliplatin, 759–760
oxazaphosphorines (cyclophosphamide), 237, 566, 759
oxazolidinones, 745–746
oxcarbazepine, 190, 774–775
oxycodone, 786–787
oxygen

anoxic encephalopathy, 27–28
hyperbaric, 141–142
hypoxia, 293–294

paclitaxel, 761
Paget's disease of bone, 451
pain
  back
    degenerative disc disease, 142, 342
    disc herniation, 261
    discitis, 157
    lumbar stenosis, 344
    strain/sprain, 54, 343–344
  catamenial, 180
  complex regional pain syndrome, 124
  facial
    atypical, 47–48
    glossopharyngeal neuralgia, 233–234, 605
    Gradenigo syndrome, 236
    Raeder's paratrigeminal neuralgia, 560–561
    trigeminal neuralgia, 605, 667–668
  headache, *see* headache; migraine
  neck
    arthritis, 109
    disc disorders, 109–110
    facet syndrome, 110–111
    myofascial pain syndrome, 111
  post-herpetic neuralgia, 503
  psychogenic, 542
  radiculopathy, 560
    diabetic, 153
pain relief, *see* analgesics
palatial myoclonus, 451–452
paliperidone, 796–797
pallidal degeneration, 551–552
Pancoast syndrome, 72
pancreatic cancer, 452–453
pancreatitis, 453–454
PANDAS (pediatric autoimmune neuropsychiatric disorders associated with streptococcal infections), 427, 635–636, 658
panic attacks, 454–455
panic disorder, 455–457
pantothenate kinase-associated neurodegeneration (PKAN), 410, 457
Paracoccidioides brasiliensis, 457–458
paraganglioma, 458–459
  pheochromocytoma, 484–485
paragonimiasis (lung fluke), 459–460
parainfluenza, 460
paramyotonia congenita, 477

paraneoplastic syndromes
  anti-Hu syndrome, 30
  autonomic neuropathy, 461
  in breast cancer, 74
  carcinoid, 82–83
  encephalomyelitis, 461–462
  LEMS, 329–330, 463, 550
  in leukemia, 337
  limbic encephalitis, 177–178,
    462–463, 695–696
  myasthenia gravis, 396–397, 463–464,
    550, 624, 743
  opsoclonus–myoclonus, 464
  optic neuropathy–retinopathy, 465
  pancreatic cancer, 452–463
  POEMS syndrome, 494
  renal cancer, 568
  sensory neuronopathy
    (ganglionopathy), 465–466
  stiff person syndrome, 621
paraparesis (HTLV-1 associated
    myelopathy), 274–275
paraplegia
  flaccid, see flaccid paralysis
  spastic, 259–260
paraproteinemia
  anti-MAG polyneuropathy, 30–31,
    418–419
  cryoglobulinemia, 134–135
  MGUS, 383
  plasma cell dyscrasias, 492
parasitic infections
  angiostrongyliasis, 25–26
  cysticercosis, 139
  echinococcosis, 170–171
  fascioliasis, 208
  loiasis, 342, 432
  onchocerciasis, 432–433
  paragonimiasis, 459–460
  schistosomiasis, 588–589
  strongyloidosis, 628–629
  trichinosis, 665–666
parasomnias
  NREM-related, 424
    confusional arousal, 125–126
    periodic limb movement disorder,
      475–476
    sleep-related eating disorder, 606
    sleep terrors, 606–607
    sleepwalking, 607–608
  REM-related
    nightmare disorder, 420–421
    recurrent isolated sleep paralysis, 564
    REM behavior disorder, 566–567

parasympathetic anticholinergic
    blockade, 29
parathyroid hormone (PTH)
  hyperparathyroidism, 283–284
  hypoparathyroidism, 292–293, 725
parietal lobe epilepsy, 466–467
parietal lobe ischemia (MCA
    occlusion), 377
Parinaud (dorsal midbrain) syndrome,
    197, 467, 652
parkinsonism, see also antiparkinsonian
    drugs
  hemiparkinsonism–hemiatrophy
    syndrome, 246–247
  manganese toxicity, 359–360
  Parkinson's-plus syndromes, 48–51
    ALS-PDC, 21–23
    CBD, 49–50, 128–129
    LBD, 48, 50, 337–338
    MSA, 48, 49, 50, 391–393
    PSP, 48, 49, 197, 529–530
  rapid-onset dystonia–parkinsonism,
    561–562
  X-linked dystonia–parkinsonism, 703
Parkinson's disease, 467–469, see also
    antiparkinsonian drugs
  dementia, 337
  depression, 354–355
  psychosis, 544–545
parotid cancer, 469
paroxysmal exercise-induced dyskinesia,
    471
paroxysmal hemicrania, 470, see also
    hemicrania continua
paroxysmal kinesigenic dyskinesia,
    470–471
paroxysmal nocturnal
    hemoglobinuria, 471–472
paroxysmal non-kinesigenic
    dyskinesia, 471
Parsonage–Turner syndrome (brachial
    neuritis), 5, 417
patent ductus arteriosus (PDA), 472
patent foramen ovale (PFO), 472–473
PCA (posterior cerebral artery)
    infarction, 500–501, 663
PCP (phencyclidine), 483
pediatric conditions, see children;
    neonates
peduncular hallucinosis, 473
pellagra (niacin deficiency), 419–420,
    537
penicillins, 746
perampanel, 777

perilymphatic fistula, 473–474
perineuritis, 474–475
periodic limb movement disorder,
    475–476
periodic paralysis, 476–478
  Andersen–Tawil syndrome, 23, 477
  hyperkalemic, 477
  hypokalemic, 291, 476–477
  paramyotonia congenita, 477
  thyrotoxic, 477, 657
periodontal disease, 147–148
perioperative nerve injuries, 86, 267–268,
    634
pernicious anemia, 226, 686, 688
peroneal neuropathy, 152, 418, 478–479
persistent depressive disorder (dysthy-
    mia), 479–480, see also major
    depressive disorder
persistent idiopathic (atypical) facial
    pain, 47–48
persistent vegetative state, 480–482
personality disorders
  antisocial, 306
  borderline, 204
  schizotypal, 593–595
pertussis, 156, 482–483
petit mal epilepsy, 3, 317
petrous apicitis (Gradenigo syndrome),
    236, 624
phaeohyphomycosis (dematiaceous
    fungi), 145–146
phagophobia (psychogenic dysphagia),
    540–541
pharmacokinetic boosters, 748, 750
phencyclidine (PCP), 483
phenothiazines, 781
phenylephrine, 735
phenylketonuria, 484
phenytoin, 692, 777
pheochromocytoma, 484–485, see also
    hyperadrenalism
phosphate (hypophosphatemia), 293
phosphodiesterase-5 (PDE-5)
    inhibitors, 725
phospholipase A-associated
    neurodegeneration, 485–486
phytanic acid oxidase deficiency (Refsum
    disease), 259, 573
pica, 486–487
Pickwickian syndrome (obesity hypoven-
    tilation syndrome), 425
pilocytic astrocytoma, 42–43
pineoblastoma, 487–488
pineocytoma, 488–489

pioglitazone, 721
piriformis syndrome, 489
pituitary gland disorders
    adenoma, 13, 490–492, 624
        prolactinoma, 284, 532–533
    adrenal insufficiency, 10
    pituitary apoplexy, 242, 489–490
    in pregnancy, 242
    third ventricle tumors, 652
PKAN (pantothenate kinase-associated neurodegeneration), 410, 457
plantar fasciitis, 207
plasma cells
    dyscrasia, 492–493
    multiple myeloma, 389
plasma exchange/plasmapheresis, 7, 505, 507, 622, 696
Plasmodium spp. (malaria), 356–357, 764
platelets
    antiplatelet drugs, 711–712
    essential thrombocythemia, 195
    thrombocytopenia, 654
        HIT, 250–251
        HUS, 247
        ITP, 297–298
        TTP, 655–656
platinum analog drugs, 759–760
platybasia, 493–494
PLERM (probable *Loa* encephalopathy temporally related to Mectizan treatment), 432
PML (progressive multifocal leukoencephalopathy), 271, 527
    immunosuppressant drugs, 752, 753
pneumococcus (*Streptococcus pneumoniae*), 626–627
POEMS syndrome, 494
poisoning, *see* toxins/toxicity
poliovirus, 182, 494–495
polyarteritis nodosa, 255, 495–496
polychondritis, 565–566
polycythemia vera, 496–497
polydipsia, psychogenic, 542–543
polymyalgia rheumatica, 497–498
polymyositis, 255, 274, 498–499
polyneuropathy, *see also* Guillain–Barré syndrome
    anti-MAG, 30–31, 418–419
    axonal, 500
    CANOMAD syndrome, 81
    CIDP, 116–117
        multifocal, 387
    critical illness, 132–133
    diabetic, 153

diphtheric, 155
GALOP syndrome, 224
HIV, 270
POEMS syndrome, 494
polyradiculopathy, *see* radiculopathy
pomalidomide, 761
post-concussion syndrome, 187
postencephalitic symptoms, 179
posterior cerebral artery (PCA) infarction, 500–501, 663
posterior ciliary artery thrombosis, 41, 501
posterior cortical atrophy, 18
posterior fossa syndrome, 367
posterior reversible encephalopathy syndrome (PRES), 285, 501–503, 575–576
    in HUS, 247
    medication-associated, 502, 509, 570, 752, 753, 762
    in pregnancy, 108, 172, 416
post-herpetic myelitis/neuralgia, 265–266, 503
post-immunization encephalomyelitis, 503–505
post-infectious syndromes, *see* Guillain–Barré syndrome; post-viral syndromes
post-intensive care syndrome (PICS), 511–512
post-lumbar puncture headache, 242, 243, 507–508
postoperative nerve injuries, 86, 267–268, 634
    post-transplant, 276, 508–509
postoperative psychosis, 305
post-transplant acute limbic encephalitis, 276
post-transplant encephalopathy, 508–509
post-traumatic stress disorder (PTSD), 160, 589, 510–512, *see also* acute stress disorder
postural orthostatic tachycardia syndrome, 512–513
post-viral syndromes, *see also* Guillain–Barré syndrome
    ADEM, 5–6, 146, 178, 364, 505–507
    poliovirus, 494
    subacute sclerosing panencephalitis, 364
potassium
    hyperkalemic periodic paralysis, 281–282, 477
    hypokalemia, 281–282
    hypokalemic periodic paralysis, 291, 476–477

myotonia syndromes, 513–514
potassium-sparing diuretics, 713
Prader–Willi syndrome, 514–515, *see also* Angelman syndrome
pramlintide, 719
prazosin, 421, 722
prednisone, 752
pre-eclampsia, 515–516, *see also* eclampsia
pregabalin, 560, 778
pregnancy
    bipolar disorders, 64, 65
    chorea gravidarum, 115–116, 383
    drug recommendations/contraindications
        AEDs, 190–191, 692, 779
        amiodarone, 710
        antiparkinsonian drugs, 384
        antipsychotics, 116
        heparin, 108
        immunosuppressants, 397, 695
        leflunomide, 765
        lithium, 64, 65
        lorcaserin, 800
        methotrexate, 765
        tPA, 108
        vitamin A, 685, 731
        vitamin supplements, 190
    eclampsia, 108, 172–173, 190–191, 397
    epilepsy, 189–191
    headache, 241–243
    listeriosis, 339–340
    lumbosacral plexopathy, 346, 417
    movement disorders, 383–385
    multiple sclerosis, 390–391
    myasthenia gravis, 396–397
    neuro-ophthalmic disorders, 415–417
    neuropathies common in, 417–418, 675–676
    nicotine replacement therapy, 801
    pre-eclampsia, 515–516
    rubella, 582
    stroke, 107–108
    Zika virus, 704
premature ejaculation, 516–517
premenstrual dysphoric disorder, 517–518, *see also* menstrual psychosis
premenstrual syndrome, 518
PRES, *see* posterior reversible encephalopathy syndrome
priapism, 794, 800
primary amebic meningoencephalitis, 20

primary carnitine deficiency, 518–519
primary central sleep apnea, 519–520
primary CNS angiitis, 521
primary CNS lymphoma, 270–271, 521–523
primary lateral sclerosis, 525
primary progressive aphasia, 219, 525–526
    logopenic variant, 18–19
primary torsion dystonia, 526–527
primidone, 196
prion diseases
    BSE/vCJD, 70–71
    CJD, 130–131
    fatal familial insomnia, 209
procainamide, 710
progesterone/progestins, 565, 724
progressive epileptic aphasia (Landau–Kleffner syndrome), 330
progressive multifocal leukoencephalopathy (PML), 271, 527
    immunosuppressant drugs, 752, 753, 771
progressive myoclonic epilepsy, 528–529
    DRPLA, 148, 528
    Lafora disease, 328–329, 528
    MERRF, 400–401, 528
progressive myoclonus epilepsy–ataxia syndrome, 528
progressive supranuclear palsy (PSP), 48, 49, 197, 529–530
progressive systemic sclerosis (scleroderma), 530–532, 596–598
prolactin (hyperprolactinemia), 284, 532–533
prolonged QT syndrome, 533, 743, 744
pronator syndrome, 533–534
propranolol, 196, 712–713
propriospinal myoclonus, 534–535
prostate cancer, 535–536
prostenoids, 717
prosthetic heart valves, 536
protease inhibitors, 750
proteasome inhibitors, 700, 760
protein-calorie malnutrition, 536–537
    refeeding syndrome, 27, 53
protein C deficiency, 537–538
protein S deficiency, 538
proton pump inhibitors, 728–729
protozoal infections
    amoebiasis, 20
    babesiosis, 54
    malaria, 356–357, 764
    sarcosporidiosis, 587

    toxoplasmosis, 271, 572
    trypanosomiasis, African, 277–278
    trypanosomiasis, American, 113
Pseudallescheria boydii, 538
pseudoephedrine, 735
Pseudomonas aeruginosa, 538–539
pseudotumor cerebri, see idiopathic intracranial hypertension
psilocybin, 539
psoas abscess, 539–540
psoas hemorrhage, 540
PSP (progressive supranuclear palsy), 48, 49, 197, 529–530
psychogenic amnesia (dissociative), 159–161
psychogenic dysphagia, 540–541
psychogenic non-epileptic seizures, 541–542
psychogenic pain (psychalgia), 542
psychogenic polydipsia, 542–543
psychogenic vertigo, 544
psychogenic vision loss, 221
psychosis/psychotic disorders, see also antipsychotic drugs
    brief psychotic disorder, 74–75
    delusional disorder, 144–145
    depression with psychotic features, 546–548, 589
    due to another medical condition, 548–549, 777, 792
    ICU/postoperative, 305
    menstrual, 564–565
    Parkinson's disease, 544–545
    PTSD, 511
    schizoaffective disorder, 589–590
    schizophrenia, 590–592, 689
    schizophreniform disorder, 592–593
ptosis, 549–551
PTSD (post-traumatic stress disorder), 160, 510–512, 589, see also acute stress disorder
pupillary defects
    afferent defect (Marcus Gunn), 13–14
    diabetic autonomic neuropathy, 151
    efferent defect (tonic), 662–663
    miosis, 378–379
pure autonomic failure, 551
pure pallidal degeneration, 551–552
purine metabolism
    Lesch–Nyhan syndrome, 335–336
    molybdenum cofactor deficiency, 382–383
pyomyositis, 552–553

pyrazinamide, 746
pyridostigmine, 104
pyridoxine
    deficiency, 553
    toxicity, 214, 554, 732
pyridoxine-dependent seizures, 553–554

quetiapine, 796–797

rabbit syndrome, 555–556
rabies virus, 556
radial nerve, 556–557, 587–588
radiculopathy, 560
    diabetic, 153
    HIV, 270
    HSV-II, 265
    Lyme radiculoneuritis, 348
radiochemotherapy, 557, 559
radiosurgery (gamma knife), 196, 370
radiotherapy
    CNS, 450, 557–558
        and AVMs, 41
        in children, 184
    cranial/spinal nerves, 559–560
    peripheral nerves/plexuses, 649, 675
    pituitary tumors, 492
Raeder's paratrigeminal neuralgia, 560–561
raloxifene, 760–761
raltegravir, 748
ramelteon, 801
rapid-onset dystonia–parkinsonism, 561–562
rasagiline, 355
Rasmussen encephalitis, 562–563
Rathke cleft cysts, 490
rat lungworm (angiostrongyliasis), 25–26
Raymond syndrome, 624
reactive arthritis, 563–564
rebound headache, 366
recreational drugs, see substance abuse
recurrent isolated sleep paralysis, 564
recurrent menstrual psychosis, 564–565
red blood cells
    acanthocytosis, 409–411
    polycythemia vera, 496–497
refeeding syndrome, 27, 53
reflex sympathetic dystrophy (complex regional pain syndrome), 124
Refsum disease, 259, 573
Reiter's syndrome, 563–564
relapsing polychondritis, 565–566
release visual hallucinations, 92, 352, 436
REM behavior disorder, 566–567

renal disease
  action myoclonus–renal failure syndrome, 528
  acute renal failure, 568–569, 577
  cancer, 567–568
  chronic renal failure, 569–570
  HUS, 247
repaglinide, 721
repetitive hand use, 570–571
reserpine, 717
respiratory failure
  ARDS, 294
  chronic, 118–119
restless leg syndrome, 383, 384, see also periodic limb movement disorder
retina
  detachment, 99, 571–572
  diabetic retinopathy, 416, 572
  macular degeneration, 352–353
  paraneoplastic retinopathy, 465
  pregnancy-associated conditions, 416
retinal artery occlusion, 98, 416
retinal migraine, 572–573
retinal vein occlusion, 98–99
retinitis pigmentosa, 573–574
retinoblastoma, 440
retinol (vitamin A), 573, 685–686, 731
retrobulbar hemorrhage, 438–439
Rett syndrome, 574
reversible cerebral vasoconstriction syndrome (RCVS), 574–575
reversible posterior leukoencephalopathy syndrome, see posterior reversible encephalopathy syndrome
rhabdomyolysis, 301, 576–577, 684
rheumatic fever, 577–578
  chorea gravidarum, 116
  mitral stenosis, 380
  Sydenham chorea, 635–636
rheumatoid arthritis, 109, 578–579, 764–766
rhino-orbito-cerebral mucormycosis, 386–387
rickettsial infections, 579–580
Ridoch phenomenon, 103
rifampin, 746–747
Riley–Day syndrome, 319
riluzole, 772
ring chromosome 20 syndrome, 580
risperidone, 796–797
ritonavir, 750
rituximab, 31, 237, 696, 700
rivastigmine, 769
river blindness (onchocerciasis), 432–433
rizatriptan, 788–789

Rocky Mountain spotted fever, 579–580
rolandic epilepsy (BECTS), 58
Rosai–Dorfman disease, 581
rosiglitazone, 721
rt-PA (recombinant tissue plasminogen activator), 377, 416, 582
  in pregnancy, 108
rubella virus, 582
Rubenstein–Taybis syndrome, 582–583
rubeola (measles), 364–365
rufinamide, 778

sadness, 354
safeguarding, 204
SAH (subarachnoid hemorrhage), 23–24, 108, 629–630, 693
  spinal, 618
salbutamol (albuterol), 736–737
salicylates, 711–712, 787
salivary gland cancer, 469
salmeterol, 469
Sanfilippo syndrome, 584
sarcoid myopathy, 584–585
sarcoidosis, 677
sarcoma, 447–448, 585–587
sarcosporidiosis, 587
Saturday night palsy, 587–588
saxagliptin, 720
SBMA (spinal and bulbar muscular atrophy), 613
schistosomiasis, 588–589
schizoaffective disorder, 589–590
schizophrenia, 590–592, 689, 765
schizophreniform disorder, 592–593
schizotypal personality disorder, 593–595
schwannoma
  facial nerve, 200
  vestibular, 595
sciatic nerve
  hip pathology/surgery, 267–268
  piriformis syndrome, 489
  in pregnancy, 418
  uterine mass compression, 675–676
scleritis, 595–596
scleroderma (progressive systemic sclerosis), 530–532, 596–598
scoliosis, 598
scopolamine, 729
Segawa disease, 163
seizures, see also epilepsy
  absence, 3
  Alpers disease, 17, 18
  atonic, 45
  eclampsia, 172–173, 190–191, 397
  febrile, 210–211

psychogenic nonepileptic, 541–542
  tonic–clonic, 228
selective mutism, 598–599
selective serotonin receptor modulators (SSRMs), 760–761
selective serotonin reuptake inhibitors (SSRIs), 204, 354–355, 793–794
  hypoactive sexual desire, 357
selegiline, 355
selenium deficiency, 599–600
self-harm, see also suicide risk
  Lesch–Nyhan syndrome, 335
  non-suicidal, 486
sella turcica (empty sella syndrome), 177
semicircular canal dehiscence, 633–634
sensory neuronopathy (ganglionopathy), 465–466
sensory neuropathy
  anti-Hu, 30
  Charcot–Marie–Tooth disease, 258
  CIDP, 116–117, 387
  Dejerine–Sottas disease, 258–259
  hepatitis A, 254
  hepatitis B, 255
  meralgia paresthetica, 418
  Refsum disease, 259, 573
sepsis/septic shock, 600
septic embolism, 600–601
serotonin 1D/1B selective agonists (triptans), 788–789
serotonin–norepinephrine reuptake inhibitors (SNRIs), 793
serotonin receptor antagonists, 782
serotonin syndrome, 601–602
  ergotamines, 785
  lorcaserin, 800
  MAOIs, 355, 480
  other antidepressants, 792, 793, 795, 796
  triptans, 788
sexual activity headache, 524–525
sexual dysfunction
  and antidepressants, 357, 794, 795–796
  erectile disorder, 192–193, 725
  female sexual interest/arousal disorder, 211
  male hypoactive sexual desire disorder, 357–358
  premature ejaculation, 516–517
  priapism, 800
shift work disorder, 602–603
short-acting beta agonists (SABAs), 736–737

Shy–Drager syndrome (multiple system atrophy), 48, 49, 50, 391–393
   MSA-C, 49, 393–394
SIADH (syndrome of inappropriate antidiuretic hormone secretion), 174, 292, 543
sialidosis, 528, 603–604
sickle cell disease, 705
siderosis, 633
sildenafil, 725
simultagnosia, 55
sinus histiocytosis (Rosai–Dorfman disease), 581
sirolimus, 753
sitagliptin, 720
Sjögren's syndrome, 604–606
skull
   basilar invagination, 56–57
   glomus jugulare tumor, 233
   platybasia, 493–494
   temporal bone fracture, 645–646
sleep disorders
   advanced sleep–wake phase disorder, 12
   central sleep apnea
     Cheyne–Stokes respiration, 101–102, 114
     high altitude, 99–100
     medications/substance abuse, 100–101
     primary, 519–520
   confusional arousal, 125–126
   delayed sleep–wake phase disorder, 142–143
   hypersomnia
     idiopathic, 295–296
     Kline–Levine syndrome, 301, 321–322
   insomnia
     chronic, 302–303
     fatal familial insomnia, 209
     short-term, 303–304
     treatment, 302–303, 304, 801, 802, 804
   insufficient sleep syndrome, 304
   irregular sleep–wake rhythm disorder, 311–312
   jet lag, 316–317
   narcolepsy, 405–406
   nightmare disorder, 420–421
   NREM-related parasomnias, 424
   obstructive sleep apnea, 428
     obesity hypoventilation syndrome, 425
   periodic limb movement disorder, 475–476

recurrent isolated sleep paralysis, 564
REM behavior disorder, 566–567
shift work disorder, 602–603
sleep-related eating disorder, 606
sleep terrors, 606–607
sleepwalking, 607–608
sleeping sickness (African trypanosomiasis), 668–669
smallpox, 609
   vaccination, 608–609
small vessel disease, *see also* diabetes mellitus
   HUS, 247
   Susac syndrome, 635, 676
   TTP, 655
smoking, 660–661
smoking cessation, 801, 804–805
Sneddon's syndrome, 609–610
SNRIs (serotonin–norepinephrine reuptake inhibitors), 512, 793
sodium
   hypernatremia, 282–283
   hyponatremia, 292, 542–543, 774
sodium glucose cotransporter-2 inhibitors, 721
sodium oxybate, 405, 406, 802–803
solvent abuse, 13, 234–235, 267, 610
somatization, 610–611
   conversion disorder, 204, 220–221, 511
     loss of vision, 221
   factitious disorder, 160, 202–204, 486
   illness anxiety disorder, 298–299
   malingering, 160, 203–204, 359
   somatic symptom disorder, 90
     with predominant pain, 542
somnambulism (sleepwalking), 607–608
spasmodic dysphonia, 611–612
spastic paraplegia/paraparesis
   hereditary, 259–260
   HTLV-1 associated myelopathy, 274–275
speech difficulties
   aphasia, *see* aphasia
   spasmodic dysphonia, 611–612
spider venom, 66–67
spina bifida occulta, 612–613
spinal muscular atrophy (SMA)
   distal, 162
   type III, 616
spine/spinal cord, *see also* brachial plexopathy; lumbosacral plexopathy
   AAA repair, 36
   arachnoiditis, 38–39
   arthritis, 109
   atlantoaxial subluxation, 44–45

back strain/sprain, 54, 343–344
cauda equina syndrome, 94, 618
cerebrotendinous xanthomatosis, 107
compression fractures, 124–125
decompression sickness, 141–142
disc disorders
   cervical, 109–110, 142, 260
   degenerative, 142, 342
   discitis, 156–157
   herniation, 260–261
   lumbar, 142, 261, 342
DISH, 154–155
dural AV fistula, 39
epidural abscess, 614
epidural hemorrhage, 614
epidural lipomatosis, 615
extradural hematoma, 187
facet syndrome, 110–111
fungal infections, 222
hemangioblastoma, 615–616
HIV-associated myelopathy, 270
HTLV-1 associated myelopathy, 274–275
hyperlordosis, 282
ischemia/infarction, 29, 313–314, 613–614
kyphosis, 326
lumbar stenosis, 344
myelitis, *see also* encephalomyelitis
   Lyme disease, 348
   neuromyelitis optica, 414, 605
   transverse, 254
   viral, 182, 254, 264–266, 494, 684
neural tube defects, 612–613
neurolathyrism, 413
odontoid process fractures, 111–112
perimedullary fistula, 617–618
poliomyelitis, 182, 494
propriospinal myoclonus, 534–535
radiation myelopathy, 557
SBMA, 613
scoliosis, 598
spinal muscular atrophy
   distal, 162
   type III, 616
spondylitis, 618
spondylolisthesis, 343
spondylolysis, 343
spondylosis
   cervical, 112
   lumbar, 343
stroke
   ischemic, 29, 313–314, 613–614
   SAH, 618
subdural hematoma, 631–632

syringobulbia, 638–639
syringomyelia, 244
tethered cord syndrome, 650
trauma (cervical), 111–113
tumors, 188, 616–617
vitamin B12 deficiency, 537, 687
spondylitis, 618
spondylolisthesis, 343
spondylolysis, 343
spondylosis
cervical, 112
lumbar, 343
Sporothrix schenckii, 619
sports injuries
back injuries, 54, 343–344
brachial plexopathy, 71–72
epicondylitis, 185
SSRIs (selective serotonin reuptake
inhibitors), 204, 354–355, 512,
793–794
hypoactive sexual desire, 357
Staphylococcus aureus, 619
statins, 715
status epilepticus, 620–621
epilepsia partialis continua, 191–192
ESES, 175–176
nonconvulsive, 424, 736
stavudine, 749–750
Stevens–Johnson syndrome, 774,
775–776, 777, 778, 779, 780
stiff person syndrome, 235–236, 621–622
stimulants, 803–804
St. Louis encephalitis virus, 622–623
Stokes–Adams attacks, 623
strabismus, 623–625
Streptococcus spp.
group A (rheumatic fever), 116, 379,
577–578, 635–636
group B, 625
microaerophilic, 625–626
PANDAS, 635–636, 658
S. pneumoniae, 626–627
stress, 627
acute stress disorder, 7–8
adjustment disorder, 10, 354, 511
PTSD, 160, 510–512, 589
striatal nigral degeneration (MSA-P), 49
stroke, 627–628
ACA infarction, 28, 331–332
AChA infarction, 28–29
atherosclerosis, intracranial, 308–309
cardioembolic, 46, 85
carotid artery endarterectomy/stent-
ing, 88–89
central visual loss, 103

depression following, 354
hemorrhagic
AVM rupture, 40–41
intraventricular, 310, 340–341
lobar, 340–341
in pregnancy, 107–108
SAH, 23–24, 108, 618, 629–630,
693
vitamin K deficiency, 692
hemorrhagic transformation,
248–249
lacunar, 327–328
MCA infarction, 375–377
moyamoya disease, 385
PCA infarction, 500–501
in pregnancy, 107–108
spinal
ischemic, 29, 313–314, 613–614
SAH, 618
TIAs, 385, 664–665, 682–683
top of the basilar syndrome, 663
venous sinus thrombosis, 95, 106
vertebral artery dissection, 681–682
strongyloidosis, 628–629
Sturge–Weber syndrome, 232, 571, 629
subacute combined degeneration, 537, 687
subacute necrotizing encephalomyelopathy (Leigh disease), 332
subacute sclerosing panencephalitis, 364
subarachnoid hemorrhage (SAH), 23–24,
108, 629–630, 693
spinal, 618
subclavian steal syndrome, 630
subcortical leukoencephalopathy
Binswanger's disease, 61–62, 312
CADASIL, 105, 312
subdural hematoma
acute cerebral, 630–631
chronic cerebral, 631
spinal, 631–632
substance abuse, *see also* toxins/toxicity
alcohol, *see* alcohol abuse
and amnesia, 160
cannabis, 79–80
withdrawal, 80–81
cocaine, 122–123
ecstasy, 173–174
and impulsive/aggressive behavior,
306
ketamine, 320–321
LSD, 349–350
mescaline, 371
methamphetamine, 373–374
nitrous oxide, 421–422, 687
opioids, 433–434

central sleep apnea, 100–101
heroin, 261–263
withdrawal, 262–263, 434–435
and panic attacks, 454
phencyclidine, 483
psilocybin, 539
solvents, 13, 234–235, 267, 610
tobacco/nicotine, 660–661
cessation therapy, 801, 804–805
sudden unexpected death in epilepsy
(SUDEP), 189, 190
suicide risk
ADHD, 47
Alzheimer's disease, 10
bipolar disorders, 64, 65
body dysmorphic disorder, 69
depression, 353, 354, 355, 547
dissociative amnesia, 160
epilepsy, 189, 354, 646
gender dysphoria, 226–227
Huntington's chorea, 277, 773
medication-associated
AEDs, 774
alemtuzumab, 752
antidepressants, 791, 792, 793,
794, 795, 796
antipsychotics, 797
atomoxetine, 797
clonidine, 790
isotretinoin, 731
leukotriene antagonists, 735
lorcaserin, 800
metoclopramide, 728
suvorexant, 804
psychogenic pain, 542
psychogenic seizures, 541–542
psychosis, 75
schizoaffective disorder, 589
tardive dyskinesia, 642
sulfamethoxazole–trimethoprim, 747
sulfasalazine, 766
sulfatide autoantibodies, 419
sulfite oxidase deficiency, 334, 382–383
sulfonylureas, 721
sumatriptan, 788, 789
SUNCT/SUNA headaches, 632–633
superficial siderosis, 633
superior orbital fissure, 661–662
superior semicircular canal dehiscence,
633–634
surgery
nerve injuries during, 86, 267–268, 634
postoperative psychosis, 305
post-transplant neuropathies, 276,
508–509

Susac syndrome, 635, 676
suvorexant, 804
swallowing difficulties
    botulinum toxin, 110, 783
    psychogenic, 540–541
Sydenham chorea, 635–636
sympathectomy, 35
symptomatic palatial myoclonus, 451–452
syncope, 636–637
    cardiogenic, 86–87
    carotid sinus hypersensitivity, 90
    Stokes–Adams attacks, 623
syndrome of inappropriate antidiuretic
        hormone secretion (SIADH),
        174, 292, 543
synovial cyst (ganglion cyst), 225
syphilis, 32, 271, 637–638, 662
syringobulbia, 638–639
syringomyelia, 244
systemic lupus erythematosus, 639–640
systemic sclerosis (scleroderma),
        530–532, 596–598

tacrolimus, 752
tadalafil, 725
Takayasu arteritis, 641
tamoxifen, 760–761
tapeworms
    cysticercosis, 139
    echinococcosis, 170–171
tardive dyskinesia, 555, 589–590,
        641–642
tardive dystonia, 642–643
tasimelteon, 801
taxanes, 761
Tay–Sachs disease, 643–644
TCAs (tricyclic antidepressants), 355,
        480, 794–795
tedizolid, 745–746
telangiectasia, 81–82
temporal arteritis (giant-cell arteritis),
        32, 644–645
    AION, 41, 501
temporal bone fracture, 645–646
temporal lobe epilepsy, 646–647
    with febrile convulsions, 210
    mesial temporal sclerosis, 371–372
temporal lobe ischemia (MCA occlu-
        sion), 376, 377
temporomandibular joint syndrome,
        647–648
tendonitis
    de Quervain's tenosynovitis, 149–150
    epicondylitis, 185
tennis elbow, 185

tenofovir, 749–750
tension headache, 242, 648–649
teratogens
    AEDs, 190–191, 779
    amiodarone, 710
    azathioprine, 695
    leflunomide, 765
    lithium, 64, 65
    vitamin A, 685, 731
teriparatide (parathyroid hormone), 725
Terson's syndrome, 693
testicular cancer, 228, 229–230, 649
testosterone, 323, 358, 722–723
tetanus, 120, 121, 649–650
    vaccine, 156
tethered cord syndrome, 650
tetrabenazine, 773
tetracyclines, 747
thalidomide and analogs, 761–762
theophylline, 736
thiamine (vitamin B1)
    deficiency, 323–324, 537, 569–570,
        651–652, 700–701
    supplements, 701, 732
thiazide diuretics, 281, 714
thiazolidinediones, 721
third ventricle tumors, 652–653
thirst, psychogenic, 542–543
thoracic outlet syndrome, 653–654
thoracic radiation myelopathy, 558
threadworm (strongyloidosis), 628–629
thrombocythemia, essential, 195
thrombocytopenia, 654
    HIT, 250–251
    HUS, 247
    ITP, 297–298
    TTP, 655–656
thromboembolism, see embolism;
        thrombophilia
thrombolysis, 108, 377, 416, 582
    and hemorrhagic transformation of
        stroke, 248–249
thrombophilia, 654–655
    antithrombin deficiency, 31
    essential thrombocythemia, 195
    factor V Leiden, 204
    HIT, 250–251
    in pregnancy, 108
    protein C deficiency, 537–538
    protein S deficiency, 538
thrombophlebitis, cavernous sinus, 95
thrombotic thrombocytopenic purpura
        (TTP), 655–656
thunderclap headache, 575, 656
thymus gland, and myasthenia gravis,

397, 463
thyroid disease
    and amiodarone, 710
    Hashimoto's thyroiditis, 241
    hyperthyroidism, 286–287
        Graves' eye disease, 197, 439, 624,
            656
        thyrotoxic periodic paralysis, 477,
            657
L-thyroxine, 565, 726
tiagabine, 778
TIAs, see transient ischemic attacks
tick-borne diseases
    babesiosis, 54
    ehrlichiosis, 174–175
    Lyme disease, 347–348
    Rocky Mountain spotted fever,
        579–580
    tick-borne encephalitis virus, 213
tick paralysis, 660
tics, 201–202, 426–427, 657–659
tipranavir, 750
tissue plasminogen activator (tPA), 377,
        416, 582
    in pregnancy, 108
tizanidine, 785
tobacco use, 660–661
    cessation, 801, 804–805
tocopherol (vitamin E), 690–692,
        732–733
tolcapone, 768–769
Tolosa–Hunt syndrome, 661–662
tonic–clonic seizures, 228
tonic pupil, 662–663
tooth disease, 147–148
top of the basilar syndrome, 663
topiramate, 191, 778–779
Tourette's syndrome, 201, 426–427,
        657–659
toxic epidermal necrolysis, 774, 775–776,
        777, 778, 779, 780
toxins/toxicity, 663–664, see also sub-
        stance abuse
    aluminum, 153–154, 570, 727
    anticholinergic agents, 29
    black widow spider venom, 66–67
    botulism, 70, 120, 550
    buckthorn fruit, 76
    carbon disulfide, 82
    carbon monoxide, 82
    cassava root, 91
    ciguatoxin, 119
    ethylene oxide, 196
    grass pea, 413
    hexane, 267

lead, 330–331
manganese, 359–360
methotrexate, 374, 765
opioids, 100–101, 261–262, 433–434,
   786–787
pyridoxine, 214, 553, 732
radiation, *see* radiotherapy
tick paralysis, 660
vitamin A, 685–686, 731
vitamin D, 689
zinc, 705
toxoplasmosis, 271, 572
trace elements
copper, 127–128, 705
iron, 310–311, 730
selenium, 599–600
zinc, 704–706, 733
transient global amnesia, 664
transient ischemic attacks (TIAs),
   664–665
amaurosis fugax, 20
moyamoya disease, 385
vertebrobasilar insufficiency,
   682–683
transplants, post-transplant neuropathies, 276, 508–509
transverse myelitis
hepatitis A, 254
neuromyelitis optica, 414, 605
trauma
aortic, 36–37
cervical, 111–113
dissociative amnesia after, 159–161
facial nerve, 201, 645
head, *see* head injuries
humeral fracture, 276–277
lumbosacral plexopathy, 346
trazodone, 794
tremor
drug-induced, 165–167
essential, 195–196
facial, 130
FXTAS, 216
orthostatic, 442
trichinosis, 665–666
trichotillomania, 486, 666–667
tricyclic antidepressants (TCAs), 355,
   427, 480, 794–795
trigeminal nerve (CN V), *see also* atypical
   facial pain
and corneal injuries, 319
hemimasticatory spasm, 246
neuralgia, 605, 667–668
Raeder's paratrigeminal neuralgia,
   560–561

trinucleotide repeat disorders
DRPLA, 148, 528
fragile X syndrome, 214–216
Friedreich's ataxia, 216–218
FXTAS, 216
Huntington's chorea, 277, 383, 384,
   773
myotonic dystrophy, 92, 402–403
SBMA, 613
triptans (serotonin 1D/1B selective agonists), 788–789
trisomy 21 (Down syndrome), 44–45,
   163–164, 765
trochlear nerve (CN IV), 624
tropical ataxic neuropathy, 668
tropical spastic paraparesis, 274–275
trypanosomiasis, African (sleeping sickness), 668–669
trypanosomiasis, American (Chagas
   disease), 113
TTP (thrombotic thrombocytopenic
   purpura), 655–656
tuberculosis, 271, 669
anti-tubercular drugs, 742, 743–744,
   746–747
tuberous sclerosis, 571, 670
tumor necrosis factor-alpha (TNF-α)
   inhibitors, 766
tumors, *see also* chemotherapy
angioma, 94–95, 680–681
astrocytoma, 42, 44
bladder, 67–68
bone, 230, 445, 447–448
and brachial plexopathy, 72
brain metastases, 72–73
breast, 72, 73–74, 83
carcinoid, 82–83
carcinomatous meningitis, 83–84
cavernous sinus, 96
ependymoma, 183–184
epidermoid, 185–186
facial nerve, 200
ganglioglioma, 224–225
gastrointestinal, 82–83, 225–226
germ cell, 228, 230, 491, 649
gliomatosis cerebri, 232–233
glomus jugulare, 233
gynecologic, 228, 229–230, 238–239,
   449–450, 674–675
hemangioblastoma, 243–244, 571,
   615, 697–698
hemorrhage into, 249
kidney, 567–568
leukemia, 336–337, 754, 758
lung, 72, 346, 347

lymphoma
Burkitt, 77
intravascular, 309–310
lymphoplasmacytic, 699–700
orbital, 440
primary CNS, 270–271, 521–523
medulloblastoma, 367
melanoma, 368, 757
meningioma, 369–370, 440, 491
multiple myeloma, 389
nasopharyngeal, 406
neck, 406–407
neurofibromatosis, 411–412, 440
oligodendroglioma, 431–432
optic glioma, 436
orbital, 440–441
ovarian, 228, 229–230, 238–239,
   449–450
pancreatic, 452–453
paraganglioma, 458–459
parotid gland, 469
pheochromocytoma, 484–485
pineal gland, 487–489
pituitary adenoma, 13, 490, 492,
   624
prolactinoma, 284, 532–533
prostate, 535–536
sarcoma, 447–448, 585–587
spine, 188, 616–617
testicular, 228, 229–230, 649
third ventricle, 652–653
uterine, 238–239, 674–675
vestibular schwannoma, 595
Turner syndrome, 671
tympanic membrane perforation,
   117–118
typhoid fever, 671–672
tyramine cheese reaction, 355, 480

ubiquinone (coenzyme Q_{10}) deficiency,
   520–521
Leigh disease, 332
NADH CoQ reductase deficiency,
   404–405
ulcerative colitis, 673
ulnar nerve, 673–674
unconsciousness, *see also* locked-in
   syndrome
medication-associated, 754, 758
persistent vegetative state, 480–482
syncope, 636–637
cardiogenic, 86–87
carotid sinus hypersensitivity, 90
Stokes–Adams attacks, 623
Unverricht–Lundborg disease, 528

upper limb, *see also* brachial plexopathy
  carpal tunnel syndrome, 90–91, 417, 418, 533
  de Quervain's tenosynovitis, 149–150
  diabetic mononeuropathy, 152
  epicondylitis, 185
  ganglion cyst, 225
  humeral fracture, 276–277
  ischemic monomelic neuropathy, 313
  pronator syndrome, 533–534
  radial neuropathy, 556–557, 587, 588
  repetitive hand use, 570–571
  subclavian steal syndrome, 630
  thoracic outlet syndrome, 653–654
  ulnar neuropathy, 673–674
  vascular insufficiency to hand, 679–680
urea cycle disorders, 8–9
uremia, 569
uric acid excess (Lesch–Nyhan syndrome), 335–336
urinary incontinence (enuresis), 183
uterine cancer, 238–239, 674–675
uterine mass causing sciatic nerve compression, 675–676
uveitis, 676–677, 694

vaccines
  diphtheria, tetanus, and pertussis, 156
  MMR, 365–366
  pneumococcus, 626–627
  polio, 495
  post-immunization encephalomyelitis, 503–505
  smallpox, 608–609
valacyclovir, 739
valgancyclovir, 739
valproate (depakote), 779
  in bipolar disorder, 64
  in MERRF, 199
  teratogenicity, 191, 779
valves, prosthetic, 536
valvuloplasty, 678
vancomycin, 743
vardenafil, 725
varenicline, 804–805
variant Creutzfeldt–Jakob Disease (vCJD), 70–71
varicella (herpes) zoster virus, 265–266, 503
variola (smallpox), 609
  vaccination, 608–609
vascular claudication, 307–308, 678–679
vascular dementia, 388, 679
  Binswanger's disease, 61–62, 312

vasculitis
  aortic arteritis, 32–33
  giant-cell arteritis, 32, 41, 501, 644–645
  granulomatosis with polyangiitis, 237–238
  Henoch–Schönlein purpura, 249–250
  neuropathy, 680
  polyarteritis nodosa, 255, 495–496
  primary CNS angiitis, 521
  Takayasu arteritis, 641
vasodilators, 717–718
vasogenic edema, *see* posterior reversible encephalopathy syndrome
vasopressin, *see* antidiuretic hormone (ADH)
vasovagal (cardiogenic) syncope, 86–87
VEGF signaling inhibitors, 352, 762
venous angioma, 680–681
venous sinus thrombosis, 106–107
  in mastoiditis, 364
  in pregnancy, 107, 108
  thrombophlebitis, 95
ventilation, assisted
  central alveolar hypoventilation syndrome, 126
  central sleep apnea, 102
  chronic respiratory failure, 118–119
  obesity hypoventilation syndrome, 425
ventricular drains/shunts, 37, 310, 341
ventricular hemorrhage, 310, 340–341
ventricular septal defect (VSD), 681
vertebral artery dissection, 681–682
vertebral osteomyelitis (discitis), 156–157
vertebrobasilar insufficiency, 682–683
vertigo
  BPPV, 60–61
  lacunar stroke, 328
  Meniere's disease, 369
  otosclerosis, 449
  ototoxic drugs, 738, 743, 747, 759
  perilymphatic fistula, 473–474
  psychogenic, 544
  semicircular canal dehiscence, 633–634
  temporal bone fracture, 645–646
  vestibular degeneration, 683
  vestibular neuritis, 683–684
vestibulocerebellar ataxia, 207
vestibulocochlear nerve (CN VIII)
  vestibular neuritis, 683–684
  vestibular schwannoma, 595
vigabatrin, 779–780

vilazodone, 795
vildagliptin, 720
vinca alkaloids, 762–763
viral infections, *see also* antiviral drugs; post-viral syndromes
  adenovirus, 8
  coxsackie, 129–130
  cytomegalovirus, 139–140, 271
  dengue, 146–147, 213
  eastern equine encephalitis, 169–170
  echovirus, 171–172
  encephalitis workup, 178
  enteroviruses, 129–130, 171–172, 182–183
  Epstein–Barr, 192, 349
  flaviviruses, 212–214
  hepatitis (acute), 252–253
  hepatitis A, 253–255
  hepatitis B, 255–256, 257
    chronic, 253
  hepatitis C, 256–257
    chronic, 253
    cryoglobulinemia, 134–135, 257
  hepatitis neuropathy, 257–258
  herpes simplex I, 263–264
  herpes simplex II, 264–265, 381
  herpes/varicella zoster, 265–266, 503
  herpesvirus 6 (HHV-6), 275–276
  HIV, *see* HIV-positive patients
  HTLV-1, 274–275
  influenza, 300–302, 745
  Japanese encephalitis, 213, 315–316
  JC virus, 271, 527
  La Crosse, 327
  lymphocytic choriomeningitis, 348–349
  measles, 364–365
  mumps, 394–395
  myelitis, 182, 254, 264–266, 494, 684
  myositis, 301, 684–685
  parainfluenza, 460
  poliovirus, 182, 494–495
  rabies, 556
  rubella, 582
  smallpox, 609
  St. Louis encephalitis, 622–623
  Zika, 704
vision, loss of, *see also* blepharospasm; strabismus
  afferent pupillary defect, 13–14
  amaurosis fugax, 20, 644
  cataracts, 91–93
  central visual impairment, 102–103
  functional (nonphysiologic), 221

glaucoma, 231–232
intracranial hypertension, 296, 297
Leber's hereditary optic atrophy, 331
lens subluxation, 333–334
macular degeneration, 352–353
medication-associated, 710, 731, 739, 742, 758, 764, 779–780
microphthalmos, 374–375
onchocerciasis, 432–433
optic nerve
    AION, 41, 423, 501
    atrophy, 435–436
    compression, 437–438
    glioma, 436
    neuritis, 416, 436–437, 465, 504, 742
    perineuritis, 475
orbital hemorrhage, 438–439
paraneoplastic retinopathy/neuropathy, 465
pregnancy-associated conditions, 415–417
retinal artery occlusion, 98, 416
retinal detachment, 99, 571–572
retinal migraine, 572–573
retinal vein occlusion, 98–99
retinitis pigmentosa, 573–574
temporal arteritis, 644
uveitis, 676–677, 694
vitamin deficiencies, 685, 687
vitreous hemorrhage, 693–694
visual hallucinations, see hallucinations
visual phenomena in occipital lobe epilepsy, 429
vitamins
    A (retinol), 573–574, 685–686, 731
    B12 (cobalamin), 226, 537, 686–688, 732
    B complex supplements, 731–732
    D, 688–690, 732
    E (tocopherol), 690–692, 732–733
    folate, 190, 214, 537, 732
    K, 692–693
    multivitamin deficiencies, 16, 97, 136
    niacin (B3), 419–430, 537, 716
    in pregnancy, 190, 731
    pyridoxine, 553
        seizures, 554
        toxicity, 214, 553, 732

thiamine (B1)
    deficiency, 323–324, 537, 569–570, 651–652, 700–701
    supplements, 701, 732
vitreous hemorrhage, 693–694
Vogt–Koyanagi–Harada disease, 676, 694–695
voltage-gated potassium channel antibody syndrome, 695–696
volume depletion, 697
vomiting
    antiemetic drugs, 728, 729, 781–782
    cyclic vomiting syndrome, 137–138
von Hippel–Lindau disease (VHLD), 697–698
    hemangioblastoma, 243–244, 571, 615–616
voriconazole, 739
vortioxetine, 795–796

Waldenström's macroglobulinemia, 699–700
warfarin, 46, 377, 711, 783
Watchmen® device, 46
Waterhouse–Friderichsen syndrome, 408
Weber syndrome, 624
Wegener's granulomatosis, 237–238
weight management, see obesity management
Weil's disease (leptospirosis), 335
Wernicke aphasia, 376
Wernicke disease/encephalopathy, 537, 569–570, 651, 700–701
    Korsakoff syndrome, 323–324, 537
West Nile virus, 213
West syndrome, 299
Whipple's disease, 702
white matter disease
    adrenoleukodystrophy, 11–12
    Binswanger's disease, 61–62, 312
    CADASIL, 105, 312
    in eclampsia, 172
    ischemic, 312–313
    metachromatic leukodystrophy, 372–373
    PML, 271, 527, 752, 753
    PRES, see posterior reversible encephalopathy syndrome

whooping cough (pertussis), 156, 482–483
Wilson's disease, 92, 384
withdrawal
    alcohol, 16–17
    cannabis, 80–81
    opioids, 262–263, 434–435
wrist
    carpal tunnel syndrome, 90–91, 417, 533
    de Quervain's tenosynovitis, 149–150
    ganglion cyst, 225

xanthomatosis, cerebrotendinous, 107
X chromosome aneuploidy
    Klinefelter syndrome (47, XXY), 322–323
    Turner syndrome (45, X), 671
X-linked disorders
    adrenoleukodystrophy, 11–12
    centronuclear myopathy, 103–104
    dystonia parkinsonism, 703
    Fabry disease, 198–199
    fragile X syndrome, 214–216
    FXTAS, 216
    Hunter syndrome, 350–351
    hydrocephalus, 37
    Lesch–Nyhan syndrome, 335–336
    McLeod syndrome, 409–410
    Menkes disease, 370–371
    muscular dystrophy
        Becker, 57
        Duchenne, 167
    Norrie's disease, 571
    Rett syndrome, 574

zafirlukast, 735
zaleplon, 316, 802
zidovudine, 749–750
Zika virus, 704
zinc, 704–706, 733
zolmitriptan, 789
zolpidem, 316, 802
zonisamide, 780